Davidson's
Principles and Practice of
Medicine

The Editor

JOHN MACLEOD

M.B. Ch.B., F.R.C.P.(Edin)

Formerly:
Chairman of University Department of Medicine, Western General Hospital, Edinburgh;
Consultant Physician, Western General Hospital, Edinburgh;
Consultant Physician, Royal Edinburgh Hospital;
Consultant Physician, Clinic for Rheumatic Diseases, Royal Infirmary, Edinburgh.

The Contributors

Primarily from the Departments of Medicine and Therapeutics, University of Edinburgh, but also from other University Departments in Britain, Africa and Australia

Davidson's Principles and Practice of Medicine

A TEXTBOOK FOR STUDENTS AND DOCTORS

EDITED BY

John Macleod

FOURTEENTH EDITION

CHURCHILL LIVINGSTONE

EDINBURGH LONDON MELBOURNE AND NEW YORK 1984

CHURCHILL LIVINGSTONE
Medical Division of Longman Group Limited

Distributed in the United States of America by Churchill
Livingstone Inc., 1560 Broadway, New York, N.Y. 10036,
and by associated companies, branches and representatives
throughout the world.

First Edition 1952
Second Edition 1954
Third Edition 1956
Fourth Edition 1958
Fifth Edition 1960
Sixth Edition 1962
Seventh Edition 1964
Eighth Edition 1966
Ninth Edition 1968
Tenth Edition 1971
Eleventh Edition 1974
Twelfth Edition 1977
Thirteenth Edition 1981
Fourteenth Edition 1984
Reprinted 1985
Reprinted 1986

ISBN 0 443 03003 0 (Cased)
ISBN 0 443 03002 2

British Library Cataloguing in Publication Data
Davidson, Sir Stanley
   Davidson's principles and practice of medicine. — 14th
   ed.
   1. Pathology   2. Medicine
   I. Title   II. Macleod, John, 1915–
   616   RB111

Library of Congress Cataloging in Publication Data
Davidson, Leybourne Stanley Patrick, Sir, 1894–
   Davidson's Principles and practice of medicine.

   Includes bibliographical references and index.
   1. Internal medicine.   I. Macleod, John George.
II. Title.   III. Title: Principles and practice of medicine.
[DNLM: 1. Principles and practice of medicine.
2. Medicine.   WB 100 D252p]
RC46.D24   1984   616   84-4932

Typeset by H Charlesworth & Co Ltd, Huddersfield
Printed in Great Britain
at the University Printing House, Oxford
by David Stanford
Printer to the University

Preface to the Fourteenth Edition

With this new production, *Davidson's Principles and Practice of Medicine* will have appeared in 14 editions since it was first published 32 years ago. The book has established an international reputation; it is used extensively throughout the English speaking world and has also been translated into Spanish, Portuguese, Italian, Greek, Malay and Serbo-Croatian. Since 1965 it has been published in Africa and Asia in a paperback edition under the auspices of the English Language Book Society. This continuing success is a remarkable tribute to the genius and vision of the late Sir Stanley Davidson and the progressive editorial policy he instituted, but we are acutely aware that, if the book is to retain its unique place in the field of medical education it must be kept completely up to date in relation to the evolution of medical science and technology.

In pursuit of this aim, the regular recruitment of younger authors in place of those who have retired from clinical practice has always been a main feature of editorial policy. On this occasion there are six new contributors, namely Drs G.K. Crompton and D.P. de Bono, Professor C.R.W. Edwards, Dr Anne Lambie, Professor J.F. Smyth and Dr R.N. Thin.

There are more changes in this than in any previous edition. Prominent among them is a new introductory chapter on oncology which includes a consideration of terminal care. Sections which have been rewritten include recombinant DNA technology, diseases of the heart, respiratory failure, the treatment of asthma, sexually-transmitted disease, the acquired immunodeficiency syndrome, diseases of the pituitary gland, the aetiology of diabetes mellitus, the physiology of bone and the prevention of acute poisoning.

There has been a major reorganisation in the presentation of diseases due to infection, whereby those not appropriately placed in one of the systems have been brought together in a single chapter. The remainder of the book has been thoroughly revised and extensive alterations made, including the introduction of new diagrams, e.g. the pathology of glomerulonephritis.

There is an obvious change in the format of the book, which is now printed in double columns on slightly bigger pages to facilitate reading. The book is still of an easily manageable size and, although larger, is not longer, if the short new chapter is excluded. This containment has been achieved mainly by discarding material that has been superseded. The end result, we believe, is a textbook of medicine which will continue to meet the needs of the 1980s.

The opening chapters provide an overall view of fundamental general factors such as genetics, immunology, infection, nutrition, electrolyte balance and oncology. This is followed by accounts of diseases of the various systems and by outlines of psychiatry and acute poisoning. Emphasis has been placed on the more important (i.e. commoner) conditions and on those of educational value. A chapter on tropical disease and climatic disorders is included so that Western readers will have at least some knowledge of medical problems and human needs in countries other than their own and will be alerted to the dangers of imported disease. Next there is a major chapter on diseases due to infection with particular reference to those encountered in the tropics. A final short chapter deals on a global basis with the promotion of health and prevention of disease, re-emphasising the prominence given to prophylaxis throughout the book. In recognition of the fact that education must be a continuing process, many of the chapters conclude with brief comments on prospects for the immediate future. Guidance is given about further reading, most of the references being briefly annotated to encourage students to use medical libraries.

A close interrelationship has been maintained with the 6th edition of *Clinical Examination* in which several of the contributors and the editor participate. In addition, for the reader who wishes to test his or her understanding of the material included in both these books, an MCQ Companion is also available.

Our primary objective, as in previous editions, has been to ensure that the book provides a *rational and easily comprehensible basis for the practice of medicine.* We hope that 'Davidson' will continue to make as substantial a contribution to the education of medical students, both undergraduate and postgraduate, in the future as it has done in the past.

Edinburgh, 1984   John Macleod

Acknowledgements

We have had generous help from many colleagues, and students and doctors from all over the world have provided the challenge of constructive criticism. We are particularly indebted to Dr G.M. Fraser for the radiographs of the alimentary tract and to Mr J.E. Pizer for line drawings. Miss Susan Hunter of Churchill Livingstone has skilfully guided the manuscript through its critical later stages. Other acknowledgements are made in the text.

List of Contributors

Allan, N.C., M.B., Ch.B., F.R.C.P.(Edin.), F.R.C.P.Path.
Senior Lecturer, University Department of Medicine, Western General Hospital, Edinburgh and formerly of University of Ibadan, Nigeria; Consultant Haematologist, Western General Hospital, Edinburgh
Diseases of the Blood

Baird, Joyce D., M.A., M.B. Ch.B.(Aberd.), F.R.C.P.(Edin.)
Senior Lecturer, University Department of Medicine, Western General Hospital, Edinburgh and Honorary Consultant Physician, Western General Hospital, Edinburgh
Diabetes Mellitus and other Metabolic Disorders
Obesity

Bryceson, A.D.M., M.D., F.R.C.P.(Edin.), D.T.M. and H.
Senior Lecturer, London School of Hygiene and Tropical Medicine; Consulting Physician, Hospital for Tropical Diseases; Consultant in Tropical Dermatology, St John's Hospital for Diseases of the Skin, London
Tropical Diseases and Climatic Disorders
Diseases due to Infection

Crean, G.P., Ph.D., F.R.C.P.(Edin.), F.R.C.P.(Glasg.),
Honorary Lecturer in Medicine, University of Glasgow (Western Infirmary); Consultant Physician, Southern General Hospital, Glasgow; Physician-in-charge, Gastrointestinal Centre, Southern General Hospital, Glasgow
Diseases of the Alimentary Tract and Pancreas

Crompton, G.K., M.B., Ch.B., F.R.C.P.(Edin.)
Senior Lecturer, University Department of Medicine, Western General Hospital, Edinburgh; Senior Lecturer, University Department of Respiratory Medicine, City Hospital, Edinburgh; Consultant Physician, Respiratory Unit, Northern General Hospital, Edinburgh
Diseases of the Respiratory System

de Bono, D.P., M.D.(Cantab.), F.R.C.P.(Edin.)
Consultant Physician, Department of Cardiology, The Royal Infirmary, Edinburgh
Diseases of the Cardiovascular System

Edwards, C.R.W., M.A., M.D.(Cantab.), F.R.C.P.(Edin.), F.R.C.P.(Lond.)
Professor of Clinical Medicine and Chairman, University Department of Medicine, Western General Hospital, Edinburgh and Honorary Consultant Physician, Western General Hospital, Edinburgh
Diseases of the Hypothalamus, Pituitary and Parathyroid Glands and Sexual Disorders
The Promotion of Health and Prevention of Disease

Emery, A.E.H., M.D., Ph.D (Johns Hopkins), D.Sc., F.R.C.P.(Edin.), M.F.C.M., F.R.S.E
Professor Emeritus (Human Genetics), University of Edinburgh
Genetic Factors in Disease

Finlayson, N.D.C., Ph.D., M.B. Ch.B., F.R.C.P.(Edin.), M.R.C.P.(Lond.)
Physician, Gastrointestinal and Liver Service, The Royal Infirmary, Edinburgh
Diseases of the Liver and Biliary Tract

Geddes, A.M., M.B. Ch.B., F.R.C.P.(Edin.), F.R.C.P.(Lond.)
Honorary Professor of Infectious Diseases, University of Birmingham; Consultant Physician, Department of Communicable and Tropical Diseases, East Birmingham Hospital, Birmingham
Infection and Disease
Diseases due to Infection

Grant, I.W.B., M.B. Ch.B., F.R.C.P.(Edin.)
Senior Lecturer, University Department of Medicine, Western General Hospital, Edinburgh; Consultant Physician, Respiratory Unit, Northern General Hospital, Edinburgh
Diseases of the Respiratory System

Irvine, W.J., D.Sc., M.B. Ch.B., F.R.C.P.(Edin.), F.R.C.Path., F.R.S.E.
Reader, Department of Medicine, University of Edinburgh; Consultant Physician, Royal Infirmary, Edinburgh
Immunological Factors in Disease
Diseases of the Thyroid and Adrenal Glands

Julian, D.G., M.A., M.D., F.R.C.P.(Edin.), F.R.C.P.(Lond), F.R.A.C.P.
British Heart Foundation Professor of Cardiology, University of Newcastle upon Tyne; Consultant Cardiologist, Freeman Hospital, Newcastle upon Tyne
Diseases of the Cardiovascular System

Lambie, Anne T., M.B., Ch.B., F.R.C.P.(Edin.), F.R.C.P.(Lond.),
Senior Lecturer in Medicine and Consultant Physician Royal Infirmary, Edinburgh
Disturbances in Water and Electrolyte Balance and in Hydrogen Ion Concentration
Diseases of the Kidney and Genito-Urinary System

Lawson, A.A.H., M.D., F.R.C.P.(Edin.)
Honorary Senior Lecturer in Medicine, University of Edinburgh; Consultant Physician, Milesmark Hospital, Dunfermline and to associated hospitals in West Fife District, Fife; Postgraduate Tutor for West Fife Postgraduate Board for Medicine, University of Edinburgh
Acute Poisoning

McHardy, G.J.R., M.A., B.Sc., B.M., F.R.C.P.(Edin.), F.R.C.P.(Lond.)
Senior Lecturer, Department of Respiratory Medicine, University of Edinburgh; Consultant Physician, Chest Unit, City Hospital, Edinburgh; Consultant Clinical Respiratory Physiologist, City Hospital and Western General Hospital, Edinburgh
Diseases of the Respiratory System

Nuki, George, M.B. B.S., F.R.C.P.(Edin.), F.R.C.P.(Lond.)
Professor of Rheumatology, University of Edinburgh; Honorary Consultant Physician, Northern General Hospital and Royal Infirmary, Edinburgh
Diseases of Connective Tissues, Joints and Bones

Richmond, John, M.D., F.R.C.P.(Edin.), F.R.C.P.(Lond.)
Professor of Medicine, University of Sheffield; Honorary Consultant Physician, Sheffield Area Health Authority (Teaching)
Diseases of the Liver and Biliary Tract

Robson, J.S., M.D., F.R.C.P.(Edin.), F.R.C.P.(Lond.)
Professor of Medicine, University of Edinburgh; Honorary Consultant Physician, Royal Infirmary, Edinburgh
Disturbances in Water and Electrolyte Balance and in Hydrogen Ion Concentration
Diseases of the Kidney and Genito-Urinary System

Shearman, D.J.C., Ph.D., M.B. Ch.B., F.R.C.P.(Edin.), F.R.A.C.P.
Mortlock Professor of Medicine, University of Adelaide and Head of the Professorial Medical Unit, Royal Adelaide Hospital, Australia
Diseases of the Alimentary Tract and Pancreas

Simpson,   J.A.,   M.D.(Glasg.),   F.R.C.P.(Edin.), F.R.C.P.(Lond.), F.R.C.P.(Glasg.), F.R.S.E.
Professor of Neurology, University of Glasgow; Senior Neurologist, Institute of Neurological Sciences, Southern General Hospital and Consultant Neurologist, Western Infirmary, Glasgow
Diseases of the Nervous System

Small, W.P., V.R.D., M.B. Ch.B., Ch.M., F.R.C.S.(Edin.), F.R.C.P.(Edin.)
Consultant Surgeon, Gastrointestinal Unit, Western General Hospital, Edinburgh
Diseases of the Alimentary Tract and Pancreas

Smyth,   J.F.,   M.A.,   M.D.(Cantab.),   M.Sc.(Lond.), F.R.C.P.(Edin.), F.R.C.P.(Lond.)
Imperial Cancer Research Fund Professor of Medical Oncology, University of Edinburgh; Honorary Consultant Physician, Western General Hospital and The Royal Infirmary, Edinburgh
Introduction to Oncology

Thin, R.N., M.D., F.R.C.P.(Edin.) ·
Consultant Physician, Department of Genitourinary Medicine, St Thomas' Hospital, London
Sexually Transmitted Diseases

Truswell, A.S., M.D., F.R.C.P.(Lond.), F.F.C.M.
Boden Professor of Human Nutrition, Sydney University, Australia; Head of Nutrition Section, School of Public Health and Tropical Medicine, Sydney; Honorary Consultant in Nutrition, Royal Prince Alfred Hospital, Sydney
Nutritional Factors in Disease

Walton, H.J., Ph.D., M.D., M.D. (Hon) Uppsala, F.R.C.P.(Edin.), D.P.M.
Professor of Psychiatry, University of Edinburgh; Director, University Department of Psychiatry, Western General Hospital; Honorary Consultant Psychiatrist, Royal Edinburgh Hospital
Psychiatry

Contents

1. Genetic Factors in Disease 1

Chromosomes and Chromosomal Disorders; Unifactorial and Multifactorial Inheritance; Prevention of Genetic Disease; Recombinant DNA Technology; Prospects

2. Immunological Factors in Disease 19

The Immune System; Types of Immune Reaction and their Relation to Human Disease; Autoimmune Disease; The HLA System and Disease; Suppression of Immune Reactions or of their Effects; Immunodeficiency Disorders; Prospects

3. Infection and Disease 37

General Aspects of Infection; Source, Nature, Spread, Diagnosis and Prevention of Infection; Diseases due to Infection; Antimicrobial Therapy; Bacteraemic Shock

4. Nutritional Factors in Disease 51

Classification and Aetiology; Energy-Yielding Nutrients; Undernutrition and Starvation; Protein Energy Malnutrition; Water, Electrolytes and Minerals; Vitamins and Disorders due to Vitamin Deficiency; Dietary Fibre; Biochemical Diagnosis and Prevention of Nutritional Deficiencies; Obesity

5. Disturbances in Water and Electrolyte Balance and in Hydrogen Ion Concentration 88

Normal Distribution of Water and Electrolytes. Disturbances involving Sodium, Potassium, Magnesium and Water; Diuretic Therapy; Hydrogen Ion Concentration; Metabolic and Respiratory Acidosis and Alkalosis

6. Introduction to Oncology 104

Epidemiology and Aetiology; Pathology; Tumour Markers; Clinical Features; Principles of Treatment including Staging, Radiotherapy, Chemotherapy and Endocrine Therapy; Terminal Care; Prospects

7. Diseases of the Cardiovascular System 122

Clinical Examination and Investigation; Disorders of Rate, Rhythm and Conduction; Cardiac Arrest; Heart Block; Acute Circulatory Failure; Cardiac Failure; Rheumatic Fever; Diseases of the Heart Valves; Ischaemic Heart Disease; Hypertension; Diseases of the Pulmonary Circulation; Diseases of the Myocardium and Pericardium; Congenital Heart Disease; Heart Disease in Pregnancy; Diseases of Arteries and Veins, Prospects

8. Diseases of the Respiratory System 202

Anatomy, Physiology, Clinical Features, Investigation and Treatment; Infections, including Tuberculosis; Allergic Diseases, including Asthma; Diseases of Larynx, Trachea and Bronchi. Intrathoracic Tumours. Pulmonary Fibrosis and Related Diseases; Occupational Lung Disease; Sarcoidosis; Diseases of the Pleura and Chest Wall; Prospects

9. Diseases of the Alimentary Tract and Pancreas 278

Physiology and Investigation of the Alimentary Tract; Diseases of the Mouth, Oesophagus, Stomach, Duodenum, Pancreas, Small and Large Intestine; Infective, Ischaemic and Psychogenic Disorders; Prospects

10. Diseases of the Liver and Biliary Tract 334

Anatomy, Physiology and Investigation; Jaundice; Acute and Chronic Parenchymal Disease;

Miscellaneous Diseases and Tumours of the Liver; Anatomy, Physiology and Investigation of the Gall Bladder and Bile Ducts; Gallstones; Acute Cholecystitis; Miscellaneous Diseases and Tumours of the Gall Bladder and Bile Ducts; Prospects

11. Diseases of the Kidney and Genito-Urinary System   376
Anatomy, Physiology and Investigation; Glomerulonephritis; Infections; Renal Failure; Obstruction of the Urinary Tract; Calculi; Congenital Abnormalities; Drugs and the Kidney; Tumours; Sexually Transmitted Diseases; Prospects in Nephrology

12. Endocrine and Metabolic Diseases   417
Introduction; Diseases of the Hypothalamus, Pituitary, Thyroid, Parathyroid and Adrenal Glands; Sexual Disorders; Diabetes Mellitus and other Metabolic Disorders; Prospects in Diabetes Mellitus

13. Diseases of the Blood   488
Blood Formation and Destruction; Terminology; Diseases of the Red Blood Cells, White Blood Cells and Monocyte-Macrophage System; Haemorrhagic Diseases; Thrombosis; Prospects

14. Diseases of Connective Tissues, Joints and Bones   551
Rheumatoid Arthritis; Spondarthritis; Juvenile Chronic Arthritis; Infective and Miscellaneous Arthritis; Systemic Lupus Erythematosus and other Connective Tissue Diseases; Crystal Deposition Diseases; Osteoarthrosis; Miscellaneous Lesions of Connective Tissue; Physiology and Diseases of Bone; Prospects

15. Diseases of the Nervous System   591
Anatomy and Physiology; Diseases of Cranial Nerves; Epilepsies; Tumours; Headache; Cerebrovascular Diseases; Infections; Demyelinating Diseases; Diseases of the Extrapyramidal System; Congenital and Degenerative Diseases; Nutritional Neurological Diseases; Diseases of the Spinal Cord and Peripheral Nerves; Diseases of Muscle; Prospects

16. Psychiatry   670
Mental Health; Diagnostic Decision Making; Organic and Functional Psychoses; Psychoneuroses; Personality Disorders; Alcoholism and Drug Dependence; Psychosexual Disorders; Psychosomatic Disorders; Psychiatric Disorders in Relation to Age

17. Acute Poisoning   701
Classification and Causes; Diagnosis; General Therapeutic Measures; Poisoning and Envenomation by Specific Agents; Prevention

18. Tropical Diseases and Climatic Disorders   714
Patterns of Disease in Tropical and Developing Countries; Geographical Influences on Diseases of the Main Systems; Disorders due to Climate

19. Diseases due to Infection (with particular reference to those encountered in the tropics)   726
Diseases due to Viruses and Chlamydiae, Rickettsiae, Bacteria, Spirochaetes, Protozoa, Helminths and Arthropods; Advice to Travellers

20. The Promotion of Health and Prevention of Disease   808

21. Appendices   812
Diets
Desirable Weights
Notes on SI Units
Biochemical and Haematological Values
Notes on Nomenclature and Prescription of Drugs

Index   823

Note to Readers. The policy regarding administration of drugs and advice about their dosage is given on page 822.

1. Genetic Factors in Disease

Nowadays there is an increasing awareness of the importance of genetic factors in the aetiology and pathogenesis of many disorders affecting man. Perhaps of more importance is that this knowledge has also led to possible means of prevention of such disorders through genetic counselling and antenatal diagnosis.

At the turn of the century morbidity and mortality in infancy and childhood could largely be attributed to environmental factors such as infections and nutritional deficiencies. With advances in medicine these problems are decreasing, at least in the developed countries, while others, in which genetic factors are largely or even entirely responsible, are becoming more obvious. In a survey carried out in Newcastle in 1970, no less than 42% of childhood deaths could be attributed to diseases which are genetic in causation. The contribution of genetic factors to mortality and morbidity in adults is more difficult to assess but is also increasing.

It is useful to consider human disease as forming a spectrum at one end of which we have those diseases which are entirely genetic in origin and in which environmental factors play little if any part. This group of disorders includes *chromosomal abnormalities* and so-called *unifactorial disorders*. The latter are due to single gene defects (Mendelian factors); though individually rare there are over a thousand of them. They are usually serious disorders; they often present at birth or in childhood, though notable exceptions are Huntington's chorea, myotonic dystrophy and polyposis coli. The mode of inheritance is straightforward and follows Mendelian principles, and the risks of occurrence in relatives are high. For the vast majority of these unifactorial disorders there is as yet no effective treatment and prevention is the main approach to the problem.

At the other end of the spectrum are those diseases such as infections and nutritional deficiencies which are entirely environmental in aetiology. In the middle of the spectrum are many common conditions which are partly genetic and partly environmental in causation, so-called *multifactorial disorders*. These include many congenital malformations (such as congenital dislocation of the hip, club foot, congenital pyloric stenosis, congenital heart disease, anencephaly and spina bifida), 'diseases of modern society' (diabetes mellitus, essential hypertension, coronary artery disease) and possibly certain psychiatric disorders (such as schizophrenia and manic-depressive psychosis). In multifactorial disorders the genetic component is complex, probably involving in each case many genes. The risks to relatives are usually low.

In this chapter, after a review of the chemical basis of inheritance, an outline is given of chromosomal abnormalities, unifactorial and multifactorial disorders and the prevention of genetic disease.

CHEMICAL BASIS OF INHERITANCE

In the nucleus of every cell are the chromosomes containing the genes composed of segments of deoxyribonucleic acid (DNA) within which genetic information is stored.

DNA is made up of two polynucleotide chains, twisted together to form a double helix (Fig. 1.1). Each nucleotide is composed of a nitrogenous base, a sugar molecule (deoxyribose) and a phosphate molecule. The nitrogenous bases in DNA are adenine and guanine (purines) and cytosine and thymine (pyrimidines). A purine in one chain always pairs with a pyrimidine on the other chain. There is also specific base pairing: guanine in one chain always pairs with cytosine in the other chain and adenine always pairs with thymine. At nuclear division the two strands of the DNA molecule separate and as a result of specific base pairing each chain then builds its complement. In this way, when a cell divides, genetic information is conserved and transmitted to each daughter cell.

Fig. 1.1 Protein synthesis. Sequences of bases in nuclear DNA (genes) send instructions via messenger RNA (m-RNA), to transfer RNA (t-RNA) on ribosomes in the cytoplasm, whereby amino acids are linked to form polypeptides. In these processes guanine (G) pairs with cytosine (C) and adenine (A) with thymine (T) or uracil (U).

The primary action of the gene is to synthesise protein by various combinations of 20 different amino acids. Genetic information is stored within the DNA molecule in the form of a triplet code such that a sequence of three bases specifies the structure of one amino acid.

Whereas DNA is found mainly in the chromosomes, ribonucleic acid (RNA) is found mainly in the nucleolus and the cytoplasm. RNA has a structure similar to DNA (Fig. 1.1): both nucleic acids contain adenine, guanine and cytosine but thymine is replaced by uracil in RNA and the latter contains the sugar ribose.

The information stored in the DNA code of the gene is transmitted from one strand to a particular type of RNA, so-called messenger-RNA (m-RNA). Each m-RNA is formed by a particular gene, such that every base in the m-RNA molecule is complementary to a corresponding base in the DNA of the gene: cytosine with guanine, thymine with adenine but adenine with uracil since the latter replaces thymine in RNA. The m-RNA then migrates into the cytoplasm where it becomes associated with the ribosomes which are the site of protein synthesis. In the ribosomes the m-RNA forms the template for arranging particular amino acids in sequence.

In the cytoplasm there is yet another form of RNA referred to as transfer-RNA (t-RNA). Each amino acid in the cytoplasm becomes attached to a particular t-RNA. The other end of the t-RNA molecule consists of three bases which combine with complementary bases on the m-RNA. Thus a particular triplet in the m-RNA is related through t-RNA to a specific amino acid. The ribosome moves along the m-RNA in a zipper-like fashion, the assembled amino acids linking up to form a polypeptide chain.

There are essentially two types of genes: structural genes which are responsible for the synthesis of specific proteins such as haemoglobin, collagen and enzymes, and control genes which are thought to modify the action of structural genes.

A change (mutation) of a base pair of the DNA molecule may result in any one of a number of possible effects. If the altered triplet codes for the same amino acid then of course the change will go undetected. Possibly 20 to 25% of all possible single base changes are of this type. Alternatively a single base mutation may result in a triplet which codes for a different amino acid resulting in an altered protein. The latter may retain its biological activity (e.g. enzyme activity) but have altered physico-chemical properties such as electrophoretic mobility or stability so that it is more rapidly broken down. This is the case in many of the abnormal haemoglobinopathies in which the aberrant haemoglobin may be detected by its altered electrophoretic mobility. However the substitution of a different amino acid may result in reduced or even absent biological activity. In inborn errors of metabolism therefore the level of a particular enzyme may be reduced because it is not synthesised, or it is synthesised but has reduced activity or because of its instability it is more rapidly broken down.

CHROMOSOMES AND CHROMOSOMAL DISORDERS

Chromosome Structure and Number. Among higher animals each species bears within the nucleus of its cells a set of chromosomes which is characteristic both in number and in morphology for that species. Each nucleus in the somatic cells of man contains a set of 46 chromosomes. Two of these chromosomes determine the sex of the individual and are therefore known as *sex chromosomes*; the remaining 44 chromosomes are known as *autosomes*.

The DNA of higher organisms is coated with histone and non-histone proteins. This produces a deoxyribonucleoprotein fibre (chromatin) which forms the basic unit of chromosome structure. Chromosomes are in a suitable state for detailed study only during specific intervals within the period of cell division, for it is during these periods that the chromosomes become contracted, thicker and more readily stained. Chromomosomes in the resting nucleus do not take up most stains in a satisfactory way.

Each chromosome has a point along its length, a constriction, known as the *centromere* which divides the chromosomes into two arms which are usually unequal in length. The chromosomes also differ in their overall length. Further by using certain stains each chromosome can be shown to have a specific banding pattern. By these criteria it is now possible to identify individual chromosomes.

The chromosomal complement of any nucleus is composed of two sets of chromosomes which are arranged in pairs. Because the two members of any given pair (with the exception of the sex chromosomes) resemble one another they are said to be *homologous*. One homologue of any pair is derived from one parent and its partner from the other parent. Thus man has 22 pairs of homologous chromosomes (autosomes) and one pair of sex chromosomes.

During gametogenesis the number of chromosomes is halved in order that the number of chromosomes remains constant and is not doubled at each conception. Thus somatic cell nuclei contain twice as many chromosomes as gametes and with respect to their chromosome complement are said to be *diploid*, whereas gametes are said to be *haploid*.

The two sex chromosomes of the female are identical and are referred to as *X chromosomes*. The sex chromosomes of the male, however, are not identical. One of the pair resembles the X chromosomes seen in females while the other is much smaller, differs considerably in morphology and is referred to as a *Y chromosome*. Thus the sex chromosome constitution is XX in a female and XY in a male. In the female each ovum bears one or other of the X chromosomes, whereas in the male the sperms bear either an X or a Y chromosome. At fertilisation an ovum therefore has an equal chance of being fertilised by either an X or a Y bearing sperm. It is for this reason that the sex ratio is approximately (not exactly) unity at birth.

Mitosis. Unlike highly differentiated cells such as neurones, the cells of many tissues in the body repeatedly undergo division. In fact some cells, such as those of the intestinal tract and bone marrow, continue to divide throughout the life of an individual. For the error rate in cell division to remain as low as it is, nuclear division must be extremely well regulated. The process by which nuclei divide to produce two identical daughter nuclei is known as mitosis.

During mitosis each chromosome divides into two so that the number of chromosomes in each daughter nucleus is the same as in the parent cell. Though mitosis is a continuous process, one step merging imperceptibly into the next, it can be divided into stages for ease of description. These stages are known as interphase, prophase, metaphase, anaphase and telophase (Fig. 1.2).

Interphase is the resting stage between nuclear divisions when the chromosomes are loosely

Fig. 1.2 Stages of mitosis and meiosis

coiled and difficult to visualise. By the end of interphase each chromosome has divided longitudinally into two daughter chromosomes, or *chromatids*, which remain attached to each other at the centromere.

During *prophase*, the chromosomes take up stains more readily and therefore become easier to visualise. By the end of prophase the nucleoli are no longer visible and each chromatid is a tightly coiled structure which is closely aligned to its partner.

Metaphase begins with the disappearance of the nuclear membrane and the formation of the spindle apparatus, which consists of a number of

minute 'threads' which run from one pole (centriole) of the spindle to the other. The chromosomes become orientated around the centre of the cell in the equatorial plane. Each chromosome is attached to the spindle by means of its centromere. The spindle is responsible for the movement of the chromosomes during mitosis.

During *anaphase* the centromere of each chromosome divides into two, each half 'repels' the other and the chromatids move apart towards opposite poles of the spindle. When the chromatids reach the poles they form two separate but identical groups.

Telophase begins as the daughter chromosomes

arrive at the poles of the spindle. The two groups of chromosomes become surrounded by a new nuclear membrane and gradually become less visible. Cell division is completed by cleavage of the cytoplasm. New cell membranes develop and the nuclei of the two daughter cells re-enter the interphase stage. Thus at the end of mitosis a cell has divided into two daughter cells each with an identical genetic constitution.

Meiosis. The process by which the chromosome number is halved during gametogenesis is known as meiosis. Although meiosis involves two division stages, the chromosomes divide only once, each gamete normally receiving either of a pair of homologous chromosomes.

Each of the two steps in meiosis has a prophase, metaphase, anaphase and telophase stage as in mitosis (Fig. 1.2). The prophase of the first stage is very long. It is thought that DNA replication has already taken place by the onset of this stage, although each chromosome still appears morphologically to be a single thread. During prophase the chromosomes become more contracted, as a result of tighter coiling, and homologous chromosomes come together and pair along their length. Then a process known as *crossing-over* may occur in which there is an exchange of genetic material between chromatids of homologous chromosomes.

Following prophase the sequence of events is essentially similar to that occurring in mitosis, except that during this first meiotic division the centromere does not divide. Instead the members of each pair of homologous chromosomes migrate to opposite poles of the nucleus so that each daughter nucleus receives only one member of each pair and therefore bears a haploid chromosome complement.

In the second stage of meiosis the centromere divides and the chromatids of each chromosome separate and migrate into different nuclei. Thus each daughter cell from the first meiotic division has in turn divided to form two identical cells. Meiosis therefore results in each gamete having a haploid number of chromosomes and receiving one or the other member of each homologous pair of chromosomes and the genes it bears. This forms the cytological basis for Mendelian inheritance.

Methods of Studying Chromosomes. There are a variety of ways in which the study of chromosomes can be approached. Broadly these fall into two categories: those techniques which are used to study the complete chromosome complement of an individual, or those which enable information to be gained about the sex chromosome constitution of a person without having to do a complete chromosome analysis.

Since it is only during critical stages of the mitotic or meiotic cycle that the chromosomes are in a suitable state to study, chromosome analysis requires the provision of a large number of cells which are actively dividing. Meiotic studies can of course be done only on specimens of tissue obtained from the gonads. Mitotic studies, on the other hand, can be made on a variety of different and more easily available tissues, e.g. directly from cells which are rapidly dividing *in vivo*, as in bone marrow. More commonly, however, specimens are obtained from tissues which are not rapidly dividing *in vivo* but are much more accessible to study, such as skin and blood leucocytes, and the cells are stimulated to divide *in vitro* by the addition of phytohaemagglutinin. The addition of colchicine arrests cell division at the metaphase stage when the chromosomes are most suitable for study. The use of hypotonic solutions causes the cells to swell, disperses the chromosomes and makes them easier to identify and count (Fig. 1.3). Finally the material is stained (e.g. with Giemsa) to demonstrate the banding patterns of the chromosomes. A suitable meta-

Fig. 1.3 Preparation of a karyotype

phase spread is then photographed through a high power microscope and the individual chromosomes are cut out from the photograph. The chromosomes are then arranged in an orderly fashion, in homologous pairs, to produce a standard arrangement known as a *karyotype*.

Methods are available for studying the sex chromosome constitution of an individual without having to resort to the costly and time-consuming process of preparing and analysing the complete karyotype. These include the study of sex-chromatin and fluorescent bodies in buccal smears and 'drumsticks' in polymorphonuclear leucocytes.

Female nuclei contain a distinctive mass of nuclear chromatin characteristically situated close to the nuclear membrane, the *sex chromatin* or 'Barr-body', which represents a genetically inactive X chromosome. In the female inactivation of one X chromosome in normal cells is a random process so that either the paternal or maternal X chromosome can be inactivated in any particular cell of the same person. The cell nuclei of all the tissues in a human female contain a sex-chromatin body, but for convenience the most suitable cells for study are those of the buccal mucosa.

The inside of the cheek is gently scraped with a spatula and the cells obtained spread onto a glass slide (*buccal smear*). These cells are then fixed and stained and can be examined for the presence of sex-chromatin bodies which are seen in 30 to 60% of nuclei of a normal female. Since only one X chromosome is active per cell, then the number of sex-chromatin bodies (inactivated X chromosomes) is one less than the total number of X chromosomes. Thus a normal female has one sex chromatin body, a patient with XO Turner's syndrome (p. 9) has no sex-chromatin bodies (chromatin negative) and a patient who has Klinefelter's syndrome (p. 9) with three X chromosomes (XXXY) has two sex chromatin bodies.

In suitably stained smears of peripheral blood about 3% of the polymorphonuclear leucocytes of females show a small accessory nuclear lobule, which resembles a drumstick and projects from the main mass of the nuclear lobes. This is not seen in polymorphs from normal males, or females with an XO sex-chromosome constitu-

tion. The number of drumsticks is not, however, related to the number of X chromosomes.

Interphase nuclei of cells from males exhibit a fluorescent spot called the *F body* (or Y chromatin) when stained with quinacrine; the number of F bodies represents the number of Y chromosomes. The technique can be adapted for use with buccal smears and so provides a method of assessing the number of Y chromosomes comparable with the sex-chromatin method of studying X chromosomes.

It can be seen, therefore, that these techniques are complementary and by combining them the sex chromosome constitution of an individual can be determined with ease, speed and accuracy. This is extremely useful clinically in the investigation of patients with abnormalities of sexual development or infertility, or for use in large-scale population surveys. Apart from these more common applications these techniques are also being used in new fields such as the separation of X and Y bearing sperm (half of human sperms contain an F body and are presumably Y bearing) and the determination of the sex of an unborn child.

Chromosome Nomenclature. A shorthand notation is used to describe a karyotype in the simplest way. This consists first of the total number of chromosomes (in numerals), followed by the sex chromosome constitution, and finally by any abnormalities that are present. Thus a normal male is 46, XY; a normal female is 46, XX. A girl with Turner's syndrome may be 45, XO and a boy with Klinefelter's syndrome, 47, XXY. The short and long arms of any chromosome are designated 'p' and 'q' respectively. A (+) or (−) sign is placed before an appropriate symbol where it means an additional or missing whole chromosome, but after a symbol when it refers only to part of a chromosome. Thus a boy with Down's syndrome is 47,XY, + 21 and a boy with part of the short arm of chromosome 5 missing is 46,XY,5p − .

Chromosomal Disorders

Specific chromosomal abnormalities are associated with recognised diseases or clinical syndromes in man. These include Down's syndrome (mongolism), abnormalities of sexual development (Turner's and Klinefelter's syndromes), syndromes of multiple congenital malformations (13- and 18-trisomies), spontaneous abortions, personality disorders (XYY and XXX etc.), chronic myeloid leukaemia and ataxia telangiectasia.

It has been found that 1 in every 200 live-born babies has a gross abnormality of chromosome number or structure. High as this figure is, it does not indicate fully the frequency with which chromosomal anomalies occur at fertilisation, for in a study of early spontaneous abortions chromosomal aberrations occurred in over 50%. Many of these chromosomal anomalies are rarely found in live-born babies and are therefore presumably lethal and the cause of a significant number of early abortions.

Chromosomal abnormalities can be divided into those which involve the autosomes and those which involve the sex chromosomes. These can be further divided into abnormalities of number and of structure. Numerical abnormalities arise when one or more chromosomes are either lost or gained, a phenomenon referred to as *aneuploidy*. When a whole set of chromosomes is gained the phenomenon is known as *polyploidy* and is not compatible with survival in man. The loss of a whole autosome, *monosomy*, also appears to be lethal in man. The addition of an extra chromosome, so resulting in three chromosomes instead of two (*trisomy*), seems, however, to result in less severe effects.

Autosomal Abnormalities. Trisomy of a number of different autosomes have now been reported in man; the most common is trisomy-21 which results in Down's syndrome. The two other well-recognised syndromes (trisomy-13 and trisomy-18) occur far less frequently than Down's syndrome. They are both more severe in effect and usually result in death within the infant period.

DOWN'S SYNDROME occurs in about 1 in 700 live-births and is characterised by a flat face with widely spaced and upward slanting eyes, epicanthic folds, brachycephaly, malformed ears, broad and/or short neck, and a single, transverse palmar crease. Patients with Down's syndrome are invariably mentally retarded, but have a pleasant, quiet personality and show a great fondness for music. The condition is also associated with an increased frequency of both congenital visceral anomalies, particularly congenital heart disease, and acute leukaemia. Although the mortality rate of these patients is high within the first year of life, many now survive into adulthood and there are several reports of women with Down's syndrome having children; on average half their offspring are normal and half have Down's syndrome.

About 95% of cases of Down's syndrome are due to regular trisomy-21 which arises as a result of non-disjunction during meiosis. Normally during meiosis the two homologous chromosomes of any pair separate and pass into different gametes. Occasionally an accident occurs and the chromosomes fail to separate, both members of the pair passing into the same gamete. If such a gamete is then fertilised by a normal gamete the resulting zygote will possess an additional chromosome.

All the trisomy syndromes are found to have a significant relationship to maternal age, the frequency of trisomic births increasing with increasing maternal age. It is thought that perhaps some effect of ageing in the ova of older mothers makes them more prone to non-disjunction. There have been reports, however, of trisomy-21 recurring in some families, which suggests that the phenomenon of non-disjunction may be under genetic control at least in these rare families.

About 1% of cases of Down's syndrome are *mosaics*, that is, they possess two different cell lines, one of which has a normal chromosome constitution, the other an extra chromosome 21. This arises as a result of non-disjunction occurring at or after the first zygotic division and is very rarely inherited. The clinical picture may often be considerably modified in some of these cases.

About 4% of cases of Down's syndrome result from a phenomenon known as *translocation*, in which there is an exchange of segments between different chromosomes. The mechanism is thought to be that two chromosomes lying close to one another suffer simultaneous breaks followed by an exchange of chromosomal material. For example, in Down's syndrome a large part of chromosome 21 may be united with part of chromosome 15. A carrier of such a translocation (who has only 45 chromosomes) produces four types of gametes. A gamete may contain a normal chromosome 15 and a normal chromosome 21, in which case the resulting offspring will be normal. Or a gamete may contain a translocation (15/21), in which case the resulting offspring will have only 45 chromosomes and will be a carrier like the parent. Or a gamete may contain the translocation and a normal chromosome 21, in which case the offspring will have 46 chromosomes but in effect will be trisomic for chromosome 21 and will therefore have Down's syndrome. Finally a gamete may contain a chromosome 15 but no chromosome 21; this would produce a zygote monosomic for chromosome 21 which is lethal and would presumably result in an abortion. Theoretically, therefore, a carrier of such a translocation has a 1 in 3 chance of having a child with Down's syndrome, but for reasons which are not clear, the actual risk is much less. In Down's syndrome the translocation usually involves an exchange of material between chromosomes 13, 14 or 15 and chromosome 21. Rarely there may be an exchange between chromosomes 21 and 22 or even between two 21s. In the case of a parent who carries a translocation involving two 21s, all the offspring will have Down's syndrome.

OTHER AUTOSOMAL ABNORMALITIES. *Deletions* arise when a segment of a chromosome has been lost. New techniques have led to the demonstration of deletions involving a number of autosomes and an increasing number of these are being associated with clinically recognisable syndromes, examples of which are summarised in Table 1.1. Other rarer forms of chromosomal abnormalities are *ring chromosomes* and *isochromosomes*. Ring chromosomes involving both autosomes and sex chromosomes have been described; they are thought to be formed when two ends of a chromosome have been deleted and the broken (more 'sticky') ends fuse to form a ring. In effect ring chromosomes are manifest as deletions and in shorthand they are represented as an 'r'. An isochromosome is formed when the centromere divides horizontally instead of longitudinally resulting in a chromosome consisting of either two long arms or of two short arms.

The *Philadelphia chromosome* (Ph') is an *acquired* chromosomal abnormality associated with chronic myeloid leukaemia. It is a deleted chromosome 22, the long arm being translocated to another autosome, usually chromosome 9.

Sex Chromosome Abnormalities. Numerical abnormalities of the sex chromosomes are

Table 1.1 Autosomal abnormalities associated with recognised clinical syndromes

Chromosome abnormality	Syndrome	Clinical features
trisomy-21 translocation 13-15/21 translocation 22/21 translocation 21/21	Down's	characteristic facies mental retardation hypotonia congenital heart disease Simian palmar crease
trisomy-8	——	moderate mental retardation concomitant strabismus clinodactyly other skeletal defects
trisomy-9	——	abnormal facies skeletal abnormalities hypoplastic genitalia congenital heart disease
trisomy-13	Patau's	motor and mental retardation microcephaly microphthalmia cleft palate/hare lip polydactyly congenital heart disease
trisomy-18	Edwards'	motor and mental retardation flexion deformities of fingers micrognathia 'rocker-bottom' feet congenital heart disease
trisomy-22	——	mental and motor retardation microcephaly abnormal facies and ears
trisomy-4p	——	abnormal facies digital anomalies foot deformities
trisomy-9p	——	abnormal facies large, low-set ears mental retardation incurved and short V digit
4p-	——	mental retardation abnormal facies cleft palate coloboma epilepsy hypospadias scalp defects

Table 1.1 (continued)

Chromosome abnormality	Syndrome	Clinical features
5p-	Cri du chat	mental retardation microcephaly hypertelorism characteristic cry
13q-	——	mental and motor retardation
13r		abnormal facies microcephaly abnormal thumbs abnormal ears
18q-	De Grouchy's	mental retardation 'carp-mouth' abnormal ears tapering fingers
18p-	De Grouchy's	mental retardation ocular abnormalities abnormal ears dental decay CNS abnormalities
18r	——	combination of 18p- and 18q- features
21q- (G deletion syndrome I)	'anti-mongolism'	antimongoloid slant of eyes hypertonia micrognathia growth retardation skeletal malformations
22q- (G deletion syndrome II)	——	epicanthic folds hypotonia syndactyly retarded development

more common than with the autosomes, and in general they produce less severe effects. They are brought about by the same phenomenon of non-disjunction. As with the autosomes, abnormalities of structure also occur although they are far less common than the numerical anomalies.

KLINEFELTER'S SYNDROME was the first sex chromosome aneuploidy to be demonstrated in man. Affected males have an extra X chromosome resulting in an XXY sex chromosome constitution or as many as four X chromosomes may be present; an extra Y chromosome may also be present on occasions resulting in an XXYY sex chromosome constitution. The main clinical features are eunuchoid body proportions, sterility (due to azoospermia), hypogonadism, gynaeco-mastia and often mental retardation.

There appears to be a relationship between mental retardation and the number of X chromosomes in both males and females. In Klinefelter's syndrome all individuals with an XXXY sex chromosome constitution are mentally retarded, whereas this is so in only about one-quarter of those with XXY sex chromosome constitution. Like the autosomal trisomies, Klinefelter's syndrome is found to occur more frequently in the sons of older mothers.

THE XYY CONSTITUTION is another sex chromosome aneuploidy in the male. Such men are reported to occur with increased frequency amongst inmates of institutions for the mentally retarded with criminal tendencies. It has been shown by various surveys that between two and five per cent of such populations may be XYY. However, the exact relationship of this chromosomal anomaly with either mental retardation or criminal tendencies is uncertain especially as XYY individuals have been found amongst the normal general population.

TURNER'S SYNDROME was the first aneuploidy to be described in females. An XO sex chromosome constitution is the commonest abnormality, but clinical features of Turner's syndrome may also result from iso-chromosomes, deletions, and rings involving the X chromosome. This abnormality must arise by non-disjunction, but unlike Klinefelter's syndrome, Turner's syndrome does not show a relationship with maternal age.

The main clinical features are shortness of stature, primary amenorrhoea, lack of secondary sex characteristics and a variety of congenital abnormalities such as webbing of the neck, increased carrying-angle of the forearm (cubitus valgus) and coarctation of the aorta. Although, overall, patients with Turner's syndrome have a significantly lower I.Q. than normal, marked retardation is uncommon and the discrepancy is mainly in the performance aspect of their I.Q.

Females have also been described with three or even four X-chromosomes (XXX, XXXX); they may occasionally be mentally subnormal or have psychiatric disorders, but in all other respects appear to be healthy. Usually children born to XXX females are normal.

UNIFACTORIAL INHERITANCE

These disorders are due to defects of a single gene, i.e. to a primary error in the DNA code.

They are inherited in a simple fashion, following Mendelian laws. The risk of their recurring in a family may therefore be accurately predicted on theoretical grounds making genetic counselling more straightforward.

These disorders may be subdivided according to the chromosome on which the abnormal (or mutant) gene is situated and also by the nature of the trait itself. Thus a trait which is determined by a gene situated on an autosome is said to be inherited as an *autosomal* trait, and this may be either *dominant* or *recessive*. A trait determined by a gene situated on one of the sex chromosomes is said to be *sex-linked* and may also be either dominant or recessive.

Autosomal Dominant Inheritance. A dominant trait is one which is manifested in the *heterozygote*. In other words a person exhibiting an autosomal dominant trait possesses both the mutant gene and the normal gene, the presence of only one mutant gene being necessary for the trait to be manifested in the carrier. If the disorder is common, then some affected individuals could be *homozygotes* (i.e. have a 'double dose' of the mutant gene), but if the disorder is rare (as is usually the case), then affected individuals are almost always heterozygotes. It should be noted that the normal and abnormal genes are known as *alleles*, i.e. they are alternative forms of the same gene.

Usually persons affected with an autosomal dominant trait are found to have an affected parent, the trait being transmitted from one generation to the next in a family, as illustrated in Figure 1.4. This is not always the case, however; sometimes the disorder may appear suddenly in a family when no members of previous generations have been affected. This may be due to illegitimacy, to one parent being minimally affected and the disorder not recognised, or more commonly to the occurrence of a new mutation. This may complicate genetic counselling and is a problem which arises particularly in conditions inherited in a dominant fashion.

In diseases which are severe, affected individuals seldom have children because they are either infertile or do not survive to reach reproductive age. In such conditions the disease will eventually become extinct in affected families and

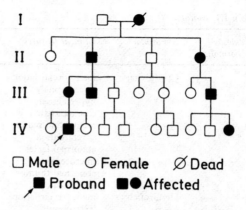

Fig. 1.4 Characteristic pedigree: autosomal dominant trait.

is maintained in the population only by fresh mutations. Achondroplasia is one of the forms of short-limbed dwarfism and is inherited as an autosomal dominant trait. In one large study it was shown that affected individuals exhibited a marked reduction in reproductive fitness. It is not surprising, therefore, that a high proportion of cases are the result of new mutations.

In conditions which do not have much effect on survival it is often possible to trace the conditions through many generations of a family. Such a condition is the adult form of polycystic disease of the kidneys. Although affected individuals may eventually die from chronic renal failure, they often show no symptoms or signs of the disease until early middle life when they have already had their family and run the risk of transmitting the trait to their children.

In autosomal dominant conditions, if an affected individual marries a normal person, then on average half their children will be similarly affected. This arises because the affected individual produces gametes, half of which contain the normal gene and the other half contain the mutant gene. The normal partner produces gametes all of which contain the normal gene. Thus at fertilisation the normal partner's gametes have an equal chance of uniting with a gamete carrying either a normal or an abnormal gene with the result that at conception there is a 1 in 2 chance of producing an affected individual. Because of the smaller size of modern families, by chance all the children of an affected individual may be normal, or similarly by chance again all his children may be affected. It is on average that half the offspring of an affected individual will be affected.

Some autosomal dominant traits are extremely variable in severity, this variability in clinical manifestation being referred to as *expressivity*. Osteogenesis imperfecta, for example, is an autosomal dominant condition in which affected individuals may have only blue sclerae, whereas others may exhibit the full syndrome of blue sclerae, deafness and multiple fractures.

Occasionally an individual may carry a mutant gene and yet not exhibit any of its effects; the gene is then said to be non-penetrant, *penetrance* being the probability that an individual with the genetic predisposition will express clinical disease. This phenomenon explains situations where dominant mutant traits appear to have 'skipped' generations in certain families. This variation in expression of a mutant gene results both from the modifying influence of other genes and from environmental factors. The degree of penetrance of a gene is that proportion of heterozygotes who express the gene in any degree, however mild. For a gene to be *fully penetrant* its effects must be manifest to some degree in all individuals who carry the gene.

The phenomenon of varying penetrance can give rise to problems when estimating recurrence risks in order to give genetic advice. For example, tuberous sclerosis (epiloia) is inherited as a dominant trait but is not always penetrant. This condition is characterised by adenoma sebaceum (small papules over the cheeks and nose), epilepsy and mental retardation of varying severity. Some individuals carrying the gene may be so mildly affected as to pass as normal and so produce an apparently 'skipped' generation. However, it is unusual to find a proven carrier (e.g. with an affected child and an affected parent) who does not show at least some evidence of the disease, such as a few typical papules on the face.

Autosomal Recessive Inheritance. Autosomal recessive traits also affect both males and females. Unlike dominant traits, recessive traits are manifest only in the homozygous state, that is, in those individuals who possess a double dose of the mutant gene. Heterozygotes who possess only one mutant gene are usually perfectly healthy.

Similarly the offspring of an affected person are usually normal, because most recessive conditions are so rare that it would be most unlikely that an affected person would marry a person heterozygous for the same mutant gene. In the even more unlikely event of two persons homozygous for the same recessive trait marrying, all their children would be affected. In general, however, both parents and offspring of a person homozygous for a rare recessive gene will be healthy. Characteristically in recessive traits, affected individuals cannot be traced from one generation to the next and if more than one member of a family is affected they are usually sibs, i.e. brothers and sisters. The pedigree of an autosomal recessive trait (Fig. 1.5), therefore, differs from that of a dominant trait.

Fig. 1.5 Characteristic pedigree: autosomal recessive trait.

At conception there is a 1 in 4 chance that any child of two heterozygous parents will be affected. Each parent produces gametes of two types, one bearing the normal gene and the other bearing the mutant gene. At conception, therefore, one-quarter of the offspring will be normal, one-half will be healthy heterozygotes and one-quarter will be affected. These are average figures; by chance all the offspring of such a couple might be affected, or similarly all their offspring might be normal. It has been calculated theoretically that in marriages between two heterozygotes, in 75% of families with only one child that child will be unaffected, in 56% of families with two children both children will be unaffected, but in only 32% of families with four children will all four children be unaffected.

When dealing with rare recessive diseases the

parents of affected individuals are often found to be related, because such individuals are more likely to have inherited the same mutant gene from an ancestor they have in common. The chance that first cousins will carry the same recessive gene is 1 in 8, but the chance that two unrelated individuals will carry the same recessive gene is very much lower and depends on the frequency of the particular gene in the population. In general the rarer the gene the greater the frequency of consanguinity amongst the parents of affected individuals.

At present roughly 1 in 200 marriages in Britain is between first cousins, so that giving advice on the genetic consequences of cousin marriages is a problem with which geneticists are frequently faced. Several extensive studies have shown that among the offspring of consanguineous matings there is an increased perinatal mortality rate together with an increased frequency of both congenital abnormalities and mental retardation, but the actual risks are small and in fact only slightly greater than in the general population. The situation is quite different, however, if there is a family history of a recessive disorder, when the risks will be greatly increased.

Many conditions show an autosomal recessive mode of inheritance and include, for example, many inborn errors of metabolism, some types of deaf-mutism and some types of congenital blindness. The commonest autosomal recessive trait known in Western Europe is cystic fibrosis which affects one in every 2000 births.

Sex-linked Inheritance. Conditions determined by genes situated on either of the sex chromosomes are said to be inherited as sex-linked traits. Genes carried on the X chromosome are said to be X-linked, those on the Y chromosomes being Y-linked. Y-linkage of a gene implies that only males would be affected and that all the sons of an affected male would inherit the gene. With the possible exception of hairy ears, there are no proven examples of Y-linked single gene disorders in man. Thus all known sex-linked conditions are due to genes on the X chromosome. As with autosomal traits these conditions may be either dominant or recessive.

X-linked dominant conditions are manifest both in females who are heterozygous for the mutant

gene and in males who carry the mutant gene on their single X chromosome. The pedigree of an X-linked dominant trait (Fig. 1.6) can superficially resemble that of an autosomal dominant trait, but there is a fundamental difference. Although an affected female will transmit the trait to half her offspring of either sex, an affected male will transmit the trait to all of his daughters but to none of his sons. There will therefore be an excess of females in families exhibiting such conditions. There are few X-linked dominant disorders but a notable example is one form of vitamin D resistant rickets.

Fig. 1.6 Characteristic pedigree: X-linked dominant trait.

An *X-linked recessive condition* is caused by a gene carried on the X chromosome and is manifest in females only when the gene is in the homozygous state. In males, a mutant gene present on the single X chromosome is always manifest because it is unopposed by the modifying effect of a normal gene on the second X chromosome, as happens in females. As with autosomal recessive conditions, the heterozygous carrier is usually healthy. Conditions inherited in this way therefore predominantly affect males and are transmitted by healthy female carriers (Fig. 1.7). In those conditions where affected males may survive to have children, the condition will also be transmitted by affected males (Fig. 1.8).

Haemophilia is the best known example of an X-linked recessive trait. Whereas in the past most boys with this disease died at an early age, with improvements in treatment most now survive. If an affected man marries a normal woman, then all his daughters will be carriers but none of his sons will be affected. An X-linked trait is never transmitted from father to son. This is because a man

Fig. 1.7 Characteristic pedigree: X-linked recessive trait — when affected males do not reproduce (e.g. Duchenne muscular dystrophy).

Fig. 1.8 Characteristic pedigree: X-linked recessive trait — when affected males do reproduce (e.g. haemophilia).

transmits his only X-chromosome (which if he is affected bears the mutant gene) to each of his daughters but his Y chromosome to each of his sons.

If a woman carrying an X-linked recessive trait marries a normal man, then half of her sons will be affected and half of her daughters will be carriers because each of her children has an equal chance of inheriting from her either the normal X chromosome or the one bearing the mutant gene.

Duchenne muscular dystrophy is inherited as an X-linked recessive trait and because affected boys die young, it is transmitted solely by healthy female carriers.

Very rarely a female may exhibit an X-linked recessive trait. This situation may arise in several different ways. Firstly, she may have an abnormal chromosomal constitution resulting in her having only one X chromosome, such as in Turner's syndrome (XO). Secondly, she may be homozygous for the mutant gene, but this is very unlikely with rare recessive disorders because she would have to have inherited the disorder from both her parents. The third possibility is that she may be a 'manifesting heterozygote'. If, by chance, in the majority of her cells it is the normal X chromosome which is inactivated, then a

Table 1.2 Mode of inheritance of some unifactorial disorders

Autosomal dominant	Autosomal recessive	X-linked recessive
Achondroplasia	Albinism	Christmas disease
Facioscapulohumeral muscular dystrophy	Ataxia telangiectasia	Duchenne muscular dystrophy
Gilbert's syndrome	Congenital adrenal hyperplasia	Glucose-6-phosphate dehydrogenase deficiency
Hereditary spherocytosis	Congenital goitrous cretinism	Haemophilia
Huntington's chorea	Crigler-Najjar syndrome	Hunter's syndrome
Hyperlipoproteinaemia Type II	Cystic fibrosis	Lesch-Nyhan syndrome
Marfan's syndrome	Dubin-Johnson syndrome	Nephrogenic diabetes insipidus
Myotonia congenita	Fanconi's syndrome	
Myotonic dystrophy	Friedrich's ataxia	
Neurofibromatosis	Galactosaemia	
Osteogenesis imperfecta	Gaucher's disease	
Polycystic disease of kidneys (adult form)	Glycogen storage diseases	
	Hurler's syndrome	
Polyposis of colon	Limb girdle muscular dystrophy (Erb)	
Porphyria, acute intermittent	Niemann-Pick disease	
Tuberous sclerosis	Phenylketonuria	
von Willebrand's disease	Pendred's syndrome	
	Tay-Sachs disease	
	Wilson's disease	

female heterozygote may exhibit the trait. Careful examination of carriers of Duchenne muscular dystrophy sometimes reveals varying degrees of weakness in the same group of muscles that are weak in affected boys.

The modes of inheritance for some unifactorial disorders are given in Table 1.2.

MULTIFACTORIAL INHERITANCE

Many human characteristics can be measured and if the values are plotted against the number of individuals in the population with each particular value then a bell-shaped or normal frequency distribution curve is found (Fig. 1.9). This applies to such charactersitics as intelligence, stature, weight, skin colour and blood pressure. Some of these traits may be largely environmentally determined, such as weight, whereas others are largely genetically determined, such as stature and intelligence. In each case many genes are probably involved. Characteristics which are due to many genes plus the effects of environment are said to be inherited on a multifactorial basis.

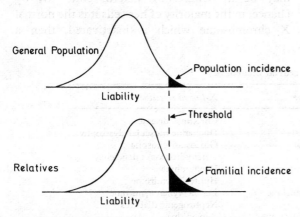

Fig. 1.9 Liability Hypothetical curve of liability in the general population and in relatives for a hereditary disorder in which the genetic predisposition is multifactorial.

It is now believed that many common disorders are inherited in this way. In such conditions it is assumed that there is some underlying graded attribute which is related to causation. This is referred to as the individuals' *liability*, which includes not only their genetic predisposition but also the environmental factors which render them more or less likely to develop the disease. It is assumed that the curve of liability has a normal distribution in the general population.

In one simple model (Fig. 1.9), it is believed that there is a *threshold* value such that all affected individuals have a liability above this value and all unaffected individuals have a liability below this value. Relatives of affected individuals have a higher average liability than the population average so the curve of liability for relatives is shifted to the right. In the general population the proportion above the threshold is the population incidence and among relatives the proportion above the threshold is the familial incidence. Such a model can be used to explain the familial incidence of such disorders as essential hypertension, coronary artery disease, peptic ulceration and many of the commoner congenital malformations.

There are several consequences of such a model. Familial incidence will be greater among the relatives of more severely affected individuals because presumably they are more extreme deviants along the curve of liability and the number of abnormal genes segregating in such families is greater than in families in which individuals are less severely affected. Thus in hare lip with or without cleft palate the proportion of affected sibs and children is roughly 6% when the index patient has double hare lip and cleft palate, but only 2.5% if the index patient has a single hare lip. By similar reasoning it would be expected that the incidence among sibs born subsequent to the index patient would be greater the more affected relatives there were in the family. In spina bifida, for example, the incidence of this condition, or the related disorder anencephaly, in sibs born after one affected child is roughly 5%, but the incidence rises to 10% after the birth of two affected children. This is quite different from the situation in unifactorial disorders where the risk to subsequent sibs remains constant irrespective of the number of affected individuals in the family (e.g. 1 in 4 for an autosomal recessive trait). Finally as a consequence of this model it might be expected that when there is a sex difference in the population incidence, the relatives of the less frequently affected sex would be more often affected. The reason for this is that in the less frequently affected sex, when individuals are affected they are presumably more extreme deviants along the curve of liability and possess more abnormal genes. Thus in congenital pyloric stenosis, which is 5 times commoner in boys than girls, the proportions of affected relatives of male index patients are roughly 5.5% for sons and 2.4% for daughters, but 19.4% for sons and 7.3% for daughters when the index patient is a female.

Though it is not possible to measure liability to a particular disease it is possible to estimate how much of the aetiology can be ascribed to genetic factors as opposed to environmental factors. This is referred to as the *heritability* which is calculated from the known incidences of the disorder in the general population and in relatives. Some estimates of heritability are given in Table 1.3. The values, though approximate, do indicate that genetic factors are of more importance in aetiology in asthma and schizophrenia than in, for example, peptic ulcer.

Table 1.3 Estimates for heritability for various multi-factorial disorders

Disorder	Incidence (%)	Heritability (%)
Schizophrenia	1	85
Asthma	4	80
Cleft lip ± cleft palate	0.1	76
Pyloric stenosis (congenital)	0.3	75
Ankylosing spondylitis	0.2	70
Club foot (congenital)	0.1	68
Coronary artery disease	3	65
Hypertension (essential)	5	62
Dislocation of hip (congenital)	0.1	60
Anencephaly and spina bifida	0.5	60
Peptic ulcer	4	37
Congenital heart disease (all types)	0.5	35

PREVENTION OF GENETIC DISEASE

Since there is at present no effective treatment for most genetic disorders the role of the medical practitioner lies mainly in the prevention of such conditions through genetic counselling. This involves providing advice on the chances of recurrence of a genetic disorder in the children of either healthy parents who already have an affected child, or when one of the parents or a near relative is affected with a disease which is known to be inherited.

In chromosomal disorders if the parents have normal karyotypes, i.e. do not carry a translocation which in the unbalanced state would cause abnormality, then the chances of recurrence are usually low. The most important chromosomal disorder from this point of view is Down's syndrome. The risk of having a child with Down's syndrome is about 1 in 100 in women who have previously had an affected child, and at least 1 in 50 in women over the age of 40. However, the risks are higher if one of the parents carries a chromosome translocation (Table 1.4).

Table 1.4 Recurrence risks of Down's syndrome (C = Carrier, N = Normal).

Patient	Father	Mother	Recurrence risk (%)
Translocation			
21/13-15	N	C	10-15
	C	N	5
21/22	N	C	10-15
	C	N	5
21/21	N	C	100
	C	N	100
Trisomy 21	N	N	1
Translocation or mosaic	N	N	1

In unifactorial disorders the chances of recurrence are based on Mendelian principles. As we have seen, for example, for a fully penetrant autosomal dominant disorder there is a 1 in 2 chance of recurrence in any child of an affected parent. However, if both parents are healthy an affected child must be the result of a new mutation and the chances of recurrence in subsequent children are negligible. If parents have had a child with an autosomal recessive disorder the chance of recurrence in subsequent children is 1 in 4. Should such a child survive there is very little chance of its having affected children. Finally, with X-linked recessive disorders there is a 1 in 2 chance that any son of a known carrier will be affected and a 1 in 2 chance that any daughter will be a carrier. All the daughters of an affected male will be carriers. A major advance in the prevention of X-linked disorders has been the development of tests for detecting healthy female carriers of such disorders as Duchenne muscular dystrophy and haemophilia. An important problem is the need for reliable methods of detecting symptomless, preclinical cases of autosomal dominant disorders such as Huntington's chorea, polyposis coli, polycystic kidney disease and myotonic dystrophy in which symptoms often do not develop until the third or fourth decade of life. Such tests would make it possible for individuals likely to become affected, and therefore transmit the disease to their children, to receive advice before they had a family. Developments in recombinant DNA technology may soon make possible preclinical detection of many of these disorders (p. 18).

In multifactorial disorders risk of recurrence cannot be predicted from Mendelian principles but have to be determined by studying the frequency of the condition among the relatives of affected individuals. Examples of risk figures, derived in this way (so-called *empiric* risks), for some relatively common conditions are given in Table 1.5.

Table 1.5 Empiric risks for some common disorders (in percent)

Disorder	Incidence	Sex ratio M:F	Normal parents having a second affected child	Affected parent having an affected child	Affected parent having a second affected child
Anencephaly	0.20	1:2	5*	—	—
Asthma	3–4	1:1	10	26	—
Cerebral palsy	0.20	3:2	1†	—	—
Cleft palate only	0.04	2:3	2	7	15
Cleft lip ± cleft palate	0.10	3:2	4	4	10
Club foot	0.10	2:1	3	3	10
Congenital heart disease (all types)	0.50	1:1	1–4	1–4	10
Diabetes mellitus (juvenile, insulin-dependent)	0.20	1:1	6	1–2	—
Dislocation of hip	0.07	1:6	6	12	36
Exomphalos (omphalocoele)	0.02	1:1	< 1	—	—
Epilepsy ('idiopathic')	0.50	1:1	5	5	10
Hirschsprung's disease	0.02	4:1			
short segment			3	2	—
long segment			12	—	—
Hydrocephalus (isolated, not XR)	0.05	1:1	3**	—	—
Hypospadias (in males)	0.20	—	10	10	—
Manic-depressive psychosis	0.40	2:3	10–15	10–15	—
Mental retardation ('idiopathic')	0.30–0.50	1:1	3–5	10	20
Profound childhood deafness	0.10	1:1	10	8	—
Pyloric stenosis	0.30	5:1			
male index			2	4	13
female index			10	17	38
Renal agenesis (bilat.)	0.01	3:1			
male index			3	—	—
female index			7	—	—
Schizophrenia	1–2	1:1	10	16	—
Scoliosis ('idiopathic, adolescent')	0.22	1:6	7	5	—
Spina bifida	0.30	2:3	5*	4*	—
Tracheo-oesophageal fistula	0.03	1:1	1	1	—

* Risk for anencephaly or spina bifida
† If associated with ataxia, or symmetrical spastic paraplegia or athetosis risk approx. 10%
** Additional 1–2% risk of other neutral tube defects.

Genetic Advice

The procedure for giving genetic advice is first to establish a precise diagnosis, second to be certain that the disorder in question is genetic and third to verify the presence or absence of the disease in relatives. Without a precise diagnosis it is not possible to give reliable genetic counselling since certain disorders though superficially similar may be inherited differently. For example Hunter's syndrome and Hurler's syndrome both present similar clinical features of 'gargoylism' but whereas clouding of the cornea does not occur in the former condition it is present in the latter. Further, Hunter's syndrome is an X-linked recessive trait and therefore the unaffected sister of an affected boy may be at risk of having affected children. Hurler's syndrome on the other hand is an autosomal recessive disorder and only affects sibs. In this condition there is therefore no chance of an unaffected sister having affected children, provided she does not marry a near relative who might also carry the mutant gene.

It is always advisable to check that the disease in question is in fact genetic and not due to some environmental factor (i.e. a *phenocopy*). For example congenital deafness is often due to a rare recessive gene but it may also result from intrauterine infection with rubella during the first three months of pregnancy which may also cause abnormalities in the fetus such as congenital heart disease and eye defects. If it can be shown in a particular case that congenital deafness was due to maternal rubella then there would be no chance of recurrence in subsequent children. It is therefore important before giving genetic advice to ask about the possibility of maternal exposure to radiation, drugs or infections during pregnancy and details of any birth trauma which might possibly account for the disorder in question.

Factors which influence the parents' decision whether or not they will accept a risk of having an affected child include the severity of the abnormality, whether or not there is an effective treatment, the actual risk, their religious attitude and possibly their socioeconomic status. In general, however, parents usually accept the risk of having an affected child if this is less than one in 20 but do not accept a risk of greater than one in 10 if the disease is serious.

Antenatal Diagnosis. Family limitation is not the only course of action open to parents who are found to be at high risk of having a child with a serious genetic disorder. Other possibilities include (i) artificial insemination by donor (if the father is affected with a dominant disorder or carries a chromosome translocation or if both parents are heterozygous for a rare recessive gene) and (ii) antenatal diagnosis with selective abortion of affected fetuses. The second procedure is possible by studying cells present in amniotic fluid or the amniotic fluid itself. About 5 to 10 ml of fluid is removed by transabdominal amniocentesis around the 16th week of gestation. The specimen is centrifuged and the uncultured cells (which are derived largely from the fetal skin) may be studied to determine the sex of the fetus by fluorescent (F-body) and sex-chromatin studies, though it is advisable to confirm the sex of the fetus by also culturing the cells for full karyotype analysis.

Fetal sexing is valuable in X-linked disorders which cannot yet be diagnosed *in utero* (e.g. Duchenne muscular dystrophy). In this way a known carrier mother can be guaranteed a daughter who will not be affected (though she might be a carrier), for if the fetus is a male the parents may decide on termination since there is a one in two chance the fetus could be affected. Amniotic fluid cells can also be cultured and from the study of this material it is possible not only to sex the fetus but also to diagnose cytogenetic abnormalities and certain inborn errors of metabolism in the fetus. At present the main application of such studies is in the antenatal diagnosis of Down's syndrome and many centres now offer amniocentesis to all pregnant women over the age of 40 because of their increased risk of having a child with this disorder. Finally anencephaly and open spina bifida are associated with raised levels of alpha-fetoprotein in amniotic fluid and these disorders may therefore also be diagnosed *in utero*.

Conclusion. The main contribution which genetics can make to medicine is in understanding more about the aetiology of certain disorders and in preventing such disorders through genetic counselling. But it is not sufficient merely to quote risk figures. As far as possible the nature and cause of the disease should be explained to parents and any feelings of guilt should be removed. Since genetic counselling may have profound long-term effects on a family such advice must never be given without careful appraisal of all the factors involved if the needs of the individual are to be met. Genetic counselling, like many other aspects of medicine, is as much an art as a science.

RECOMBINANT DNA TECHNOLOGY

A major advance in the last few years has been the introduction of genetic engineering, or more precisely recombinant DNA technology which consists essentially of generating fragments of DNA containing specific genes of interest. This is done by using enzymes called restriction endonucleases which cleave DNA at sequence-specific sites. These fragments are incorporated into the DNA of a vector such as a plasmid which is a small circle of DNA. This is the recombinant part of the process. The vector is then introduced into a microbial host usually *Escherichia coli* which is grown in culture to produce clones with multiple copies of the incorporated gene. The cloned gene may be labelled with ^{32}P and used as a probe to detect homologous DNA sequences in DNA from various tissues by means of hybridization and autoradiography on electrophoresis gels, a method known as the Southern blot. A probe may be a piece of genomic DNA, an artificially synthesised piece of DNA, or a complementary DNA copy (cDNA) produced from mRNA using RNA-dependent DNA polymerase (reverse transcriptase) as shown in Figure 1.10.

These techniques have wide applications in medicine, the most important being the synthesis of biologically important molecules (such as human insulin, growth hormones and interferon), carrier detection, preclinical diagnosis and the antenatal diagnosis of certain genetic diseases. In the case of several of the haemoglobinopathies antenatal diagnosis is possible because it has been found that the normal and abnormal genes are carried on DNA fragments of unequal size which can be recognised by their different mobilities on an electrophoresis gel (Fig. 1.10).

PROSPECTS IN GENETICS

In the future recombinant DNA technology may be used in the treatment of genetic disease by the direct replacement of defective genes (gene therapy). This technology will also help us to understand more about the molecular basis of human disease, and its prevention through advances in antenatal diagnosis. We are also likely to see the development of presymptomatic treatments for those who are healthy but would otherwise develop a genetic disorder. In the case of congenital defects it may one day be possible to treat the affected fetus before birth.

A.E.H. EMERY

Fig. 1.10 Technique used in the antenatal diagnosis of haemoglobinopathies. (*From* Emery, A.E.H., 1981. *Lancet* ii: 1406–1409, with permission).

FURTHER READING:

Emery, A.E.H. (1983) *Elements of Medical Genetics*, 6th edn. Edinburgh: Churchill Livingstone. An introductory textbook.

Emery, A.E.H. & Rimoin, D. (1983) *Principles and Practice of Medical Genetics*. Edinburgh: Churchill Livingstone. A more detailed textbook.

Emery, A.E.H. (1976) *Methodology in Medical Genetics*. Edinburgh: Churchill Livingstone. A textbook concerned with the more statistical aspects of medical genetics.

Emery, A.E.H. (1981) Recombinant DNA technology. *Lancet* ii: 1406–1409. An outline of genetic engineering.

Gerbie, A.B. (1980) *Antenatal Diagnosis of Genetic Defects* (Clinics in Obstetrics & Gynaecology Vol. 7). London: W.B. Saunders.

Old, R.W. & Primrose, S.B. (1981) *Principles of Gene Manipulation: An Introduction to Genetic Engineering*, 2nd edn. Oxford: Blackwell Scientific Publications. More detailed information about recombinant DNA technology.

2. Immunological Factors in Disease

The science of immunology arose from the study of man's resistance to infection. The most striking feature of this resistance is the specific nature of its enhancement in individuals following infection. Thus, antigenic stimulation and antibody production began to be elucidated in the context of infectious disease and immunity to it. Terms such as 'immunology', 'immunisation' and 'specific immune response' are derived from these origins.

It soon appeared that such specific 'immune' responses might also confer unpleasant and sometimes dangerous hypersensitivity to subsequent exposure to the provoking antigen. Resistance to infection is not an essential feature of the immune response; for example, bacteria may induce antibodies which have no obvious protective value and immune responses are often evoked by injection of intrinsically harmless non-living organic substances, such as serum protein from another individual or species. After exposure to antigen the individual develops a changed reactivity or *allergy*, a term which originally included immunity and hypersensitivity but which is now restricted to the latter.

The ability to develop specific immunity to infection is only one consequence of a wider capacity in the individual to recognise and to respond specifically to the foreignness of an extensive range of biological substances that are not normally present. Immunology is the study of what this 'changed reactivity' is in terms of cellular biochemistry, how it is brought about, and how it is regulated both quantitatively and qualitatively.

In the present chapter an account is given of current concepts of the physiology of the immune system in order that the clinical application of immunology may be understood in such diverse conditions as infection, asthma, drug reactions and certain endocrine, gastrointestinal, haematological, connective tissue, neurological and other disorders.

THE IMMUNE SYSTEM

Cellular Components — Lymphocytes and Macrophages

The antigenicity of a substance (i.e. its ability to induce an immune response) is determined by one or more specific molecular groups on its structure known as *antigenic determinants*. When lymphocytes recognise a foreign substance (antigen) they respond by transforming into lymphoblasts and then into antibody-producing plasma cells or lymphocytes as indicated in Figure 2.1.

If antigenic material (either part of self or a foreign substance) comes into contact with the cells of the antibody-forming system at the stage before the cells have reached maturity, e.g. in fetal life, the result is a failure of response rather than stimulation of antibody formation or other form of immune reaction against the antigen concerned. This is referred to as *immune tolerance* to the antigen. Probably for this reason individuals do not normally show a significant immune response against components of their own tissues. In the abnormal situation where an immune reaction does occur, the reaction is referred to as *autoimmune*.

Immune reactions are mediated by *humoral* or *cellular mechanisms*. Included among the humoral factors is antibody (immunoglobulin) secreted by plasma cells. The cellular component is made up

19

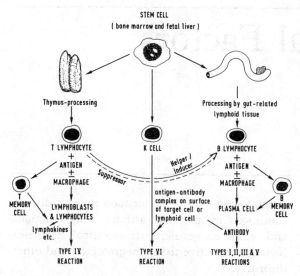

Fig. 2.1 Role of T lymphocytes, B lymphocytes and K cells in immunological responses. Many of these events involve active cell proliferation, but for clarity this has not been shown.

of lymphocytes sensitised to specific antigens and reactive with those antigens without the presence of free antibody. Stem-cells originating in the bone marrow differentiate to form two main lymphocyte populations known as T and B lymphocytes or cells.

T lymphocytes are dependent upon a hormone or factor produced by the epithelial cells of the thymus for becoming immunologically competent from non-competent predecessors originating in the bone marrow.

B lymphocytes are independent of the thymus but are dependent on the bursa of Fabricius in birds; its equivalents in man are probably the tonsils and the lymphoid tissue of the gut. B lymphocytes are responsible for the synthesis of humoral antibody.

The *recognition of antigen* by B lymphocytes is mediated by antibody synthesised in the cell and bound into the surface membrane, the specificity of the antibody being determined by the genetic characteristics (programming) of the individual lymphocyte. The precise molecular nature of the antigen-specific receptors on T lymphocytes is unclear. Although the same variable region genes that serve as the antigen-binding sites on conventional immunoglobulin molecules (Fig. 2.3) seem

to function as the antigen-binding sites on T cells, that portion of the T cell receptor corresponding to the constant region of the immunoglobulin molecule has yet to be defined.

The *induction of mitosis in T lymphocytes* and their transformation to larger 'blast' cells may be effected both by specific antigens and by non-specific mitogens which include agents such as phytohaemagglutinin. It is likely that stimulation of mitosis in some T lymphocytes involves processing of the antigen by macrophages, possibly leading to presentation of antigen determinants at the surface of the macrophage. For example, lymphocyte preparations largely freed of phagocytic cells are unresponsive to certain antigens but activity can be restored by addition of macrophages. Lymphocytes in tissue-culture can be seen to wander incessantly and presumably identify the antigens of the cells over which they move in terms of their degree of 'fit' with the antibody or antibody-like receptor on the lymphocyte surface. Likewise, in the body the lymphocytes migrate through the tissues (*immunological surveillance*) permitting their sensitisation or transformation to blast cells by contact with antigen with or without the help of macrophages.

The T lymphocyte sensitised to a specific antigen undergoes blast transformation and proliferation on contact with the antigen. In addition, the interaction of antigen with T lymphocytes leads to the release of non specific factors, *lymphokines*, which bring about a number of tissue changes associated with cell-mediated hypersensitivity (p. 28). One of these factors inhibits the migration of macrophages in tissue culture. *In vivo* the effect of this factor would be to immobilise randomly wandering macrophages at the site of reaction with antigen, where they might exert a cytotoxic action or merely act as scavengers of cells already damaged by lymphocytes. Other lymphokines can increase vascular permeability or cause inhibition of growth or death of tissue cells. Transfer factor is a dialysable substance produced by normal lymphocytes and can apparently pass the 'information' necessary for specific cell-mediated hypersensitivity responses to be mounted by previously unsensitised lymphocytes. Another lymphokine, interferon, blocks the reproduction of viruses. The release of lymphokines is an example of an amplification mechanism, like the complement system, that augments the specific response initiated by relatively few cells. In addition to lymphokines, specific macrophage arming factor is released which renders macrophages cytostatic to cells bearing that particular antigen.

The induction of mitosis in B lymphocytes to become the antibody-forming plasma cells is not yet fully understood. A possible sequence of events is shown in Figure 2.2. Certain antigens are apparently capable of reacting directly with the corresponding antibody on the surface of a B lymphocyte to induce it to transform and proliferate into active antibody-producing plasma cells. Such antigens generally have many antigenic determinants of the same specificity so that they can simultaneously trigger a number of receptors on the surface of the same B lymphocyte. Other antigens, or small doses of antigen, may have to be taken on to the surface of a macrophage, as mentioned in relation to T lymphocytes, thus being more readily available for stimulating a B lymphocyte either directly or through the co-operation of a helper T lymphocyte. In this way a high local concentration of antigen is achieved during cell to cell contact with the B lymphocyte, thereby stimulating a greater number of receptor sites in a given cell than if the antigen were uniformly dispersed throughout the body fluids. Once stimulated, the cell undergoes division and produces the antibody that it is genetically programmed to do.

There is negative in addition to positive control of immunological mechanisms as indicated in Figure 2.2. A sub-population of T cells (*suppressor T lymphocytes*) exists which can exert an inhibitory effect on the synthesis of antibody by B cells. Relaxation of this control may play an important role in the development of autoimmunity.

Subsets of T Lymphocytes. T cells may be subdivided into effector cells and regulatory cells. Effector cells are lymphocytes involved in delayed hypersensitivity (p. 28) and cytotoxic T lymphocytes which destroy cells infected with virus (p. 31). Regulatory cells are helper (or inducer) cells and suppressor cells. The definition and quantification of the various subsets is being greatly facilitated by the development of monoclonal antibodies (p. 550) to the surface markers

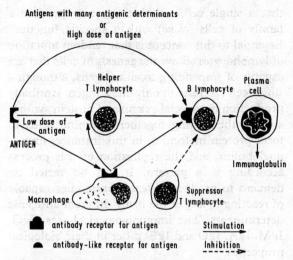

Fig. 2.2 Possible sequence of events in immunoglobulin formation, illustrating co-operation between T lymphocytes, B lymphocytes and macrophages and the role of suppressor T lymphocytes.

on lymphocytes (e.g. OK T4 for helper/inducer cells). About 75% of lymphocytes in the peripheral blood are T cells, about one third of which are helper/inducer cells.

The activity of T lymphocytes is restricted by the HLA system (p. 31).

Immunological memory is achieved by the existence of long-lived T and B cells (Fig. 2.1).

Killer Cells. Certain lymphoid cells and monocytes, although not themselves specifically sensitised, can gain specificity in the presence of antibody or antigen-antibody complexes on the surface of the target cells or on their own surface. This is known as antibody-dependent cell-mediated cytotoxicity (p. 28). The cells involved are referred to as killer or K cells.

Natural killer (NK) cells are large granular lymphocytes from nonimmune persons with the capacity to lyse rapidly (within hours) tumour cells, virally infected cells, or certain undifferentiated normal cells. They may play a part in host surveillance against tumour development, in resistance to viral infections, and, possibly, in haemopoietic regulation.

Immunoglobulin

It is considered that the population of antibody-producing cells arises by random mutation and that a single cell will then react to produce a family of cells (*clone*) with a specific function. Essential to this concept is that random mutation of lymphocytes allows the genesis of cells that are capable of responding to all antigens, although a single cell can react to only one antigen. Antibody production is a special example of protein synthesis, i.e. the putting together of amino acids to form protein molecules, in this instance, immunoglobulins, and the replication of this process according to a pattern. It can be varied on demand to produce different antibodies capable of reacting to any of the many different antigenic determinants. The immunological classes (IgG, IgM, IgA, IgD and IgE) differ in their biological properties.

Structure. Immunoglobulins are made up of distinct sub-units held together in the whole molecule by disulphide (S-S) bonds (Fig. 2.3). The bonds can be broken by reducing agents, so that the molecule falls apart into pairs of polypeptide chains called light and heavy chains as determined by their molecular weights. Two types of light chain exist, kappa and lambda, of which individual immunoglobulins have only one type.

The enzyme papain splits the immunoglobulin molecule into two antigen binding (Fab) fractions and one Fc fragment which fixes and activates

Fig. 2.3 Structure of immunoglobulin IgG. Disulphide bond cleavage produces two light chains and two heavy chains. Papain cleavage produces two Fab fractions and one Fc fragment. The amino acids that vary in sequence for different antibodies are shown as interrupted ends of the light and heavy chains.

complement. With the exception of erythrocytes, all circulating blood cells have specific receptors for the Fc component, resulting, for example, in macrophage binding and in fixation to the killer (K) lymphoid cells of Type VI reactions (p. 28). The Fc component is also responsible for the antigenic differences between the classes of immunoglobulin which enables their ready quantitation by antisera.

Within the variable (V) regions of the Fab components are the hypervariable areas, each of approximately 5 amino acids in size, where the major differences between V regions are localised. These hypervariable areas are widely spread out in the open V-region chain structure but are brought together by the three dimensional folding of the molecule so that they are directly involved in the antibody-combining site. The unique antigenic structures within the variable region are called *idiotypes*. An individual can develop anti-idiotype responses and these determine, at least in part, the magnitude and duration of antibody production to a given antigen.

Classification and Functions. *IgG*. In healthy adults, the total IgG accounts for 73% of the immunoglobulins in normal serum and is distributed equally between the blood and interstitial fluids, about a quarter passing across the capillary walls each day and the same amount returning via the thoracic duct. In man, IgG is the only immunoglobulin that is transported across the placenta to reach the fetal circulation and provide the baby with passive immunisation during its early life. IgG is particularly suited to neutralising soluble toxin such as that of *Clostridium diphtheriae*. IgG also has an opsonic effect on bacteria, coating them so that their ingestion by phagocytes is facilitated.

IgM. The macro-molecular IgM is predominantly intravascular. It constitutes only 7% of the serum immunoglobulins and is made up of five immunoglobulin units linked with disulphide bonds to provide ten identical combining-sites instead of the two of IgG. IgM is especially effective in activating complement to produce immune lysis of foreign cells by digesting holes in the cell membranes at the sites where antibody has reacted. IgM antibodies are much more efficient than IgG antibodies in linking particulate antigens together for agglutination and phagocytosis and would seem to be specially adapted for dealing with cell debris or bacteria in the bloodstream.

IgA accounts for 19% of the total serum immunoglobulins and is preferentially secreted into colostrum, saliva, intestinal juice and respiratory secretions. The major sites of IgA synthesis are the laminae propriae underlying the mucous membranes throughout the respiratory tract and the gut. The monomer produced locally by plasma cells is taken up as a dimer by the epithelial cells of the gut, and a secretory piece is added which protects the immunoglobulin from digestive enzymes. Secretory IgA is available right through to the colon and these antibodies are vital in the defence of the gut against enteroviruses, e.g. poliomyelitis. In general, IgA plays a major role as part of an antiseptic secretion over the mucous surfaces of the body.

IgD has some of the properties of IgG, although little is known of its exact role.

IgE has a very low serum level and a distinctive affinity for cell surfaces. It is also known as reaginic antibody and constitutes an integral part of immediate hypersensitivity reactions such as occur in hay fever. The physiological function of IgE antibodies is obscure but they may possibly have a role in the defence against helminths.

Complement System

The principal activities of the complement system are directed at protection against infectious diseases. Complement belongs to the group of plasma systems termed 'triggered enzyme cascades', which also include the coagulation, fibrinolytic and kinin generating systems. They are all effector mechanisms which can produce a rapid and amplified response to a trigger stimulus. They are complex both in their reaction pathways and in the homeostatic mechanisms which have been evolved to control them. The complement system is activated classically by antigen-antibody interactions; the sequence of events involved consists of three stages (Fig. 2.4):

1. The first is the generation of C3 splitting enzymes by the classical and by the alternative

Fig. 2.4 The complement system. The bar over a component represents an activated state, usually enzymatic, generated during the complement sequence. B represents factors of unknown nature which activate the alternative pathway.

pathways. The latter is activated by factors other than an antigen-antibody reaction and provides another line of defence against microbial infection.

2. The second stage is the activation of C3, which is the central event of the complement sequence and its bulk reaction, analogous to the conversion of fibrinogen to fibrin in blood coagulation. The fixation of C3 at complement fixation sites (e.g. the Fc component of IgG after reaction with antigen) is probably the system's most important activity. Bound C3 reacts with various receptors on phagocytic cells, platelets, erythrocytes and certain lymphocytes and retention of cells at complement fixation sites contributes largely to the activity of the complement system in inflammation. The generation of C3b leads to the activation of a self-amplifying positive feedback cycle which is damped by the action of the C3b inactivator (Fig. 2.4).

3. The activation of the terminal components is initiated by the activation of C5 and is the last enzymic reaction in the complement sequence. Thereafter the remaining components (C6-C9) combine to form a membrane attack complex which mediates the most characteristic *in vitro* event of the complement system: the generation of membrane lesions leading to cell lysis.

Excessive activity is prevented by the rapid decay of several components of the complement system and by inhibitor proteins.

TYPES OF IMMUNE REACTION AND THEIR RELATION TO HUMAN DISEASE

Immune reactions result primarily in defensive inflammatory changes in the tissues but these can be augmented or misdirected to such a degree that immunologically-mediated disease becomes apparent. The different types of immune reaction that may be involved are described here under six headings, (types I-VI), although there is no general agreement as to how they should be labelled. They are illustrated in Figure 2.5 and are:

Type I — anaphylactic (immediate hypersensitivity);

Type II — antibody-mediated cytotoxic or blocking;

Type III immune complex;

Type IV T cell-mediated (delayed hypersensitivity);

Type V stimulating antibody;

Type VI antibody-dependent cell-mediated cytotoxicity (ADCC).

Type I — Anaphylactic (Immediate Hypersensitivity) Reactions

In man, only IgE antibodies are able to produce anaphylactic reactions. As IgE antibodies adhere strongly to tissues (and particularly to mast-cells in the tissues) they are often called tissue-sensitising antibodies. Anaphylactic phenomena are caused by antigen-antibody reaction on the surface of the mast cell activating a series of enzymes leading to the release of vasodilators from the mast cells (Fig. 2.5). These agents are histamine, leukotrienes, serotonin and the plasma kinins, bradykinin and kallidin. The kinins cause increased capillary permeability, vasodilatation and a fall in blood pressure. Another effect is to cause polymorphonuclear leucocytes to migrate from blood vessels and accumulate in the tissues (chemotaxis). Once they are formed the kinins are rapidly broken down by kininases present in the blood. Thus their accumulation at any site is controlled.

Previously the term anaphylaxis emphasised the clinically severe form, anaphylactic shock, but

Fig. 2.5 Immune reactions which may be harmful to the tissues.

current usage refers to the underlying mechanism and not to clinical severity. Anaphylactic reactions depend on whether the portal of entry of the antigen is local, systemic or via the intestine. Relatively mild symptoms occur when antigen-antibody reactions take place on an exposed mucosal surface. These reactions occur most commonly to pollens or animal dander and the symptoms may be limited to rhinorrhoea and conjunctivitis. However, intense bronchospasm may be produced as a result of inhalation of the antigen. Patients with asthma induced by contact with antigens in this manner have levels of IgE immunoglobulin that may be much higher than those found in patients with asthma that is not induced in this way. Individuals who have a hereditary predisposition to produce high levels of IgE are said to be atopic.

Systemic anaphylaxis consists of a group of much more severe reactions which may occur rapidly if the antigen is injected, as in the case of a drug such as penicillin, foreign sera, or the sting of an insect. The features are bronchospasm, laryngeal oedema resulting in extreme dyspnoea and cyanosis and a marked fall in blood pressure (anaphylactic shock). There may also be nausea, vomiting and diarrhoea. Systemic anaphylaxis is a potentially fatal condition if not treated promptly with adrenaline (500–1000 μg i.m.) and an antihistamine (e.g. chlorpheniramine 10–20 mg slowly i.v.) followed, in severely ill patients, by intravenous corticosteroids.

Urticaria, the formation of weal and flare lesions in the skin, is an anaphylactic phenomenon which can develop as a result of absorption of antigen through the intestinal tract. Common allergens are present in strawberries, nuts, eggs and shellfish. Urticaria often occurs alone, but may be associated with other signs of anaphylaxis. Not all urticaria is caused by an immune reaction; the pharmacological agents which cause urticaria can be released by other means, especially physical agents such as trauma or cold.

Diagnostic Methods. Intradermal testing in sensitised individuals is the most convenient *in vivo* method for the detection of specific IgE antibodies. A simple, rapid, radioallergosorbent test is available for the *in vitro* detection and quantitation of antigen specific IgE.

Type II — Antibody-mediated Cytotoxic or Blocking Reactions

Here antigen on the cell's surface combines with antibody and complement to destroy the cell (Fig. 2.5). The clearest example of a Type II reaction as a cause of disease occurs in autoimmune haemolytic anaemia; this can be demonstrated *in vitro* by the antiglobulin (Coombs') test. When antihuman globulin is added to a suspension of the patient's red cells that have antibody on their surfaces, agglutination of the cells occurs. *In vivo*, the altered or damaged red cells are destroyed by the monocyte–macrophage system in the spleen or liver. Both IgG and IgM antibodies have been implicated.

Another example of IgG antibodies being directly pathogenic is antibody to glomerular basement membrane in a rare type of glomerulonephritis (Goodpasture's syndrome, p. 385). This mechanism may result in damage to a kidney transplant in a patient whose own kidneys had previously been destroyed by glomerulonephritis.

In other instances, IgG antibodies may have only a weakly pathogenic effect. Thus, the occurrence of intrinsic factor antibodies in the circulation of a patient shows a strong correlation with Addisonian pernicious anaemia, but the role of the antibody in causing the gastric atrophy characteristic of this condition is not clear. For example, pernicious anaemia may occur in patients with marked hypogammaglobulinaemia. However, antibody reactive with the vitamin B_{12} binding site of intrinsic factor has been shown to be present in the gastric juice of some patients with pernicious anaemia; it may block the action of any remaining secretion of intrinsic factor with consequent malabsorption of vitamin B_{12}.

Antibodies which react with antigens close to the site of the acetylcholine receptors impair neuromuscular transmission, which is characteristic of myasthenia gravis (p. 665). Antibodies that react with insulin receptors may produce a very severe form of insulin resistant diabetes. Blocking antibodies are not associated with complement fixation.

There are circumstances in which IgG antibodies may be pathogenic only when combined with cell-mediated hypersensitivity or other forms of tissue damage. Thus complement-fixing IgG antibodies to thyroid secretory epithelium are a frequent occurrence in autoimmune thyroid disease but they seem to have little or no pathogenic role by themselves. These antibodies can be transmitted across the placenta with no evidence of damage to the fetal thyroid. Although at least one of these antibodies can bring about rapid destruction of trypsinised human thyroid cells *in vitro* in the presence of complement, *in vivo* it seems to have difficulty in reaching the intracellular antigens in the absence of some other damaging agent.

Finally, in other situations, antibodies detectable in the serum and often useful diagnostically, seem to have no discernible pathogenic role when acting on their own. For example, antibody to thyroglobulin is harmless to thyroid cells in tissue culture and infusion into animals produces at most a weak granulomatous reaction in the thyroid. However, antibody to thyroglobulin may play an important role in pathogenesis when part of a type VI reaction (p. 28). A second example is the mitochondrial antibodies with no tissue specificity which occur most commonly in patients with primary biliary cirrhosis.

Diagnostic Methods. *The indirect immunofluorescence technique* is used to detect autoantibodies to nuclei, to the cytoplasm of thyroid, gastric parietal, adrenocortical, steroid-producing ovarian and pancreatic islet cells and to glomerular basement membrane. Cryostat sections of the appropriate tissue are incubated with serum and, after thorough washing, with fluorescein labelled antihuman Ig serum. They are then examined by fluorescence microscopy.

Complement Fixation Tests. Certain antigen-antibody reactions fix complement and the occurrence of such a reaction *in vitro* can be detected by determining whether complement, which had been added in a critical amount, is still present in the free form. An indicator system is used consisting of sheep red cells coated with horse or rabbit antibodies against the red cells. If complement has been fixed before the addition of the indicator system, it is no longer available to permit lysis of the sheep red cells. This technique forms the basis of the Wassermann reaction for syphilis; it is also used in the demonstration of

antibodies against certain viruses and also for thyroid and gastric autoantibodies in serum.

Precipitation testing may be used, for example, in the detection of antibodies to thyroglobulin in the differential diagnosis of thyroid disorders.

Tanned Red Cell or Latex Particle Agglutination. Sheep red cells are treated with tannic acid so that they can be coated with antigens (e.g. thyroglobulin). In the presence of the corresponding antibody the cells undergo agglutination. This provides a very sensitive and semi-quantitative method for the detection of certain serum antibodies, e.g. to thyroglobulin. Latex particles coated with human γ-globulin are used to detect the presence of the rheumatoid factor in patients' serum (p. 556).

Type III — Immune Complex Reactions

Immune complex reactions are induced by deposition of antigen and antibody in the tissues, causing the activation of complement; this results in a polymorphonuclear inflammatory response and also damage to the cell membranes of adjacent tissues (Fig. 2.6). In addition to the effect of complement, macrophages and lymphocytes are activated by attachment to the Fc component of the immunoglobulin molecule. Hydrolytic enzymes released from the granules of the leucocytes also contribute to the vascular damage which is the hallmark of this type of immune reaction.

The immune complex reaction can be induced in man by the intradermal injection of antigens if there is a high level of circulating IgG antibodies, for example in pulmonary aspergillosis (p. 240) and 'farmer's lung' (p. 249). Red and oedematous changes reaching maximum intensity between 4–12 hours appear at the site of injection of the antigen. This is known as the *Arthus reaction*.

Glomerulonephritis can be caused by an immune complex reaction. Thus, in the clinical entity of glomerulonephritis, there are at least two immune pathogenic mechanisms and, in all probability, numerous aetiological factors capable of initiating each. As described on page 25, in the rare glomerulonephritis produced by a Type II immune reaction, antibodies react with glomerular basement membrane. In glomerulonephritis produced by an immune complex reaction the specificity of the

Fig. 2.6 The role of components of the complement system in the production of inflammation. Amplification of the immune response is achieved by the action of the complement system as an enzyme cascade. Thus one C1 complex generates many C42 complexes which in turn activate many molecules of C3b and so on to cell lysis. When the antigen is not part of an intact cell wall the biological effects are the same apart from cell lysis.

antibodies is irrelevant; what is important is that antigen-antibody complexes of appropriate size are present in the circulation and are deposited in the glomerular capillary walls.

The only property of antigen-antibody complexes presently known to affect the localisation in vessels is size and this depends on the ratio of antigen and antibody in the complexes. Small complexes in great antigen excess tend to remain in the circulation whereas frank precipitates formed at equivalence or at antibody excess are rapidly taken up and disposed of by phagocytes. The intermediate-sized complexes formed in moderate antigen excess are still soluble but large enough to react with complement and are the most likely to be deposited in vessel walls and so induce inflammation. The vessel walls of the renal glomeruli are particurlarly vulnerable. Morphologically the trapped antigen-antibody complexes appear under the electron microscope as heaped-up lesions on the glomerular basement membrane (p. 387).

The antigen involved may be foreign to the body or it may be autogenous. Thus, as an example of the former, post-streptococcal proliferative glomerulonephritis, at least as seen in children, is caused by the deposition of circulat-ing non-glomerular antigen-antibody complexes. The best example of an autogenous immune complex reaction causing glomerulonephritis in man is that occurring in systemic lupus erythematosus. It is associated with the formation of anti-nuclear antibodies (particularly to DNA) and the deposition of these antibodies, nuclear antigens and complement in the renal glomerulus (p. 573).

The systemic syndrome known as *chronic serum sickness* is based on an immune complex reaction and can be produced by a wide range of different antigens, such as antitetanus serum and especially drugs such as penicillin and streptomycin. It consists of rashes, fever, joint pains and often swelling of the regional lymph nodes. The duration of symptoms varies greatly. The illness is seldom serious, though it may give rise to much discomfort.

Other conditions in which lesions occur due to immune complexes include rheumatoid arthritis (p. 552), polyarteritis, viral hepatitis, the renal manifestations of infective endocarditis, the nephrotic syndrome in children with *P. malariae* infections and in lepromatous leprosy. Immune complex reactions thus occur in response to diverse antigens related particularly to micro-organisms, drugs and autogenous sources.

Type IV — Cell-mediated (Delayed) Hypersensitivity Reactions

Type IV reactions are those mediated by T lymphocytes and in which free antibody plays no part (Fig. 2.5). Antigen stimulates the T cell to produce lymphokines (p. 20). Type IV reactions are characteristically induced by infectious agents which are predominantly intracellular in the infected host, e.g. many viral infections and some bacterial infections such as tuberculosis, brucellosis, pertussis, and syphilis. The classical example of this reaction is the tuberculin test (p. 232). Homograft rejection is believed to be predominantly produced by cell-mediated hypersensitivity.

Type IV reactions can also occur by skin contact with a variety of substances notably drugs, including penicillin. These substances are not themselves antigenic but become antigenic by co-valent binding to proteins in the skin. The hypersensitivity of the skin is generalised and may be detected by a small patch test containing the substance applied anywhere on the body.

Cell mediated hypersensitivity is a main factor in the pathogenesis of autoimmune disease (see below).

Type V — Stimulating Antibody Reaction

Certain IgG antibodies have the ability to stimulate their target cells rather than to inhibit or kill them (Fig. 2.5). Human specific TSH receptor antibodies are the likely cause of thyrotoxicosis when there is diffuse involvement of the thyroid (Graves' disease p. 430). The transfer across the placenta of these thyroid stimulating antibodies is the most probable explanation for neonatal hyperthyroidism.

Type VI — Antibody Dependent Cell-Mediated Cytotoxicity (ADCC)

Killer (K) cells may be defined as belonging to a subpopulation of lymphoid cells or monocytes which *in vitro* are able to lyse target cells coated with antibody. The cytotoxic reaction is complement-independent and is initiated through contact of the K cell with the Fc portion of the antibody molecule complexed with antigen on the surface of the target cells (Fig. 2.5). K cells may also be 'armed' through the Fc receptor with antigen-antibody complex which, if present in antibody excess, will be cytotoxic to target cells coated with that specific antigen. Should immune complexes be produced in the presence of excess antigen, there would be no free combining sites left on the antibody moiety to react with antigen on target surfaces so that this type of K cell would be ineffective (blocked).

K cell mediated cytotoxic mechanisms may be important in the pathogenesis of autoimmune disease and in tumour rejection. K cells are also involved in the defence against helminthic infections such as schistosomiasis where the size of the parasite is too large for effective phagocytosis.

Autoimmune Disease

Immune mechanisms may simply be part of a chain of events that leads to the final end product, the clinical manifestation of disease. Thus a viral infection may initiate tissue damage or combine with a cell constituent to act as a hapten and thereby engender an autoimmune response in a susceptible individual. This may occur for example in insulin-dependent diabetes. The interactions of immune mechanisms in the production of autoimmune disease are shown in Figure 2.7.

Evidence suggesting the importance of cell-mediated hypersensitivity as a main factor in autoimmune disease can be summarised as follows:

1. The histology of the affected organs shows lymphocytic infiltration and atrophy, e.g. in Hashimoto thyroiditis, atrophic gastritis of Addisonian pernicious anaemia and idiopathic (autoimmune) adrenal failure. 2. Similar histological changes can be produced in animals by sterile methods that cause cell-mediated hypersensitivity. 3. When such diseases have been induced immunologically in experimental animals they can be transferred to normal animals by means of lymphocytes alone. 4. Positive *in vitro* tests for cell-mediated hypersensitivity have been obtained with the lymphocytes from the peripheral blood of patients or of experimental animals with certain autoimmune diseases. These tests include

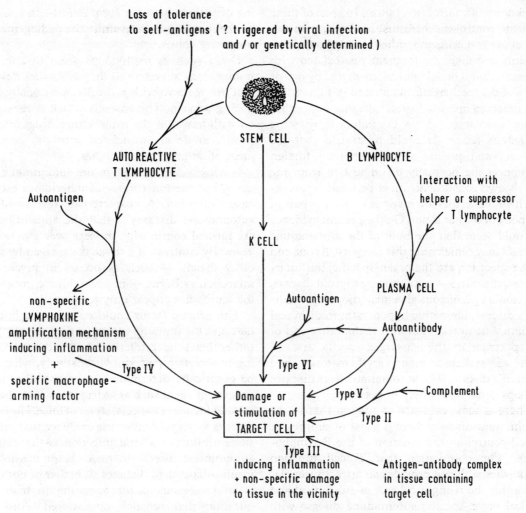

Fig. 2.7 Interactions of immune mechanisms types II-VI in the production of autoimmune disease. The different mechanisms may have greater importance in some disease than in others. Thus type II reactions are predominant in autoimmune haemolytic anaemia, while types II, IV and VI are predominant in Hashimoto's thyroiditis, and type V in thyrotoxicosis.

the leucocyte migration inhibition test, transformation and cytotoxicity tests.

Aetiology. *Defect in Immunological Tolerance*. Normally a person or animal does not mount a significant immune response against its own body constituents because intricate controlling and suppressor mechanisms exist to prevent this happening. For example, it has been suggested that clones of immunocompetent cells capable of reacting with self-antigens are either eliminated or rendered unresponsive by early and continued exposure to antigen (p. 19).

Unresponsiveness may exist either at the level of the helper T lymphocyte or at the level of the antibody-producing B lymphocyte or at both. If unresponsiveness exists only at the level of the helper T cell, autoantibody synthesis will occur when the requirement for T cell help is bypassed. As discussed on page 21 a subpopulation of T lymphocytes can suppress the synthesis of antibody by B cells which however would be increased if the function of these suppressor cells became impaired. The dose of antigen presented to the immune system is also relevant to the breakdown of control (tolerance). In spite of these intricate control mechanisms, however, man can and does synthesise antibodies against body components and these are frequently associated with disease (clinical or subclinical) mediated by one or more of the mechanisms illustrated in Figure 2.7.

A defect in immunological tolerance may either occur spontaneously or be induced by some exogenous factor. It could be argued that the intricate and precise system whereby foreign substances are normally distinguished from the body's own constituents must be liable to breakdown so that errors are made as to what is part of the body and what is not. On the present evidence it would seem that the bulk of the autoimmune diseases may come under this category. At one end of the spectrum are the organ-specific, but interrelated, disorders — autoimmune thyroid disease, Addisonian pernicious anaemia, idiopathic Addison's disease, idiopathic hypoparathyroidism and autoimmune ovarian failure. At the other end of the spectrum are the non-organ-specific diseases such as systemic lupus erythematosus and Sjögren's disease. The autoimmune liver diseases perhaps come somewhere in between.

There is some evidence to suggest that in the autoimmune diseases there is a loss of suppressor T cell control on the function of the B lymphocytes. The observation that T cell function diminishes with age provides an attractive explanation for the rising incidence of subclinical and clinical organ-specific autoimmune disease with advancing years.

Sequestrated Antigen. There are some antigens that do not normally come into contact with the immunological system so that there has been no opportunity for immunological tolerance of self-recognition to develop. For example, sperm, if extravasated following unilateral blockage of the vas deferens, may induce antibody formation and contribute to sterility. Sperm antibodies may also be produced following vasectomy in normal men.

Infection. In the hypersensitive host, invading micro-organisms may share antigen with certain of the host's tissues and induce the formation of antibodies which cross-react with these tissues. Thus the sharing of antigen between some Group A haemolytic streptococci and the heart may be relevant to rheumatic carditis. Likewise, the sharing of antigen between *Esch. coli* 014 and colonic epithelium may be relevant to the pathogenesis of ulcerative colitis.

Drugs such as methyldopa seem to alter the immunological system so that antibodies develop that are reactive with red cells occasionally producing a haemolytic anaemia which is reversible on withdrawal of the drug. Other drugs such as procainamide are associated with the development of antinuclear antibodies.

Genetic factors operate in the autoimmune diseases, but the exact mode of inheritance escapes clear definition. A characteristic feature of the autoimmune diseases is that the autoantibodies are formed continually, at least over a period of years. By contrast, if a tissue is damaged by some other means — such as occurs in myocardial infarction or burns — in general the corresponding antibodies appear only temporarily.

The genetic factor could operate as a built-in defect in the immune system so that, usually later rather than sooner, tolerance breaks down according to a certain pattern. Alternatively, what may be genetically determined is susceptibility to an exogenous agent such as a virus, for which there is some evidence in a special strain of mice. However, there is as yet no convincing evidence that genetic susceptibility to a viral infection is the basis of autoimmune disease in man except possibly in insulin-dependent diabetes. Whether or not there is an exogenous factor operating in man is a question that remains unanswered. Also unanswered is why immunological tolerance should break down according to patterns that clinicians recognise as interrelated diseases in which immune mechanisms play an important part.

The HLA System and Disease

The antigens causing the immune response that results in rejection of a tissue allograft are known as human leucocyte antigens (HLA). They are genetically determined and situated on chromosome 6 where they constitute the major histocompatibility complex (MHC). Histocompatibility antigens are found in most tissues, but differ quantitatively in their distribution on these tissues; they can be detected either by serological techniques or in lymphocyte culture.

The antigens which are detected serologically can be divided into four series, HLA-A, HLA-B, HLA-C and HLA-DR (D related) (Fig. 2.8). Another series of antigens, HLA-D, can be determined by their ability to stimulate lymphocytes in culture. The D and DR antigens may be the same. Well-defined antigens in each series are given a number, e.g. HLA-A1, while less well defined antigens are given the letter W, e.g. HLA-AW19. The possible number of combinations of alleles on a chromosome (haplotypes) is enormous, although certain alleles tend to occur together on the chromosome, e.g. HLA-A1 and HLA-B8. Nevertheless the chance of two unrelated people being identical for HLA is very low.

Fig. 2.8 The HLA region. (International Workshop, 1980). Complement components (Class III) are among the other products of this region.

Renal allografts between HLA identical siblings have very few rejection episodes and a 95% survival at three years. However, in unrelated cadaver renal transplantation, true HLA identity is rare and a partial matching for HLA can offer only a modest improvement in survival figures.

Some strong associations between HLA and susceptibility to certain diseases especially to the autoimmune diseases, have been described, e.g. ankylosing spondylitis (B27); rheumatoid arthritis (DR4); idiopathic Addison's disease (B8, DW3); insulin-dependent diabetes (B8, DR3, B15, DR4); thyrotoxicosis (B8, DR3); myasthenia

gravis (B8); narcolepsy (DR2) and haemochromatosis (A3).

Certain HLA antigens occur together more commonly than would be expected by chance (*alleleic association* or *linkage disequilibrium*); e.g. A1, B8, DW3 and DR3; A2, CW3, B15, DW4 and DR4; A3, B7, DW2 and DR2. In some instances the presence of an HLA antigen (or group of antigens in linkage disequilibrium) are protective or confer resistance to acquiring the disease (e.g. B7, DW2 and DR2 in insulin-dependent diabetes).

HLA-RESTRICTION. It has become clear that the high degree of polymorphism at the loci of the major histocompatibility complex is concerned with immunity to infection and particularly to viral infection. Thus T helper/inducer cells may respond only to antigen which is presented in association with the HLA-DR antigens on the surface of the individual's own monocytes and macrophages. In this linked recognition of antigen by T cells the HLA-DR antigens are referred to as the restricting elements of the response.

Human suppressor and cytotoxic T lymphocytes are stimulated to divide in tissue culture by viral antigens and by foreign histocompatibility antigens. Cytotoxic T cells lyse targets which have antigens such as viral-encoded proteins in association with an HLA antigen on their surface. This linked recognition resembles that of helper T cells except that the restricting elements belong to the A, B and C series of HLA antigens rather than the DR.

Viral infections may be related to a number of HLA associated diseases (e.g. insulin dependent diabetes) or it may be that the MHC has other effects on the immune response relevant to auto-immune disease that have not yet been elucidated. The fact that there is not a clear association between autoantibody formation and HLA is likely to be due to the heterogeneity of genetic mechanisms that may influence the development of significant autoimmunity, including idiotype antibodies (p. 22).

SUPPRESSION OF IMMUNE REACTIONS OR OF THEIR EFFECTS

Antihistamines. When anaphylaxis presents as an acute clinical problem the immediate aim is to give drugs which antagonise the effects of the mediators. These antagonists are the antihistamines and various drugs which have opposite actions to the mediators.

The antihistamines occupy the same tissue receptors as histamine without providing any stimulus to the effector cells. In man, the intravenous injection of an antihistamine quickly produces adequate tissue concentrations. The weal, the erythema and the itch of acute urticaria are reduced but there is no consistent improvement in lung function in acute bronchial asthma.

The failure of the antihistamines to relieve airway obstruction caused by an anaphylactic reaction has been attributed to high concentrations of histamine close to the smooth muscle cells. It may also be due to the presence of other mediators of the anaphylactic response. Bradykinin is rapidly inactivated in plasma by a kininase but its effects are not inhibited by antihistamines. No specific antagonists of bradykinin or leukotrienes are known.

Sodium cromoglycate is believed to inhibit the release of the mediators from mast cells following the interaction of antigens with IgE antibodies. It is partially effective in preventing the induction of asthma by specific antigens. If inhaled by an asthmatic subject before exposure to the antigen, protection may last for several hours, but if given after exposure to the antigen it has little effect.

Adrenaline and related drugs act by producing effects which oppose the mediators and are more effective in emergencies than the antihistamines. Adrenaline, isoprenaline and aminophylline are efficient bronchodilators in bronchial asthma. Urticaria is relieved and where oedema threatens the airway, the risk of asphyxia is lessened.

Despite their effectiveness these non-specific antagonists have serious disadvantages. They act on receptors which differ from those occupied by the mediators, and their effects never precisely counteract those of the mediators. The dose of a sympathomimetic amine which relieves airflow obstruction may produce tachycardia and palpitations even when the amine is administered as an aerosol. Salbutamol does not have these disadvantages as it is more specific in its action on β-adrenergic receptors in the bronchi.

Corticosteroids. Hydrocortisone or prednisolone produce improvement in status asthmaticus in a few hours. The mechanism is not known but is probably related to their anti-inflammatory actions and not to selective interference with any particular stage in the development of the anaphylactic response. Their use in Types II, III and IV immune reactions is discussed below.

Hyposensitisation. Anaphylactic individuals can be made less sensitive by multiple subcutaneous injections of antigen in gradually increasing dosage. Pollen antigens can be used to prevent the development of hay fever and asthma in some patients. The patient develops IgG antibodies against the antigen; these antibodies have a higher avidity for the antigen than do IgE antibodies and are able to compete successfully for the antigen sites on the pollen, or whatever has induced the anaphylactic response. As reactions with the IgG antibodies do not take place at cell surfaces, anaphylactic phenomena are not produced and there is no harmful effect as the amount of IgG antibodies produced is not sufficient to cause an immune complex reaction. In this context the IgG antibodies are referred to as blocking antibodies.

Immunosuppressive Drugs. The production of immunoglobulins and the cellular immune response are dependent upon the division of lymphoid cells. Drugs which interfere with dividing cells are therefore all potentially immunosuppressive. Such drugs were originally developed as antitumour agents and are referred to as cytotoxic drugs. Of these azathioprine, cyclophosphamide and methotrexate have been used for immunosuppression. In organ transplantation the use of azathioprine has become almost universal and it is under trial in the treatment of diseases such as systemic lupus erythematosus, rheumatoid arthritis and ulcerative colitis.

Immunosuppressive drugs may have serious adverse effects, including bone marrow suppression and the promotion of tuberculous, viral or fungal infection.

A further possible hazard is an increased incidence of malignant tumours, such as lymphomas, possibly on account of the suppression of immunological surveillance of the body tissues which is part of the normal mechanism for the control of spontaneous tumours (p. 33).

Cyclosporin is a potent immunosuppressive drug which inhibits activation of both B and T cells and in particular helper and cytotoxic T lymphocytes. Its role is limited by nephrotoxicity but it is being used increasingly in organ transplantation.

Anti-D Immunoglobulin. The clearest example of interference with a specific immune response is the use of human anti-D immunoglobulin to prevent haemolytic disease of the newborn (p. 514).

Anti-inflammatory Agents. Drugs which interfere with the unwanted consequences of Types II, III and IV immune reactions include the corticosteroids and, to a lesser extent, salicylates. The corticosteroids may also partially suppress the development of immune responses, but in high dosage they have serious side-effects (p. 453). Use is therefore made of non-steroidal anti-inflammatory drugs (p. 558).

Plasmapheresis. Apheresis is the generic term for removal of a component from the blood; a prefix indicates whether this is plasma, leucocytes etc. Plasmapheresis (plasma exchange) has been used beneficially in myasthenia gravis and Goodpasture's syndrome, removing acetylcholine-receptor and glomerular basement membrane antibodies respectively. It is used in conjunction with cytotoxic drugs and corticosteroids in order to check the rate of resynthesis of antibody. Controlled trials are in progress in relation to the removal of immune complexes in diseases such as rheumatoid arthritis and systemic lupus erythematosus.

Thymectomy as a treatment for autoimmune diseases other than myasthenia gravis may be effective only in childhood when the influence of the thymus on the immunological system is particularly important.

Cancer Immunology. Cancer cells lose some of the normal tissue-specific antigens and appear to gain some tumour-associated antigens which were not previously present in the cells from which they were derived. It used to be thought that the process of immunological surveillance destroys many early cancers by virtue of the recognition by the normal immune system of the 'foreignness' of tumour-associated antigens. However, immunodeficiency, either primary or induced by immunosuppressive drugs is mainly associated with lymphomas and not with cancer generally. It is more likely that the immune system is important in relation to the control of oncogenic viruses, rather than immune surveillance *per se*. Attempts have been made to augment the normal immune response so as to help ablate malignant growth after the bulk of the tumour has been removed or killed by conventional means. Thus allogeneic irradiated malignant cells may be beneficial in acute myeloid leukaemia.

IMMUNODEFICIENCY DISORDERS

So important are the immunological mechanisms for survival that it is not surprising that patients are rarely seen suffering from major defects. Deficiences of the humoral and cellular components of the immunological system may occur separately or together. Figure 2.9 shows the probable sites of the primary defects in the immune system for a number of clinical patterns that have been recognised. The more precise analysis of immunodeficiencies is being greatly aided by the monoclonal antibody markers for the different T cell subsets, for the different stages of maturity of B cells, and for monocytes.

Combined Deficiency States

A block in the development of the stem-cell leads to deficiency in both the T and B lymphocyte systems and therefore to impairment of cell-mediated hypersensitivity and of synthesis of humoral antibody (Fig. 2.9, lesion 1). A failure of stem-cell development at an even earlier stage leads to the additional feature of agranulocytosis although the red cells and platelets are normal. About half the infants with the autosomal recessive form of severe combined immunodeficiency have a concomitant deficiency of adenosine deaminase which has enabled prenatal diagnosis by finding the enzyme deficiency in cultured amnion cells. Infants with either the autosomal or the X-linked type are incapable of limiting the most benign viral infections. Death has resulted from generalised chickenpox, or measles or from cytomegalic or other viral infections. Vaccination results in progressive, ultimately fatal vaccinia

Site of Defect	Clinical Syndrome
1	*Severe combined immunodeficiency*: thymic hypoplasia, lymphopenia and agammaglobulinaemia. Autosomal recessive or X-linked inheritance. Do not survive infancy, but variable therapeutic success has been achieved with fetal liver cell or fetal thymus transplants.
2	*X-linked recessive agammaglobulinaemia*: normal thymus, no lymphopenia and normal cell-mediated hypersensitivity. Recurrent infection with extracellular pyogenic pathogens. Treated effectively with gammaglobulin to maintain a serum level of 200 mg per 100 ml.
3	*Defective synthesis of immunoglobulins.*
4, 5 & 6	*Thymic hypoplasia and lymphopenia*: normal immunoglobulins. Frequent fungal or viral infections. Usually die in infancy. In 5, *Di George syndrome*, absence of parathyroids presenting as tetany in the newborn can be dramatically reversed by transplants of fetal thymic tissue.
7	*Thymic hypoplasia-ataxia telangiectasia.* May be part of a more widespread mesenchyme deficiency. Thymus fails to develop. Autosomal recessive inheritance. Difficult to classify.
8	*Various defects of helper, suppressor and cytotoxic cells.* These include impaired suppressor T cells in autoimmunity and excessive suppressor T cell activity resulting in hypogammaglobulinaemia.

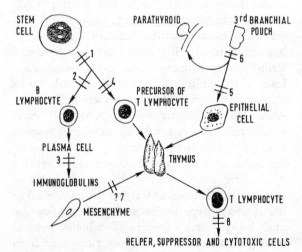

Fig. 2.9 Immunodeficiency syndromes. Sites of some of the developmental and other defects.

infection. Following successful bone marrow transplantation, 10 year survivals with maintenance of normal T and B cell function have been recorded.

Deficiency of Humoral Immunity

Primary Immunoglobulin Deficiency. Selective deficiency of the B lymphocyte system occurs in X linked recessive hypo- or a-gammaglobulinaemia (Fig. 2.9, lesion 2). The lack of immunoglobulins is not absolute but the patient fails to respond to antigenic stimuli. However, cell mediated hypersensitivity is normal. This disorder is not incompatible with survival for many years, though the patient is very susceptible to bacterial infections, particularly to pyogenic cocci.

Most patients with immunoglobulin deficiency have 'acquired' or 'late onset' agammaglobulinaemia known as '*common, variable, unclassifiable immunodeficiency*'. B lymphocytes are usually, but not always present in contrast to their absence in the X-linked form of agammaglobulinaemia. Deterioration of T cell function may also be observed. Primary acquired agammaglobulinaemia is associated with an unusually high incidence of autoimmune disease, such as pernicious anaemia or haemolytic anaemia. A prominent and frequent complication is a sprue-like syndrome and *Giardia intestinalis* infection (p. 775) is common. Another distinguishing feature of the acquired form is the frequent occurrence of non-caseating granulomas, e.g. in lungs, liver, and skin.

As the different immunoglobulins have different functions, deficiencies might be expected to produce different clinical pictures. Thus IgM deficiency is possibly associated with meningococcal meningitis and lack of IgA with gastrointestinal or respiratory tract infections. In the absence of IgA the lowered resistance permits invasion of the normally sterile upper gut by bacteria, some of which could produce decomposition of bile salts and thus affect the absorption of fat.

Immunoglobulin injections (300 mg/kg body weight) consisting mainly of IgG can provide effective protection against severe, recurrent pyogenic infections in patients with various types of hypo- or a-gammaglobulinaemia. Since the half-life of the gamma globulin injected is 30 days or more, these patients must receive at least a monthly injection of 100 mg per kg to maintain the desired level of approximately 200 mg per 100 ml. Smaller doses are ineffective.

Secondary Immunoglobulin Deficiency. Maternal IgG is transferred across the placenta by active secretion to the fetus during the third trimester of pregnancy. Premature babies may thus have some degree of hypogammaglobulinaemia and prophylactic IgG treatment may reduce the incidence of infections. The production of immunoglobulins in the early years of life is well below that of adults and this may well explain the greatly increased susceptibility of the young to infection, particularly gastrointestinal and respiratory tract infection because of IgA deficiency. IgA is present in colostrum and there is evidence that breast feeding provides the infant with intestinal immunity.

Immunoglobulin deficiency may arise also in adults as a result of abnormal metabolism of serum proteins as occurs in uraemic patients in whom susceptibility to infection is increased. Drugs may also depress the immune system; for example phenytoin or penicillamine may induce IgA deficiency.

Deficiency of Cellular Immunity

Primary Cellular Deficiency. This condition is a selective primary deficiency of T lymphocytes (Fig. 2.9, lesions 4, 5 and 6). There is severe lymphocytopenia and a predominance of reticulum cells in the lymphoid tissue. The patient's lymphocytes are unable to respond by transformation into lymphoblasts following stimulation with antigens. On account of the deficiency in cell-mediated hypersensitivity, affected children do not respond in the normal way to antigens such as monilia. Infants with thymic aplasia in whom the cell-mediated aspect is completely lacking are highly susceptible to viral infections, which usually prove fatal.

The fact that there are deficient humoral antibody responses to some antigens in conditions associated with lesions at sites 4, 5 and 6 of Figure 2.9 exemplifies the existence of co-operation between T and B lymphocytes in relation to certain antigens.

The transplantation of fragments of human fetal thymus has been effective in replacing the cellular immune deficiency in congenital thymic aplasia. Tissue matched bone marrow transplantation or transfer factor (p. 20) has been used in the Wiskott-Aldrich syndrome; this is a hereditary cellular immunodeficiency disorder, characterised by thrombocytopenia, but difficult to classify.

Secondary Cellular Deficiency. Secondary T cell defects may occur in Hodgkin's disease or sarcoidosis, following infections such as leprosy, miliary tuberculosis or measles, or may be induced by cytotoxic drugs.

An *acquired cellular immunodeficiency syndrome* (AIDS) has been described mainly in young homosexual males who frequently are addicted to the intravenous use of drugs. The probable cause is a retrovirus — human T cell lymphotrophic virus type III (HTLV-III), also known as lymphadenopathy-associated virus (LAV), isolated from blood, semen and saliva. AIDS is transmitted by close sexual contact (particularly passive anal intercourse) and by parenteral transmission of infected blood and plasma products. A decrease in helper T cells ensues.

There is often a prodromal illness characterised by fever, loss of weight, oral thrush, diarrhoea and lymphadenopathy. The virus can penetrate the brain and may cause encephalitis. The syndrome is frequently complicated by opportunist infections, notably pneumonia due to *Pneumocystis carinii* (p. 225). The mortality is about 40% but rises even higher in the presence of a further complication, Kaposi's sarcoma of the skin (p. 722). The detection of antibodies to HTLV-III indicates that there has been exposure to the virus. There is no specific treatment. Great care must be taken to avoid spread of infection.

Deficiency of Complement

Study of complement deficiency indicates that the principal function of the complement system is related to protection against infectious disease. In the case of failure of C3 activation, syndromes are produced that are basically very similar to those of the antibody deficiency syndrome. Absence of the components of the classical pathway C3 convertase seem to cause a more subtle immunity deficiency where infection with essentially non-virulent organisms may give rise to immune complex disease. Deficiency of the late-acting complement components may be associated with an increased susceptibility to certain forms of bacterial infection, particularly those due to *Neisseria*. Hypocomplementaemia is also associated with some types of glomerulonephritis.

PROSPECTS IN IMMUNOLOGY

The development of monoclonal antibodies is leading to the better recognition and quantitation of the different lymphocyte subsets and to how they can be modified to produce selective immunosuppression. Experience with new immunosuppressive drugs, such as cyclosporin, is increasing.

The next few years will see the HLA association with disease being largely rewritten as the more precise and detailed analysis of the HLA region on chromosome 6 is achieved, again with the help of monoclonal antibodies. Exciting new developments can be expected from the further study of the role of the HLA system in determining the individual's immune responses.

With improved genetic and immunological markers for disease susceptibility, it should be possible within the not too distant future to initiate effective immunosuppressive therapy at an earlier stage in a range of disabling immunological disorders.

W.J. IRVINE

FURTHER READING:

Irvine, W.J. (ed.) (1979) *Medical Immunology*. Edinburgh: Teviot Scientific Publications; New York: McGraw Hill.

Roitt, I.M. (1980) *Essential Immunology*, 4th edn. Oxford: Blackwell Scientific Publications.

Weir, D.M. (1983) *Immunology. An outline for students of medicine and biology*, 5th edn. Edinburgh: Churchill Livingstone.

More detailed texts:

Andreani *et al.* (eds.) (1984) *Immunology in Diabetes*. London: Kimpton.

Holborow, E.J. & Reeves, W.G. (eds.) (1983) *Immunology in Medicine*, 2nd edn. New York: Grune & Stratton.

Lachmann, P.J. & Peters, D.K. (1982) *Clinical Aspects of Immunology*, 4th edn. Oxford: Blackwell Scientific Publications.

3. Infection and Disease

General Aspects of Infection

Infection can involve any organ or system of the body and thus embraces all medical disciplines. It will therefore be referred to in each chapter. In this introductory chapter an account is given of general aspects, spread, diagnosis, prevention and treatment of infection. The term infectious disease is commonly used to denote infections that are contagious or communicable i.e. transmissible from man to man. However, there has been a trend, especially in North America, to refer to all diseases caused by micro-organisms as infectious diseases.

Infection differs from other diseases in a number of aspects; the most important is that it is caused by a living micro-organism, which can frequently be identified, thus establishing the aetiology of the disease early in the illness. Many of these organisms, including all bacteria, are sensitive to antibiotics and most infections are therefore curable, unlike many non-infective diseases such as those of the cardiovascular or nervous systems which frequently become chronic and are not amenable to specific therapy. The communicability of infections is another factor which differentiates them from non-infective diseases; this leads to the transmission of pathogenic organisms to other people and if large numbers are involved an epidemic may result. Finally, many infections are preventable by hygienic measures or by vaccines. In certain circumstances, infection may be prevented by the judicious use of antibiotics (chemoprophylaxis).

During the past 50 years there has been a dramatic fall in the incidence of communicable diseases in developed countries. This is due to several factors such as immunisation, antimicrobial chemotherapy, improved nutrition, and better sanitation and housing. Infections which have decreased, and in some instances almost disappeared in these countries include diphtheria, poliomyelitis, tuberculosis, brucellosis and bacillary dysentery. In less advanced countries, however, especially in the tropics, infection continues to be one of the commonest causes of death, particularly in children; measles, for example, has a high mortality in malnourished infants in many African countries.

Even in developed countries certain infections continue to pose problems and some are even increasing in incidence. Sexually transmitted diseases have become common as a result of sexual 'liberation' and promiscuity both heterosexual and homosexual. Food poisoning caused by Salmonellae and Campylobacter species has increased due commonly to the modern practice of battery-rearing and deep-freezing of poultry. Patients in hospitals have always been at risk of acquiring infection as Lord Lister and Florence Nightingale recognised over a hundred years ago. In spite of the availability of antiseptics and antibiotics, however, hospital-acquired (nosocomial) infection remains a major problem which has increased in recent years in parallel with the introduction of new techniques of patient care, the grouping together of susceptible patients in specialized units, and the number of patients with decreased resistance to infection (compromised hosts).

A patient's resistance to infection may be reduced as a result of extremes of age, disease, medical or surgical therapeutic regimes, or a combination of several of these factors. A person whose resistance to infection is decreased as a result of abnormality in the immune response is referred to as an immunocompromised host.

Examples of immunocompromised patients are provided by a recipient of a renal transplant or a patient suffering from leukaemia. Both have serious diseases and are usually being treated with immunosuppressive and corticosteroid drugs and are thus very susceptible to infection which is not infrequently fatal. Infections in immunocompromised patients are caused by a wide variety of micro-organisms including those which are common human pathogens such as *Staphylococcus aureus* and the varicella/zoster virus. However, these patients are also very susceptible to organisms which rarely cause serious infections in healthy people, for example *Staphylococcus epidermidis* and *Pseudomonas aeruginosa* and fungi such as *Candida albicans* (opportunist organisms).

By the end of the present decade, approaching one thousand million passengers will travel by air each year, and it is now possible to circumnavigate the world in 48 hours. As a result there has been an increase in the number of imported infections in developed countries. These commonly originate in areas of the world with tropical or sub-tropical climates. Returning travellers may suffer from a wide variety of infections, the commonest being diarrhoeal diseases and malaria. For example, between 1970 and 1980 there was a tenfold increase in the number of notifications of malaria in England and Wales.

Within the past 10 years a number of 'new' infections have been recognised, principally as a result of improved laboratory diagnostic techniques, but also due to improved epidemiological methods including the establishment of national communicable disease surveillance centres which monitor incidents and outbreaks of infection and exchange information with similar organizations in other countries. These 'recently recognized' infections are: *Campylobacter enteritis* (p. 753), *rotavirus enteritis* (p. 727), *non-A, non-B hepatitis* (p. 353), *legionnaires' disease* (p. 224), *viral haemorrhagic fevers* (p. 733), *Chlamydia urethritis* (p. 412), *anti-biotic-associated colitis* (p. 46), *group B streptococcal neonatal infections* (p. 742), *toxic shock syndrome* (p. 743) and the *acquired immune deficiency syndrome* (AIDS, p. 35).

Source and Spread of Infection

Infection may originate from the patient (autogenous) usually from the skin, nasopharynx or colon, or from outside sources (exogenous), commonly from another person who may either be suffering from an infection or carrying a pathogenic micro-organism. Carriers are usually healthy and may harbour the organism in the throat (diphtheria) or stool (salmonella infection). Non-human sources of infection include animals (rabies), soil (tetanus) and water (typhoid fever). Fomites is the term used to describe inanimate articles such as blankets, furniture and crockery which can be reservoirs of infection.

Micro-organisms may be transmitted by several routes. Autogenous infection may develop as a result of local spread e.g. from bowel to peritoneum, or by the blood stream. An example of the latter is infective endocarditis caused by *Streptococcus viridans* originating in the patient's mouth and entering the blood during meals or dental procedures. Exogenous infection may be acquired directly or indirectly by one of the following routes:

1. *Direct Contact*. Venereal and skin infections are transmitted by contact between body surfaces.
2. *Airborne Transmission*. This includes transmission by droplets and dust particles. Infected droplets originate in the nasopharynx and mouth and are expelled during talking, breathing and sneezing, carrying micro-organisms with them. Respiratory tract infections and many of the common infectious diseases of childhood such as measles are airborne-spread.
3. *Faecal-oral Spread*. Infections transmitted by this route are usually acquired by the ingestion of food and drink contaminated by human faeces. This often occurs during preparation of meals as a result of a low standard of personal hygiene in kitchen workers. Large outbreaks of hepatitis or cholera may follow pollution of domestic water supplies. Other diseases spread by the faecal-oral route include dysentery and enterovirus infections such as poliomyelitis. Hand washing is the vital factor in the prevention of infection transmitted by this route.
4. *Mammal, Bird or Insect Borne*. Mammals and birds may transmit infection directly (rabies

and psittacosis) or indirectly via food and drink (salmonella infection and brucellosis). Blood sucking insects are important vectors in the transmission of many important infections such as malaria, yellow fever, plague and rickettsial diseases.

5. *Transmission by Medical and Nursing Procedures*. Infection may be transmitted by inadequately sterilized instruments, faulty nursing techniques or contamination of transfused blood or other liquid.

Incubation period is the period of time which elapses between the invasion of the tissues by pathogens and the appearance of clinical symptoms and signs of infection.

Diagnosis of Infectious Disease

A knowledge of infections prevailing in the locality may be a valuable guide to diagnosis, e.g. when mumps is prevalent, the occurrence, without apparent cause, of acute epididymo-orchitis in an adult may be attributed to mumps with some confidence, a diagnosis which could not be made on clinical evidence alone. It is wise to enquire about contacts among the family, friends and workmates. Persons following certain occupations may be exposed to infection, e.g. leptospirosis occurs in coal miners, pig farmers, sewerworkers and fish-cleaners; anthrax occurs in tanners and in handlers of imported bone meal.

A recent history of laparotomy or of obscure abdominal pain should suggest subphrenic or intrahepatic abscess as a cause of unexplained fever.

Residence or travel abroad within the previous year or two raises the possibility of malaria, amoebic abscess of the liver or other exotic disease.

In many infections a diagnosis beyond all reasonable doubt may be made on clinical grounds, e.g. measles or chickenpox. In others there may be doubt about the identity of the causal organism and demonstration of its presence is essential for diagnosis.

Differential Diagnosis of Pyrexia. Most febrile illnesses are due to infection and often the diagnosis can be made by clinical examination alone. In other instances a diagnosis may require confirmation by haematological examination, radiography, scanning, bacteriological or serological investigation of blood or other body fluids, discharges or excreta. Often, detection of specific antibodies in the serum may have to be undertaken before the diagnostic problems may be solved. Occasionally the cause of a febrile illness remains uncertain in spite of investigation and such a case is categorised PUO (pyrexia of unknown origin).

In order to establish the diagnosis the following measures should be undertaken:

1. Retake the history; a symptom may have been overlooked or misinterpreted; enquire again whether the patient has lived or travelled overseas.
2. Repeat the examination of the patient; new signs may have appeared while others could have been missed or their significance not appreciated.
3. Examine the urine repeatedly for protein, white and red blood cells and micro-organisms.
4. Inspect the temperature charts for evidence of some characteristic appearance such as the undulations seen in some cases of lymphoma or the periodicity of malaria.
5. Review the results of laboratory investigations, thoroughly rescrutinise any radiographs and repeat such examinations as may seem necessary.

If the diagnosis is still uncertain further tests will be required. These will be indicated by any new information obtained as a result of the clinical reassessment. It should be borne in mind that most cases of PUO are due to a common disorder with an unusual presentation. In Britain the more common causes of PUO are tumours (such as carcinoma with or without metastases, or lymphomas), infections (among which tuberculosis is important), connective tissue disorders and drug hypersensitivity. In the tropics and elsewhere a wide variety of infections must be considered, as a glance at the map on page 717 will demonstrate.

Mysterious fevers, particularly in patients who have some knowledge of medicine or nursing, may be due to deceit (factitious fever). Doubts should be raised if the skin of a supposedly febrile patient does not feel hot or if the general health does not deteriorate in spite of persistent fever. The occurrence of some bizarre symptom or sign may arouse suspicion that the temperature is being falsified. There are both subtle and simple techniques for doing this. The latter include holding the thermometer close to a hot water bottle or other source of heat, dipping it into a hot drink, applying friction to the bulb, or shaking it in a retrograde manner.

If the diagnosis remains obscure another opinion should be obtained, as reconsideration of the evidence by an unbiased observer may throw new light on the problem.

When a diagnosis still cannot be established and the patient's condition is deteriorating, various remedies, e.g. antibiotics, may be tried empirically in the hope of influencing the course of the disease. A therapeutic trial should not be regarded as a satisfactory diagnostic test and it can further obscure the diagnosis by suppressing but not curing the infection. It is most useful in suspected tuberculosis.

The Prevention of Infection

The prevention of infection depends on three concepts which may be inter-related:

1. *Elimination of the Source.* Successful examples of this include the eradication of tuberculosis and brucellosis from cattle in many countries and the world-wide elimination of smallpox. The laboratory screening of donated blood for syphilis and hepatitis B virus has virtually eliminated these sources of infection.

2. *Prevention of Transmission of Infection.* This may be accomplished by the isolation of infected patients (source isolation) and of those such as the immunosuppressed who are particularly susceptible to infection (protective isolation). Strict antisepsis in operating theatres and good nursing practices in wards are essential if transmission of infection is to be prevented. Hand-washing is of paramount importance.

   Insect control by the elimination of breeding grounds and the use of insecticides, is a major factor in malaria prevention programmes. Individuals who have been in close contact with serious infectious diseases such as diphtheria or Lassa fever are placed in quarantine — a term derived from the period of 40 days of compulsory isolation of ships after leaving a port where life-threatening infections such as plague were rife. The duration of quarantine depends on the incubation period of the disease. For the common infectious diseases of childhood strict quarantine is not necessary although the child should normally be kept away from school until non-infectious.

3. *Protection of Susceptible Persons.* This involves the judicious use of prophylactic antibiotics (p. 50) and of active or passive immunization.

   Active Immunisation. In Britain parents should be advised to have their children immunised against whooping-cough, diphtheria, tetanus, measles and poliomyelitis (Table 3.1). Because of the risk of damage to the developing embryo or fetus if rubella should occur during pregnancy, it is recommended that rubella vaccine be given to all girls between 11 and 14 years and to non-pregnant women of child-bearing age who are found to be serologically negative for this antigen. Similarly, immunisation against tuberculosis should be given to all non-reactors to tuberculin during adolescence.

   The indications for immunisation against influenza, enteric fevers, cholera, plague, typhus, yellow fever and rabies depend upon the likelihood of exposure or international health regulations (p. 807). Acute demyelinating encephalomyelitis (p. 647) is a rare complication of immunisation.

   Passive Immunisation. An injection of immunoglobulin will provide temporary protection against certain infectious diseases. Human normal immunoglobulin (pooled) is indicated for prevention of measles (p. 727) and virus A hepatitis (p. 351), and human specific immunoglobulin for chickenpox (p. 730), virus B hepatitis (p. 353), tetanus (p. 745) and rabies (p. 731).

Diseases Due to Infection

Diseases due to infection are the commonest cause of ill health throughout the world. The organisms involved are viruses, chlamydia, rickettsia, bacteria, spirochaetes, protozoa, helminths and fungi. The term infestation is limited to ectoparasites, usually arthropods such as lice and fleas, which remain on the surface of the body but which may transmit a systemic infection.

Table 3.1. Immunisation schedule recommended in Britain.

Age	Visits	Vaccine	Intervals
3–12 months	3	Three administrations of DTP + OPV	6–8 weeks and 4–6 months
12–24 months	1	Measles vaccination	
First year at school	1	Booster DT + OPV	
10–13 years	1	BCG for the tuberculin negative	
Girls: 11–13 years	1	Rubella vaccination	
15–19 years or on leaving school	1	TT + OPV	

DTP = Diphtheria, tetanus, pertussis ('triple') vaccine.
OPV = Oral poliomyelitis vaccine.
DT = Diphtheria, tetanus vaccine.
TT = Tetanus toxoid.

As yet few specific therapeutic measures are available for viral diseases, among which are the exanthemata — chickenpox, measles and rubella; mumps and infectious mononucleosis; respiratory illnesses such as the common cold and influenza; viral hepatitis and diseases of the nervous system such as rabies, poliomyelitis and meningitis. The problem of chemotherapy is to control the growth and propagation of the virus without damage to the host cell on which it is dependent. The number of viral infections for which prophylaxis, using vaccines, is available is increasing in parallel with modern advances in virology and now there is preventative treatment for rabies, hepatitis B, yellow fever, poliomyelitis, measles, mumps and rubella. Several viral infections may be prevented temporarily by passive immunisation with human immunoglobulin.

Organisms smaller than true bacteria, the rickettsiae which cause typhus fevers, and the chlamydia of psittacosis, lymphogranuloma, urethritis and trachoma are widespread and susceptible to antimicrobial therapy.

The range of diseases caused by bacteria is large; streptococci and staphylococci are widespread and produce similar diseases throughout the world. Others such as the cholera vibrio and plague bacillus are locally endemic but may produce epidemics from time to time. Some bacterial infections may be acute such as diphtheria and tetanus, others chronic such as tuberculosis, syphilis and leprosy.

Protozoal infections such as malaria, amoebic dysentery, sleeping sickness and leishmaniasis and helminthiasis (worms) are of great importance in the tropics. Fungi causing ringworm and thrush occur all over the world but systemic infections with other fungi, such as coccidioidomycosis, histoplasmosis and the blastomycoses, are rare except in certain geographical locations.

Most bacterial, protozoal and fungal infections can be successfully treated with antimicrobial agents provided that the appropriate drug is prescribed early in the disease. This emphasises the need for rapid and accurate diagnosis supplemented where necessary by specific tests to indicate the most effective therapeutic agent.

Diseases due to infection which involve one system predominantly are described in the appropriate chapters in this book, e.g. infective endocarditis (p. 165), respiratory infections (p. 219), viral hepatitis (p. 349), sexually transmitted disease (p. 408), infectious mononucleosis (p. 519), and meningitis (p. 637). Other infectious diseases are described in Chapter 19.

Students should familiarise themselves first with infections which are common in their own countries. In Britain these include streptococcal and staphylococcal infections (p. 743), the childhood infectious diseases such as measles (p. 727), whooping cough (p. 748), and chickenpox (p. 730), food poisoning (p. 753) and the serious imported infections, e.g. typhoid fever (p. 751) and malaria (p. 768).

ANTIMICROBIAL THERAPY

The ability of one micro-organism to interfere with the growth of another is called antibiosis and is due to specific diffusible metabolic products termed *antibiotics*. Since the introduction of penicillin in 1940, research has produced a wide range of antibiotics. A variety of chemotherapeutic agents such as metronidazole, trimethoprim, dapsone and isoniazid has also followed the demonstration of the therapeutic effect of sulphanilamide in 1935. A general term for all of these substances is *antimicrobial agent*.

Effective therapy is now available against all known bacteria, rickettsiae, mycoplasmas and chlamydia. Specific antiprotozoal compounds are used in the treatment of diseases such as sleeping sickness, kala azar, malaria and amoebic dysentery. Topical antifungal agents are widely prescribed, but fully effective, non-toxic, anti-fungal drugs have not yet been found for use in systemic infection. Antimicrobial agents active against viruses have also been discovered but few have been successful therapeutically.

THE SULPHONAMIDES

Although the sulphonamides have been superseded in many countries by antibiotics, their usefulness has been greatly extended by the introduction of co-trimoxazole, a combination of a sulphonamide and trimethoprim. The preparations most suitable for clinical use are the short-acting sulphonamides, e.g. sulphadimidine, which is rapidly absorbed and quickly excreted in the urine in a soluble form. Administration is every 4 to 8 hours, by mouth; a preparation is also available for intravenous or intramuscular administration.

The most common indication for the use of sulphonamides is cystitis. A dose of 1 g, 8 hourly is adequate. Sulphonamides have long been used in the treatment of meningococcal infection, particularly meningitis; unfortunately the incidence of resistant strains is increasing and therefore penicillin is now used in treating this condition.

Adverse Effects. Sulphonamides have a wide range of potential hazards including rashes, fever and agranulocytosis. Serious but rare complications are haemolytic anaemia, purpura, pancytopenia and renal lesions (p. 406). Glucose-6-phosphate dehydrogenase deficiency (p. 507) is a contraindication to the use of sulphonamides, as haemolysis may be induced. The Stevens-Johnson syndrome (erythema multiforme and ulceration of mucous membranes) may be induced by sulphonamide and can be fatal. When any of the above complications develop the drug must be stopped immediately.

Sulphonamides can detach protein-bound drugs such as warfarin and sulphonylurea antidiabetic agents and thereby cause overdosage.

Sulphonamide preparations applied to the skin are liable to cause light sensitivity which may persist for a number of years; they should not be used topically.

Co-trimoxazole. The two components of this compound, trimethoprim and sulphamethoxazole, act by inhibiting enzymes at two successive stages in the synthesis of para-aminobenzoic acid to folic acid and DNA. Co-trimoxazole is particularly useful in exacerbations of chronic bronchitis and infections of the urinary tract. It is also effective in the treatment of invasive salmonella infections and typhoid carriers. The adult dose is 2 tablets twice daily and there is a preparation for injection. Trimethoprim is also available in combination with sulphamoxole (co-trifamole).

The adverse effects are those of the sulphonamides but the clinician must also be on the alert for possible haematological reactions to trimethoprim including thrombocytopenia and megaloblastic anaemia due to folate deficiency (p. 503).

Trimethoprim alone is now available for the treatment of urinary tract infection for which it is given in a dose of 200 mg twice a day, or 100 mg each evening for long-term chemoprophylaxis. It is also used for the treatment of respiratory tract infections. Side-effects are less than with co-trimoxazole.

THE BETA-LACTAM ANTIBIOTICS

These are the *penicillins* and *cephalosporins* and are so called because of the 4 membered beta-lactam ring which forms part of their basic structure. Resistance is commonly due to bacterial enzymes called beta-lactamases (penicillinases and cephalosporinases) which can inactivate the antibiotics by opening the beta-lactam ring. The plasmids (p. 18) which code for these enzymes are transmissible between bacteria.

The Penicillins

All penicillins are bactericidal and the range of activity of the group is wide as both Gram-positive and certain Gram-negative organisms are sensitive to individual penicillins. The outstanding adverse effect is the risk of inducing a hypersensitivity reaction. Even so the penicillins are the most useful antibiotics at present available. The principal penicillins are:

1. *Benzylpenicillin*, which is the original and most active penicillin; it must be given by injection. Its action can be prolonged by combining it with procaine — *procaine penicillin* and an even longer-acting form is *benzathine penicillin*.
2. *Phenoxymethylpenicillin* is absorbed when administered by mouth.
3. *Cloxacillin* and *flucloxacillin* are not inactivated by staphylococcal penicillinase and are reserved for the treatment of severe staphylococcal infections resistant to benzylpenicillin.
4. *Ampicillin*, its esters and its analogue *amoxycillin* are effective against Gram-negative bacilli, in contrast to most other penicillins whose activity is largely limited to Gram-positive organisms and Gram-negative cocci.
5. The *acylureidopenicillins*, mezlocillin, azlocillin and piperacillin are ampicillin derivatives which have a broader spectrum than ampicillin but, like ampicillin, are susceptible to beta-lactamases.
6. *Carbenicillin*, *ticarcillin* and *azlocillin* are used in pseudomonas infections.

Benzylpenicillin is rapidly absorbed following intramuscular injection and is excreted by the kidneys within a few hours. A dose of 300 mg (half a million units) 6- or 8-hourly will suffice for most infections due to sensitive organisms. Large intramuscular or intravenous doses (up to 12 million units daily) may be required to achieve therapeutic concentrations within deep-seated or walled-off foci of infection, as occurs in infective endocarditis or lung abscess. The intramuscular injection of large doses is painful. Probenecid, 2 g daily by mouth, will raise the blood level of penicillin by delaying its excretion by the kidney and allow smaller doses to be used.

Benzylpenicillin remains the antibiotic of choice for the treatment of pneumococcal, meningococcal and streptococcal infections, gonorrhoea and syphilis, yaws, diphtheria, tetanus, gas gangrene, anthrax and actinomycosis. It is also indicated for infections caused by penicillin-sensitive strains of *Staph. aureus*.

Penicillin is also used prophylactically. Benzylpenicillin is given to patients with valvular heart disease before a dental extraction to reduce the risk of infective endocarditis (p. 166). It is also given to prevent gas gangrene and tetanus after high amputations of ischaemic legs and for wounds containing dirt and devitalised tissue.

Benzylpenicillin passes in very small quantities into cerebrospinal fluid or pleural, pericardial or joint spaces. In the presence of inflammation its diffusion to these sites is greater.

Procaine Penicillin and Benzathine Penicillin. These are long-acting penicillins given by injection and used in the treatment of gonorrhoea and the treponemal diseases, syphilis and yaws. *Procaine penicillin* in aqueous suspension, in a dose of 300 mg once a day intra-muscularly, is relatively painless and will maintain an adequate blood level for 24 hours.

Benzathine penicillin has a duration of action of 3 to 4 weeks. It can be used for the prophylaxis of rheumatic fever in patients who cannot be relied upon to take oral penicillin. The dose varies from 229–916 mg once a week. For rheumatic fever prophylaxis the dose is 916 mg every 3 weeks.

Phenoxymethylpenicillin is incompletely absorbed from the stomach and frequent oral administration will produce reasonable blood levels. The usual dose is 500 mg every 4 to 6 hours, taken half an hour before meals to ensure maximum absorption. In patients who are ill or vomiting, intramuscular benzylpenicillin is essential because of uncertainties in absorption. During recovery oral therapy may be substituted in such patients.

Phenoxymethylpenicillin is indicated for minor streptococcal infections and for pneumococcal pneumonia after initial therapy with benzylpenicillin. It is used prophylactically on a long-term basis following an attack of rheumatic fever to prevent recurrences.

Cloxacillin and Flucloxacillin. These semisynthetic penicillins are stable to staphylococcal beta-lactamases. The only indications for their use are infections caused by penicillin-resistant *Staph. aureus* and *Staph. epidermidis*. For oral therapy flucloxacillin is superior to cloxacillin as it is almost twice as well absorbed from the gut. The dose is 500 mg 6-hourly but this can be increased to 1 g every 4 hours for seriously ill patients.

Ampicillin. This is a semisynthetic penicillin which is effective by mouth and which has a bactericidal action against Gram-positive organisms and also a variety of Gram-negative organisms, including salmonellae, shigellae, *Haemophilus influenzae* and certain strains of *Esch. coli* and *Proteus*. It is inactivated by staphylococcal penicillinase. Ampicillin is of value in urinary tract infections due to *Esch. coli* and *Proteus* and in exacerbations of chronic bronchitis.

The dose is 250 mg to 1 g, 4- to 8-hourly by mouth. Preparations for injection are also available. Maculopapular rashes occur in approximately 5% of all patients given ampicillin and in over 90% of patients with infectious mononucleosis; this antibiotic should not therefore be prescribed for sore throats which may be due to glandular fever.

There are a number of ampicillin esters including talampicillin, bacampicillin and pivampicillin. These improve the absorption of ampicillin thus producing higher blood levels of the antibiotic.

Amoxycillin is an analogue of ampicillin which has a similar antibacterial range but is better absorbed from the gastrointestinal tract. It is effective in typhoid fever.

Clavulanic acid is a new beta-lactam agent with only weak antibacterial activity. It is, however, a potent inhibitor of many beta-lactamases and can protect beta-lactamase-susceptible antibiotics, such as amoxycillin, from inactivation by these enzymes. A combination of amoxycillin plus sodium clavulanate is available.

Carbenicillin and Ticarcillin. Carbenicillin was initially the only penicillin with activity against *Ps. aeruginosa*. This organism, however, is only moderately sensitive to carbenicillin which has been replaced by its more active analogue ticarcillin.

Mezlocillin, Azlocillin and Piperacillin. These acylureidopenicillins have a wider range of activity than ampicillin and are also more effective against many Gram-negative bacilli. Azlocillin is more active than ticarcillin against *Ps. aeruginosa*. The acylureidopenicillins are generally used in combination with one or more antibiotics for the treatment of undiagnosed infections in immunocompromised patients. They have activity against anaerobic Gram-negative bacilli such as *Bacteroides fragilis*, a common pathogen in intra-abdominal sepsis (p. 330).

Ps. aeruginosa is usually of relatively low virulence but it is an important cause of disease in patients with impaired defence mechanisms. Treatment is with either ticarcillin or an acylureidopenicillin but in pseudomonas septicaemia a combination of an aminoglycoside with a penicillin is required; tobramycin plus ticarcillin (5 g t.i.d.) or azlocillin is probably the best choice.

Adverse Effects of the Penicillins. An increasing number of patients have acquired hypersensitivity to the systemic administration of the penicillins. This takes the form of urticaria and pyrexia or of an acute anaphylactic reaction which has occasionally proved fatal. Ampicillin commonly produces a maculopapular rash which differs from penicillin-induced urticaria and is specific for ampicillin. It is almost certainly unrelated to true penicillin allergy and is not a contraindication to future treatment with other penicillins. The patient should always be asked about previous allergy to any form of penicillin before treatment is commenced as a severe reaction may be provoked by the administration of only a few milligrams. Patients who suffer from bronchial asthma or are hypersensitive to other drugs are particularly liable to become allergic to penicillin.

Skin sensitisation may result from topical applications of any antibiotic, but is so frequent with penicillin that it should never be applied locally.

Although penicillin is otherwise a safe antibiotic, its accumulation in patients with renal failure may lead to encephalopathy, so that dosage in these circumstances must be guided by the blood levels. The injectable preparations of all penicillins are formulated as sodium or potassium salts and hypernatraemia or hyperkalaemia can also result if large doses are given to patients with renal failure. Great care should be taken with the intrathecal administration of penicillin as fatal encephalopathy can occur if the dose is excessive.

It is important to avoid accidental intravenous administration when injecting procaine penicillin intramuscularly as this may result in a very severe reaction consisting of a sensation of impending death, paraesthesiae and confusion lasting up to an hour and followed by exhaustion and anxiety. The reaction may be fatal.

The Cephalosporins

The cephalosporins have a wide range of activity against many, but not all, important Gram-positive and Gram-negative bacteria and are therefore of value for the initial 'blind' therapy of undiagnosed infections. *Cephalexin, cefaclor* and *cephradine* are all absorbed from the gut but the other available cephalosporins such as *cefuroxime, cephamandole* and *cephazolin* must be given by injection. *Cefóxitin*, also known as a cephamycin antibiotic, has the additional advantage of activity against *B. fragilis*. Cefuroxime and cefoxitin are very resistant to degradation by many beta-lacta-mases.

Cefotaxime, latamoxef, ceftizoxime and *ceftazidime* are expensive cephalosporins which are especially stable in the presence of beta-lactamases and have greater intrinsic activity against many Gram-negative bacilli than the earlier cephalosporins. They also have varying degrees of activity against *Ps. aeruginosa* and *B. fragilis* but are less active than cefuroxime or cephamandole against Gram-positive organisms especially *Staph. aureus. Cefsulodin* is a cephalosporin with only one indication i.e. infection caused by *Ps. aeruginosa*.

The dose of the cephalosporins ranges from 250–1000 mg 6-hourly depending on the size of the patient, renal function, and severity of infection. For abdominal sepsis the dose of cefoxitin is 2 g. Cefuroxime is probably the best cephalosporin for general use.

Adverse reactions are similar to those of the penicillins. A small number of penicillin-sensitive patients may also be allergic to the cephalosporins which should be avoided if there is a history of significant hypersensitivity to the penicillins. Nephrotoxicity is discussed on page 406.

ERYTHROMYCIN

Erythromycin has a similar although not identical antibacterial spectrum to penicillin and is commonly used to treat infections caused by Gram-positive organisms in penicillin-allergic patients. It is also effective in whooping cough, Campylobacter enteritis and Legionnaires' disease provided it is given early enough in the course of these illnesses. It is a safe and effective antibiotic for the treatment of respiratory infections in children in domiciliary practice. Erythromycin is prescribed in a dosage of 250–500 mg by mouth every 6 hours. There is a preparation for intravenous injection. Diarrhoea is the principal side effect although cholestatic jaundice may rarely develop if the course of treatment exceeds 10 days.

THE TETRACYCLINES

Tetracycline, oxytetracycline and *chlortetracycline* are very closely related bacteriostatic agents which for practical purposes have an identical range of activity. The adult dose is 250–500 mg 6-hourly before meals. *Doxycycline* has the advantage that it is given only once daily, 200–300 mg on the first day and 100–200 mg thereafter.

The tetracyclines inhibit the growth of a wide range of Gram-positive and Gram-negative bacteria and are particularly useful in the treatment of exacerbations of chronic bronchitis, but their value is limited by an increase in tetracycline-resistant pneumococci and *H. influenzae*. The tetracyclines are also active against rickettsiae (typhus fevers), *Coxiella burneti* (Q-fever), *Mycoplasma penumoniae* and chlamydia (lymphogranuloma venereum, psittacosis and non-gonococcal urethritis) and are effective in brucellosis.

The tetracyclines are employed systemically in the treatment of acne vulgaris and rosacea where their beneficial effect is almost certainly not due solely to their antibacterial action. Chlortetracycline is used for the local treatment of skin infections as it does not cause cutaneous sensitisation.

Adverse Effects. The tetracyclines are safe antibiotics with few side-effects. The commonest is diarrhoea which usually stops when the antibiotic is discontinued. Tetracyclines chelate with calcium and are deposited in developing bone and teeth causing a brown discoloration. They should not therefore be given to children or pregnant women. With the exception of doxycycline, the tetracyclines can exacerbate renal failure and should not be given to patients with kidney disease.

CHLORAMPHENICOL

Chloramphenicol has a range of activity similar to that of the tetracyclines with the important difference that it is effective in enteric fever. It is more active than the tetracyclines against *H. influenzae* and is the antibiotic of choice in meningitis due to this organism. The daily dose for an adult is 1–3 g. Preparations for parenteral administration are also available. Chloramphenicol eye drops and ointment are indicated for purulent conjunctivitis.

Adverse Effects. Chloramphenicol has in its chemical structure a benzene ring of the type known to cause bone marrow aplasia. Although pancytopenia due to chloramphenicol is very uncommon, it is almost invariably fatal; this antibiotic should be used systemically only for the treatment of typhoid fever and *H. influenzae* infections and in other conditions if there is no alternative therapy.

Chloramphenicol should never be given to premature infants and very rarely to the newborn because of the risk of the development of the frequently fatal '*grey baby syndrome*'. This is a state of acute circulatory failure caused by the very high blood levels of chloramphenicol due to its inadequate conjugation in the liver at this age.

CLINDAMYCIN

Clindamycin (7-chlorolincomycin) has a similar antibacterial spectrum to penicillin against most Gram-positive organisms including penicillin-resistant staphylococci. It penetrates well into bone and is therefore useful for osteomyelitis caused by *Staph. aureus*. The other principal indication is for the treatment of infections caused by *B. fragilis* (p. 330). The dose is 300 mg 6 hourly, orally or by injection.

Clindamycin is the commonest cause of *antibiotic-associated pseudomembranous colitis*. This adverse reaction, which can also complicate treatment with other antibiotics, especially ampicillin, is due to selective overgrowth of *Clostridium difficile* which produces a toxin detectable in the faeces and is the direct cause of the disease. Treatment is with vancomycin or metronidazole, the latter being less costly.

SODIUM FUSIDATE

This sodium salt of fusidic acid is highly bactericidal against *Staph. aureas* and is useful in infections caused by penicillin-resistant staphylococci. Like the lincomycins it is well concentrated in bone. Sodium fusidate is given orally in doses of 250–500 mg thrice daily, is rapidly absorbed, attains high tissue levels and is reasonably well tolerated, although nausea and vomiting are not uncommon during therapy. An intravenous preparation is available. Jaundice has occasionally been associated with its use. This antibiotic is expensive and is principally indicated for serious infections due to staphylococci especially osteomyelitis and endocarditis.

THE AMINOGLYCOSIDE ANTIBIOTICS

Streptomycin, Kanamycin, Gentamicin, Tobramycin, Netilmicin, Amikacin and Neomycin

These have similar chemical structures, pharmacological actions and adverse effects. They are not absorbed and for systemic treatment must be given by injection.

The outstanding property of *streptomycin* is its bactericidal effect on the tubercle bacillus. It is given in conjunction with two other antituberculous drugs and this triple therapy prevents the emergence of resistant strains (p. 238). For long-term therapy the daily dose of streptomycin should not exceed 1 g. Its use in infections due to Gram-negative bacilli is restricted by the rapid development of bacterial resistance.

Kanamycin is active against many Gram-negative bacilli and resistance develops much more slowly than with streptomycin. It has been mainly replaced by gentamicin for infections caused by Gram-negative bacilli.

Gentamicin has a range of activity similar to kanamycin but has the very important additional advantage of being effective against *Ps. aeruginosa*. It is also active against penicillin-resistant staphylococci but inactive against anaerobes and streptococci with the exception of *Strep. faecalis*; in serious infections caused by this organism gentamicin is combined with ampicillin. The dose depends on renal function and the age and weight of the patient. Up to 7·5 mg per kilogram body weight per 24 hours in divided doses is required for serious infections but 2 mg per kg is sufficient for uncomplicated urinary tract infections. Therapeutic blood concentrations of gentamicin are given on page 820.

Tobramycin is more active than gentamicin against *Ps. aeruginosa* but has no other advantage.

Netilmicin, a gentamicin derivative, is stable to three of nine aminoglycoside-inactivating enzymes, and like amikacin, should be reserved for infection caused by gentamicin-resistant organisms. Netilmicin may be less nephrotoxic than gentamicin.

Amikacin, a derivative of kanamycin has less intrinsic antibacterial activity than gentamicin, but has the advantage of being stable to eight of nine aminoglycoside-inactivating enzymes, in contrast to gentamicin which is susceptible to six of the nine. For this reason amikacin is active against many gentamicin-resistant Gram-negative bacilli and should be reserved for the treatment of infections caused by these organisms. The dose is 500 mg 12 hourly — this may have to be increased for serious infections.

Neomycin is too toxic to be given parenterally but local applications containing neomycin are used in infections of the skin and eye. Neomycin is used in hepatic encephalopathy to reduce the numbers of colonic bacteria.

Adverse Effects. The aminoglycosides are all nephrotoxic (p. 406) and ototoxic. The commonest adverse effect of the aminoglycosides is on the eighth cranial nerve. With streptomycin and gentamicin the vestibular division is initially affected with resultant vertigo and incoordination. Later, deafness may also occur. Kanamycin tends to cause deafness first. Aminoglycosides, especially gentamicin, should not be administered together with the diuretic frusemide, as both can cause eighth nerve damage and additive ototoxicity may result from the combination.

The ototoxicity of the aminoglycosides is related to the age of the patient, the serum level of the antibiotic and the duration of administration. The aminoglycosides are principally excreted from the body by the kidneys and the risk of toxicity is increased when there is impairment of renal function. In such cases serum levels of the antibiotic must be monitored and the frequency of dosage adjusted accordingly. Serum concentrations of the antibiotic should be measured in all seriously ill patients to prevent toxicity and also to ensure therapeutic blood levels.

Spectinomycin

Spectinomycin is an aminocyclitol compound with certain structural similarity to streptomycin although it is not an aminoglycoside. Its only clinical use is for the treatment of gonorrhoea if penicillin is contraindicated because of allergy or bacterial resistance.

METRONIDAZOLE

This imidazole compound has high activity against anaerobic bacteria and protozoa but none against aerobic organisms. It is the drug of choice for infections due to *Trichomonas vaginalis* and *Entamoeba histolytica* (p. 775) and is widely used for the treatment and prophylaxis of infections caused by anaerobic bacteria, notably *B. fragilis* (p. 330).

Metronidazole is a non-toxic drug but should not be given to women during the first trimester of pregnancy as fetal abnormalities have been reported in animals given high doses for prolonged periods. Alcohol should be avoided during therapy with metronidazole which has a similar action to disulfiram (p. 695). The oral dose varies from 200–400 mg given 3 or 4 times a day. Up to 800 mg 3 times a day is required for amoebic infections. There is a preparation for intravenous infusion.

Tinidazole is similar to metronidazole but has a longer serum half-life (12 hours as compared with 7 hours) allowing less frequent administration.

ANTIFUNGAL AGENTS

For therapeutic purposes, fungal infections are classified as superficial (skin or mucous membranes) and systemic. The former are commonly caused by *Candida albicans* and usually respond readily to topical applications of any anti-fungal agent. Systemic fungal infections often occur in a compromised host and can be extremely difficult to cure.

Nystatin is the most commonly prescribed agent for the treatment of Candida infections of skin and mucous membranes (thrush). It is not absorbed when given by mouth and cannot be administered parenterally because of its low solubility and toxicity. A suspension, tablets and pessaries are available for the treatment of oral, intestinal and vaginal thrush.

The imidazole antifungal agents include *clotrimazole, econazole, miconazole* and *ketoconazole*. They are effective against a wide range of fungi. The first two agents are used for the topical therapy of superficial fungal infections. Miconazole and ketoconazole are absorbed from the gut and have been successfully used for the treatment of systemic fungal infections as well as for superficial mycoses. There is also an intravenous formulation of miconazole. Hepatotoxicity has been reported during ketoconazole therapy. Liver function tests should, therefore, be carried out during long-term therapy.

Amphotericin remains the most important antibiotic for the treatment of systemic fungal infections. It is a moderately toxic drug and side-effects are relatively common. These include fever, vomiting, thrombophlebitis and nephrotoxicity (p. 406). The antibiotic is given by intravenous infusion in gradually increasing daily doses commencing with 1 mg.

Flucytosine is well absorbed from the gut and side-effects are relatively uncommon although bone-marrow depression can occur. It is active only against yeasts and has been used for the treatment of systemic candidiasis, sometimes in combination with amphotericin. *C. albicans* can develop resistance to flucytosine.

Griseofulvin is selectively concentrated in keratin and is the drug of choice for widespread or chronic dermatophyte infections such as ringworm. It is well absorbed from the gut and is given in a daily dose of 250 mg (child) and 500 mg (adult). Skin lesions respond quickly but infection of the nails requires several months of therapy. Localised and minor ringworm lesions usually respond to topical application of Whitfield's ointment or miconazole.

ANTIVIRAL AGENTS

The main problem with antiviral chemotherapy is to find an agent which will arrest the replication of the virus without interfering with the metabolism of the host cell. Another difficulty is that by the time a viral infection has been diagnosed much of the damage has already been done to the host tissues. The following is an outline of the present position.

Idoxuridine is effective in herpes zoster (shingles) and *H. simplex* keratitis if applied early; it is too toxic for parenteral administration.

Vidarabine (adenine arabinoside) has been used for *H. simplex* encephalitis with variable effect.

Acyclovir is an antiviral agent which is highly active against herpes simplex viruses types I and II (p. 729) and varicella-zoster virus (p. 730). It is licensed in Britain only for the treatment of *H. simplex* infections although it has been used successfully for life-threatening chickenpox and shingles in immunocompromised patients. There is a preparation for intravenous injection and eye drops for ophthalmic herpes infections. Oral and topical formulations are also available for the treatment of *H. simplex* infections of the skin and mucous membranes including genital herpes. Side-effects are uncommon, the only notable adverse reaction being a rise in serum urea if the intravenous injection is given too quickly.

Interferon is a lymphokine produced by T cells in response to viral infections (p. 20). It is not yet available commercially but possible uses include the treatment of hepatitis and influenza, and exotic diseases such as Lassa fever. It also has anti-tumour activity.

SELECTION OF ANTIMICROBIAL AGENT

In addition to knowledge about the properties of the available antimicrobial agents, important considerations in the choice of effective chemotherapy are the nature and site of the infection, adverse effects and cost.

The Nature and Site of the Infection. In instances where the nature of the infection can usually be predicted from the clinical features of the illness, treatment can proceed without isolation of the causative organism. For example, acute follicular tonsillitis and lobar pneumonia are sufficiently characteristic on clinical examination to allow the causative organism and its antibiotic sensitivity to be assumed with a high degree of probability and the appropriate antibiotic (penicillin) given. In exacerbations of chronic bronchitis the causative organisms are almost always pneumococci and *H. influenzae* and the use of ampicillin or co-trimoxazole is indicated without specific laboratory diagnosis.

Where there is uncertainty about the nature of the infection a bacteriological diagnosis should be made so that the appropriate antibiotic can be given. If the organism is one such as *Streptococcus pyogenes*, which has a predictable susceptibility to the generally used antimicrobial agents, no further laboratory sensitivity tests are necessary.

Sensitivity tests will be required for bacteria known to vary in their susceptibility to antimicrobial agents. The acquisition of resistance occurs particularly with staphylococci, Gram-negative bacilli and tubercle bacilli. Once the sensitivity of the organism has been determined, it is relatively rare for this to change in the course of treatment. However, there is not a complete correlation between the results of sensitivity tests and the response to chemotherapy and sometimes clinical judgement may indicate a different drug from that recommended by the bacteriologist.

When sensitivity tests indicate that several antimicrobial agents are effective it is advisable in the first instance to select one that is bactericidal in order that the organisms are killed rapidly; bacteriostatic drugs suppress the growth of the organism while the natural defence mechanisms of the body dispose of it. The choice is probably of no great significance in the majority of infections but may be important in the treatment of bacteraemia and in patients with deficient defence mechanisms.

Antibiotics with a relatively limited range of activity such as benzylpenicillin are usually preferable to broad-spectrum compounds like one of the new cephalosporins, so as to reduce the danger of superinfection.

The use of two or more antibacterial drugs is only occasionally of proven value. Thus in tuberculosis three agents are prescribed, at least initially, so as to reduce the emergence of resistant strains. Combinations of antibiotics with differing ranges of activity may also be used to treat infections due to more than one species of microorganism or where it is believed that the effect of the combination of drugs is more potent than an equivalent amount of any one of the compounds acting alone. This has been described as 'synergy'; an example of this is co-trimoxazole. Unfortunately there have been relatively few clinical trials which have compared the efficacy of combinations of antibiotics with single drugs so that the use of combinations remains somewhat empirical. Whenever possible their choice should be specifically directed by bacteriological diagnosis and accompanying sensitivity tests.

The selection of an antimicrobial agent is also determined by the site of the infection. This is discussed with the treatment of individual diseases and in the management of bacteraemia (p. 50).

Selection of Antimicrobial Agents in Relation to Adverse Effects. Before prescribing an antimicrobial agent enquiry should be made about any previous allergic reactions. Pregnant women and children should not be given tetracyclines. Co-trimoxazole is also best avoided in pregnancy and this compound, together with other sulphonamides, must not be given to patients with glucose-6-phosphate dehydrogenase deficiency as haemolysis may be precipitated (p. 507). Chloramphenicol should be prescribed only in the circumstances described on page 46 and is contraindicated in the neonate. Ampicillin must not be given to patients suffering from glandular fever and the aminoglycoside antibiotics should be used with caution in patients with renal disease and in the elderly. Clindamycin should not be used for trivial infection because of the risk of colitis.

Prophylactic Use of Antibiotics. The indications for this are limited. They include the prevention of meningococcal infections (p. 747) and diphtheria (p. 743) in susceptible contacts. Chemoprophylaxis is also indicated in patients with heart valve lesions undergoing dental or urological procedures (p. 166), for the prevention of tetanus (p. 745) and gas gangrene, and to prevent infective complications following gastrointestinal and gynaecological surgery.

Cost. The chemotherapy of infections can be very expensive, especially when newly introduced preparations are used. Unusual antibiotics should not be prescribed without good reason as the difference in cost can be over a hundred-fold.

Bacteraemia, Septicaemia and Bacteraemic (Septic) Shock

Spread of infection to the blood stream is known as *bacteraemia* and, if the organisms multiply there, as *septicaemia*. Further dissemination may result in 'metastatic' foci of infection especially in bone, liver, brain or heart valves. The site of the primary infection varies but can be in diverticular disease, the gall bladder or the urinary tract, especially in the compromised host.

Bacteraemic shock occurs in up to one third of episodes of Gram-negative septicaemia: it is due to potent bacterial endotoxins which affect cell walls, promote the release of vasoactive substances such as histamine and bradykinin and cause endothelial damage.

Initially there is a hyperdynamic reaction with high cardiac output, vasodilatation and low peripheral resistance followed by fluid loss from the vascular compartment as a result of extensive capillary leakage; this leads to hypovolaemia, peripheral vasoconstriction and acute circulatory failure (p. 147). The endotoxin may initiate disseminated intravascular coagulation (D.I.C. p. 548) by endothelial injury activating the clotting mechanisms and leading to tissue damage and organ failure.

Clinical Features. The pyrexia of the infection may be overtaken by the hypothermia of acute circulatory failure. Leucopenia, thrombocytopenia and a prolonged bleeding time point to D.I.C. Progressive impairment of blood flow may then lead to organ failure, particularly of the brain, kidneys, liver and lungs (shock lung). Mortality can be over 60% in Gram-negative sepsis causing severe hypotension and a low cardiac output.

Treatment. Antimicrobial therapy must be commenced immediately with a combination such as gentamicin and an agent active against Gram-positive cocci (e.g. penicillin or flucloxacillin) plus possibly a third against anaerobes (e.g. metronidazole). This is adjusted when the nature of the infection has been determined.

Where Gram-positive cocci are the cause of the infection, benzylpenicillin should be given if the organism is known to be sensitive to penicillin. Flucloxacillin is indicated if penicillinase-producing staphylococci are responsible for the infection. If the patient is allergic to penicillin or the organism is resistant to cloxacillin, the next choice is clindamycin. Metronidazole is indicated for anaerobic infections. Gentamicin alone will suffice for other Gram-negative infections but not for pseudomonas (p. 45). Amikacin is reserved for gentamicin-resistant organisms.

Two doses of corticosteroid (e.g. dexamethasone 1·5 mg/kg) given early may be beneficial by suppressing the damage caused by the exaggerated inflammatory response. They inhibit prostaglandin production and possibly act as endotoxin mediators. Acute circulatory failure (p. 149) and D.I.C. (p. 548) must also be treated.

A.M. GEDDES

FURTHER READING:

Christie, A.B. (1980) *Infectious Diseases: Epidemiology and Clinical Practice*, 3rd edn. Edinburgh: Churchill Livingstone.

Duguid, J.P., Marmion B.P. & Swain, R.H.A. (1978) *Medical Microbiology*, 13th edn. Edinburgh: Churchill Livingstone.

Garrod, L.P., O'Grady, F. & Lambert, H.P. (1981) *Antibiotic and Chemotherapy*, 5th edn. Edinburgh: Churchill Livingstone.

4. Nutritional Factors in Disease

Although man has used foods for ritual purposes and attributed magical properties to some of them since the beginning of history, the science of nutrition has nearly all originated in the twentieth century. The concept of vitamins was introduced around 1912; the cure of human rickets with vitamin D was established in 1922; nicotinamide was first used to treat pellagra in 1938. Kwashiorkor was originally reported in 1932 from an obscure African hospital, but medical science did not become aware of its importance until 1952. Human zinc deficiency was not established until 1972.

The world's population is estimated to have reached about 4 500 000 000 and presents the greatest threat to mankind. This explosive growth in population is due not to increased fertility but to the remarkable reduction in the death rate that has been achieved in recent decades.

The most obvious effects of overpopulation are actual shortage of food for many poor people in underdeveloped communities and ever rising food costs in industrial countries. Some 450 million people are under-nourished, many of them children. Famines are occurring most of the time in one part of the world or another. Agricultural production is hampered by bad climates, soil erosion, lack of fertilisers, antiquated farming methods, political upheavals and war. The situation will deteriorate unless national programmes of population control and family planning based on modern contraceptive techniques are effectively put into operation. Food production can be further increased by the application of science to peasant agriculture but nothing will be gained if machines displace people from the land and increase the numbers of unemployed in cities of the developing countries.

A knowledge of nutrition has three uses in clinical medicine:

1. Elsewhere in this book diseases are described the multiple causes of which may include what or how people eat over long periods; among these are dental caries, coronary heart disease, diabetes mellitus, and even some of the carcinomas, e.g. of the liver and of the colon. These diseases take a long time to develop and the precise importance of one factor such as diet involves discussion and sometimes controversy. Details are not appropriate to a clinical primer and may be sought in a textbook of nutrition (p. 87).

2. For some diseases, modification of the diet is valuable treatment. In gluten enteropathy and phenylketonuria the correct diet is of vital importance. For other diseases like chronic renal failure and diabetes mellitus appropriate adjustment of the diet forms a major aspect of the management. Principles of therapeutic diets are discussed with the diseases concerned. Space does not allow inclusion of a full set of diet sheets; those for obesity and diabetes appear on pages 812–814. For other diet sheets the reader is referred to a textbook of nutrition (p. 87).

3. There are diseases which result primarily from disturbed nutrition; these are described in this chapter. It should be stressed that these primary nutritional diseases seldom present in pure form. Where food is short in quantity or defective in quality all the members of a community are not equally affected. People with physical (or mental) diseases are likely to succumb first. Nutritional diseases thus often have a predisposing illness and when this is prominent the resulting malnutrition is spoken of as conditioned or secondary.

Someone who has one type of malnutrition is likely to have another; sometimes it is possible to find clinical or biochemical signs of six or more nutrient deficiencies in the same patient. For this reason treatment should never be confined to large intakes of the nutrient whose deficiency is the most prominent clinical feature.

Lastly, malnourished patients are liable to complications, particularly certain infections. These may be the presenting illness or they may occur in modified form because the malnutrition has suppressed some of their characteristic features. Complications must be sought out and treated.

Much of the skill in diagnosing patients with malnutrition consists in being aware of and disentangling predisposing illnesses, other types of malnutrition and complicating illnesses. Only when this is done can treatment be fully effective.

Classification and Aetiology of Nutritional Disorders

Classification. Nutritional disorders can be thought of in five groups.

1. UNDERNUTRITION. This is not enough food energy (calories or joules). Severe forms are starvation in adults or marasmus in children. If secondary to disease this may be called cachexia. Epidemic undernutrition is famine.

2. MALNUTRITION. This is a deficiency of protein or of one or more of the 35 other essential nutrients. Most foods lack several of these nutrients. The full number is normally provided by a variety of different kinds of foods. Deficiency diseases like kwashiorkor and rickets are examples but malnutrition can also be subclinical.

3. OBESITY. Excess of body fat results from a prolonged positive energy balance, an energy (calorie or joule) intake greater than energy expenditure.

4. QUALITATIVE OVERNUTRITION. This is due to too much of one food component. This may be an essential nutrient, e.g., hypervitaminosis D or siderosis (iron overload), or a non-essential nutrient, e.g., high intakes of saturated fats raise the plasma cholesterol and may predispose to coronary heart disease.

5. EFFECTS OF NATURAL TOXINS IN FOODS. Some foods contain small amounts of toxic substances which can lead to disease if a person or community has to rely too heavily on a single foodstuff, e.g., lathyrism (p. 656).

Social and Economic Causes of Nutritional Disorders. Even in countries where the overall food supply is adequate, cases of malnutrition may occur because of unequal distribution of income or because of ignorance or social disorganization. The old, the solitary and the children are most often affected.

Pathological Causes of Nutritional Disorders. SECONDARY MALNUTRITION. Even with an ample income, an adequate home and some knowledge of dietetics, a patient may develop a nutritional disorder secondary to disease. The main ways in which this may happen are:

1. DEFECTIVE INTAKE OF FOOD. *(a) Loss of appetite* may be an important symptom of organic disease, e.g. cancer of the stomach, and also of psychogenic disease, e.g. anxiety, depression and anorexia nervosa. *(b) Persistent vomiting* from any cause. *(c) Food fads*, e.g. in very strict vegetarians (vegans). *(d) Alcohol* provides calories but no essential nutrients. Chronic alcoholics suffer from malnutrition more often than undernutrition. *(e) Unbalanced therapeutic diets*, can omit the usual dietary source of a nutrient unless care is taken to provide it. *(f) Prolonged intravenous fluids* with only glucose and saline solutions may precipitate acute deficiencies of the vitamin B complex or of trace elements.

2. DEFECTIVE DIGESTION AND ABSORPTION. *(a) Achlorhydria* is a factor in the causation of iron deficiency anaemia. *(b) Steatorrhoea* leads to malabsorption. *(c) Intestinal hurry* due to surgical short circuits, etc. may impair digestion. In starving people the ingestion of unsuitable foods often causes intestinal hurry and intensifies their plight. *(d) Antibiotics*, if their administration is prolonged, may interfere with the synthesis of certain vitamins by intestinal bacteria e.g. vitamin K.

3. DEFECTIVE UTILISATION. *(a) Cirrhosis* of the liver may interfere with the utilisation of ingested nutrients, e.g. of amino acids and vitamin K. *(b) Malignancy*, in some unknown ways, may produce a state of undernutrition despite an adequate diet. *(c) Prolonged infections* cause undernutrition through a combination of anorexia and increased metabolism. *(d) In renal failure*

vitamin D is not converted to the active metabolite (p. 66). *(e)* Some *drugs*, e.g. antiepileptics, are antagonists of folate and of vitamin D. *(f) Inborn errors of metabolism* may interfere with nutrients, e.g. Hartnup disease in which tryptophan absorption is impaired (p. 77).

4. LOSS OF NUTRIENTS FROM THE BODY. *(a)* In the *nephrotic syndrome* protein is lost in the urine. *(b)* In *diabetes mellitus* uncontrolled glycosuria causes undernutrition. *(c)* In *excessive menstrual bleeding* secondary iron deficiency anaemia is common. *(d)* In severe or chronic *diarrhoea* potassium is lost.

5. INCREASED NUTRITIONAL NEEDS. *(a)* In *pregnancy*, *lactation* and *adolescence* (especially after an illness in the last named), and for those engaged in hard physical work, particularly in cold climates, the usual diet may be insufficient. *(b)* In *fevers* and *hyperthyroidism* the increased metabolism calls for more calories. *(c)* After *burns*, *trauma* and *major surgery*, there is an increased catabolism of protein and ascorbic acid.

Nutrients can be sub-divided into four groups:
1. Energy-yielding nutrients (carbohydrates, fats and proteins)
2. Water, electrolytes and minerals
3. Vitamins
4. Fibre

In this chapter the related disorders will be described under these headings and thereafter overnutrition will be considered.

ENERGY-YIELDING NUTRIENTS

Carbohydrates (4 kcal/g) usually provide the greater part of the energy in a normal diet, but no individual carbohydrate is an essential nutrient in the sense that the body needs it but cannot make it for itself from other nutrients. If the carbohydrate intake is less than 100 g per day ketosis is likely to occur.

Fats. With their high caloric value (9 kcal/g) fats are useful to people with a large energy expenditure; moreover they are helpful in cooking and making food appetising.

Essential fatty acids are precursors for the synthesis of prostaglandins but clinical deficiency in man is rare. It has been demonstrated in patients who have been fed intravenously for long periods without fat emulsions. They develop a scaly dermatitis and eicosatrienoic acid accumulates in plasma lipids.

Proteins provide some 20 amino acids, of which eight are essential for normal protein synthesis and for maintaining nitrogen balance in adults. These *essential amino acids* are methionine, lysine, tryptophan, phenylalanine, leucine, isoleucine, threonine, and valine. Histidine and perhaps arginine are also needed for growth in infants.

The 'biological value' of different proteins depends on the relative proportions of essential amino acids they contain. Proteins of animal origin, particularly from eggs, milk and meat, are generally of higher biological value than the proteins of vegetable origin which are deficient in one or more of the essential amino acids. However it is possible to have a diet of mixed vegetable proteins with high biological value if the principle of *complementation* is used. For example cereals, e.g. wheat, contain about 10% protein and are relatively deficient in lysine. Legumes contain around 20% of protein which is relatively deficient in methionine. If two parts of wheat are mixed (or eaten) with one part of legume, a food results which contains 13% protein of high biological value. This happens because cereals contain enough methionine and legumes enough lysine to supplement the other component of the mixture.

The usual recommended allowance for an adequate protein intake is 10% of the total calories i.e. about 65 g per day for the average adult. The minimum requirement is around 40 g of protein of good biological value.

Energy Requirements

Requirements for energy (calories) vary widely, even among apparently similar individuals. 'Recommended Allowances' provide only an approximation for an individual. WHO recommend that 3000 kcal for man and 2200 kcal for women are adequate for a life of moderate activity. Slightly lower figures are suitable in the affluent countries where most people are sedentary.

The population of Britain, including infants,

children and adults, probably needs an average *intake* of 2500 kcal/head/day. In order that the population may actually consume this amount, the food retailed must provide more to allow for household wastage, pets, tourists etc. The food supplies of Britain ordinarily provide around 3000 kcal/head/day. It is this gross value of our food supplies that is sometimes discussed in the Press and Parliament and often confused with average physiological requirements.

There are two units in use for energy: calories and joules. Though both are metric, joules are SI units and are gradually replacing calories in scientific usage.

1 kcal = 4·184 kJ.

UNDERNUTRITION AND STARVATION

Starvation may conveniently be defined as undernutrition of sufficient severity to warrant inpatient treatment in hospital; the body weight is reduced to less than 75% of normal. What follows here describes undernutrition as it affects adults and older children. In infants and pre-school children a similar process is called marasmus. This is described on pages 59 and 60 under protein-energy malnutrition.

Aetiology. Undernutrition and starvation arise (1) when there is not enough food to eat, for instance in times of famine, (2) when there is severe disease of the digestive tract, preventing the absorption of nutrients, as in the malabsorption syndrome and cancer of the oesophagus or (3) when there is a condition which prevents normal metabolism of nutrients by the tissues, e.g. in chronic renal or hepatic failure or protracted infections. In all these circumstances there is wasting of the body with much loss of both muscle and fat.

Clinical Features. When the energy (caloric) value of the diet is inadequate, adults lose weight and children cease to grow or even lose weight. The loss may be rapid at first, but tends to slow down and stabilize at a lower weight because the body is able to adapt, at least partly, to an insufficient intake of food because (a) the bulk of the muscles and glands is reduced in size, requiring less energy for maintenance, (b) the basal metabolism is reduced, (c) the lighter body requires less work to move it about, and (d) unnecessary voluntary movements are curtailed.

The patient becomes thin and the skin lax, most noticeably over the upper arm and abdomen. The skin is thin, dry, inelastic and often cyanosed at the extremities. The hair becomes dull, dry and inflexible. The eyes are dull and sunken, yet the wasting of orbital tissues may give them an unusual prominence. The heart is reduced in size and there is often bradycardia and a fall in systolic blood pressure. Atrophy of the small intestine is present and may be severe, in which case the inability to digest and absorb nutrients requires great care during refeeding. In severe cases, the onset of diarrhoea causes disturbances in water and electrolyte balance.

Loss of 2–4 kg of body water in the urine is a characteristic immediate response to severe calorie or carbohydrate restriction. It is probably related to depletion of glycogen which has water-holding properties and explains why reducing diets for obesity can be so successful for the first few days. After prolonged intake of insufficient food, dependent 'famine' oedema begins to appear. It is often preceded by a period of nocturnal polyuria. Famine oedema is not necessarily associated with any fall in the level of plasma proteins, but is due rather to wasting of tissues without a corresponding loss of body water. Mild normocytic, normochromic anaemia is common, due to a reduction in the red cell population without a corresponding alteration in the plasma volume.

Seriously underfed patients are weak and sometimes suffer from syncope. Hypothermia should be looked for with a low-reading thermometer. Psychological symptoms frequently occur in starving people. Mental restlessness, irritability and indifference to the troubles of others may be combined with physical apathy. Under-nourished individuals are susceptible to infections. With respiratory muscles weakened by wasting, bronchopneumonia carries an increased mortality. Diarrhoea is very common and starving groups in famines have often had high mortalities from epidemics, e.g. of typhus or cholera.

The severity of the starvation can be assessed by working out the patient's weight for height as a percentage of the estimated normal for the population (Table 21.2, p. 816). Starvation is severe and dangerous when weight is less than 70% of normal.

Treatment. In mild undernutrition, all that is needed is suitable food. Management is more an administrative than a medical problem. When the patient is seriously ill, treatment must depend on the facilities available.

Most famine victims, because of alimentary dysfunction, cannot deal with large quantities of food. The patient's appetite may be immense but is no guide to digestive capacities. Limitation of the food intake is essential if there is diarrhoea or a severe degree of cachexia.

The choice of foods needs care. It is advisable to give those with which the patient is familiar. In advanced cases only bland food can be tolerated by the thin-walled intestines lacking essential digestive enzymes. Skimmed milk may not be well tolerated if the patient has deficient intestinal lactase activity.

The ideal initial diet is one based on the patient's staple cereal and some sucrose or glucose together with moderate amounts of bland, protein-rich food, e.g. milk powder, and some fat or oil. Small feeds should be given at frequent intervals and new foods added one at a time to ensure that they do not increase diarrhoea. It is advisable to give a multivitamin preparation. With refeeding there may be some increase in oedema, unless salt is restricted.

There may come a time when a patient with severe starvation refuses all food, although fully rational. Feeding of homogenized liquid/food mixtures through a nasogastric tube then provides the only hope.

Physical and psychological recovery usually appears to be complete if sufficient calories are provided for cases of primary undernutrition. When irreversible changes have developed in the heart and small intestine in severe starvation, the prognosis is poor.

Prevention rests with legislators and administrators. Famines from crop failure can be greatly alleviated by advanced contingency planning. Those caused by a natural disaster like an earthquake are unexpected: the outcome depends on how well the country's administration stands up to the strain. Famines resulting from war present the most difficult problems.

PROTEIN-ENERGY (CALORIE) MALNUTRITION

Aetiology and Classification. Protein-energy malnutrition (PEM) in early childhood is a spectrum of disease. At one end there is *kwashiorkor* in which the essential feature is deficiency of protein with relatively adequate energy intake. At the other end is *nutritional marasmus* which is total inanition of the infant, usually under 1 year of age, and which is due to a severe and prolonged restriction of all food, i.e. energy sources and other nutrients in addition to protein. In the middle of the spectrum is *marasmic kwashiorkor* in which there are clinical features of both disorders.

Some children adapt to prolonged energy and/or protein shortage by *nutritional dwarfism*. The most prevalent of all the varieties is *mild to moderate PEM* or the underweight child (Table 4.1). Children with one form of PEM often shift to another form. Thus a child with mild to moderate PEM may develop kwashiorkor after an

Table 4.1 Classification of PEM in young children.

	Body weight as percentage of international standard for age	Oedema	Deficit in weight for height
Kwashiorkor	80–60	+	+
Marasmic kwashiorkor	<60	+	++
Marasmus	<60	0	++
Nutritional dwarfing	<60	0	minimal
Underweight child	80–60	0	+

Based on Joint FAO/WHO Committee on Nutrition. 8th Report, 1971 (with modifications in weight/height column).

infection. Such a child when treated loses oedema and may look marasmic.

The incidence of PEM in its various forms is high in India and Southeast Asia, in most parts of Africa and the Middle East, in the Caribbean Islands and in South and Central America. PEM is the most important dietary deficiency disease in the world. Severe forms affect around 2% and mild to moderate PEM affects around 20% of young children in the Third World; hence PEM will be described in detail.

Kwashiorkor

Cicely Williams in 1933 was the first to record that 'some amino acid or protein deficiency' might be an aetiological factor in kwashiorkor, the name given to this disease by the Ga tribe living in and around Accra, the capital of Ghana.

Aetiology. Kwashiorkor typically arises when, after prolonged breast feeding, the child is weaned on to a traditional family diet, which is low in protein, such as cassava, plantain or yam, or to a cereal that has been refined and diluted (Fig. 4.1, p. 60). There is little milk and custom, sometimes reinforced by taboos, determines that the limited supply of foods of animal origin is given to the men of the family, or the small amount of high protein food is in a sauce, which is made with hot peppers or spices and unsuitable for young children. In many rural areas, where kwashiorkor is endemic, the food supply becomes scarce each year before the harvest; at this 'hungry season' the incidence of kwashiorkor and other nutritional diseases increases.

If the customary diet of a population is limited in protein and in energy to around the levels of minimum requirements, a child may be in moderate health until the protein requirements are raised by an infection. Gastroenteritis, measles and malaria are all notorious precipitating causes of kwashiorkor.

Pathology. The insufficient supply of amino acids leads to inadequate protein synthesis, which impairs tissue replacement and development of organs and reduces synthesis of enzymes and plasma proteins. Some enzymes and tissues, particularly those with a rapid turnover, are more severely affected than others.

The total protein content of the body may be as low as 60% of normal for height, while the water content is increased. The failure to synthesise plasma albumin reduces the concentration to around 15 g/l. By contrast the plasma gammaglobulin is usually well maintained. Synthesis of digestive enzymes is usually impaired, including those secreted by the pancreas and in the mucosa of the small intestine (especially lactase). This may be partially responsible for the diarrhoea which is so commonly present and which leads to loss of potassium and magnesium in the stools. The protein content of the liver is reduced, while its lipid content is much increased. Subnormal cell-mediated immunity makes the child susceptible to infections like measles, tuberculosis and herpes.

Clinical Features. *Failure of Growth*. The child's weight is usually well below standard for the age (Table 21.1, p. 815) but the deficit may be masked by *oedema* often due to hypoalbuminaemia. This usually affects the feet but may also be found in the hands and face. Ascites and pleural effusions are usually slight and, if detected clinically, suggest the presence of an infection such as tuberculosis.

Muscles and Fat. The muscles are wasted. This is particularly noticeable around the chest and the upper arm; the wasting of the legs and around the hips is frequently concealed by oedema. Subcutaneous fat is often plentiful in children whose diets have provided sufficient energy but little protein. If the disease has resulted from a restriction of both calories and protein, an almost complete lack of subcutaneous fat and muscle wasting are the most striking features, but the feet are oedematous ('marasmic kwashiorkor').

Mental Changes. The child is apathetic and miserable.

Hair. This is nearly always affected in African children; in Asiatics the changes are less frequent. The hair becomes fine, straight and often sparse. The hair of African children may show a variety of pigmentary changes from brown and reddish to grey, blond or even white. Children with long straight black hair may show a pale band across the hair, corresponding to an earlier episode of kwashiorkor, the 'flag sign'. The extent of these changes in the hair is an indication of the duration rather than the severity of the disease.

Skin. Alterations in the skin are usually present, especially in severe cases. These include pigmentation, desquamation and ulceration. In moderate cases the dermatosis resembles crazy paving. A severe case may look like an extensive burn. The legs, buttocks and perineum are most frequently involved, but any region may be affected. This is in contrast to pellagra in which the dermatosis occurs mainly on the exposed surfaces. The skin lesions are determined in part by associated vitamin deficiencies and in part by infections and trauma.

Mucous Membranes. Angular stomatitis, cheilosis and a smooth tongue are commonly seen, as is ulceration around the anus.

Liver. This may be enlarged but it can be histologically fatty without being clinically remarkable. Hepatosplenomegaly from malaria and other causes is common in the tropics.

Gastrointestinal System. Anorexia is usually present and sometimes vomiting. There is nearly always diarrhoea, with the passage of stools containing undigested food. The diarrhoea may be due to impaired secretion of digestive enzymes, to intestinal mucosal atrophy or to an intestinal infection.

Anaemia. Some degree of anaemia is frequently present. It often becomes worse during treatment. The degree of anaemia and its nature are largely determined by associated infections and other dietary deficiencies.

Associated Vitamin Deficiencies. Vitamin A deficiency with xerophthalmia and keratomalacia (p. 66) occurs in from one to 70% of severe cases of PEM. It is a major cause of preventable blindness in developing countries. Biochemical signs of thiamin and niacin deficiencies are commonly associated with kwashiorkor in countries where rice and maize respectively are the staple weaning foods. Folate deficiency is also fairly frequent. Children with PEM have often been indoors out of the sun for weeks and a minority of cases have signs of rickets (p. 67). Deficiency of vitamin K may result in purpura or bleeding.

Treatment. GENERAL MEASURES. An easily digested diet which provides adequate amounts of protein, minerals and vitamins with extra calories for 'catch-up growth' is essential. Milk is a good base, and the most convenient locally available form may be used. If skimmed milk is given, however, it is necessary to include additional fat. Plant protein mixtures, such as corn-soya-dried milk, may also be used.

Severely ill children may be unable to maintain their body temperature even in the tropics, especially where there is a large fall of atmospheric temperature at night. Heated rooms or electric blankets are useful for such cases.

If dermatosis is severe the skin should be cleaned and carefully protected. The child's weight tends to fall during the first days of treatment due to loss of oedema. Initiation of cure is indicated by returning appetite, improvement in general condition, loss of oedema and rise of plasma albumin.

DIETS FOR ACUTE CASES. The major units with research experience of kwashiorkor have each evolved somewhat different therapeutic diets, depending on local availability of and preferences for weaning foods. The principle of all the regimes is to work up to protein intakes of 3 to 4 g/kg/d and energy intakes of 150 kcal/kg/d or more. For the first day or two, if the child is unable to feed from a spoon, nasogastric intubation will be necessary.

A recipe successfully used in Jamaica is: dried, skimmed milk 60 g, flour 20 g, butter 15 g, and water to make 250 ml. This is offered freely in five to six feeds daily. The mixture contains 22 g protein and 250 kcal per 250 ml. A child recovering from kwashiorkor, unless progress is retarded by infection, will accept very high calorie intakes until the weight approaches the normal value for height.

Anorexia may be serious, but often can be overcome by feeding the child very slowly in the mother's lap and by giving frequent feeds. Food may be taken better cold than hot. If the diarrhoea appears to be made worse on feeds containing skimmed milk, lactose intolerance may be present (p. 314). Such a child should respond to a mixture such as Casilan, cream, glucose and cereal.

As the clinical condition improves and the child attains normal weight for height, the local diet should be given in frequent feeds, care being taken to introduce a variety of plant and animal protein foods and maintain the fat content of the diet.

SUPPLEMENTS. Vitamins A and D, B complex and C and therapeutic doses of iron should be given routinely. If there is any suspicion of xerophthalmia, 30 mg vitamin A should be given for 3 days.

Infants may lose 20–30 mmol of potassium in the stools in one day if there is severe diarrhoea. The effect of the resulting potassium depletion on the myocardium may cause sudden death. Potassium should be given by mouth as a routine to all infants admitted with kwashiorkor. Depending on the age and weight of the child and the severity of the diarrhoea, the dose should be from 0.5 to 1 g of potassium chloride dissolved in water and added to three or four feeds each day. There is little or no danger of potassium intoxication when the mixture is given by mouth in these doses. Some centres also give magnesium, and zinc may accelerate the healing of skin lesions.

PARENTERAL THERAPY. For very ill patients in a well-equipped and well-staffed hospital, who are suffering from marked dehydration, hypoglycaemia, acid-base disturbance or electrolyte imbalance, parenteral therapy with solutions such as half isotonic Darrow's solution with 2.5% glucose may be a life-saving measure which should be started before dietetic treatment. Likewise, for severe anaemia from any cause, small slow transfusions of packed erythrocytes are of great value. In developing countries facilities for these measures are not available for the majority of severe cases of PEM.

COMPLICATIONS. Early recognition and prompt specific treatment of infection is crucial. Patients with PEM have increased susceptibility to (i) gastrointestinal infections and Gram-negative bacteraemia (ii) respiratory infections (iii) certain viral diseases, especially measles and herpes simplex (iv) tuberculosis (v) streptococcal and staphylococcal skin diseases (vi) helminthic infections. The usual signs of pyrexia and leucocytosis may not appear. The possibility of tuberculosis must always be considered, particularly if the child does not make the expected progress to recovery.

Antimalarial drugs are well tolerated whereas all anthelmintics are potentially toxic and must be used with due care in patients who are seriously ill. If anaemia from hookworm is so severe as to endanger life, small transfusions of packed cells should be given and will probably restore the child's condition sufficiently to permit appropriate treatment later.

Iron-deficiency anaemia, which is frequently present due to associated dietary deficiency of iron and as a consequence of infections, requires appropriate treatment. Less commonly a megaloblastic anaemia is present which responds to folic acid.

CONVALESCENCE. Children who have had severe kwashiorkor are still usually well below normal weight and height for their age when the time comes to return home. At this stage 'catch-up' (supernormal) growth is possible and obviously desirable, but it will not occur unless the children are in a favourable environment and getting all the food they will eat. If home conditions are difficult some simple convalescent home or nutritional rehabilitation centre would be ideal where available. In any case follow up should be arranged to see that the child does not deteriorate.

MILD KWASHIORKOR AND FOLLOW-UP PATIENTS. Most children have to be treated outside hospital. Dried skimmed milk is sprinkled over the food or if not available a local protein-rich food mixture is recommended. Mothers should be given realistic advice on foods to give and on hygienic ways to prepare them. The doctor should try to arrange help for socio-economic problems where possible. A well-run nutrition rehabilitation centre can be very effective in treating these children at modest cost.

Prognosis. Severe kwashiorkor has a mortality of around 20% even in a well equipped hospital. Most deaths occur in the first 10 days. Jaundice, petechiae and stupor are bad signs. The usual causes of death are intercurrent infections and severe malnutrition, including potassium deficiency. Availability of medical care is another factor influencing prognosis.

In the long term, follow-up studies have shown that the fatty liver of acute kwashiorkor does not progress to cirrhosis. Physical growth of the brain is retarded in children who suffer from severe PEM in the first two years of life. There is circumstantial evidence that intelligence may be impaired, particularly if the child goes home to an environment in which catch-up growth cannot occur. Hence the great importance of trying to arrange the best possible conditions for a child's nutritional needs to be met after leaving hospital.

Prevention. Poverty and ignorance are two main factors responsible for kwashiorkor. Every effort should be made to alleviate these causes. Education in nutrition, the introduction of improved farming methods and measures to reduce infections in young children, are all important. In each country careful thought must be given to the provision of protein-rich foods made from local crops which are suitable both for infant feeding and for supplementing diets low in protein. Cameron and Hofvander (p. 87) recommend weaning recipes suited to the conditions of various developing countries.

Even small amounts of food of animal origin, such as dried milk, egg, a little meat or concentrates of fish protein, are of great value when mixed with high protein vegetable foods. Although milk powder is a convenient source of protein it is essential only for treating severe kwashiorkor. The disease can, and often has to be, prevented by appropriate combinations of local foods, e.g. cereals and legumes or groundnuts.

Education of parents, particularly mothers, in regard to the value of foods and best methods of preparing them, especially at the time of weaning, is invaluable. Much is being done by the establishment or extension of Child Welfare Clinics and Health Centres where free or subsidised skimmed milk powder or a protein food mixture is supplied, advice on diet given, and diseases liable to lead to kwashiorkor are prevented by immunisation or treated. At the same time the advantages to mother and child of wider spacing of births should be explained and contraceptives provided.

Nutritional Marasmus

In some developing countries marasmus is of greater clinical importance than kwashiorkor. It affects principally infants under 1 year of age in contrast to kwashiorkor which is chiefly encountered between 1 and 4 years of age. Marasmus is more likely to occur in poor people who live in cities in underdeveloped countries while kwashiorkor occurs more frequently in those living in rural areas.

The factors which predispose to marasmus are a rapid succession of pregnancies, and early and often abrupt weaning, followed by dirty artificial feeding of the infants with very dilute milk or milk products given in inadequate amounts to avoid expense. Thus the diet is low in both calories and protein. In addition unsatisfactory home conditions make the preparation of uncontaminated feeds almost impossible. Repeated infections therefore develop, especially of the gastrointestinal tract, which the mother often treats with water, rice water or some other non-nutritious fluid (Fig. 4.1).

The most important cause of marasmus, early weaning, is in contrast to the late weaning, often extending over 2 years, which is characteristic of kwashiorkor. The mother may be induced to stop breast feeding for various reasons, including the presence of infection in herself or in the infant. She may have been influenced by advertisements which advocate the advantages of artificial food products. One reason for stopping breast feeding is economic pressure on the mother to go out and work. Another reason is pregnancy; there is widespread belief among uneducated women in developing countries that the milk of a pregnant woman is bad for her child.

Clinical Features. The two constant features of marasmus are: (1) retardation of growth and reduction of weight which is much more marked than that of length, and (2) wasting of subcutaneous fat and muscles which gives the infant a wizened, old appearance. There is usually watery diarrhoea or semi-solid, bulky, acid stools. In contrast to kwashiorkor, oedema is absent and the characteristic changes in the hair and skin, apathy and anorexia are not usually present. The abdomen may be distended with gas but the liver is not fatty.

A careful search must be made for chronic infection like tuberculosis which predisposes to marasmus. The features of associated vitamin disorders such as angular stomatitis or keratomalacia, may develop, as may a deficiency of minerals, especially potassium and magnesium. Dehydration frequently occurs as a consequence of gastrointestinal infection.

Treatment and Prevention. In the acute stage of marasmus survival depends primarily on

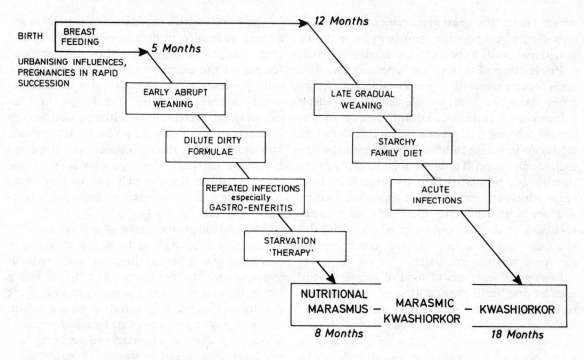

Fig. 4.1 Nutritional marasmus and kwashiorkor Paths leading from early weaning to nutritional marasmus and from protracted breast feeding to kwashiorkor. (By courtesy of Dr D.S. McLaren and the editor of the *Lancet*.)

the efficiency with which measures can be applied to combat dehydration and restore electrolyte balance. In addition the child must be given a satisfactory diet along similar lines to those described for kwashiorkor. A longer refeeding period is usually required because the marasmic child is more severely wasted. The mortality rate during treatment is similar to that of kwashiorkor.

Prevention is a complex and difficult problem. A more equal distribution of land and wealth in developing countries and employment for all who can work is the ideal solution. Failing or pending that, education of mothers about birth spacing and about continuing breast feeding for as long as possible is of great importance.

Further research is urgently needed into improved methods of feeding both healthy and ill infants in developing countries. It is probable that in the future marasmus will become of increasing clinical importance in developing countries as a consequence of a continuing decline in breast feeding and the urbanisation of uneducated families, socially insecure and living in poor, insanitary houses and with insufficient money to buy adequate supplements of nutritious food.

Nutritional Dwarfism

Some children adapt to very prolonged mild to moderate calorie and/or protein deficiency by a proportional failure of growth. They are light in weight and short in stature but have superficially normal body proportions and subcutaneous fat. Such children are more prone to infections than normal. Unless the weight for age of such a child is checked against normal standards (Table 21.1, p. 815) it is easy for the doctor in a busy clinic to miss this form of PEM.

Mild to Moderate PEM (The Underweight Child)

For every florid case of kwashiorkor or marasmus there are several children in the community with mild to moderate PEM. The situation is like an iceberg. There is more malnutrition below the surface than is recognisable on clinical inspection.

The children with subclinical PEM can however be detected by their weight for age, which is less than 80% of the international standard (Table 21.1).

In areas where kwashiorkor is the predominant florid form of PEM, subclinical cases have reduced plasma albumin and sometimes other biochemical signs of protein deficiency ('prekwashiorkor'). In parts of many developing countries surveys may show up to 5% of children under 5 years with signs and symptoms of kwashiorkor or marasmus while up to 50% are underweight.

The great importance of mild to moderate PEM is that these children are growing up smaller than their potential and they are very susceptible to gastroenteritis and respiratory infections, which in turn can precipitate frank malnutrition. Mild to moderate PEM is probably the major underlying reason why the 1 to 4 year mortality in a developing country can be 30 to 40 times higher than in Europe or North America. Official statistics record most of these deaths as due simply to infections.

Protein-energy Malnutrition in Adults

Medical nutritionists, working in some larger hospitals in North America and in Europe have realised that a proportion of medical and surgical patients have features of protein-energy malnutrition resulting from the factors listed on pages 55 and 56. Malnutrition is not an inevitable accompaniment of severe or prolonged disease but can be largely prevented or treated by giving more attention to the patient's nutrition, including parenteral feeding where oral feeding is impossible or inadequate (p. 285).

The energy status can be assessed from a history of loss of weight, by clinical non-instrumental appraisal of subcutaneous fat, by weight in relation to height and by measuring skinfold thickness. Mid-arm circumference and urinary 24 hour creatinine can be used to assess muscle mass. Concentrations of several plasma proteins are sensitive to protein status — albumin, transferrin, retinol-binding protein and pre-albumin. Of these the plasma albumin is usually the most reliable, though it is lowered in liver disease and the nephrotic syndrome.

Micronutrient deficiencies are also likely. In acute illness the critical nutrients tend to be different from those seen where there is food shortage. Potassium deficiency is very important and folate deficiency common.

WATER, ELECTROLYTES AND MINERALS

The normal distribution of water and electrolytes in the body and the disturbances which result when their intake or output is diminished or increased are discussed in detail on pages 88 to 103.

Twelve or more elements are essential for man, as they are for other animals; deficiency disease is known for each but may not always result from an inadequate diet but from other causes such as excessive losses. The elements are sodium (p. 89), potassium (p. 91), magnesium (p. 94), calcium, phosphorus, iron, sulphur, iodine, zinc, copper, chromium, selenium and molybdenum. Fluoride appears to be essential for rats and optimal intakes reduce dental caries in man. Cobalt is physiologically active only in the form of vitamin B_{12}.

In addition manganese, tin, vanadium, nickel and silicon have been shown, by artificial isolator systems, to be essential for animals. Human deficiency disease is not known for any of these minor trace elements.

Elements of Importance in Human Nutrition

Calcium. The body of an adult normally contains about 1200 g of calcium. At least 99% of this is present in the skeleton, where calcium salts (chiefly hydroxyapatite), held in a cellular matrix, provide the hard structure of the bones and teeth.

Obviously all of this calcium comes from the diet. Among common foods, the calcium-containing protein of milk (caseinogen) is much the richest source, which is one reason why milk and cheese are especially valuable for growing children. Half a litre of cow's milk contains about 0.6 g of calcium. Most other foods contribute much smaller amounts. However, peas, beans, other vegetables and particularly cereal grains are frequently the chief contributors because of the large amounts eaten.

Drinking water can provide significant amounts of calcium. In Britain the average intake from this source is about 75 mg Ca/day; but the variations are large: from none in water from peaty, acidic hill lochs in Scotland to 200 mg or even more in water obtained from wells sunk in chalk or limestone.

Absorption. 70 to 80% of the calcium in the food is normally excreted in the faeces. Calcium absorption may be impaired either by lack of vitamin D, by any conditions causing small intestinal hurry, by the combination of calcium with excess fatty acids to form insoluble soaps in steatorrhoea, or by certain substances in the diet which can form insoluble salts with calcium. These include foods rich in oxalic acid (e.g. spinach) and phytic acid which is present in the outer layers of cereal grains. Hence 'wholemeal' bread contains more phytic acid than white.

Recommended Intakes of Calcium. WHO (1974) recommends a daily intake of 500 mg for adult men and women, rising to 1200 mg during pregnancy and lactation. For adolescent boys and girls the recommended intake is 600 to 700 mg daily.

In many parts of Africa and Asia children develop healthy bones and adults remain in calcium balance despite calcium intakes which may be no more than half the above recommendations. Abundant sunshine possibly produces this effect and calcium requirements may be lower where the protein intake is smaller than in affluent countries. However a daily intake of 1000 mg should be taken during pregnancy and lactation.

Deficiency of calcium and vitamin D go hand in hand and are best considered together (p. 66).

Phosphorus. 85% of the phosphorus is normally present in the bones in combination with calcium. The remainder is chiefly in the cells. Phosphorus is essential for most metabolic processes.

Phosphorus is present in all natural foods, though in refined and processed foods the content may be greatly reduced. Primary dietary deficiency is not known to occur in man.

Phosphorus depletion can occur from prolonged and excessive intake of aluminium hydroxide antacids which bind dietary phosphate in the gut. The features are weakness, anorexia, malaise and bone pains. Plasma inorganic phosphorus and urinary phosphate are very low.

Iron. A good mixed diet with average amounts of meat and vegetable contains about 12–15 mg of iron. Cheap, monotonous high carbohydrate diets based on refined wheat flour contain much less. Foods rich in iron are meat, liver, wholemeal cereals, oatmeal, peas, beans and lentils.

An account of iron metabolism and of the measures for the prevention and treatment of iron deficiency anaemia is given on page 495. This is one of the most important nutritional causes of ill-health in Britain and other prosperous countries.

Siderosis. Dietary iron overload is seen in South African men who cook and brew beer in iron pots. They may ingest as much as 100 mg of iron per day. Iron accumulates in the liver and when severe can lead to cirrhosis. A similar condition has been described in other countries following excessive indulgence in cheap wines which can contain 30 mg of iron per litre.

Iodine. Simple enlargement of the thyroid gland attributed to lack of iodine in the diet occurs particularly in mountainous regions far from the sea where it is known as endemic goitre. Other factors may also contribute to the causation of simple goitre (p. 439).

Sources. Iodine in small amounts is widely distributed in living matter. Seafoods are the best natural source but most people eat only small quantities. Vegetables and milk may contain useful amounts. One of the food colours, erythrosine, is very rich in iodine and some medicines also contain the element.

Prophylactic Uses. The recommended intake for adults and adolescents is 150 μg/day. Endemic goitre is now rare in Britain. Some countries have largely eradicated goitre by compulsory iodisation of salt, e.g., Switzerland, Canada and much of Central and South America. The most severe endemic goitre, with associated cretinism, occurs in underdeveloped mountainous countries with bad roads in which packaged salt is not widely distributed, e.g., Ethiopia, Nepal, Bolivia and Papua New Guinea. In such areas, where almost everyone has a goitre, periodic injections of iodised oil to all young women can reduce the incidence of cretinism.

Fluoride. The regular presence of fluoride in minute amounts in human bones and teeth and its influence on the prevention of dental caries justifies its inclusion as an element of importance in human nutrition.

Sources. Most adults ingest between 1 and 3 mg of fluoride daily. The chief source is usually drinking water, which, if it contains 1 part per million (p.p.m.) of fluoride, will supply 1–2 mg/day. Soft waters usually contain no fluoride, whilst very hard waters may contain over 10 p.p.m.

Compared with that in water, the fluoride in foodstuffs is of little importance. Very few contain more than 1 p.p.m.; the exceptions are sea-fish which may contain 5–10 p.p.m. and tea. In Britain, Australia and China, where people drink tea frequently, the adult intake from this source may be as much as 3 mg daily.

Use of Fluoride in the Prevention of Dental Caries. Epidemiological studies in many parts of the world have established that where the natural water supply contains fluoride in amounts of 1 p.p.m. or more, the incidence of dental caries is lower than in comparable areas where the water contains only traces of the element.

Fluoride becomes deposited in the enamel surface of the developing teeth of children. Such teeth are unusually resistant to caries. It may be that traces of fluoride in the enamel interfere with glycolysis by acid-forming bacteria; alternatively, the calcium hydroxyapatite of the enamel may be rendered more resistant to organic acids by combination with traces of the element.

Fluoride is not deposited in fully developed adult teeth, so that less benefit to adults can be expected when they begin for the first time to drink water containing traces of fluoride.

The deliberate addition of traces of fluoride (at 1 p.p.m.) to those public water supplies which are deficient is now a widespread practice throughout North America where about 100 million people are now drinking fluoridated water. In at least 30 other countries similar projects have been started. In Britain regrettably some local authorities are not yet adding fluoride to their water supplies in those areas in which the element is lacking.

Fluorosis. In parts of the world where the water fluoride is high (over 3 to 5 p.p.m.) *mottling of the teeth* is common. The enamel loses its lustre and becomes rough, pigmented and pitted. The effect is purely cosmetic; fluorotic teeth are resistant to caries and not usually associated with any evidence of skeletal fluorosis, or impairment of health.

Chronic fluoride poisoning occurs in several localities in India, China, Argentina, East and South Africa, where the water supply contains over 10 p.p.m. fluoride. Fluorine poisoning has also occurred as an industrial hazard among workers handling fluorine-containing minerals such as cryolite, used in smelting aluminium. The main clinical features are referable to the skeleton which shows sclerosis of bone, especially of the spine, pelvis and limbs, and calcification of ligaments and tendinous insertions of muscles.

Zinc. Although human deficiency was not clearly established before 1972, zinc is emerging as a nutrient of clinical importance. In PEM, associated zinc deficiency causes thymic atrophy and zinc supplements may accelerate the healing of skin lesions.

In adults a negative zinc balance and low plasma zinc can occur secondary to intestinal disease, chronic alcoholism, diabetes mellitus, nephrotic syndrome, burns, haemodialysis and chronic febrile illness. In some cases poor wound healing has responded to treatment with zinc.

Acute zinc deficiency has been reported in patients receiving prolonged intravenous alimentation without added zinc. Diarrhoea, mental apathy, a moist eczematoid dermatitis especially round the mouth and loss of hair were accompanied by a very low plasma zinc concentration.

Chronic deficiency has been described in association with dwarfism and hypogonadism.

The recommended intake in adults is 15 mg/day. The best dietary sources are meats, whole grain cereals and legumes. Oysters are outstandingly rich in zinc, while white bread, fats and sugar contain negligible amounts.

Other Minerals. *Sulphur* is mainly supplied by the S-containing amino acids in the diet — methionine and cysteine; effects of its deficiency are therefore inseparable from those of protein. *Copper* metabolism is abnormal in Wilson's disease (p. 366). Deficiency occasionally occurs in young children; the main features are anaemia, retarded growth and skeletal rarefaction. *Chromium* facilitates the action of insulin. Deficiency has been reported in some children with PEM and as a rare complication of prolonged parenteral nutrition, presenting as hyperglycaemia.

The roles of *sodium*, *potassium* and *magnesium* are discussed in the next chapter.

THE VITAMINS

Disorders due to vitamin deficiency are still widespread in many parts of the world. Even in industrial countries certain types of people are known to be at risk of developing some vitamin deficiency. Doctors should be ready to diagnose these treatable conditions in their early stages.

Vitamins are organic substances in food which are required in small amounts but which cannot be synthesised in adequate quantities. 12 vitamins have, so far, been demonstrated to have clinical effects in man. These are:

Fat-soluble	*Water-soluble*	
Vitamin A	Vitamin C—Ascorbic acid	
Vitamin D		Thiamin (B₁)
Vitamin E		Niacin
Vitamin K		Riboflavin
	Vitamin B	Pyridoxine (B₆)
	complex	Biotin
		Cobalamins (B₁₂)
		Folate

Pantothenic acid, a major component of coenzyme A, also appears to be essential, but human deficiency disease has not been reported, perhaps because the vitamin is widely distributed in foods, as its name implies.

Factors Influencing the Utilisation of Vitamins

Availability. Fat-soluble vitamins may be deficient if dietary fat is not eaten or absorbed. Not all of a vitamin may be in absorbable form; for instance niacin in maize is bound in such a way that it is not absorbed from the gut unless the food is specially treated.

Antivitamins are known to be present in some natural foods, e.g. thiaminase in raw fish. Some synthetic antagonists of the vitamins are used as drugs in the therapy of neoplasms (e.g. methotrexate p. 113) or of infections (e.g. pyrimethamine, p. 772). Neoplastic cells and micro-organisms are much more sensitive than normal cells but with high doses of the antivitamin a secondary vitamin deficiency can occur in the host.

Provitamins. Substances occur in foods which are not themselves vitamins but are capable of conversion into vitamins in the course of digestion. Thus some of the carotenes are provitamins of vitamin A and, to some extent at least, the amino acid tryptophan can be converted to niacin.

Bacteria in the Gut. The normal bacterial flora of the gut is capable of synthesising significant amounts of vitamin K. Bacteria are also capable of extracting vitamins from the ingested food and retaining them until excreted in the faeces. Except for vitamin K and probably biotin, for both of which the requirements are very small (about 0·1 mg per day) bacteria are more likely to reduce than to increase the amounts of vitamins available for absorption, as is demonstrated in bacterial colonisation of the small intestine (p. 311).

Biosynthesis in the Skin. Vitamin D need not be provided in the diet if the skin is regularly exposed to adequate sunshine (p. 67).

Interactions of Nutrients. If the diet is rich in carbohydrates or alcohol more thiamin is needed for their metabolism. The requirement for vitamin E is increased when the intake of polyunsaturated fats is high. Sodium and potassium are one example of a pair of elements that are partly antagonistic, and copper and zinc are another such pair.

These considerations indicate how difficult it may be in practice to define the nutritive value of a diet simply from chemical analysis of its vitamin content.

VITAMIN A (RETINOL)

On the world scale vitamin A deficiency is one of the seven most common causes of blindness (the others being trachoma, onchocerciasis, gonococcal ophthalmia, accidents, cataract and glaucoma). WHO estimates that 250 thousand children become blind every year from keratomalacia.

Retinol is found only in foods of animal origin. Herbivores obtain the vitamin from its precursors or provitamins — some of the carotenoid pigments in plants. The conversion of even the best of these, β carotene, into retinol in the human small intestinal wall is only 30% efficient. The absorption of both retinol and carotene is facilitated by fats and bile salts. Retinol has a place in the function of the retina and of epithelial and probably other cells. It may be a protective factor against cancer of the lung and possibly other epithelial sites.

Dietary Sources. Retinol is chiefly found in milk, butter, cheese, egg yolk, liver and some of the fatty fish. The liver oils of fish are the richest natural sources but these are used as nutritional supplements rather than foods.

Carotene is found chiefly in green vegetables in association with chlorophyll; the green outer leaves of cabbage and lettuce are good sources. Other useful sources are some of the yellow and red fruits.

Vegetable oils are devoid of vitamin A activity except red palm oil which is a rich source of carotene. In Britain and some other countries retinol is added artificially to margarine to provide the same concentration as in good quality summer butter. Both retinol and carotene are stable to ordinary cooking methods, though some loss may occur at temperatures above 100°C.

Healthy adults in Britain have large stores of retinol in their livers (p. 338).

Recommended daily intakes of retinol are 300 μg for infants and young children, 500–750 μg for children of 9 to 15 years, 750 μg for adolescents and adults, and 1200 μg for lactating women (1 μg retinol = 3 of the old i.u.). In many parts of the world most or all of the requirements are obtained from carotenoids in vegetable foods.

Because only approximately $\frac{1}{3}$ of β carotene is absorbed into the intestinal wall and then only $\frac{1}{2}$ of this is converted into retinol, 1 μg retinol equivalent (= 1 μg retinol) is now taken as = 6 μg β carotene.

Pathology. Deficiency of the vitamin results in morphological changes in the epithelial surfaces of all parts of the body. The cells undergo squamous metaplasia whereby they become flattened and heaped one upon another. The sebaceous glands and hair follicles of the skin and the tear glands of the eye become blocked with horny plugs of keratin so that their secretions diminish. The lack of tears and the heaping up of epithelium on the scleral conjunctiva and cornea produce xerophthalmia. If softening, ulceration and necrosis of the cornea develop, the condition is referred to as keratomalacia.

Night Blindness

Retinol is an essential component of the pigment rhodopsin (visual purple) on which rod vision in dim light depends. Hence lack of retinol may result in impairment of 'dark adaptation' which can be measured by means of an adaptometer. Night blindness is common, as also is vitamin A deficiency, in poor people living in underdeveloped countries; it can occur in the malabsorption syndrome in affluent countries.

Fatigue and anxiety states may cause persons to complain of night blindness. It may also result from organic disease of the eye such as retinitis pigmentosa. The diagnosis of vitamin A deficiency is supported by low plasma vitamin A concentration and is confirmed by marked improvement in dark adaptation following therapeutic doses of retinol.

Xerosis Conjunctivae, Bitôt's Spots and Xerophthalmia

The earliest sign of xerosis conjunctivae is a dry, thickened and pigmented bulbar conjunctiva with a peculiar smoky appearance. Bitôt's spots are glistening white plaques formed of desquamated thickened conjunctival epithelium, usually triangular in shape and firmly adherent to the underlying conjunctiva. Xerosis conjunctivae and Bitôt's spots are certainly common in children whose diet is deficient in vitamin A but they can also occur in children whose intake of the vitamin is satisfactory. When dryness spreads to the cornea it takes on a dull, hazy, lacklustre appearance due to keratinisation, and xerophthalmia is said to be present.

In young children, xerophthalmia is almost always attributable to recent vitamin A deficiency and is usually associated with PEM. In older children and in adults its interpretation is less simple. Exposure to dust and glare may produce similar changes. They should, however, always call attention to the diet. Xerophthalmia is very important in young children because once the cornea is involved the process can rapidly progress to keratomalacia.

Keratomalacia

This disease causes blindness among Indians, Indonesians and other rice-eating people of Asia; it also occurs in parts of Africa, the Middle East and Latin America. In Europe and North America it is very rare. Children between the ages of 1 and 5 years are most commonly affected. It occurs only in persons who have been living for a long period on diets almost entirely devoid of vitamin A. The disease is frequently associated with PEM.

The earliest manifestations are night blindness and xerophthalmia. Later the cornea undergoes necrosis and ulceration. Unless early and adequate treatment is given, there is a grave risk of blindness or death from associated diseases.

Treatment. Immediately on diagnosis 110 mg retinol palmitate or 66 mg retinol acetate (200 000 iu) should be given orally, or, if there is vomiting or severe diarrhoea 55 mg retinol palmitate (100 000 iu) by intramuscular injection. The oral dose should be repeated the next day and again prior to discharge or at a follow-up visit.

Underlying conditions such as PEM and other nutritional disorders, diarrhoea, dehydration and electrolyte imbalance and infections must be treated appropriately.

For the secondary bacterial infection, antibiotics are of value. Local treatment of the eye will be required only if disorganisation is already present, in which case the services of an ophthalmic surgeon should be obtained.

Prevention. Doctors and nurses working in the tropics, who may have been trained in Europe or North America, should make sure they are familiar with the appearances of xerophthalmia. If in doubt it is better to give a short course of vitamin A treatment.

Pregnant women should be advised to eat dark green leafy vegetables. This helps to build up stores of retinol in the fetal liver. They should also be taught to give such vegetables or locally available yellow or orange fruits to their babies. In some countries where keratomalacia is a major cause of blindness, e.g. in India, single prophylactic oral doses of 60 mg retinol (200 000 iu) are being tried in young children.

Follicular Keratosis

In this condition the hair follicles are blocked with horny plugs of keratin, rendering the skin surface rough and dry like the skin of a toad. The typical distribution is over the backs of the upper arms and the fronts of the thighs. Therapeutic trials in Africa have shown a striking clinical improvement in follicular keratosis when patients are given halibut liver oil or red palm oil. Nevertheless, it is not a specific sign of vitamin A deficiency, since it occurs not uncommonly in people who, by every other criterion, are adequately nourished in respect of vitamin A.

VITAMIN D

The material originally described as *vitamin D₁* was subsequently found to be an impure mixture of sterols. *Vitamin D₂ (ergocalciferol)* is manufactured by the action of ultraviolet light on ergosterol, a sterol found in fungi and yeasts. When the term 'calciferol' is used in clinical practice it refers to ergocalciferol. Although widely used in therapeutics, it occurs very rarely in nature. *Vitamin D₃ (cholecalciferol)* is the natural form of the vitamin which occurs in man and other animals. It is formed in the skin by the action of ultraviolet light on 7-dehydrocholesterol.

Cholecalciferol is not the active form of the vitamin. It is converted in the liver to 25-hydroxycholecalciferol (25-OH-D_3) which is further hydroxylated in the kidney, mainly to 1,25 dihydroxycholecalciferol ($1,25\ (\text{OH})_2\text{D}_3$). Most of the hydroxylated forms of vitamin D in human plasma are based on vitamin D_3 (cholecalciferol) derived from synthesis in the skin or from fish liver oils. A smaller proportion is based on vitamin D_2 (ergocalciferol) from calciferol tablets or fortified milk (e.g. in USA). Though plasma 25-OH-D_3 and 25-OH-D_2 can be distinguished by immunoassay, they and their corresponding derivatives appear to have identical activities.

1,25(OH)$_2D_3$ is many times more potent than cholecalciferol and can be regarded as a hormone. It is transported in the blood to target organs, notably gut and bone and is regulated by a complex feedback system. The main function of 1,25(OH)$_2D_3$ is to increase calcium absorption to meet the demands of growth, pregnancy and lactation. An adequate concentration of calcium is thus ensured for the formation of calcium phosphate in bone where calcium comes in contact with inorganic phosphates, liberated from organic phosphates under the influence of phosphatase produced by osteoblasts.

Alfacalcidol, 1α hydroxycholecalciferol (1α OH-D_3) is a synthetic analogue which is converted into 1,25 (OH)$_2D_3$ in the liver without the need for hydroxylation in the kidney. It is used in treating hypocalcaemia and osteomalacia due to renal disease.

The main reasons for impaired production of 1,25 (OH)$_2D_3$ are: (1) deficiency of 25-OH-D_3 due to lack of sunlight, an inadequate diet or malabsorption; (2) disturbed metabolism in liver or renal disease, notably chronic renal failure and (3) depression of the feedback system as in hypoparathyroidism.

Dietary Sources. The richest sources are fatty fish and their liver oils, some of which contain thousands of micrograms of vitamin D per 100 g. Vitamin D is also present in much smaller quantities in dairy products such as butter and eggs. In Britain vitaminised margarine is the most reliable food source of the vitamin for adults: 28 g (1 oz) contains nearly the daily requirement. Milk has a very small content of vitamin D; meat and white fish have insignificant amounts and cereals, vegetables and fruit have none. Unlike vitamin A, stores of vitamin D in the body are not large; only a little is stored in the liver and moderate amounts in adipose tissue.

The recommended daily intake (WHO) for infants and children up to 5 years of age and for pregnant or lactating women is 10 μg. For older children and adults about 2.5 μg is adequate (1 μg = 40 iu). People who regularly have ad-equate exposure of their skin to sunlight do not normally need vitamin D in their diet.

Rickets

Rickets is a disease of calcium and phosphorus metabolism which occurs when infants or children obtain insufficient vitamin D. It can affect infants in some developing countries, especially in large towns and cities.

Infants in their first year are mainly affected due to an inadequate intake of vitamin D because of the low content of this vitamin in both human and animal milk and the failure to provide them with a supplement of vitamin D in any form. In addition, for various social and cultural reasons, their mothers wrap them up in clothes which prevents their exposure to sunlight. By the second year the infant is able to crawl about in the sunshine and spontaneous healing usually occurs.

The disease is now uncommon in countries where vitamin D is freely available. In Britain clinical rickets occurs in Asian immigrant children, often of schoolgoing age, from a combination of little exposure of the skin to sunlight and very low dietary intakes of vitamin D. High phytate intake in chapatti flour may contribute by inhibiting calcium absorption. The disease is also liable to occur in premature babies.

Patients on long-term antiepileptic drugs are liable to develop rickets in childhood or osteomalacia in adult life; these drugs induce changes in liver microsomal enzymes which lead to the conversion of vitamin D to inactive metabolites.

Clinical Features. The infant with rickets has often received sufficient calories and may appear well nourished, but is restless, fretful and pale, with flabby muscles. Sweating of the head is common. The abdomen is distended. The infant is prone to respiratory infections and gastrointestinal upsets. Development is delayed; the teeth often erupt late and there is failure to sit, stand, crawl and walk at the normal ages.

The bony changes are the most characteristic signs of rickets. The earliest lesion is often craniotabes — small round unossified areas in the membranous bones of the skull, yielding to the pressure of the finger, with a crackling feeling. This sign is of particular value in the diagnosis of rickets in developing countries where the disease is common in infants under 1 year of age. It usually disappears within 12 months of birth.

Two other early signs are enlargement of the epiphyses at the lower end of the radius and swelling of the costochondral junctions of the ribs, ('rickety rosary'). Later there may be 'bossing' of the frontal and parietal bones and delayed closure of the anterior fontanelle. Later still, there may be deformities of the chest such as pigeon chest and Harrison's sulcus.

If rickets continues into the second or third year of life, deformities such as kyphosis develop as a result of the new gravitational and muscular strains, caused by sitting up and crawling. At the same time there may be enlargement of the epiphyses at the lower ends of the femur, tibia and fibula. When the rachitic child begins to walk, deformities of the shafts of the leg bones develop, so that 'knock knees' or 'bow legs' are seen. Pelvic deformities may follow and lead later to serious difficulties at childbirth.

When there is a reduction in ionised plasma calcium, infantile tetany may result, with spasm of the hands and feet and of the vocal cords. The latter causes a high-pitched distressing cry and great difficulty in breathing. Epileptic fits may also occur.

Investigation. Radiological examination of the wrist will show characteristic changes in the epiphyses at the lower ends of the radius. The zones of epiphyseal cartilages are thickened and the distal ends of the shafts are widened. In older children this shows as a typical 'saucer' deformity.

Chemical Pathology. Plasma calcium tends to fall from its normal level (p. 817). More commonly the serum phosphate falls due to the parathyroid glands responding to a slight reduction in calcium by increasing the excretion of phosphate in the urine.

Clinical rickets may occur when the levels of calcium and phosphorus in the plasma are still within normal limits but an increase in alkaline phosphatase is of diagnostic value. This enzyme is formed by the osteoblasts which, unable to make bone without a sufficient supply of calcium, liberate into the circulation the excess of this enzyme which they cannot use. Plasma 25-hydroxychole-calciferol, the main circulating form of vitamin D, is absent or very low in rickets.

Treatment. The two essentials of treatment are the provision of a supplement of vitamin D and an ample intake of calcium.

A therapeutic dose of vitamin D varies from 25 to 125 μg (1000–5000 i.u.) daily, depending on the severity of the disease and age of the child. In contrast, the prophylactic dose is 10 μg or less daily depending on the sunlight. Children can be given halibut-liver oil in a very small dose (1 ml) since it contains 30 times the vitamin D concentrations of cod-liver oil. For severe cases needing 125 μg or more daily, synthetic calciferol is useful.

In times of social upheaval, such as may be occasioned by war or disasters, when a young child may be seen once by an emergency medical service and perhaps not again for months, a single massive dose of vitamin D, e.g. 3·75 mg, can be given by mouth with reasonable safety and curative effects. The daily administration of small doses is the method recommended for normal practice, because of the danger of overdosage (p. 69).

In addition to vitamin D, rachitic infants and children require an ample supply of calcium, the best source of which is milk. At least half a litre should be taken daily by a young child with rickets. For a severe case a supplement of calcium tablets should also be given.

Treatment of tetany is described on page 442.

PROGRESS . The earliest evidence of healing in rickets is provided by radiological examination of the growing ends of the bones. The levels of calcium and phosphorus in the serum provide an unreliable guide. Decrease in the raised serum alkaline phosphatase does not usually occur for several weeks after treatment is initiated. The therapeutic dose of vitamin D should be continued so long as the alkaline phosphatase remains elevated; thereafter it may gradually be reduced to the prophylactic dose of 10 μg daily.

Rickets is not a fatal disease *per se*, but the untreated rachitic child is always at risk of infections, notably bronchopneumonia. The skeletal changes, if mild in degree, usually tend to heal spontaneously as the child gets older, but in severe cases pigeon chest, spinal curvature, knock knees, bow legs or contracted pelvis persist.

VITAMIN D RESISTANT RICKETS. Occasionally cases of rickets are encountered which are resistant to ordinary therapeutic doses of vitamin D. The disease persists into late childhood ('late rickets') or even adult life, producing the clinical appearance of osteomalacia, unless adequately treated.

One cause is defective reabsorption of phosphate as occurs in uncommon congenital disorders of the renal tubules e.g. the Fanconi syndrome (p. 379). A similar state may sometimes arise as a conditioned deficiency resulting from malabsorption of vitamin D or from chronic renal failure in which renal formation of $1,25 (OH)_2 D_3$ is impaired.

Whatever the cause, treatment consists in giving large doses of vitamin D by mouth together with calcium salts. The initial dose of calciferol may be 1·25–3·75 mg daily but it should be reduced at the first suspicion of toxic symptoms.

HYPERVITAMINOSIS D. In the case of vitamin D it is possible to have too much of a good thing. Large doses are toxic and cause hypercalcaemia. The symptoms include nausea, vomiting, constipation, drowsiness and signs of renal failure; metastatic calcification in the arteries, kidneys and other tissues may occur.

Since renal damage may develop before clinical signs of toxicity appear, all patients on large doses of vitamin D should have their serum calcium level checked regularly at 3 monthly intervals and if this is found to be above 2·6 mmol/l (10·5 mg/100 ml) it is an early indication of overdosage.

Prevention. The provision of adequate milk for children, the clearing of slums, the building of new housing estates and smoke abatement schemes are basic prophylactic measures which must be continued. In addition mothers must be educated in the need to keep their infants and children in the sunshine as much as possible. Nevertheless, in northern countries, the supply of the vitamin from this source is uncertain and attention must be paid to the dietary supply.

None of the common foods in a child's diet is a good source of vitamin D and children may benefit from a daily supplement of about 10 μg from cod-liver oil, continued at least in the winter for the first 5 years of life or more.

It is necessary to consider how much vitamin D an infant is getting from other sources. Some proprietary cereal foods for infants are 'fortified' with vitamin D by the manufacturers, as is margarine (p. 67). Not only is there no advantage in giving infants and young children more than 10 μg of vitamin D daily from all sources for prophylactic purposes, but higher doses given over a long period could predispose to infantile hypercalcaemia, a form of hypervitaminosis D.

The prophylactic dose of vitamin D for premature infants should be twice that for full-term infants and it should be started within 2 weeks of birth.

OSTEOMALACIA AND OSTEOPOROSIS

Osteomalacia, which means softening of bone, is primarily due to a deficiency of vitamin D, and to a lesser extent of calcium, or both. This results in a failure to replace the turnover of calcium and phosphorus in the organic matrix of bone. Hence the calcium phosphate content is reduced and bony substance becomes replaced by soft osteoid tissue.

Osteoporosis, which is atrophy of bone, is believed to be due to predominance of resorption over formation of the cellular matrix of bone which leads to a reduction in the total mass of bone. In other words osteoporosis is too little bone of normal mineral content. In contrast to osteomalacia the ratio of calcium phosphate to matrix is normal.

Osteomalacia

Aetiology. Osteomalacia is the adult counterpart of rickets. It was formerly common in women in purdah in oriental countries, living on poor cereal diets devoid of milk, kept indoors and seldom seeing the sun. Symptoms occurred with pregnancy.

In Scotland and in other countries where osteomalacia is a relatively common disease in old people, especially women, the disease may be due to malabsorption from any cause, including operations like partial gastrectomy, or to direct dietary deficiency of vitamin D. Chronic renal disorders are a less important cause. Adults who have to take antiepileptic drugs for years are likely to develop osteomalacia (p. 67).

Clinical Features. Skeletal pain is usually present and persistent and ranges from backache to severe pain. Bone tenderness on pressure is common. Muscular weakness is often present and the patient may find difficulty in climbing stairs or getting out of a chair. A waddling gait is not unusual. Tetany may be manifested by carpo-pedal spasm and facial twitching. Spontaneous fractures may occur, independent of the pseudo-fractures described below. The biochemical changes in the blood are the same as in rickets.

Radiological examination shows rarefaction of bone and commonly translucent bands (pseudo-fractures, Looser's zones), often symmetrical, at points submitted to stress. Common sites are the ribs, the axillary border of the scapula, the pubic rami and the medial cortex of the upper femur. Looser's zones are pathognomonic when well-developed.

Histological examination of stained undecal-cified sections of bone obtained by biopsy may be required as this shows unequivocally the presence of excess osteoid tissue.

Treatment. When osteomalacia is primarily due to defective intake, treatment is essentially the same as for rickets, namely 25 to 125 μg vitamin D daily. The response is usually dra-matic. If there is evidence of malabsorption the dose should be 1·25 mg daily and it may have to be given intramuscularly at weekly intervals. If the disease is secondary to renal disorders double or treble this dose may be necessary.

Maintenance treatment with vitamin D will be required for all cases of osteomalacia in which the cause cannot be removed. In addition a good diet should be given which includes milk. A sup-plement of calcium should be given orally, e.g. one to two tables of calcium gluconate thrice daily. Within 4 to 8 weeks of starting treatment the pain and weakness have usually disappeared.

The decision to reduce or discontinue the dose of vitamin D and calcium is based on the improve-ment in the clinical features and the disappearance of biochemical and radiological abnormalities. The dangers of vitamin D intoxication should be kept in mind.

Prevention. With improved education and better standards of living the disease is now much rarer in many Asian towns where previously it was common. Free access to sunshine and an adequate intake of dairy produce, supplemented when necessary with prophylactic vitamin D (10 μg/day), will prevent nutritional osteomalacia. Particular attention to these prophylactic mea-sures should be given to inmates of geriatric and mental hospitals and to old people living alone whose exposure to sunshine is limited and also to those who have had gastric surgery. Patients on long-term antiepileptic therapy should be given prophylactic doses of vitamin D.

Osteoporosis

Osteoporosis is the commonest metabolic disease of bone and is found most frequently in elderly women when it is known as postmenopausal osteoporosis. It may occur in elderly men (senile osteoporosis) and rarely in younger people (idio-pathic osteoporosis). There is a wide variation in the geographical and racial incidence of general-ised osteoporosis. For example, in the United States it is more prevalent in Caucasians than in Negroes.

Aetiology. A physiological decrease in skeletal mass occurs in all persons from the age of 40 to 50 onwards; the process is more marked in women, and in some individuals it would appear to be accelerated by factors which are largely unknown. In postmenopausal women a failure of oestrogen secretion and in men diminished androgen forma-tion may contribute.

In women with postmenopausal osteoporosis calcium absorption is reduced; serum 1,25 $(OH)_2D$ tends to be low. Calcitonin secretion is lower in women than men and declines with age. A major function of this hormone appears to be prevention of unwanted bone resorption. Calci-tonin levels are strikingly increased by oestrogens in postmenopausal women.

Inadequate physical activity promotes general-ised osteoporosis and may, in part at least, ac-count for the high incidence of this condition in affluent societies. Immobilisation by splinting, inflammation or pain is the main cause of local osteoporosis.

Generalised osteoporosis may be secondary to prolonged treatment with adrenal corticosteroids; it occurs in various endocrine disorders, notably Cushing's syndrome and hypogonadism, and also in severe malnutrition and chronic renal disease. Osteoporosis, like anaemia, may therefore be the end result of a number of diverse processes.

Clinical Features. The patient is usually an elderly woman who is otherwise healthy. There may be no disability despite obvious radiological abnormality. In others there are episodes of severe pain usually due to fractures of the brittle bones often occurring after minimal trauma. The lumbar and thoracic vertebrae, the neck of the femur, the upper end of the humerus and the lower end of the radius are the commonest sites of fracture. Healing is not impaired and as it occurs pain usually subsides. More persistent backache is a later feature of osteoporosis due to progressive compression or collapse of several vertebrae. This may result in loss of stature and in kyphosis. Persistent pain elsewhere is not a feature of osteoporosis but is more characteristic of osteomalacia, Paget's disease or skeletal metastases. In contrast to these conditions there is also a tendency for spontaneous improvement to occur in osteoporosis. Idiopathic osteoporosis is occasionally found in younger persons in whom it also tends to be self-limiting.

The radiological changes are more marked in the bones of the axial skeleton than in the limbs; they consist of loss of bone density, reduction in the number and size of trabeculae and thinning of the cortex. The upper and lower surfaces of the lumbar and thoracic vertebral bodies become biconcave, and later compression or collapse causes anterior wedging.

The calcium, phosphorus and alkaline phosphatase levels in the blood are normal in contrast to osteomalacia.

Treatment. Any primary factor such as excessive corticosteroid therapy or endocrine disease should be corrected if possible. The physiological decline in skeletal mass, the obscure aetiology of idiopathic osteoporosis and its tendency to remission, together with the need for long-term assessment, make therapeutic measures very difficult to evaluate.

The patient should know that the natural history of the disease is characterised by spontaneous improvement and that suitable regular exercise is beneficial. The patient should remain ambulant if symptoms permit. The use of spinal supports is undesirable. Immobilisation following a fracture should be limited to the part involved and accompanied by graduated remedial exercises. It should be borne in mind that osteomalacia can coexist with osteoporosis especially in patients with a fracture of the neck of the femur.

Cyclical oestrogen therapy may be prescribed for otherwise healthy post-menopausal women. At least an adequate intake of vitamin D and calcium should be ensured. Cows' milk is the best source of the latter, half a litre providing about 600 mg of calcium. Obesity must be avoided and, if present, corrected. There is evidence that calcium supplements are beneficial. The use of sodium fluoride to stimulate osteogenesis and also 1α OH-D are under investigation.

VITAMIN E

Alpha-tocopherol is the most potent of eight related substances with vitamin E activity. Good sources include vegetable oils, wholegrain cereals and fatty fish.

Vitamin E prevents oxidation of polyunsaturated fatty acids in cell membranes. The first feature of human deficiency is a mild haemolytic anaemia which has been described only in premature infants and in a few cases of malabsorption. In chronic deficiency, e.g., in cystic fibrosis, ataxia and visual scotomas occur which respond to vitamin E. Early administration reduces the severity of retrolental fibroplasia in premature infants given oxygen.

There is no scientific justification for self-medication with vitamin E in the belief that this will increase energy or virility. Pharmacological doses of vitamin E have produced surprisingly few side effects but they do appear to interfere with thyroid function and potentiate the action of coumarin anticoagulants.

VITAMIN K

Vitamin K is required for the formation in the liver of factors necessary for the normal clotting of blood (p. 539). It exists in nature in two forms, vitamin K_1 and vitamin K_2. Vitamin K_1 (phytomenadione) is soluble in fat solvents but only slightly in water. It is found in leafy vegetables and is available for oral and parenteral use.

Foods of animal origin (including fish-liver oils) are poor sources unless they have undergone extensive bacterial putrefaction, with formation of one of the vitamin K_2 series. Adequate amounts are normally supplied in the average diet and bacterial synthesis occurs within the colon.

Primary vitamin K deficiency is not uncommon in the newborn and 1 mg vitamin K_1 with the first feed is a safe prophylactic measure against the development of haemorrhagic disease of the newborn.

Secondary vitamin K deficiency occurs in obstructive jaundice, malabsorption and in patients given prolonged courses of intestinal antibiotics. The coumarin anticoagulants owe their therapeutic action to interference with the role of vitamin K in synthesis of the clotting factors in the liver.

The clinical features and treatment of vitamin K deficiency are discussed on page 546.

VITAMIN C (ASCORBIC ACID)

Ascorbic acid is a simple sugar. It is the most active reducing agent found in living tissues and is easily and reversibly oxidised to dehydro-ascorbic acid. Its highest concentrations are in the adrenal cortex and in the eye. Stress and corticotrophin secretion lead to a loss of ascorbic acid from the adrenal cortex. The presumption, therefore, is that ascorbic acid is intimately concerned in bodily reactions to stress. Man is one of the few animals that cannot synthesise ascorbic acid from glucose.

Dietary Sources. Blackcurrants, guavas, citrus fruits, berries and green vegetables are the richest sources. Foods of animal origin contain very little except for liver and glandular tissue. Dried cereals and pulses contain no ascorbic acid.

Ascorbic acid is very easily destroyed by heat, alkalies such as sodium bicarbonate, traces of copper or by an oxidase liberated by damage to plant tissues. Ascorbic acid is very soluble in water. For these reasons many traditional methods of cooking reduce or eliminate it from the diet. The recommended intake is 60 mg in the USA. Body stores last for about $2\frac{1}{2}$ to 3 months on a deficient diet.

Scurvy

Aetiology. In 1497 when Vasco da Gama sailed round the Cape of Good Hope 100 out of his 160 men died of scurvy. For the next 300 years scurvy was a major factor determining the success or failure of all sea ventures even after it was recognised by Lind (1753) and by Cook (1755) that it results from the prolonged consumption of a diet devoid of fresh fruit and vegtables. Final proof and isolation of vitamin C were not possible until the guinea pig was found to provide a suitable animal model (1907).

Sporadic cases of scurvy continue to arise in infants as a result of ignorance, poverty and maternal neglect and also amongst old people, especially men living alone who are not feeding themselves properly. Scurvy appears to be rare in most tropical countries but is more likely to occur in arid regions in times of drought.

Pathology. Ascorbic acid deficiency results in defective formation of collagen in connective tissue because of failure of hydroxylation of proline to hydroxyproline, the characteristic amino acid of collagen. There is in consequence delayed healing of wounds. There are also capillary haemorrhages and subnormal platelet stickiness.

Clinical Features. ADULT SCURVY. The pathognomic sign is the swollen and spongy gums particularly of the papillae between the teeth, sometimes producing the appearance of 'scurvy buds'. These are bluish-grey and bleed easily. The teeth may become loose and even fall out in severe cases. There is always some infection; indeed this seems necessary for the production of the scorbutic gingival appearances since volunteers suffering from experimental deficiency did not develop it if their gums were previously healthy. Associated with the infection there is an offensive fetor. In patients without teeth the gums appear normal.

The first sign of cutaneous bleeding is often found on the lower thighs. These are perifollicular haemorrhages—tiny points of bleeding around the orifice of a hair follicle. There is a heaping-up of keratin-like material on the surface around the mouth of the follicle, through which a deformed 'corkscrew' hair characteristically projects. Perifollicular haemorrhages are often followed by petechial haemorrhages, developing independently of the hair follicles, which are usually first seen on the feet and ankles. Thereafter large spontaneous bruises (ecchymoses) may arise almost anywhere in the body, but usually first in the lower extremities, producing the characteristic 'woody leg'. Haemorrhage may occur into joints, into a nerve sheath, under the nails or conjunctiva or into the gastrointestinal tract; there may be epistaxis. Scurvy can present with any of these features. By the time the disease is fully developed the patient is usually anaemic.

Before the changes in the gums and skin appear, the patient has usually felt feeble and listless for some weeks. A patient with scurvy may die suddenly and without warning, apparently from cardiac failure. Another characteristic of scurvy is that fresh wounds fail to heal—a possibility that the surgeon has to bear in mind.

The dietary and social history is helpful in doubtful cases. Old, solitary people may insist that they fend very well for themselves, but careful questioning will reveal that they do not bother to buy fresh fruit or vegetables. In other instances the proper foods may be purchased but they are so badly cooked that the diet loses all its vitamin C.

Plasma ascorbate is very low (p. 817); a fresh sample of plasma is needed because the vitamin can decompose in a few hours at warm room temperatures. Probably a better index of tissue reserves of the vitamin is its concentration in the buffy layer or in the platelets.

INFANTILE SCURVY. The main clinical features are lassitude, anaemia, painful limbs and enlargement of the costochondral junctions. Until the teeth have erupted, scorbutic infants do not develop gingivitis. The first sign of bleeding is usually a large subperiosteal haemorrhage in one of the long bones. This gives rise to intense pain, especially on movement.

Treatment. Because of the danger of sudden death, ascorbic acid should be given at once in adequate amounts. The aim should be to saturate the body quickly with ascorbic acid. The normal body contains about 1·5 g of the vitamin, so that a dose of 250 mg by mouth four times daily should achieve this within a few days, despite a considerable loss in the urine which quickly follows each dose. Parenteral treatment has little advantage over oral administration.

Attention should be paid to correcting the general deficiencies of the patient's former diet. A liberal mixed diet should be given. If the patient is anaemic iron and sometimes folic acid are indicated.

With adequate treatment no patient dies of scurvy and recovery is usually rapid and complete.

Prevention. In breast milk the vitamin C content responds to maternal intake. Fruit juice should be given to bottle-fed infants.

No simple administrative means has been found of preventing scurvy among the old and solitary, who are largely unresponsive to education. Should the physician be unable to persuade such a person to eat fruit or vegetables, 50 mg synthetic ascorbic acid should be taken daily. Alternatively a massive dose can be given at longer intervals—say, 500 mg every month.

Trauma, surgery and burns, infections, smoking and certain drugs—adrenocortical steroids, aspirin, indomethacin and tetracycline—all increase the requirement for vitamin C. Consequently any sick patients in hospital require considerably more than the recommended allowance of 60 mg/d.

ASCORBIC ACID AND THE COMMON COLD. It has been claimed that ascorbic acid in doses of 1–2 g daily will prevent the common cold. If it does, this is a pharmacological and not a vitamin effect as coryza is not a manifestation of scurvy. In the largest controlled trial, in Toronto, two placebo groups were included. One of these had fewer colds than those taking 0·25, 1 or 2 g vitamin C per day prophylactically. It is inadvisable for people to dose themselves with large quantities of ascorbic acid as this favours the formation of oxalate stones in the urinary tract.

THIAMIN (VITAMIN B₁)

Thiamin pyrophosphate (TPP) is an essential coenzyme for the decarboxylation of pyruvate to acetyl coenzyme A. This is the bridge between anaerobic glycolysis and the tricarboxylic acid

(Krebs) cycle. TPP is also the coenzyme for transketolase in the hexose monophosphate shunt pathway and for decarboxylation of α-ketoglutarate to succinate in the Krebs cycle.

Consequently when thiamin is deficient (a) the cells cannot utilise glucose aerobically; this is likely to affect the nervous system first, since it depends entirely on glucose for its energy requirements; (b) there is accumulation of pyruvic acid and of lactic acid derived from it, which produce vasodilatation and increase cardiac output. High carbohydrate diets, heavy alcohol intake or intravenous glucose infusions predispose to and aggravate thiamin deficiency.

In man thiamin deficiency can produce cardiomyopathy and/or peripheral neuropathy and/or encephalopathy. These occur in various combinations in wet and dry beriberi, infantile beriberi and Wernicke's encephalopathy.

Dietary Sources. Legumes, pork, liver, nuts, the germ of cereals and yeast, are the only rich sources. Green vegetables, roots, fruits, flesh foods and dairy produce (except butter) contain small amounts of the vitamin. It is not found in fats or oils. In sugar and many cereal products (wheat, rice) nearly all the naturally occurring vitamin may be removed; there is little or none in most alcoholic drinks.

As thiamin is readily soluble in water, considerable amounts may be lost when vegetables are cooked in an excess of water which is afterwards discarded. It is relatively stable below 100°C provided that the medium is slightly acid, as in baking with yeast. But if baking powder is used, or if soda is added in cooking vegetables, almost all the vitamin may be destroyed. The loss of thiamin in cooking an ordinary mixed diet is usually around 25%. Modern processes for freezing, canning and dehydrating food result in only small losses. Thiamin is not stored in the body to any appreciable extent; hence symptoms due to deficiency may develop within a few weeks.

The recommended daily intake is 0.4 mg per 1000 kcal or about 1·2 mg in an adult man.

Beriberi

Beriberi is a nutritional disorder formerly widespread in South and East Asia. The word comes from the Singhalese language and means 'I cannot' (said twice), signifying that the patient is too ill to do anything. Beriberi has almost disappeared from prosperous Asian countries such as Japan, Taiwan and Malaysia and from big cities such as Hong Kong, Manila and Singapore.

Oriental beriberi is usually caused by eating diets in which most of the calories are derived from polished, i.e. highly milled, rice. The disorder is often precipitated by infections, hard physical labour or pregnancy and lactation. In Britain and North America occasional cases of beriberi heart disease are seen, usually in alcoholics who have been consuming little but alcohol for some weeks.

Chemical and Pathological Findings. Owing to a lack of thiamin, glucose is incompletely metabolised and pyruvic and lactic acids accumulate in the tissues and body fluids. These metabolites cause dilatation of peripheral blood vessels, as in normal exercise. In beriberi this vasodilatation may be extreme, so that fluid leaks out through the capillaries, producing oedema. At the same time the blood flows rapidly through the dilated peripheral circulation. There is a high cardiac output and as the disease progresses the heart dilates because the myocardium is both overworked and unable to use glucose efficiently as an energy substrate. Cardiac failure accentuates the oedema. Sudden death may result. Microscopic examination usually shows loss of striation of myocardial fibres, which are also finely vacuolated and often fragmented and separated by oedema.

In dry beriberi there is severe wasting of muscles. In long-standing cases there is degeneration and demyelination of both sensory and motor nerves. The vagus and other autonomic nerves may be affected. In dry beriberi the level of blood pyruvate is usually within normal limits.

In Wernicke's encephalopathy there are foci of congestion and petechial haemorrhage in the upper part of the mid-brain, the hypothalamus, and the walls of the third ventricle. Involvement of the mamillary bodies is a pathognomonic finding at post-mortem.

Clinical Features. The *early* symptoms and signs are common to wet and dry beriberi. The onset is usually insidious, though sometimes precipitated by unaccustomed exertion or a febrile illness. There is anorexia and malaise, associated with heaviness and weakness of the legs. There may be a little oedema of the legs or face and the patient may complain of precordial pain and palpitations. The pulse is usually full and moderately increased in rate. There may be complaints of 'pins and needles' and numbness in the legs. The tendon jerks are usually reduced and the calf muscles may be tender on pressure. Hypoaesthesia or anaesthesia of the skin, especially over the tibiae, is common.

In areas where beriberi is endemic such a condition may persist for months or even years with only minor alterations in the symptoms. The patients are only mildly incapacitated and many continue to earn their living even as manual labourers, but at a very low level of efficiency. At any time this chronic malady may develop into either of the severe forms.

WET BERIBERI. Oedema is the most notable feature and may develop rapidly to involve not only the legs but also the face, trunk and serous cavities. Palpitations are marked and there may be pain in the legs after walking, probably due to the accumulation of lactic acid. The neck veins become distended and pulsate freely. There is usually tachycardia and an increase in pulse pressure. The heart is enlarged.

While the circulation is well maintained, the skin is typically warm owing to the vasodilatation; as heart failure advances, the skin of the extremities becomes cold and cyanotic. The mind is usually clear. Electrocardiograms often show no changes except sinus tachycardia but in some cases there are inverted T waves or conduction defects.

DRY BERIBERI. The essential feature is a polyneuropathy (p. 662). The muscles become progressively weak and wasted, and walking is increasingly difficult. The thin, even emaciated patient needs at first one stick, then two, and may finally become bedridden. The disease is essentially a chronic one, which may be arrested at any stage by improving the diet. Bedridden patients and those with severe cachexia are very susceptible to infections. Patients with dry beriberi are always liable to a sudden onset of oedema which may be due to a variety of dietary causes, e.g. lack of thiamin or protein, or to starvation.

INFANTILE BERIBERI. This is seen in areas where adult beriberi is endemic. It occurs in breast-fed infants, usually between the second and fifth months. Although the mothers of such infants must have been eating a diet and secreting milk with a low thiamin content, classical signs of beriberi are stated to be absent in 50% of them.

The illness usually starts acutely and is rapidly fatal, if not promptly treated. The mother may have noticed that the infant is restless, often cries, is passing less urine than normal and shows signs of puffiness. The infant then may suddenly become cyanosed with dyspnoea and the physical signs of acute cardiac failure and die within 24 to 48 hours. Other serious signs are convulsions and coma. In severe cases partial to complete aphonia is characteristic and is usually preceded by the infant's cry becoming thin with a plaintive whine.

Infantile beriberi was formerly the chief cause of death between 2 to 6 months of age in rice-eating rural areas in S.E. Asia, and it may still occur in isolated areas.

WERNICKE'S ENCEPHALOPATHY AND KORSAKOFF'S PSYCHOSIS. This cerebral form of thiamin deficiency occurs in Europe and North America. It often presents acutely, usually in an alcoholic but it is sometimes seen in people with malnutrition, e.g. persistent vomiting; it occurred in prisoners of war on small rations of polished rice.

The patient is quietly confused and the most valuable clinical sign is some form of bilateral, symmetrical ophthalmoplegia. This may be in one or more than one direction and accompanied by abnormal pupillary reflexes and/or nystagmus. Ataxia is also present. The confusion is liable soon to progress to stupor or death if treatment is delayed. There may be permanent memory defect, *Korsakoff's psychosis*, the characteristic bedside feature of which is confabulation. The patient is disorientated and psychological tests show a severe defect of memorising, i.e. storing new information.

Wernicke's encephalopathy and Korsakoff's psychosis are often associated with polyneuropathy and/or with superior midline cerebellar degeneration (p. 656) but it is surprising how uncommon these cerebral forms are in S.E. Asia and that beriberi cardiomyopathy is seldom seen with Wernicke/Korsakoff disease.

Investigation. Plasma pyruvic or lactic acids are not elevated in the more chronic forms of beriberi and if they are increased are not specific. The best laboratory test is measurment of transketolase activity in red cells with and without added thiamin pyrophosphate (TPP) *in vitro*. The test requires fresh heparinised whole blood and this must be taken before thiamin treatment is started. A TPP effect above 30% is to be expected in beriberi or Wernicke's encephalopathy.

Treatment. *Wet Beriberi*. Treatment must be started as soon as the diagnosis is made, because fatal heart failure may occur suddenly. Complete rest is essential and 50 mg thiamin should be given intramuscularly for three days. Thereafter 10 mg three times a day should be continued by mouth until convalescence is established.

The response of a patient with beriberi to thiamin is one of the most dramatic events of medicine. Within a few hours the breathing is easier, the pulse rate slower, the extremities cooler and a rapid diuresis begins to dispose of the oedema. In a few days the size of the heart is restored to normal. Muscular pain and tenderness are also dramatically improved. The ECG may show characteristic paradoxical changes while the patient improves. In a typical case the tracing is normal while heart failure is severe, then as recovery starts T wave inversions appear over the right ventricle for a few days.

Dry Beriberi. The treatment is that of a nutritional polyneuropathy as described on page 657.

Wernicke's encephalopathy should be treated without delay with 50 mg thiamin hydrochloride by slow intravenous injection followed by 50 mg intramuscularly daily for a week.

Infantile Beriberi. The simplest way to treat infantile beriberi is via the mother's milk. The mother should receive 10 mg thiamin hydrochloride twice daily—in severe cases by injection. In addition the infant must be given thiamin starting with 20 mg intramuscularly.

Associated Deficiencies. Other deficiencies in the patient's diet may include protein, niacin, riboflavin and other micronutrients. In the early stages the other B vitamins should be supplied, e.g. as tablets, and a good protein intake given.

Thereafter a mixed diet with less emphasis on rice is needed.

Prevention. In principle all that is necessary in endemic areas is to prevent the production of over-milled rice or wheat. In practice, however, there are many difficulties in the control of milling processes and in persuading people to change their customary diet. Much can sometimes be done with small gardens properly cultivated. The substitution of parboiled rice for highly milled rice keeps some of the thiamin in the rice as eaten. Parboiling is the term used to indicate that unhusked rice has been steamed or boiled after preliminary soaking before it is milled. Beriberi is much less common in Asia than it used to be.

In Western countries the prevention of beriberi and Wernicke's encephalopathy is related to the control of alcoholism. In a chronic alcoholic vitamin B complex tablets can at least prevent the complications of thiamin deficiency.

NIACIN (*Nicotinic Acid and Nicotinamide*)

Nicotinamide is an essential part of the two important pyridine nucleotides, NAD and NADP which are hydrogen-accepting coenzymes for dehydrogenases at many steps in the pathways of glucose oxidation. NAD is also the coenzyme for alcohol dehydrogenase. Nicotinic acid is readily converted in the body into the amide. For nutritional purposes the two have equal biological activity and are considered together in foods under the generic term 'niacin'. Both are water-soluble and resistant to heat.

Dietary Sources. Niacin is widely distributed in plant and animal foods, but only in relatively small amounts, except in meat (especially the organs), fish, wholemeal cereals and pulses. Removal of the bran in milling cereals reduces their niacin to low levels. A cup of good coffee provides about 1 mg of niacin. In a normal Western European diet about half the nicotinic acid content is provided by meat and fish.

Cooking causes little destruction of niacin but 15 to 25% may be lost in the cooking water and 'drippings' from cooked meat if these are discarded. Commercial processing and storage of foodstuffs cause little loss.

A special feature of this vitamin is that it is

normally synthesised in the body in limited amounts from the amino acid tryptophan; 60 mg of tryptophan yields 1 mg of nicotinamide. For this reason niacin equivalents in a diet are calculated by adding together the niacin plus 1/60 of the tryptophan intake (in mg). As a rule of thumb it can be assumed that tryptophan is about 1/100th of the protein intake. The recommended daily intake is 18 mg of niacin equivalents in adult men.

Pellagra

Pellagra is a nutritional disease endemic among poor peasants who subsist chiefly on maize (American corn). The greater part of the niacin in maize is in a bound form, niacytin, which is unavailable to the consumer. Moreover the principal protein of maize, zein, is deficient in the essential amino acid tryptophan, the alternative source of niacin.

Pellagra is a relatively new disease, unknown to classical and mediaeval physicians. It has occurred all over the world, wherever maize is the staple cereal, e.g. the southern states of the USA, Africa and Southern Europe and also in certain regions in India, Asia and Latin America. In recent years pellagra has disappeared from many countries where it was once endemic; in areas where it remains the incidence is much less than formerly. An exception is southern Africa where outbreaks still occur in the spring and summer in certain Bantu homelands.

Isolated cases of pellagra occur among people who are not dependent on maize. It is occasionally seen in alcoholics and in the malabsorption syndrome. Pellagra has been reported as a complication of very low protein diets used in patients with renal failure if supplementary B vitamins are forgotten. In the rare inborn error of metabolism, *Hartnup disease*, tryptophan absorption is impaired and there is a pellagrous dermatitis with neurological abnormalities which respond to nicotinamide.

Pathology. There is dermatitis and the mucous membranes of the alimentary tract and vagina usually show abnormal epithelium with underlying inflammation. Small mucous cysts are seen in the colon and sometimes ulcers. In the nervous system there may be chromatolysis of ganglion cells.

Clinical Features. *General*. Pellagra can develop in only 6 to 8 weeks on diets very deficient in niacin and tryptophan. The patient is often underweight, and presents the general features of poor nutrition. Pellagra has been called the disease of the three D's: dermatitis, diarrhoea and dementia.

Skin. The diagnosis is generally first suggested by the appearance of the skin. Characteristically, there is an erythema resembling severe sunburn, appearing symmetrically over the parts of the body exposed to sunlight and especially on the neck. Local trauma or irritation of the skin may also determine the site of the lesion. The affected areas are well demarcated from normal skin. They are at first red and slightly swollen; they may itch and burn. In acute cases the skin lesions may progress to vesiculation, cracking, exudation and crusting with ulceration and sometimes secondary infection; but in chronic cases the dermatitis occurs as a roughening and thickening of the skin with dryness, scaling and a brown pigmentation. Dermatitis of the vulva, perineum and perianal area is usually present. Nasolabial seborrhoea is occasionally seen (p. 79).

Pellagra may sometimes occur without skin lesions if the patient has been confined indoors. This variety has been called 'pellagra sine pellagra' and should be remembered if unexplained delirium or dementia is found in a housebound person who has been taking a poor diet for a prolonged period.

Alimentary Tract. Diarrhoea is common but not always present. There may be anorexia, nausea and dysphagia. The tongue characteristically has a 'raw beef' appearance — red, swollen and painful. Glossitis is an early symptom and may precede the skin lesions. The mouth is sore and often shows angular stomatitis and cheilosis (p. 79). It is probable that a non-infective inflammation extends throughout the gastrointestinal tract and accounts for the diarrhoea which is usually watery, sometimes with blood and mucus in the stools.

Nervous System. In the milder cases the symptoms consist chiefly of weakness, anxiety, depression, irritability and failure of concentration; in severe cases delirium is the most common mental disturbance in the acute form of the disease and dementia in the chronic form. Because of these changes, chronic pellagrins may be admitted to mental hospitals.

Treatment. Nicotinamide is given in a dose of 100 mg every 4 to 6 hours by mouth, although a smaller dose is likely to be effective. The vitamin is rapidly absorbed, despite severe digestive disorders. There is therefore no indication for giving it parenterally. The response to nicotinamide is usually rapid; within 24 hours the erythema of the skin diminishes, the tongue becomes paler and less painful and the diarrhoea ceases. Often there is also striking improvement in the patient's behaviour and mental attitude.

Nicotinamide alone is usually insufficient to restore health. Some of the features found in pellagra are clearly the result of associated nutritional deficiencies. First, a relatively low intake of protein including tryptophan is an essential condition for development of the disease, and hypoalbuminaemia is common. Second, anaemia may coexist, either of iron or folate deficiency type. Third, deficiencies of other B complex vitamins are to be expected. Peripheral neuropathy may be caused by thiamin or pyridoxine deficiency, nasolabial seborrhoea and angular stomatitis by riboflavin deficiency and spinal cord lesions, when present, by vitamin B_{12} deficiency. Lastly the patient has usually lost weight. Nicotinamide treatment should therefore be supplemented with a nutritious diet, high in protein. Vitamin B complex tablets should be given and iron, folic acid and vitamin B_{12} may be necessary in addition for some cases. Alcohol should be forbidden.

Prognosis. In endemic areas most cases are mild, improving in the winter and relapsing with the increased sunshine in the spring. In long-standing cases there may be persistent mental, spinal cord and digestive disorders.

Occasionally a fulminating form develops, with fever and prostration, and may be fatal. In the past, most of the deaths arose from secondary infections, or from emaciation due to PEM intensified by the diarrhoea.

Prevention. The disappearance from the southern states of America of pellagra which before the Second World War afflicted tens of thousands of poor country folk, demonstrates that the disease is preventable. Fortification of bread and maize meal with nicotinic acid, is only one of several factors which have produced this satisfactory result. General improvement in the economic state, education and nutrition of the population appears to have had more effect.

In Central America the peasants eat a staple diet of maize but pellagra is unusual. This is because of the traditional method of boiling the maize in lime water (dilute calcium hydroxide) before they make tortillas. It has been found that the indigestible niacytin is hydrolysed to free niacin in dilute alkali.

In areas where pellagra is still endemic less dependence on maize and instead more animal husbandry and cultivation of legumes should be encouraged. Patients in endemic areas with a poor dietary history or skin signs suggesting early pellagra may benefit from vitamin B complex tablets.

RIBOFLAVIN

Riboflavin is a constituent of the flavoproteins which are concerned with tissue oxidation. It is a yellow-green fluorescent compound soluble in water. Though stable to boiling in acid solution, in alkaline solution it is decomposed by heat. It is also destroyed by exposure to light.

Dietary Sources. The best sources of riboflavin are liver, kidney, milk, meat, cheese and eggs. Green vegetables contain moderate amounts. It differs from other components of the vitamin B complex in that it occurs in good amounts in dairy produce, but is relatively lacking in cereal grains, especially when highly milled. It is also present in beer. Ordinary methods of cooking do not destroy the vitamin apart from losses that occur when the water in which vegetables have been boiled is discarded. If foods, especially milk, are left exposed to sunshine, large losses may occur. The recommended daily intake is 1·7 mg in adult men.

Disorders Due to Riboflavin Deficiency

When human volunteers have been given diets very low in riboflavin, the most consistent clinical manifestations were angular stomatitis, cheilosis and nasolabial seborrhoea; these responded to the addition of pure riboflavin in the deficient diet.

Angular stomatitis is not specific for lack of riboflavin. Deficiencies of niacin, pyridoxine and iron can all produce it. It can follow herpes febrilis at the angle of the mouth. A common cause is ill-fitting dentures, associated with candidiasis.

Cheilosis is the name given to a zone of red, denuded epithelium at the line of closure of the lips. It has occurred in experimental pure niacin deficiency. It is often associated with angular stomatitis and frequently seen in pellagrins.

Nasolabial seborrhoea or dyssebacea is the term given to enlarged follicles around the sides of the nose which are plugged with dry sebaceous material. This occurs in primates on a diet deficient only in riboflavin. It is seen in some patients with pellagra.

Other Abnormalities. Vascularisation of the cornea, scrotal dermatitis, a magenta-coloured tongue and anaemia have been attributed to riboflavin deficiency but they may have alternative explanations. Riboflavin clearly plays a vital role in cellular oxidation and there are communities and individuals who have both minimal dietary intakes and very low concentrations in urine or blood. Yet it is surprising that the clinical effects of riboflavin deficiency are trivial and mainly nonspecific. Features of riboflavin deficiency are most likely to be found in pellagrins and in malnourished rice-eaters in Southeast Asia. In the first situation they are overshadowed by niacin deficiency and in the second by thiamin or protein deficiency.

Treatment. The therapeutic dose of riboflavin is 5 mg three times a day by mouth. It gives the patient's urine a green fluorescence. As discussed above, other B complex vitamins should also be given.

PYRIDOXINE (VITAMIN B_6)

Pyridoxine, pyridoxal and pyridoxamine are three closely related compounds with similar physiological actions. The active form of the vitamin in man is pyridoxal phosphate, the coenzyme for over 60 different enzyme systems involved in the metabolism of the amino acids including aminotransferases. Vitamin B_6 is widely distributed in plants and animal tissues. Liver, whole grain cereals, peanuts and bananas are good sources. The normal adult requirement is 2 mg per day.

Disorders Due to Vitamin B_6 Deficiency

Although a series of pathological changes in the skin, liver, blood vessels, nervous tissue and bone marrow have been produced experimentally in various animals, disorders due to deficiency of vitamin B_6 rarely occur in man, and then very seldom as a result of dietary deficiency.

A minor epidemic of convulsions in infants in the USA in the 1950s was traced to a milk formula which provided little vitamin B_6 because of a manufacturing error. In adults dermatitis, cheilosis, glossitis and angular stomatitis have been produced by means of the pyridoxine inhibitor, 4-desoxy-pyridoxine. The peripheral neuropathy associated with isoniazid therapy is due to a secondary vitamin B_6 deficiency. Certain drugs such as isoniazid and penicillamine, act as chemical antagonists to pyridoxine. Some cases of sideroblastic anaemia respond to treatment with pyridoxine (p. 499).

Biochemical features of vitamin B_6 deficiency can occur in women taking oral contraceptives, and the mild depression which affects a small proportion of such women may be relieved by pyridoxine.

Megavitamin doses of vitamin B_6 (2000 mg/day) have been reported to cause a sensory polyneuropathy.

BIOTIN

Biotin functions as coenzyme for several carboxylases. It is present in a number of different foods; the requirement is small (about 100 μg/day) and it can be synthesised by intestinal bacteria. Human deficiency is rare; it has occurred in adults who have taken for long periods large amounts of raw egg which contain the antagonist avidin. The clinical features include dermatitis and hypercholesterolaemia. A form of seborrhoeic dermatitis of infants responds to biotin.

VITAMIN B$_{12}$ AND FOLATE

These vitamins and disorders due to their deficiency are discussed on page 500 and page 503.

DIETARY FIBRE

This is the natural packing of plant foods. It can be defined as those parts of foods which are not digested by human enzymes. The principal classes of dietary fibre are cellulose, hemicelluloses, lignins, pectins and gums. These are all polysaccharides (i.e., carbohydrates) except lignin, which occurs with cellulose in the structure of plants. Pectins and gums are viscous, not fibrous.

Some types of dietary fibre, notably the hemicellulose of wheat, increase the water-holding capacity of colonic contents and the bulk of the faeces. They relieve simple constipation, appear to prevent diverticulosis and may reduce the risk of cancer of the colon. Other, viscous indigestible polysaccharides like pectin and guar gum have more effect in the upper gastrointestinal tract. They tend to slow gastric emptying, contribute to satiety, may flatten the glucose tolerance curve and reduce plasma cholesterol concentration.

Dietary fibre is in fact partly digested in the large intestine, by resident bacterial flora, not endogenous enzymes, with flatus formation, and a small quantity of volatile fatty acids is absorbed through the colonic mucosa. There are as yet no official recommended intakes because analyses for the different types of dietary fibre in foods are not complete, but the present average intakes of about 15 to 20 g/day in affluent countries are thought to be too low.

BIOCHEMICAL DIAGNOSIS OF NUTRITIONAL DEFICIENCIES

Biochemical methods are an integral part of modern medical diagnosis. For example, plasma sodium and potassium concentrations are essential for the diagnosis and treatment of difficult electrolyte problems and plasma or red cell folate and plasma vitamin B$_{12}$ concentrations are desirable before treating a patient with megaloblastic anaemia. Likewise with the other vitamins, biochemical tests have been developed which are

more or less valuable, (a) for confirming the diagnosis of a deficiency disease in places where it is uncommonly seen or if the clinical picture is complicated or (b) in community surveys, for identifying individuals with subclinical vitamin deficiencies.

The tests which can be used for the major nutrients are listed in Table 4.2. As with other tests in chemical pathology there can be false positives and false negatives. Each result needs to be evaluated with critical understanding; for example, serum vitamin B$_{12}$ is increased in acute hepatitis and alkaline phosphatase may not be elevated if rickets is accompanied by PEM.

In general when the dietary intake of a nutrient is inadequate the individual goes through three stages. The first stage is that of adaptation to the low intake. For example, urine excretion falls but there is no evidence of abnormal function or of depletion of the cells.

In the second stage there are in addition biochemical changes indicating either impaired function, e.g. reduced red cell transketolase activity in thiamin deficiency, or cellular depletion, e.g. reduced white cell ascorbic acid. But clinical manifestations of deficiency are absent or non-specific.

The third stage is that of clinical deficiency disease.

Most clinical biochemistry laboratories provide only some of the methods as a routine but others could be set up in special circumstances or, alternatively, a laboratory specialising in nutrition research could be asked to help.

PREVENTION OF NUTRITIONAL DEFICIENCIES

There are broadly three ways of approaching prevention:

1. *Increasing Food Consumption Per Head.* This requires increased production of food in the country or increased export earnings with which to import food. However, an overall increase of food in a country will be of little value unless the majority of people have jobs which provide sufficient money to buy the food they need. In addition effective national programmes of population control must be implemented in many countries. Doctors are likely to have more of a role to play in

Table 4.2. Biochemical methods for diagnosing nutritional deficiencies (protein, major vitamins and minerals)

Nutrient	Principal methods		Supplementary methods
	Indicating reduced intake	Indicating impaired function (IF) or cell depletion (CD)	
Protein	Urinary nitrogen	Plasma albumin (IF)	Fasting plasma amino acid pattern
Vitamin A	Plasma vitamin A (retinol) and plasma carotene		
Thiamin	Urinary thiamin	RBC transketolase and TTP effect★ (IF)	Plasma pyruvate and lactate★
Riboflavin	Urinary riboflavin	RBC glutathione reductase and FAD effect (IF)★	RBC riboflavin
Niacin	Urine N'methyl nicotinamide and 2-pyridone		Fasting plasma tryptophan
Vitamin B_6	Urinary 4-pyridoxic acid	RBC glutamic oxal-acetic transaminase and PP effect (IF)★	Urinary xanthurenic acid after tryptophan load★ Plasma pyridoxal phosphate
Folate	Plasma folate (*Lactobacillus casei*)	Red cell folate (CD)	Urinary FIGLU after histidine load★
		Haemoglobin, PCV and smear (IF)	Bone marrow morphology
Vitamin B_{12}	Plasma vitamin B_{12} (*e.g. Euglena gracilis*)	Haemoglobin PCV and smear (IF)	Schilling test. Bone marrow morphology
Vitamin C	Plasma ascorbate	Leucocyte ascorbate (CD)	Urinary ascorbate
Vitamin D	Plasma 25-hydroxy-cholecalciferol	Plasma alkaline phosphatase (IF)★	Serum calcium and inorganic phosphorus
Vitamin E	Plasma tocopherol	RBC haemolysis with H_2O_2 *in vitro*	
Vitamin K		Plasma prothrombin (IF)	
Sodium	Urinary sodium	Plasma sodium	
Potassium	Urinary potassium	Plasma potassium	Total body potassium by ^{40}K
Iron	Plasma iron and transferrin	Haemoglobin, PCV and smear (IF)	Plasma ferritin (CD)
Iodine	Urinary (stable) iodine	Plasma thyroxine and T_3(IF)	
Zinc	Plasma zinc	Leucocyte zinc	Hair zinc

Asterisk(★) indicates value *increased* in deficiency.

helping with birth control than with agricultural or economic planning.

2. *Nutrition Education and Food Enrichment.* Education in nutrition consists of teaching and motivating people to make a healthy choice of foods. It ranges from advising agricultural planners which crops should be encouraged, to teaching mothers how to feed their children and distribute food sensibly in the family using what is available to them.

Where vitamin or mineral deficiencies occur, or could occur, food enrichment is one possible solution. This is used mostly in industrial countries; it is difficult to organise in developing countries where there are many small farmers who grow their own food.

To be effective the enriched food should reach the potentially deficient segment of the population, so the choice of which staple food to enrich needs careful consideration. Addition of vitamins

A and D to margarine and iodisation of salt are examples of worthwhile food enrichment. The use of nutrients which are toxic in large amounts must be limited.

Food enrichment should be supervised and monitored by the appropriate government ministry. It is not the answer to every nutritional deficiency even in industrial countries; for example, further enrichment of bread with iron will not solve the problem of iron deficiency anaemia. This kind of deficiency is better dealt with by the third strategy.

3. *Health and Medical Action for Vulnerable Groups.* Many countries provide nutritious lunches for school children. Pregnant mothers should be given prophylactic doses of iron and folic acid; mothers should expose young children to sunlight regularly or give them small prophylactic doses of vitamin D. Women with menorrhagia and patients who have had gastric surgery should be given iron tablets periodically. The housebound elderly should be given prophylactic amounts of vitamin D and sometimes other nutrients. Patients receiving diuretics should have a good intake of potassium and magnesium. Doctors should be trained to anticipate the possibility of certain types of malnutrition in association with particular diseases.

In developing countries where most people do not have direct access to a doctor, maternal and child health clinics provide a centre for therapeutic, preventive and educational services at moderate cost, aimed at the most vulnerable sections of the community. In this setting nutrition and infection must be treated in an integrated way and can often be combined with family planning.

A.S. TRUSWELL

OBESITY

Obesity is the most common nutritional disorder in affluent societies. Its significance requires constant emphasis because it is associated with increased mortality, predisposes to the development of important diseases and diminishes the efficiency and happiness of those affected.

Obesity may be defined as a condition in which there is an excessive amount of body fat. This simple definition gives rise to two questions: how can body fat be measured, and what is 'excessive'?

All methods of measuring the fat content in the living subject are, to a greater or lesser degree, indirect. The simplest, but also the least direct, is the measurement of body weight and this is the method almost exclusively used in clinical practice. In the clinical context the 'desirable' or 'ideal' weight for height (p. 816) is that associated with the lowest mortality in actuarial terms and excessive weight that associated with increased mortality.

Aetiology. Excess fat accumulates because there is imbalance between energy intake and expenditure. This can arise in different ways and obesity is a clinical sign with several possible causes. There is no satisfactory aetiological classification of obesity, but a number of factors are known to be associated with its development.

Age. Obesity is most prevalent in middle-age, but can occur at any stage of life. Obesity in childhood and adolescence is likely to be followed by obesity in adult life.

Socio-economic. In affluent countries obesity is more common in the lower socio-economic groups. In developing countries it can occur only in the prosperous elite. Some occupations predispose to obesity, e.g. cooks and barmen, whilst jockeys, fashion models and airline pilots have to keep themselves slim. In some societies fat men are respected and fat women considered beautiful; in others they are not.

Heredity. A familial tendency exists in many cases, but it is difficult to disentangle environmental and genetic components. Patterns of eating and activity are influenced by social, cultural and economic factors which may be handed on from one generation to another. However, studies involving twins and adopted children indicate the importance of genetic factors in influencing both total body fat and its distribution. There is no evidence in man of obesity produced by a single gene, as in the genetically obese strains of rodents.

Endocrine Factors. An endocrine influence on body fat is seen both in normal physiological situations and in pathological states. The normal fat content of young adult women is about twice that of young men and pregnancy is characterised by an increase in body fat. Obesity in women commonly begins at puberty, during pregnancy or at the menopause. Obesity frequently, but not invariably, accompanies hypothyroidism, hypogonadism, hypopituitarism and Cushing's syndrome. However, the overwhelming majority of obese patients show no clinical evidence of an endocrine disorder. The plasma concentration of insulin and cortisol is commonly raised and that of growth hormone reduced in obese subjects, but these changes probably result from, rather than cause the obesity, since they disappear when weight is lost.

Energy Intake. A very small excess of calories, if habitual, can lead eventually to a large accumulation of fat. If a person eats a slice (20 g) of bread that is not needed each day or goes by car instead of walking for 20 minutes, the daily extra 48 kcal (200 kJ) will build up over 10 years to 20 kg of fat deposited.

Social factors, such as advertising and business lunches, may contribute to overeating and some people overeat because they are unhappy. There is some evidence that in obese people eating is determined less by 'internal cues', i.e. hunger and satiety, than by external influences like the availability, appearance and taste of food or the environment in which the food is served.

However, while some obese subjects, for one reason or another, eat more than those who are not obese, undoubtedly many do not and the presumption must be that many obese subjects have an unusually low energy expenditure.

Energy Expenditure. Physical inactivity has an important role in the development of obesity. Affluence is commonly associated with reduced energy expenditure. It is well recognised that physical activity is less in the obese than in the lean, but this may result from, rather than cause, the obesity. Moreover, the amount of energy expended by an obese person on most tasks is likely to be more because of the extra weight to be moved.

Little is understood about the control of energy balance in man, but there can be no doubt that some individuals gain weight more readily than others. Apart from possible alterations in the efficiency of basal metabolism there is some evidence that the thermic response to food may be less than normal in obese subjects, leading to greater conservation of energy. The possible roles of brown adipose tissue and of the sodium pump are being investigated.

Drugs. The use of steroids, oral contraceptives, phenothiazines and insulin is commonly followed by obesity, mainly because appetite is stimulated.

Clinical Features. In most cases the diagnosis will be apparent from the patient's appearance but the degree of obesity should also be assessed, usually by measurement of height and weight and reference to a table such as that on page 816 where the weight of the patient can be compared with that of an 'ideal' subject of the same age, sex, height and frame. In addition, the skinfold thickness over the triceps muscle can be measured using special spring-loaded calipers. Obesity is indicated by a reading above 20 mm in a man, and above 28 mm in a woman.

This very common disorder is frequently overlooked because the doctor is preoccupied by one of its many complications or ignores it because it is so familiar.

Obesity must be distinguished from a gain in weight due to fluid retention associated with cardiac, renal or hepatic disease, bearing in mind the fact that oedema does not become manifest clinically until the extracellular fluid has increased by about 15%.

Complications. *Psychological*. Obese patients are often psychologically disturbed, but it is difficult to distinguish between cause and effect. Depressed or anxious patients or the emotionally deprived may seek solace in food. Many obese people, especially younger adult females, are ashamed of their unattractive appearance and develop psychosocial and sexual problems.

Mechanical Disabilities. Flat feet and osteoarthrosis of the knees, hips and lumbar spine are more common in obese people. The abdominal muscles supporting the viscera and the leg muscles, whose contractions promote venous return, are less efficient, predisposing to the development of abdominal and diaphragmatic hernias and varicose veins. Adipose tissue round the trunk interferes with the mechanics of respiration resulting in exertional dyspnoea and increased susceptibility to respiratory infection. Fat people are more likely to suffer from accidents.

Metabolic Disorders. Non-insulin dependent diabetes mellitus, hyperlipidaemia (with elevation of both cholesterol and triglyceride), gallstones, hyperuricaemia and gout are all more common among the obese than in the general population.

Cardiovascular Disorders. Obesity increases the work done by the heart, which enlarges with rising body weight. The cardiac output, stroke volume, and blood volume all increase. Hypertension is common but, in the obese, blood pressure recorded with a standard sphygmomanometer cuff may be higher than direct intra-arterial measurements. The major source of error is failure of the blood pressure cuff completely to encircle the arm.

The contribution which obesity alone makes to the aetiology of ischaemic heart disease is controversial. There is little doubt that obesity is associated with this disease, but it is difficult to separate the contribution of obesity from that of other risk factors which may be causally associated, such as diabetes, hypertension and hyperlipidaemia, or from that of independent risk factors, such as smoking. Special mention should also be made of physical inactivity, which may be both a cause and an effect of obesity and also plays an important role in the genesis of ischaemic heart disease.

Life Expectancy. With all these possible complications it is not surprising that overweight is associated with an increased rate of mortality at all ages. The level of excess mortality varies more or less in proportion to the degree of obesity. Thus subjects 30% overweight incur a 30% increase in mortality and for those 40% overweight the increase rises to 50%.

There is also evidence that a substantial reduction of the body weight of obese people is alone sufficient to diminish the greater death rate. In the Society of Actuaries Build and Blood Pressure Study of 1959, the mortality was reduced to normal in those who successfully lost and maintained weight within the desirable range. Thus the diagnosis and effective treatment of obesity is literally of vital importance, and recording the patient's height and weight must be just as much a routine part of clinical examination as taking the blood pressure or testing the urine.

Treatment. Whatever the ultimate cause of obesity in the individual case the immediate cause is energy imbalance, and weight reduction can be achieved only by reducing energy intake or by increasing output, or by a combination of the two. This involves change in the individual's life-style. Thus treatment is difficult and the patient needs motivation. Rewards must be seen ahead and psychological understanding and behavioural advice are essential weapons. It is most important for success that patients should be educated and informed about their disorder and misconceptions corrected. There are no 'slimming foods' or 'slimming tablets', which do not depend on a reduced energy intake.

Long-term results are best where patients are well motivated and educated, follow structured diets designed to provide 800 to 1600 kcal daily (p. 812) and are being seen and weighed regularly, every 1 to 2 weeks initially, by the same person. The number of patients requiring supervision is so great, the need for support is so prolonged and the success of some lay organisations such as 'Weight Watchers' compares so favourably with conventional medical methods, that it is justifiable to take advantage of the facilities provided by these groups. Most refer members to their own doctors at the first suggestion of any untoward developments.

However supervision is arranged, it is most important for success that obese patients should be given precise instructions as to how they should reorganise their dietary and other habits, a target weight to aim for and an indication of the rate of weight loss expected.

Among the important lessons to be learned by obese people is the need to manage the disorder themselves. Unlike many conditions for which patients seek help, success does not depend upon operations, drugs, injections or other manipulations undertaken by the therapist but rather on the ability of the patient to accept advice, to act upon it, and to persist indefinitely with some restriction on dietary freedom.

The physician's role is to provide advice and continuing support. Many doctors find obese people unattractive, have difficulty in sympathising with their problems and fail to establish satisfactory rapport with them. Such attitudes contribute to the frequent lack of success in treatment.

THE CONSTRUCTION OF A WEIGHT REDUCING DIET. A weekly weight loss of 0·5 to 1 kg should be the general aim. An obese middle-aged housewife will usually lose weight satisfactorily on a diet providing 800 to 1000 kcal per day, such as the example on page 812. An obese man engaged in active physical work will not tolerate a diet as low as 1000 kcal per day but a satisfactory weight loss can be expected from a diet containing about 1500 kcal per day.

Protein. Dietary protein of 50 g/day is sufficient to maintain nitrogen balance. High protein diets may satisfy appetite more effectively than high carbohydrate diets, but they are expensive, may not be particularly palatable after a time, or may have a high incidental content of fat, and are therefore seldom practicable.

Carbohydrate. Obese people seldom develop more than a trace of ketosis and never sufficient to cause symptoms as long as they consume small amounts of carbohydrate. In a diet of 1000 kcal/day, 100 g of carbohydrate is a suitable allowance and this should be taken as foods providing complex carbohydrates and dietary fibre (such as fruits and vegetables and whole grain cereals) rather than as foods containing glucose and sucrose.

Fat. A 1000 kcal diet containing 100 g of carbohydrate and 50 g of protein, cannot include more than 40–45 g of fat. This allowance of fat, though small, is sufficient to make the diet palatable.

Vitamins. The diet should contain plenty of green vegetables and fruits, since they contain few calories, while their bulk helps to fill the stomach and relieve hunger; they also help to minimise the constipation common with a low food intake. Their vitamin A activity and vitamin C content will be sufficient to meet the body's needs. With meat, fish and eggs in the diet and little or no refined cereals and sugar, it is improbable that deficiency of any component of the vitamin B complex will arise.

Minerals. The only minerals that need serious consideration are calcium and iron. Provided the diet incudes 300 ml of skimmed milk, there is little likelihood of a negative calcium balance developing in an adult. The supply of iron is less sure and may call for the prescription of iron supplements.

Fluids and Salt. At one time, patients were often advised to restrict their intake of water, but there is no logical reason for keeping fat patients thirsty. Sweetened 'juices' must be avoided, except those sold for diabetic patients, which have a low caloric content.

The obese are susceptible to water and salt retention but diuretics must be used with care because potassium depletion is particularly liable to occur while patients are on a reducing regimen. Salt restriction alone may be sufficient to alleviate oedema, but when diuretics are considered essential, potassium supplements should be given.

Alcoholic drinks are also a source of calories and hence are best avoided, but if taken, a corresponding reduction in the diet is necessary. A 100 ml glass of dry wine or 30 ml whisky and water provide 70 kcal and half a pint of lager 80 kcal.

General. This diet is suitable for treatment of obese persons in Britain but it may be unsuitable in other circumstances and in other climates. Dietitians with knowledge of local eating customs can devise diets which are socially acceptable and which provide about 1000 kcal made up from about 100 g carbohydrate, 50–60 g protein and 40–45 g fat.

In the absence of oedema or any endocrine disorder, failure to respond to such a diet nearly always indicates non-compliance, despite protestations to the contrary! In such cases, treatment in hospital under strict supervision for 1 or 2 weeks may be beneficial to demonstrate that the prescribed regimen is effective if carefully followed and to allow a period of intensive education.

THERAPEUTIC STARVATION. A period of several weeks of starvation in hospital with only water, non-caloric drinks with vitamin and mineral supplements being allowed, has been recommended for very obese patients who have failed to respond to orthodox treatment.

Although the initial loss of weight may be marked, the long-term results are no more satisfactory than with other systems since many patients regain most of the weight lost when strict measures are discontinued. Such a regimen is contraindicated for older patients, especially if they have cardiovascular complications, since deaths have occasionally occurred. Ketosis may be troublesome in the early stages and hyperuricaemia, sometimes accompanied by gout, can develop.

EXERCISE. Most obese patients lead sedentary lives and benefit from physical activity such as walking, swimming and gardening, provided it does not exceed their cardiovascular capacity. Regular daily exercise is much more valuable than episodic activity.

An hour's walk at 3 miles per hour will expend about 300 kcal (or more for a heavy person). This may seem a small amount, equivalent to about 30 g of fat, but if the daily walk becomes a habit it will add up, other things being equal, to a weight loss of 9 kg in a year. Doctors should suggest, discuss and work out with each patient an increasing programme of exercise which is within the physical capacity and which will add to the quality of life of the individual.

DRUG THERAPY. This is no substitute for a dietary regimen but has a limited use as an adjunct in carefully selected patients with refractory obesity. Some of the more effective drugs used in the past, notably amphetamine, are addictive and have been so widely abused that they should not be prescribed for the treatment of obesity.

Amphetamine-like drugs with similar anorectic properties but causing less central nervous stimulation include diethylpropion (75 mg in a single dose daily) and phentermine (15–30 mg before breakfast). They may be given intermittently for periods of about a month to help attain a short-term goal. They should not be used in patients with hypertension or coronary heart disease.

Fenfluramine, which increases release of serotonin in the brain, probably acts by stimulating satiety rather than inducing anorexia. It may cause nausea, diarrhoea, lethargy, breathlessness due to pulmonary hypertension, excessive dreaming and, particularly if suddenly withdrawn, depression. It must be given only under careful medical supervision in a dose of 20 mg b.d., gradually increased to a maximum of 120 mg daily, unless adverse effects intervene. Treatment can be continued as long as weight is being lost.

None of these drugs must be given to a patient with a history of psychiatric illness.

The administration of thyroxine to euthyroid patients is not only useless but is potentially dangerous, especially if heart disease is present. It should be prescribed only if hypothyroidism co-exists with obesity.

FIBRE-RICH PRODUCTS. There is evidence that some foods rich in fibre have an effect on satiety. Methylcellulose is an indigestible substance which adds bulk to the diet. It distends the stomach and so may help to allay hunger. In clinical trials it has been shown to have little if any effect in promoting weight loss.

SURGICAL TREATMENT. Wiring the jaws together to prevent eating has been used to treat those who have found it impossible to adhere to a low-energy diet. Although this usually results in marked loss of weight, many patients regain weight when the procedure is reversed. Operations such as small intestine bypass, aimed at inducing malabsorption, have been undertaken in some centres for the treatment of intractable cases of severe 'morbid' obesity. Complications can be severe and sometimes fatal. An alternative and safer procedure is to reduce the size of the stomach, for example by stapling, which, it is claimed, can be reversed.

It seems unlikely that these experimental techniques will contribute substantially to the management of obesity in more than a very small minority of the most resistant cases.

Prognosis. It is easy for an obese person to lose up to 5 kg in weight. This accounts for the temporary successes of numerous popular 'slimming cures'. How difficult it is to achieve further losses is not generally realised. The published records of seven obesity clinics in the USA showed that satisfactory results ranged only from 12 to 28% if the index of success was the loss of 12 kg or more.

Experience in many clinics has also shown that it is difficult for patients to maintain their reduced weight since this requires some restriction of energy intake on a long-term basis.

Prevention. This must depend in part on the doctor who discerns when patients, be they infants, children or adults, are gaining too much weight. For this purpose alone, among the most useful information that a doctor can keep about patients is a record of body weight, measured at regular intervals. The doctor's responsibility with an overweight patient, at any time, is advisory and educational; the attention of patients must be drawn to the dangers of obesity and to the appropriate methods of correcting it.

All the health agencies available should be mustered to support a steady campaign of education and persuasion of patients and potential patients on the need to avoid obesity. The antenatal services, infant welfare clinics, school health authorities, health visitors and many others to whom the public look for advice when they are in difficulties should contribute to this educational programme. The media also play an increasingly important role.

JOYCE D. BAIRD
A.S. TRUSWELL

FURTHER READING:

General Nutrition
Davidson, Sir Stanley, Passmore, R., Brock, J.F. & Truswell, A.S. (1979) *Human Nutrition and Dietetics*, 7th ed. Edinburgh: Churchill Livingstone. The standard text-book. Covers the whole field of nutrition in 64 chapters.

Paul, A.A. & Southgate, D.A.T. (1978) *McCance & Widdowson's The Composition of Foods*, 4th ed. London : H.M.S.O. British food tables : data on many nutrients readily available in a single volume.

Committee on Dietary Allowances, Food and Nutrition Board (1980) *Recommended Dietary Allowances*, 9th revised edition. Washington, D.C.: National Academy of Sciences. Most of the major countries have their own recommended dietary intakes. The latest American ones cover 30 different nutrients, are kept up to date and well documented.

Turner, M.R. (ed.) (1982) *Nutrition and Health: A perspective*. Lancaster: MTP Press. The current status of research on diet-related diseases.

Infants and children
Cameron, M. & Hofvander, Y. (1983) *Manual on Feeding Infants and Young Children (for application in the developing areas of the world with special reference to home-made weaning foods)*, 3rd edn. Delhi: Oxford University Press.

Jelliffe, D.B. & Jelliffe, E.F.P. (1979) *Human Milk in the Modern World. Psychosocial, Nutritional and Economic Significance*. Oxford : Oxford University Press. 488 readable pages on all aspects of breast feeding and human milk.

McLaren, D.S. & Burman, D. (eds.) (1982) *Textbook of Paediatric Nutrition*, 2nd edn. Edinburgh : Churchill Livingstone. A systematic textbook with 25 international contributors.

The Elderly
Exton-Smith, A.N. & Caird, F.I. (eds.) (1980) *Metabolic and Nutritional Disorders in the Elderly*. Bristol : John Wright. A collection of straightforward chapters by different specialists.

Dietary Fibre
Spiller, G.A. & Kay, R.M. (eds.) (1980) *Medical Aspects of Dietary Fiber*. New York : Plenum Press. Chapters by different specialists on various aspects of dietary fibre.

Obesity
Garrow, J.S. (1981) *Treat Obesity Seriously. A Clinical Manual*. Edinburgh : Churchill Livingstone. The author has translated his research and clinical practice on obesity into a book with emphasis on management.

Royal College of Physicians (1983) *Obesity*. London : Royal College of Physicians. A comprehensive report.

5. Disturbances in Water and Electrolyte Balance and in Hydrogen Ion Concentration

The chemical events collectively called metabolism require the concentration of hydrogen ions and electrolytes to remain within narrow limits in the tissue cells and in the fluid which bathes them. Derangement of water and electrolyte balance and disturbances in hydrogen ion concentration occur in a wide variety of clinical conditions which are separately described in the appropriate chapters of this book. It is convenient, however, to summarise here the relevant physiological facts and to describe briefly the more common abnormalities.

The kidney plays an important part in maintaining water, electrolyte and acid base balance; the details of the movements of ions that occur in the nephron are given on pages 376 and 377.

NORMAL DISTRIBUTION OF WATER AND ELECTROLYTES

Water. The body of a normal man of 65 kg contains approximately 40 litres of water. About 28 litres of this is intracellular, and 12 litres extracellular. The latter is composed of 9–10 litres of interstitial fluid and 2–3 litres of plasma.

Water readily passes through almost all membranes of the body and permeates easily into all fluid compartments. Its final distribution between the compartments is determined by osmotic and hydrostatic pressures and under normal conditions the total amount of water in the body is kept remarkably constant.

Electrolytes. The inorganic ions dissolved in the body water include sodium, potassium, calcium, magnesium, chloride, phosphate, bicarbonate and sulphate. These are not dispersed in the same concentrations throughout the various body fluid compartments.

Sodium and chloride are confined mainly to the extracellular fluids where they are present in average concentrations of 142 mmol/l and 100 mmol/l respectively. These ions contribute the major part of the total osmolal concentration of the plasma and extracellular fluids.

Potassium, magnesium, phosphate and sulphate are present in highest concentration inside the cells where they maintain the osmolal concentration analogous to that of sodium and chloride in the extracellular fluids. In extracellular fluid potassium is present in a mean concentration of only 4·5 mmol/l and magnesium in a concentration of about 1 mmol/l.

Bicarbonate is found in the fluid outside the cells and in the tissue cells themselves in concentrations of 25 mmol/l and 10 mmol/l respectively.

Hydrogen ions are present in a concentration of only 40 nmol/l. They are present within cells at a higher concentration than in the extracellular fluids.

Because of the permeability of the capillaries, the concentration of electrolytes in the plasma and in the extracellular fluids in the tissue spaces is very similar. Interchange between these extracellular compartments is limited, however, in respect of protein molecules, the concentration of which is many times greater in the plasma than in the interstitial fluid.

The volume of the plasma is largely determined by the balance between capillary hydrostatic pressure which tends to force water and electrolytes outwards, and the colloid osmotic pressure of the plasma proteins which draws the water and salts back into the vascular bed. In spite of the differences in the ionic pattern inside the cells as compared with that of the fluid which bathes them, in health the osmotic pressure is believed to be identical in extracellular and intracellular fluids. The differences in composition are established and maintained by the activity of ionic pumps within the cell membrane and are essential to life.

DISTURBANCES IN WATER AND ELECTROLYTE BALANCE

Changes in the volume and composition of body fluids occur both as a result of disease and as a consequence of therapeutic endeavour and drug administration. Such disturbances not only contribute to the clinical picture of many diseases, but are themselves a hindrance to recovery.

For this reason it is important to maintain the volume and the chemical composition of the body fluids and to correct as far as possible any derangements that may arise. It is also essential that specific disturbances are recognised and appropriately treated. The labelling of such abnormalities in fluid and electrolyte balance simply as 'dehydration' and the indiscriminate use of intravenous isotonic NaCl solution, i.e. 'normal' saline in an attempt to correct them is to be deprecated.

The more important disturbances of water and electrolyte balance are described below. It is convenient to discuss the disorders separately but in practice two or more often coexist.

Sodium Depletion

Normal sodium balance depends upon an equality between the amounts of sodium excreted and ingested. In health in temperate climates negligible amounts of sodium are lost in the stools and from the skin. In the absence of renal disease the kidneys possess considerable power to conserve sodium in the face of reduced intake and normal sodium balance may be maintained with a very small daily intake. For these reasons sodium depletion generally occurs because of excessive loss of salt from the body rather than because of inadequate intake.

Because of the intimate relation of salt to water balance, loss of sodium is usually accompanied by a reduction in the water content of the body. *Pure sodium depletion* unattended by significant water deficit is uncommon and occurs only as a result of abnormal loss of salt and water when an unrestricted intake of water has been permitted or encouraged. This may arise, for example, from excessive sweating in unfavourable environments when fluid loss is replenished by salt-free liquids.

In these circumstances the change in total body water may be negligible in spite of a considerable deficit of body salt. More commonly, however, conditions giving rise to sodium depletion are attended by some degree of water loss and unless large amounts of salt-free fluids have been given, a *mixed depletion* exists, though the sodium loss usually predominates over the water loss.

Causes of Sodium Depletion. In temperate regions predominant sodium depletion arises as a result of excessive loss of sodium in the urine or because of increased loss of sodium-containing fluids from the gastrointestinal tract.

Failure of the kidney to conserve sodium may develop because of intrinsic renal disease or inadequate hormonal control. Examples are found in some patients with chronic pyelonephritis (i.e. 'salt-losing nephritis'), or cystic disease of the kidney, in the diuretic phase of acute renal failure of ischaemic origin, and sometimes immediately after the relief of obstruction of the urinary tract. It also occurs in Addison's disease. Excessive loss of sodium and water in the urine occurs in the osmotic diuresis of uncontrolled diabetes mellitus and chronic uraemia. If diabetic ketoacidosis develops, urinary sodium loss is further increased because sodium is excreted along with the anions of the ketoacids until the production of renal ammonia increases (p. 378). Sodium depletion may also result from the excessive or prolonged use of diuretics.

Gastrointestinal causes of sodium depletion include all conditions involving external loss of sodium-containing fluids, i.e. acute or chronic diarrhoea, intestinal fistulae, aspiration of gastrointestinal contents and vomiting. Considerable degrees of sodium loss also occur if sodium containing fluid is sequestered in dilated loops of intestine as in ileus or in the peritoneal cavity as in ascites.

Sweating is a well-known cause of sodium depletion in tropical countries and often aggravates the degree of sodium depletion caused by disease (p. 723). Loss of sodium from the skin is also important and occurs in extensive burns, severe generalised dermatitis and in children suffering from cystic fibrosis.

Consequences of Predominant Sodium Depletion. As sodium is mainly extracellular, depletion reduces the volume of the extracellular fluids. When proportionately more sodium than water is lost, the extracellular fluids become hypotonic and the plasma sodium concentration falls.

This trend is mitigated by two events, (1) initially secretion of antidiuretic hormone (ADH) is inhibited and the proportion of water relative to solute excreted in the urine is increased, and (2) some extracellular water migrates into the cells. As a result there is a further diminution in the volume of extracellular fluid, including plasma, while the water content of the cells may increase.

The fact that predominant salt depletion chiefly affects the volume of the extracellular fluid is responsible for many of the clinical features such as loss of elasticity of the skin, diminution of intra-ocular pressure and dryness of the tongue. Thirst is not a prominent complaint, and its absence may be due to the hypotonicity of the body fluids. The decrease in blood volume leads to a reduction in cardiac output and a fall in blood pressure. The pulse rate rises. Glomerular filtration falls and, oliguria occurs; the capacity to excrete urea diminishes and uraemia develops. Selective vasoconstriction diminishes the circulation through the skin so that the extremities become pale and cold. Although the plasma sodium concentration may be within normal limits, it may be reduced to 120 mmol/l or less in severe cases or in those in whom the deficit of water has been partly made good; in such patients muscle cramps are common.

Treatment. Administration of water or of glucose in water in conditions associated with sodium depletion is fraught with danger because the hypotonicity may be further aggravated. As more salt-free fluid is given, much of the water passes into cells and initially the kidneys respond by excreting dilute urine in an attempt to restore normal osmolal concentrations; thus the extracellular fluid volume remains low. The ill-effects of such treatment, moreover, are all too easily obscured by the conventional fluid balance chart which records only fluid intake and urine output, without reference to sodium balance.

Adequate treatment consists of giving salt and water by mouth or an isotonic NaCl solution intravenously. The latter is required in all but mild cases with normal recumbent blood pressure. In adults with moderately severe depletion 2–4 litres of isotonic NaCl solution intravenously in 6–12 hours represents the usual requirements.

In severe cases with marked circulatory impairment, deficits equivalent to 4–8 litres of isotonic NaCl solution occur. Such deficits should be repaired largely by isotonic sodium chloride solution but when acidosis is present some of the sodium should be given as isotonic $NaHCO_3$ (p. 101). The first 2–3 litres should be given rapidly within the first 2–3 hours, the remainder being given within 24–48 hours.

The best guides to the amount required are the disappearance of the signs of sodium depletion and the restoration of normal blood pressure and pulse rate. Plasma sodium determinations are useful in controlling the treatment of severe cases, especially when the causative disease is likely to lead to a continued salt loss, (e.g. severe and persisting diarrhoea) and in regulating the relative amounts of sodium and water to be given. Excessive administration of salt is to be avoided; the bases of the lungs should be frequently examined for crepitations, and the jugular venous pressure assessed. In severe cases it is often helpful to monitor the right atrial (central venous) pressure or the pulmonary capillary (wedge) pressure.

Severe sodium depletion is almost invariably associated with water depletion and disturbance in acid-base balance. Frequently potassium balance, and occasionally magnesium metabolism, are also disturbed. In these circumstances appropriate amounts of other electrolytes need to be added to the intravenous fluid once the circulation has been restored.

Primary Water Depletion

Pure or predominant water depletion is one of the simplest of chemical disorders. The water content of the body is reduced both absolutely and relative to the sodium content, and the osmolal concentration of the extracellular fluids rises.

In a temperate climate an adult loses between 0·5–1 litre of water daily in the expired air and by evaporation from the skin. This loss continues irrespective of the water intake. The urine is the other main channel of excretion of water but the volume of urine can be reduced if water is in short supply by increasing its concentration up to a limit determined by renal concentrating ability and the amount of solute to be excreted.

Causes of Water Depletion. Primary water depletion occurs less commonly in clinical practice than sodium depletion and usually arises because water intake is reduced below an amount necessary to maintain balance.

Water deficiency is liable to occur in patients who suffer from dysphagia or have obstructive lesions of the oesophagus or in those who are comatose, depressed or apathetic, as is common for example in the aged. It then occurs because the intake falls below the amount being lost from the lungs, skin and urine. This obligatory daily loss of water from the lungs and skin is increased by hyperpnoea, hyperthyroidism and in fever.

Excessive loss of water in the urine is a less common cause of water depletion but occurs in patients in whom the renal power of concentration is markedly restricted, as for example in diabetes insipidus or hyperparathyroidism.

Water deficiency may be induced by giving patients liquid feeds containing large amounts of protein or salt mixed with insufficient water. Newborn infants are especially susceptible to this danger as their power to concentrate the urine is not fully developed.

Consequences of Water Depletion. As water is lost from the body the extracellular fluid becomes hypertonic and the concentration of plasma sodium rises. Water then migrates from the cells until osmotic equilibrium is re-established and intracellular dehydration occurs. The overall body water loss is thus shared by the extracellular and intracellular fluids. For this reason the circulatory signs of dehydration are not so obvious as those of salt depletion.

Thirst is usual unless the patient is senile or confused. The migration of water from the cells to the extracellular fluids helps to maintain the volume of the extracellular fluid nearly within normal limits temporarily, so that the blood pressure, haemoglobin, and plasma electrolyte concentrations remain unaltered until considerable depletion has occurred. The patient, however, may exhibit mental confusion or complain of vertigo and have difficulty in swallowing. In severe cases the skin and tissues acquire a curious 'doughy' consistency.

Ultimately renal blood flow is reduced and the blood urea concentration rises. At this stage the plasma sodium concentration and the haemoglobin concentration then become elevated.

Treatment. Water depletion can often be prevented if the need to maintain an adequate intake is recognised in patients who are unable to swallow or who do not drink enough of their own accord.

Established depletion should be treated by giving salt-free fluids. The use of isotonic NaCl solution is contraindicated. If the patient is conscious and is not vomiting, water should be given by mouth until thirst is quenched and thereafter amounts of between 1·2 to 2·5 litres per day are usually sufficient. If the patient is unable to swallow fluids in sufficient amounts, 5% glucose in water should be given by intravenous infusion.

The amount required varies with the degree of depletion. In moderately severe cases 2–4 litres of 5% glucose in the course of 24 hours is usually sufficient. In severe water depletion 5–10 litres may be needed and such a deficit should be replaced over 2–3 days to avoid sudden shift of water into cells. The best guides to the amount of fluid required are the clinical improvement of the patient and the increase in the volume of urine, which should rise to at least 1·5 litres per 24 hours.

When water depletion is associated with salt loss, isotonic NaCl solution and water are both required and should both be given in amounts determined by clinical assessment of the relative degrees of the two deficiencies.

Potassium Depletion

Maintenance of potassium balance depends largely on the regulation of urinary excretion of this ion, since in health over 85% of the daily potassium intake is excreted in the urine and the remainder in the stools.

Causes of Potassium Depletion. Potassium depletion usually occurs as a result of excessive loss of potassium from the gastrointestinal tract or in the urine. Alimentary losses occur as a result of severe acute or chronic diarrhoea, vomiting, fistulous drainage or gastric aspiration. The habitual use of laxatives is sometimes a factor which is easily missed and a potassium secreting villous adenoma of the rectum is an important but uncommon cause. In the malabsorption syndrome excessive potassium loss can occur even when the stools are well formed.

Renal wastage of potassium is more complex. Since most filtered potassium is reabsorbed in the upper nephron, urinary potassium is largely determined by the rate at which the ion enters the tubular fluid in the distal nephron into which it diffuses passively down a luminal negative, transepithelial, electrochemical gradient. The magnitude of this gradient increases (i) when the intracellular concentration of potassium rises, (ii) when the rate of flow through the distal nephron increases, (iii) when the rate of reabsorption of sodium in the distal tubule increases and (iv) when negatively charged anions are present in excess in the distal tubules. In most cases in which renal wastage of potassium occurs, one or more of these factors augment diffusion of potassium into the urine. The clinical conditions in which these factors operate are considered under the two categories, extrarenal and renal.

1. *Disorders in which Extrarenal Factors Increase the Rate of Potassium Excretion*. In primary aldosteronism, Cushing's syndrome and in patients receiving corticosteroids or carbenoxolone the uptake of potassium into the tubular cells and the intracellular potassium concentration are increased; this encourages the diffusion of potassium into the tubular lumen. A similar mechanism probably operates in secondary aldosteronism occurring in the course of heart failure, liver disease, the nephrotic syndrome or renovascular hypertension.

Loss of potassium in the urine in metabolic or respiratory alkalosis is well recognised and is thought also to be due to an increase in the concentration of potassium in tubular cells. This loss is further augmented by the presence of poorly reabsorbed negatively charged bicarbonate ions in the distal tubular fluid. Cell potassium is reduced in acidosis but paradoxically in long-standing metabolic acidosis, urinary excretion of potassium is often increased because of an accompanying increase in the delivery of sodium and water to the distal nephron. Diuretics, including osmotically active substances such as mannitol and glucose, which increase delivery of sodium and water to the distal nephron also facilitate potassium loss by this means.

In diabetic ketoacidosis the delivery of both poorly reabsorbable anions of ketoacids and increased amounts of sodium and water to the distal tubule result in loss of potassium in the urine.

2. *Renal Diseases in which the Rate of Potassium Excretion is Increased*. Occasionally potassium is lost in the urine as a result of a primary renal disease. Thus, renal potassium wastage occurs in renal tubular acidosis, probably because of a change in the permeability to potassium of the luminal membrane of the distal tubular cells and because of the alkaline urine. Loss of potassium also occurs in the recovery phase of acute tubular necrosis and after relief of severe urinary tract obstruction.

It should be appreciated that circumstances which encourage transfer of potassium from the cells to the extracellular fluid lead to increased urinary loss and ultimately to potassium depletion. These include impaired carbohydrate metabolism, severe water depletion, shock, hypoxia and acidosis of metabolic or respiratory origin in which buffering of H^+ in cells leads to loss of potassium ions from them.

Many elderly people who take a diet inadequate in potassium become mildly potassium-depleted. The precise mechanism is unknown but it is most likely due to continued urinary loss.

Consequences and Clinical Features of Potassium Depletion. Clinically significant depletion of potassium may occur without alteration in the plasma potassium concentration and the diagnosis of intracellular potassium deficit is made difficult by the inaccessibility of the intracellular fluid to analysis. Potassium lack may be suggested biochemically by an associated elevation in plasma bicarbonate concentration. This effect is believed to be due to the migration of hydrogen and sodium ions from the extracellular into the intracellular fluids.

The most important features of potassium depletion are due to changes in electrical potential across cell membranes. Symptoms attributable to potassium deficiency include apathy, muscular weakness, mental confusion and abdominal distension. It is clear that such features arise in the course of many diseases. Nevertheless, their occurrence in circumstances which are known to lead to potassium deficiency, and their relief after potassium administration, justify the diagnosis.

Potassium depletion reduces the ability of the kidney to concentrate urine, hence polyuria and thirst commonly occur. Potassium depletion may induce cardiac arrhythmias such as atrial tachycardia; it also increases susceptibility to intoxication with digitalis. Severe potassium depletion lowers the cardiac output and this may give rise to oedema.

Potassium deficiency sufficiently severe to be associated with reduction of the plasma concentration is more easily recognised, but is less common than simple intracellular depletion. It may occur in any of the conditions mentioned above if the deficiency is sufficiently severe and is particularly liable to develop in cases of diabetic ketoacidosis which have been vigorously treated with solutions of sodium salts or glucose and insulin; this therapy causes a migration of potassium from the extracellular to the intracellular space with resulting hypokalaemia.

The clinical picture of extracellular potassium deficit is characterised by generalised muscular weakness with paresis or flaccid paralysis and ileus. Paraesthaesiae are also frequently present and loss of memory, disorientation and mental confusion may occur. The electrocardiogram commonly shows a small T wave and ST depression. Death may occur from respiratory paralysis or cardiac arrest if potassium depletion is unrelieved or if treatment is inadequate.

Treatment. Potassium depletion should be treated by giving a potassium salt orally or intravenously. The former route is more commonly used and carries less risk of inducing hyperkalaemia than parenteral administration. The normal daily intake of potassium is about 2–3 g (50–80 mmol).

1. Established deficiencies of moderate severity (about 400 mmol) can be remedied by giving 10–15 g/day of potassium chloride, in divided doses, for some days and a diet rich in potassium, i.e. containing fruit juices, coffee and milk based food and meat.

Potassium chloride tablets sometimes cause gastrointestinal ulceration especially if there is delay in intestinal transit. 'Slow release' tablets of potassium chloride are less troublesome in this respect; each tablet contains 600 mg (8 mmol) of KCl. Some patients tolerate effervescent potassium tablets more readily as these appear to be less nauseating. Each tablet contains 250 mg of potassium and some also contain chloride. The latter is useful in correcting the metabolic alkalosis which is associated with potassium depletion and which is frequently due to concurrent chloride depletion (p. 101).

2. Intravenous infusions of potassium chloride are needed for patients who are unable to take potassium by mouth, but should be given only when there is hypokalaemia as established by chemical analysis. Such infusions should rarely be used in the presence of significant sodium depletion, anuria or oliguria and only when facilities for repeated chemical analysis are available. Associated water and salt depletion should be treated first.

For intravenous administration, potassium chloride (1·5 g in sterile ampoules) can be conveniently added to 500 ml of isotonic NaCl or 5% glucose solution. The solution then contains 40 mmol/l and should be given slowly over 2 to 3 hours. Repeated measurements of the plasma potassium are necessary to determine whether further infusions are required.

Administration of potassium by mouth should be started as soon as possible, as most of the deficit is best corrected by this means. When the depletion of potassium has arisen because of persistent vomiting and is associated with alkalosis due to loss of gastric hydrochloric acid, potassium is conveniently given with sodium and ammonium chloride as described on page 102.

Prophylactic administration of potassium chloride (3–4 g daily) or effervescent potassium tablets should be given to patients who are being treated by drugs known to increase urinary loss of potassium. These include corticosteroids and many diuretics.

Potassium Excess

Causes. An increased concentration of potassium in the blood and extracellular fluid most often occurs in association with severe oliguria or anuria. It is commonly found in conditions leading to acute renal failure, e.g. circulatory failure from blood loss or injury and in severe cases of adrenal insufficiency. It may occur in diabetic ketoacidosis prior to adequate treatment with insulin and intravenous solutions. Some patients with severe chronic renal failure develop hyperkalaemia especially if potassium supplements, spironolactone or potassium conserving diuretics (p. 97) are given.

Consequences of Potassium Excess. Patients with hyperkalaemia develop muscular weakness which may progress to flaccid paralysis with loss of tendon reflexes. Abdominal distension due to ileus also occurs. These features are indistinguishable from those of hypokalaemia. In addition tingling of the face, hands and feet is common.

Cardiac disturbances are often the first and only manifestation of hyperkalaemia. The pulse becomes irregular and heart block of variable degree occurs. Typical electrocardiographic changes include increase in the amplitude of the T wave, atrioventricular and intraventricular conduction defects and ultimately ventricular fibrillation or asystole.

Hyperkalaemia is of considerable clinical importance because of the danger of cardiac arrest with concentrations of plasma potassium above 7·5 mmol/l. The diagnosis is made more frequently by knowing the circumstances in which intoxication is likely to arise and confirming the suspicion by measuring plasma potassium than from any specific clinical feature.

Treatment. It is important to prevent the occurrence of potassium intoxication in conditions associated with oliguria and anuria. The recommendations made with regard to the diet in acute renal failure (p. 401) are designed with this aim in view. When dealing with an established case of hyperkalaemia, the following measures are advised:

1. Migration of potassium into cells should be encouraged by giving glucose and insulin and alkali. 5 to 10 units of soluble insulin and 50 ml of a 50% solution of glucose should be given intravenously and repeated if hyperkalaemia recurs. Alternatively 20% glucose solution containing 6–12 units of insulin is infused slowly over 6–12 hours. Provided there is no evidence of circulatory overload, isotonic sodium bicarbonate solution should be infused slowly until the plasma bicarbonate is in the upper reference range.

2. When severe electrocardiographic changes are present, 10 ml of 10% calcium gluconate should be injected intravenously to reduce the cardiotoxic effects of the potassium ion. The ECG is monitored throughout the procedure.

3. Any deficit of sodium or water should be replaced in order to restore normal circulation. Metabolic and respiratory acidosis should be corrected (pp. 101 and 103).

Measures to prevent recurrence of hyperkalaemia include (1) the dietary restriction of foods rich in potassium, and (2) administration of sodium or calcium loaded resins which absorb potassium in the intestine from the blood and intestinal secretions and contents. 30 g suspended in a small volume of water is given by mouth or by retention enema as required, usually 3 or 4 times a day.

If these methods fail or if the rise of concentration of potassium is rapid, removal of potassium by peritoneal dialysis or by haemodialysis is indicated.

Magnesium Deficiency and Excess

Disorders of magnesium metabolism are occasionally responsible for otherwise puzzling clinical features and are susceptible to therapeutic control.

Magnesium Deficiency. The most frequent cause of magnesium deficiency is prolonged diarrhoea or vomiting, which has been treated with parenteral fluid without magnesium supplements. It is associated with chronic diarrhoea and severe undernutrition, such as occurs in protein-energy malnutrition and the malabsorption syndrome. Uncontrolled diabetes mellitus, aldosteronism, hyperparathyroidism, the diuretic phase of acute renal failure and chronic alcoholism lead to magnesium deficiency from excessive urinary loss. It occasionally follows long continued diuretic therapy.

Clinical features are predominantly neuromuscular, with tremor, choreiform movements and aimless plucking of the bedclothes. Mental depression, confusion, agitation, epileptiform convulsions and hallucinations also occur. The diagnosis can be confirmed by finding the concentration of magnesium in the plasma to be less than 0.75 mmol/l.

Magnesium deficiency is best treated parenterally; 30–50 mmol of magnesium chloride may be added to 1 litre of 5% glucose or other isotonic solution and given over a period of 12 to 24 hours. The infusion should be repeated daily until the plasma concentration remains within the normal range.

Magnesium excess mainly occurs in acute and chronic renal disease and contributes to the central nervous features associated with uraemia. Its treatment is that of the primary disorder.

Water Excess

Healthy individuals can safely drink very large volumes of water and respond to this by a vigorous water diuresis. The capacity of the kidney to excrete water when given without electrolytes is dependent upon many factors which include the rate of glomerular filtration and the power of the distal tubules to produce a dilute urine.

Many patients who are ill have, for a variety of reasons, a restricted ability to dilute the urine when given large amounts of water. These include patients suffering from acute and chronic renal disease, severe heart failure, hypopituitarism, adrenocortical insufficiency, severe hypothyroidism and hepatic cirrhosis or liver failure. Occasionally tumours of the lung, pancreas or ovaries secrete a polypeptide with antidiuretic properties which leads to water intoxication. Post-operative patients are also incapable of diluting the urine because of the liberation of antidiuretic hormone by the stress of the operation. In addition, a number of drugs induce water retention by releasing pituitary vasopressin and can lead to water intoxication. These include carbamazepine, and morphine. Chlorpropamide, phenylbutazone, and indomethacin exert a similar effect by enhancing the action of the hormone on the distal nephron.

In all these circumstances even a modest water intake reduces the plasma osmolality and the concentration of sodium and produces symptoms which are primarily those of disordered cerebral function; these are partly due to cerebral oedema and include dizziness, headache, nausea and mental confusion. Severe water intoxication can produce convulsions, coma and death. Diagnosis depends upon being aware of the circumstances in which water intoxication is likely to occur and the demonstration of a plasma sodium concentration below 130 mmol/l.

Treatment consists of restricting water intake for a few days. In severe cases 100 ml 5% sodium chloride solution should be given intravenously and repeated in a few hours if there is little or no clinical improvement. The use of fludrocortisone is beneficial in cases of hyponatraemia due to tumours and is also indicated in the treatment of Addison's disease in which it is given with cortisone.

Sodium and Water Excess

In health, the total amount of sodium in the body is kept within narrow limits in spite of great day-to-day variations in the amount ingested. Positive sodium balance with consequent accumulation of sodium results from renal excretion that is inadequate in relation to the amount ingested. The accumulation is generally accompanied by the retention of water so that the concentration of sodium in the extracellular space is usually not materially altered. When the distribution of the retained fluid is generalised, the expansion in the volume of the extracellular space does not become clinically detectable until the increase is of the order of 15%.

The primary mechanisms responsible for the accumulation of water and salt which lead to oedema, vary with the nature of the disease and they are discussed in the appropriate sections of this book. They include (i) reduction in the colloid osmotic pressure from hypoproteinaemia as occurs in the nephrotic syndrome; (ii) an increase in venous hydrostatic pressure with migration of fluid from the vascular space to the tissue spaces as in heart failure and (iii) primary inability to eliminate salt and water in the urine as in acute glomerulonephritis. In addition several compensatory reactions occur which promote further retention of water and salt. These include a rise in the level of circulating antidiuretic hormone and also an increased secretion of aldosterone mediated by the renin-angiotensin system (p. 379).

The therapeutic use of corticosteroids, androgens or oral contraceptives with a high oestrogen content may also give rise to water and sodium retention by virtue of their action on the kidney. Other drugs which do so include carbenoxolone and phenylbutazone.

Some oedema is not uncommon in normal women during the premenstrual stage of the menstrual cycle. Oedema is commonly present in normal pregnancy but is more severe and is associated with proteinuria when renal disease or pregnancy hypertension is present.

Other disorders associated with generalised oedema include nutritional oedema and thiamin deficiency. In some diseases several mechanisms appear to be operating simultaneously. This is exemplified particularly in the oedema and ascites of hepatic cirrhosis in which portal hypertension, hypoproteinaemia and possibly salt retaining and antidiuretic hormones all contribute.

The clinical features of water and salt accumulation depend to some extent upon the distribution of the retained fluid. These are described under the various diseases.

Principles of Treatment. These are:

1. The use of measures designed to remedy specific factors leading to the oedema, e.g. digitalis in heart failure, corticosteroids in some forms of glomerulonephritis, intravenous administration of plasma proteins or salt-free albumin in conditions associated with hypoproteinaemia, and a high protein diet in oedema of nutritional origin, hepatic cirrhosis and the nephrotic syndrome.

2. The restriction by dietary means of the raw materials necessary for the formation of extracellular fluid, i.e. water and salt.

3. Increasing the excretion of salt and water by the use of effective diuretics.

Diuretic Therapy. Drugs which block reabsorption of sodium or chloride by the renal tubules also increase the urinary volume because of the osmotic effect of the extra solute. The following are the most important diuretics discussed in order of their potency.

HIGH POTENCY DIURETICS. The diuresis induced by these agents is rapid, intense and of short duration. They include frusemide and bumetanide. They are sometimes called *loop diuretics* because their predominant action reduces the reabsorption of sodium and chloride in the ascending limb of the loop of Henle (Fig. 11.1 p. 377). As a result they reduce the renal concentrating power and so eliminate a greater volume of water than do other diuretics; because they deliver an increased amount of sodium and water to the distal tubules they also lead to increased potassium loss in the urine. Occasionally a precipitate diuresis may cause acute retention of urine, particularly in elderly men with prostatic obstruction.

Frusemide may be given orally (40–80 mg) or intravenously (20–40 mg). On a weight basis *bumetanide* is more potent than frusemide, comparable oral doses being 1–2 mg, but is otherwise similar in its action. Frusemide and bumetanide are drugs of great value in the treatment of generalised oedema and severe pulmonary oedema. They have few adverse effects but in susceptible subjects may lead to a rise in blood sugar or in plasma urate with the risk of precipitating an attack of gout. Tinnitus and myalgia may occur in renal failure. Adverse effects on electrolytes are discussed below.

MEDIUM POTENCY DIURETICS. Thiazide diuretics have two separate effects on renal function. They have a variable influence on the activity of carbonic anhydrase and so of sodium bicarbonate reabsorption in the proximal renal tubules, but their main action is to depress tubular reabsorption of sodium and chloride in the early distal convoluted tubules. Potassium depletion occurs both because of the reduction of H^+ secretion and because of the delivery of increased amounts of sodium and water to the late distal tubules.

Chlorothiazide was the prototype but the drugs most commonly used now are *bendrofluazide* (10 mg) and *hydrochlorothiazide* (100 mg). *Chlor-*

thalidone (100–200 mg) is similar in its action to chlorothiazide and its analogues but it produces a slower and more prolonged diuresis extending over 48 hours. Adverse effects of thiazides include impotence, postural hypotension and allergic rashes. Hyperuricaemia and diabetes may also be produced in susceptible patients. Adverse effects on electrolytes are discussed below.

LOW POTENCY DIURETICS. These consist of several agents which are not sufficiently potent by themselves but, because of other properties, are sometimes valuable when combined with more potent diuretics.

Amiloride (20 mg) and *triamterene* (200 mg) antagonise the effects of aldosterone. Neither has a steroid structure and they do not compete for aldosterone binding sites. Their very mild natriuretic effect is due to inhibition of sodium reabsorption in the distal tubule; potassium secretion is not increased and so they do not lead to potassium deficiency.

Spironolactone (100–400 daily) is a specific antagonist to aldosterone and reverses the renal effect of the hormone. Its important clinical effect is the reduction in the capacity of the kidney to excrete potassium which it shares with the low potency diuretics. These diuretics should not be given in the presence of renal failure or with potassium supplements as dangerous hyperkalaemia may develop.

ADVERSE EFFECTS OF DIURETIC THERAPY ON ELECTROLYTES. *Potassium Depletion.* High potency and thiazide diuretics produce potassium depletion, especially when given repeatedly over long periods and when combined with diets low in sodium. Symptoms of potassium deficit may arise before satisfactory loss of oedema has been achieved and are then superimposed upon the clinical features of water and sodium accumulation.

This state of affairs is especially prone to develop in the treatment of severe cardiac failure (p. 154) and is particularly serious since it may be responsible for increased sensitivity to digitalis, with the development of toxic manifestations to this drug before control of the heart failure has been attained.

In hepatic disease with oedema and ascites the potassium depletion may seriously aggravate or precipitate the neurological features of hepatic insufficiency. Prophylactic administration of potassium is therefore essential when diuretics are being given frequently, e.g. on alternate days. Between 3 and 4 g potassium chloride is required daily given either as slow release or effervescent tablets.

Sodium Depletion and Oligaemia. Overtreatment with diuretics is likely to occur when high potency diuretics are given over prolonged periods. These patients exhibit the features of sodium depletion although paradoxically some, in whom the plasma albumin is low, may still be oedematous.

The circulatory characteristics of sodium depletion, due to oligaemia, are present, namely hypotension with an increase in the pulse rate. The blood urea is increased and the plasma sodium is reduced to 130 mmol/l or less. Such patients usually suffer from advanced cardiac or hepatic disease associated with hypoproteinaemia. In these circumstances persistent attempts to reduce the oedema lead to further deterioration. Relief may sometimes be achieved by infusion of 25–100 g plasma protein fraction to restore the blood volume. Diuretics should be withheld temporarily and a diet unrestricted in its salt content permitted.

Hyponatraemia. In cardiac and hepatic diseases associated with severe oedema hyponatraemia sometimes develops without oligaemia. This is due to inability to excrete water normally because of poor renal perfusion and increased ADH release. It is exacerbated particularly by thiazide diuretics.

In these circumstances the water intake should be restricted to a volume equal to or less than the output and a loop diuretic substituted. Occasionally, when symptoms of water intoxication are present and the plasma sodium is less than 125 mmol/l, slow infusion of 100–200 ml of 5% saline may be needed to relieve symptoms.

DIAGNOSIS OF DISTURBANCES IN WATER AND ELECTROLYTE BALANCE

It is apparent from this summary of the consequences of body depletion of sodium, water, potassium and magnesium and of potassium and magnesium excess, that these disturbances present considerable diagnostic difficulty and are not characterised by pathognomonic signs or symptoms. The neuromuscular abnormalities of potassium depletion are clinically indistinguishable from those of hyperkalaemia; severe sodium depletion is attended in the majority of instances by considerable water deficit and is not readily distinguishable on clinical grounds from severe degrees of water deficit. Furthermore, it is not uncommon for dual electrolyte deficits to develop simultaneously. For example, in diabetic keto-acidosis, potassium depletion may occur in conjunction with predominant sodium depletion. In addition the symptoms of lethargy, apathy and mental confusion are common accompaniments both of major electrolyte disorders and of many diseases in which no significant body fluid disturbance exists.

It should also be recognised that the results obtained from biochemical analysis of blood and urine are of limited diagnostic value. Potassium or magnesium deficit may occur without significant alteration in their plasma concentrations, and serious sodium depletion commonly develops with plasma sodium concentrations within the recognised limits of the reference range. A low plasma sodium may not even indicate salt depletion, and hyponatraemia is frequently seen in conditions of water excess; it also occurs in the late stages of malignant disease and in generalised tuberculosis.

The measurement of electrolytes in the urine without knowledge of the dietary intake is also obviously of limited value. In the majority of conditions in which there is a reduced blood or ECF volume the urinary loss of sodium is less than 10–20 mmol/day. However, the presence of larger amounts in the urine of patients who are volume-depleted strongly suggests a renal salt wasting disorder. Urinary potassium determination is also of limited value but is sometimes helpful in patients who are found unexpectedly to have hypokalaemia. Then the finding of a urinary K^+ of more than 20 mmol/day indicates that the kidney is responsible unless extrarenal losses are of recent and sudden onset. In contrast the finding of a urinary K^+ of less than 10 mmol/l in the presence of hypokalaemia indicates that the route of the loss is extrarenal and is usually gastro-intestinal.

Accurate diagnosis largely depends upon a knowledge of the conditions and diseases which may give rise to abnormalities in water and electrolyte balance. In patients with such diseases, the suspicion that these abnormalities may exist is strengthened by the presence of the clinical features known to occur with them and possibly by the results of appropriate biochemical and electrocardiographic examinations.

By understanding the mechanism by which the economy of the fluids of the body becomes disturbed and by the intelligent use of the reparative fluids which have been described, much can be done to restore the distortions of body fluid balance wrought by disease.

HYDROGEN ION CONCENTRATION

Life is possible only if the blood is kept within a narrow range of alkalinity, and, in health, a physiological hydrogen ion concentration of 36–44 nmol/l corresponding to a pH between 7·37 and 7·45 is maintained by two widely different mechanisms which are closely integrated. Some understanding of these mechanisms is necessary to appreciate the clinical implications of acidosis and alkalosis.

The blood is alkaline because it contains bicarbonate, phosphate and proteins which are quite strong bases. It also contains carbonic acid and the $[H^+]$ of the blood depends principally upon the ratio of the main acid component, carbonic acid and the main base, bicarbonate.

The concentration of carbonic acid in the plasma is determined by the partial pressure of carbon dioxide (P_{CO_2}) in the alveoli. The latter is normally about 5·3 kPa (p. 204) which gives rise to little over 1 mmol/l of carbonic acid in physical solution in the plasma. The alveolar partial pressure of carbon dioxide is itself maintained steady by the equality between its rate of production by the tissues and the rate at which ventilation eliminates it from the body. On the other hand, the concentration of bicarbonate is regulated by the tubular epithelium of the kidneys and in health is kept at about 22–27 mmol/l by the mechanism described on page 378.

A great many metabolic processes result in the production of acids and these must be eliminated from the body if the reaction of the tissues and the blood is to remain within the normal range. The route of disposal of acids depends upon whether or not they are capable of being oxidised completely to carbon dioxide and water. Carbon dioxide forms carbonic acid within the body and is eliminated as carbon dioxide by ventilation. Other acids such as acetoacetic acid or sulphuric acid which are derived from the oxidation of fatty acids or sulphur-containing proteins respectively are excreted by the kidneys.

At the site of their production in the tissues and during their carriage in the blood all acids increase the hydrogen ion concentration. The extent of this increase is minimised by the stabilising power of the blood and tissues and this in turn depends on the presence of the physiologically important buffers.

Carbonic acid is produced by metabolic reactions in far greater amounts than any other acid. A small part of the carbon dioxide is transported in the blood reversibly bound to haemoglobin as a carbamino compound. A greater part is converted to carbonic acid in the red blood cells which are rich in carbonic anhydrase, and is then buffered by haemoglobin after it has given its oxygen to the tissues and has been converted to deoxyhaemoglobin (Fig. 5.1). The hydrogen ions of the carbonic acid are taken up by the haemoglobin in the red cells while the bicarbonate ions move out from the red cells to the plasma in exchange for chloride ions (chloride shift). Most of the carbonic acid added to the blood therefore appears not as acid but as bicarbonate ion. When the blood passes through the lungs and the haemoglobin is reoxygenated this process is reversed and the carbon dioxide formed is exhaled by ventilation.

In health, on a normal diet, 40–80 mmol of non-volatile acid are excreted in the urine daily. However in some disorders, notably diabetic ketoacidosis, a large amount of acetoacetic acid is formed. The tissues and blood are buffered against these acids by a different mechanism which involves in particular the sodium bicarbonate and carbonic acid buffer system in the plasma.

The addition of acid to the plasma results in a

Fig. 5.1 Transport of CO_2

movement of the reactions in the direction indicated by the broad arrow (Fig. 5.2). As a result of this and of a similar reaction on the part of the other buffer systems, many of the hydrogen ions which would otherwise increase the acidity of the plasma are removed to form increased amounts of carbonic acid. There is a corresponding diminution in the concentration of bicarbonate ions. By this means the $[H^+]$ of the plasma rises far less than it would do if the buffers were not present.

Fig. 5.2 Effect of acid on the blood buffer system.

The rise in $[H^+]$ stimulates ventilation and the excess carbonic acid is removed from the body as carbon dioxide. The anion of the acid (e.g. acetoacetate) and the depleted body bicarbonate are dealt with simultaneously by the kidney. The renal tubules form carbonic acid, much of the hydrogen ion of which is excreted in the form of ammonium ions along with the acid anion. The bicarbonate ion generated in this process is returned to the blood and reconstitutes the depleted blood buffer (p. 378).

These buffering and excreting mechanisms are continually in operation in response to the normal production of acids derived from food and its metabolism. It is clear from this simplified description that the important limiting factor in the buffering power of blood is the available haemoglobin and bicarbonate. The excreting power of the kidneys is the limiting factor in the body's ability to rid itself of the hydrogen ions and anions derived from inorganic and organic acids other than carbonic acid.

DISTURBANCES IN HYDROGEN ION CONCENTRATION

Abnormalities in the reaction of the body fluids are reflected in changes in the concentration of carbonic acid (i.e $Paco_2$) and by alterations in body base, notably that of bicarbonate. The estimation of $Paco_2$ is of particular value in respiratory disorders and its use in these conditions is described on page 214.

As there is no entirely satisfactory method available for the determination of $[HCO_3^-]$, it is usually calculated from a knowledge either of $Paco_2$ or total co_2 and pH using the Henderson Hasselbach equation or a nomogram based upon it. Since the concentration of bicarbonate is itself influenced by $Paco_2$ it is common practice to express the $[HCO_3^-]$ as the concentration which would exist at a standard value of $Paco_2$ of 5.3 kPa. It is then known as standard bicarbonate and normally ranges betwen 22 and 26 mmol/l.

Metabolic Acidosis

Metabolic acidosis arises as a result of the production or ingestion of acids other than carbonic acid, or as a consequence of body depletion of the base bicarbonate. The condition is characterised by a rise in $[H^+]$ and a marked reduction in the concentration of bicarbonate in the plasma. The $Paco_2$ is reduced secondarily by the hyperventilation produced by stimulation of respiration; this mitigates to some extent the increased $[H^+]$ which arises from the fall in $[HCO_3^-]$.

The production of large amounts of lactic acid in vigorous exercise is probably the most common cause of acidosis and is to be regarded as physiological. Shock from any cause, notably severe myocardial infarction or cardiac arrest, causes metabolic acidosis because of hypoxia of the tissues and the accumulation of organic acids, particularly lactic acid. Lactic acid acidosis is also a recognised complication of treatment with oral hypoglycaemic biguanides such as phenformin; it is also seen in acute alcoholic intoxication and severe liver failure. In all these circumstances the accumulation of lactic acid is related to a rise in the ratio of cellular NADH:NAD.

Other important causes of acidosis are diabetic ketoacidosis and renal failure. In the former condition, β-hydroxybutyric acid and acetoacetic acid are produced in abnormally large amounts, and at a rate which is greater than the capacity of the body to oxidise them. In patients with acute or chronic renal failure and renal tubular acidosis, the ability of the kidneys to conserve and generate bicarbonate ions and to produce and secrete hydrogen and ammonium ions is impaired.

A number of ingested substances may also be responsible. Salicylate intoxication produces metabolic acidosis as well as respiratory alkalosis (p. 102). Intoxication with methanol or ethylene glycol may also do so because their oxidation results in the formation of formic acid and oxalic acid respectively.

Depletion of body bicarbonate occurs from direct loss of sodium bicarbonate in the stools in chronic or severe acute diarrhoea or from loss of intestinal contents from fistulae or by intestinal aspiration.

Consequences of Metabolic Acidosis. The most obvious consequence of acidosis is the stimulation of respiration by the abnormally high blood concentration of hydrogen ions. In severe cases the respirations become deep and rapid (Kussmaul's respiration).

It is clear, however, from the list of causes given above that the clinical picture in the individual case is largely determined by the underlying condition and by the presence of other concomitant disturbances in water and salt balance. By the time acidosis is severe in diabetic ketoacidosis, considerable water and salt depletion has usually occurred. The acidosis of chronic diarrhoea is similarly associated with salt loss and especially with potassium deficit. The failure of ammonium and hydrogen ion production by the kidney in chronic nephritis, which leads to acidosis, is commonly accompanied by abnormal loss of sodium and potassium in the urine.

As in the case of disturbances in water and electrolyte balance, the diagnosis of metabolic acidosis is facilitated by an awareness of those pathological conditions in which it is likely to arise. The diagnosis should be confirmed by the determination of the concentration of $[H^+]$ and of bicarbonate in the blood. In acidosis of moderate degree plasma bicarbonate is reduced to 15 mmol/l, while concentrations below 10 mmol/l represent severe degrees of acidosis.

Treatment. Since metabolic acidosis is commonly associated with some degree of sodium depletion and water deficiency, it is reasonable to correct these disturbances, in the first instance, by the administration of isotonic NaCl solution (p. 90); this is a neutral solution and by itself might be expected to have only a little influence on the reaction of the blood and tissues. In fact, provided the kidneys are not primarily diseased and provided the degree of sodium and water depletion is not so severe as to impair renal function seriously, its intravenous administration is usually effective in correcting metabolic acidosis of moderate severity. Its success depends upon the capacity of the kidneys to generate bicarbonate from carbon dioxide and water and to retain this with the infused sodium, rejecting the chloride in the urine (p. 379).

In the presence of renal disease, severe acidosis and severe sodium depletion giving rise to uraemia, it is unwise to depend upon the collaboration of the kidney for the alkalising effect of sodium chloride. In these circumstances, isotonic sodium bicarbonate should be given by intravenous infusion in addition to isotonic sodium chloride.

The two solutions should be given in a ratio of 1 to 2 and need not be mixed. The total volume of the combined solutions required varies with the severity of the sodium depletion and with the degree of acidosis. A moderately severe case of diabetic acidosis, for example, may require as much as 4–6 litres in the first 24 hours, of which 1–2 litres should be the isotonic bicarbonate solution.

The latter infusion should be given for as long as there is evidence of acidosis, as determined by the estimation of blood $[H^+]$ and of the bicarbon-

ate concentration. When this has returned to normal levels, it may be necessary to continue the intravenous infusion of isotonic sodium chloride alone. This is indicated if there is still evidence of predominant sodium depletion.

In severe shock or cardiac arrest, acidosis develops without sodium depletion. In these circumstances it is best to give sodium bicarbonate in a small volume of hypertonic concentration, i.e. 50–100 ml 8·4% solution intravenously as a bolus. The treatment of lactic acid acidosis in diabetes is given on page 477.

Metabolic Alkalosis

Metabolic alkalosis arises most commonly as a result of the abnormal loss of hydrochloric acid in the course of prolonged or severe vomiting. Chloride deficiency itself also leads to alkalosis because it stimulates the renal tubular reabsorption of bicarbonate. This is especially liable to occur with the use of high potency diuretics which block chloride reabsorption. Potassium depletion also gives rise to alkalosis as this encourages the transfer of hydrogen ions into cells as well as their excretion in urine (p. 92).

Consequences of Alkalosis. The sequence of events which occurs when hydrochloric acid is lost from the body as a result of vomiting is shown in Figure 5.3. The loss of hydrogen ions in severe and continuous vomiting lowers the hydrogen ion concentration of the blood and leads to alkalosis. The effect is mitigated by an increase in the ionisation of blood carbonic acid to hydrogen and bicarbonate ions, as indicated by the broad arrow. The former tends to restore the hydrogen ion concentration towards normal, and the latter replaces the chloride which has also been lost in the gastric contents. For as long as the chloride

Fig. 5.3 **Effect of alkalosis on the blood buffer system.**

deficiency persists increased tubular conservation of bicarbonate sustains the alkalosis.

Alkalosis is commonly unattended by specific clinical disturbances. However acute alkalosis produces tetany which occurs spontaneously or may be induced by the Trousseau manoeuvre and which is due to a reduction in the concentration of plasma ionised calcium.

Severe alkalosis of some duration is often associated with significant depression of renal function with uraemia. Protein and casts are found in the urine, and the diagnostic error of attributing vomiting due to pyloric stenosis to primary renal disease must be avoided.

In spite of the existence of metabolic alkalosis, the urine may remain acid. There are two causes for this paradoxical aciduria. The alkalosis is frequently associated with chloride depletion, and under these circumstances alkaline urine may not be elaborated. Secondly, respiratory compensation for the alkalosis results in a rise in $Paco_2$ which is also known to increase renal tubular reabsorption of bicarbonate. Apathy, personality changes, delirium and stupor occur; since the patient usually suffers from associated water and potassium depletion, it is probably wrong to attribute these features solely to the effect of alkalosis.

The diagnosis of alkalosis may be made with certainty only by estimation of the concentration of plasma bicarbonate. In moderately severe alkalosis this is elevated to 35 mmol/l. The pH of the blood is also elevated.

Treatment. In patients with mild or moderate alkalosis in whom the bicarbonate concentration is not elevated above 35 mmol/l, it is often possible to correct the abnormality by the intravenous administration of isotonic sodium chloride. This treatment is effective only if there is normal renal function. In this event the chloride is retained and excess bicarbonate in the plasma is excreted in the urine. 2 to 4 litres may be required in the course of 24 hours.

In severe cases the administration of ammonium chloride by intravenous infusion has been found effective and is conveniently prepared in a solution which is designed also to repair the commonly associated potassium deficit. This is called the 'gastric solution'. One litre of a solution containing 63 mmol/l of sodium chloride, 17 mmol/l of potassium chloride and 70 mmol/l of ammonium chloride may be given in 4 to 6 hours and repeated as indicated by blood analysis. The use of this solution is of particular benefit in those patients who are being prepared for operation for relief of gastric outlet obstruction and in whom continuous gastric aspiration is needed to prevent vomiting and reduce the size of a dilated stomach.

Ketosis without Acidosis

The excessive production of β-hydroxybutyric acid and acetoacetic acid in diabetic ketoacidosis has already been described as a cause of acidosis. Abnormal amounts of acetoacetic acid also arise in the body when the carbohydrate in the food is inadequate and increased amounts of fat are being utilised for energy. This is found in cases of cyclical or severe vomiting in children, severe vomiting of pregnancy, starvation, and in postoperative vomiting.

Two opposing tendencies are obviously in operation, the ketosis tending to increase, and vomiting tending to decrease the concentration of hydrogen ions in the blood. In these cases it is not uncommon, therefore, to find that metabolic alkalosis coexists with ketosis. Thus, the presence of acetoacetic acid in the urine does not necessarily imply the existence of acidosis, and the existence of metabolic acidosis is established only by the determination of the blood pH or bicarbonate concentration.

Apart from the possible need to treat concomitant acidosis or electrolyte disturbances, ketosis is best remedied by restoring the consumption of carbohydrate to normal. In cases of diabetic ketosis the administration of insulin is essential. In other forms of ketosis this need not be given. Ample supplies of glucose should be provided; if this cannot be taken by mouth an intravenous infusion of 5% glucose in water may be given. 2 to 4 litres of this solution may be needed in the course of the day.

Respiratory Acidosis and Alkalosis

Respiratory acidosis arises when the effective alveolar ventilation does not keep pace with the rate of production of carbon dioxide (p. 210). As a result the Pa_{CO_2} and carbonic acid concentration of the blood increases, and the pH falls. The distinction between respiratory acidosis and metabolic alkalosis is usually easily made from a knowledge of the cause of the disturbance. The reaction of the arterial blood is decisive; in both the Pa_{CO_2} is increased, but in respiratory acidosis $[H^+]$ is increased, whereas in metabolic alkalosis the $[H^+]$ is reduced.

The kidney responds to an increase in Pa_{CO_2} by excreting an acid urine and conserving sodium bicarbonate. The causes and consequences of respiratory acidosis are given on page 209.

Respiratory alkalosis occurs when there is excessive loss of carbonic acid by overventilation of the lungs. Most commonly this occurs in hysterical overbreathing or in overventilation during the course of assisted respiration, though it may arise also in the course of lobar pneumonia, pulmonary embolism, meningitis, encephalitis, salicylate intoxication and liver failure. As a result the Pa_{CO_2} of the blood falls. Renal compensatory mechanisms result in the excretion of sodium bicarbonate which mitigates the fall in blood $[H^+]$.

The distinction between respiratory alkalosis and metabolic acidosis is usually clear from the clinical circumstances. In both, the concentration of plasma bicarbonate is reduced and the reaction of the blood is again decisive. In respiratory alkalosis the plasma $[H^+]$ falls while in metabolic acidosis it rises.

Electrolyte repair solutions play no part in the treatment of respiratory acidosis or alkalosis, and therapy should be directed to the underlying disorder. The treatment of hypercapnia is described on page 217 and that of respiratory alkalosis due to hysterical overbreathing on page 442. Tetany may be treated by an intravenous injection of 10 ml of 10% calcium gluconate if necessary. The underlying causative factors should receive appropriate attention.

ANNE T. LAMBIE
J.S. ROBSON

FURTHER READING:

Brenner, B. & Stein, J.H. (1978) (1) *Sodium and Water Homeostasis*, (2) *Acid-base and Potassium Homeostasis*. Edinburgh: Churchill Livingstone.

Passmore, R. & Robson, J.S. *Companion to Medical Studies*, 3rd edn. Vol. I (1984), Chs 2, 27 & 31; 2nd edn. Vol. II (1980), Ch. 12; Vol. III (1974), Ch. 49. Oxford: Blackwell.

Robinson, J.R. (1975) *Fundamentals of Acid-Base Regulation*, 5th edn. Oxford: Blackwell.

Clinical Pathophysiology of electrolyte and acid-base metabolism I & II 1977. Reviews in Clinical Nephrology, vol. 7.

6. Introduction to Oncology

Oncology is the study of tumours. *Neoplasia* means abnormal new growth, which may be benign or malignant. *Cancer* is a term that is used to describe a wide variety of malignant diseases, the management of which requires several medical disciplines. Traditionally physicians have played a lesser role than surgeons or radiotherapists in the treatment of these diseases but the development of cytotoxic drugs has resulted in the greater involvement of physicians in the overall management of malignancy. The use of cytotoxic drugs requires specialised knowledge and experience but since cancer impinges on every medical discipline, it is necessary for all doctors to be aware of the basic principles of investigating and managing malignant diseases. This chapter reviews these basic principles and outlines some aspects of the aetiology and pathology of tumours, the assessment of tumour burden, the use of radiotherapy, chemotherapy and hormone therapy, and possible approaches to the prevention of these diseases, many of which may be associated with avoidable causes.

EPIDEMIOLOGY AND AETIOLOGY

Cancer is second only to coronary artery disease as being the commonest cause of death in the Western world. The age standardised mortality in England and Wales for the years 1976–1978 was 283·7 and 178·4 per 100 000 population for men and women respectively, with even higher figures for Scotland (373·5 and 274·2 per 100 000). There is considerable geographical variation in the incidence of malignant diseases around the world but as Figure 6.1 shows, British countries are amongst the highest for mortality rates, with

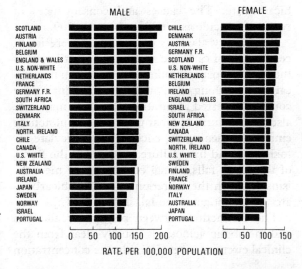

Fig. 6.1 Age-adjusted mortality rates for all cancers in various countries 1966–67.

Scotland actually leading the world tables for its incidence of cancer in men. In many developed countries the incidence is steadily increasing (Fig. 6.2).

Throughout the Western world the commonest sites of malignant disease are the lung, large bowel and breast. Over the past 25 years the incidence of lung cancer in men has increased by 125%, and even more significantly in women concomitant with their increased consumption of cigarettes. The incidence of colonic, prostatic and bladder cancer has also shown an increase but during the past decade there has been a decrease in the incidence of carcinomas arising in the stomach, uterus, rectum and oesophagus.

Age has a bearing on the incidence of specific cancers. In children, cancer is the leading cause of

Fig. 6.2 Death rates from cancer in Scotland 1930–80.

death between the ages of 3–13 years, about half of these being due to acute lymphoblastic leukaemia. For the age group in the third and fourth decades, cancer is three times as common in women as in men but men are at greater risk than women between the ages of 60–80.

The aetiology of many malignant diseases remains unknown but studies of the geographical distribution of their incidence gives some leads as to the possible influence of particular environmental or social factors in causation. The best documented aetiological factor is cigarette tobacco which is unquestionably associated with the considerable increase in lung cancer in countries where cigarette smoking has increased over the past 30 years.

The incidence of carcinoma of the oesophagus varies greatly from country to country (over a 200 fold range) with a particularly high incidence in a geographical band covering eastern and southern Africa, Iran, Afghanistan, Soviet and central Asia, Mongolia and northern China. Suggestions that diet or cooking practices are involved are as yet unconfirmed.

The incidence of carcinoma of the pancreas is increasing in most of the developed countries but is relatively rare in Japan, whereas the reverse is true for stomach cancer which is particularly prevalent in Japan.

It has been known for a long time that the incidence of breast cancer varies appreciably in different parts of the world, being high in the USA and low in the Orient but increasing over two generations of orientals who emigrate to the USA. Population migration represents a natural experiment where the assumption of incidence levels of the host country strongly suggests an environmental rather than a genetic aetiology. For both large bowel and breast cancer, the environmental factors are thought to be dietary in origin but specific carcinogens have not been clearly identified.

The incidence of carcinoma of the uterine cervix has increased in recent years particularly amongst younger women. This has coincided with changing social patterns of greater sexual freedom and the use of oral contraception, suggesting that a sexually transmissable agent may be the aetiological factor responsible.

There is evidence that both environmental and genetic factors are important in the pathogenesis of malignant melanoma. In the USA, figures for 1975 show an incidence of 4·2 cases per 100 000 population, but of great concern is the fact that the incidence is rising rapidly, doubling every 10–15 years. Melanoma is rare in black and oriental people suggesting that skin pigment plays a genetic role in protecting against the development of melanoma. Although not proven, there is support for the fact that sunlight is environmentally involved in the aetiology of this disease. Although the incidence between the sexes is equal, women tend to develop melanoma in the legs and exposed parts of the limbs more frequently than men who have a higher incidence of lesions on the trunk. Furthermore, studies from Norway, Canada, the USA and Australia show that the incidence of melanoma increases as one approaches the equator, consistent with greater exposure to ultraviolet light.

It has long been suspected that viruses may be involved in the pathogenesis of human neoplasms, but there is as yet no conclusive evidence of a direct aetiological relationship. There is however indirect evidence to suggest the hypothesis that viruses may act as cofactors in the development of some malignant diseases. This evidence includes the fact that viral particles can be demonstrated in the cells of certain malignancies, the enzyme reverse transcriptase (of oncornavirus-type) has been demonstrated in human cancer cells, and the nuclei of some malignant cells have been shown to contain DNA base sequences complementary to the base sequences of known tumour viruses.

The integration of viral information into the genome of the human cell that subsequently becomes malignant has led to the concept of 'oncogenes', whereby cancer results from the de-repression of these viral oncogenes to permit malignant transformation. De-repression may be caused by exposure to an external carcinogen, or by spontaneous mutation. This hypothesis is the subject of intensive research at the present time.

PATHOLOGY

A fundamental principle of oncology is to establish the pathological nature of any lesion suspected of being neoplastic before making decisions about management. This usually entails biopsy of the tumour for histological examination.

The first distinction to be made is between benign and malignant lesions. Benign tumours represent the accumulation of cells which have been transformed to reproduce in abnormal numbers but under circumstances where they remain within the tissue of origin. Malignant tumours are comprised of cells which are capable of invading adjacent tissues and leaving the tissue of origin to disseminate and form metastases. The histological distinction between benign and malignant lesions will depend, amongst other factors, on the pleomorphism of the cells, the presence of aberrations in the nucleus, increased numbers of mitoses and whether or not there is evidence of invasion into surrounding tissues.

Cancers are classified into three major groups: the 'carcinomas' which arise in endodermal or ectodermal tissue, the 'sarcomas' of mesodermal origin, and the leukaemias and lymphomas which are derived from the white blood cells and the monocyte–macrophage system. Within a given tissue there may be major differences in the cell type from which the tumour has arisen. Thus for example bronchogenic carcinomas are classified histologically into four major groups: squamous carcinomas, adenocarcinomas, small cell and large cell undifferentiated carcinomas.

Such distinctions are essential to clinical management since the choice between surgery, radio-therapy and chemotherapy will depend on whether or not the lesion is benign or malignant, and whether or not the particular histological subtype is sensitive to radiotherapy or chemotherapy. As regards the latter, there is great variation in the sensitivity of different tumours to different cytotoxic drugs, and therefore appropriate therapy can be prescribed only when the tumour tissue has been accurately classified.

Although there is evidence to support the concept that many human tumours arise from the transformation of a single cell, i.e. are clonal in origin, it is not unusual to find a mixed histological picture; for example in the testis, teratomas and seminomatous tissue may occur together, and in the lung, squamous and small cell undifferentiated tumour may present in the same biopsy specimen.

In addition to defining whether the tumour is benign or malignant and from which cell type it arises, it is useful to define the degree of differentiation or anaplasia of the cancer cell since for many tumour types this has been shown to correlate with prognosis and response to treatment of differing forms.

Whilst most histology is performed on tissue that is obtained by surgical biopsy, in certain circumstances it is possible to achieve excellent classification from cytology alone. Thus for example sputum may be examined for malignant bronchogenic cells, pleural or peritoneal effusions may provide suitable cells for diagnostic purposes and smears can be prepared from the uterine cervix. Increasing use is being made of needle aspiration for cytological diagnosis. A fine gauge needle can be inserted into breast lumps, subcutaneous deposits, intrathoracic or hepatic lesions, and a smear for cytological evaluation can be made from the aspirated material. In experienced hands, this technique has many advantages over the more conventional surgical biopsy technique, mainly because of speed and simplicity.

TUMOUR MARKERS

Malignant cells appear different histologically and vary biochemically from their normal counterparts but attempts to identify biochemical abnormalities unique to the cancer cell have proved unrewarding. Nevertheless it is now appreciated that the presence of viable tumour tissue in the body may be detectable by the presence in the blood of biochemical products known as 'tumour markers'. These are normal metabolic constituents that are found either in abnormal amounts or at an inappropriate time of life, for example fetal proteins being re-expressed in adult life.

Tumour markers of this type can be useful in a number of different clinical situations. In theory tumour markers might be useful for screening whole populations for undetected cancers but in practice this has not proved useful for the following reasons. The predictive value of a screening test depends on the sensitivity of the test, its specificity and the prevalence of the particular disease. Sensitivity refers to the number of times a test is positive for patients known to have the disease, i.e. true positives, and specificity refers to the incidence of true negatives, i.e. that the test should prove negative in people known to be free of the disease. Unfortunately sensitivity is inversely related to specificity. For example it is known that some gastrointestinal tumours contain carcinoembryonic antigen (CEA), a substance that is present in the gut during fetal life but which is not found in normal adult gastrointestinal tissues. Radio-immunoassays of CEA in blood have shown an overall 67% positivity in patients with colorectal carcinoma but the test is also positive in alcoholic cirrhosis (70%), emphysema (57%) and diabetes mellitus (38%) amongst many other diseases. Screening the population at large for subclinical carcinomas of the colon would therefore fail because of lack of specificity.

However the presence of a tumour marker can be of clinical value in monitoring the progress of individual patients known to have a given malignancy. For example testicular teratomas not infrequently secrete another oncofetal protein — alpha-fetoprotein (AFP). Figure 6.3 illustrates a typical case where during the months following surgical resection of the primary tumour, a rising level of AFP was associated with (and preceded) the clinical appearance of metastases. The successful use of chemotherapy was associated with a disappearance of the abnormal tumour marker.

Human chorionic gonadotrophin (normally produced only by placental tissue) is another

Fig. 6.3 Serum alpha-fetoprotein (AFP) levels in a young man with testicular teratoma. The levels of AFP fluctuate with disease state and can be used to monitor the effects of the treatment.

tumour marker seen in testicular teratoma whereas the production of placental alkaline phosphatase is associated with approximately 40% of testicular seminomas.

A variety of hormones can be produced ectopically by small cell anaplastic lung tumours including antidiuretic hormone (ADH) and ACTH. The levels of these hormones, or the biochemical consequences of their production — such as hyponatraemia resulting from inappropriate ADH secretion — can be useful markers of the viability of residual tumour following treatment, therefore indicating whether or not further therapy is required.

CLINICAL FEATURES

Malignant diseases manifest themselves in a variety of ways. The presence of an abnormal accumulation of cells may, by virtue of its physical bulk alone, produce clinical symptoms and signs. Thus for example painless swellings in the breast or in muscle may indicate an underlying carcinoma or sarcoma respectively. Lymphomas usually present as painless enlargements of lymph nodes or spleen. Space-occupying lesions in the brain will cause symptoms of raised intracranial pressure such as headache, vomiting or visual disturbance in association with papilloedema. Tumours in the distal colon may partially obstruct the lumen of the bowel with a resulting change in bowel habit. Bronchogenic tumours may cause shortness of breath or cough resulting from partial or complete occlusion of an airway.

Malignant tumours not infrequently present as haemorrhage from an eroded epithelial surface. For example bronchogenic carcinomas may present with haemoptysis, gastric carcinomas with haematemesis, colonic carcinoma with bleeding per rectum, and renal and bladder carcinomas as haematuria.

Pain is often thought to be an inevitable accompaniment of malignant disease but in fact pain is not a common symptom especially at presentation of most cancers. When it does occur, it is due either to nerve compression or to distension of an organ. The most common peripheral nerve compressions are due to involvement of the brachial plexus (carcinomas of the lung or breast), the sacral plexus (carcinomas of the rectum or cervix) or the paraspinal nerves (carcinoma of the pancreas). Metastatic tumours in the liver may cause pain as a result of distension and stretching of its capsule. Bone pain resulting from primary, or more commonly, secondary deposits usually occurs in the weight bearing bones, and results from compression secondary to weakening of the structural component of the bone. Pathological fractures may arise as a consequence. Patients may present with referred pain, most frequently in the shoulder, hip or knee, as when a nerve root is involved directly or by metastases.

Cachexia is a clinical feature of many malignant diseases, especially carcinomas of the gastrointestinal tract, lung, ovary and testis. It is however not a universal phenomenon and is rare in breast cancer and in tumours of the central nervous system, and uncommon in leukaemia and lymphomas.

Cachexia may arise as a direct result of malnutrition from a tumour in the gastrointestinal tract. This malabsorption may arise rarely as a consequence of tumour replacing the absorptive epithelia but more commonly from reduced exocrine function (from carcinomas of the pancreas), or loss of bile from carcinomas of the upper gastrointestinal tract that obstruct biliary outflow. Loss of taste and the malaise that accompanies many malignant diseases may contribute to poor food intake but all of these factors in promoting malnutrition do not of themselves fully explain the cachexia of malignancy. Although many patients will have a negative nitrogen balance, others who are in positive balance may show a caloric deficit. It has been shown that in the cachexia accompanying malignant disease, caloric expenditure remains high with an elevated basal metabolic rate despite reduced dietary intake (the reverse of the situation that follows starvation) which indicates that this phenomenon results from a profound systemic derangement of host metabolism, the pathogenesis of which remains unclear.

In addition to these generalised clinical features that are commonly associated with the presentation of a malignant disease, there are a variety of syndromes for which the term 'paraneoplastic' has been used. These syndromes include many that arise as a result of the secretion into the blood of tumour products (usually polypeptide hormones) which produce clinical signs as a consequence of their action on target organs remote from the primary tumour. Although relatively rare, these syndromes are important since they may precede the clinical presentation of the primary tumour, facilitating early detection. In addition they may mimic metastatic disease and thus confuse management decisions. They may also serve as tumour markers to monitor therapy. The ectopic production of ADH and ACTH (p. 261) are most commonly associated with an underlying small cell anaplastic carcinoma of the bronchus. Squamous cell lung cancers may produce parathyroid hormone manifesting as hypercalcaemia.

A number of neurological paraneoplastic syndromes (p. 668) have been described for which the tumour product remains unknown. These include peripheral neuropathies, a myasthenia-like syndrome and subacute cerebellar degeneration. Whilst all of these syndromes may improve with successful treatment of the primary tumour, complete resolution is rare.

Dermatomyositis and polymyositis present as gradually progressive muscle weakness predominantly affecting the proximal musculature, coming on over a period of months. Whilst these disorders are not universally associated with malignancy, patients suffering from them have a greatly increased risk of an underlying neoplasm compared with the general public, and malignancies of the breast, lung, and gastrointestinal and genitourinary tract should be considered.

Acanthosis nigricans is a rare condition characterised by the appearance of black velvety verrucose lesions in the flexures around the neck, axillae and groin. It is particularly seen in patients with carcinomas of the stomach.

PRINCIPLES OF TREATMENT

In order to plan the optimal management for an individual patient, it is necessary to consider two essential questions: (1) Is the tumour still localised to its site of origin? and (2) Is it a realistic aim to 'cure' the patient, or should treatment be focused on palliation of symptoms? Tumours that have not metastasised are amenable to local forms of treatment, surgery or radiotherapy, whilst tumours that have already disseminated require systemic treatment with chemotherapy or hormonal therapy. Not infrequently it is necessary to use a combination of these measures, particulary if it is appropriate to aim for complete eradication of the tumour. Surgery, radiotherapy and chemotherapy all cause some degree of host toxicity and this may be enhanced by combining the treatments.

For this reason it is important to decide whether or not cure is feasible and desirable in order to minimise any treatment-related toxicity in circumstances where an aggressive therapeutic approach would be inappropriate. Thus for example lymphoma arising in a young person may require a protracted course of combination chemotherapy and radiotherapy but cure is attained in a significant proportion of patients and will be the initial intention in planning management. If the same disease presents in an 80 year old then management should be planned to relieve symptoms as effectively as possible but to minimise hospital attendances and any treatment-related toxicity. Such an example may appear obvious but more subtle decisions are frequently required in planning management for patients with carcinomas of breast, stomach or ovary.

The patient's history and physical examination provide a starting point for planning treatment but it is usually necessary to perform specialised investigations to determine the extent of dissemination of the tumour prior to selecting treatment — the process of 'staging' the tumour. Staging investigations take time and inevitably the delay in announcing a decision about treatment causes anxiety for the patient. For this reason it cannot be overemphasised that the first interview with a patient suspected of having a malignant disease is of particular importance. It is essential to perform this interview in a quiet and unhurried manner. In addition to a routine history of symptoms and previous illnesses, it is important to ascertain whether patients already know that they have malignant disease and what this means to them. For many patients the word 'cancer' is automatically associated with an incurable disease and very distressing death. This myth of universal hopelessness is slowly being destroyed, helped by greater public interest in health and medical progress generally but the patient who holds such beliefs will be helped very considerably by positive assurance that symptoms can almost always be improved, if not completely resolved, even if the underlying disease cannot be eradicated. At the first interview the physician may not have sufficient facts to know the likelihood of cure but at this stage it is important to explain to the patient that the first aim of treatment will be to control the disease, whether or not cure can ultimately be achieved.

Whether or not to tell patients that they have malignant disease is a matter of individual circumstances but as a general rule it is recommended that patients should be informed of this, whilst it is not necessarily appropriate to inform them of the exact prognosis which in any case may be uncertain. The first interview may not be the time to discuss these matters but it is recommended that they should always be discussed prior to starting treatment. If it is necessary to arrange a series of staging investigations, patients should be informed of the purpose of these so that their natural anxiety is not accentuated. Time should be taken to counsel the patient at the earliest opportunity about these matters so that they can have confidence in those who are going to be responsible for therapy and follow-up which by the nature of these diseases need to be continued for a long period.

Staging

The concept of staging arose from the fact that survival rates were better for malignancies that were localised than for those which had metastasised at the time of clinical presentation. This was associated with the concept of 'early' and 'late' presentation, implying a regular progression with time. It is now known that the stage of disease at diagnosis is much more complex than this, and is a reflection not only of the degree of malignancy of the particular tumour but also of the tumour-host relationship. However, staging is still an essential part of oncological management since in addition to its contribution towards selecting appropriate treatment, it may give an indication of prognosis, assist in the monitoring and evaluation of treatment, and allow comparison of different treatments.

The internationally recognised staging system is known as the TNM classification in which T defines the extent of the primary tumour, N defines the extent of regional lymph node involvement and M defines the presence or absence of metastases. To T, N or M, the addition of numbers indicates the extent of the disease, thus for example TO refers to an excised tumour, T1, 2 or 3 to (defined) increases in primary tumour size. N1, N2 and N3 apply similarly to increasing involvement of nodes, and the suffix I indicates the presence of metastases where MO indicates that metastases are not present. For T and N the exact criteria of size and regions of nodal involvement have been defined for each anatomical site, for example for lung cancers:

T1   < 3 cm with no invasion
T2   > 3 cm ± extension to hilar region
T3   Gross extension/effusion/atelectasis
N1   Hilar nodes
N2   Mediastinal nodes
M0   Metastases absent
M1   Metastases present

The TNM system is a clinical staging system but if supplemented by the pathological examination of biopsied or resected specimens the suffix p is added. Having defined the T, N and M status of the tumour, it is then possible to group patients into different stages. Thus for example in lung cancers the stage groupings are as follows:

Occult Cancer	Tx*	NO	MO
Stage Ia	T1	NO	MO
	T2	NO	MO
Stage Ib	T1	N1	MO
Stage II	T2	N1	MO
Stage III	T3	NO,N1	MO
	Any T	N2	MO
Stage IV	Any T	Any N	M1

*Tx refers to tumour proven by the presence of malignant cells in bronchopulmonary secretions but not visualised by radiography or bronchoscopy.

For certain diseases it has proved useful to define specific staging systems which differ from the TNM classification, as for example the Ann Arbor staging for Hodgkin's lymphoma (p. 531), and Dukes' classification for carcinomas of the rectum. Nevertheless increasing use of the TNM system for the majority of malignant diseases is being encouraged particularly in order to facilitate comparisons of the results of treatments in different centres internationally.

The investigations required to define the T, N or M status of a tumour differ for different diseases. Primary tumours may be assessed by palpation or inspection (fibreoptic bronchoscopy, cystoscopy, etc.) or by radiography (conventional or computed tomography [CT]); nodes are assessed by palpation, excision, lymphangiography or CT scanning; and metastases are evaluated by a variety of techniques such as biochemical screening of liver function, radionuclide scans of bone, liver or brain, ultrasound of the liver, peritoneoscopy or laparotomy.

Performance Status

In addition to the anatomical assessment of tumour extent evaluated by staging procedures, it is important to assess the overall degree of functional impairment that the disease is causing the patient at the time of diagnosis. A variety of 'performance status' scales have been devised such as the Eastern Cooperative Oncology Group (ECOG) scale shown in Table 6.1. The complications of disease which impinge on a patient's life and therefore affect his or her performance status are multiple and variable but these simple divisions into major groups have been found useful in prognosis in assessing the efficacy and toxicity of

Table 6.1 Performance Status Scale (ECOG).

0 Fully active, able to carry on all usual activities without restriction and without the aid of analgesics.
1 Restricted in strenuous activity but ambulatory and able to carry out light work or pursue a sedentary occupation. This group also contains patients who are fully active, as in grade 0, but only with the aid of analgesics.
2 Ambulatory and capable of all self-care but unable to work. Up and about more than 50% of waking hours.
3 Capable of only limited self-care, confined to bed or chair more than 50% of waking hours.
4 Completely disabled, unable to carry out any self-care and confined totally to bed or chair.

treatment, and in research studies comparing different forms of treatment.

Evaluation of Response

With presently available therapies most methods of cancer treatment are associated with significant morbidity. For this reason alone, it is essential to evaluate the response to therapy as accurately as possible but since research into new methods of treatment is so widespread, properly defined criteria for evaluating response are necessary in order to make valid comparisons between different treatments. The concept of 'survival time', particularly the long hallowed 'five year survival' concept, places too much emphasis on cure as the only objective of treatment. Since palliation is a much commoner objective in management planning, more subtle criteria are required than crude survival figures.

The terms universally accepted for evaluating treatment are those of 'objective response', 'complete response', 'partial response', 'no response' and 'progressive disease'. These are defined as follows:

Objective response:	any response that fulfils the criteria of complete or partial response.
Complete response:	complete disappearance of all known disease in the absence of any new lesions appearing.
Partial response:	a reduction in size by at least 50% of the tumour in the absence of any new lesions appearing.
No response:	no change, or an increase or decrease of 25% in the size of the tumour in the absence of new lesions.
Progressive disease:	increase in the size of the tumour by 25% or the development of any new lesions.

The term 'complete response' may or may not indicate true eradication of the tumour and for any given disease these terms can only reflect the ability to detect viable tumour.

Principles of Radiotherapy

Whilst it is outside the scope of this chapter to consider details of the radiobiological aspects of radiotherapy, it is important that physicians should be familiar with an outline of the procedures involved when their patients are referred for this form of treatment.

Radiotherapy involves the exposure of a defined area of the body to a source of ionising radiation under carefully controlled conditions. Treatment planning involves accurate localisation of the tumour and prescription of multiple daily fractions of irradiation for a specified period of time. The biological effect of radiation depends on the amount of energy absorbed per unit mass. The unit of absorbed dose is the gray and is equivalent to 1 joule per kilogram.

Ionising radiation damages cells by interaction with nuclear DNA thus preventing the normal reproduction of that cell. As with cytotoxic drugs there is only a relative selectivity in this process, and normal (non-malignant) cells are readily damaged by radiation. For this reason radiotherapy planning must take into account the exact anatomical distribution of the tumour in order to minimise the exposure of normal tissues whilst at the same time ensuring that all of the diseased tissues are included in the treated area. Great care is taken to ensure that the patient can be accurately and reproducibly repositioned whilst radiotherapy is being undertaken.

Patients are usually treated in the supine position although the prone position may be more suitable for some abdominal and pelvic tumours, and in certain situations patients may be treated seated or standing with horizontal beams rather than supine with vertical or oblique beams. In order to immobilise the area to be treated, moulds, casts and shells are constructed for the individual patient.

With the patient comfortably positioned and the treatment area immobilised, the tumour is localised by a variety of techniques such as the placement of radio-opaque seeds in the tumour or the use of contrast media as in conventional radiography. Increasingly computed tomography is being used to assist in planning radiotherapeutic treatment, especially since CT can provide information about tumour margins in the transverse plane in which most radiotherapy is administered.

Radiotherapy localisation is usually carried out on specialised equipment known as a simulator which is designed to allow isocentric rotation and thus to simulate the exact axis distance of the treatment machine. In most centres computers are now available to integrate the information obtained from simulators in order to select the optimum configuration, energy and variable loading of different treatment beams. This ensures that the least possible dose of radiation will be given to critical normal tissues and that a homogeneous high level of dose will be given to the tumour.

To maximise the absorbed dose within the tumour area and minimise the dose to normal tissues, treatment is given through multiple portals, for example as a four-field box technique for the pelvis, or through fields at right angles to each other with compensating wedge filters to even the dose distribution where the beams overlap. Compensating filters are used to overcome variations in thickness of the areas to be treated through multiple ports. Since the human body is not a symmetrical cube, the routine use of these filters compensates for the lack of consistent tissue thickness and ensures a more homogeneous dose distribution throughout the target.

Most radiotherapy is performed with 'teletherapy' techniques i.e. where a beam of photons is used to irradiate the tumour from outside the patient. Alternatively for specific sites, 'brachytherapy' is used whereby a source of radiation is implanted in a body cavity or within the tumour itself. Teletherapy techniques include the use of low energy ortho- or kilovoltage sources and the more widely used megavoltage sources. Low energy radiation (50–100 kVp range) is useful for treating carcinomas of the skin and lip, and orthovoltage (250–300 kVp) machines are sometimes used for the palliative treatment of bone metastases and lesions of the chest wall. However,

orthovoltage machines are unsuitable for the treatment of more deep seated tumours.

^{60}Cobalt machines and linear accelerators are the most widely used teletherapy equipment. Both of these types can be used isocentrically i.e. the radiation source can be mounted in a gantry which can be rotated around the axis of the patient thus allowing direction of multiple beams to the centre of the target volume with great accuracy. ^{60}Cobalt machines which give radiation of a quality similar to that from a 4 MV linear accelerator are less expensive to operate and easier to maintain but provide a less well defined beam of radiation, lower dose rates and poorer depth doses. In general, ^{60}cobalt or 4MV linear accelerators are used for treating carcinomas of the head and neck and breast, 6 MV linear accelerators for lymphomas and lung cancers, and higher energy accelerators for some deep seated abdominal and pelvic tumours. In addition to producing X-rays, the higher energy linear accelerators can be used to produce accelerated electrons. The latter are charged particles which are absorbed within a finite range of tissue and can be useful in the treatment of superficial lesions where it is desirable to spare underlying tissues. Thus, for example, electrons may be employed (with advantage) for the treatment of some lesions of the head and neck, lymph nodes near the spinal cord, and lesions of the chest wall such as occur in breast carcinoma.

Brachytherapy is performed with sealed sources of radioactivity introduced for a few days into a body cavity or tumour, for example the insertion of ^{137}caesium into the uterus for treating carcinoma of the cervix, or the use of ^{192}iridium wire placed within breast tumours. The advantages of brachytherapy are that a relatively high dose of radiation can be administered to a very limited volume of tissue thereby sparing any adverse effects on normal adjacent tissues. Brachytherapy is applicable only when the tumour is accessible and when its size can be accurately defined. Such treatments are often supplemented by teletherapy to treat the larger volume where microscopic disease may be present.

Radiotherapy is most frequently prescribed in daily fractions of 200 centigray (cGy) for 5 days a week where, depending on the tumour type and management plan, treatment may continue for 3–6 weeks. During and after this time a number of side-effects may occur. Many patients, particularly those treated with target volumes greater than 500 cm³, will experience some malaise and fatigue. Nausea and anorexia are common but vomiting is a frequent problem if it is necessary to irradiate very large volumes, particularly in the upper abdomen. Acute skin reaction usually consists of mild erythema best treated by keeping the skin dry. Oral and pharyngeal mucosal reactions are common if the area receives high radiation doses. Particular attention to oral hygiene is required and close inspection for candidiasis essential.

Radiation effects on the bone marrow may occur if large volumes are treated. Minor decreases in lymphocyte count are common but a frequent check on the peripheral blood must be made throughout treatment to adjust this if significant marrow suppression occurs. Maintenance of adequate haemoglobin is important to the outcome of therapy since hypoxia may render the tumour less sensitive to radiation damage. Irradiation of the gastrointestinal tract may result in temporary dysphagia, diarrhoea, tenesmus or production of mucus per rectum. Management depends on the severity and duration of the symptoms but antacids and reduction of residue in the diet may be beneficial.

Principles of Chemotherapy

During the second world war, research into the action of mustard gas showed that sulphur and nitrogen mustard could destroy dividing cells in lymph nodes and the bone marrow. The potential harnessing of this effect for therapeutic benefit was explored in treating some lymphomas with nitrogen mustard which was then developed as the first clinically useful cytotoxic drug. Study of the effects of folic acid metabolism on leukaemic cells resulted in the second cytotoxic drug of therapeutic value — the antifolate, methotrexate. Thereafter many naturally occurring substances were tested for antitumour activity in experimental systems, resulting in the present availability of some 30 effective antineoplastic drugs (Fig. 6.4).

Fig. 6.4 **Anticancer drugs**. The year that clinical effectiveness was established for some of the commonly used anticancer drugs. TG = thioguanine, Ara C = cystosine arabinoside, DIC = dimethyl triazeno-imidazole carboxamide (DTIC), VCR = vincristine, VLB = vinblastine, Act D = actinomycin D, MP = mercaptopurine, MTX = methotrexate, HN₂ = nitrogen mustard.

A classification of anticancer drugs into 6 main groups is given in Table 6.2.

1. Methotrexate acts to inhibit folate metabolism by preventing the cell from replenishing its source of reduced folates necessary for purine and pyrimidine synthesis (p. 500). The term 'antimetabolite' is used for this group of drugs which includes mercaptopurine, thioguanine, fluorouracil and cytosine arabinoside.

2. Nitrogen mustard is thought to destroy cells by the process of alkylation — the addition of an alkyl group to constituents of DNA, thus interfering with replication and transcription of further nucleic acid. Busulphan, chlorambucil, cyclophosphamide and melphalan are other clinically useful alkylating agents.

3. The plant alkaloids inhibit cell division by binding to tubulin and disrupting the mitotic spindle.

4. The compounds grouped altogether as antibiotics include adriamycin and actinomycin which act by intercalating between base pairs in DNA, and bleomycin which causes breaks in both single and double-stranded DNA.

5. The mechanism of action of the nitrosoureas probably involves alkylation.

6. With the miscellaneous synthetic compounds, alkylation and other metabolic lesions

Table 6.2 Classification of anticancer drugs.

Antimetabolites	Methotrexate	– acts by interfering with the metabolism of –	folic acid
	6-Mercaptopurine		hypoxanthine
	6-Thioguanine		guanine
	5-Fluorouracil		uracil
	Cytosine arabinoside		cytidine
Alkylating agents	Nitrogen mustard (mechlorethamine)		
	Cyclophosphamide		
	Chlorambucil		
	Busulphan		
	Melphalan		
	Thiotepa		
	Iphosphamide		
Plant alkaloids	Vinblastine		
	Vincristine		
	Vindesine		
	VP 16–213		
	VM 26		
Antibiotics	Adriamycin		
	Daunorubicin		
	Actinomycin D		
	Bleomycin		
	Mitomycin C		
Nitrosoureas	BCNU		
	CCNU		
	Methyl CCNU		
	Streptozotocin		
Miscellaneous synthetic compounds	DTIC		
	Cis-diammine-dichloroplatinum		
	Procarbazine		
	Hexamethylmelamine		
	Hydroxyurea		

may be involved. The site of action of the main groups of anticancer drugs is shown in Figure 6.5.

Unfortunately none of these biochemical events is of unique importance to the metabolism of malignant cells. Systemic exposure to these cellular poisons therefore must inevitably result in some damage to normal host tissues, particularly to those which rely on rapid cell division such as the bone marrow and gastrointestinal tract. In addition to their relative lack of selectivity, these drugs are very potent because they act at low concentrations. Together with a tendency towards steep dose-response curves, these factors all account for the narrow 'therapeutic index' of cytotoxic drugs. This is illustrated in Figure 6.6 which demonstrates that too low a dose is ineffective, but the dose range for optimal treatment is narrow before an increased dose produces unacceptable toxicity.

The narrow therapeutic index of antineoplastic

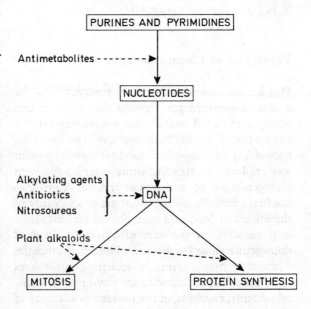

Fig. 6.5 Anticancer drugs: site of action of major groups.

Fig. 6.6 Dose response curve for cyclophosphamide in mice bearing the L1210 leukaemia. Too low a dose is ineffective but beyond a narrow therapeutic range too high a dose kills the animals from haematological toxicity.

drugs is the major reason for emphasising that the greatest care is required in their administration. Certain specific toxicities are mentioned later but it is a general principle that whenever these drugs are used, it is necessary to monitor the peripheral blood count and be aware of any functional disturbances such as dysphagia or diarrhoea produced by damage to the gastrointestinal tract. Since the maximum dose of any cytotoxic drug that can be prescribed on any one occasion is governed by its toxicity to normal cells, it is found that only partial tumour shrinkage results from any single treatment. It is therefore necessary to administer these drugs repeatedly, the total duration of treatment varying from a few months to several years. In order to prevent unacceptable or cumulative damage to host tissues, intermittent administration is necessary thus allowing an interval for host tissue to recover between treatments. Damage to bone marrow cells results in temporary depression of the blood counts between 10 and 14 days following drug administration. The therapeutic programme varies with different drugs but many cytotoxic drug regimens are given on 21 day cycles to preserve bone marrow integrity.

Choice of Drug. In order to select the most appropriate drug for any individual clinical problem, it is necessary to know the spectrum of activity against disease for the various drugs, and to select a drug which has the minimum toxicities in relation to the particular patient. This information is obtained through a sequence of three phases of clinical trials. Having demonstrated some antineoplastic activity in an experimental system and having been screened by conducting toxicology studies in animals, the new drug enters phase I clinical trials to establish its toxicological properties in man. For ethical reasons, phase I studies are usually performed in patients with advanced disease which has proved refractory to conventional treatment. Since the effects of the new drug are unknown, it is necessary to start phase I trials with very low doses of the drug, and increase the dose until some toxicity is observed. Pharmacokinetic studies are performed during phase I trials to establish if possible the distribution, metabolism and elimination of the compound. Then phase II trials are performed in patients with a wide variety of different malignant diseases in order to determine the spectrum of activity of the drug. If activity is demonstrated for a particular tumour type, then phase III trials are performed. The latter are larger scale randomised trials where the new drug is compared with the best previously known treatment either alone or in combination with other drugs.

Combination Chemotherapy. When in the early 1960s it was first appreciated that a variety of different types of chemical could influence the progression of malignant diseases, the concept of combining drugs in twos, threes and fours was first explored. The theory behind combination chemotherapy was to evaluate the hypothesis that simultaneous disruption of the metabolism of a tumour cell at more than one site might have far more profound effects on the cell than a single metabolic lesion. Dramatic results were produced by treating lymphomas in this way. The four-drug combination of nitrogen mustard, vincristine, procarbazine and prednisolone yielded complete remissions in more than 80% of patients with advanced Hodgkin's disease whereas these same drugs used singly rarely produced remissions in 15–20% of cases. Similarly combination chemotherapy for acute leukaemia increased the remission rates from 20% to 90%. Over the past 20 years it has been shown that combination chemotherapy is valuable in many other malignant diseases including carcinomas of the breast, ovary, lung, testis and several of the childhood tumours. The five general principles governing the use of combination chemotherapy are:

1. Each drug in the combination should have been demonstrated to have some activity on its own against the tumour type for which the combination is being used.

2. Drugs with a similar mechanism of action should not be combined.

3. As far as is possible the major dose-limiting toxicity of each drug should differ from that of the other components of the combination.

4. Since it is rarely possible to avoid some overlap in toxicity to host tissues, it is usually necessary to reduce the dose of each of the component drugs compared with the optimal dose which would be used if the drugs were prescribed individually.

5. There should be no known adverse interaction between the drugs.

Multimodality Treatment. With the development of combination chemotherapy, it became apparent that the clinical course of many different malignant diseases could be influenced by cytotoxic drugs, with cure in some and useful palliation in many others. Nevertheless, since in so many situations cytotoxic drugs are capable of shrinking only a proportion of the tumour, increasing attention has been paid to the use of chemotherapy in conjunction with surgery or radiotherapy to lessen the total tumour load. Thus chemotherapy can be used to reduce tumour bulk prior to local therapy with surgery or radiotherapy, as for example in treating head and neck tumours, or drug treatment can be introduced after primary resection or irradiation to prevent the growth of subclinical micrometastases. The latter use of chemotherapy is frequently referred to as 'adjuvant' chemotherapy, and is now widely used for treating breast carcinomas, lymphomas, and several tumours in children.

Caution must be exercised to prevent additive damage to host tissues, particularly the bone marrow if radiotherapy and chemotherapy are used together, but the principle of combining local and systemic therapy has many potential advantages since as a general principle small tumours are much more susceptible to chemotherapy than large ones. This is explained in part by the fact that drugs penetrate small tumours more effectively but also by the fact that the emergence of drug resistance may be related to the frequency of mutations in the tumour, and the potential number of such events increases with the growth of a tumour.

One major difficulty with adjuvant chemotherapy is to decide for how long it should be continued. In obvious advanced tumours, it is possible to measure tumour shrinkage and continue treatment for as long as benefit lasts. Conversely drug resistance is detectable and thus further inappropriate chemotherapy can be avoided. However in the 'adjuvant' setting where there is no measurable tumour, it is not possible to be certain in the short term whether or not treatment is proving effective. Clinical trials have demonstrated that, for curable tumours in children, it is necessary to continue chemotherapy for 1–2 years. For lymphomas and carcinomas in adults, the optimum duration of adjuvant chemotherapy is less certain and is the subject of continuing study.

It is possible to rank many malignant diseases into groups comprising those for which chemotherapy contributes to cure, those for which effective control prolongs useful life and those for which benefit is less certain or unproven (Table 6.3). Not all patients in any of these groups prove sensitive or resistant to chemotherapy and there is considerable variation between patients in the degree of responsiveness even amongst the most favourable tumours, but such a classification gives an indication of the diseases where further research is particularly needed.

The Side-Effects of Chemotherapy. Due to the relatively poor selectivity of presently available anticancer drugs, it is impossible to avoid some damage to normal host tissues. Nevertheless, when properly administered and monitored, many cytotoxic drugs can be given without producing side-effects which cause symptoms. For example, reversible decreases in haemoglobin, leucocytes and platelet counts should not cause significant symptoms provided adequate time is allowed between cycles of treatment and the blood count is monitored prior to subsequent treatment, thus preventing any cumulative effect.

Acute damage to the gastrointestinal tract may cause mouth ulceration, nausea, vomiting or diarrhoea. Mouth ulceration and diarrhoea result

Table 6.3 Contribution of Chemotherapy to various Malignant Diseases.

Tumours for which chemotherapy can be curative:
Acute lymphoblastic leukaemia in children
Burkitt's lymphoma
Hodgkin's lymphoma
Wilms' tumour
Rhabdomyosarcoma
Testicular teratoma
Choriocarcinoma
Diffuse histiocytic lymphoma
Ewing's sarcoma

Tumours that are highly sensitive to chemotherapy, resulting in remissions that prolong life:
Breast carcinoma
Ovarian carcinoma
Small cell anaplastic lung carcinoma
Non-Hodgkin's lymphoma
Chronic lymphocytic leukaemia
Acute myeloid leukaemia
Medulloblastoma

Tumours that are sensitive to chemotherapy where life is sometimes prolonged:
Gastric carcinoma
Pancreatic carcinoma
Myeloma
Soft tissue sarcoma
Bladder carcinoma
Thyroid carcinoma

Tumours that are usually refractory to currently available chemotherapy:
Squamous cell lung carcinoma
Colorectal carcinoma
Carcinoma of oesophagus
Melanoma

from necrosis of the rapidly dividing epithelial cells lining the gut. Appropriate timing of chemotherapy can prevent this but sometimes it is necesary to adjust the dose of the drug if an individual is particularly sensitive. The complex physiological events leading to nausea and vomiting almost certainly include a direct central nervous system response to many cytotoxic drugs, or their metabolites, but the nature and anatomical site of such chemoreceptors are uncertain. For the cytotoxic drugs which are known to cause nausea and vomiting, it is necessary to prescribe antiemetics, prior to and following administration of the cytotoxic drug, and skilled use of compounds such as metoclopramide (p. 289) can ameliorate these symptoms very successfully.

Nevertheless, despite the fact that it is possible to minimise many of these acute side-effects, there are several subacute and chronic toxicities

which are less susceptible to control. Alopecia, resulting from interruption in the normal proliferation of the hair follicle, is associated with the administration of some of the cytotoxic drugs particularly adriamycin and cyclophosphamide. If such drugs are to be prescribed, it is important to warn the patient in advance and, if appropriate, to arrange for a wig to be fitted. Alopecia is almost always reversible on cessation of therapy.

The pyschological effect of having to receive chemotherapy over a period of many months is another adverse effect of which the physician must be constantly aware. If properly counselled, many patients tolerate the impact of being informed of their diagnosis and their early treatment remarkably well, only to become anxious and depressed as treatment continues even though their tumour may be obviously responding to treatment. Awareness of this problem is essential and constant reassurance and support are necessary to help patients with the disruption in their lives occasioned by repeated visits to hospital, venepunctures and treatment.

The chronic toxicity of cancer chemotherapy is an area of increasing importance now that this form of treatment is becoming more widely available, and increasing numbers of patients are surviving for longer periods. Data from the follow-up of children cured of malignant disease have shown that physical growth can be stunted by the use of combinations of cytotoxic drugs with radiation but there is conflicting evidence as to whether or not these agents cause significant intellectual impairment.

Fertility is preserved for the majority of pre-pubertal children who have to be treated with cytotoxic drugs but for adults, fertility may be lost. This is particularly the case for men. For women the problem is more variable depending on their premorbid menstrual pattern and the length of time prior to the expected menopause. Many patients suffering from malignant diseases may be subfertile at the time of diagnosis and for women amenorrhoea is common for the months during which they are receiving treatment. Nevertheless, this is not a universal finding and since cytotoxic drugs are potentially teratogenic, patients of both sexes should be advised to use contraceptive measures whilst they are receiving chemotherapy.

With the increasing success of chemotherapy and long-term survival, it has become apparent that cytotoxic drugs may be associated with the development of a second malignancy in a small proportion of patients. The cases described have usually been of acute myelomonocytic leukaemia developing 5–10 years following the use of alkylating agents. For example in a study of over 5000 cases of ovarian cancer treated with alkylating agents, it has been shown that the risk of developing acute leukaemia was 36 times that of the population at large. Nevertheless, it should be emphasised that only certain classes of anticancer drug are associated with this phenomenon which is rare and which has arisen only as a result of developing therapies which may cure the primary tumour.

Some anticancer drugs have accumulative toxicities which are organ specific. For example the use of adriamycin beyond a total cumulative dose of $550 \, mg/m^2$ is associated with a greatly increased risk of developing cardiac failure due to the generation of free radicals that damage cardiac tissue by causing the peroxidation of cardiac lipid. This drug should therefore be prescribed only very exceptionally above this total dose. Cis-diammine-dichloroplatinum (cisplastin) causes a progressive impairment of renal function (predominantly tubular) and in addition to monitoring patients for the common side-effects mentioned above, it is necessary to assess renal function prior to subsequent doses of this drug. Bleomycin may cause pulmonary fibrosis in a proportion of patients and the vinca alkaloids, especially vincristine, can cause a neuropathy with cumulative effect. This manifests itself initially as peripheral sensory impairment but later involves motor function and may cause autonomic damage usually presenting as constipation or even intestinal obstruction. The neuropathy due to the vinca alkaloids is reversible on withdrawal of the drug but the cardiac effect of adriamycin, the renal toxicity of cis-diamminedichloroplatinum and the pulmonary fibrosis caused by bleomycin are usually irreversible.

Principles of Endocrine Therapy

Tumours which develop in organs that are known to be under hormonal control sometimes retain hormonal dependency. This can be used therapeutically either by withdrawing the source of the hormone, by prescribing an anti-hormone or by the administration of another hormone. Carcinomas of the breast, prostate, endometrium and thyroid are the diseases amenable to endocrine therapy. The therapeutic use of adrenal corticosteroids is exceptional in that these compounds influence non-endocrine-related tumours, for example the lymphomas and leukaemias.

The biological effect of hormones such as oestrogen and progesterone is dependent on the hormone binding to a cytoplasmic receptor protein that transports the hormone to the nucleus where it interacts with DNA to modulate gene expression. Oestrogen-binding protein can be assayed in biopsies of breast tumours or lymph nodes containing metastases. It has been found that for about 65% of patients whose tumours possess a significant amount of this protein, removal of the source of oestrogen drive will be therapeutically useful whilst for those in whom this protein is absent, hormonal therapy is usually of no benefit. The presence of progesterone-binding protein further increases the likelihood of hormone sensitivity. The development of techniques to predict hormone sensitivity has had a major influence on the management of patients with breast carcinomas. If oestrogen receptor activity is present then premenopausal patients may benefit from oophorectomy and both pre- and postmenopausal patients may respond to the administration of tamoxifen, a compound that blocks oestrogen binding.

The use of ablative procedures such as adrenalectomy is now being superseded by the availability of compounds like aminoglutethamide which achieves the same result by 'medical' rather than surgical means. Aminoglutethamide inhibits the desmolase that catalyses the conversion of cholesterol to delta-S-pregnenolone, thus preventing the synthesis of corticosteroids, oestrogens and androgens. It also inhibits the aromatase that converts androgens to oestrogens in peripheral tissues. In order to prevent excess secretion of ACTH (as a result of the failure to produce the 11-hydroxycorticosteroids), it is necessary to prescribe hydrocortisone together with aminoglutethamide. Tumour response to tamoxifen and aminoglutethamide may not be manifest for 6–12 weeks from the start of therapy and it is therefore necessary to wait for this period before making decisions about further management. Androgen may produce responses in about 20% of patients with breast cancer, particularly in postmenopausal women with bone metastases.

Oestrogens are useful in the palliation of prostate cancer, and have a similar response rate (c. 80%) to that of orchidectomy which removes the major source of testosterone.

Progestogens are compounds related to the progesterone produced by the corpus luteum and placenta. Some women with metastatic endometrial carcinoma benefit from these drugs, particularly patients with well differentiated tumours.

Some papillary carcinomas of the thyroid remain under the influence of thyroid-stimulating hormone (TSH) and the administration of thyroid hormone may be useful as a result of its inhibiting pituitary secretion of TSH.

The major advantage of hormonal therapy over chemotherapy is that the side-effects of endocrine treatment are usually less severe than those associated with cytotoxic drugs. Tamoxifen rarely causes toxicity but aminoglutethamide can cause drowsiness, depression and transient skin rashes in some patients. The use of oestrogen in elderly men with prostate cancer warrants special caution in view of its known propensity to exacerbate the fluid retention that may be associated with cardiovascular disease. Research is currently in progress to evaluate compounds that inhibit pituitary gonadotrophin, thus mimicking the effects of castration but doing so in a reversible way, and in a manner that is free of important side-effects.

Terminal Care

An essential component of oncological medicine is the management of patients in the terminal phase of their illness. When it becomes apparent that active measures to arrest further tumour growth are no longer proving effective, or for those patients in whom it is not appropriate to embark on such therapy, it is more important than ever to provide support and attention to the alleviation of distressing symptoms. Psychological support is the most important aspect but this can be provided only if positive measures are taken to relieve pain, to ensure adequate and appropriate nutrition and treat specific symptoms such as cough, pruritus, nausea, etc. Successful symptomatic treatment allows patients to prepare themselves mentally for death, and the relief of physical distress in the patient will also help the patient's family to cope with impending bereavement.

An individual patient's reaction to the inevitability of death from a malignant disease depends on a host of interrelated variables including his or her cultural and religious background, age, education, the duration of the illness, reactions of dependents, etc. Nevertheless certain common patterns of behaviour are recognisable and an awareness of these is important in order to provide appropriate counselling and support at different stages of the patient's progression towards death. A period of initial disbelief and denial is often replaced by resentment and anger. This in turn is followed by a period of depression which is almost universal but many patients, with or without medical intervention, enter a final phase of peacefully accepting the inevitability of death.

When to tell patients that they have a terminal illness is a matter of experience and judgement that cannot easily be summarised. Death does not necessarily represent a failure of treatment and it is essential that those caring for the terminally ill do not avoid discussion of the processes of terminal illness for fear of this being seen as professional failure. Avoiding such discussions can only enhance the patient's sense of loneliness and isolation.

It is not always appropriate to present all of the facts to a patient, most especially on a single occasion, and time must be spent to determine the patient's awareness of their situation, and their expectations. Non-committal, even ambiguous statements about the future may be appropriate but the patient should never be told what is known to be untrue.

Preparation for death is not the sole responsibility of the medical profession and, especially for patients dying in hospitals, it is important to make provision for the adequate access of relatives, friends and other professionals such as the clergy when patients request their support. Religious belief does not necessarily make death any easier and even for patients who hold such beliefs it should not be forgotten that fear of the unknown, most especially the unknown of death, is something shared by patients and all those who are caring for them.

The most important principle of managing terminal illness is to provide adequate time for talking with the patient. In a busy world this is difficult to find but it is sometimes easier to use the lack of time as an excuse for avoiding demanding consultations that drain the doctor's emotional resources. Nevertheless, to develop the ability to listen to patients and to learn from them how best to provide psychological support during terminal illness can be one of the most rewarding experiences in medicine.

PROSPECTS IN ONCOLOGY

It is to be hoped that continued research into the cause of different malignant diseases will identify either environmental factors that can be avoided or populations at particular risk for whom screening for malignant disease would become cost-effective. In a recent survey of the trend in American mortality from cancer it has been estimated that up to 90% of all cancer deaths could be attributed to potentially avoidable factors such as tobacco, alcohol, diet, reproductive and sexual behaviour, occupation, pollution and geophysical factors.

The only cause whose effect is large and which has been reliably identified is tobacco which is estimated to have been responsible for 130 000 — 140 000 deaths in the USA in 1981. Despite the indisputable association between cigarette tobacco consumption and lung cancer, public health measures have been only modestly successful in reducing cigarette consumption and much remains to be done, especially amongst the young to reduce and eliminate this carcinogen.

It appears easier to influence dietary habits but future research is needed to identify the specific agents responsible for the development of tumours where diet appears to play a role, such as gastrointestinal carcinomas.

The recent increase in carcinoma of the cervix appears to be related to changing patterns of sexual behaviour and the screening of women who have started sexual activity at an early age or have had multiple partners should be encouraged since early detection can be curative.

As further aetiological factors are identified, it is reasonable to predict that other screening exercises will become useful for certain groups although at present there is no indication for screening the entire population.

Unfortunately early detection does not guarantee cure for any malignant disease but generally it is easier to treat small tumours than large ones. Similarly early detection does not necessarily guarantee that tumours are less likely to have metastasised but the treatment of localised tumours is likely to continue to yield better long-term results than those for widely disseminated lesions. Technological advances are still required to improve tumour localisation and surgical or radiotherapeutic eradication but without doubt the area that is most in need of further improvement is the systemic treatment for metastatic tumours.

With the exception of endocrine therapy for hormonally-dependent tumours, the only systemic therapy of proven value is cytotoxic chemotherapy. Attempts to modify the immune response with non-specific agents such as BCG or corynebacterium parvum ('immunotherapy') have not proven therapeutically useful. Research currently in progress to evaluate the antiviral compound interferon is as yet too preliminary for critical evaluation.

The major problem with cytotoxic drugs is their relatively low selectivity for tumour tissues, and much research is being pursued to develop less toxic drugs that still maintain their antineoplastic efficacy. Such research is beginning to show results and a number of 'second generation' compounds are now available. Thus, for example, analogues of cis-diammine-dichloroplatinum with less nephrotoxicity and analogues of adriamycin with less cardiotoxicity are currently entering clinical trials. Alternative approaches to overcome host toxicity are also being explored such as the harvesting of bone marrow prior to administering highly marrow-toxic chemotherapy so that unexposed marrow can be reinfused after the drug or drugs have been given. To minimise the unwanted exposure of host tissues, research is being carried out to use monoclonal antibodies raised against the tumour to target cytotoxic drugs exclusively to the malignant cells but the efficacy of this attractive idea awaits clinical evaluation. Further research is needed to understand the gastrointestinal side-effects of many cytotoxic drugs but increasing knowledge of the physiological mechanisms controlling nausea and emesis is being used to improve antiemetic therapy.

With such a wide spectrum of clinical problems created by malignant diseases, it is unwise to make specific predictions about the future. Nevertheless it is a fact that at no time in the past has so much attention been focussed on the management of these diseases. With the significant progress that has been achieved over the past 20 years, it is reasonable to be cautiously optimistic about the future. This applies most especially to the changing emphasis away from the ultimate objective of cure to the more practical issues of ameliorating symptoms, controlling further disease progression and relieving the anxieties so frequently created by malignant disease.

J.F. SMYTH

FURTHER READING:

DeVita, V.T., Hellman, S. and Rosenburg, S.A. (1982). *Cancer, Principles and Practice of Oncology*. Philadelphia: Lippincott. This is a comprehensive textbook.

Chabner, B. (1982). *Pharmacologic Principles of Cancer Treatment*. Philadelphia: W.B. Saunders. A detailed account both preclinical and clinical.

Calman, K.C., Smyth, J.F. and Tattersall, M.H.N. (1980). *Basic Principles of Cancer Chemotherapy*. New York: MacMillan. A brief introduction to the subject.

Doll, R. and Peto, R. (1981). *The Causes of Cancer*. Oxford: Oxford Medical Publications. This is a short resumé of the known epidemiological factors.

Saunders, C.M. (1978). *The Management of Terminal Disease*. The Management of Malignant Disease, vol. 1. London: Edward Arnold. A summary of the theory and practice of terminal care by the Medical Director of St Christopher's Hospice, London.

7. Diseases of the Cardiovascular System

At all ages and in all countries, diseases of the cardiovascular system are major causes of death and disability, but the pattern of cardiovascular disease varies strikingly between different countries and age groups. For example, rheumatic fever, still a major cause of morbidity in young adults in many parts of the world, is now exceedingly rare in Britain. In contrast, ischaemic heart disease is an increasing problem in many countries where it was formerly uncommon, though in the United States and Australia its contribution to mortality seems to be declining. As more people live on into old age, degenerative causes of valvular disease and cardiac conduction problems become increasingly prevalent, while at the other extreme of life a reduction of infant mortality from infective and nutritional causes focusses attention on morbidity from congenital heart disease.

Patients with heart disease present not only with breathlessness, swollen ankles and chest pain, which are its cardinal symptoms, but also with other symptoms less obviously related to the heart, such as stroke resulting from thrombo-embolism, or fever and anaemia from endocarditis. The presentation of cardiovascular disease is thus protean.

The Symptoms of Heart Disease

Dyspnoea. Awareness of undue breathlessness on exertion is frequently the first symptom of heart failure. From the history alone it is usually hard to distinguish this from the dyspnoea which is due to lung disease (p. 208) but the differentiation is often possible if the patient is observed at the time. Typically, patients with cardiac failure take rapid, shallow breaths, and wheezing or the excessive use of accessory respiratory muscles is uncommon. Occasionally, in the presence of pulmonary oedema (see below) wheezing does become prominent; this is sometimes called cardiac asthma.

Orthopnoea is the name given to breathlessness which prevents the patient lying flat. On lying down, there is a rise in right atrial pressure and hence in right ventricular output, forcing more blood into the lungs, a tendency for the redistribution of oedema fluid, and perhaps an alteration in the pattern of bloodflow within the lungs. The sensation of breathlessness is probably due partly to increased stiffness of the congested lungs and partly to direct stimulation of fine nerve endings around the alveoli.

Accumulation of excess fluid in the lungs at night may reach a critical level before the patient is wakened by breathlessness and has to sit up to gain relief. There is often a repetitive cough which, initially at least, is unproductive. This *paroxysmal nocturnal dyspnoea* is an alarming experience causing tachycardia and temporary hypertension, which may make matters worse. Usually the attack subsides within a few minutes. If the breathlessness continues, the cough becomes productive of watery and often bloodstained sputum, *pulmonary oedema* has supervened. The patient sits up gasping for breath. Respiration often becomes bubbly and sometimes wheezy. There is often intense vasoconstriction, as a result of which the skin is cold and cyanosed.

Cheyne Stokes respiration (periodic breathing), in which there is waxing and waning of ventilation from hyperventilation to apnoea, is common in severe cardiac failure. It may also occur in elderly people without evidence of cardiac failure, particularly during sleep.

Oedema occurs in cardiac failure as a consequence of excessive salt and water retention (p. 95). Pulmonary oedema has already been described. Peripheral oedema is found mainly in the feet and ankles in ambulant patients, as its site is largely determined by gravity. Pressure with the thumb, if sustained, will displace the fluid and leave a pit. On going to bed the oedema is redistributed, principally to the sacrum and thighs. In severe cardiac failure fluid may accumulate in the abdominal cavity (ascites) and as pleural effusions. Oedema resulting from cardiac failure needs to be distinguished from that caused by chronic venous insufficiency in the legs or the nephrotic syndrome (p. 390).

Pain. The cardinal symptom of cardiac ischaemia is the pain known as angina pectoris (p. 167). The pain of pericarditis is described on page 187. Precordial catch is the name given to a stabbing pain felt momentarily at the cardiac apex; it is often indicated by a finger pointing below the left breast. It is not associated with cardiac pathology but frequently causes undue concern to the anxious. Hepatic pain felt in the epigastrium is sometimes a feature of acute or worsening cardiac failure. It is due to hepatic distension resulting from a rise in central venous pressure. Pleuritic pain is a feature of pulmonary infarction, which often complicates cardiac failure. A sudden 'tearing' pain in the back, between the shoulder blades, may be due to a dissecting aneurysm of the aorta.

Palpitation is awareness of the heart beat; it is a common result of exercise or anxiety and occurs with increased catecholamine secretion or with sympathomimetic drugs. Patients often feel the thump of an ectopic beat or, more often, of the more powerful beat which follows a compensatory pause. Palpitation may be the only symptom of paroxysmal tachycardia; often the patient can indicate its rate, and usually is able to say whether the heart beat is regular as in supraventricular tachycardia or irregular as in atrial fibrillation.

Syncope ('fainting') is loss of consciousness resulting from a fall in blood pressure. The latter may be due to decreased cardiac output, decreased peripheral resistance, or a combination of the two. *Simple* or *vasovagal* syncope is the product of a complex reflex which causes bradycardia and peripheral vasodilatation. It usually occurs in circumstances where venous return to the heart is not adequately maintained, e.g. with prolonged standing, particularly when it is hot or when there is a loss of fluid, as from diarrhoea. Simple syncope may also occur as a result of a frightening, unpleasant or painful experience. A feeling of nausea and sometimes a failure of vision and a ringing in the ears may herald its onset. Pallor, sweating and a slow pulse are characteristic. Recovery is usually rapid when venous return is restored by raising the patient's legs. If the patient is kept upright, convulsions and occasionally brain damage may ensue.

Syncope can also occur when a rise in intrathoracic pressure reduces venous return sufficiently, as in the Valsalva manoeuvre. This may happen with prolonged vigorous coughing (*cough syncope*) or when elderly men strain to empty the bladder (*micturition syncope*). Syncope on standing, *postural syncope*, is a feature in some patients with an unusually low blood pressure as in adrenal insufficiency. More commonly it is due to antihypertensive or vasodilator drugs, and it sometimes results from a failure of the normal vasomotor reflexes as in diabetic autonomic neuropathy. Dizziness on moving the neck suggests a reduction in vertebrobasilar blood flow.

Cardiac causes of syncope should be suspected when syncope occurs on exertion (*exercise syncope*) or when it occurs in the absence of obvious precipitating circumstances. Exercise syncope may be due to cardiac arrhythmias, or to exercise-induced vasodilatation in patients unable to increase their cardiac output appropriately, perhaps because of severe coronary artery or valvular heart disease. It may be a feature of aortic stenosis, severe pulmonary stenosis or hypertrophic cardiomyopathy. Syncope which occurs without obvious precipitating circumstances needs to be distinguished from epilepsy (p. 617). It is frequently due to cardiac arrhythmias, either excessive bradycardia or tachycardia.

Other Symptoms. Tiredness is a common complaint with severe heart failure and with ischaemic heart disease. Sometimes it is the consequence of treatment rather than the disease itself, e.g. beta-blockade or hypokalaemia from diuretics. In those with valvular disease without heart failure it should lead to a suspicion of infective endocarditis.

Nocturia, or a reversal of the usual diurnal rhythm of diuresis, sometimes occurs in ambulant patients with cardiac failure. It probably reflects improved renal perfusion during bed-rest rather than a simple mobilisation of oedema fluid from the ankles. Cough is a feature of pulmonary oedema. Anorexia, nausea and vomiting are all common in severe protracted heart failure; they may also be manifestations of digitalis intoxication (p. 142).

Physical Examination

While taking the history and before proceeding to the examination of the heart, certain pertinent observations may be made. The presence should be noted of any anaemia, obesity, breathlessness or cyanosis.

Peripheral cyanosis is due to an excessive extraction of oxygen from the blood when the circulation is impaired from vasoconstriction, low cardiac output or stasis; it occurs in healthy people when the extremities are cold, and warmth abolishes it.

Central cyanosis is due to oxygen under-saturation of the arterial blood from poor gaseous exchange in the lungs resulting from respiratory failure or pulmonary oedema, or when there is a right-to-left shunt as in congenital heart disease. If the tongue is cyanosed it may be deduced that the cyanosis is central in origin. A combination of central and peripheral cyanosis is often seen in cardiac failure.

Other Observations. The temperature of the skin varies with the skin blood flow. In cardiac failure, except in those rare forms where the cardiac output is increased, the extremities are abnormally cold, even in a warm environment. Unduly moist palms suggest anxiety if they are cold or thyrotoxicosis if they are warm. Clubbing of the fingers occurs in cyanotic congenital heart disease and in advanced infective endocarditis, as well as in a variety of respiratory and other diseases (p. 210). Subungual or 'splinter' haemorrhages may result from trauma and occur in normal individuals, but they are also a feature of infective endocarditis.

The arterial pulse should be examined for rate, rhythm and volume, and for the character of the pulse wave. The radial pulse is traditionally used, but the carotid is more reliable for assessing the pulse wave because its form is less altered by transmission. Bradycardia (p. 133) describes a heart rate of 60 per minute or less, and tachycardia (p. 133) a heart rate of 100 or more. In health the pulse is normally regular, but a slowing of the pulse in expiration is common (sinus arrhythmia p. 133), particularly in children. The other causes of irregularity are discussed on pages 134–138.

A pulse of small volume is a feature of reduced cardiac output, as in major haemorrhage or pulmonary embolism, or with severe obstruction to bloodflow at a cardiac valve. A pulse of large volume, sometimes called a collapsing pulse, is found where there is rapid flow of blood out of the arterial system with peripheral vasodilatation as in fever or hyperthyroidism, or with aortic regurgitation. A pulse of large volume may also accompany bradycardia, as in complete heart block.

Pulsus paradoxus is a name given to a variation of pulse volume with breathing, in which systolic pressure diminishes with inspiration. A small variation of this nature is physiological (so the 'paradox' is misnamed), but it is abnormal for there to be more than 5 mm Hg difference between inspiratory and expiratory systolic blood pressures during ordinary quiet breathing, or for the difference to be readily palpable. An exaggerated fall in systolic pressure during inspiration may occur in asthma or, for a different reason, in patients with constrictive pericarditis or pericardial tamponade from a tense pericardial effusion (p. 187).

In *pulsus alternans* the pulse is regular but its amplitude is alternately large and small. It is best detected with the sphygmomanometer; there may be a difference of 10–40 mm Hg between the strong and weak beats. It is a sign of left ventricular failure.

In aortic stenosis the pulse is characteristically slow-rising, with a shudder or vibratory feel to the upstroke. A pulse with a double peak, *pulsus bisferiens*, is suggestive of combined aortic stenosis (usually mild) and regurgitation.

In old age, arteries become more rigid, and this may affect the way they transmit the pulse wave. They also elongate and become more tortuous. In elderly patients, particularly hypertensive women, an arterial pulsation may be seen above the right clavicle because of 'kinking' of a tortuous carotid artery.

Arterial pulsation in the neck is increased in aortic regurgitation and sometimes in coarctation of the aorta. A bruit heard over a major artery with the stethoscope bell is an important sign of partial obstruction but needs to be distinguished from a murmur conducted from the aortic valve.

In hypertensive patients, and in children suspected of having congenital heart disease, the radial and femoral pulses should be palpated simultaneously in order to detect coarctation of the aorta. In this condition the femoral pulse is seldom absent, but it is of small volume, delayed after the radial pulse, and measurement of the arterial pressure in the legs with a suitably large cuff shows it to be lower than in the arms.

Jugular Venous Pulse. With the patient reclining against pillows at about 45°, and with the neck muscles relaxed, the jugular venous pulse may be examined from movement of the skin overlying the internal jugular vein, although the vein itself is not visible. Unlike arterial pulsation, jugular venous pulsation represents the zone of transition between distended and collapsed segments of vein, and the height of this above the level of the right atrium is a measure of the right atrial, or central venous, pressure. In normal subjects, or in those with a low central venous pressure, jugular pulsation is often hidden behind the clavicle in this position, and rarely extends for more than 2 or 3 cm above the sternal angle. When venous pressure is transiently increased by pressure on the abdomen, the level of pulsation moves upwards in the neck: this is called *hepato-jugular reflux* and is one of the ways in which the jugular pulse can be distinguished from arterial pulsation.

The venous pulse varies with the patient's position and the phase of respiration; it frequently exhibits two peaks to every one of the arterial pulse (Fig. 7.1), and the most prominent movement is often an inward one. It is often taught that the venous pulse is impalpable and that it can be

Fig. 7.1 Carotid and jugular pulses. Simultaneous central arterial and venous pulses to demonstrate carotid and jugular pulse wave form. a = atrial contraction, c = onset of ventricular contraction, v = pressure peak immediately prior to opening of tricuspid valve, c-x = x descent, v-y = y descent.

abolished by pressure on the root of the neck, but these criteria are not infallible.

It is usual to express *jugular venous pressure* (which is equivalent to central venous pressure) as the vertical distance in centimetres between the zone of jugular pulsation and the sternal angle. Sometimes the jugular pressure is so high that pulsation is apparent only when the patient sits or stands upright. The commonest and most important cause of a raised jugular venous pressure is cardiac failure. Sometimes it is possible to find out more about the cause of the failure by analysing the wave-form of the pulse.

The *wave form of the jugular venous pulse* in a patient in sinus rhythm is shown in Figure 7.1. The *a* wave is due to atrial systole. It is absent in atrial fibrillation, and may be abnormally large when there is obstruction to right atrial discharge, as in tricuspid stenosis, or when the right ventricle is hypertrophied and stiff, as in pulmonary stenosis or pulmonary hypertension. With tricuspid regurgitation there are prominent waves in the venous pulse in time with ventricular systole; these are often called *v* waves but the mechanism and timing are different from the physiological *v* waves shown in Figure 7.1.

In patients with atrio-ventricular dissociation (p. 143) intermittent large volume systolic waves may be seen in the venous pulse; these are called *cannon waves*, and occur when the atrium contracts against a closed tricuspid valve.

Examination of the Heart. The methods employed are inspection, palpation, percussion and auscultation; at each stage the intelligent use of one of these methods often makes the deployment of the next easier.

INSPECTION. In children, enlargement of the right ventricle during the growing period may show as a prominence to the left of the sternum. The apical impulse (see below) may be visible, and its position may give a clue to cardiac enlargement. The sustained apical impulse of left ventricular hypertrophy, and the diffuse pulsation over a left ventricular aneurysm can often be seen as well as felt. Occasionally an aneurysm of the aortic arch can be seen to move the upper sternum with each systole; when the heart is very much enlarged, as with advanced valvular disease, the whole chest may move with each beat.

Systolic pulsation in the epigastrium caused by aortic pulsation is quite common in thin healthy individuals. Pulsation in the epigastrium and right hypochondrium may also be due to hepatic pulsation in tricuspid regurgitation; correct interpretation is enabled by recognising the accompanying systolic jugular venous pulsation.

PALPATION. It is best briefly to palpate the whole of the precordium with the flat of the hand before attempting to localise the apex beat, and then to return to areas of special interest for detailed analysis.

The *apex beat* is the furthest outward and downward point where the finger is lifted during systole; localisation may be impossible if there is obesity or emphysema. In health the apex beat is within the mid-clavicular line in the fifth intercostal space. Significant displacement of the apex beat to the left usually indicates cardiac enlargement, but more reliable evidence is provided by a chest radiograph. If the mediastinum is displaced by fibrosis, collapse or removal of the lung on the left side or by a large pleural effusion on the right, the apex beat may lie to the left in the absence of cardiac enlargement.

The quality of the cardiac impulse should be noted. In left ventricular hypertrophy it is forceful and sustained, while abrupt closure of the mitral valve, either with anxiety or when associated with mitral stenosis, may give it a tapping quality. When the heart is dilated, as for example in dilated cardiomyopathy or advanced ischaemic heart disease, the apex is displaced to the left but the impulse is diffuse rather than forceful.

With right ventricular hypertrophy a pulsation may be imparted to the hand on the chest to the left of the sternum. This may also result when the heart is displaced forward by a dilated left atrium. A dilated pulmonary artery under abnormally high pressure may cause a pulsation in the second left intercostal space beside the sternum. Closure of the semilunar valves under abnormal pressure may give a diastolic shock, or palpable second heart sound.

Turbulent blood flow may impart a vibration to the hand; this *thrill* is the palpable equivalent of a murmur. Usually only loud murmurs are associated with thrills, but a low-pitched vibration is sometimes felt as readily as it is heard. A systolic thrill at the apex usually indicates mitral regurgitation, and a diastolic thrill mitral stenosis. A systolic thrill can often be felt at the lower left sternal edge with a ventricular septal defect, and at the upper sternal edge in aortic or pulmonary stenosis. An aortic diastolic thrill is very rare and usually indicates rupture of an aortic valve cusp.

PERCUSSION is seldom used except when seeking abnormal dullness to the right of the sternum in a patient with a suspected pericardial effusion. One of the physical signs of emphysema is a loss of the normal area of cardiac dullness.

AUSCULTATION. It is essential to use a satisfactory stethoscope with both diaphragm and bell. The diaphragm, firmly pressed against the chest, preferentially conveys high pitched sounds and murmurs, whereas the bell, lightly applied to the skin, favours the transmission of those that are lower pitched.

Sounds. The *first heart sound* results particularly from the closure of the mitral, and to a lesser extent of the tricuspid valve. It is loudest at the apex and may be diminished in the presence of obesity or emphysema. It is accentuated by tachycardia, as in anxiety or thyrotoxicosis, and is often abnormally loud in mitral stenosis (p. 159). The first sound may be diminished when the valve fails to close properly in mitral regurgitation, or when left ventricular function is impaired by myocarditis or cardiomyopathy. It may be obscured by the murmur of mitral regurgitation. Both mitral and tricuspid components may be audible (as a 'split' first heart sound) when contraction of one ventricle is delayed, as in bundle branch block and also in some healthy individuals.

The *second heart sound* is due to closure of the aortic and pulmonary valves. Normally, closure is synchronous in expiration, but in inspiration the pulmonary component is delayed because of increased right ventricular filling and the aortic component is advanced because of decreased left ventricular filling, so the second heart sound becomes split. This *physiological inspiratory splitting* is most prominent in children and young adults. Abnormally delayed closure of one of the semilunar valves may result from conduction or mechanical factors. An example of the former is when aortic closure is delayed by left bundle branch block. This leads to *reversed splitting* of the second heart sound, splitting being heard in expiration rather than in inspiration. Increased right ventricular stroke volume from a left to right shunt, together with equalisation of left and right atrial pressures, leads to wide, *fixed splitting* of the second heart sound throughout the respiratory cycle in atrial septal defect.

Various added sounds may also be significant. In the young a low pitched mid-diastolic *third heart sound*, at the end of the rapid phase of diastolic left ventricular filling, is often heard at the apex. In older patients this sound is associated with abnormal left ventricular filling, either from an increased stroke volume as in mitral regurgitation, or from altered left ventricular compliance, as in cardiomyopathy. In the latter case it usually implies actual or incipient cardiac failure.

A *fourth heart sound* indicates an abnormally forceful left ventricular distension as a result of atrial discharge; it occurs just before the first heart sound, and may be palpable as well as audible. It is a feature of long-standing hypertension, hypertrophic cardiomyopathy, ischaemic heart disease and other conditions associated with left ventricular hypertrophy or reduced compliance.

The *opening snap* is a feature of mitral stenosis with a pliant mitral valve. It is best heard with the diaphragm of the stethoscope to the left of the lower sternum.

An *ejection sound* is an early systolic click which occurs at the time of opening of the relevant semilunar valve in aortic or pulmonary stenosis or when there is dilatation of the proximal aorta or pulmonary artery. A systolic click, or sometimes multiple clicks, may be a feature of mitral valve prolapse.

Prosthetic Sounds. Mechanical replacement heart valves also produce added heart sounds; there is usually a loud click indicating valve closure and a quieter one indicating valve opening. With a mitral prosthesis the closing sound accompanies the first heart sound, and the opening click has the same timing as an opening snap.

Murmurs are associated with turbulent blood flow. When cardiac output is greatly increased, as with pregnancy or severe anaemia, the blood flow through a normal pulmonary or aortic valve may become turbulent and give rise to a systolic murmur, usually best heard in the second left intercostal space at the sternal border. Murmurs also arise when blood is projected through, or leaks back through, abnormal valves; the murmurs then usually radiate in the direction of the abnormal flow.

In coming to a decision as to the cause of a murmur it is important to note whether it occurs in systole or diastole, where it is best heard, and the direction in which the sound of the murmur is conducted. The pitch and quality of the murmur are also important. The characteristics of the main murmurs are shown in Figures 7.29, 7.30 and 7.32. As a general rule a harsh murmur, like a saw, is usually systolic; this should be confirmed by simultaneous palpation of the carotid artery or by identifying that the murmur precedes the second heart sound. The murmur of regurgitation through either of the semilunar valves is usually best heard down the left sternal edge. Because of its quality it is easily confused with a breath sound, and it is often best heard with the patient leaning forward and the breath held in expiration. The murmur of mitral stenosis, on the other hand, is low pitched and is most likely to be heard if the bell of the stethoscope is lightly pressed at or near the apex with the patient turned half towards the left side, particularly after exercise.

Blood Pressure. The inflatable cuff of a sphygmomanometer is wrapped carefully round the upper arm with the bag over the brachial artery and is connected with a mercury or aneroid manometer. The bell of the stethoscope is applied over the brachial artery and the cuff is inflated to a level well above that which abolishes the Korotkov sounds. The pressure in the cuff is then allowed to fall slowly and the point of return of the sounds is taken as the systolic pressure. As the pressure falls further the sounds become louder, and then usually quite suddenly they become muffled (phase 4) and later disappear (phase 5). In some people a phase 5 endpoint cannot be reached. Although it has been traditional in Britain to use the phase 4 reading to indicate diastolic pressure, there is less observer variation with the phase 5 end-point. It is good practice to record both, e.g. 140/90–85, where 140 mmHg is the systolic and 90 and 85 mmHg the phase 4 and 5 diastolic readings respectively.

When the blood pressure is to be recorded in the leg the patient lies prone, a special large cuff is applied to the thigh, and the stethoscope diaphragm is placed over the popliteal fossa.

The *pulse pressure* is the difference between the systolic and diastolic pressures; it tends to be abnormally high in the elderly who have rigid arteries and in patients with conditions that give rise to an increased stroke volume.

Arterial pressure is difficult to measure by the cuff method when there is severe peripheral vasoconstriction, or when there is marked beat to beat variation as in atrial fibrillation.

Blood pressure varies throughout the day, falling to low levels during sleep and rising with stress or anxiety. Isolated blood pressure records can therefore prove misleading, particularly in those who are unduly anxious. Sometimes this is manifest from tremor, sweating or tachycardia. In nervous patients repeated blood pressure estimations tend to result in progressively lower figures, but not invariably.

It would be helpful if normal blood pressure could be clearly defined, but this is not feasible because it varies according to circumstances, particularly age. In an infant, levels of 90/60 would be normal; in the 20 year old age group, blood pressure taken at rest in most normal subjects varies between about 140/90 and 95/55, and there is a tendency for systolic, and to a lesser extent diastolic, pressures to increase with age. The problem is further discussed in the section on hypertension.

Investigation

Electrocardiography plays an essential role in the diagnosis and investigation of heart disease. Its main value lies in the elucidation of cardiac arrhythmias and conduction defects, and in the diagnosis and localisation of myocardial infarction. It also provides important information about problems such as digitalis toxicity, electrolyte disturbances and hypertrophy of the various chambers of the heart. However difficulties with interpretation are common and the electrocardiogram (ECG) must always be viewed in the light of the clinical findings and the results of other investigations.

The normal resting cardiac cell is polarised as a result of an ionic gradient across the cell wall produced by a sodium pump which reduces the intracellular and increases the extracellular sodium concentration; the ionic balance is preserved by a high intracellular and low extracellular potassium concentration. It is the potassium gradient across the cell membrane which is mainly responsible for the electrical potential difference across it.

When the membrane is electrically stimulated, there is a sudden inrush of sodium ions, and the cell becomes depolarised. Although impermeability to sodium is rapidly restored, a slow inward flux of calcium ions is also triggered, and helps to prolong the depolarisation. Repolarisation is finally achieved by inactivation of the calcium flux and a transient increase in potassium permeability. Since cardiac cells are connected by electrically-conducting junctions, membrane depolarisation

Fig. 7.2 ECG leads. The ECG is recorded using electrodes attached to each of the limbs and a mobile electrode which is moved to different positions to record the chest leads. The electrode attached to the right leg is used as an earth connection. The standard (bipolar) leads record the potential difference between the two limbs (lead I: left arm — right arm; lead II: left leg — right arm; lead III: left leg — left arm). Unipolar leads, designated by the letter V, use an exploring electrode placed on a chosen site and linked with an indifferent electrode whose potential is close to zero. The indifferent electrode is formed by connecting all three limb electrodes (i.e. both arms and left leg) in the case of the chest leads, or in the case of the augmented (a) unipolar limb leads (aVR, aVL, aVF) by connecting the two limb electrodes which are not being used as the exploring electrode.

Fig. 7.3 Activation of septum and ventricles. Activation of the septum is from left to right by the left branch of the bundle of His and is followed by spread of the impulse throughout both ventricles. The lower illustration also shows the placement of the chest leads and how each 'looks at' the heart.

spreads as a wave through the whole myocardium. It is principally the movement of the depolarisation wave, and the ensuing wave of repolarisation, which are detected by the surface electrocardiogram.

It is conventional to use a series of different electrode positions to record the ECG. Each pair of electrode positions is called a *lead*. Usually, 12 leads are recorded, called leads I, II, III, aVR, aVL and aVF (the limb leads) and V1 to V6 (the chest leads). Further details on the placement of the electrodes and the names of the leads are given in Figure 7.2. It is a useful simplification to im-

agine each lead 'looking at' electrical activity in the heart from a specific direction (Fig. 7.3). The machine is connected so that movement of the depolarisation wave towards the 'observer' causes an upward deflection and movement away from the observer a downward one. As depolarisation proceeds in many directions simultaneously, the ECG represents the summation of these events.

Normally cardiac activation starts in the sino-atrial (SA) node, but this cannot be detected by the ECG. The impulse then flows through the atrium producing the P wave. The only point at which it can pass to ventricular tissue is at the atrioventricular (AV) node, through which conduction is relatively slow. It then goes rapidly through the right and left branches of the bundle of His to the Purkinje fibres of the ventricles. The next part of the ECG — the QRS complex — represents various components of ventricular depolarisation. The interventricular septum is first activated by the left bundle branch from left to right, producing an initial upward deflection (R wave) in leads V1 and V2, and an initial downward deflection (Q wave) in leads V4–V6 (Fig. 7.3). The impulse then spreads out simultaneously through both ventricles from the endocardial to the epicardial surfaces. The amplitude and duration of the QRS complexes depend to some extent on the bulk of the muscle through which the impulse is passing; as the left ventricle is normally much thicker than the right, most of the QRS complex is dominated by activation of the left ventricle. For example, lead V1 normally shows an S wave because the left ventricular activation wave moves away from this electrode, whereas V5 usually shows a large R wave. Atrial repolarisation is usually obscured by the QRS complex. There is a short period of inactivity after the QRS complex, during which the whole ventricular mass is depolarised (the ST segment). Repolarisation then takes place, producing the T wave. This is normally upright in all leads except aVR and sometimes leads III or V1. Examples of abnormal ECGs are given on pages 134–138, 143, 145, 149, 173 and 174.

AMBULATORY ECG (HOLTER) MONITORING. Continuous recordings of one or two ECG leads may be obtained by attaching them to a small portable tape recorder. This technique is useful in detecting transient episodes of arrhythmia or ischaemia, which seldom occur at the time of routine 12-lead ECG recordings.

Radiological examination is important for determining the size and shape of the heart, and the state of the pulmonary blood vessels. Most information is given by a postero-anterior (PA) projection taken in full inspiration. Antero-posterior (AP) projections are less useful because the heart outline is distorted owing to its distance from the film.

A rough estimate of overall heart size can be made by comparing the maximum width of the cardiac outline with the transverse diameter of the thoracic cavity at the same level. The cardiothoracic ratio so determined should be less than 0·5. Dilatation of individual cardiac chambers can be

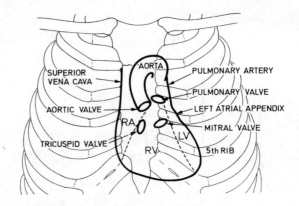

Fig. 7.4 **The radiological outline of the heart** and the surface projection of its valves.

recognised by the characteristic alterations they cause to the cardiac silhouette (Figs. 7.4 and 7.5 and also the sections on valvular heart disease). A barium swallow to outline the oesophagus coupled with a lateral or oblique projection sometimes helps to determine the size of the left atrium. Lateral or oblique projections are also useful in detecting aortic or mitral valve calcification, which may be obscured by the spine on the PA view.

Fig. 7.5 **Radiological cardiac outlines associated with different cardiac lesions.** A: normal; B: Mitral stenosis with enlarged left atrial appendage; C: Aortic stenosis with left ventricular hypertrophy and post-stenotic dilatation of the aorta (significant mitral or aortic stenosis can sometimes occur without any visible abnormality of the postero-anterior chest radiograph); D: Dilatation of the main pulmonary artery and its proximal branches in pulmonary hypertension; E: Generalised cardiac enlargement (or pericardial effusion); F: Tetralogy of Fallot. Note lack of prominence of pulmonary artery and its branches, and elevation of cardiac apex by enlarged right ventricle.

Fig. 7.6 Principles of M-Mode echocardiography. The reflected echoes of ultrasound are converted into blips of light on a cathode-ray tube. The blips can be used to plot a 'graph against time' of the position of cardiac structures on a moving strip of paper.

A rise in pulmonary venous pressure from left-sided cardiac failure first shows on the chest radiograph as an abnormal distension of the upper lobe pulmonary veins in the erect position. Subsequently, interstitial oedema causes thickened septa and dilated lymphatics which show as horizontal lines in the costophrenic angles (Kerley 'B' lines). More advanced changes are a hazy opacification spreading from the hilar region, and pleural effusion. An increased pulmonary blood flow, as in congenital heart disease with a left-to-right shunt, causes enlargement of the pulmonary artery and a generalised increase in pulmonary vascular markings. Pulmonary arterial hypertension also causes an enlargement of the main pulmonary artery and of the proximal pulmonary arteries, but the peripheral lung vascular markings tend to be diminished.

Radioscopy (screening) of the heart, using an image intensifier, may help in the detection of abnormal cardiac pulsations and of valvular calcification. Its main use, however, is during cardiac catheterisation and pacemaker implantation.

Echocardiography uses ultrasound to study the disposition and movement of valves and other structures within the heart. It depends on the reflection of ultrasound waves at interfaces between blood and more solid tissues.

In *M-mode echocardiography* the ultrasound is focused into a narrow beam, and the output is a graph against time of the movement relative to the chest wall of those structures through which the beam passes (Fig. 7.6). Characteristic patterns of movement are produced in, for example, mitral stenosis and pericardial effusions are easily recognised. Accurate measurements can be made of cardiac dimensions.

In *two-dimensional (2D) real-time echocardiography*, the ultrasound beam is swung rapidly back and forth over an arc or sector and the resulting information synthesised into a two-dimensional map or picture of the position of the reflecting structures on a television screen (Fig. 7.7). The picture is the equivalent of a 'slice' through the heart, and the structures shown will depend on the position and orientation of the ultrasound crystal. Because the beam oscillates very rapidly, the ultrasound image accurately reproduces the movement of structures in the

Fig. 7.7 Principles of two-dimensional (2D) real time echocardiography. A moving, two-dimensional image of the echoes detected from a 'slice' of heart can be built up by swinging the ultrasound beam rapidly back and forth.

living heart. This type of echocardiography is particularly good at detecting intracardiac masses, such as thrombi or tumours, or endocarditic vegetations. It is also very useful in sorting out complex structural abnormalities in congenital heart disease.

Phonocardiography records heart sounds and murmurs and may help to elucidate difficult problems of auscultation. Examples of phonocardiograms are given in Figure 7.29 (mitral stenosis), Figure 7.30 (aortic stenosis), Figure 7.32 (aortic regurgitation), Figure 7.39 (persistent ductus arteriosus), Figure 7.41 (atrial septal defect) and Figure 7.42 (ventricular septal defect).

Cardiac Catheterisation and Angiocardiography. In contrast to the preceding investigations, these are invasive techniques. A catheter inserted into a vein can be advanced into the right atrium, and then manipulated into the right ventricle and pulmonary artery. In the presence of an atrial septal defect or patent foramen ovale, venous catheters can also enter the left atrium and left ventricle. If the atrial septum is intact, access to the left ventricle is usually by retrograde passage of a catheter across the aortic valve. Left atrial pressure can be measured directly by puncturing the interatrial septum with a special long, curved needle via a catheter passed up the femoral vein to the right atrium. For many purposes, however, a satisfactory approximation to left atrial pressure can be recorded by 'wedging' an end-hole venous catheter in a branch of the pulmonary artery.

Cardiac catheters are usually manipulated under radiographic control using an image-intensifier, but if a venous catheter is provided at its distal end with a small balloon which can be inflated when the catheter is in the right atrium then the blood stream itself will guide the catheter through the right ventricle and into the pulmonary artery. The balloon also makes it easy to 'wedge' the catheters so as to estimate left atrial pressure. These Swan-Ganz catheters (p. 150) are being used in increasing numbers in intensive and coronary care units, where they can be inserted without the need to transfer the patient to a radiology department.

Pressure measurements obtained through cardiac catheters can be used to assess the severity of valvular stenoses, and measurement of ventricular end-diastolic pressures gives an indication of ventricular compliance and indirectly of ventricular function. Measurement of oxygen saturation in samples withdrawn via the catheters at different sites in the heart allow the detection of intracardiac left to right or right to left shunts, and also allows calculation of pulmonary and systemic blood flow. Cardiac output can also be measured by dye-dilution or thermodilution techniques.

Catheters allow the injection of radio-opaque contrast medium into individual chambers of the heart, the aorta or pulmonary artery, or, using specially shaped catheters, into either coronary artery.

Radionuclide Scanning. The availability of radionuclides of short half life emitting gamma rays, together with sophisticated equipment (the gamma camera) for detecting this radiation has made it possible to use radionuclides for studying cardiac function. Two basic types of technique are available:

1. BLOOD POOL SCANNING. The isotope is injected into the bloodstream and mixes with the circulating blood. The gamma camera detects the amount of isotope-emitting blood in the heart at different phases of the cardiac cycle, and also the size and 'shape' of the cardiac chambers. By linking the gamma camera to the ECG it is possible to collect information over several cardiac cycles. The principal use of blood pool scanning is as an accurate and reproducible measure of left ventricular function, and for detecting left ventricular aneurysms.

2. MYOCARDIAL SCANNING. Although this uses the same gamma camera, both the radionuclides used and the concepts involved differ from blood pool scanning. The object is usually to distinguish between ischaemic and non-ischaemic myocardium (using radioactive thallium) or between normal and damaged myocardium (using radioactive pyrophosphate).

Radionuclide scanning is also of great value in detecting pulmonary embolism, particularly if the injection of an isotope into the bloodstream is combined with a study of the distribution of an inhaled radioactive gas (ventilation-perfusion scanning).

DISORDERS OF CARDIAC RATE, RHYTHM AND CONDUCTION

The Control of Cardiac Rate. Some cardiac cells have the faculty of self excitation. The pacemaking of the heart is due to this activity, and it is normally controlled by the cells with the fastest natural rate. These are usually in the sinoatrial node. The SA node has its own intrinsic rate but it is also under nervous control; vagal activity slows it and sympathetic activity accelerates it. If the sinus rate becomes unduly slow, lower centres may take over the pacemaking, e.g. either the AV node, (junctional rhythm) or sometimes an ectopic ventricular focus. At other times the natural rate of lower centres may be increased as a result of disturbances of cellular metabolism, such as occur with electrolytes disorders, digitalis excess, or as a result of cellular damage from myocardial disease.

Sometimes, as a consequence of congenital abnormality or acquired disease, there are alternative pathways for the conduction of the impulse. A premature, ectopic impulse may find the normal pathway refractory, and then has to take a different course. It may arrive when the distal end of the normal pathway is no longer refractory, and may then travel through it retrogradely. This short-circuit, or re-entry phenomenon, can lead to a rapid circus movement and is one of the causes of paroxysmal tachycardia (Fig. 7.8).

Fig. 7.8 Mechanism of re-entry tachycardia. In this example there are two alternative pathways, A and B, through the AV node. B has a longer refractory period than A. The atrial ectopic beat E finds pathway B refractory, but travels through A. On reaching the end of A, the impulse finds that B has now completed its refractory period, so the impulse can now travel retrogradely to give a further premature atrial beat, which repeats the process. The result is a re-entry or reciprocating tachycardia.

Sinus Rhythms

Sinus arrhythmia is a phasic alteration in heart rate in time with breathing; the rate increases in inspiration and slows in expiration. It is a manifestation of normal autonomic nervous activity, and is often particularly pronounced in children. A complete absence of variation in heart rate with breathing or with changes in posture may be a feature of autonomic neuropathy.

Sinus bradycardia is arbitrarily defined as a sinus rate of less than 60 per minute. This may occur in normal people during sleep, and is a common finding in athletes. It can be caused by several drugs, most commonly by beta-adrenoceptor antagonists. It may also be a feature of myxoedema, jaundice or raised intracranial pressure, and occurs in some patients after myocardial infarction.

Sinoatrial disease (the sick sinus syndrome) is characterised by inappropriate bradycardia, episodes of sinus arrest (with absent P waves on the ECG), an increased liability to *paroxysmal tachyarrhythmias*, and a tendency to delayed or absent return of sinus node activity following termination of a tachyarrhythmia. The underlying pathology is uncertain but SA node fibrosis or degeneration may occur. There may be associated AV node dysfunction.

Sinoatrial disease may occur at any age, but is most common in the elderly. It is an important cause of syncope, but its prevalence was underestimated before the widespread use of ambulatory ECG monitoring, which is the best way of detecting it. Symptomatic patients may require a cardiac pacemaker; there is no evidence this is needed in those who have the ECG abnormality without symptoms. An artificial pacemaker may also be required, for safety, if drugs are used to control the tachycardia.

Sinus tachycardia is defined as a resting sinus rate of more than 100 per minute. It is a feature of anxiety, fever, hyperthyroidism and acute circulatory or cardiac failure. Except in infants, the rate seldom exceeds 160 per minute. Apart from the rapid rate, the ECG is normal.

Ectopic Rhythms

When the impulses arise elsewhere than in the SA node the rhythm is called ectopic; it may be regular or irregular. Ectopic rhythms arise either because of increased automaticity of pacemaker cells, or because of re-entry circuits (Fig. 7.8). They can broadly be classified into supraventricular (arising in the atria, AV node or other AV junctional tissue) and ventricular.

Supraventricular Ectopic Rhythms

Ectopic Beats (*Extrasystoles, Premature Beats*). These usually cause no symptoms but can give the sensation of an extra or thumping beat. The rhythm is basically regular, but premature beats may occur either at regular intervals or apparently randomly. If sufficiently premature they may produce no pulse, but their presence can usually be detected with the stethoscope. The ECG (Fig. 7.9) shows a premature beat with a normal QRS complex; the conformation of the P wave is often different because the impulse starts at an abnormal site.

Fig. 7.9 Atrial ectopic beats. The QRS complexes of the two ectopic beats are similar to those of the normal beats and are preceded by a P wave.

Supraventricular Tachycardia (Fig. 7.10). Paroxysmal tachycardia may occur with a rate of between 140 and 220 as a result of re-entry or a rapidly firing ectopic focus. This usually occurs in hearts which are otherwise normal and may last from a few seconds to a day or two when untreated. The patient is usually aware that the heart has suddenly started to beat fast, and may feel faint or breathless. With prolonged attacks polyuria is sometimes a feature. Particularly if the heart is otherwise abnormal, cardiac pain or left ventricular failure may occur. Coffee, alcohol, tobacco, anxiety or hyperthyroidism may be precipitating factors.

The ECG confirms the tachycardia and shows a QRST of normal configuration; occasionally, bundle branch block develops at rapid rates.

Fig. 7.10 Atrial tachycardia. The rate is 190 per min. The QRS complexes are normal.

Massage of the carotid sinus on one side for a few seconds may terminate an attack. If it does not do so, a sedative and retiring to bed may be all that is required; many patients then awake to find that the attack is over. If the attack is causing severe symptoms it can usually be terminated by intravenous verapamil, by a beta-adrenoceptor antagonist or disopyramide, or in an emergency by cardioversion (p. 145). Digoxin is also effective but takes longer to work. If attacks are frequent or otherwise disabling, oral therapy with any of the above drugs may help to reduce their frequency. In resistant cases amiodarone is helpful. Further information about antiarrhythmic drugs is given on page 139.

The Wolff-Parkinson-White (WPW) syndrome results from the presence of an abnormal band of atrioventricular conducting tissue which can bypass the AV node. In normal sinus rhythm conduction takes place partly through the AV node and partly through the more rapidly conducting bypass, which produces a shortening of the PR interval and a slurring of the QRS complex called a delta wave (Fig. 7.11). Because the AV node and the bypass pathway have different conduction speeds and refractory periods, a re-entry circuit can develop causing paroxysms of tachycardia. During the tachycardia the QRS is usually normal. Because the bypass pathway lacks the rate-limiting properties of the normal AV node, patients are at risk from very rapid ventricular rates, and sometimes ventricular fibrillation and death, should they develop atrial fibrillation or a rapid atrial tachycardia.

Treatment is aimed at reducing conduction rate and increasing the refractory period of the bypass, using disopyramide, quinidine or amiodarone (p. 141).

Atrial Tachycardia with Atrioventricular Block. In this condition there is an atrial tachy-

PR 0·12 – 0·20 SEC   PR < 0·12 SEC

Fig. 7.11 A normal ECG complex (left) compared with one from a patient with the Wolff-Parkinson-White syndrome (right). In this syndrome, premature excitation of part of the ventricles through an accessory atrioventricular conduction pathway produces the delta wave, which gives the appearance of a short PR interval and a broad QRS complex. These patients are prone to re-entry tachycardias — during such a tachycardia the QRS usually becomes normal, since ventricular activation is taking place only through the AV node, and the accessory pathway is conducting the impulses back to the atria.

cardia of 140–220 per minute accompanied by atrioventricular block, usually either 2:1 or variable (p. 143). Carotid sinus massage may slow the pulse by increasing the degree of block (Fig. 7.12), but seldom terminates the attack. Atrial tachycardia with block seldom occurs in otherwise normal hearts, and it is sometimes a manifestation of digitalis toxicity. If the latter is suspected, digitalis should be stopped, potassium supplements given (the intracellular potassium is often low even if plasma potassium is normal) and the heart rate controlled if necessary, with a beta-adrenoceptor antagonist. If this arrhythmia develops in a patient not already taking a digitalis preparation, then digoxin is, paradoxically, the drug of choice for controlling the ventricular rate.

CSP

Fig. 7.12 Atrial tachycardia with atrioventricular block induced by carotid sinus pressure (CSP).

Atrial Flutter. This is also a condition in which a rapid atrial rate is associated with two, three or four to one atrioventricular block. The atrial rate however tends to be more rapid, usually about 300 per minute, and the aetiology resembles that of the commoner atrial fibrillation.

The ECG shows characteristic saw-toothed flutter waves (Fig. 7.13). With a regular 2:1 AV block it may be difficult to distinguish atrial flutter from supraventricular or even sinus tachycardia, but carotid sinus pressure may help by temporarily increasing the degree of block.

Fig. 7.13 Atrial flutter. ECG showing saw-toothed atrial flutter waves and 4:1 atrioventricular block.

Digoxin is traditionally used to control the ventricular rate, and as prophylaxis in patients with paroxysmal atrial flutter. In some patients atrial flutter is difficult to control without inducing digitalis toxicity, and cardioversion may be preferable (p. 145). If digoxin alone does not give adequate prophylaxis, quinidine or disopyramide may be added (p. 140).

Atrial Fibrillation. In this arrhythmia the atria beat rapidly, chaotically and ineffectively; the ventricles respond at irregular intervals giving the characteristic 'irregularly irregular' pulse. The ECG (Fig. 7.14) shows no change in the QRS complexes and an absence of P waves; sometimes the baseline shows irregular fibrillation waves. These are most obvious in atrial fibrillation of recent onset.

Fig. 7.14 Atrial fibrillation. The ventricular complexes are irregular, there are no P waves and irregular oscillations (f waves) disturb the base line.

Atrial fibrillation may result from any stimulus which produces atrial dilatation. Mitral valve disease is the commonest cause in young and middle aged patients; in older patients the reason is often obscure, though many have hypertension or ischaemic heart disease. Atrial fibrillation may occur temporarily with myocardial infarction, with pericarditis, or after thoracic operations. It is rare in congenital or pulmonary heart disease, and it is a late complication of isolated aortic valve disease. Thyrotoxicosis, which increases atrial excitability, is an important and often undetected cause, particularly in the elderly.

'Lone' atrial fibrillation may be found in the absence of any other evidence of heart disease, and then may be intermittent at first, but later is often permanent; it is frequently a component of the sick sinus syndrome. Episodes of atrial fibrillation can be provoked, in those who are prone to it, by alcohol or infections.

Atrial fibrillation may be asymptomatic, more commonly in the elderly. Patients with paroxysmal atrial fibrillation are more aware of the arrhythmia than those in whom it is established. Atrial fibrillation frequently precipitates or aggravates cardiac failure in those with an abnormal heart, particularly with mitral stenosis. The ventricular rate at the onset of atrial fibrillation is usually rapid, diastole is shortened, and the left atrial pressure rises, sometimes leading to pulmonary oedema. The absence of the contribution of atrial systole to ventricular filling is another adverse factor.

Ineffective atrial contraction coupled with left atrial dilatation predisposes to stasis, thrombosis, and a risk of systemic thromboembolism. The risk is greatest when atrial fibrillation coexists with mitral valve disease, in patients with paroxysmal atrial fibrillation, and in the weeks immediately following the onset of fibrillation; however there is some risk of systemic embolism in all patients with atrial fibrillation.

Digoxin is used to reduce the ventricular rate by increasing the degree of AV block, and this alone may result in a striking improvement, particularly in patients with mitral stenosis. When atrial fibrillation persists after correction of hyperthyroidism, sinus rhythm can often be restored by cardioversion (p. 145). In chronic rheumatic heart disease such therapy is pointless, because the arrhythmia is almost certain to return unless the valve lesions can be improved by surgery. In patients with paroxysmal atrial fibrillation in the absence of an obvious predisposing factor, quinidine, disopyramide or amiodarone (p. 140) may help to preserve sinus rhythm.

Long-term anticoagulant therapy with warfarin reduces the risk of systemic embolism in patients with mitral valve disease, and is probably also indicated in patients with paroxysmal atrial fibrillation and to cover elective cardioversion. The potential benefits have to be weighed against the risks of anticoagulant therapy in each case. Although patients with lone atrial fibrillation have an increased risk of stroke, there is no evidence that this is reduced by anticoagulation.

Ventricular Ectopic Rhythms

Ectopic Beats. The symptoms and signs are the same as those of atrial ectopic beats, from which they can be distinguished by their abnormally widened QRS complex on the ECG (Fig. 7.15). They are fairly frequent in normal people, and their prevalence increases with age. They are sometimes precipitated by excessive tea, coffee or alcohol consumption. Ectopic beats in patients with otherwise normal hearts are often more prominent at rest, and tend to disappear with exercise. Ventricular ectopic beats often occur at a fixed interval after a sinus beat, and together with the compensatory pause after the ectopic beats produce a coupled or bigeminal pulse rhythm.

Fig. 7.15 Ventricular ectopic beats. Alternate beats have an abnormally wide QRS complex with no preceding P waves, i.e. coupling of the pulse results.

Ventricular ectopic beats are sometimes a manifestation of underlying heart disease, particularly disease of ventricular muscle which enhances ventricular excitability and increases the scope for ventricular re-entry circuits. Examples include acute myocardial infarction and myocarditis. Under these conditions an unusually premature ectopic beat falling on the T wave of a normal beat ('R on T') may initiate ventricular tachycardia or ventricular fibrillation.

Frequent ventricular ectopic beats, often against a background of bradycardia, are a feature of digitalis intoxication, and here too they may be a herald of more serious arrhythmias. Hypokalaemia may cause ventricular ectopic beats on its own, and will potentiate other causes. Ventricular ectopic beats are sometimes a feature of mitral valve prolapse, and occasionally they occur as 'escape beats' in the presence of an underlying bradycardia.

Treatment of ventricular ectopic beats should be directed at the underlying causes. The use of lignocaine to suppress ventricular ectopic beats after myocardial infarction has not been shown to improve survival. If frequent ectopic beats are causing annoyance in an otherwise healthy patient, beta-adrenoceptor antagonists, quinidine, disopyramide or mexiletine may help to suppress them (pp. 140–141).

Ventricular tachycardia (Fig. 7.16) is a grave arrhythmia because it is nearly always associated with serious heart disease, because the ventricular rate may be very rapid, and because it may degenerate into ventricular fibrillation. Patients sometimes complain of palpitation, but more often the symptoms are those of a low cardiac output — dizziness and dyspnoea, or even loss of consciousness. The ventricular rate is usually between 140 and 220 per minute, and carotid sinus pressure is ineffective. The ECG shows broad, abnormal QRS complexes; P waves are difficult to see, and when visible they may bear no regular relationship to the QRS complex. Ventricular tachycardia is sometimes difficult to distinguish from supraventricular tachycardia with bundle branch block; when there is doubt, it is usually safer to treat for ventricular tachycardia.

Fig. 7.16 Ventricular tachycardia. The rate is 220 per min. The complexes are broad and abnormal.

The commonest cause of ventricular tachycardia is acute myocardial infarction. It may also be due to myocarditis, cardiomyopathy, or chronic ischaemic heart disease, especially when the last is associated with a ventricular aneurysm. In a few individuals a predisposition to ventricular arrhythmia is associated with abnormal prolongation of the QT interval of the ECG, a trait which is sometimes hereditary. Hypokalaemia, hypomagnesaemia or digitalis excess are also predisposing factors.

Patients recovering from myocardial infarction sometimes have periods of idioventricular rhythm ('slow' ventricular tachycardia) at a rate only slightly above the preceding sinus rate. These episodes are usually self limiting, asymptomatic, and do not require treatment. Most other instances of ventricular tachycardia, if they last for more than a few beats, will require treatment, often as an emergency.

Intravenous lignocaine is the treatment of choice in urgent cases, given as a bolus (1·5 mg per kg) followed by an infusion of 4 mg per minute reducing to 2 mg per minute over a period of 2 to 4 hours. The dose may need to be reduced in the elderly, the frail and those with liver disease. Lignocaine toxicity is manifested by confusion, paraesthesiae and twitching; if these are observed the dose should be curtailed. Mexiletine or disopyramide may be effective, either as alternatives to lignocaine or when lignocaine has failed, but if the patient is gravely ill then cardioversion is preferable to polypharmacy. Hypokalaemia, hypomagnesaemia and acidosis must be corrected. Cardioversion should be avoided if digitalis toxicity is likely; if it is considered necessary in these circumstances the first attempts should be made at low energy settings.

Urgent treatment of ventricular tachycardia should be followed by oral prophylaxis with mexilitine, disopyramide, procainamide or quinidine (p. 140). Slow release preparations may help in maintaining adequate plasma concentrations. Treatment can usually be stopped after 6 weeks in patients who develop ventricular tachycardia as a complication of acute infarction, but it may need to be continued indefinitely in patients with recurrent attacks. Procainamide should be avoided for long term treatment (p. 140). Amiodarone (p. 141) may be helpful in difficult cases.

Ventricular fibrillation is the commonest immediate cause of sudden death. It results from critical anoxia or ischaemia of ventricular muscle, most commonly as a result of coronary artery disease, or from inappropriate electrical stimulation, as in electrocution. Susceptibility to ventricular fibrillation can be enhanced by underlying heart disease, by hypokalaemia or by drugs such as the catecholamines. The ventricles have a rapid, ineffective uncoordinated movement which produces no pulse, and the ECG (Fig. 7.17) has broad, bizarre, irregular complexes.

Fig. 7.17 Ventricular fibrillation. The change from sinus rhythm to ventricular fibrillation occurs when a ventricular ectopic beat falls on the T of the previous complex.

Within seconds of the onset of the attack the patient loses consciousness. Respiration ceases and the pupils begin to dilate. Death is virtually inevitable unless treatment is started promptly. If a defibrillator is available, the immediate application of a direct current shock may restore sinus rhythm within seconds. Under other circumstances the circulation has to be maintained by the resuscitation procedures described on page 139. Failure of circulation causes acidosis, and sodium bicarbonate should be given intravenously (p. 102). If sinus rhythm is restored, lignocaine should be given to reduce the likelihood of recurrence, followed by oral prophylaxis as described for ventricular tachycardia.

Ventricular asystole is another arrhythmia which can cause sudden death. It may be due either to a localised failure of impulse-conducting tissue, with delay in the emergence of a ventricular escape rhythm, or to massive ventricular damage complicating myocardial infarction. With the former, cardiac massage or a blow to the chest will often restore cardiac activity, although an artificial pacemaker may be needed to prevent recurrent attacks. When asystole occurs as a consequence of massive myocardial damage, it is nearly always resistant to treatment. Sometimes,

electrical activity returns but is not accompanied by effective ventricular contraction.

Cardiac Arrest

Cardiac arrest is the sudden and complete loss of cardiac function. It is usually due to ventricular fibrillation, less often to asystole. These can usually be distinguished only by an ECG, or during cardiac surgery when the heart is visible. Most attempts at resuscitation have to be commenced before an ECG is available. The development of the technique of closed-chest cardiac massage together with mouth-to-mouth ventilation, has improved the outlook immeasurably, and all doctors, nurses, ambulance drivers and attendants should receive instruction in this vitally important form of first aid.

The indication for resuscitation is clearest when the arrest has occurred as a result of an accident, such as electrocution or drowning, or when it occurs during an investigation such as cardiac catheterisation. One of the problems in hospital practice is to determine when it is inappropriate to attempt resuscitation because the nature of the patient's illness is such that recovery would be unprecedented. Inevitably it is sometimes necessary to institute resuscitation until someone familiar with the patient can make the decision as to whether the attempt should continue.

Treatment. The brain suffers irreversible damage unless some circulation of oxygenated blood can be achieved within 2 or 3 minutes. A smart blow should be given to the left of the sternum with the hand or fist, and both legs should be elevated to 90 degrees. If the heart does not start immediately, as indicated by the return of the carotid or femoral pulse, closed-chest cardiac massage (external cardiac compression) and mouth-to-mouth ventilation (expired air resuscitation) should be commenced.

TECHNIQUE OF CARDIOPULMONARY RESUSCITATION. The patient is laid on the back on the floor or some other firm surface. The operator places the hands one on top of the other (Fig. 7.18) on the patient's lower sternum and commences forceful, rhythmic compressions at the rate of 60 — 100 per minute. The danger of fracturing ribs is reduced if the pressure is transmitted through the ball of the hand onto the sternum. Previous practice with a dummy or mannikin is very helpful. At the same time, ventilation must be ensured. The head is extended, and the jaw pulled forward. Mouth-to-mouth, mouth-to-nose or mouth-to-airway ventilation is employed until a face mask and bag are available. When there are two operators the lungs should be inflated after every fifth compression of the sternum. If there is only one operator, two inflations are alternated with 15 compressions of the sternum.

Meanwhile an intravenous infusion of 50 — 100 mmol of sodium bicarbonate should be set up to combat acidosis. Where a defibrillator is available it should be used as soon as possible, for no harm is done if the patient proves to have asystole rather than ventricular fibrillation. 200 Joules (Watt-seconds) is an adequate energy level for all but the largest adults. Repeated attempts at defibrillation should be interspersed with periods of massage and ventilation. Intravenous lignocaine (100 mg) may make refractory fibrillation more amenable to correction. Intravenous adrenaline (1 ml of 1:1000) can be given if asystole fails to respond to massage alone, but the outlook in these cases is poor.

Resuscitation is most likely to be successful in cardiac arrest resulting from accidents, or from myocardial infarction without severe heart failure. If it transpires that the acute circulatory failure was due to cardiac rupture following myocardial infarction, cardiac tamponade or massive pulmonary embolism, resuscitation will nearly always be unsuccessful. Such a cause can be suspected from failure to produce a satisfactory carotid or femoral pulse during massage. Nowadays those who have simple syncope are increasingly at risk of overenthusiastic resuscitation measures.

Anti-Arrhythmic Drugs

Some of the drugs used to treat individual arrhythmias have already been mentioned. However the increasing number of antiarrhythmic agents available makes it important to have some form of classification for the drugs and some guidelines to a rational strategy for their use. For

1. Head hyperextended and chin raised

2. Direct mouth-to-mouth breathing

3. Indirect mouth-to-mouth breathing

4. Cardiac massage

Fig. 7.18 Emergency resuscitation.

practical purposes there are three important characteristics of any antiarrhythmic drug — its mode of action, its pharmacokinetics (how an adequate blood and tissue concentration can be

Table 7.1 Classification of antiarrhythmic drugs (adapted from Singh, B., & Vaughan Williams E.M. Cardiovascular Research 6, 109, 1972).

Class	Action	Examples
I	Slow fast-rising phase of ventricular action potential (by inhibiting 'fast sodium current')	Quinidine Lignocaine Mexiletine
II	Beta-adrenoceptor antagonists	Propranolol
III	Delay repolarisation; prolong 'plateau' of ventricular action potential	Amiodarone
IV	Calcium-channel antagonists	Verapamil

achieved and maintained), and its side effects.

The mode of action is the basis for the classification of antiarrhythmic drugs shown in Table 7.1.

Class I Drugs. These act principally by depressing excitability and slowing conduction in atrial or ventricular muscle. Lignocaine and mexiletine are used mainly for ventricular arrhythmias; procainamide, quinidine and disopyramide can be used for both atrial and ventricular arrhythmias. Phenytoin is claimed to be particularly useful in digitalis induced arrhythmias.

Lignocaine has to be given parenterally, and has a very short plasma half-life, so its concentration will depend on the rate of infusion. It is mainly used for the urgent treatment or prophylaxis of ventricular tachycardia or fibrillation (p. 137).

Procainamide can also be given intravenously, but tends to cause hypotension. It is effective orally, and has been used in the prophylaxis of ventricular arrhythmias. The plasma half-life is short, and it is best given as a sustained-release preparation. With prolonged usage there is a risk of a systemic lupus erythematosus like syndrome (p. 574), which is usually reversible on withdrawal of the drug.

Mexiletine can be given intravenously or orally in the treatment or prophylaxis of ventricular arrhythmias. It is tending to supersede procainamide as it seems to have fewer side effects. These mainly take the form of nausea and vomiting but ataxia can also be troublesome. The usual oral dose is 200 to 250 mg 8-hourly; the manufacturer's literature should be consulted for the parenteral dosage schedule. Metabolism is mainly hepatic, and can be impaired in liver disease.

Disopyramide can be used for the treatment or prophylaxis of both atrial and ventricular tachyarrhythmias. It can be given intravenously or orally. If it is used in patients with atrial flutter and AV block, there is a risk of a parodoxical increase in heart rate as the atria slow and 2:1 block changes to 1:1 conduction; this can be prevented by previous administration of digoxin.

Disopyramide and mexiletine are of similar efficacy in treating ventricular arrhythmias, but differ in their side effects and metabolism. Disopyramide has weak atropine-like effects and may cause urinary retention or precipitate glaucoma. It has a depressant effect on ventricular function and should be avoided in cardiac failure. Metabolism is renal as well as hepatic. The plasma half-life is quite short, and the oral dose is 100 to 150 mg every six hours, or as slow-release disopyramide 250 mg twice a day. The manufacturer's instructions should be consulted for the intravenous dose schedule.

Quinidine gained a bad reputation when it used to be given in large doses to convert atrial fibrillation to sinus rhythm. In more modest doses (e.g. oral slow release quinidine 500 mg b.d.) it is of similar efficacy and safety to disopyramide in the prophylaxis of atrial arrhythmias and to disopyramide or mexiletine in the prevention of ventricular arrhythmias. In practical terms, a choice between these drugs will often be determined by personal experience, patient tolerance and availability. Quinidine tends to cause abdominal discomfort and diarrhoea; rarely an autoimmune thrombocytopenia or haemolytic anaemia may occur. It is a myocardial depressant, and should be avoided in patients with poor left ventricular function. Excretion is almost entirely renal, and the drug will accumulate in renal failure.

Phenytoin can be given by slow intravenous injection at a dose of up to 5 mg per kg to patients with a refractory ventricular tachycardia, particularly if this is due to digitalis toxicity. It is seldom used for the long-term treatment of arrhythmias.

Class II Drugs. These comprise the beta-adrenoceptor antagonists. They are useful in controlling supraventricular arrhythmias, and as an adjunct to digoxin in controlling the ventricular rate in atrial fibrillation. They can be useful in treating ventricular arrhythmias, but are seldom the drugs of first choice for this purpose. Their tendency to depress ventricular function is a disadvantage. Choice is determined by availability, duration of action, and side effects.

Propranolol is an effective drug but needs to be taken three times a day, or as a sustained release preparation, in order to maintain adequate plasma concentrations. Because it is extensively metabolised the effective dose is unpredictable; 10 mg is a safe starting dose, but some patients need up to 320 mg daily, or more in thyrotoxicosis. Intravenous propranolol is very potent, and an initial dose should not exceed 1 mg. Intravenous metoprolol, atenolol or sotalol are preferable.

Metoprolol is a cardioselective β_1-antagonist (p. 182), which may have fewer side effects than propranolol. Oral metoprolol needs to be given twice or thrice daily, or as a slow-release preparation. The usual oral starting dose is 50 mg b.d. Intravenous metoprolol (or atenolol or sotalol) may be used to treat supraventricular tachycardia.

Atenolol is a cardioselective beta-adrenoceptor antagonist with a long duration of action. It is usually given once daily. The oral dose is usually 100 mg daily, but 50 mg is a safer starting dose in the elderly. Intravenous atenolol is also available.

Sotalol is not cardioselective, but has a long half-life and also has some class III antiarrhythmic activity. The oral dose is usually 80 mg twice daily, increasing to 320 mg daily or more if necessary. The intravenous dose is 10-20 mg given slowly.

Other adverse effects of these beta-blockers are discussed on page 182.

Class III Drugs. These act by prolonging the plateau phase of the action potential, thus lengthening the refractory period. Although both disopyramide and sotalol have class III activity *amiodarone* is the principal drug in this class. Amiodarone also has unusual pharmacokinetics, and it is unclear whether these or its mode of action contribute more to its undoubted efficacy as an antiarrhythmic agent. It is effective against a wide variety of atrial arrhythmias, and is probably the most potent drug in controlling paroxysmal atrial fibrillation and the arrhythmias of the Wolff-Parkinson-White syndrome. It is also useful in preventing recurrent ventricular tachycardia.

Tissue levels are built up slowly, and with oral therapy it may take two weeks or longer to achieve therapeutic concentrations. Conversely, it is a very persistent drug, and traces can still be detected weeks or months after treatment has ceased. The recommended oral dosage is 200 mg thrice daily for 1 or 2 weeks, reducing thereafter to 200 or 400 mg daily. After several months it may be possible to reduce the dosage further.

Side effects are numerous, and have to be balanced against the advantages of therapy. Corneal deposits are virtually universal, but do not affect vision and seem to regress after withdrawal of the drug. Photosensitisation of the skin is also very common. Gastrointestinal problems tend to get better when the dose is reduced. Amiodarone is an iodine-containing compound, and both hypo- and hyperthyroidism have been reported. Hepatitis and allergic alveolitis are other potentially serious complications. Drug interactions may be a problem, particularly with digoxin and with warfarin. Patients taking amiodarone should be kept under review and have regular examination of the eyes, thyroid liver and lung function.

Class IV Drugs. These block the 'slow calcium channel' (p. 170) which is particularly important for impulse generation and conduction in atrial and nodal tissue, although it is also present in ventricular muscle.

Verapamil is the only widely used antiarrhythmic drug in this class; nifedipine (p. 170) has no significant antiarrhythmic effect in man. Verapamil may be given intravenously, in 5 mg aliquots to a maximum of 20 mg, to patients with supraventricular tachycardia. Although very effective, bradycardia and hypotension may occur and this treatment is not recommended outside hospital. Intravenous verapamil must not be combined with a beta-adrenoceptor antagonist, or given to patients who have taken such drugs within 48 hours. Oral verapamil (40–120 mg t.i.d.) can be used to control recurrent atrial arrhythmias, or as an adjunct to digoxin in treating atrial fibrillation. It is not used for ventricular arrhythmias. Side effects include dizziness, constipation, and sometimes myocardial depression.

Digoxin. This is an important anti-arrhythmic drug which does not feature in the above classification. Its principal value lies in its ability to slow conduction and prolong the refractory period in the AV node. This effect helps to control the ventricular rate in atrial fibrillation or paroxysmal atrial tachycardia, and will often interrupt re-entry tachycardias involving the AV node. On the other hand the effect of digoxin on sodium and potassium pumping tends to enhance excitability and conduction, and shorten the refractory period, in other parts of the heart; therefore atrial or ventricular tachycardias may be features of digoxin toxicity.

Digoxin is a purified glycoside from the European foxglove, *Digitalis lanata*. Digitalis is a less precise term sometimes used for the powdered leaves of *D. lanata*, sometimes as a generic term for the whole family of cardiac glycosides. The absorption of digoxin from the bowel depends on the formulation of the tablets. An alteration in formulation during the past decade has led to enhanced absorption and dose recommendations have had to be revised.

Digoxin is widely distributed in body tissues, and to achieve a rapid therapeutic effect it is best to give a loading dose of approximately 0·02 mg per kg over the first 48 hours, followed by a maintenance dose of 0·25 mg daily. Digoxin is largely excreted by the kidneys, and the maintenance dose should be reduced in children, the elderly and those with renal impairment. In an emergency, digoxin can be given intravenously as an infusion of 0·5 mg in 100 ml saline over 30 minutes, repeated every six hours until the required loading dose has been given. Digoxin has a long plasma half-life, and effects may persist 24–36 hours after the last dose. Measurements of plasma digoxin concentrations (p. 820) are useful, (i) in determining that the dose being used is inadequate and (ii) in confirming a clinical impression of toxicity. Treatment of suspected toxicity should not be delayed pending concentration measurements, particularly as a fall in plasma potassium concentration may induce digoxin toxicity without a change in plasma digoxin concentration.

Digoxin Toxicity. Extracardiac manifestations of digoxin toxicity include anorexia, nausea, vomiting, diarrhoea and altered colour vision (xanthopsia). Cardiac manifestations include bradycardia, ventricular ectopic beats, often multiple or coupled, paroxysmal atrial tachycardia and ventricular tachycardia or fibrillation. Digoxin administration should be stopped, and blood taken for plasma digoxin levels, urea and electrolyte estimation. Fluid loss should be replaced, intravenously if necessary, and potassium supplements given as required. Symptomatic bradycardia should be treated with atropine and if necessary an artificial pacemaker. Symptomatic atrial tachycardia can be controlled with a beta-adrenoceptor antagonist. Ventricular tachycardia is treated with lignocaine, or if this fails with phenytoin. Cardioversion carries an increased risk of provoking ventricular fibrillation, but will be required for refractory ventricular tachycardia or for ventricular fibrillation. Treatment with antibodies to digoxin has been used with success for digoxin overdosage in self-poisoning.

Strategy in Anti-arrhythmic Therapy. The availability of many agents is an invitation to overtreatment. Many arrhythmias are benign, asymptomatic or self limited, and best left alone. Simple measures such as rest, reassurance, analgesia and sedation must not be forgotten. If treatment is needed it is best to use as few drugs as possible, and to give them in the maximum possible dose before discarding them as ineffective. Acidosis, hypokalaemia and hypomagnesaemia need to be corrected. If a patient's condition is deteriorating because of a tachyarrhythmia then cardioversion should not be delayed; even if the relief is only temporary it will buy time for a review of drug therapy and correction of adverse factors. Perseverance is often rewarded, particularly after myocardial infarction where arrhythmias tend to settle with time. When it is considered necessary to use a combination of drugs, it would seem sensible to combine drugs with different modes of action, though objective evidence for this is scanty. Patients on long term anti-arrhythmic drugs should be reviewed regularly, and attempts made to withdraw therapy if it appears that the factors which precipitated the arrhythmias are no longer operative.

HEART BLOCK

Sinoatrial (SA) Block

In this condition a complete cardiac cycle is missed so that a gap appears in the pulse. The electrocardiogram shows that both atrial and ventricular complexes are absent. Sinoatrial block is one of the features of the sick sinus syndrome (p. 133).

Sinoatrial block does not require treatment if it is asymptomatic. Sinoatrial disorders causing symptoms may require the implantation of an artificial pacemaker.

Atrioventricular (AV) Block

In this condition conduction between the atria and ventricles is impaired.

1. In *first degree heart block* (delayed AV conduction) the PR interval is prolonged beyond the upper limit of normal (0.20 second) (Fig. 7.19).

Fig. 7.19 First degree heart block. The PR interval is 0.26 sec.

2. In *second degree heart block* (partial heart block) some impulses from the atria fail to get through to the ventricles, i.e. dropped beats occur. Sometimes there is progressive lengthening of successive PR intervals followed by a dropped beat. This is known as *Wenckebach's phenomenon* (Fig. 7.20) and is due to progressive fatigue of the AV bundle with recovery following the rest period when the dropped beat occurs. Second degree heart block sometimes occurs with atrial tachyarrhythmias.

Fig. 7.20 Second degree heart block (Wenckebach's phenomenon). The first beat in the cycle has a PR of 0.28 sec; it lengthens with the next two beats and the fourth P wave is not followed by a QRS — the dropped beat.

3. In *complete heart block* no impulses from the atria reach the ventricles. Cardiac action is maintained by an escape rhythm arising in the bundle of His or elsewhere in the ventricles (Fig. 7.21).

Fig.7.21 Complete heart block. There is complete dissociation of atrial and ventricular complexes. The atrial rate is 90 and the ventricular rate 40 per min.

Aetiology. Depression of atrioventricular conduction may be due to ischaemia, fibrosis or inflammation of the atrioventricular node or proximal part of the bundle of His, to vagal stimulation or to drugs. Myocardial infarction is the most frequent cause of heart block which develops suddenly. Idiopathic fibrosis of the bundle of His is a common cause of chronic heart block in the elderly. The bundle of His runs close to the aortic and mitral valves and may be affected by calcification extending from a valve, by an abscess cavity resulting from endocarditis, or by surgical trauma. Other causes of complete heart block include congenital maldevelopment of the bundle of His, digitalis poisoning, sarcoidosis and Chagas' disease (p. 780).

Clinical Features. *First degree heart block* can be diagnosed only by ECG.

Second Degree Heart Block. When the atrial and ventricular contractions bear a simple ratio to one another such as in 2:1 and 3:1 block, the pulse is slow and regular. Change in the degree of partial heart block may give rise to sudden changes in the pulse rate. More complex ratios such as 3:2 or 4:3 block give rise to dropped beats. Partial heart block is usually transient and may occur during an acute infection, from digitalis overdose, or after myocardial infarction. It is sometimes observed at rest or during sleep in athletic young adults with a high vagal tone.

Complete heart block may be chronic or intermittent. Chronic complete heart block should be suspected when the pulse is slow (30 to 40 per minute) and regular, and does not vary with exercise. It may be possible to see dissociation between jugular venous pulsation, reflecting atrial activity, and the carotid pulse. Venous cannon waves may occur (p. 125). The arterial pulse volume is large, and the increased stroke volume may produce a systolic murmur.

Intermittent complete heart block may cause fairly prolonged ventricular asystole because of a delay in establishing a ventricular escape rhythm. It is one of the causes of cardiac syncope. Temporary ventricular asystole, resulting from prolonged sinoatrial block in the sick sinus syndrome or from transient failure of the ventricular escape rhythm in chronic complete heart block, produces the same clinical picture, called the *Adams-Stokes syndrome*. Attacks frequently occur without warning, although some patients describe a prodrome. Consciousness is rapidly lost and the patient may fall. Convulsions may occur if the heart does not begin to beat again within about 10 seconds, and death will result if the arrest is prolonged. The skin blanches at the beginning of the attack, but when the heart starts beating again there is a characteristic flush as the emptied vessels are filled with blood.

Treatment. *First degree heart block* does not require treatment, but may be an indication of underlying heart disease, a warning of drug toxicity, or a contraindication to the use of drugs which might further impair conduction.

Asymptomatic *second degree heart block* does not require treatment, but the patient should be observed in case it progresses to complete heart block. 24 hour ECG monitoring may be helpful. Symptomatic second degree block following inferior myocardial infarction usually responds to atropine (0.3 mg i.v., repeated to a maximum of 1.2 mg). If it does not, a temporary pacemaker may be needed. Chronic symptomatic second degree block may be an indication for a permanent artificial pacemaker.

Complete heart block complicating acute inferior myocardial infarction is often accompanied by an escape rhythm at a satisfactory rate; it may need no treatment, or it may respond to atropine. If the latter is unsuccessful a temporary pacemaker may be needed. Complete heart block following acute anterior infarction requires a temporary pacemaker. If the patient presents with asystole, atropine and isoprenaline (1–5 mg in 500 ml glucose,

infused intravenously at the minimum rate needed to produce a satisfactory heart rhythm) may help to maintain the circulation until a temporary pacing electrode can be inserted.

Most cases of chronic complete heart block, or of intermittent complete heart block unrelated to myocardial infarction or to drug administration, require a permanent artificial pacemaker. An exception may be made in young asymptomatic patients with congenital complete heart block or in frail and asymptomatic elderly patients. Sustained release isoprenaline (30 mg or more four times daily) may help to relieve heart failure and reduce the frequency of Adams-Stokes attacks in patients for whom pacemaker implantation is impracticable or unacceptable.

Bundle Branch Block and Hemiblock

Interruption of the left or right branches of the bundle of His causes delay in the activation of the appropriate ventricle, broadening of the QRS complex on the ECG to 0.12 seconds or more, and characteristic alterations to QRS morphology shown in Figures 7.22 and 7.23.

Right bundle branch block is occasionally congenital, sometimes results from gross hypertrophy or dilatation of the right ventricle or from surgical damage, and is usually (in adults) a manifestation of ischaemic heart disease.

Left bundle branch block is most commonly due to ischaemic heart disease; it is sometimes a feature of cardiomyopathy or of calcific infiltration of the bundle of His from a calcified aortic valve. The left branch of the bundle of His rapidly divides into a fan-like array of conducting tissue on the left side of the interventricular septum. Partial interruption of the bundle at this point (hemiblock) does not broaden the QRS complex, but alters the mean direction of ventricular depolarisation (cardiac axis). Damage to the anterior part of the system (*left anterior hemiblock*) shifts the axis to the left (large R in leads I and aVL, large S in II, III, aVF). Damage to the posterior part (*left posterior hemiblock*) shifts the axis to the right (S in I, aVL, large R in III, aVF).

The treatment and prognosis of bundle branch block are in general those of the underlying disease. The development of left bundle branch

Fig. 7.22 Right bundle branch block. Note that in V1 the late secondary R wave indicates a delay in depolarisation of the right ventricle.

Fig. 7.23 Left bundle branch block. The wide QRS in V6 and aVL indicates a delay in depolarisation of the left ventricle.

block, or of right bundle branch block plus anterior or posterior hemiblock after myocardial infarction indicates extensive myocardial damage, and often a poor prognosis.

Electrical Treatment of Cardiac Arrhythmias

Defibrillation and Cardioversion. The heart can be completely depolarised by passing a sufficiently large electrical current through it from an external source. When the current has stopped there is a period of asystole followed, usually, by the resumption of normal sinus rhythm. Modern 'defibrillators' use direct current (d.c.) stored in a bank of electrical capacitors to deliver a shock of high energy but short duration. The current is transmitted to the chest wall by large-area electrodes which must be coated with electrically-conducting jelly. One electrode is applied over the sternum and the other is pressed against the chest wall beneath the left scapula or in the left axilla.

The precise timing of the discharge is unimportant in ventricular fibrillation, but when the technique is used to treat supraventricular or ventricular tachycardia or atrial fibrillation discharge should be synchronised with the R wave of the ECG. The reason for this is that if a current, not large enough to cause total depolarisation, is applied during a critical period at the end of the T wave it may provoke ventricular fibrillation.

In *ventricular fibrillation* neither preparation, anaesthesia nor synchronisation are required. Discharge energy should be set at 200 Joules (Watt-seconds) and the sooner the shock is applied the more likely it is to succeed. For other arrhythmias there is less urgency, a synchronised discharge should be used, and the patient should be anaesthetised. *Atrial fibrillation* often requires energies of 150 to 200 J to restore sinus rhythm but lower energies of 50 J or less may suffice in *atrial flutter* or *supraventricular tachycardia*.

Digitalis intoxication increases the risk of untoward arrhythmias after cardioversion, and ideally digitalis therapy should be withdrawn 36 hours before elective cardioversion. Patients with long-standing atrial arrhythmias are at risk of systemic embolism after cardioversion, unless this is preceded by a period of anticoagulation.

Artificial Pacemakers. In an emergency it is sometimes possible to stimulate the heart by passing an electric current through electrodes placed on the chest wall, or passed down the oesophagus, or inserted directly through the chest wall into the myocardium. None of these methods is satisfactory for longer than a few minutes, if at all, and the most effective technique for *temporary artificial pacemaking* is to insert a bipolar pacing electrode via an antecubital, subclavian or femoral vein and position it under radioscopic control in the apex of the right ventricle. The electrode is connected to an external pulse generator. The threshold for reliable ventricular stimulation should be less than 1 volt, and the pulse generator should be set to deliver at least three times this figure – usually 3 to 4 volts.

The ECG of a patient whose rhythm is controlled by an artificial ventricular pacemaker shows regular broad QRS complexes with a left bundle branch block pattern and left axis deviation (Fig. 7.24). Each complex is immediately preceded by a small 'pacing spike'. Nearly all pulse generators are used in a 'demand' or 'ventricular-inhibited' mode whereby a spontaneously generated QRS complex can inhibit the artificial impulse. In other words, if the patient's spontaneous rhythm recovers and its rate exceeds that at which the artificial pacemaker is set, the latter is inhibited, but if the patient's spontaneous rate drops below that set on the pulse generator then artificial pacing will be resumed.

Fig. 7.24 ECG of a patient with a ventricular pacemaker. The QRS complexes are broad and each is immediately preceded by a narrow pacemaker 'spike'.

It is also possible to pace the atria, using a J-shaped electrode inserted percutaneously and positioned in the right atrial appendage. Sequential pacing of atria and ventricles, using a special pulse generator, reproduces the physiological sequence of atrial and ventricular contraction, and gives a better cardiac output than ventricular pacing alone. This may be important when there is impaired left ventricular function, e.g. after myocardial infarction.

Temporary pacemakers are invaluable where heart block is transient, as is usually the case after myocardial infarction, but their long term use is inconvenient and the insertion site is prone to infection. Only in very exceptional circumstances should one be used for longer than 2 weeks.

Permanent artificial pacemakers utilise the same principles, but the pulse generator is smaller, completely enclosed, and can be implanted under the skin. The electrode passed to the heart is usually unipolar, the body of the pulse generator providing the other terminal for the current. The battery capacity of the pulse generator will usually sustain it for 5 to 10 years, after which it needs to be replaced. A longer lifespan can be achieved either by using a larger and bulkier battery, or by providing a facility for 'programming' the pacemaker, i.e. controlling its rate, output etc. by external radio frequency or magnetic stimuli so as to minimise the drain on its resources. Programming can also be used to increase output in the face of an unexpected increase in threshold, or to alter sensitivity if the pacemaker is inappropriately inhibited by electrical potentials generated in the pectoral muscles. It is still controversial whether these benefits of programmability outweigh the considerable increase in cost.

Atrial electrodes can also be used with permanent pacemakers. One of their more important roles is to detect the atrial P wave and use it to initiate the impulse delivered to the ventricle. This has the dual advantage that atrioventricular synchrony is preserved and that the ventricular rate can increase together with the atrial rate during exercise. Although the physiological advantages of these more sophisticated pacemakers are widely canvassed, their increased complexity and cost call for careful selection and assessment of patients.

ACUTE CIRCULATORY FAILURE

Acute circulatory failure, shock and *low output state* are terms used to describe a clinical syndrome of hypotension, peripheral vasoconstriction, oliguria, and often impairment of consciousness. The basic cause is an inadequate cardiac output with compensatory vasoconstriction and renal and cerebral hypoperfusion.

Onset may be sudden or gradual. The skin is cold, pale and sweaty. In advanced or neglected cases there may be peripheral cyanosis or gangrene. The systolic blood pressure is usually low, often under 100 mmHg. With peripheral constriction the blood pressure, measured by cuff, is often an underestimate of central pressure. There is usually tachycardia, and the heart sounds may be difficult to analyse. Urine output is often less than 30 ml per hour. There may be Cheyne-Stokes breathing. Consciousness may be superficially preserved, but frequently there is confusion and irritability.

If treatment is not prompt and effective,

systemic consequences may ensue (Fig. 7.25). Oliguria may progress to acute tubular necrosis (p. 400). A rising plasma potassium concentration and progressive acidosis both from renal failure and ischaemic necrosis of skeletal muscle cause cardiac arrhythmias which may eventually be intractable. Even if recovery occurs, permanent cerebral damage or loss of peripheral tissues may be inevitable.

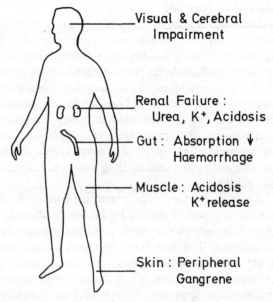

Fig. 7.25 Systemic consequences of acute circulatory failure.

Successful treatment of acute circulatory failure is absolutely dependent on identification of the cause; this requires meticulous assessment of the history and physical signs, and efficient use of investigation. While this is being done the patient should be protected from fuss, unnecessary disturbance and hypothermia; anxiety and pain should be relieved using small intravenous doses of morphine if necessary. Oxygen should be administered by facemask or nasal prongs. A catheter should be inserted to monitor urine output, and great care taken to protect ischaemic skin from damage.

Aetiology. The causes of acute circulatory failure can basically be divided into those associated with a low central venous pressure (hypovolaemic shock) and those characterised by a raised venous pressure (cardiogenic shock). Central venous pressure can be difficult to assess with the patient lying flat, and if there is doubt a central venous catheter should be inserted and the pressure measured with a saline manometer.

The commonest cause of hypovolaemia is haemorrhage — external, into the bowel, or into a body cavity. Gastrointestinal haemorrhage can often be diagnosed on the basis of history and rectal examination; its further assessment is considered on page 297.

Intra-abdominal haemorrhage, from a leaking aortic aneurysm in the elderly or a ruptured spleen or ectopic gestation sac in younger patient, is often insidious in its presentation, and atypical in its physical signs. Less common causes of hypovolaemia include plasma loss in severe burns, or into the abdominal cavity in acute pancreatitis, inappropriate vasodilatation in bacteraemic shock (p. 50) and anaphylactic shock (p. 25), and excess urinary fluid loss as in diabetic ketoacidosis.

Acute circulatory failure with a raised central venous pressure is caused by problems affecting the left or right side of the heart or the pulmonary circulation. The two most common causes are acute myocardial infarction and acute massive pulmonary embolism. When the diagnosis is not immediately apparent, it is useful to consider possible causes in a methodical order (Fig. 7.26).

Dissecting aneurysm of the aorta (p. 197) presents with severe pain, often between the shoulders. There may be an inappropriate bradycardia and an early diastolic murmur may be heard. Chest radiography and echocardiography are helpful.

Pericardial tamponade (p. 187) is an important cause of acute circulatory failure because it carries a high mortality if neglected and because it usually responds dramatically to treatment. Possible causes are discussed on page 188. Characteristically there is severe circulatory failure with oliguria, a grossly elevated venous pressure, and pulsus paradoxus. The chest radiograph shows an enlarged cardiac shadow. Echocardiography, which may be done at the bedside, is the best way of confirming the diagnosis, and helps to indicate the best site for paracentesis.

Aortic valve disease may precipitate acute circulatory failure by causing left ventricular failure

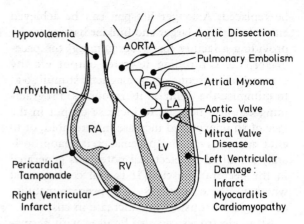

Fig. 7.26 Some possible cardiac causes of acute circulatory failure.

and pulmonary oedema. The signs of *aortic stenosis* (p. 161) may be masked by a low cardiac output, the characteristic murmur becoming quiet. Acute severe *aortic regurgitation*, from cusp rupture or endocarditis, may also be atypical, with an unimpressive murmur and little cardiac enlargement on the chest radiograph. Echocardiography is helpful.

Myocardial infarction extensive enough to cause acute circulatory failure is usually obvious from the ECG, but occasionally ECG changes of ischaemia are a secondary result of circulatory failure from some other catastrophe such as pulmonary embolism. Usually, circulatory failure from myocardial infarction is associated with pulmonary oedema, but if the infarct predominantly affects the right ventricle (see below) this is not always the case.

Progressive *myocarditis*, including that of rheumatic fever, sometimes presents as acute circulatory failure; the chest radiograph usually shows an enlarged heart and echocardiography reveals severely impaired left ventricular function.

Tachyarrhythmias are usually obvious clinically and from the ECG. The onset of atrial fibrillation may precipitate acute circulatory failure, often with severe pulmonary oedema, in patients with impaired left ventricular function or *mitral stenosis*. The murmur of mitral stenosis (p. 159) is difficult to hear in the presence of tachycardia, but the history, chest radiograph and echocardiogram will confirm the diagnosis.

Acute massive pulmonary embolism (p. 184) is a sequel to leg or pelvic vein thrombosis. Collapse is sudden, often with extreme breathlessness. A tachycardia and elevated jugular venous pressure are invariable; other physical signs such as a parasternal lift, wide splitting of the second heart sound and a third sound over the right ventricle are helpful but unreliable. The ECG may show signs of acute right ventricular strain (Fig. 7.27) or may be normal apart from a tachycardia. The chest radiograph is of value mainly in excluding other diagnoses. Echocardiography shows a dilated right ventricle and, often, a small vigorously contracting left ventricle. Radionuclide perfusion lung scanning is helpful provided it can be done quickly enough. Pulmonary angiography is the definitive diagnostic procedure, but is not without risks — including those of moving a severely ill patient and of delay in instituting treatment.

Apart from pulmonary embolism, pure 'right sided' causes of acute circulatory failure are rare. Probably the most common is the combination of a right ventricular infarct with excessive diuretic therapy; this can be suspected if cardiac output and urine production decline after an inferior infarct in the absence of pulmonary congestion, and confirmed by demonstrating a high central venous pressure but a low pulmonary artery wedge pressure (measured with a Swan-Ganz catheter (p. 150). Other causes include right atrial or right ventricular tumours, or right atrial tamponade from a localised pericardial effusion.

Treatment. The immediate objective is to restore and maintain cardiac output at a satisfactory level until the cause of the circulatory failure can be identified and specifically treated or allowed to resolve. In hypovolaemic circulatory failure the most important step is to replace fluid lost from the vascular compartment. Initially, it matters little whether isotonic saline, plasma or plasma substitutes are used, but when large quantities are required the nature of the fluid lost should determine the nature of its replacement. The rate of fluid replacement is judged according to estimates of the fluid lost, the clinical state of the patient, observation of the jugular venous pressure, and in severely ill patients by manometer measurement of the central venous pressure. Vasoconstrictor drugs are of little use, except in cases where inappropriate vasodilatation is the cause of the hypovolaemia. Where large

Fig.7.27 ECGs from a patient before and immediately after a massive pulmonary embolism (the embolus was successfully removed surgically shortly after this record was taken). Right ventricular dilatation and strain are manifested by the development of an S wave in lead I and a Q wave plus T inversion in lead III (the '$S_1Q_3T_3$' pattern). There is also acute T wave inversion in V1 and a shift from a left ventricular to a right ventricular pattern in V3. Note that many of these features can be seen in ECGs from normal subjects, and it is only by taking the pattern as a whole, and particularly by comparison with a previous ECG, that the full significance is appreciated.

transfusions are needed rapidly it is important to warm the fluid used to body temperature.

Hypovolaemic shock sometimes occurs in patients with pre-existing cardiac disease. Under these conditions central venous or right atrial pressure may be an unreliable guide to fluid replacement, and it is better to obtain an estimate of pulmonary venous or left atrial pressure by bedside haemodynamic monitoring. This can be done using a *Swan-Ganz catheter*, which is a flexible double-lumen tube with a small balloon at the distal end. The catheter is introduced into a vein and advanced to the right atrium. One lumen is then used to inflate the balloon with about 1 cm³ of air; the force of the bloodstream carries the balloon and attached catheter through the right ventricle to the pulmonary artery, the changing pressures measured through the other lumen indicating its progress. Ideally the tip of the catheter is positioned in a peripheral branch of the pulmonary artery. When the balloon is deflated it records pulmonary artery pressure, but when the balloon is inflated the tip is isolated from the main pulmonary artery and instead registers left atrial pressure. The mean left atrial pressure is normally between 5 and 10 mmHg; in left sided cardiac failure it may rise as high as 30 mmHg. In managing patients with acute circulatory failure a left atrial pressure of about 15 mmHg is usually aimed at; this is high enough to give good left ventricular filling but carries a low risk of pulmonary oedema.

Acute pulmonary oedema (p. 122) is usually a feature of circulatory failure caused by left sided cardiac problems. The three initial steps in its management are the administration of (i) morphine, to alleviate breathlessness and reverse reflex peripheral vasoconstriction, (ii) a powerful diuretic such as frusemide (40–80 mg i.v.) both for its diuretic effect and also as a vasodilator, and (iii) a high concentration of oxygen.

If these immediate measures are inadequate, one may try to stimulate the heart using inotropic agents, or to reduce left ventricular load by using more powerful vasodilators.

INOTROPIC AGENTS. These increase ventricular output for a given filling pressure, but at the cost of increased oxygen consumption. Digoxin, though an inotrope, is of little immediate value because of the time taken to achieve a therapeutic level; it may have a role in persistent circulatory failure.

Noradrenaline, adrenaline and isoprenaline all have effects on peripheral resistance as well as inotropic properties. These range from vasoconstriction for noradrenaline to vasodilatation for isoprenaline. They all cause a tachycardia and increase the risk of arrhythmias. For this reason they are tending to be superseded by dobutamine and dopamine. Dobutamine is an inotropic agent with little effect on peripheral resistance, and less tendency to produce tachycardia than isoprenaline. It may be given by continuous intravenous infusion. Dopamine has an inotropic action and complex effects on peripheral resistance. In low doses (2–4 micrograms per kg per minute) it has a selective renal vasodilating effect, in larger doses it produces more widespread vasodilatation, while in very large doses it causes vasoconstriction.

CONTROLLED VASODILATATION. This is an important concept in the management of pulmonary oedema and of left-sided cardiac failure in general.

Venodilatation reduces central venous pressure and right ventricular output, and slows the accumulation of pulmonary oedema, while *arteriolar dilatation* improves left ventricular function by reducing the afterload against which it has to work. Glyceryl trinitrate and isosorbide dinitrate are predominantly venodilators, hydralazine, nifedipine and salbutamol predominantly arteriolar dilators, and sodium nitroprusside does both very powerfully. These distinctions become blurred in patients with severe circulatory failure. Small doses of vasodilating drugs improve cardiac output and reduce pulmonary oedema but have little effect on blood pressure — the increased efficiency of left ventricular contraction more than compensating for the fall in peripheral resistance. Larger doses may however cause dangerous hypotension. It is therefore essential, if vasodilators are used in treating acute circulatory failure, that their administration should be carefully controlled (e.g. by slow intravenous infusion using a pediatric burette or infusion pump) and their effects carefully monitored, if possible by measurement of left atrial as well as systemic arterial pressure.

There is no hard and fast rule about the order in which inotropic agents and vasodilators should be used. Dopamine is useful because at low doses it combines the benefits of both, and in severely ill patients inotropes and vasodilators are frequently used in combination.

The management of massive pulmonary embolism is discussed on page 185. In pure right sided cardiac failure it is important to maintain an adequate filling pressure for the right side of the heart, and the left atrial pressure may be a better guide to this than the central venous pressure. Inotropic agents may be helpful, but diuretics should be used with care and venodilators are contraindicated.

CARE OF OTHER SYSTEMS. Renal failure (p. 399) is a common complication of acute circulatory failure. The kidney responds to a severe fall in blood pressure by vasoconstriction and by redistribution of blood flow between medulla and cortex. If this vasoconstriction persists, tubular necrosis may ensue. Inducing a diuresis with frusemide or the osmotic diuretic mannitol may help protect the kidney from vasoconstriction, but perhaps the most effective antidote to renal vasoconstriction is low-dose dopamine. Once tubular necrosis has occurred it is important to restrict fluid intake, or pulmonary oedema will follow. Correction of the acidosis which often accompanies circulatory failure presents a dilemma in the presence of tubular necrosis, because of the sodium and fluid load involved. Peritoneal or haemodialysis are sometimes needed.

Hypoxaemia is common in acute circulatory failure, particularly when there is pulmonary oedema. If it does not respond rapidly to oxygen and diuretic therapy, early consideration should be given to endotracheal intubation and positive-pressure ventilation. This often has a strikingly beneficial effect on pulmonary oedema, by reducing right ventricular output.

Prognosis of acute circulatory failure is determined by the underlying cause. No amount of medication can compensate for massive and irretrievable myocardial damage, and the prognosis for circulatory failure complicating extensive myocardial infarction is poor. In contrast the prognosis after drainage of a pericardial effusion,

replacement of a diseased valve, or dissolution of a pulmonary embolus may be exellent.

CARDIAC FAILURE

Acute circulatory failure is at one end of the spectrum of possible manifestations of cardiac failure. The other manifestations are less dramatic, but can be responsible for a great deal of ill health. The common factor in all forms of cardiac failure is the inability of the heart to produce an output sufficient for the needs of the patient. In the mildest forms of cardiac failure, cardiac output is adequate at rest and becomes inadequate only during exercise. In most patients, however, it is possible to detect at least some features of cardiac failure and of the complex haemodynamic, endocrine and renal compensatory mechanisms it evokes even when the patient is examined at rest. The successful management of cardiac failure depends both on an understanding of its pathophysiology and on an accurate diagnosis of its cause.

Pathophysiology. It is convenient to consider separately the consequences of impaired function of the left and the right sides of the heart. The left side of the heart is a term for the functional unit of the left atrium and left ventricle together with the mitral and aortic valves, and the right side stands for the right atrium and ventricle and the tricuspid and pulmonary valves.

Left sided cardiac failure is characterised by a reduction in effective left ventricular output for a given pulmonary venous or left atrial pressure, or conversely, an increase in the left atrial pressure needed to sustain a given cardiac output. An acute increase in left atrial pressure may cause pulmonary congestion or pulmonary oedema; with a more gradual increase in left atrial pressure there tends to be, for reasons at present poorly understood, reflex pulmonary vasoconstriction which protects the patient from pulmonary oedema at the cost of increasing pulmonary hypertension. This is one reason why right sided and left sided failure often occur together, another is that the same disease process (e.g. ischaemic heart disease) frequently affects both ventricles.

In right sided cardiac failure there is similarly a reduction of right ventricular output for a given right atrial pressure, or a need for an increased right atrial pressure to maintain a given output. The increased right atrial pressure is manifested as an increase in jugular venous pressure and as hepatic engorgement.

In both left and right sided cardiac failure the body attempts to compensate for the drop in cardiac output by activation of the sympathetic nervous system, causing tachycardia and vaso-constriction, and retention of salt and water by the kidneys. Fluid retention is accompanied by the development of oedema; in pure left sided failure this is principally pulmonary, and a small accumulation may cause prominent symptoms. In right sided failure, or in a combination of right and left sided failure, most of the oedema is peripheral and its site is determined mainly by gravity. It affects the ankles in ambulant patients, and the thighs or sacrum in the bed-bound. Considerable quantities of peripheral oedema may accumulate without causing distress. Massive accumulation of fluid may cause ascites or pleural effusions (p. 271).

CAUSES OF LEFT OR RIGHT SIDED CARDIAC FAILURE. Nearly all causes of these can be accounted for under four headings: (1) ventricular outflow obstruction, (2) ventricular inflow obstruction, (3) impaired ventricular function and (4) volume overload.

1. *Ventricular Outflow Obstruction*. Obstruction to the outflow of blood from either ventricle causes an increase in ventricular afterload. It may occur as a result of systemic or pulmonary hypertension or of aortic or pulmonary valve stenosis. The initial response is ventricular hypertrophy, the size of the ventricular cavity remaining the same. The increased muscle bulk makes the ventricle stiffer, and higher atrial pressures are needed for diastolic filling. This leads to atrial hypertrophy, and on the left side may precipitate pulmonary oedema. Eventually the increase in afterload may reach a point where the muscle fibres are no longer able to contract fully with each systole. The ventricle then begins to dilate, and as a result, a higher wall tension is needed to maintain the same systolic pressure. (Laplace's law states that the wall tension required to counteract a given pressure in a spherical cavity is proportional to the radius of the cavity). At the same time, it becomes increasingly difficult for the coronary vessels to supply the hypertrophied muscle, and fibres begin to die and to be replaced by fibrous tissue. It is characteristic of this cause of cardiac failure that it is initially well tolerated, but that once deterioration begins it progresses rapidly.

2. *Ventricular Inflow Obstruction*. The commonest cause is mitral or tricuspid valve stenosis; rarer causes include cardiac tumours, external pressure or constriction as in constrictive pericarditis, and occasionally endomyocardial fibrosis. The ventricle itself remains small and usually contracts vigorously; however the chamber upstream, the atrium, often becomes dilated. With obstructed ventricular inflow, atrial contraction becomes increasingly important, and the onset of the atrial fibrillation may cause a striking deterioration.

3. *Impaired Ventricular Function*. This can be divided into two subgroups: (i) cases where ventricular muscle is diffusely affected, as in myocarditis, and (ii) cases where part of the ventricle is virtually normal and part has been damaged, usually by myocardial infarction and subsequent fibrosis.

In the first group cardiac enlargement is usually observed as a result of ventricular dilatation. The damaged muscle fibres require to be stretched more in diastole (i.e., they need an increased preload) to enable them to exert the same contractile effort. Unfortunately as in accordance with Laplace's law the dilated ventricle requires an even greater tension to be developed, so a vicious circle may be set up. The pericardium initially tends to limit the amount of ventricular dilatation, but it stretches in response to prolonged pressure. The stroke volume divided by the ventricular end-diastolic volume is called the *ejection fraction*; it is less than 0·5 in patients with impaired ventricular function. A global reduction in ventricular function of this type may result not only from primary disease of the ventricular muscle, but as the end stage in ventricular outflow obstruction or volume overload.

Areas of ventricular muscle which have been damaged or converted to scar tissue contract less well than adjacent normal muscle, and are called *akinetic areas or segments*. They may impede the function of the normal segments by distorting their contraction pattern. An extensive area of scar tissue may actually bulge outward while the rest of the ventricle is contracting; this is called dyskinetic movement. A circumscribed dyskinetic segment constitutes a ventricular aneurysm.

4. *Volume overload* occurs as a consequence of a chronically increased cardiac output, as in patients with an arteriovenous fistula, because of leakage of the mitral or aortic valves (or their right-sided equivalents), or as a result of left-to-right intracardiac shunting, as in atrial septal defect. In all cases there is an increase in diastolic filling or preload, which in turn causes an increase in the diastolic volume of the ventricle. Healthy muscle responds by contracting vigorously, causing the large stroke volume and hyperdynamic cardiac impulse characteristic of these conditions. Eventually however progressive ventricular dilatation occurs, together with a reduction in ejection fraction and impairment of ventricular function.

Clinical Features. The symptoms of cardiac failure have been considered (p. 122), as have the clinical features of acute circulatory failure, pulmonary oedema and massive pulmonary embolism. This section considers the ways in which the pathophysiological mechanisms involved in a particular patient can be deduced from the clinical examination and investigation.

The first priority is to decide whether the patient has left sided or right sided failure, or a combination of the two. Symptoms of orthopnoea or paroxysmal nocturnal dyspnoea, or the crepitations heard during inspiration over the lung bases in pulmonary oedema, indicate a left sided problem. They may however not occur in the presence of pulmonary vasoconstriction (p. 158). The chest radiograph is often a more sensitive indicator of pulmonary venous congestion than the clinical signs, and shows characteristic abnormalities (p. 131) even in the presence of pulmonary vasoconstriction. The most characteristic features of right sided cardiac failure are a raised jugular venous pressure and the presence of peripheral oedema.

Palpation of the precordium often gives a clue to the presence of left or right ventricular hypertrophy or dilatation, and this can be confirmed by the ECG, chest radiograph, and echocardiography. The detection of ventricular hypertrophy demands a search for signs of systemic or pulmonary hypertension, or a murmur indicating aortic or pulmonary stenosis. Ventricular hypertrophy in the absence of hypertension may be due to hypertrophic cardiomyopathy. A hyperdynamic, rather than a hypertrophic, character to the cardiac impulse should concentrate attention on causes of volume overload.

The detection of a murmur or murmurs suggests the possibility of a valvular lesion, or less probably, an intracardiac shunt. It is sometimes difficult to be sure whether a valve lesion is the cause of the cardiac failure, a minor incidental finding, or the consequence of some other mechanism of cardiac failure; for example, dilatation of the left or right ventricle may cause mitral or tricuspid regurgitation respectively. Echocardiography is often of great value in assessing valve lesions.

Cardiac failure in the absence of murmurs or ventricular hypertrophy is most commonly due to impaired ventricular function, and if necessary this can be confirmed by echocardiography or by radionuclide ventriculography. The ECG may provide clues to the aetiology, for example evidence of previous infarction. Other less common causes include pericardial effusion or a peripheral cause for volume overload.

High output cardiac failure is a term applied to situations where signs of cardiac failure coexist with peripheral vasodilatation and an increased cardiac output, as in severe anaemia, beri-beri and thyrotoxicosis. In many of these cases there are other reasons for the cardiac failure, and the high output requirements may be a precipitating rather than a causative factor.

HEPATIC IMPAIRMENT. Liver function is disturbed by a combination of increased hepatic venous pressure and reduced hepatic artery perfusion. Both the synthesis of coagulation factors and the metabolism of warfarin are affected early, leading to a potentiation of anticoagulant therapy. Later, there may be a rise in plasma bilirubin, alkaline phosphatase and alanine aminotransferase, but severe jaundice or hepatic failure are very unusual.

URAEMIA, HYPOKALAEMIA, AND HYPONATRAEMIA are discussed on page 156.

Treatment. There are three aspects to the treatment of cardiac failure, the eradication of the precipitating cause, the improvement of cardiac output and efficiency, and the treatment of complications such as pulmonary oedema. The cause of the failure can be tackled only in a selected group of patients by eliminating arrhythmia, correcting structural defects and repairing or replacing damaged valves. The other two aspects are interrelated, and the principles of treatment involved are common to different causes and varieties of cardiac failure.

As discussed under acute circulatory failure (p. 147), the main ways in which cardiac function can be improved are by increasing ventricular contractility, by optimising preload and by decreasing afterload. It is more convenient however to discuss the treatment of chronic cardiac failure under the headings of the principal classes of therapeutic agents which may be employed: digoxin, diuretics, and vasodilator drugs.

DIGOXIN. There is general agreement that digoxin is the agent of choice for controlling the ventricular rate in patients with atrial fibrillation and that it is a useful drug for treating certain supraventricular arrhythmias (p. 141). There is less certainty concerning its use as an inotropic agent, and in particular its value for the long term treatment of patients with cardiac failure who remain in sinus rhythm. Digoxin and other digitalis glycosides seem to exert their inotropic action by increasing intracellular calcium availability, and it has been suggested that with long-continued use some form of adaptation occurs to lessen the effect.

Some clinical trials support, and others deny, the long-term efficacy of digoxin as an inotrope. The most likely explanation is that the effect is selective, but there are no well-validated rules for deciding whether an individual patient will benefit or not from long-term digoxin therapy. In general, digoxin is often particularly effective when myocardial function is depressed by drug therapy, e.g. with beta-adrenoceptor antagonists or quinidine, and largely ineffective in the presence of extensive ventricular damage from ischaemic heart disease. In practice, digoxin therapy should be given a trial in patients whose heart failure can be attributed to impaired ventricular function, but discontinued if there is no evidence of benefit. Because of the possibility of digoxin toxicity, the long-term use of digoxin in patients who remain in sinus rhythm should be subject to periodic review. Digoxin dosage and toxicity are discussed on page 142. Attempts have been made to produce other inotropic drugs suitable for long term use, but such agents are not at present generally available.

DIURETICS. This therapy is extensively used in cardiac failure. All diuretics cause an increased urinary output of sodium, chloride and water, by inhibiting the reabsorption of these substances from the glomerular filtrate. The main effects are:

1. A reduction in oedema, both pulmonary and peripheral. This improves the patient's comfort and relieves breathlessness.

2. A reduction in blood, and especially plasma, volume. This reduces right and left ventricular preload, lowers jugular and pulmonary venous pressure, and relieves hepatic congestion. Although a reduction in ventricular filling pressure will, by Starling's law, tend to reduce cardiac output, the curve relating output to filling pressure is 'flat' in cardiac failure, so unless excessive doses of diuretics are used, the reduction in output will be minimal (Fig. 7.28). At the same time, ventricular size tends to diminish and the ventricles contract more effectively.

3. There is also often a small but significant reduction in left ventricular afterload as a result of peripheral arteriolar dilatation, which also helps to improve cardiac function.

Commonly used diuretics have been classified in three groups (p. 96), (i) high potency, loop diuretics e.g. frusemide and bumetanide; (ii) medium potency thiazide diuretics e.g. bendrofluazide and hydrochlorothiazide. Chlorthalidone, though not chemically a thiazide is similar; and (iii) low potency, potassium sparing diuretics e.g. amiloride, triamterene and spironolactone. Dosage, mode of action and adverse effects are described on pages 96 to 97.

It is logical to combine diuretics from different classes if an increased effect is desired, but the use of multiple agents increases the responsibility of the prescriber for monitoring potentially dangerous upsets of fluid or electrolyte imbalance. Combining a thiazide or a loop diuretic with a potassium sparing diuretic will give an increased

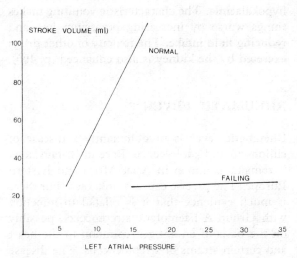

Fig. 7.28 Starling curves relating stroke volume to filling pressure in a normal subject and one with a failing ventricle. The curves shown are for the left ventricle; right ventricular curves show a similar relationship but at lower filling pressures. Because the 'curve' for the failing ventricle is very flat, preload reduction (lowering the filling pressure) makes little difference to output, but enables left atrial pressure to be lowered so that pulmonary oedema does not accumulate.

diuresis while helping to conserve potassium. Even though thiazides are less potent than loop diuretics, the addition of a thiazide to a combination of loop diuretic and potassium sparing diuretic will often produce a further increase in diuretic effect.

Several diuretic combinations are commercially available. They tend to be expensive, and the use of a theoretically balanced combination is no substitute for electrolyte monitoring. Occasionally however they may help by reducing the number of pills the patient is expected to take.

VASODILATORS. The rationale for the use of vasodilators in cardiac failure has been discussed in the section on acute circulatory failure. Vasodilators suitable for prolonged oral administration include *isosorbide dinitrate* (predominantly a venodilator), *hydralazine* (predominantly an arteriolar vasodilator) and *prazosin* (dilates both arteries and veins). *Captopril* (p. 183) is a powerful vasodilator and also reduces aldosterone production. In theory, vasodilator therapy can be related to the patient's requirements by using a venodilator for relieving pulmonary congestion and arteriolar

dilators to improve cardiac output. In practice the choice of vasodilator is often affected by tolerance of the patient. Apart from experiencing side effects such as headache or postural hypotension, most patients adapt to vasodilators and require increasing doses over the first few weeks of therapy. Vasodilator therapy sometimes causes, or increases, peripheral oedema, partly because of increased vascular leakage, partly because of fluid retention by the kidneys; higher doses of diuretic may be needed. Vasodilators are much less widely used than digoxin or diuretics in the long-term treatment of cardiac failure. Captopril, because of its ability to inhibit the effects of renin, is particularly valuable in the management of severe chronic cardiac failure, where plasma renin levels tend to be high. It is a potent drug and accordingly its haemodynamic effects should be carefully monitored; until there is greater experience of its possible long-term side effects the use of captopril in milder forms of cardiac failure is not encouraged.

OTHER TREATMENT. Physical rest is a valuable aid to the management of cardiac failure. Bed rest increases renal blood flow and will often initiate a diuresis in an oedematous patient without any adjustment of diuretic therapy. Conversely, patients often need a larger dose of diuretic when they are up and about than when in bed. Patients with left ventricular failure may be unable to lie flat, and prefer to rest and sleep in a chair or raised on pillows.

Patients should be discouraged from adding extra salt to food, or consuming salty foods or drugs containing or retaining sodium (p. 363), but there is little place for special low salt diets. Fluid restriction is necessary only in exceptional cases.

Obesity seriously impairs effort tolerance, and should be vigorously treated. In contrast, patients with severe cardiac failure become cachectic, and it is difficult to reverse this unless the cardiac failure can be controlled. Anaemia must also be corrected.

Complications of Cardiac Failure and their Treatment. Patients with advanced cardiac failure often exhibit complex metabolic and endocrine upsets which are partly the consequence of the cardiac failure and partly the result of therapy.

URAEMIA. Renal function is impaired by a reduction in renal blood flow. This may be caused by reflex vasoconstriction, by severe damage to cardiac function, or most commonly by excessive use of potent diuretics. A rising plasma urea concentration is an indication for reviewing the patient's state of hydration, and perhaps reducing the dose of diuretic. When renal function is deteriorating in spite of adequate hydration a renal vasodilator such as dopamine may help, but the possibility of acute tubular necrosis should also be considered (p. 400).

HYPOKALAEMIA. Under conditions of reduced renal blood flow, renin production is increased and leads in turn to increased aldosterone production. Renin output is further enhanced by the salt-depleting effects of diuretics, and aldosterone metabolism is hindered by hepatic congestion. The resulting *secondary hyperaldosteronism* may in itself cause hypokalaemia and alkalosis, and it potentiates the potassium depleting properties of diuretics. Most of the body's potassium is intracellular, and there may be substantial depletion of potassium stores even when the plasma concentration is in the normal range. Potassium depletion should be treated by replacement therapy with potassium chloride and/or a potassium sparing diuretic. If cardiac failure is so severe as to cause renal failure, hyperkalaemia may become a problem, and potassium supplements must be stopped.

HYPONATRAEMIA. A falling plasma sodium concentration may sometimes be encountered in severely ill patients on large doses of diuretics. If the patient is oedematous and has a high venous pressure this usually represents inappropriate water retention and responds to a moderate restriction of water intake (p. 95). On the other hand if there is no oedema and the venous pressure is low it is more likely to reflect severe sodium depletion, and oligaemia. This calls for diuretic withdrawal and perhaps fluid replacement (p. 97). In very ill patients the ion pump of the cell membrane may fail to function normally, leading to a falling plasma sodium and a rising potassium concentration.

DRUG TOXICITY. Digoxin toxicity is often a feature of worsening cardiac failure, as renal function becomes impaired. It is potentiated by hypokalaemia. The characteristic vomiting makes things worse by increasing potassium loss and reducing fluid intake. The toxicity of other drugs excreted by the kidney is also enhanced (p. 406).

RHEUMATIC FEVER

Rheumatic fever is predominantly a disease of childhood and adolescence. Rare in Britain now, it remains common in Asia, Africa and Eastern Europe. The precise cause is unknown, but there is much evidence that it is related to infection with Group A haemolytic streptococci, possibly on the basis of an antigen common to the heart and certain strains of streptococcus. The disease is often preceded by tonsillitis or pharyngitis 1 to 3 weeks before. Rheumatic fever is characterised by acute arthritis and/or carditis, sometimes with involvement of the nervous system. Recurrences are frequent unless prophylactic treatment is given. After the acute attack, which may sometimes be mild or subclinical, progressive damage to the heart valves may occur, often not manifesting itself until several years later. This is called chronic rheumatic heart disease.

Pathology. In the acute attack the connective tissues of the myocardium, pericardium, synovial membranes and tendons are affected by inflammation, with oedema, hyperaemia and leucocyte infiltration. The hallmark of rheumatic fever is the Aschoff nodule, a central area of necrosis surrounded by small round cells, histiocytes and giant cells. The mitral, and to a lesser extent the aortic valves, have pinhead-size warty vegetations. In some aggressive forms of rheumatic fever, valve tissue is rapidly destroyed. Subsequent scarring leads to the valve changes of chronic rheumatic heart disease.

Clinical Features. The onset may be sudden with pain, swelling and stiffness in one or more joints, fever, sweating and tachycardia, or it may be insidious with fatigue, and loss of weight. The large joints are principally affected. Characteristically there is a migrating polyarthritis, one joint improving as another becomes worse. In severe cases the joints become hot, swollen, red and very tender; effusions may develop. The joints return to normal when the attack is over.

Tachycardia tends to be out of proportion to the degree of fever, and may persist after the latter has settled.

Although pancarditis probably occurs to some extent in all cases of rheumatic fever, only about half of them have later evidence of chronic rheumatic heart disease. In the early stages, endocarditis may be suspected from the diminished intensity of the first heart sound or from the development of a systolic murmur. A transient mitral diastolic murmur may be heard (Carey Coombs murmur). Aortic regurgitation can also occur. Myocarditis may be assumed to be present if there is endocarditis or pericarditis. Its presence is also suggested by undue tachycardia, decreased intensity of the first heart sound, increasing enlargement of the heart, evidence of cardiac failure and abnormalities in the ECG (see below).

Pericarditis is characterised by retrosternal pain and pericardial friction may be heard. An effusion may develop. Pericarditis is not in itself a serious manifestation of rheumatic fever.

Rheumatic nodules occur most often in childhood, and their significance lies in the almost invariable association with active carditis. They are painless, subcutaneous, not attached to skin and tend to occur over bony prominences such as elbows, knees, scapulae, occiput and vertebrae, or on tendons. Erythema marginatum (erythema annulare) consists of transient pink patches which appear mainly on the trunk and rapidly enlarge to form irregular crescents which join to form larger areas with a pale centre. The margins are slightly elevated.

Sydenham's chorea is described on page 651. The majority of children with chorea subsequently develop evidence of chronic rheumatic valvular disease.

A raised ESR is usually present and may persist as evidence of the activity of the rheumatic process when all other manifestations have subsided. In about a quarter, a group A streptococcus can be grown from the throat. A high ASO (antistreptolysin 'O') titre rising or raised to above 300 units provides evidence of recent streptococcal infection. The chest radiograph often shows cardiac enlargement. Echocardiography may confirm ventricular dilatation or demonstrate a pericardial effusion. The commoner ECG changes are prolongation of the PR interval and abnormalities of the ST segments and T waves.

Diagnosis. Since there is no single diagnostic test, diagnosis depends on an assessment of the whole clinical picture together with the laboratory findings. The Duckett Jones criteria have been proposed as an aid to diagnosis. They classify the clinical manifestations into major criteria (carditis, arthritis, nodules, erythema marginatum and chorea) and minor criteria (fever, arthralgia and a previous history of rheumatic fever). A raised ESR and a prolonged PR interval also qualify as minor criteria. It is suggested that a diagnosis should be based on two major criteria or one major and two minor criteria plus in each case evidence of previous streptococcal infections.

Treatment. Rest in bed is indicated until symptoms and fever have subsided, the sleeping pulse rate, white count and haemoglobin level have returned to normal, and weight is being regained. Thereafter the return to activity should be gradual. The ESR is a useful guide to progress. Phenoxymethylpenicillin should be given, routinely for 7 to 10 days, to kill any remaining haemolytic streptococci in the nose or throat. Erythromycin is an alternative in penicillin-sensitive patients.

Aspirin is effective in combating pain and fever. The daily dose is 50 mg per kg body weight divided into 4-hourly doses, with a double dose at night to avoid waking the patient. This dose should be continued until fever and symptoms have been controlled for at least 10 days and then gradually reduced. Should rheumatic manifestations return, larger quantities will have to be resumed. If toxic symptoms develop the dose must be reduced to a level which can be tolerated. Nausea, headache, dizziness, tinnitus and deafness are the early toxic symptoms, followed by vomiting, hyperventilation and confusion. Aspirin relieves symptoms but probably does not shorten the course of the disease or reduce the incidence of cardiac complications.

Corticosteroids such as prednisolone (60–80 mg per day, or 3 mg per kg in children, tailing off after 10 days) may help to relieve severe symptoms, but there is little convincing evidence they affect long-term results. Heart failure is treated in the usual way with digoxin and diuretics. Mitral or aortic valve damage may be severe enough to warrant valve replacement.

Convalescence in a suitable environment will be required when the acute attack is over and before return to school or work. Its length will depend on the duration of the preceding illness and the severity of any complications.

Prevention is important. Apart from public health measures to reduce the risk of streptococcal infection, children who have had rheumatic fever should have continuous antibiotic prophylaxis until about 20 years of age. Intramuscular benzathine penicillin 1·2 mega units per month is more effective, though less convenient, than phenoxymethylpenicillin (125 mg b.d.) or sulphadimidine (550 mg b.d.).

DISEASES OF THE HEART VALVES

A diseased valve may be narrowed (stenosed) or it may fail to close adequately and thus permit regurgitation of blood. The term incompetence may be used synonymously with regurgitation but the latter is preferable as a stenosed valve is obviously not 'competent'. Regurgitation may be present without structural change in the cusps, e.g. from dilatation of the mitral valve ring in left ventricular failure, the tricuspid valve ring in right ventricular failure, the pulmonary valve ring in pulmonary hypertension or the aortic valve ring in aortic aneurysm.

The principal worldwide cause of symptomatic valvular disease is rheumatic endocarditis, but in many countries it is being overtaken by congenital and degenerative causes. Chronic rheumatic disease most commonly affects the mitral valve, next the aortic valve, comparatively infrequently the tricuspid valve and very rarely the pulmonary valve.

Mitral valve prolapse is possibly the most common valvular abnormality; it has been claimed to be present in about 5% of the young adult population. About one child in 80 is born with a bicuspid aortic valve; initially this is asymptomatic, but it may become the seat of infective endocarditis, and in middle or old age degeneration and calcification may result in aortic stenosis or regurgitation. Congenital aortic stenosis may occur, but is much less common. Congen-

ital lesions are responsible for most cases of pulmonary valve disease. Infective endocarditis may transform a trivial valve lesion into a major one; it usually affects valves deformed by congenital abnormality or rheumatic disease. Syphilis may cause aortic regurgitation from dilatation of the aorta. Exceptionally, a cusp may rupture spontaneously or as a result of external trauma.

Mitral Stenosis

In about half the patients there is a history of rheumatic fever or chorea. The gradual scarring process in the heart takes many years to develop fully. The commissures of the mitral valve become adherent and the chordae are often short and deformed. The mitral valve orifice is about 5 cm² in diastole in health, and is reduced in severe mitral stenosis to about 1 cm². With the reduction in the size of the valve orifice, cardiac output can be maintained only by a rise in left atrial, pulmonary venous and pulmonary capillary pressures with a resultant loss of lung compliance. A sudden increase in pulmonary venous pressure, caused perhaps by the onset of atrial fibrillation, may precipitate pulmonary oedema. With a more gradual rise in pressure, there tends to be an increase in pulmonary vascular resistance which provides some protection against pulmonary oedema.

In about 80% of cases left atrial dilatation is prominent, and may be accompanied by atrial fibrillation. In a minority, the left atrium remains small but becomes hypertrophied and sinus rhythm tends to persist in spite of severe stenosis. All cases may develop pulmonary hypertension and right ventricular hypertrophy, but this is often more severe in those who remain in sinus rhythm. All patients with mitral stenosis are at risk from left atrial thrombosis and systemic thromboembolism, particularly those with atrial fibrillation. Mitral stenosis is frequently associated with mitral regurgitation or disease of the aortic or tricuspid valves.

Clinical Features. The gradual reduction in the mitral valve orifice usually produces breathlessness in about the third decade. The extra demands of pregnancy, or the impairment of function brought about by tachycardia or atrial

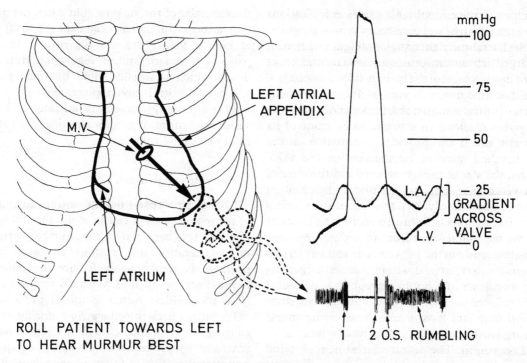

ROLL PATIENT TOWARDS LEFT
TO HEAR MURMUR BEST

Fig. 7.29 Mitral stenosis. O.S. = opening snap.

fibrillation may precipitate a deterioration, and may bring on breathlessness even at rest. Pulmonary congestion may cause a cough, and pulmonary hypertension lead to haemoptysis. Systemic embolism is sometimes the presenting feature.

In some patients with mitral stenosis the face may have a malar flush but this is not specific. The major signs are those which are due to the abnormal valve. It closes with an unusually loud sound which may be palpable — the tapping apex beat. The turbulent flow, which is heralded by the opening snap, causes the characteristic diastolic murmur, and often a thrill (Fig. 7.29). The murmur may be accentuated during atrial systole, and in early or asymptomatic patients this presystolic murmur may be the only auscultatory abnormality. In patients with symptoms the murmur usually extends from the opening snap to the first heart sound. The opening snap may be inaudible if the valve is heavily calcified. Accompanying mitral regurgitation may cause a pansystolic murmur.

An abnormal pulsation is often felt to the left of the sternum; this may be due either to right

ventricular hypertrophy or to forward displacement of the heart by a dilated left atrium. Pulmonary hypertension may cause a loud pulmonary component of the second heart sound, and right atrial hypertrophy may produce a prominent *a* wave in the jugular venous pulse. Tricuspid regurgitation secondary to right ventricular dilatation causes a systolic murmur and systolic waves in the venous pulse.

The physical signs of mitral stenosis are often found before symptoms develop, and their recognition is of particular importance in the obstetric department, since the identification of mitral disease allows appropriate decisions to be made about its management.

Investigation. The ECG may show either the bifid P waves associated with left atrial hypertrophy or atrial fibrillation. There may be evidence of right ventricular hypertrophy; one of the earliest signs is a reduction in the size of the usual QS complex in lead V1. Enlargement of the left atrium and its appendage and of the main pulmonary artery may be seen on the chest radiograph (Fig. 7.29). There may be enlargement of the upper pulmonary veins and horizontal shadows in the costophrenic angles as indications of a high left atrial and pulmonary venous pressure. In the lateral and right anterior oblique position an enlarged left atrium causes a characteristic backward displacement of the barium-filled oesophagus.

Echocardiography is very useful in the evaluation of mitral stenosis; apart from confirming the diagnosis it allows an estimate to be made of its severity and it also provides information on the rigidity and state of calcification of the valve cusps, the size of the left atrium, and the state of left ventricular function. Cardiac catheterisation has been extensively used to confirm the severity of mitral stenosis by measurement of the gradient across the mitral valve from recording pressures simultaneously in the left ventricle and left atrium (or pulmonary arterial wedge position). Increasing confidence in echocardiography has considerably reduced the need for this, although catheterisation may still have a role in assessing mitral regurgitation and associated coronary disease.

Treatment. The definitive treatment of mitral stenosis is surgical, in the form either of mitral valvotomy or mitral valve replacement, but since surgery is not without risk and its long-term results somewhat unpredictable, asymptomatic or mildly symptomatic patients should be treated medically. Pregnancy or contemplated pregnancy is an exception to this rule: it nearly always causes a deterioration in symptoms, and elective mitral valvotomy is indicated, before pregnancy if possible.

Medical treatment of mitral stenosis consists of anticoagulation (p. 547) to reduce the risk of systemic embolism, digoxin to control the ventricular rate in atrial fibrillation (or to protect against a rapid rate if fibrillation should develop), diuretics to reduce pulmonary congestion and antibiotic prophylaxis against infective endocarditis (p. 166).

Mitral valvotomy remains the surgical treatment of choice in patients with significant symptoms, pure mitral stenosis, no mitral regurgitation, and a thin, mobile and noncalcified mitral valve. It may be done with a dilator introduced into the mitral valve through the left ventricle under guidance from a finger inserted into the left atrium, or under direct vision using cardiopulmonary bypass. The results are dependent on the expertise of the surgeon, but when the operation is successful patients can expect 5 to 20 years of benefit before the stenosis recurs. In some patients traumatic mitral regurgitation is produced which is usually slight but may require subsequent mitral valve replacement.

Mitral valve replacement is indicated if there is substantial mitral regurgitation, or if the valve is rigid or heavily calcified.

Mitral Regurgitation

Mitral prolapse ('floppy' mitral valve) is one of the more common causes of mild mitral regurgitation. It is caused by a congenital abnormality or degenerative myxomatous changes. Mitral prolapse is sometimes a feature of connective tissue disorders such as Marfan's syndrome.

In the mildest forms of mitral prolapse the valve bulges back into the atrium during systole, causing a mid-systolic click, but remains competent and so produces no murmur. Frequently however the click is followed by a late systolic murmur, and the combination of mid-systolic click and late systolic murmur is the clinical hallmark of mitral prolapse. Sometimes multiple clicks are heard, while in other cases prolapse occurs at the start of systole, the click is obscured by the first heart sound, and the pansystolic murmur is indistinguishable from other causes of mitral regurgitation. The physical signs may vary with posture or respiration. The diagnosis can be confirmed by echo- or angio-cardiography.

Progressive elongation of the chordae tendineae may lead to increasing mitral regurgitation, while if chordal rupture occurs, regurgitation may suddenly become severe. These complications are rare before the fifth or sixth decade.

Mitral prolapse is associated with an increased incidence of arrhythmias; these are usually benign but a small minority of patients have frequent and bizarre arrhythmias and perhaps an increased risk of sudden death. Many patients found to have mitral prolapse present with atypical chest pain but the specificity of this association is uncertain. Telling a patient there is an abnormal valve sometimes exacerbates or perpetuates a cardiac neurosis. Mitral prolapse is more common than would be expected in young people with embolic stroke or transient cerebral ischaemic attacks, but the overall risk of the complication is very small and prophylactic treatment unwarranted in the absence of previous embolic symptoms. Mitral prolapse can predispose to infective endocarditis but overall, the long term prognosis is good.

Other Causes of Mitral Regurgitation. This can also result from dilatation of the mitral valve ring in association with diseases involving the myocardium, such as rheumatic fever, diphtheria, myocarditis or cardiomyopathy. Papillary muscle dysfunction or papillary muscle rupture may follow myocardial infarction. The valve cusps may be damaged gradually from chronic rheumatic heart disease, in which case there is often coexisting mitral stenosis and/or aortic valve disease. Mitral regurgitation may develop quickly with infective endocarditis.

Clinical Features. The symptoms depend on how suddenly the regurgitation develops. When the valve damage is a slow process the symptoms are similar to those in mitral stenosis. In myocardial disease, the mitral regurgitation exacerbates an already serious situation.

The physical signs arise from the regurgitant jet which causes an apical systolic murmur. This often radiates into the axilla, and may be accompanied by a thrill. The apex beat is usually displaced to the left as a result of dilatation of the left ventricle. The abnormal valve closure is often associated with a quiet first heart sound, and the increased forward flow through the mitral valve may give rise to a loud third heart sound or a short mid-diastolic murmur.

Investigation. The radiograph and ECG often give evidence of left atrial or left ventricular hypertrophy. Atrial fibrillation is common as a consequence of atrial dilatation. Echocardiography provides information about the state of the mitral valve, but does not give a direct measurement of the severity of regurgitation. At cardiac catheterisation the severity of mitral regurgitation may be indicated by the size of the v waves in the left atrial or pulmonary artery wedge trace, or by left ventricular angiography. In practice, the usual problem lies in deciding the extent to which cardiac failure is due to mitral regurgitation and the extent to which it reflects impaired left ventricular function.

Treatment. If mitral regurgitation is due to myocardial disease, treatment, when available, is directed to the latter. When the valve disease is predominant and the symptoms severe, mitral valve replacement is indicated. Infective endocarditis should be treated, if possible, prior to surgery. Mitral regurgitation of moderate severity can often be managed medically, using a diuretic, digoxin and perhaps a vasodilator. Anticoagulation should be considered if there is atrial fibrillation.

Aortic Stenosis

Stenosis of the aortic valve may be a congenital fault, may arise from fusion of the valve cusps from rheumatic damage, or it may be a late development from an accelerated aging process in a congenital bicuspid aortic valve. Rarely congenital aortic stenosis may be due to a subvalvar diaphragm or more rarely still to a supravalvar stenosis. Except in the congenital forms, aortic stenosis develops slowly; the cardiac output is maintained at the cost of a steadily increasing gradient across the aortic valve. The left ventricle becomes increasingly hypertrophied and fibrotic changes may follow. The coronary blood flow may become inadequate, particularly if there is concomitant coronary atheroma. There is often accompanying aortic regurgitation.

Clinical Features. Symptoms arise from restriction of the cardiac output on exercise, which may cause syncope; inadequate coronary blood-flow may cause angina or arrhythmias, and left ventricular failure may give rise to dyspnoea on exertion or nocturnal dyspnoea. Breathlessness does not develop until left ventricular hypertrophy fails to compensate for the obstruction and is therefore a late feature of the disease. Sudden death is common with severe aortic stenosis.

The physical signs arise from the jet through the aortic valve (Fig. 7.30) which causes a systolic murmur and often a thrill which may be transmitted to the carotid pulse as the 'carotid shudder'. There is sometimes an ejection sound (ejection click) from movement of the stenotic aortic valve prior to the onset of the murmur; this is absent when the valve is rigid and calcified.

The sustained, thrusting, apical impulse of left

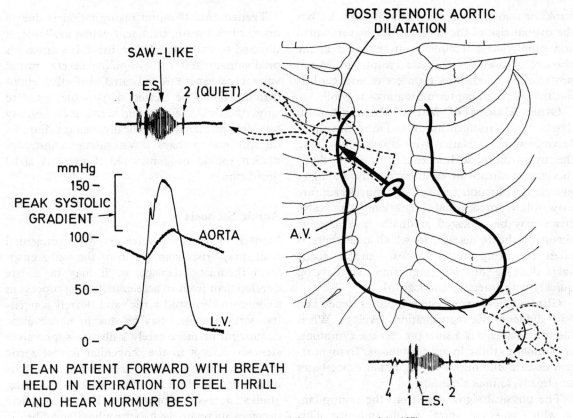

Fig. 7.30 **Aortic stenosis**. E.S. = ejection sound (p. 127).

ventricular hypertrophy is characteristic. The combination of a stiff left ventricle and hypertrophied left atrium may cause a fourth heart sound. The restricted cardiac output is often reflected in a small volume, slow-rising arterial pulse. The physical signs are usually diagnostic, the slow-rising pulse helping to distinguish aortic stenosis from hypertrophic cardiomyopathy (p. 186) or mitral regurgitation.

Investigation. The radiographic changes are shown in Fig. 7.30. Under the image intensifier calcification of the aortic valve can often be seen. The ECG may show left atrial and left ventricular hypertrophy, and in advanced cases changes of the latter are gross (Fig. 7.31). Echocardiography may demonstrate a disorganised aortic valve, left ventricular hypertrophy or left ventricular dilatation. Cardiac catheterisation can be used to measure the gradient across the aortic valve, and together with a measurement of cardiac output this can be used to calculate the aortic valve area.

As with mitral stenosis, echocardiography has tended to reduce the need for catheterisation, but it is still valuable for assessing the state of the coronary arteries.

Fig. 7.31 **Left ventricular hypertrophy**. Note: (1) tall R waves over left ventricle (V5–6); (2) deep S waves over right ventricle (V1–2); (3) ST depression and asymmetrical inversion of T wave in leads I, aVL and V4–V6.

Treatment. Unlike patients with mitral stenosis, it is often necessary to recommend surgical replacement of the valve when symptoms are slight or even absent if the aortic stenosis is severe. To wait too long may result in irreversible damage to the left ventricle. The valve is replaced, under cardiopulmonary bypass, with a prosthetic or heterograft valve. Postoperatively there is usually ECG and other evidence of reduction in the left ventricular hypertrophy. In some cases of severe congenital aortic stenosis, valvotomy may be required as an intermediate measure until an adult-size valve can be inserted. Long-term medical treatment of symptomatic aortic stenosis is justified only if extreme age or intercurrent illness preclude surgery.

Aortic Regurgitation

This results from abnormal aortic cusps as in congenital bicuspid valves, or when valves have been damaged by rheumatic heart disease or infective endocarditis. Aortic regurgitation may also be due to dilatation of the first part of the aorta in cystic medial necrosis, Marfan's syndrome, late syphilis or atheroma. When the leak is large the stroke output of the left ventricle may be doubled or trebled. The major arteries are then conspicuously pulsatile; the left ventricle dilates and hypertrophies and initially compensates for the fault in the valve. The left ventricular diastolic pressure rises, at first only with exercise; the pulmonary vascular pressures then also increase and breathlessness develops.

Clinical Features. Until the onset of breathlessness the only symptom may be an awareness of the heartbeat, particularly when lying on the left side. Paroxysmal nocturnal dyspnoea may be the first symptom. Peripheral oedema may follow. Angina may occur particularly when there is coexisting coronary atheroma or when the coronary ostia are involved in syphilitic aortitis.

The characteristic murmur is illustrated in Figure 7.32; although it is usually best heard to

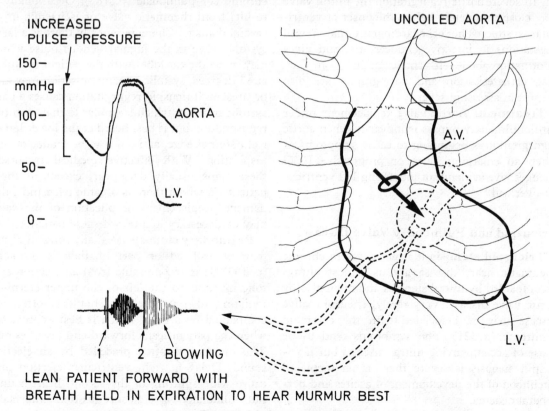

Fig. 7.32 Aortic regurgitation.

the left of the sternum it is sometimes louder to the right, particularly with syphilitic aortitis. A thrill is uncommon. When the leak is small the murmur will be heard only if the steps shown in Figure 7.32 are followed; this is of crucial importance in the early detection of infective endocarditis affecting the aortic valve. A systolic murmur due to the increased stroke volume is common and should not be regarded as due to accompanying stenosis without other evidence of the latter. When the leak is large the diagnosis is usually easy, with gross pulsation in the large arteries, a collapsing pulse, a low diastolic and an increased pulse pressure. There is usually a thrusting apical impulse and often a presystolic impulse and a fourth heart sound as evidence of left atrial hypertrophy.

Investigation. An example of the change in the radiographic outline is shown diagrammatically in Figure 7.5. The ECG usually shows left ventricular hypertrophy (Fig. 7.31). Echocardiography in aortic regurgitation often shows fluttering of the anterior mitral leaflet in the regurgitant jet. In severe aortic regurgitation the mitral valve may close completely before the onset of ventricular systole. The echocardiogram may reveal vegetations in infective endocarditis, and gives information about left ventricular function. Cardiac catheterisation and aortography are also helpful in assessing severity.

Treatment. Aortic valve replacement under cardiopulmonary bypass is indicated when aortic regurgitation is beginning to cause symptoms or when an enlarging heart or progressive ECG changes give evidence of increasing left ventricular overload.

Tricuspid and Pulmonary Valve Disease

Tricuspid stenosis is usually due to chronic rheumatic heart disease and is almost always accompanied by mitral stenosis and often also by aortic valve disease. Very rarely, tricuspid valve disease may be associated with the carcinoid syndrome (p. 321). The symptoms tend to be those of accompanying mitral disease, but if tricuspid stenosis is severe there is an increased likelihood of the development of ascites and peripheral oedema.

With sinus rhythm the *a* wave in the jugular venous pulse is conspicuous and there may be presystolic hepatic pulsation. There may be mid-diastolic and presystolic murmurs similar in timing to those in mitral stenosis but lacking the rumbling quality and increased in inspiration. Tricuspid murmurs are best heard at the lower left or right sternal edge rather than at the apex. The radiograph may show disproportionate enlargement of the right atrium, but this is unreliable; in the ECG there may be the peaked P waves of right atrial hypertrophy. The echocardiogram is often helpful.

Occasionally tricuspid valve replacement is required, but the operation is often less satisfactory than those for mitral and aortic valve disease, partly because tricuspid stenosis tends to occur in those patients who have had severe rheumatic pancarditis and who often have multiple valve lesions.

Tricuspid regurgitation is common in the presence of right ventricular dilatation, particularly with rheumatic heart disease and chronic cor pulmonale (p. 184). Occasionally it results from rheumatic valve or ischaemic myocardial damage. Characteristically there is a large systolic wave in the jugular venous pulse which may move the ear lobes with the patient reclining at 45 degrees; systolic hepatic pulsation may also be present. Tricuspid regurgitation causes a pansystolic murmur which is similar to that of mitral regurgitation but is best heard at the lower left or right sternal edge, and tends to be louder during inspiration. With effective medical treatment these signs usually disappear, except in those patients in whom there is organic tricuspid valve damage. Replacement or plication of the valve may be necessary in a few of these patients.

Pulmonary stenosis is usually congenital and may be isolated or part of Fallot's tetralogy (p. 193). It is recognisable from an ejection systolic murmur to the left of the upper sternum, radiating towards the left shoulder, often accompanied by a thrill which is best appreciated when the patient leans forward and breathes out. The murmur is often preceded by an ejection sound. Delay in right ventricular ejection may cause wide splitting of the second heart sound, but pulmonary valve closure is often abnormally quiet and the splitting may be recognised only on phonocardiography. Mild pulmonary stenosis is fairly common and does not require treatment.

Severe pulmonary stenosis is characterised clinically by a loud, harsh murmur, an increased right ventricular thrust, prominent *a* waves in the jugular pulse, ECG evidence of right ventricular and right atrial hypertrophy, and post-stenotic pulmonary artery dilatation on the chest radiograph. The severity of stenosis can be further assessed by cardiac catheterization. Pulmonary valvotomy is indicated for patients with severe stenosis; it is carried out under cardiopulmonary bypass, and the overall long-term results are very good.

Pulmonary regurgitation is rare and is usually a feature of pulmonary hypertension. The murmur is decrescendo and heard in early diastole at the left sternal edge (Graham Steell murmur). The distinction from aortic regurgitation can generally be made from other evidence.

INFECTIVE ENDOCARDITIS

Endocarditis may result from infection by many different micro-organisms and by fungi. It occurs at all ages and is increasingly being recognised in the elderly.

In the rarer acute form the disease is fulminating, may affect normal valves and if untreated may result in death in a few days, e.g. in staphylococcal septicaemia. At the other end of the spectrum the disease is insidious and may have been present for many months before diagnosis. Abnormal valves such as bicuspid aortic, rheumatic or prosthetic valves, or various forms of congenital heart disease, e.g. ventricular septal defect or persistent ductus arteriosus, are the usual underlying lesions. Regurgitant mitral and aortic valves are the commonest to be affected. Normal valves, particularly the tricuspid, are liable to become infected in 'main line' drug addicts.

Pathology. Damage to the delicate endothelial covering of the heart valves leads to the deposition of platelets and fibrin. The process is exaggerated with abnormal valves, or where an abnormal jet impinges on the endocardium. Colonisation of such deposits by blood borne organisms may occur and cause infective endocarditis. The structure of the valve cusps, and the presence of fibrin aggregates may serve to protect the organisms from the usual defence mechanisms of the host.

Streptococcus viridans, a common cause of periodontal infections, is liable to enter the bloodstream at the time of a dental extraction. Staphylococci and *Streptococcus faecalis* are other common causative organisms; with the latter there may be a history of urethral or pelvic surgery. *Coxiella burnetii* endocarditis is more common in, but not peculiar to, those who work with sheep or with carcasses.

Affected valves develop vegetations composed of organisms, fibrin and platelets which may be exuberant and a source of embolism. Regurgitation may develop or increase owing to the perforation of a cusp. Weeks or months after the onset, mycotic aneurysms may develop in systemic arteries, and rupture. At postmortem it is common to find infarction of the spleen and kidneys as well as other organs. Glomerulonephritis is also found, possibly associated with an immune complex reaction.

Clinical Features. Infective endocarditis should be suspected when a patient known to have congenital or valvular heart disease develops a fever or complains of unusual tiredness. Often however infective endocarditis occurs in patients whose heart disease has been hitherto unsuspected and the diagnosis may be dangerously delayed because it has not been considered. Persistent fever, often recognisable from a history of sweating at night, unexplained arterial occlusion, or the discovery of anaemia or splenomegaly may be presenting features. The disease is almost invariably fatal if untreated, and even if the infection is controlled there is a high mortality. Delay in diagnosis may result in an embolic stroke, progressive valve damage, heart failure and death.

In the early stages the patient looks well but later pallor may be obvious. Other features commonly listed should nowadays be regarded as evidence of delay in diagnosis; these include purpura and petechial haemorrhages in the skin and mucous membranes and splinter haemorrhages under the finger nails. Osler's nodes consist of painful tender swellings at the fingertips; they probably result from vasculitis rather than embolism, and are rare. Finger clubbing is a late sign. The spleen is frequently just palpable, but in coxiella (Q fever) infections both it and the liver may be considerably enlarged. Microscopic haematuria is common. The finding of any of these features in a patient with fever or malaise requires re-examination for hitherto unrecognised heart disease such as trivial aortic regurgitation.

Investigation. Elevation of the ESR is usual; a normocytic, normochromic anaemia and a leucocytosis are common but not invariable. Blood culture is the crucial investigation. Multiple e.g. six, preferably paired, cultures should be taken in the first 6 hours and incubated aerobically and anaerobically. No advantage is gained by waiting for an elevation of temperature. The administration of antibiotics before taking the blood may prevent laboratory diagnosis of the causative organism. Fungi should normally be detected by standard methods of culture. Q fever endocarditis can be diagnosed by showing high titres to coxiella antigens (p. 741). It is commonly associated with thrombocytopenia and abnormal liver function, particularly an elevation of plasma alkaline phosphatase.

Echocardiography is of value for detecting and following the progress of vegetations. It is however possible for these to be too small for echocardiographic detection.

Treatment. The basic objective is to give a suitable antibiotic in adequate dosage for a long enough period. Both the choice of antibiotic and the monitoring of its plasma bactericidal titre against the causative organism require close cooperation between the clinician and the bacteriologist. Benzylpenicillin is still the drug of choice for penicillin-sensitive *Streptococcus viridans* (1.2–2.4 g i.v. every 6 hours for 4 weeks). It is sometimes combined with gentamicin, which may help to improve the bactericidal titre but also increases toxicity. Oral treatment regimes with ampicillin or phenoxymethyl penicillin plus probenecid have been described, but the consequences of inadequate treatment are so serious that there is a strong incentive to use the most effective regime. *Streptococcus faecalis* is more difficult to treat, and may require a combination of penicillin or ampicillin or a cephalosporin with gentamicin. Metronidazole is of value in endo-carditis caused by anaerobes. Staphylococcal endocarditis is often penicillin resistant and requires treatment with cloxacillin or flucloxacillin plus gentamicin.

Plasma concentrations of gentamicin (p. 820) need to be measured to ensure an adequate dose without the risk of renal or ototoxicity. The dose required varies according to renal function. Coxiella endocarditis responds to tetracycline combined with clindamycin.

Any source of infection should be removed if possible, for example a tooth with an apical abscess should be extracted. Cardiac surgery is indicated if valve damage causes progressive cardiac failure, if the endocarditis involves a prosthetic valve, or if active infection persists in spite of adequate treatment, as evidenced by continuing fever, raised ESR and changing murmurs. Antimicrobial therapy should be started before surgery.

Prevention. Every patient with heart disease susceptible to infective endocarditis should be warned of the absolute necessity of taking special care of the teeth, and of having antibiotic cover for dental extractions or other dental procedures which go below the gum margin. For outpatient dental procedures, oral amoxycillin (3 g as a single dose one hour before) is effective and practical. Erythromycin is an alternative for those allergic to penicillin. Patients undergoing operations on the gastrointestinal or urinary tracts should be given ampicillin (1 g i.m. preoperatively and 500 mg t.d.s. for 48 hours afterwards). Prolonged antibiotic therapy prior to the procedure may encourage the overgrowth of resistant organisms.

ISCHAEMIC (CORONARY) HEART DISEASE

Atheromatous disease of the coronary arteries is the most important single cause of death in the Western world. Although its global incidence is still increasing there has been a recent marked fall in the United States and elsewhere. Atheroma is the commonest cause of angina pectoris, and leads also to myocardial infarction and its complications, to cardiac failure and to sudden death.

The Coronary Circulation. The right coronary artery arises from the right sinus of Valsalva and passes in the right atrioventricular groove to supply the right ventricle, part of the interventricular septum and the inferior part of the left ventricle; a branch supplies the AV node. The left coronary artery arises from the left sinus and divides into (1) an anterior descending branch, which supplies part of the septum and the anterior and apical parts of the heart and (2) the circumflex branch, which passes in the left atrioventricular groove and supplies the lateral and posterior surfaces of the heart. In health there are small anastomoses between the coronary arteries; these enlarge under the influence of ischaemia if the flow through a neighbouring coronary artery is compromised. With advancing years an extensive network of anastomotic vessels develops.

Aetiology. Ischaemic heart disease probably has multiple causes; strong correlations have been shown between it and cigarette smoking, hypertension, diabetes mellitus and plasma lipid abnormalities (p. 485). Other contributory factors may be lack of exercise, soft water, and psychological characteristics but proof of each of these is lacking. The possible roles of diet are further discussed under the heading of prevention (p. 178).

Pathology. The process of reduction in the lumen of a coronary artery may be due to atheroma affecting the intima, fibrin and platelet deposition on the intima, haemorrhage under the intima, thrombosis or a combination of these factors. When angina develops one or more coronary arteries is usually already critically reduced in lumen or even occluded. The anterior descending coronary artery is especially vulnerable to atheroma and sudden occlusion of this vessel is particularly dangerous.

In myocardial infarction there is usually complete, but sometimes temporary, occlusion of a coronary artery. There is usually an atheromatous plaque at the site of occlusion, but the final obliteration of the lumen may be due to vascular spasm, thrombosis, or haemorrhage into the plaque. This may result in subendocardial or transmural infarction. Following acute infarction there is an inflammatory reaction, and if the epicardial surface is involved there is usually overlying pericarditis; if the endocardium is affected there may be intraventricular thrombosis. Over a period of 1 to 2 months the area damaged by infarction is replaced by fibrosis; it

may ultimately become difficult to find which area was involved even at post mortem.

Angina Pectoris

Angina pectoris is the name for a clinical syndrome rather than a disease. The term is used to describe a discomfort due to transient myocardial ischaemia. It is likely to occur when the coronary bloodflow is less than is required. Coronary atheroma is the commonest cause. Factors which increase myocardial oxygen requirement include any which add to the ventricular preload such as exercise, anaemia or hyperthyroidism, and those which increase afterload such as hypertension, aortic stenosis or obstructive cardiomyopathy. Increased tension of the ventricular wall, as occurs in dilatation or hypertrophy, may also reduce coronary flow. Tachycardia increases cardiac work and often brings on pain. A rapid arterial run-off during diastole reduces coronary arterial pressure and flow in aortic regurgitation. Coronary artery spasm is increasingly recognised as causing or exacerbating angina pectoris.

Clinical Features. The history is by far the most important factor in making the diagnosis. Angina pectoris is usually experienced as a sense of oppression or tightness in the middle of the chest — 'like a band round the chest'; when describing it the patient commonly places the hand or clenched fist on the sternum, or both hands on the lower chest with the fingers touching at the sternum. It is usually induced by exertion and relieved by rest, lasting only a few minutes. Angina is likely to be worse when walking against a wind, uphill, on a cold day, and particularly after meals. Some patients find that the pain comes when they start walking and that later it does not return despite greater effort. Others can 'walk it off'. Some experience the pain when lying flat (*angina decubitus*), and some are awakened by it (*nocturnal angina*) particularly with 'energetic' or alarming dreams. Rarely, pain may come capriciously as a result of coronary arterial spasm, and be accompanied by transient ST elevation in the ECG (*Prinzmetal's or variant angina*).

The pain is often accompanied by discomfort in the arms, more commonly the left, the wrists and sometimes the hands; the patient may describe a feeling of uselessness in the limbs. Angina may more rarely be epigastric or interscapular or may radiate to the neck and jaw, or occur at any of these places of reference without chest discomfort. The precipitation by effort or anxiety, and the relief by rest or with the use of glyceryl trinitrate, should allow the pain to be recognised. There may be accompanying breathlessness. Pain may sometimes be induced by a cardiac arrhythmia.

Physical examination is frequently negative, but evidence of contributory or concomitant disease should be sought. The presence of tendon xanthomas, thickening of the achilles tendons and an arcus lipidus in a young patient may indicate a hereditary hyperlipidaemia. Aortic valve disease, particularly aortic stenosis, may cause angina. The patient should be examined for anaemia, obesity, diabetes, thyroid and peripheral vascular disease.

Investigation. *Electrocardiography*. The ECG is normal in most patients at rest between attacks. Occasionally T wave flattening or inversion may be seen in some leads; this is non-specific evidence of myocardial ischaemia or damage. A few patients may show ECG signs of established infarction (p. 172). The most convincing ECG evidence is the demonstration of reversible ST segment depression or elevation, with or without T wave inversion, at the time the patient is experiencing symptoms — whether spontaneous or induced by exercise testing. Formal exercise testing is usually done using a treadmill or bicycle ergometer and a standard procedure which ensures a progressive and reproducible increase in work load. Exercise testing should be done only where resuscitation facilities are available and the test should be stopped if the patient develops significant chest pain or discomfort or suffers arrhythmias or a fall in blood pressure. The amount of exercise which can be tolerated under these conditions is a useful guide to the extent of coronary disease.

Scanning. Myocardial perfusion scanning using radioactive thallium may be helpful, in conjunction with exercise testing, in evaluating the minority of patients with an atypical history, or the small group who have severe symptoms but no significant ECG abnormality on exercise testing. Echocardiography or radionuclide bloodpool scanning provide information about ventricular function, which may be relevant in making a decision about coronary arteriography.

Coronary arteriography provides detailed information about the extent and site of coronary artery stenosis. It is usually performed with a view to subsequent coronary bypass grafting (p. 170). In a small minority it may be indicated when a full range of noninvasive tests have failed to elucidate the cause of atypical chest pain.

Differential Diagnosis. This includes musculoskeletal, pericardial and oesophageal pain. Musculoskeletal pains are provoked by specific movement rather than by walking, and background pain often persists at rest. There may be marked tenderness over the costal cartilages and manubriosternal angle. The pain of pericarditis is occasionally provoked by exercise, but its other characteristics (p. 187) should help to make the distinction. Angina occurring at rest may be confused with oesophagitis, with or without a hiatus hernia, but pain due to oesophagitis usually has a burning quality and is relieved by alkalis. Oesophageal spasm however causes a different type of pain which may be difficult to distinguish from variant angina.

Treatment of angina pectoris involves three phases: a proper assessment of the severity of the symptoms and the likely extent of the disease; the use of measures to control symptoms; and treatment which will improve life expectancy. The first phase has been discussed under diagnosis, and a suggested sequence of investigation is shown as a flow chart in Figure 7.33.

Control of symptoms should start with an explanation of how they are caused. Patients usually respond to a careful presentation of the problem as what it is — a mismatch between coronary supply and cardiac needs. The natural process of repair by development of anastomoses should be stressed. Patients can then learn how to help themselves, e.g. by avoiding walking after meals, particularly in the cold or against a wind, and by avoiding severe unaccustomed exertion. They may need encouragement and support in their endeavours to stop smoking and to lose weight. In a few patients hyperlipidaemia re-

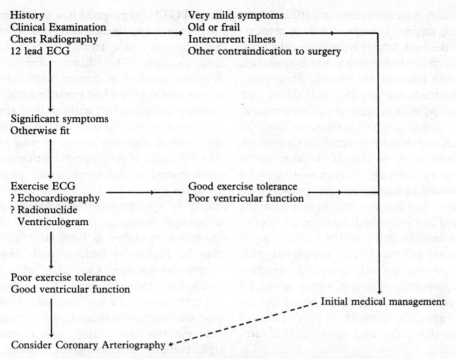

History
Clinical Examination
Chest Radiography
12 lead ECG

Very mild symptoms
Old or frail
Intercurrent illness
Other contraindication to surgery

Significant symptoms
Otherwise fit

Exercise ECG
? Echocardiography
? Radionuclide
   Ventriculogram

Good exercise tolerance
Poor ventricular function

Poor exercise tolerance
Good ventricular function

Initial medical management

Consider Coronary Arteriography

Fig. 7.33 Angina pectoris — sequence of investigation.

quires treatment by diet and other measures (p. 486).

DRUG TREATMENT. There are three principal groups of drugs which help to relieve or prevent the symptoms of angina: nitrates, beta-adreno-ceptor antagonists (beta-blockers) and calcium antagonists.

Nitrates. Fresh glyceryl trinitrate (GTN 500 micrograms), allowed to dissolve under the tongue or crunched for more rapid effect and retained in the mouth, usually relieves the pain in 2 to 3 minutes, and about the same time it often produces a slight headache. The headache may become severe in some patients if the tablet is left in the mouth, so the patient should be instructed to spit it out or swallow it once the angina is relieved. The best use of GTN is prophylactically before exercise known as liable to produce pain. The good effect comes from venous and arteriolar dilatation, which lowers the blood pressure and also dilates the coronary vessels provided their disease does not prevent this. Patients can be reassured that GTN is not dangerous or habit forming, and that it does not lose its effect. The tablets themselves have a limited shelf life,

particularly if kept in a warm place. Not more than about two tablets per hour should be used; if the requirement for it increases significantly the patient should seek medical advice. The appropriate use of GTN (or other drugs) allows more exercise to be taken; this should be encouraged because physical activity promotes the formation of collateral vessels. As sublingual GTN has a short duration of action, there has been much interest in ways of giving more prolonged nitrate therapy. GTN can be given percutaneously as a paste or plasters, or as a slow-release buccal tablet. Some patients find these helpful, but they are much more expensive than sublingual tablets. GTN is virtually ineffecti!e when swallowed, but other nitrates such as sosorbide dinitrate (10 mg or more, 3–6 per day) can be given by mouth. Headache is common when patients are started on oral nitrates, but tends to improve on persevering with the therapy. Tolerance frequently occurs, and the dose needs to be increased to maintain efficacy. The use of slow-release preparations may make it possible for the patient to accept large doses. Intravenous nitrates may have a role in treating unstable angina.

Beta-blockade is an important and effective way of preventing angina. It helps to reduce myocardial oxygen demand, largely by reducing the heart rate for a given level of exercise, and by reducing the heart rate response to anxiety. *Propranolol* can be prescribed initially in small doses (e.g. 20 mg 6-hourly) with progressive increments until benefit is obtained, which is often not until the resting heart rate has been significantly slowed. There is considerable individual variation and as much as 160 mg 6-hourly or even more may be required. Other beta-blockers are probably no more effective than propranolol but may have the advantages of less individual dose variation, once daily administration and possibly, in the case of cardioselective agents, fewer peripheral side effects. These matters are discussed, together with other properties of beta-blocking drugs, on page 182. A beta-blocking drug should not be withdrawn abruptly because of the risks of dangerous arrhythmias and myocardial infarction.

Calcium antagonists, or more correctly 'slow calcium channel inhibitors' are a group of drugs whose common pharmacological property of inhibiting calcium entry into cardiac and smooth muscle gives little clue to the diversity of their clinical effects. *Nifedipine* is a powerful coronary and systemic arteriolar dilator, and most of its antianginal effects can be explained by its action on calcium. The initial dosage is one 10 mg capsule t.i.d. with food. For rapid effect, a capsule may be bitten before swallowing it. Side effects are headache, dizziness, flushing, itching skin and mild fluid retention. It is often given in combination with a beta-blocker. *Verapamil* is enjoying a resurgence of popularity as an antianginal agent, at doses considerably higher than originally used (120–240 mg t.i.d.). It seems less likely to cause side effects related to vasodilatation than nifedipine, but should be used cautiously in patients suspected of a cardiac conduction defects. Its commonest unwanted effect is constipation.

Although each of these groups of drugs can be shown to be superior to placebo in treating symptoms of angina, there is little convincing evidence that one group is more effective than another. The authors' present policy is to start with sublingual GTN, to progress to a beta-blocker unless there are contraindications and then to add nifedipine or a long acting nitrate such as isosorbide dinitrate. The ultimate aim of achieving excellent control of angina with minimal side effects and the simplest possible tablet regime is unlikely to be reached without trial and error.

SURGICAL TREATMENT. This principally takes the form of coronary artery bypass grafting, in which lengths of the patient's saphenous vein are anastomosed to the aorta at one end and to a coronary vessel distal to a stenosis at the other. There is symptomatic improvement, which is frequently dramatic, in over 80% of patients. Operative mortality is between 1 and 2%, but may be higher in patients with impaired left ventricular function. Controlled trials have indicated that coronary grafting in patients with left main coronary artery stenosis, or with significant stenosis in the three major coronary vessels (left anterior descending, left circumflex and right coronary arteries) gives a better chance of survival over a 5 year period than medical treatment. There is as yet no clearcut evidence of improved survival in patients with less extensive disease, although they may benefit symptomatically.

Coronary arteriography is a necessary preliminary to coronary artery surgery, and should be considered in those patients whose severe symptoms or poor performance on exercise testing suggest extensive disease, as well as in those who continue to have unacceptable symptoms in spite of adequate medical treatment. Poor left ventricular function (which may be assessed by echocardiography or radionuclide scanning) or intercurrent illness are relative contraindications.

Coronary angioplasty is an alternative to coronary artery bypass grafting. It is mainly used for patients with single vessel coronary disease.

Prognosis. Overall, more than half of a group of patients with angina will live for 5 years, and a third for 10 years from the time of diagnosis. Spontaneous recovery, which may prove temporary, may occur in as many as a third, a fact which is useful to remember in talking to patients about their disease. Prognosis is worse in the patient who has had multiple cardiac infarcts or who has cardiac failure.

Unstable Angina

The term 'unstable' is used to describe angina which has become abruptly more severe or more prolonged in the absence of evidence of infarction. Many different factors may be responsible, including the natural progression of coronary atherosclerosis, thrombus formation or the development of coronary artery spasm. Affected patients are often admitted to hospital under suspicion of myocardial infarction. Most patients will respond to rest, mild sedation, nitrates and adrenergic blocking drugs. Calcium antagonists such as nifedipine may also be useful. The persistence of symptoms in spite of these measures should lead to consideration of coronary arteriography and the possibility of surgical treatment.

Myocardial Infarction

Myocardial infarction is myocardial necrosis occurring as a result of a critical imbalance between coronary blood supply and myocardial demand. The necrosis may be confined to the subendocardial region, or may affect the full thickness of the myocardium (transmural infarction). The latter is usually associated with the total, but sometimes transient, occlusion of the coronary artery supplying the area. This usually occurs at the site of a pre-existing atheromatous plaque; it is difficult to be certain of the precise factors causing occlusion in individual cases, but fissuring and dissection of the plaque, coronary spasm, and thrombosis probably all play a part.

In its mildest form the infarct may go unrecognised and be disclosed subsequently only by ECG evidence; at the other end of the range there is permanent severe disability or death. At the onset of the illness, sudden death, presumably from ventricular fibrillation or asystole, may occur immediately, and many of the patients who die do so within the first hour. If the patient survives this most critical stage, the liability to dangerous arrhythmias remains, but diminishes as each hour goes by. The development of cardiac failure reflects the extent of myocardial damage; its severity may range from slight reduction in skin perfusion and basal lung crepitations at one end to acute circulatory failure at the other. Cardiac failure is the major cause of death in those who survive the first few hours of infarction.

Clinical Features. The cardinal symptom is pain, but breathlessness, syncope, vomiting and extreme tiredness are common. The pain occurs in the same sites as for angina but is usually more severe and lasts longer. It is most often described as a tightness, heaviness or constriction in the chest. At its worst the pain is one of the most severe which can be experienced and the patient's expression and pallor may vividly convey the seriousness of the situation. Many patients are breathless and in some this is the only symptom; a few develop pulmonary oedema at the onset. Syncope may occur and the blood pressure falls particularly if the patient is upright, or from the development of a serious arrhythmia or heart block. Vomiting is common, particularly in the more severe cases. It may also result from morphine given for pain relief. At any time after the first 12 hours or so the patient may recognise that a different pain has developed, even though it is at the same site. It is worse, or only appears, on inspiration and may be altered by a change of position. It is due to pericarditis consequent on the infarct, and the diagnosis is confirmed if a pericardial rub is heard. In rare cases the infarct may go unnoticed until endocardial thrombosis resulting from it leads to systemic embolism.

The physical signs may be few in a mild attack but in severe cases there is usually pallor, sweating and breathlessness. The heart rate is usually increased, and with circulatory failure the pulse volume may be much reduced and the skin perfusion poor. Most patients seen early after myocardial infarction have a normal initial blood pressure, but transiently it may be high as a result of pain or anxiety. The blood pressure gradually falls over the first 3 or 4 days. It is low in the minority who develop circulatory failure. The jugular venous pressure is often elevated when the patient is first seen; this may be due to cardiac failure but vasoconstriction and anxiety may contribute. Later, the JVP may remain high in patients with inferior infarction even when there is no evidence of fluid overload; this is because inferior infarcts often involve the right ventricle and make it less compliant than usual. The first heart sound is often quiet and a third or a fourth heart sound may develop. Extensive anterior myocardial damage may be manifest in a diffuse apical pulsation. Pericardial friction is most often heard on the second or third day, and is usually transitory. Occasionally it persists for days, and exceptionally for weeks. Crepitations, particularly if widespread and persistent after coughing, suggest pulmonary oedema. Oliguria is common if the blood pressure is low. It is not an indication for diuretic therapy unless there are other signs of fluid overload. In many cases there is a fever, reaching a maximum on the third or fourth day, and not much higher than 38°C.

Complications. ARRHYTHMIAS. Nearly all patients with myocardial infarction have some form of arrhythmia, but in most cases this is mild and of no haemodynamic or prognostic significance.

Sinus tachycardia is the commonest; anxiety may contribute to it. If persistent, it may warn of incipient cardiac failure. Sinus bradycardia is more common after inferior infarction; it does not usually need treatment unless it is associated with hypotension. Severe bradycardia may lead to ventricular escape and the development of more dangerous rhythms. Atrial tachycardia or fibrillation occur in about 15% of patients; these arrhythmias may exacerbate hypotension or cardiac failure and require prompt treatment if the ventricular rate is excessively fast. Ventricular ectopic beats are almost invariable, and are frequently numerous. They are usually of little consequence but may indicate an increased liability to ventricular fibrillation if they fall on the T wave of the preceding beat ('R on T').

Ventricular tachycardia is also common. If it persists at a fast rate for more than a few seconds it may have serious haemodynamic effects.

Ventricular fibrillation occurs in about 5–10% of patients in hospital. The risk is much higher in the first hour after infarction, and ventricular fibrillation is thought to be the major cause of death in those who die before reaching hospital. Its potential reversibility in those patients who do not have extensive myocardial damage is one of the main foundations on which the policy of acute coronary care is built. Various degrees of heart block are also common (p. 142).

ACUTE CIRCULATORY FAILURE (p. 147). If there is a reversible arrhythmia as an important contributory factor its correction may bring about considerable improvement. In a few cases excessive diuretic therapy leading to hypovolaemia may be the cause. If neither of these is responsible, acute circulatory failure usually reflects extensive myocardial damage and indicates a bad prognosis. In its presence, all the other complications of myocardial infarction are more likely, such as dangerous arrhythmias, extension of the infarct, pulmonary oedema and renal failure.

OTHER COMPLICATIONS. *Cardiac failure* may occur, and pulmonary oedema is its commonest form. Regular examination for basal lung crepitations and chest radiography should lead to its early detection.

Rarer complications include *infarction of a mitral papillary muscle*, which leads to mitral regurgitation and may precipitate pulmonary oedema. *Rupture of the interventricular septum* is diagnosed by the development of the characteristic murmur of a ventricular septal defect (p. 192) and may be followed by severe hypotension and venous hypertension. Rupture of the ventricle into the pericardial space may lead to *cardiac tamponade* (p. 187). When a thrombus forms on the endocardium of the left ventricle, cerebral or peripheral *embolism* can occur. *Venous thrombosis* is less common now than when patients were routinely kept in bed for 6 weeks; it often first announces its presence by pulmonary embolism. Even a careful watch on the legs for the first clinical signs of thrombosis will detect only about 50%.

The *post myocardial infarction syndrome* (Dressler's syndrome), which is probably an autoimmune reaction to necrotic myocardium, is characterised by persistent fever, pericarditis and pleurisy. It occurs a few weeks or even months after the infarct and often subsides after a few days but may require aspirin, other anti-inflammatory drugs or corticosteroids for its control if symptoms are prolonged.

Ventricular aneurysm and dyskinetic or akinetic segments (p. 152) can develop later.

Investigation. ELECTROCARDIOGRAPHY. The ECG is usually a sensitive and specific way of confirming the diagnosis, but the typical changes may take some hours to develop. The ECG may also be difficult to interpret after previous infarction and occasionally it will not be significantly altered in spite of clinical and biochemical evidence of re-infarction. The earliest ECG change is usually ST elevation, which reflects acute myocardial injury. At the same time or slightly later there is diminution in the size of the R wave, and a Q wave begins to develop. One explanation for the Q wave is that the myocardial infarct acts as an 'electrical window' transmitting the changes of potential from within the ventricular cavity, and allowing the ECG to 'see' the reciprocal R wave from the other wall of the ventricle. Subsequently the T wave becomes inverted because of a change in ventricular repolarisation, and this change persists after the ST segment has returned to normal. These changes are shown diagrammatically in Figure 7.34 and their sequence is sufficiently reliable for the approximate age of the infarct to be deduced. With subendocardial infarction there is usually no Q wave or ST elevation, but symmetrical T wave inversion develops.

The ECG changes are best seen in the leads which 'face' the infarcted areas (Fig. 7.2). When there has been anteroseptal infarction the changes are found in one or more leads from V1 to V4 (Figs. 7.35 and 7.36) while anterolateral infarction produces changes from V4 to V6, in aVL and hence also in lead I. In strict anterior infarction the changes may be confined to V3 and V4. Inferior infarction is best shown in leads II, III and aVF, while leads I, aVL and the lateral chest leads show 'reciprocal' changes of ST depression (Fig. 7.37). Infarction of the posterior wall of the left ventricle is not recorded in the standard leads by ST elevation or Q waves, but the reciprocal changes of ST depression and a tall R wave may be seen in leads V1-V4 (Fig. 7.38).

PLASMA ENZYMES. Myocardial infarction leads to a detectable rise in the plasma concentration of

Fig. 7.34 **The serial evolution of ECG changes in myocardial infarction**. A: pre-infarct; B: ST elevation owing to a myocardial 'injury current', also some reduction in R wave size; C: developing Q wave and terminal T wave inversion; D: established Q wave and T inversion; E; 'old infarct' pattern — the Q wave tends to persist but T wave changes become less marked. The rate of evolution is very variable. In general stage C is usually reached in hours, stage D in days and stage E after some months. This diagrammatic representation should be compared with the actual ECGs in Figures 7.35 to 7.38.

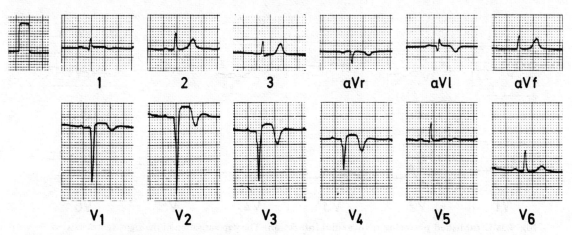

Fig. 7.35 **Recent anteroseptal myocardial infarction**. In leads V1–V4 there is ST elevation, and in these leads and in aVL inverted T and deep Q waves.

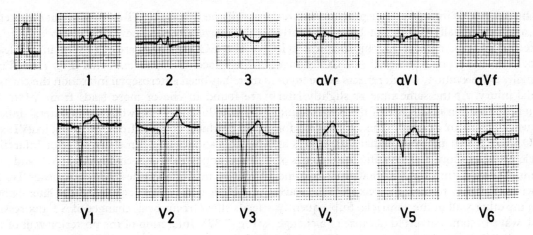

Fig. 7.36 Established anteroseptal myocardial infarction. There is a deep Q and absent R in leads V1–V5.

Fig. 7.37 Recent inferior myocardial infarction. In leads II, III and aVF there is ST elevation, inverted T and deep Q waves. In leads I, aVL and V2–V4 there is reciprocal ST depression.

Fig. 7.38 Established posterior myocardial infarction. The depolarisation of the right ventricle is no longer opposed by the depolarisation of the back of the left ventricle and hence there is a prominent R in the right anterior leads. (Q in 1, II and V6 indicate antero-lateral infarction also).

enzymes normally confined within cardiac cells. The enzymes most widely used in the detection of myocardial infarction are creatine kinase (CK), aspartate aminotransferase (AST) formerly known as glutamic oxaloacetic transaminase, and lactate dehydrogenase (LD). CK starts to rise at 4–6 hours, peaks about 12 hours and falls to normal in 48–72 hours. CK is also present in skeletal muscle, and a rise in CK may be due to an intramuscular injection or vigorous physical exercise. Measurement of the myocardial isoenzyme of CK (CK-MB) is more specific for myocardial damage. AST starts to rise about 12 hours after infarction, and reaches a peak on the first or second day. LD is also liberated from haemolysed red cells and is therefore less specific. It starts to rise after 12 hours, reaches a peak after 2 or 3 days and may be elevated for about a week. LD estimation may be useful when the diagnosis is uncertain several days after a possible infarct. Serial estimations are necessary in doubtful cases, for it is the change in enzyme levels which is of diagnostic value.

OTHER BLOOD TESTS. A leucocytosis is usual, reaching a peak on the first day. The ESR becomes raised and may remain so for several days.

CHEST RADIOGRAPHY may demonstrate pulmonary oedema which has been undetected clinically. The heart size is usually normal. Enlargement of the cardiac shadow may indicate previous myocardial damage or a developing pericardial effusion.

RADIONUCLIDE SCANNING (p. 132). A pyrophosphate scan may show the site of myocardial necrosis. A radionuclide ventriculogram indicates the extent of impairment of ventricular function and may give useful prognostic information.

Treatment. The main immediate needs are for the relief of pain and the prevention or treatment of arrhythmias and other complications. Later, efforts are concentrated on rehabilitation of the patient and the attempted prevention of further infarction.

In the first 3 or 4 hours when the risk of fatal arrhythmia is highest it is best for patients to be cared for where there is immediate access to resuscitation facilities; this will usually be in a coronary care unit. Patients seen and diagnosed after the first few hours may be cared for at home if they are free of cardiac failure or other complications and are adequately supported domestically.

RELIEF OF PAIN. The patient with a severe attack is in pain and is frightened. An effective remedy is morphine given intravenously in 5 or 10 mg aliquots titrated against the patient's response. Diamorphine (2.5–5 mg) is slightly more potent on a weight for weight basis, and produces analgesia slightly more rapidly, but has no other advantages to compensate for its expense, instability and addiction potential. Either drug may be given subcutaneously or intramuscularly (morphine 10–20 mg, diamorphine 5–10 mg) but this is less satisfactory because peripheral vasoconstriction initially delays absorption, while later vasodilation leads to rapid absorption and possible respiratory depression. The amount of analgesia needed tends to parallel the extent of myocardial damage. Opiates should be supplemented with an antiemetic such as cyclizine (50 mg i.v) or a phenothiazine. The anxiety must be recognised even if it is not overt; it is essential to reassure the patient that recovery is the most likely outcome and that the most dangerous phase of the illness is already over.

ARRHYTHMIAS. Pain relief, rest, reassurance and the correction of hypokalaemia all play a major role in preventing arrhythmias. Lignocaine (p. 140) is given after resuscitation from ventricular fibrillation or to treat ventricular tachycardia with a rapid rate. In some units lignocaine is also given if multiple ectopic beats, or the potentially dangerous 'R on T' ectopics are observed during the acute phase of the illness. If lignocaine is ineffective, mexiletine (p. 140) may be used instead; sometimes an intravenous beta-blocker (e.g. atenolol 5–10 mg or sotalol 10 mg) may be helpful.

Ventricular fibrillation should be treated with an immediate d.c. shock (p. 145). Failing this, the cardiac resuscitation procedure (p. 138) should be used until the defibrillator is available. Atrial tachycardia, flutter or fibrillation are best treated with digoxin if the ventricular rate is rapid, and spontaneous reversion to sinus rhythm is common. If the arrhythmia causes severe hypotension, synchronised d.c. shock treatment should be considered.

Sinus bradycardia does not usually require treatment, but if there is hypotension or ventricular escape, atropine may be given (0.3 mg i.v. every 5 min to a maximum of 1.5 mg). Heart block complicating inferior infarction often responds to atropine and a temporary pacemaker is needed only if this drug is ineffective in preventing hypotension. Heart block complicating anterior infarction is an indication for the prophylactic insertion of a temporary pacemaker, as asystole may suddenly supervene. Asystole sometimes responds to cardiac massage, and following this a pacemaker electrode should be inserted.

ACUTE CIRCULATORY and CARDIAC FAILURE are treated as described on pages 149 and 154.

ANTICOAGULANTS (p. 547) are indicated in the treatment of venous thrombosis and pulmonary embolism and may be used prophylactically if the patient is at risk because of prolonged immobilisation. Whether or not the long-term use of anticoagulants protects against further infarction has been controversial for many years, and is presently undergoing further evaluation.

MYOCARDIAL PRESERVATION. The concept that treatment started after the onset of the illness might limit the extent of myocardial damage, and so improve the prognosis, has attracted great interest. Measures proposed include the acute intravenous administration of beta-adrenoceptor blockers, the use of the enzyme hyaluronidase, and attempts to restore coronary patency using streptokinase. All of these are still undergoing evaluation.

REHABILITATION. There is histological evidence that an infarct takes 4–6 weeks to become replaced with fibrous tissue. Accordingly it is generally thought reasonable to restrict physical activities during this period. When there are no complications the patient can sit in a chair within a few days, be ambulant within a week, return home in 7–10 days and gradually increase activity with the prospect of a return to work after 6 weeks. When there are complications the regime has to be adjusted accordingly. Reassurance is essential at every stage because many patients are severely and even permanently incapacitated as a result of psychological rather than physical effects of myocardial infarction. The success of restoring a patient to normal life depends very much on the attitudes of the physician. The naturally vigorous person may require restraint in the early stages but more often the anxious will need encouragement. In general, patients can be reassured that exercise within the limits set by angina and tiredness will do no harm and much good. The same limits apply to sexual activity. The spouse has often to learn to stop reminding the patient of former disability. Formal rehabilitation programmes based on graded exercise and counselling may be of great psychological benefit, although it has not been possible to show convincing effects on eventual exercise ability or survival.

Prevention. The terms primary and secondary prevention are defined on page 177 where the former is described. Secondary prevention is discussed here.

Much advice given to patients after myocardial infarction is based on common sense rather than on objective demonstration of benefit, but control of obesity, regular exercise and the adoption of a less frenetic lifestyle are unlikely to do harm. Stopping smoking improves survival, more so in younger than in older patients. There is no overall evidence that control of plasma lipids, by dietary or other means, affects survival in patients who have had an infarct, but lipid control may still be worthwhile in young patients with familial hyperlipidaemias.

The beta-adrenoceptor blocking drugs, propranolol, metoprolol and timolol have all been shown in prospective controlled trials to reduce cardiovascular mortality in patients taking them on a long-term basis following myocardial infarction. Contraindications to the use of these drugs include persistent cardiac failure or heart block, and some patients are unable to tolerate them because of side effects such as breathlessness, hypotension or cold extremities. The reduction in mortality from the use of these drugs is of the order of 25% over a 1–2 year period: although this might have a considerable impact on community mortality, the improvement in survival for the individual patient is in the order of only 2–5%, so patients reluctant to take this medication should not be subjected to undue pressure to do so. Secondary prevention trials using antiplatelet drugs such as aspirin, sulphinpyrazone or dipyridamole have so far been unconvincing.

Persistent ventricular ectopic beats in the late post infarct period (2 or more weeks after infarction) are associated with increased mortality, but there is no objective evidence that anti-arrhythmic agents improve survival. Post-infarct angina is also associated with a worse prognosis, and provided ventricular function is adequate some of these patients may be helped by coronary bypass grafting.

Prognosis. In about a quarter of all cases of myocardial infarction death occurs within a few minutes without medical care. Half the deaths from myocardial infarction occur within 2 hours of the onset of symptoms and three quarters within 24 hours. About 40% of all affected patients die within the first month. Unfavourable features are old age, poor left ventricular function, heart block and persistent ventricular arrhythmias. The prognosis is worse for anterior than for inferior infarcts. Bundle branch block and high enzyme levels both indicate extensive myocardial damage. In the absence of unfavourable features, the outlook is as good for those who survive ventricular fibrillation as for the others. Of those who survive an acute attack, more than 80% live for a further year, about 75% for 5 years, 50% for 10 years and 25% for 20 years. It is therefore appropriate to be reassuring to patients about their prospects.

Sudden Death

This term can be applied when a person previously in apparent good health falls ill and dies within minutes or at most a few hours. Some of these patients have an identifiable non-cardiac cause of death such as cerebral haemorrhage or a leaking aortic aneurysm. Many have extensive coronary atherosclerosis; the proportion of these who have thrombotic occlusion of a coronary vessel is small when death is virtually instantaneous but higher in those who survive for a few hours. The explanation for this is uncertain but possibly coronary spasm may occlude a vessel for long enough to produce fatal consequences without a thrombus developing. Alternatively, death might be due to an arrhythmia in the absence of coronary occlusion. Arrhythmias are probably the immediate cause of sudden death in patients with other cardiac abnormalities such as severe aortic or pulmonary stenosis or hypertrophic cardiomyopathy. A small group of patients who die suddenly have no obvious pathological cause of death on post-mortem examination; cardiac arrhythmia seems the most likely cause in this group also, and in some cases a previous ECG has been found to be abnormal. There is evidence both from patients who have died during ambulatory ECG monitoring and from acute resuscitation services that ventricular fibrillation is the commonest arrhythmia causing sudden death, and resuscitation, if promptly applied, may restore effective cardiac action. The long-term prognosis is probably best in those who have a correctable cause for the arrhythmia.

Relatives of patients who have died suddenly often seek reassurance, and should be examined, if appropriate, for evidence of hypertrophic cardiomyopathy, Marfan's syndrome and hyperlipidaemia. A family history of sudden death in childhood or young adult life is sometimes associated with prolongation of the QT interval on the ECG, and beta-blockade may improve prognosis in this group.

Primary Prevention of Ischaemic Heart Disease

Primary prevention is the term used for measures which are applied in the absence of clinical manifestations of disease, whereas secondary prevention refers to measures put into practice after the disease has become apparent, usually as a result of the development of angina or following myocardial infarction (p. 176).

The prevalence of clinically apparent ischaemic heart disease in the United States, Australia and certain other countries reached a peak in the late 1960's and early 70's and is now falling. It is not possible to tell whether this results from reversal of a few major risk factors, or from a cumulative effect of many minor ones. While it is possible to associate an increased incidence of ischaemic heart disease with certain risk factors such as smoking or high plasma cholesterol concentrations, it is important not to confuse the absence of a risk factor with its correction by drugs, dietary manipulation or other means. Almost invariably, the results of correcting risk factors are less striking and harder to demonstrate — partly perhaps because it is difficult to maintain the 'correction' for a prolonged period, partly because the drug or diet used may have harmful effects of its own.

Cigarette Smoking. There is good evidence that non-smokers have a lower incidence of myocardial infarction, and that stopping smoking reduces the risk of subsequent infarction. The improvement is greatest for young patients and increases with the length of abstention.

Plasma cholesterol is shared among several plasma lipoprotein fractions. High-density lipoprotein (HDL) containing cholesterol appears to have a protective effect against atheroma, whereas cholesterol in the low density and very low density (LDL and VLDL) fractions appears to promote atheroma and its complications if present in excess. The reduction of very high plasma cholesterol concentrations (above 7 mmol/litre) reduces the risk of ischaemic heart disease. Dietary measures (a low cholesterol diet with an increased ratio of polyunsaturated to saturated fat) may have to be supplemented by drugs such as cholestyramine, particularly in those with familial hypercholesterolaemia. Even though the 'normal range' of plasma cholesterol concentrations in Western societies is higher than in communities with a low prevalence of atheroma, it has been difficult to show that further reduction confers any benefit.

Other Dietary Factors. These are both too numerous, and the evidence often too tenuous, to discuss in detail. The best current recommendation is for a mixed diet with not more than a third of the total energy requirement derived from fat, an adequate fruit, vegetable and fibre intake, and a low proportion of refined carbohydrate. At least a third of the fat should be polyunsaturated from fish or vegetable sources rather than animal fat.

Obesity on its own is a relatively weak risk factor for ischaemic heart disease; however its correction is often an important step in the treatment of other risk factors.

Exercise. Clinical ischaemic heart disease is more prevalent in sedentary sections of the community than in those who take regular exercise. Although there is little direct evidence that the sedentary will improve their prognosis by physical activity, regular daily exercise to the point of mild breathlessness is recommended, and is unlikely to do harm.

Blood Pressure. Even mild degrees of hypertension are strongly correlated with an increased risk of ischaemic heart disease. Unfortunately it has been difficult to show that treatment of the hypertension reduces this risk, possibly because the damage has already been done by the time it is instituted. Other reasons for treating hypertension are discussed below.

In general, primary prevention is likely to be more effective if modest and practicable measures are aimed at a wide section of the community than if rigorous ones are imposed on a small minority.

SYSTEMIC HYPERTENSION

The measurement of blood pressure has been described on page 128. In Western societies the average systolic and diastolic blood pressures gradually rise with age. Hypertension is defined arbitrarily at levels above generally accepted 'normals', for example 140/90 at the age of 20, 160/95 at the age of 50 and 170/105 at the age of 75. It is recommended that the phase V diastolic pressure be used in defining hypertension. Exercise, anxiety, discomfort and unfamiliar surroundings can all lead to a transient rise in blood pressure, and measurements should be repeated under 'basal' conditions with the patient resting and relaxed until consistent readings are obtained. Patients who have a high blood pressure on first examination which subsequently settles with rest may not require treatment but should be kept under review because they are more likely to develop sustained hypertension as time goes on. According to these criteria, some 15% of the population can be regarded as hypertensive, though only a proportion of these will be diagnosed or receive treatment.

Aetiology. In about 10–15% of cases, hypertension can be shown to be a consequence of a specific disease or abnormality. The most important of these are:

1. Coarctation of the aorta.
2. Renal disease: (a) Parenchymatous e.g. acute and chronic glomerulonephritis, pyelonephritis, analgesic-induced nephropathy,

systemic lupus erythematosus and polyarteritis nodosa; (b) Polycystic kidneys; (c) Renal artery stenosis.

3. Endocrine disorders and hormone therapy: (a) Phaeochromocytoma; (b) Cushing's syndrome, spontaneous and drug induced; (c) Primary aldosteronism (Conn's syndrome); (d) Oral contraception and oestrogen therapy.

4. Pregnancy.

These conditions give an insight into the possible mechanisms by which hypertension may be caused. In phaeochromocytoma, it results from an increased cardiac output and/or a raised peripheral resistance due to excessive catecholamines. Cushing's syndrome and Conn's syndrome are associated with increased sodium retention, and probably an alteration in the reactivity of vascular smooth muscle. Renal causes of hypertension are also often associated with sodium retention, and in many cases with high plasma concentrations of renin, which causes the production of the potent vasoconstrictor agent angiotensin II. The latter stimulates aldosterone release and thus also encourages sodium retention. In sustained hypertension it is often found that the carotid sinus baroreceptors, which help to smooth out fluctuations in blood pressure, become 'reset' to a higher level.

In the majority of patients with hypertension, although some of these mechanisms may be operating, it is not possible to define a specific underlying cause, and they are said to have *essential hypertension*. In 70% of such patients another member of the family is affected. Essential hypertension is especially frequent in some races, particularly American Blacks and Japanese. It is commoner where there is a high salt intake.

Clinical Features. In the majority of patients there are no specific symptoms attributable to hypertension, which is detected on routine examination or because of one of its complications. Acute hypertension occasionally causes headache or polyuria, but these are transient. Similarly, there are few specific physical signs unless the hypertension is severe. Long-standing hypertension leads to left ventricular hypertrophy and may be indicated by a forceful and sustained apical

impulse. Left atrial hypertrophy may accompany that of the left ventricle, and a fourth heart sound may be heard. The aortic second sound may be increased, and there is sometimes a very short aortic early diastolic murmur. Paroxysmal nocturnal dyspnoea and/or crepitations at the lung bases may give evidence of left ventricular failure. The optic fundi provide valuable evidence about the severity and duration of the hypertension.

The three main objectives of clinical examination in a hypertensive patient are to identify any underlying cause, to recognise risk factors for the development of complications and to detect any complications already present.

Patients with phaeochromocytoma sometimes give a history of panic attacks, paroxysmal headaches, or palpitation. A history of recurrent backache or undiagnosed fever is sometimes a clue to chronic pyelonephritis, and specific enquiry should be made about analgesic intake. Apart from oral contraceptives and other steroids, drugs which may cause hypertension include liquorice and carbenoxolone used for peptic ulcer and nonsteroidal anti-inflammatory drugs. Physical examination should detect the delay between radial and femoral pulses characteristic of coarctation of the aorta, and the enlarged kidneys in polycystic disease. The characteristic facies and habitus of Cushing's syndrome may be recognised, and a bruit is sometimes audible over the renal arteries in renal artery stenosis.

It is important to identify risk factors such as smoking, obesity and hyperlipidaemia which may interact with hypertension, particularly in the genesis of ischaemic heart disease.

Complications. The adverse effects of hypertension principally involve the central nervous system, the retina, the heart and the kidneys.

CENTRAL NERVOUS SYSTEM. Stroke resulting from cerebral haemorrhage or from cerebral ischaemia is a common complication of hypertension and a major cause of death in hypertensive patients. Carotid atheroma and transient cerebral ischaemic attacks are more common in hypertensive patients.

Hypertensive encephalopathy is a rare condition characterised by a very high blood pressure and neurological symptoms including transient disturbances of speech or vision, paraesthesiae, disorientation, fits and loss of consciousness. Papilloedema is common. The neurological deficit is usually reversible if the hypertension is properly controlled.

Subarachnoid haemorrhage is more common in hypertensive patients.

RETINA. The eyes are influenced by the effects of hypertension on the retinal vessels, and also provide a 'window' for observing these effects — hypertensive retinopathy (Plate I). In long-standing hypertension of moderate severity the major change is a thickening of the walls of retinal arterioles, causing the appearance of arterio-venous nipping. With more severe hypertension, retinal haemorrhages are seen, and are usually flame shaped. Retinal infarction from the occlusion of small arterioles produces soft (cotton wool) exudates (Plate I). Soft exudates fade in a few weeks, but hard exudates are small white dense deposits of lipid which may persist for years. Papilloedema indicates the most advanced stage of hypertension. In the early stages there is little effect on visual acuity, but extensive exudates or haemorrhages can cause visual field defects, or blindness if the macula is affected.

HEART. Hypertension is a major risk factor of ischaemic heart disease, and myocardial infarction is a common cause of death. Hypertension also contributes to the pathogenesis of aortic aneurysm and acute aortic dissection. The heart initially responds to hypertension with left ventricular hypertrophy (Fig. 7.31), and angina may be precipitated if there is concomitant coronary disease. Subsequently, the persistently high afterload may lead to left ventricular failure.

KIDNEYS. In addition to being a cause, renal disease may also be a result of hypertensive damage to the renal vessels. Long-standing hypertension may cause proteinuria and progressive renal failure. Sometimes, renal damage resulting from hypertension produces an increased release of renin, and a vicious circle may be set up with worsening renal failure and very severe hypertension. This is sometimes called *accelerated phase* (or *malignant*) *hypertension*, and has a bad prognosis unless the cycle is interrupted.

Investigation of the hypertensive patient has the same basic objectives as the clinical examination, but because hypertension is so common it is prudent to be selective in the use of resources. Some investigations need to be done on all patients, while others can be reserved for those with specific features of a particular condition or who are refractory to the initial treatment. The most basic investigations are urine analysis for protein (which may indicate renal disease) and sugar (diabetes mellitus may coexist with hypertension and is another important risk factor for vascular disease), and estimation of plasma urea and electrolyte concentrations. The urea or creatinine estimation is a measure of renal excretory function, and the plasma electrolytes may give a clue to the cause of the hypertension. In particular, hypokalaemia and a metabolic alkalosis may indicate hyperaldosteronism, provided diuretic therapy can be excluded as a cause. Plasma cholesterol concentration should be measured in younger patients, and plasma urate concentration is worth estimating because hyperuricaemia is associated with hypertension and gout is liable to be precipitated if diuretics are used for treatment.

A chest radiograph and ECG are not essential but are useful as a baseline in the event of subsequent complications. Screening for phaeochromocytoma is indicated in patients with clinical features of the disease (p. 454) and in other patients whose hypertension is severe or refractory to treatment.

Further investigation of the urinary tract by excretion urography or radionuclide renography is indicated: (1) in patients under the age of 40, (2) in those whose history, clinical examination or baseline investigation suggests renal pathology, and (3) in older patients where difficulty in the control of hypertension or a sudden increase in severity may indicate a renal artery stenosis. Excretion urography provides more information about urinary tract anatomy whereas radionuclide studies give a more direct estimate of renal haemodynamics. Measurement of plasma renin activity is a useful test in suspected renovascular hypertension but care is needed to ensure that samples are taken under proper basal conditions and are not affected by diuretic therapy or salt restriction. Renal arteriography provides the most detailed information about the renal vessels, and it can sometimes be combined with percutaneous balloon dilatation of a renal artery stenosis.

Treatment. The object of treating systemic arterial hypertension is to reduce the risk of complications and to improve patient survival. The benefits of treatment have to be weighed against its inconvenience and the possibility that the agents used may themselves have potentially harmful effects. In most instances, the discovery of hypertension commits the patient to a lifetime of supervision and treatment. It is important to treat the whole patient, and not just the blood pressure. Because of these considerations it is not particularly helpful to set up arbitrary levels of blood pressure at which treatment should be commenced. Decisions about treatment should also take into account the fact that the natural history of hypertension tends to be more benign in women than in men, and that black people and diabetics are more prone to hypertensive complications.

There is general agreement that hypertension should be treated if it is severe (e.g. over 160/100 at age 20, 170/110 in men aged 50) or if it is associated with retinal, cardiac or renal damage. There is less certainty concerning the benefits of treatment in mild or 'borderline' hypertensives, e.g. 140/90 at age 20, 160/95 at age 50. Although a number of clinical trials have been undertaken, they have not always been critically interpreted, and moreover the treatments used have often become obsolescent by the time the trial is complete. The trials which have shown the most consistent benefits of treatment have tended to be those in which the 'treated' group has been subject to close medical supervision, and attention has been paid to the correction of other risk factors. Perhaps it is best to regard borderline hypertensives as an 'at risk' population which requires continuing supervision, redoubled efforts at health education, and judicious intervention as determined by individual circumstances.

There is also controversy concerning the treatment of hypertension in the elderly. On one hand, hypertension sometimes develops quite rapidly in an elderly person, and responds to treatment with gratifying clinical results. On the other hand, elderly patients with long-standing hypertension often respond badly to ill-judged attempts at lowering the pressure. Clinical trials are in progress which may resolve the question, but at present it is best to assess the need for treatment on an individual basis. Rather than attempting to define 'thresholds' of blood pressure requiring treatment in the elderly, it is sensible to rely more on evidence of end-organ damage, or of a recent rise in pressure above previously recorded levels.

NON-DRUG TREATMENT OF HYPERTENSION. *Diet*. Very low sodium diets may reduce blood pressure, but there is little evidence that more socially-acceptable diets will do this consistently. Patients may be advised a 'prudent' mixed diet, and encouraged not to add excess salt at table or eat foods with a high sodium content (p. 363). Hypertensive obese patients often find that their blood pressure improves when they lose weight. There is evidence that excessive alcohol consumption may cause or exacerbate hypertension, and this should be moderated.

Smoking. The effects of cigarette smoking and hypertension on cardiovascular morbidity are additive, and smoking should be discouraged.

Exercise. Regular exercise improves physical fitness and is to be encouraged. Vigorous 'isometric' exercise, e.g. weight lifting, may cause a considerable rise in blood pressure and should be avoided.

Relaxation. It is customary to advise patients to 'avoid stress' but this is usually a pious hope. Spouses should be dissuaded from perpetually reminding patients of their hypertension. Formal relaxation classes, meditation and biofeedback have all been shown to reduce blood pressure in small groups of patients; their efficacy is usually proportional to the enthusiasm of the teacher and the commitment of the participant.

ANTIHYPERTENSIVE DRUG THERAPY. Many patients can be satisfactorily treated with a single antihypertensive drug, the choice of which will be determined by safety, convenience and freedom from side effects. Another large group will require a combination of two or three antihypertensive agents to give good control with a low level of side effects. A small minority will have severe hypertension refractory to conventional treatment and requiring intensive investigation and special treatment.

The principal agents used in single drug treatment of hypertension are thiazide diuretics, beta-adrenoceptor antagonists and methyldopa.

Thiazide diuretics and their adverse effects have

been discussed on page 96. The mechanism of their hypotensive action is incompletely understood, and it may take up to a month for the maximum effect to be observed. More potent diuretics such as frusemide have few advantages over thiazides in the treatment of hypertension unless there is substantial renal impairment, when their greater ability to cause sodium excretion may be useful.

Beta-adrenoceptor antagonists are the most widely used of the sympatholytic agents. In addition to an antihypertensive effect thay may also relieve anxiety, palpitation and angina pectoris. *Propranolol* (p. 170) is effective and reliable, but its dose has to be adjusted to the individual's needs because a large and variable proportion of the drug is destroyed in its first passage through the liver; even with equivalent blood concentrations there is some variation in response. Often twice daily dosage will suffice, but in others high doses may be required, so that treatment initiated in a dose of 40 mg b.d. may have to be increased to as much as 160 mg 6-hourly or more. The slow-release form has the advantage that the patient has to remember only a single daily dose. Many patients have no side effects but minor gastric disturbance, bradycardia, cardiac failure, bronchospasm, tiredness, bad dreams, hallucinations, cold hands and, occasionally, muscle weakness are all recognised complications.

Metoprolol and *atenolol* are appropriate if a cardioselective drug is indicated, as in patients who have airways obstruction, peripheral vascular disease or insulin dependent diabetes. Cardioselective drugs have a greater effect on the cardiac (β_1) receptors than on the β_2 receptors which subserve bronchodilatation and vasodilatation. They also delay less the return of the blood sugar to normal after hypoglycaemia.

Metabolic side effects of beta-blocking drugs include a tendency to increase plasma concentrations of cholesterol in low density lipoproteins, which could in theory have a deleterious effect on the progression of atheroma, and a tendency for nonselective beta-blockers to cause a rise in plasma potassium concentration, particularly after exercise.

Methyldopa probably works mainly through the central nervous system, causing a reduction in peripheral resistance by relaxing vasomotor tone. In divided doses up to 1 g daily, side effects are few, but they become more obvious as the dose is increased and a total daily dose of 2 g is rarely exceeded. The main central side effects are drowsiness, mental sluggishness and occasionally a depressive psychosis. The main peripheral side effect is postural hypotension. Up to 10% of patients develop a positive Coombs test, but haemolytic anaemia is rare (p. 25).

Labetalol, Prazosin and *Calcium Channel Blockers.* The acknowledged shortcomings of presently-available anti-hypertensive drugs continues to encourage the introduction of new ones. It has to be remembered that absence of reported side effects with a given drug may simply reflect limited clinical experience. Other drugs which are candidates for first-line use as anti-hypertensive agents include (i) *labetalol*, which is a combined alpha and beta adrenoceptor antagonist; (ii) *prazosin*, which is a peripheral vasodilator that also blocks alpha-adrenoceptors; and (iii) the calcium-channel blockers, *nifedipine* and *verapamil*. Prazosin in a few cases causes dramatic hypotension when first given and therefore has to be instituted in a small dose (0·5 mg t.i.d. for about 3 days) with due warning to the patient. The maintenance dose is 5–20 mg per day in divided doses.

Drug Combinations. Another approach to the problem of side effects is to use drug combinations — most commonly a thiazide diuretic together with a beta-blocker. This may allow control of hypertension refractory to either drug alone at doses insufficient to cause serious side effects. In some respects the drugs have complementary actions; thiazides increase renin production while beta-blockers depress it, and the hypokalaemic effect of thiazides may be countered by the hyperkalaemic effect of a nonselective beta-blocker. On the other hand the complexity of combination therapy may discourage compliance and the risk of side effects unrelated to the dose of drug is increased. A number of beta-blocker/thiazide combination tablets have been marketed, but the proportion of the two drugs is not necessarily optimal for every patient.

If satisfactory hypertensive control (usually defined as a phase 5 diastolic pressure of 90 or less) cannot be achieved with a beta-blocker and thiazide combination, a third drug may be added — usually a peripheral vasodilator such as prazosin or hydralazine. *Hydralazine* is rarely used alone as it tends to cause a tachycardia. The usual dose of hydralazine is 50–200 mg daily in divided doses. It is sometimes the cause of an allergic vasculitis or a syndrome resembling S.L.E. (p. 574).

Minoxidil and Captopril. These drugs are very effective in treating hypertension, but are at present reserved for more severe cases. Minoxidil is a peripheral vasodilator which is usually used in conjunction with a diuretic. It causes an increased growth of downy facial hair, which restricts its use in females.

Captopril is an inhibitor of angiotensin converting enzyme, which converts angiotensin I into the much more potent vasoconstrictor angiotensin II. It is a very effective antihypertensive agent, particularly in patients with renovascular hypertension. Care is needed in sodium depleted patients, as under these conditions captopril can cause a precipitate fall in blood pressure. Captopril sometimes causes a loss of taste sensation, a side effect it shares with the related compound penicillamine which may also cause renal damage and other adverse effects (p. 560). To date there have been no substantiated reports of similar problems with captopril, but more experience is needed before its widespread use in less severe grades of hypertension can be recommended.

The Emergency Treatment of Hypertension. It is virtually never necessary or desirable to cause an instantaneous fall in blood pressure. Even in the presence of cardiac failure or hypertensive encephalopathy a controlled reduction over a period of 30–60 minutes to a level of about 150/90 is adequate, and there is often less urgency. Too rapid a fall in pressure may cause permanent cerebral ischaemic damage, including blindness, and may sometimes precipitate coronary or renal insufficiency. The most effective agent for blood pressure reduction in an emergency is a controlled intravenous infusion of sodium nitroprusside, but this requires very careful supervision, preferably in an intensive care unit. Alternatives are intravenous or intramuscular labetalol (2 mg/min to a maximum of 200 mg) or intramuscular hydralazine (5 or 10 mg aliquots

repeated at half hourly intervals and titrated against the blood pressure response). Bed rest, sedation and a diuretic are also helpful.

Urinary output and plasma electrolytes should be monitored, and urgent enquiry made into the cause of the hypertension. Hypertensive emergencies in young patients may result from acute glomerulonephritis or from acute on chronic renal failure. The latter is also an important cause in older patients, but these are also likely to suffer from acute renal ischaemia caused by atheroma or embolism. The possibility of phaeochromocytoma should also be considered.

Refractory Hypertension. The common causes of treatment failure in hypertension are non-compliance with drug therapy, inadequate therapy, and failure to recognise an underlying cause such as renal artery stenosis or phaeochromocytoma; of these the first is by far the most prevalent. There is no easy solution to compliance problems, but a simple treatment regime, attempts to improve rapport with the patient, and careful supervision may all help.

DISEASES OF THE PULMONARY CIRCULATION

Pulmonary Arterial Hypertension

The principal cause of severe pulmonary hypertension in adults is a temporary or permanent increase in pulmonary vascular resistance. In infancy another important cause is an increased pulmonary blood flow resulting from left to right shunting, as in atrial and ventricular septal defects and in persistent ductus arteriosus. While this is initially reversible when the shunt is corrected, prolonged exposure of a child's lungs to pulmonary hypertension causes irreversible vascular damage, and a rise in pulmonary vascular resistance perpetuates the hypertension.

Pulmonary hypertension developing in adult life may be due to a reflex increase in pulmonary vascular resistance in response to a rise in pulmonary capillary pressure; to pulmonary vasoconstriction as a response to alveolar hypoxia or arterial hypoxaemia; to thromboembolic obliteration of the pulmonary vascular bed, or to a variety of disease processes directly affecting the pulmonary vessels. Any cause of left sided cardiac failure may produce pulmonary hypertension, but it is most prominent when there has been a very gradual rise in left atrial pressure, as in some cases of mitral stenosis. The combined burden of a raised left atrial pressure and an increased pulmonary vascular resistance may produce secondary right heart failure. Provided the left-sided failure is relieved, e.g by mitral valvotomy, the pulmonary hypertension will usually regress.

Pulmonary vasoconstriction in response to hypoxia is to some extent a protective reflex, which will divert blood flow away from poorly ventilated alveoli. It may be responsible however for the chronic pulmonary hypertension seen in some people who live at high altitude, and for the pulmonary hypertension and right heart failure associated with chronic alveolar hypoventilation. Another important cause of right heart failure in association with chronic lung disease (*cor pulmonale*) is a rise in pulmonary vascular resistance as the result of loss of pulmonary vessels in destructive lung diseases such as emphysema. Pulmonary thromboembolism is particularly important and is considered in the next section. Pulmonary vessels can be affected by connective tissue diseases such as systemic sclerosis, or by drugs such as fenfluramine.

In primary pulmonary hypertension the underlying cause is obscure. This is a rare disease most common in young women, and there is sometimes a family history.

Clinical Features. There may be a left parasternal impulse either from right ventricular hypertrophy, or from an enlarged pulmonary artery, or both. If there is accompanying right atrial hypertrophy a large *a* wave is to be expected in the jugular venous pulse. There may be an ejection sound and a loud second heart sound over the pulmonary valve, and pulmonary regurgitation may produce a soft early diastolic murmur. Associated conditions such as left sided cardiac failure or chronic lung disease may also produce their own clinical features.

Investigation. The ECG usually shows evidence of right atrial and right ventricular hypertrophy. The chest radiograph may show enlargement of the pulmonary artery and its main branches. Echocardiography is important to ex-

clude left sided obstructive lesions such as 'silent' mitral stenosis, and radionuclide lung scanning may suggest pulmonary embolism. Pulmonary arteriography and lung biopsy have a role in a few selected cases.

Treatment is basically that of the underlying cause. Prognosis is fairly good if the hypertension is due to correctable left heart failure, treatable hypoxia or to drugs which can be withdrawn; the outlook is poor if the cause is advanced lung disease or thromboembolism. Primary pulmonary hypertension generally has a poor prognosis; vasodilators have been tried but with inconsistent results. Very occasionally, spontaneous recovery has been reported.

Pulmonary Embolism and Infarction

Pulmonary embolism occurs when a portion of thrombus in a systemic vein, or less commonly the right side of the heart, is discharged into the circulation. It may lodge in the main pulmonary artery and cause sudden death, or in a smaller pulmonary artery and result in pulmonary infarction. Recurrent 'silent' pulmonary embolism may come to light only when pulmonary hypertension and chronic right heart failure develop.

Aetiology. Thrombosis in a pelvic vein or a deep vein of the legs (p. 200) is the most frequent source. As this is usually the result of stasis, pulmonary embolism most often affects people who have been confined to bed. It is particularly liable to occur within 10 days after a surgical operation or after childbirth. A long journey in an aircraft or car can cause thrombosis in a leg vein. The presence of phlebothrombosis is frequently not recognised until after the embolism.

In less than 10% of cases thrombi responsible for pulmonary embolism form in the right atrium in patients with atrial fibrillation, especially if cardiac failure is present.

Clinical Features. Massive pulmonary embolism has been described on page 149. In cases of lesser severity, symptoms and signs may be absent or there may be transient dyspnoea, tachycardia or syncope. In *pulmonary infarction*, which is usually due to a small peripheral embolus, the usual signs are pleural pain which may be severe, and haemoptysis which may be profuse and repetitive. There may be dyspnoea, tachycardia, central cyanosis, pyrexia and polymorphonuclear leucocytosis. Secondary infection may occur. Often, pulmonary infarction produces no symptoms.

Investigation. RADIOLOGICAL EXAMINATION. In massive pulmonary embolism the lung fields often appear normal but sometimes there is a hilar opacity from the blocked vessel and ischaemia distal to the embolus causes a reduction in the usual vascular markings of a lung or lobe. Pulmonary angiography is the most reliable method of diagnosis, but should not be allowed to delay urgent treatment.

In pulmonary infarction there may be a pulmonary opacity due to a recent infarct or a linear scar from an earlier one. A small pleural effusion is common (p. 271). The ipsilateral hemidiaphragm may be elevated. These radiological abnormalities are usually most marked at the base of one lung but are often bilateral.

Venous thrombosis can be demonstrated by bilateral ascending phlebography.

RADIONUCLIDE SCANNING. The intravenous injection of radionuclide-labelled macroaggregated albumin can be used to delineate underperfused areas of lung not detected on a plain radiograph. This technique is of value in the diagnosis of pulmonary embolism, especially if combined with ventilation scanning following the inhalation of a radionuclide labelled gas. Radionuclide lung scans may be difficult to interpret if the chest radiograph is abnormal.

ELECTROCARDIOGRAPHY may show evidence of right ventricular dilatation and strain in cases of massive pulmonary embolism, (right axis deviation, T wave inversion in the right ventricular leads and displacement of the interventricular septum to the left), or the pattern of incomplete right bundle branch block (Fig. 7.27). In cases of lesser severity the ECG is usually normal, except for a sinus tachycardia.

Course and Prognosis. Massive pulmonary embolism is frequently fatal. Minor and medium sized emboli are much less dangerous, but may herald subsequent massive embolism. Recurrent emboli may cause pulmonary hypertension and right ventricular failure. The vast majority of pulmonary infarcts resolve completely. Occasionally an infarct may become secondarily infected and result in a lung abscess.

Treatment. Intravenous heparin should be injected immediately and a heparin infusion continued for 3 days (p. 547). Thereafter oral anticoagulants should be given to prevent further venous thrombosis (p. 548). Depending on the circumstances such treatment should be continued for 6 weeks to 6 months. Pain and apprehension should be allayed but morphine must be avoided if there is severe hypotension. Oxygen should be administered if central cyanosis is present.

Massive pulmonary embolism is best managed in an area where intensive care can be provided. If there is no detectable cardiac output, cardiac massage may sometimes help by fragmenting a thrombus in the pulmonary artery. Vasodilators are contraindicated and a high venous pressure should be maintained. Pulmonary embolectomy under cardiopulmonary bypass may be life-saving, but often takes too long to organise to be helpful to those most in need of it. Thrombolytic therapy with streptokinase or urokinase produces more rapid angiographic resolution of thrombus, but its ability to improve survival has been less convincing. Heparin and oxygen therapy should not be neglected while these measures are being considered.

Prevention of pulmonary embolism and infarction consists of those measures directed at prophylaxis against venous thrombosis in the legs (p. 200). In cases of recurrent pulmonary embolism despite anticoagulation, venous interruption may be necessary either by inserting a filter into, or plicating, the inferior vena cava.

DISEASES OF THE MYOCARDIUM

The myocardium is involved in most types of heart disease, but the terms myocarditis and cardiomyopathy tend to be used, not always consistently, for diseases which primarily affect the heart muscle rather than the heart valves or coronary arteries. Myocarditis implies an inflammatory process; this is true of rheumatic myocarditis and many types of viral myocarditis, but diphtheritic myocarditis is due to a toxin, and sarcoid heart disease and that associated with systemic lupus erythematosus have in the past been classed as cardiomyopathies. An international commission has now recommended that the term cardiomyopathy should be confined to forms of chronic myocardial disease without a known cause, and that where a cause is known the term (specific) heart disease, e.g. sarcoid heart disease, should be used instead. In practice, myocarditis usually means an acute and potentially reversible illness affecting heart muscle, and it is convenient to consider together the chronic diseases, namely the cardiomyopathies and the specific conditions which often closely resemble them in their clinical presentation.

Acute Myocarditis

Acute myocarditis may occur as a complication of infections such as diphtheria, pneumonia, typhoid fever, scrub typhus fever and meningitis. Chagas' disease (American trypanosomiasis, p. 780) is the commonest cause in South America. Myocarditis may also be due to viral infection such as in influenza, poliomyelitis, infectious mononucleosis and, particularly, Coxsackie B infections. Rheumatic myocarditis is described on page 156.

Often the only evidence of myocarditis is a sinus tachycardia which is out of proportion to the severity of the infection. In more severe cases there may be a third heart sound, arrhythmias, conduction defects or acute cardiac failure. Prognosis in most types of acute myocarditis is usually good, but it may cause death in diphtheria. In Chagas' disease, the patient usually recovers from the acute phase and after a latent period of 10 or 20 years a chronic cardiomyopathy develops which is eventually fatal.

There is no specific therapy for acute myocarditis; the usual forms of treatment for cardiac failure and arrhythmias should be undertaken. Corticosteroids have been tried, but are of no proven value. Prolonged rest is sometimes necessary.

Specific Diseases of Heart Muscle and Cardiomyopathy

Damage to cardiac muscle is part of a number of systemic disorders such as haemochromatosis, sarcoidosis, amyloidosis, systemic lupus erythematosus, systemic sclerosis and polyarteritis nodosa. There are often, but not invariably, extracardiac clues to the diagnosis in these conditions. Heart muscle damage may also be associated with a variety of toxins, of which the most important is alcohol.

In the cardiomyopathies there is no generalised disorder and frequently no aetiological agent can be found, although in a proportion of such cases there is a family history. Sometimes there is a definite or suspected history of myocarditis. Cardiomyopathies are classified into three groups: dilated; hypertrophic; and restrictive or obliterative. Clinically, most cases of heart muscle disease for which a specific cause is known resemble one or other of these varieties.

Dilated cardiomyopathy is characterised by left and right ventricular dilatation, impaired ventricular contraction with a reduced ventricular ejection fraction (p. 152), and often mitral and/or tricuspid regurgitation. The ventricular end-diastolic pressure is elevated, and the clinical picture is one of progressive left sided and, later, right sided cardiac failure. The ECG usually shows nonspecific changes, but may show the changes of left ventricular hypertrophy. Arrhythmias are common. Echocardiography is useful in making the diagnosis. It is this form of cardiomyopathy which specific heart muscle disease most often resembles, and a similar picture is sometimes seen in advanced ischaemic heart disease.

The treatment of dilated cardiomyopathy is directed at the associated cardiac failure; specific treatment is possible only when there is a recognisable cause. The prognosis is usually poor, particularly when there is no known aetiology.

Hypertrophic cardiomyopathy is often familial. A similar condition is associated with the hereditary neurological disorder Friedreich's ataxia.

Hypertrophic cardiomyopathy is characterised by increased thickness of the ventricular wall; this may be generalised or may principally affect the interventricular septum. If asymmetrical septal hypertrophy is present, it may cause left ventricular outflow obstruction, but this is not essential to the diagnosis. In many cases the diagnosis is made only at autopsy following sudden death in a young person. In others, the condition may present with syncopal episodes or with angina.

On examination, there is usually palpable left ventricular hypertrophy, and there may be an apical double impulse reflecting also atrial hypertrophy. On auscultation there is commonly a midsystolic murmur over the left ventricular outflow, and there may be associated mitral regurgitation. The pulse is characteristically 'jerky' and not slow-rising. The ECG usually shows left ventricular hypertrophy; there may be bizarre T wave abnormalities and an inferior myocardial infarct may be mimicked. Echocardiography is usually diagnostic.

The natural history is variable. Sometimes patients who present with hypertrophic cardiomyopathy gradually develop features of a dilated cardiomyopathy over the course of some years. The prognosis may be better in those who have the condition discovered incidentally in adult life than in those who present with symptoms in childhood or adolescence.

No treatment is definitely known to improve prognosis, but propranolol helps to relieve angina and sometimes prevents syncopal attacks, particularly in those with ventricular outflow obstruction. Arrhythmias are common, and amiodarone is useful in their control. Digoxin and vasodilators may increase outflow obstruction and should be used with caution.

Restrictive or obliterative cardiomyopathy is characterised by an increased ventricular 'stiffness' effectively causing ventricular inflow obstruction. It is found with endomyocardial fibrosis in the tropics (p. 716) and with endocardial eosinophilia. Amyloidosis of the heart can produce a similar picture. Diagnosis can be very difficult, especially where the condition is uncommon. The combination of severe left or right heart failure with a normal heart size and no murmurs is suggestive. Endocardial biopsy may be diagnostic. Treatment is usually symptomatic, but successful excision of fibrotic endocardium has been reported.

DISEASES OF THE PERICARDIUM

Pericarditis

The most common identifiable causes of acute pericarditis in Britain are myocardial infarction and viral infections, e.g. with coxsackie B viruses. Rheumatic fever and tuberculosis are also important, but are now rare in Britain. Pericarditis may occur as a complication of bacterial infection and of malignant disease. Other causes include uraemia, trauma and connective tissue disorders such as systemic lupus erythematosus. In many cases of pericarditis it is not possible to identify a cause, and these are referred to as 'idiopathic'.

Pathology. Pericarditis may be fibrinous, serous, haemorrhagic or purulent. In the first there is a fibrinous exudate on the surface which may eventually lead to varying degrees of adhesion formation. In serous pericarditis there is in addition an exudate of anything from a few millilitres to a litre or more. The effusion is straw-coloured and often slightly turbid with a high protein content. A haemorrhagic effusion suggests a malignant origin. Purulent pericarditis is due to a pyogenic infection.

Clinical Features. The characteristic pain of pericarditis is retrosternal and often radiates to the shoulders and neck. It may be present on, or made worse by, a deep breath, movement, change of position, exercise or swallowing.

A friction rub is the diagnostic sign of pericarditis. It consists of a superficial scratching sound, best heard to the left of the lower sternum; it is usually systolic but may be audible also in diastole. It frequently has a 'to and fro' quality. Friction is often better heard when the stethoscope diaphragm is pressed firmly upon the chest, the patient's breath being held for a time in inspiration and then in expiration. If a pericardial effusion develops there is sometimes a sensation of retrosternal oppression. An effusion may be difficult to detect clinically — the heart sounds may become quieter, but pericardial friction is not always abolished.

CARDIAC TAMPONADE refers to compression of the heart by a large or rapidly developing effusion which interferes with diastolic filling. The amount of fluid which is needed to produce tamponade depends in part on the compliance of the pericardium, and is variable. In the presence of tamponade, jugular venous pressure rises and cardiac output falls. Pulsus paradoxus (p. 124) may be found, and urine output is suppressed.

The clinical picture of acute circulatory failure may develop. Pulmonary oedema is unusual but not unknown. Atypical presentations may occur when the effusion is loculated as a result of previous pericarditis or cardiac surgery.

The ECG in acute pericarditis shows ST elevation with upward concavity over the affected area, which may be widespread. Later, there may be T wave inversion. QRS voltage is often reduced in the presence of an effusion. Serial radiographs may show a rapid increase in the size of the cardiac shadow over days or even hours, and with a large effusion the heart may have a pear shaped appearance. Echocardiography is particularly useful in detecting pericardial effusion.

Treatment. The pain can usually be relieved by aspirin, but a more potent anti-inflammatory agent such as indomethacin may be required. Paracentesis of a pericardial effusion may be indicated for diagnostic purposes or to relieve symptoms from cardiac tamponade. Either of two approaches may be used depending on the experience of the operator and the configuration of the patient:

1. The needle is inserted to the left of the xiphoid process, insinuated deep to the left costal margin, and then directed towards the left shoulder.

2. The needle is inserted medial to the cardiac apex at a point where echocardiography reveals the presence of a layer of fluid lying in front of the heart.

For diagnostic purposes it is usually enough to withdraw a few millilitres of fluid. If therapeutic drainage is needed it may be safer to use a plastic cannula inserted over a needle or guidewire than to attempt aspiration of the whole effusion through a rigid needle. A viscous or loculated effusion may require surgical drainage. The main dangers of pericardiocentesis are arrhythmia, damage to a coronary artery, and exacerbation of tamponade as a result of injury to the right ventricle. It is however life saving in the presence of severe tamponade.

Viral, Tuberculous and Purulent Pericarditis

Viral pericarditis may follow an upper respiratory infection, and in about 10% of cases a Coxsackie infection can be established. Recovery usually occurs within a few days or weeks, but there may be recurrences. There is no specific treatment; corticosteroids may help suppress symptoms but there is little evidence they accelerate cure.

Tuberculous pericarditis may be secondary to manifest pulmonary or mediastinal tuberculosis, but the primary source may not be detectable. The disease sometimes begins with an acute febrile illness but is more commonly insidious in onset with vague malaise and low grade fever. The subsequent course is chronic. An effusion usually develops and the pericardium may become thick and unyielding so that the heart is compressed. Pleural effusions are often associated.

The diagnosis may be confirmed by aspiration of the fluid and direct examination or culture for tubercle bacilli. Antituberculous chemotherapy is prescribed (p. 236). Corticosteroids may help to prevent the development of constrictive pericarditis. Pericardial aspiration may be carried out as required to relieve symptoms. In the inactive stage surgical relief may be necessary.

Purulent pericarditis is rare. It occurs as a complication of septicaemia, by direct spread from an intrathoracic infection, or from a penetrating injury. Treatment is by antimicrobial therapy and if necessary surgical drainage.

Chronic Pericardial Constriction

Tuberculosis was formerly a frequent cause. Some cases accompany rheumatoid arthritis and others follow a haemopericardium or, rarely, acute pericarditis. Often the cause is obscure. A slowly progressive fibrosis of the pericardium develops and constricts the movement of the heart, so that it cannot expand in diastole. The fibrous tissue is dense and inelastic and calcification is common. The inflow to the heart is impeded, so that cardiac output is diminished and systemic venous pressure raised, with hepatic congestion, ascites and oedema.

Clinical Features. Breathlessness is not a prominent symptom as the lungs are seldom congested. A raised jugular venous pressure is usually present, with a rapid and transitory y descent (Fig. 7.1). The jugular pressure may rise on inspiration. The arterial pulse tends to be rapid, of small volume, and pulsus paradoxus may be present. Enlargement of the liver and ascites occur relatively early compared with peripheral oedema. Cardiac enlargement is usually absent both clinically and radiologically. Chest radiography may show pericardial calcification, which is sometimes better seen in the lateral view. The main differential diagnosis is from restrictive cardiomyopathy.

Treatment. The problem is primarily a mechanical one, and rapid improvement is usual if surgical resection of the pericardium is performed. However, it may take several months for maximum benefit to be obtained.

CONGENITAL HEART DISEASE

The incidence of haemodynamically-significant congenital cardiac abnormalities is about 1% of live births. In most cases the cause of the abnormality is unknown, but some fetal defects are due to maternal infections in the early weeks of pregnancy, e.g. rubella. All degrees of severity occur. Many defects are not compatible with extrauterine life, or only for a short time. Early diagnosis is important because most types are amenable to surgical treatment, but this opportunity may be lost if secondary changes, for example the development of pulmonary vascular damage, are allowed to occur.

Symptoms may be absent, or the child may be noticed to be breathless, or may fail to thrive and grow normally. In many instances the symptoms and signs of the cardiac lesion become apparent only some time after birth. Local signs vary with the anatomical lesion.

Central cyanosis occurs when desaturated blood enters the systemic circulation without passing through the lungs (i.e. there is a right to left shunt). In the neonate the commonest cause of this is transposition of the great arteries, in which the aorta derives from the right ventricle and the pulmonary artery from the left. In older children cyanosis is usually the consequence of a ventricular septal defect combined with severe pulmonary stenosis (tetralogy of Fallot, p. 193) or with pulmonary vascular disease (Eisenmenger's syndrome, p. 193).

Persistent Ductus Arteriosus

During fetal life, before the lungs begin to function, most of the blood from the pulmonary artery passes through the ductus arteriosus into the aorta just below the origin of the left subclavian artery. Normally the ductus closes soon after birth but sometimes it fails to do so. Since the pressure in the aorta is higher than that in the pulmonary artery there will be a continuous arteriovenous shunt, the volume of which depends on the size of the ductus. As much as 50% of the left ventricular output may be recirculated through the lungs, with a consequent increase in the work of the heart. The condition, which may be associated with other abnormalities, is much commoner in females.

With small shunts there may be no symptoms for years but, if the ductus is large, growth and development are retarded. There is usually no disability, but cardiac failure may eventually ensue, dyspnoea being the first symptom. A continuous 'machinery' murmur is heard with late systolic accentuation, maximal at the second left rib near the sternum (Fig. 7.39). It is frequently accompanied by a thrill. Enlargement of the pulmonary artery may be detected radiologically. The ECG is usually normal.

A large left to right shunt in infancy may cause a considerable rise in pulmonary artery pressure, and sometimes this leads to progressive pulmonary vascular damage. With the resulting rise in pulmonary vascular resistance, pulmonary artery pressure rises further until it equals or exceeds aortic pressure. The shunt through the defect may then reverse, causing central cyanosis; with a persistent ductus arteriosus this cyanosis may be more apparent in the feet and toes than in the upper part of the body. The murmur becomes quieter, may be confined to systole, or may disappear. The ECG shows evidence of right ventricular hypertrophy.

In uncomplicated cases the ductus can be divided with little risk, especially in children, and there is general agreement that this should be advised in all cases to remove the risk of endocarditis and of subsequent cardiac failure in adult life. Operation is contraindicated when the pulmonary vascular resistance is elevated and the shunt has become reversed.

Fig. 7.39 Persistent ductus arteriosus.

Coarctation of the Aorta

Narrowing of the aorta most commonly occurs in the region where the ductus arteriosus joins the aorta, i.e. just below the origin of the left subclavian artery (Fig. 7.40). The condition is more common in males, and is sometimes associated with other abnormalities, of which the most frequent is a bicuspid aortic valve. Acquired coarctation of the aorta is rare; it may follow trauma, or be a complication of a progressive arteritis (Takayasu disease, p. 199).

Aortic coarctation is an important cause of cardiac failure in the newborn, but symptoms are often absent in older children or adults. Headaches and cardiac symptoms may occur from hypertension in the upper part of the body, and occasionally weakness or cramps in the legs may result from decreased circulation in the lower part of the body. The blood pressure is raised in the arms but normal or low in the legs. Unduly large arterial pulsations may be seen in the neck. The femoral pulses are weak, and delayed after the radial. A systolic murmur may sometimes be heard over the coarctation posteriorly. There may also be an ejection systolic murmur in the aortic

Fig. 7.40 Coarctation of the aorta.

area. Evidence of a collateral circulation may be detectable in older children and adults in the form of visible or palpable dilated and tortuous arteries around the scapulae and below the ribs posteriorly.

Radiological examination in early childhood is often normal but at a later age may show changes

HARSH . NOT LOUD

1   A2   P2

RESEMBLES A
SYSTOLIC MURMUR

A.S.D.

ENLARGED
PULMONARY
ARTERY

PULMONARY
VALVE

T.V.

Fig. 7.41 Atrial septal defect.

in the contour of the aorta and notching of the undersurfaces of the ribs from tortuous loops of enlarged intercostal arteries. The ECG may show left ventricular hypertrophy.

In untreated severe cases, death may occur from left ventricular failure, dissection of the aorta or cerebral haemorrhage. Surgical correction is advisable in all but the mildest cases. If this is done early enough in childhood the risk of persistent hypertension may be avoided, but patients operated on in late childhood or adult life often remain hypertensive or become hypertensive again after an interval. Coexistent aortic valve disease is another reason for long-term follow-up.

Atrial Septal Defect

Atrial septal defect is more common in females. Since the normal right ventricle is much more compliant than the left, a large volume of blood shunts through the defect from the left to right atrium and thence to the right ventricle and pulmonary arteries (Fig. 7.41). As a result there is gradual enlargement of the right side of the heart and of the pulmonary artery and its main branches. Pulmonary hypertension and shunt re-versal sometimes complicate atrial septal defect, but are less common and tend to occur later in life than with other types of left to right shunt.

There may be no symptoms for many years and the condition is often detected after a routine chest radiograph. Dyspnoea, cardiac failure and arrhythmias such as atrial fibrillation are other possible modes of presentation. The characteristic physical signs are: (1) wide fixed splitting of the second heart sound — wide because of delay in right ventricular ejection, fixed because the septal defect equalises left and right atrial pressures throughout the respiratory cycle; and (2) a systolic flow murmur over the pulmonary valve. In children with a large shunt there may be a diastolic flow murmur over the tricuspid valve; unlike a mitral flow murmur, this is usually high-pitched.

The chest radiograph shows enlargement of the heart and of the pulmonary artery; increased pulsation of these vessels can be seen on screening. The ECG usually shows incomplete right bundle branch block because right ventricular depolarisation is delayed as a result of ventricular dilatation. Echocardiography is very useful, and two-dimensional echocardiography may directly demonstrate the defect.

Atrial septal defects large enough to be clinically recognisable should be closed surgically, and the long-term prognosis thereafter is excellent. Pulmonary hypertension and shunt reversal are contraindications to surgery.

Ventricular Septal Defect

The clinical features of ventricular septal defect depend on the size of the defect and the age of the patient. At birth, there may be little shunting through a large defect because fetal pulmonary vascular resistance and right ventricular pressure are high and may fall only gradually in the first few days of life. As right ventricular pressure falls, the left to right shunt increases, and children with a large ventricular septal defect commonly develop heart failure between 3 and 6 weeks of age. Following this, the defect may spontaneously diminish in size, or the pulmonary vascular resistance may increase, reducing the shunt at the price of progressive pulmonary vascular damage and eventually shunt reversal. Most patients seen with a congenital ventricular septal defect in late childhood or adult life therefore have either a small defect with a small or moderate left to right shunt or a large defect with shunt reversal. The latter is sometimes called Eisenmenger's syndrome (p. 193).

Small ventricular septal defects are characterised clinically by a harsh pansystolic murmur, often accompanied by a thrill, best heard in the fourth intercostal space to the left of the sternum. Symptoms are absent, and the chest radiograph and ECG are normal. The loudness of the murmur often seems out of keeping with the absence of other signs (Fig. 7.42). The natural history of this type of defect is usually benign, but there is a risk of infective endocarditis. Surgical closure is rarely justified unless there are complications, and many defects probably close spontaneously.

Large Ventricular Septal Defects with Left to Right Shunt. For reasons already given, this combination is usually seen in infants, or in adults as a complication of myocardial infarction with secondary rupture of the ventricular septum. A systolic murmur is usual, but its loudness is not a good indicator of the size of the shunt. There is often a mid-diastolic mitral flow murmur.

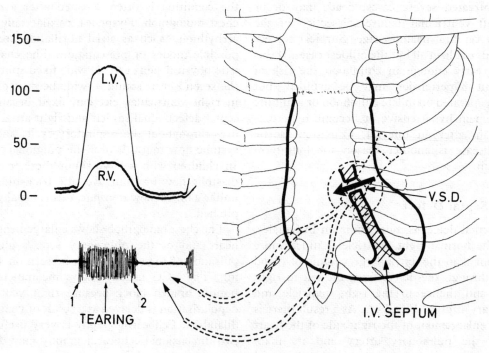

Fig. 7.42 Ventricular septal defect.

The chest radiograph shows an enlarged heart and dilatation of the pulmonary vessels. The ECG may show both right and left ventricular hypertrophy or dilatation. Cardiac catheterisation is often required to confirm the diagnosis and measure the pulmonary vascular resistance.

Cardiac failure is treated in the usual way with digoxin and diuretics, but inability to control the failure or evidence of increasing pulmonary vascular resistance are indications for early surgery. In adults with post-infarction septal defects the prognosis is poor but early investigation and surgery may be life saving.

Eisenmenger's Syndrome. This term is used for patients with pulmonary hypertension and a reversed (right to left) shunt associated with a ventricular or atrial septal defect or with a persistent ductus arteriosus. For practical purposes the management and prognosis of patients with a raised pulmonary vascular resistance, pulmonary hypertension and reversed shunting is the same whatever the site of the shunt. By this stage the time for surgery is past, and closure of the defect simply hastens death from right heart failure.

These patients usually present in childhood or early adolescence with effort intolerance or failure to thrive. Frequent respiratory infections are a common cause of complaint. The patient is centrally cyanosed with finger and toe clubbing. There is usually clinical evidence of right ventricular hypertrophy. Shunt murmurs are usually absent; there may be an early diastolic murmur of pulmonary regurgitation. The chest radiograph may show an enlarged pulmonary artery, but the heart shadow is often not enlarged. Polycythaemia is usual, and if extreme may lead to headache and neurological symptoms. The natural history is one of slow and inexorable decline; in the later stages pulmonary infarction and haemoptysis may occur.

There is no specific treatment. Periodic venesection helps symptomatically but iron deficiency is to be avoided. With the aid of venesection, diuretics and antibiotics more of these patients are reaching early adulthood, but few survive beyond the fourth decade. The prevention of Eisenmengers' syndrome by the detection and correction of large left to right shunts in infancy is an important reason for regular cardiac examination in infants and young children.

Pulmonary Stenosis

Pulmonary stenosis may occur as an isolated anomaly, in which case there is no cyanosis, or in association with an atrial or ventricular septal defect, in which case there may or may not be cyanosis depending on the relative pressures on the two sides of the defect. Stenosis may occur at the level of the pulmonary valve or in the infundibular region of the right ventricle.

Pulmonary Stenosis with Intact Interventricular Septum. Mild congenital pulmonary stenosis is fairly common, asymptomatic and rarely deteriorates. In severe pulmonary stenosis there may be dyspnoea, fatigue, or exertional syncope. The physical signs are discussed on page 164. Guides to the severity of the stenosis include the loudness of the murmur, the width of splitting of the second heart sound, and most importantly the presence of right ventricular hypertrophy on the ECG. Severe pulmonary stenosis, usually associated with a gradient of 60 mmHg or more across the right ventricular outflow tract, is an indication for surgical correction, usually by pulmonary valvotomy.

Pulmonary Stenosis with Ventricular Septal Defect (Fallot's Tetralogy). This is the most common form of cyanotic congenital heart disease in children or adults. The tetralogy comprises pulmonary stenosis, ventricular septal defect, dextroposition of the aorta which overrides this defect, and right ventricular hypertrophy (Fig. 7.43). The stenosis is predominantly in the outflow tract of the right ventricle, but the valve cusps may also be involved.

Cyanosis is usually absent at birth, and gradually develops over the next few weeks or months. In older children dyspnoea and fatigue are the principal symptoms and the child characteristically assumes a squatting position after exercise. Cyanotic spells may occur in infants or children after feeds or exertion; the child becomes deeply cyanosed and flaccid for several seconds, with gradual recovery. The principal signs are central cyanosis with a systolic murmur maximal to the left of the upper sternum. The pulmonary

Fig. 7.43 Fallot's tetralogy. The stenosis is in the infundibulum of the right ventricle.

component of the second heart sound is soft and may be inaudible. The ECG shows right ventricular hypertrophy, and the chest radiograph has a characteristic cardiac contour with absence of the usual pulmonary artery curve. Echocardiography is often diagnostic.

Propranolol may be useful as emergency treatment for cyanotic spells, but the definitive treatment is surgical. In neonates and small infants a palliative operation may be performed by anastomosing one of the subclavian arteries to the pulmonary artery (Blalock-Taussig operation) but in older and larger children it is usual to aim for total correction by closing the ventricular septal defect and resecting the right ventricular outflow obstruction under cardiopulmonary bypass.

SURGERY AND HEART DISEASE

The Surgical Treatment of Heart Disease

Surgery is playing an increasingly important role in the management of heart disease; it is now possible, for example, to correct, to varying degrees, most types of congenital heart disease and to alleviate many cases of rheumatic and ischaemic heart disease. It is not possible, short of cardiac transplantation, to replace cardiac muscle

which has been lost or irretrievably damaged.

Some operations such as mitral valvotomy and the correction of coarctation can be performed under normal circulatory conditions with blood continuing to flow through the heart. Most procedures however require an open or immobile heart, so cardiac function must be taken over by an extracorporeal circulation (cardiopulmonary bypass). With this technique, venous blood is drained from the great veins into a reservoir and is then passed through an oxygenator before being pumped back into the aorta. The heart can then be stopped for some hours though an adequate circulation is maintained to the other vital organs. The mortality of cardiopulmonary bypass should be less than 1%, but patients are nevertheless at risk from several hazards, including air embolism, trauma to the blood from the pump and oxygenator, and electrolyte and acid-base disturbances.

Some surgical procedures requires the use of prosthetic material such as a patch to close an atrial or ventricular septal defect, a tube graft for aortic repair, or an artificial heart valve. To a greater or lesser extent this material is a substrate for the ingrowth of host tissue, and with the exception of mechanical valve prostheses is eventually completely covered with host endothelium. Temporary anticoagulation may help to prevent thrombosis and embolism while this process is taking place. The choice between mechanical valves and heterograft 'tissue' valves is still controversial.

Heart transplantation has recently become a practicable procedure. The principal indication is otherwise intractable cardiac failure usually due to cardiomyopathy in a patient under 50 years of age with a normal pulmonary vascular resistance. The overall 2 year survival is approximately 50%.

It is often necessary to devote considerable effort to the physical and psychological rehabilitation of patients after cardiac surgery, particularly in those who have had a prolonged spell of disability. In contrast, patients who have had coronary artery vein grafts sometimes need reminding that their new freedom from symptoms is unlikely to be maintained unless they make efforts to correct risk factors such as cigarette smoking.

Surgery in Patients with Heart Disease

Patients with heart disease undergoing surgery are at risk from the anaesthetic and from the surgery itself. Skilled anaesthesia is particularly important. Continuous monitoring of the ECG, systemic arterial pressure, central venous pressure or pulmonary artery and pulmonary artery wedge pressure may be advisable in appropriate cases, both during surgery and in the early postoperative period.

On the whole, patients with heart disease tolerate surgery remarkably well. Exceptions to this rule are patients with recent myocardial infarction and those who have cardiac or respiratory failure. Only in exceptional circumstances should patients be operated on within 3 months of myocardial infarction; cardiac and respiratory failure should be brought under control before operation if possible. If heart block is present, a pacemaker should be inserted prior to surgery. Surgical diathermy should be avoided if possible in patients with pacemakers; if it is essential, the diathermy electrodes should be kept as far from the pacemaker as possible.

Hypertension is not usually a contraindication to surgery, but it is necessary for the anaesthetist to be aware of what antihypertensive therapy is being used, as excessive hypotension may result from interactions between antihypertensive drugs and anaesthetic agents.

In some patients it is better to defer surgery until the heart disease has been corrected or ameliorated. Thus, elective general surgery should be deferred until after mitral valvotomy, if this is indicated. On the other hand if the cardiac surgery will necessitate long term anticoagulant therapy it may be better to undertake general surgery first.

HEART DISEASE IN PREGNANCY

Pregnancy leads to increases of blood volume and cardiac output of up to 50%. These changes produce characteristic physical signs. The extremities feel warm and the pulse is of large volume. Tachycardia is present and there may be a rise in venous pressure. The arterial diastolic pressure is lower than in the nonpregnant state because of vasodilatation. The heart may be slightly enlarged and may be displaced outwards because of the high diaphragm. A pulmonary systolic murmur from increased blood flow is common and there may be a physiological third heart sound. Following delivery there is often a transient rise in venous pressure as a consequence of uterine contraction. There is also a period of blood hypercoagulability following delivery.

The increased load on the heart often provokes or worsens symptoms in patients with heart disease. These do not usually occur before about the 12th week, and tend to become maximal from the 24th week onwards. The main symptom of heart disease in pregnancy is breathlessness, but oedema may also occur. It is unusual for angina to present during pregnancy, though patients with pre-existing ischaemic heart disease tend to tolerate pregnancy badly. Symptoms are a poor guide to the severity of the heart disease as some patients are totally asymptomatic until they develop acute pulmonary oedema in late pregnancy or shortly after delivery.

The commonest major form of heart disease encountered in pregnancy is mitral stenosis; other valvular lesions are not uncommon but seldom give rise to problems. Pregnancy should be deferred in patients with severe mitral stenosis, but is usually safe after valvotomy has been performed. If a patient with advanced mitral stenosis does become pregnant either valvotomy or termination should be carried out before the 16th week. With less serious degrees of mitral stenosis and with other forms of heart disease, pregnancy can be allowed to continue and in most cases is uncomplicated. However if objective evidence of deterioration is apparent, bed rest must be enforced, combined if necessary with digoxin and diuretics. With careful management, even those with advanced heart disease can be carried successfully through pregnancy and delivery. Patients with mechanical heart valves who require continuous anticoagulation pose a particular problem during pregnancy because warfarin is capable of causing fetal abnormalities. With care and cooperation it is sometimes possible to maintain heparin anticoagulation throughout pregnancy, but a more satisfactory alternative may be to avoid this type of operation in patients likely to become pregnant.

Patients with congenital heart disease are being seen with increasing frequency during pregnancy, but usually the lesion has been corrected beforehand. In most cases no problems arise but pregnancy is a formidable hazard in those who have pulmonary vascular disease in association with congenital heart disease, and maternal mortality approaches 33% in this group if pregnancy is allowed to go to term.

DISEASES OF ARTERIES AND VEINS

For clinical purposes it is convenient to classify arterial disease under the general headings of degenerative, inflammatory and vasospastic causes.

DEGENERATIVE ARTERIAL DISEASE

Arteriosclerosis is a term which in the past has been applied rather indiscriminately to various unrelated forms of arterial disease. Its retention is justified only if it is confined to the degenerative changes which are part of the usual ageing process and which affect the whole arterial tree.

Medial or Mönckeberg's sclerosis is the name given to degenerative changes which occur in old age in the muscular coats of medium sized arteries such as the radial. Calcification of the media is the characteristic change and accounts for the 'pipe stem' arteries so commonly palpable in the elderly and of little clinical significance. Since the medium and large vessels are mainly affected and their lumina are not greatly reduced in size, clinical features are usually absent.

Atherosclerosis is a condition which principally affects the aorta, large and medium-sized vessels, particularly the coronary and cerebral arteries. It becomes increasingly common as age advances, but it is not an inevitable concomitant of ageing, and there is a great variation in its extent and severity. Although often associated with and accelerated by hypertension, atherosclerosis may be advanced even in the presence of a normal blood pressure. It may also occur in response to a persistent elevation of pressure in the pulmonary arteries.

The basic atheromatous lesion is the plaque, the most important constituents of which are cholesterol and other lipids which may be free in the intimal tissues or intracellular. At a later stage the plaque becomes sclerosed and calcified. Thrombosis is liable to occur on the surface of the plaque, particularly if it ulcerates. Embolism is frequent.

Atherosclerosis Obliterans

This condition affects males more commonly than females and usually after the age of 50. It is particularly common in diabetics and is rare in non-smokers.

Clinical Features. These are usually confined to the lower limbs. The principal symptoms which follow impairment of blood supply to the extremities are (1) pain, which occurs on exercise (intermittent claudication) and (2) cold extremities. Although the pathological changes are usually present in both lower limbs, symptoms commonly present first on one side.

Intermittent claudication appears on walking and is rapidly relieved by rest. It most commonly occurs in the calf and causes the patient to limp or stop. Pain occurs at rest with severe ischaemia. Pain which is relieved by elevation of the part suggests venous obstruction, and pain which is relieved by dependency suggests gross arterial obstruction.

Ischaemia may lead to dryness, scaling and inelasticity of the skin, loss of hair, brittle nails, ulceration or gangrene. There may be a change of colour of the skin and delay in the return of colour after blanching with light finger pressure. Ulceration or gangrene may occur. Where gross lesions are present in one limb, the lower temperature is appreciable to the touch. If the ischaemic limb is first raised 75 degrees above the horizontal, it will blanch more quickly than normal. If then placed in the dependent position, there will be delay in flushing and in venous filling.

Loss of pulsation of one or more peripheral arteries is a common and important feature of arterial disease; bruits may be heard over the larger arteries if they are partially obstructed.

Patients seldom die from peripheral vascular

disease but frequently succumb to myocardial infarction.

Investigation. A radiograph may show calcification. This is especially common in Mönckeberg's sclerosis but does not necessarily indicate that the arterial lumen is significantly narrowed. Ultrasound (Doppler) flow probes are a useful adjunct to clinical examination. Intra-arterial injection of a radio-opaque contrast medium will show the site of vascular occlusion and the extent of any collateral circulation.

Treatment. Until the pathogenesis of atherosclerosis has been clearly established and until specific therapy is discovered the treatment of peripheral vascular disease must continue to be unsatisfactory. Diabetes or obesity may require attention. The patient may need help in getting rid of the tobacco habit.

Cold should be avoided and suitable woollen clothing worn, especially on the limbs. The application of heat to the affected limb is harmful because it increases local metabolism in the ischaemic area without improving blood flow. Pain at rest may be reduced by raising the head of the bed or by lowering the limb below the horizontal and keeping it cool.

Protection against trauma and the early treatment of sepsis are most important. Fungal infection between the toes should be treated. Detailed instructions on the care of the feet and nails must be given. The feet should be kept scrupulously clean, carefully dried after washing, especially between the toes, and dusting powder containing zinc oxide and salicylic acid applied. Nails should be cut carefully and corns pared with caution. It is wise to employ the services of a chiropodist. Socks and shoes should be well fitting. Even the slightest abrasion should be taken seriously and medical advice sought. Dressings to keep the part dry are required for any breach of the surface.

Regular exercise encourages the development of collateral vessels. Patients should not be alarmed by the development of pain and they should be encouraged to believe that with exercise and the stopping of smoking improvement is expected and that the occurrence of gangrene is improbable. Vasodilators are not recommended as they act by dilating normal vessels elsewhere and may divert blood from the affected site.

Areas of gangrene should be kept clean and dry until a clear line of demarcation appears. Thereafter surgical treatment may be required. Sympathectomy may be of value when the limb is cold or rest pain is present but it seldom helps claudication. Direct arterial surgery is indicated for disabling claudication, rest pain or gangrene provided the vessels are shown by arteriography to be suitable. Balloon angioplasty, which can often be done at the same time as angiography, is an effective treatment for short stenosed segments and may avoid the need for major surgery.

Sudden Occlusion of a Major Artery

This is usually due to embolism from the heart as a result of rheumatic heart disease, myocardial infarction or, rarely, an atrial myxoma. Emboli lodge commonly at the aortic, iliac or popliteal bifurcations. The limb becomes painful, cold, numb and pale, and pulses distal to the block are absent. Surgical embolectomy should be considered without delay. A Fogarty balloon catheter is used to extract the embolus through a small arteriotomy, and the procedure is often performed under local anaesthesia. While preparations for surgery are being made, pain should be relieved and the limb kept at rest and at room temperature.

Atherosclerosis and Aneurysm Formation

Atherosclerosis is frequently present in the aorta but seldom affects its function. It may, however, be responsible for aneurysms of any part of this vessel. An aneurysm of the arch of the aorta may produce hoarseness from pressure on the left recurrent laryngeal nerve. Aneurysms of the abdominal aorta are generally due to atherosclerosis. They cause abdominal pain, backache and a pulsatile mass; their rupture leads usually to sudden death. The results of elective resection and replacement with a prosthesis are improving.

Dissecting Aneurysm of the Aorta. In this condition a tear occurs through the intima secondary to degeneraton of the media. As a result blood makes its way in a split in the media to form a new channel. Death usually occurs from rupture through the adventitia into the pericardium, pleural cavity or elsewhere. Most patients have been hypertensive. There is an increased risk of aortic dissection in pregnancy and in patients with *Marfan's syndrome*, a connective tissue disorder characterised by long, thin extremities, a high arched palate and subluxation of the lens.

The onset of dissection is sudden with severe, tearing, chest pain which often radiates into the neck, abdomen, legs or back of the chest. It may be precipitated by exertion and may simulate or include myocardial infarction. Neurological features may result from occlusion of branches of the aorta supplying the spinal cord. One or more of the peripheral pulses may be obliterated.

Diagnosis is suggested by the sudden onset of the characteristic pain and the absence of the ECG and enzyme abnormalities of myocardial infarction unless the dissection includes a coronary artery. The chest radiograph may be helpful in showing a broadened mediastinum due to widening of the aorta. CT scanning or aortography is required for precise assessment.

In the initial stages the blood pressure, if high, should be lowered by antihypertensive drugs to normal levels. Surgical treatment is usually necessary for dissecting aneurysms affecting the ascending aorta or aortic arch. Dissecting aneurysms confined to the descending aorta can often be managed medically.

INFLAMMATORY ARTERIAL DISEASE

The principal types of inflammatory arterial disease are syphilitic aortitis, polyarteritis nodosa, thromboangiitis obliterans, cranial (giant cell) arteritis and Takayasu's syndrome (pulseless disease).

Syphilitic aortitis is now very rare in Britain. There is often a latent period of 15 to 20 years following an infection before clinical manifestations are evident in the cardiovascular system. Neurosyphilis sometimes coexists.

The disease begins just above the aortic valve cusps. In the adventitia there is infiltration of lymphocytes and plasma cells round the vasa vasorum, which are obliterated by intimal proliferation. Elastic tissue is gradually replaced by fibrous tissue and this leads to dilatation and aneurysm of the aorta. Proliferation of the intima occurs and may involve the mouths of the coronary arteries leading to myocardial ischaemia, or

spread along the valve cusps which become thickened, everted and incompetent.

The diagnosis is difficult in the early uncomplicated stages. Suspicion may be aroused by an aortic systolic murmur, together with accentuation of the second sound. Later there are the characteristic signs of aortic regurgitation but the diastolic murmur is more commonly best heard to the right of the sternum. Dilatation and calcification of the ascending aorta may be demonstrated by radiological examination. The diagnosis is confirmed by serological tests (p. 410).

If adequate antisyphilitic therapy is given in the early stages of the infection cardiovascular manifestations in later life are prevented. Treatment of syphilitic aortitis consists of a course of procaine penicillin (p. 411). If cardiac failure is present this should first be controlled. Surgical treatment may be indicated for aortic regurgitation or aneurysm.

Thromboangiitis obliterans (*Buerger's disease*) is an uncommon condition of obscure origin. It usually begins before the age of 40 and is almost confined to males who smoke heavily. The limbs, especially the legs, are principally affected. The wall of the artery is infiltrated with polymorphs and the lumen may be obstructed by thrombus. The adjacent vein is often involved.

The symptoms and signs are essentially those of diminished blood supply to the limb; persistent pain in a cold, cyanosed toe is often the presenting complaint. This is followed by intermittent claudication and rest pain. In the leg, atrophic changes and finally gangrene may develop. Involvement of the veins may cause recurrent thrombophlebitis.

There is no specific treatment but it is essential that cigarette smoking is stopped.

Polyarteritis nodosa is an uncommon condition most often seen in men between the ages of 20 and 50 and thought to have an immunological basis. The characteristic lesions consist of multiple nodules on the smaller arteries. The vessel wall is infiltrated by polymorphs and necrosis follows with resultant aneurysmal dilatation. Thrombosis may occur.

Clinical features such as fever, tachycardia, wasting, sweating and generalised pain are accompanied by local manifestations of ischaemia in various parts of the body. The vessels of the kidney, gastrointestinal tract, heart, peripheral nerves and skin are particularly affected giving rise to such varied manifestations as haematuria, abdominal pain, angina, myocardial infarction, pericarditis, peripheral neuropathy, subcutaneous nodules or localised oedema. Involvement of the lungs may cause asthma. There may be leucocytosis or eosinophilia. Hypertension is common.

The course is usually progressive although mild cases may recover. There is no curative treatment, but corticosteroids, administered before vascular damage is extensive, may produce a remission.

Cranial or giant cell arteritis is a panarteritis of medium-sized vessels affecting elderly persons. The disease may be immunologically determined; it is related to polymyalgia rheumatica (p. 578).

The vessel wall is infiltrated by mononuclear cells, plasma cells and giant cells. Thrombosis may occur. The temporal arteries are usually affected and may be thickened and tender. Other arteries may also be involved, notably the ophthalmic and cerebral.

Intense headache is usual and blindness may occur. Other manifestations include fever, pain and stiffness of hips and shoulders, weakness and loss of weight. Spontaneous recovery usually occurs after several months but cranial arteritis responds promptly to prednisolone; at least 50 mg daily should be given initially because of the risk of blindness; the dose is then reduced to the minimum for control of symptoms.

Takayasu's syndrome, known also as *pulseless disease* and the *aortic arch syndrome*, is rare except in some communities, e.g. Japan. It predominantly affects young females. An arteritis, probably of immunological origin, involves the aortic arch with narrowing of its major branches. The pulses are diminished or absent in the upper extremities, neck and head. Headache, syncope, visual disturbance and muscular wasting may occur. The prognosis is poor but corticosteroids are sometimes of value.

VASOSPASTIC DISORDERS

Raynaud's disease is the name given to a peripheral vascular disturbance consisting of spasmodic contraction of the digital arteries, which is precipitated by cold, emotion and by other causative factors mentioned below. Primary Raynaud's disease is commonest in young women and is an exaggerated physiological response to cold. Secondary Raynaud's disease or phenomenon occurs in (1) disorders of connective tissue, especially systemic sclerosis, (2) obliterative arterial disease, (3) occupations in which the hands are exposed to vibration e.g. from pneumatic drills, or (4) occasionally from cold agglutinins and cryoglobulins. In the early, uncomplicated stages there are no pathological changes. Later, obliterative endarteritis may occur and result in thrombosis, ischaemic changes in the skin of the digits and nails, superficial necrosis and finally gangrene.

The disorder is usually bilateral and fingers are more affected than toes. Numbness, tingling and burning are more prominent than pain. Sensitivity to cold may be extreme and disabling. Colour changes usually consist of three phases; pallor, cyanosis and redness. If the limb is bloodless it will be pale. If blood flow is sluggish, excessive deoxygenation results in cyanosis. Redness is in some cases due to reactive hyperaemia which may follow the vasospasm.

Any primary disease should be treated and protection from cold is obviously indicated. Cigarette smoking should be stopped. Nifedipine (10–20 mg t.i.d. with food) may be helpful (p. 170).

VENOUS THROMBOSIS

A distinction may be made between *thrombophlebitis* when the endothelium is injured by inflammation, and *phlebothrombosis* when thrombosis is the primary disturbance. The latter is the more common condition and carries a much greater risk of pulmonary embolism.

Aetiology. The following factors are of importance:

1. *Slowing or Obstruction of the Blood Stream.* This may result from rest in bed, particularly if a pillow is placed under the knees, especially in the elderly or from unduly prolonged sitting, e.g. in journeys by air. Cardiac failure also leads to slowing of the circulation.

2. *Injury to the Vein.* This may be due to trauma and may follow accidents, operations, childbirth, intravenous infusions or injections.

3. *Increased Coagulability of the Blood.* Many factors may disturb the dynamic equilibrium which normally exists between coagulation and fibrinolysis, notably an increase in platelet adhesiveness. This may occur for example in malignant disease or with the use of oral contraceptives. An increased liability to thrombosis also occurs in dehydration and polycythaemia due to an increase in the blood viscosity.

Pathology. At first the thrombus consists mainly of dense layers of platelets and fibrin; later it is a loose, friable, jelly-like mass of fibrin and red cells which readily becomes detached to form an embolus. After a few days inflammatory changes occur in the wall of the vein. The thrombus may undergo lysis or organisation.

Venous thrombosis is most common in the lower limbs, particularly in the venous sinuses of the soleus muscle in the calf and in the femoral and iliac veins. It is much less frequent in the upper limb but the axillary vein may be involved as a complication of trauma, neoplasm or radiotherapy. Superficial thrombophlebitis most commonly occurs in the saphenous vein, particularly if there are associated varicosities.

Suppurative thrombophlebitis is a rare but very serious condition usually involving the veins of the pelvis following sepsis.

Tropical phlebitis is described on page 718.

Clinical Features. The patient may complain of pain in the calf but the process is often silent and undiagnosed. An unexplained slight pyrexia may be the only warning. If the lumen of a main vein is occluded, there is dilatation of the superficial veins, the skin may be warm and pink and there may be oedema at the ankle. In extensive occlusive iliofemoral thrombosis the whole lower limb is swollen and white if the collateral channels remain patent. If the collaterals are also occluded, the leg is blue — a pregangrenous condition. In contrast there are frequently no signs in the presence of an extensive non-occlusive, potentially lethal thrombus. Pulmonary embolism is often the first clinical manifestation of venous thrombosis.

The most certain way of establishing the diagnosis is by phlebography. The veins from the ankle to the inguinal ligament can be demonstrated by ascending lower limb phlebography. Percutaneous iliofemoral phlebography may also be required. Phlebography may precipitate venous thrombosis, and heparin should be given before it is undertaken. Ultrasound is used to assess the patency of deep veins in patients who present with a swollen leg or with pulmonary embolism. The uptake of ^{123}I labelled fibrinogen is used for the early detection of thrombosis, for example post-operatively; it has the advantage of being non-invasive but is less reliable than phlebography, particularly for the detection of thrombosis in the pelvic and common femoral veins.

Prevention. Efforts must chiefly be directed to the avoidance of venous stasis. This is easiest in surgical patients when the period of risk can be defined. Almost all post-operative thromboses begin during, or within 72 hours of, operation. Early ambulation should be encouraged after surgery and medical illnesses. This means more than simply transferring the patient from lying in bed to sitting in a chair. Active exercises should be prescribed and at other times the leg should be elevated. A graduated elastic support should be worn if the patient is at particular risk. If confinement to bed is unavoidable, the patient should be encouraged to move the lower limbs frequently. In hospital, exercises can be organised under the supervision of a physiotherapist. Faulty posture in bed must be corrected, constricting bandages avoided and cardiac failure and dehydration should receive attention.

For patients at particular risk other prophylactic measures include low dose subcutaneous heparin or intravenous dextran 70.

Treatment aims at preventing the propagation of thrombus and pulmonary embolism, damage to the valves of the vein and chronic venous insufficiency. Unless there is an obvious contraindication, such as active peptic ulceration or a bleeding surface as after prostatectomy, treatment is initiated with heparin and continued with warfarin (p. 547). Thrombolysis with streptokinase (p. 548) can be considered for iliofemoral thrombosis. Thrombectomy may occasionally be required for a recent non-occlusive thrombosis at this site.

The legs should be elevated to 15 degrees and physiotherapy commenced after 48 hours. Straining at stool often causes separation of venous thrombi and should be avoided. The venous flow is accelerated by the support of graduated elastic hose but care must be taken to avoid a constricting effect by the hose rolling up. The ambulant woman should wear elastic support tights and for men knee-length elastic hose is best. Support of this kind will probably be necessary permanently after a severe thrombosis to control chronic venous insufficiency. Superficial thrombophlebitis usually responds to an elastic support and a non-steroidal anti-inflammatory drug (p. 559).

PROSPECTS IN CARDIOLOGY

Detection of cardiac abnormalities in utero using two-dimensional echocardiographic examination of the fetus is now a reality, although it is too early to predict its impact on paediatric cardiology. New surgical procedures for correcting congenital heart disease continue to be introduced; they demand and usually receive critical evaluation before they are generaly accepted. In adult cardiac surgery, mechanical valve prostheses have demonstrated their durability, but some biological valves have been disappointing in this respect, and an ideal replacement valve has not yet appeared. The efficacy of coronary artery bypass grafting both in relieving symptoms and in improving survival in patients with advanced coronary disease has been further demonstrated in controlled trials; however the logistic problems of providing such surgery for everyone who might benefit have not been solved.

The incidence of ischaemic heart disease manifestations continues to fall in some parts of the world but is increasing in others. The causes are unclear, but ability and willingness to modify lifestyle, diet and smoking habits seem to be important. Acute coronary thrombolysis with streptokinase in patients with threatened myocardial infarction has proved to be practicable, but whether it is worthwhile awaits further evaluation. Platelet anti-aggregants have proved disappointing as agents of secondary prevention after myocardial infarction, but beta-blockers are more promising. There is continuing controversy over when they should be introduced and for how long they should be continued.

The introduction of new antihypertensive agents has made the treatment of severe hypertension more satisfactory, but further information about the 'cost-benefit equation' in treating mild hypertension is awaited. There is no cause for complacency concerning the efficacy and freedom from side effects of the drugs currently available for treating mild hypertension.

D.P. DE BONO
D.G. JULIAN

FURTHER READING:

Bradley R.D. (1977) *Studies in Acute Heart Failure*. London: Edward Arnold. An elegant discussion of the application of physiological principles to the management of heart failure.
Braunwald E. (1983) *Heart Disease: A Textbook of Cardiovascular Medicine* Philadelphia: W.B. Saunders. A detailed and comprehensive textbook.
De Bono D. (1983) Examination of the cardiovascular system. In: Macleod J. (ed.) *Clinical Examination*, 6th edn. Edinburgh: Churchill Livingstone.
Julian D.G. (1983) *Cardiology*, 4th edn. London: Baillière Tindall. An introduction to cardiology for the non-specialist.

8. Diseases of the Respiratory System

ANATOMY

The *upper respiratory tract*, which includes the nose, nasopharynx and larynx, is lined by vascular mucous membrane. The rich blood supply ensures that the inspired air enters the lungs at body temperature and fully saturated with water vapour. The whole respiratory epithelium down to the terminal bronchioles is ciliated. The cilia, and the thin film of mucus covering them, have the important function of trapping foreign particles including bacteria, and propelling them towards the pharynx. They contribute to the prevention of respiratory infection, as do the alveolar macrophages by means of their secretory, phagocytic and bactericidal activity.

The maxillary, frontal, ethmoidal and sphenoidal *nasal sinuses* communicate with the nasopharynx by narrow openings and are frequently involved in upper respiratory infections. Adequate drainage of infected sinuses is often prevented by oedema of the mucosa lining their narrow openings; as a result, resolution of sinus infection is often slow and sometimes incomplete.

The *larynx*, in addition to being the organ of voice production, has the function of preventing particles larger than can be dealt with by the cilia from reaching the lower respiratory tract. Together with the bronchi, the larynx is supplied with vagal receptors, which form the sensory side of the cough reflex and perhaps also of reflexes concerned with bronchoconstriction.

The larynx is often involved in disease, particularly infection. It is sometimes obstructed by oedema or exudate, or by an impacted foreign body. Laryngeal paralysis is due to a lesion of the recurrent laryngeal branch of the vagus nerve. As the left recurrent laryngeal nerve runs part of its course within the thoracic cavity, in close proximity to the aortic arch and the left pulmonary hilum, a bronchial carcinoma in the left hilar region and, less frequently, an aortic aneurysm may cause paralysis of the left vocal cord. Paralysis of the right vocal cord is rare, most cases being due to an aneurysm of the right subclavian artery. Accidental division of both recurrent laryngeal nerves in the neck during thyroidectomy and destruction of these nerves by a thyroid carcinoma are the most common causes of bilateral vocal cord paralysis.

The *trachea* begins at the cricoid cartilage and ends at the level of the sternal angle by bifurcation into the two *main bronchi*. The trachea is usually palpable in the suprasternal notch, where in normal subjects it is in the midline. Deviation of the trachea to either side, in the absence of a local lesion in the neck, is a valuable indication of displacement of the upper mediastinum.

The *right main bronchus* is more vertical than the left, with the result that a foreign body entering the trachea is more likely to lodge in that bronchus or one of its divisions than the left. The right main bronchus first gives off from its lateral wall the upper lobe bronchus and then from its anterior wall the middle lobe bronchus, after which it continues as the lower lobe bronchus. The left main bronchus gives off the upper lobe bronchus from its lateral wall and continues as the lower lobe bronchus.

The three lobar bronchi on the right side and the two on the left divide and subdivide like the branches of a tree (the term 'bronchial tree' is in common use) until the terminal bronchioles are reached. The portion of lung supplied by a terminal bronchiole is called an acinus, which is the basic functional unit of lung tissue. Each acinus contains branching respiratory bronchioles communicating with clusters of alveoli. The alveoli are lined by a single layer of flattened epithelial cells (Type I pneumocytes) which are in direct contact with the pulmonary capillaries. Exchange of the respiratory gases, oxygen and carbon dioxide, takes place between the air in the alveoli and the blood in the pulmonary capillaries. Pulmonary surfactant, a phospholipid which by reducing surface tension prevents alveolar collapse, is secreted by Type II granular pneumocytes.

The *left lung* differs from the right in having two lobes instead of three. The left lung is divided into upper and lower lobes by the oblique fissure which extends from the junction of the fourth or fifth rib with the vertebral column behind to the sixth costochondral junction in front, crossing the midaxillary line at the level of the fifth rib. As the posterior end of the fissure is at a much higher level than its anterior end, the upper lobe, as well as being above the lower lobe, is also largely in front of it. It therefore follows that upper lobe lesions produce physical signs mainly on the front of the chest and lower lobe lesions on the back.

On the *right* side the oblique fissure corresponds in position to that on the left, but the lung above it is divided into *upper* and *middle lobes* by the *transverse fissure*, which runs laterally in a horizontal direction from the junction of the fourth costal cartilage with the sternum to join the oblique fissure at the level of the fifth rib in the midaxillary line. The middle lobe is thus situated behind the lower part of the anterior chest wall. Each lobe is composed of two or more *bronchopulmonary segments*, which represent the portions of lung tissue supplied by the main branches of each lobar bronchus. The situation of the various lobes and segments in shown in Figure 8.1.

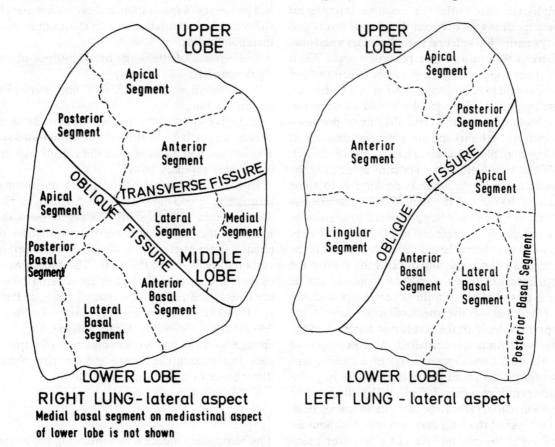

RIGHT LUNG - lateral aspect
Medial basal segment on mediastinal aspect of lower lobe is not shown

LEFT LUNG - lateral aspect

Fig. 8.1 The lobes and segments of the lungs.

In many diseases, e.g. pneumococcal pneumonia, collapse and lung abscess, the lesion is typically confined to a single lobe or segment. A knowledge of pulmonary anatomy, when applied to the interpretation of radiographs, is thus of value in determining the nature of the lesion as well as its situation.

Each lung is closely invested with *visceral pleura*. *Parietal pleura* lines the chest wall, mediastinum and diaphragm, and is continuous with the visceral pleura at the pulmonary hilum. In health the two pleural layers are separated only by a thin film of lymph, and are kept in apposition by negative (subatmospheric) pressure. This results from the natural tendency of the lung to recoil towards the hilum, because of its inherent elastic properties.

If a communication develops with the atmosphere as, for example, with a penetrating wound of the chest wall or from spontaneous rupture of an emphysematous bulla, the negative intrapleural pressure draws air between the pleural layers and the potential intrapleural space becomes a real one. There is then said to be a pneumothorax. When the space is created by the presence of serous fluid there is said to be a pleural effusion or a hydrothorax; by pus, an empyema; by blood, a haemothorax; by both serous fluid and air, a hydropneumothorax; by both pus and air, a pyopneumothorax; and by both blood and air, a haemopneumothorax.

When the pleural space contains air or fluid the elastic recoil of the underlying lung is to some extent released and the lung shrinks towards the hilum, this shrinkage being referred to as *pulmonary collapse*. The larger the amount of air or fluid between the pleural layers the more marked is the degree of pulmonary collapse and the greater the impairment of function of the collapsed lung. If the quantity of air or fluid is very large it causes displacement of the mediastinum towards the opposite side, with the result that function of the opposite lung is also impaired. A gross degree of mediastinal displacement may, in addition, embarrass the action of the heart. Mediastinal displacement is recognised clinically by alteration in position of the trachea and of the cardiac apex beat.

Collapse of the lung may also occur without air or fluid in the pleural space as a result of bronchial obstruction.

The anatomy of the *mediastinum* has an important bearing on the diagnosis of intrathoracic disease, particularly tumours and aneurysms. These lesions are liable to involve mediastinal structures and, as a result, certain readily recognisable symptoms, physical signs and radiological abnormalities may be produced (p. 263).

PHYSIOLOGY

Knowledge of the normal processes of respiration is of value in understanding the effects of disease on the lungs and airways, and is of great importance in therapy. Oxygen therapy, the treatment of respiratory failure and much of the treatment of chronic bronchitis and asthma have a rational basis in applied respiratory physiology.

The aspects of the physiology of respiration which merit special attention are:

1. *Ventilation*, which includes (a) the mechanical processes of inspiration and expiration and (b) the control of ventilation at a level appropriate to metabolic needs.

2. *Perfusion* of the lungs by the output of the right ventricle.

3. *Distribution* of ventilation and perfusion within the lungs.

4. *Diffusion* of oxygen and carbon dioxide, which occurs both within the terminal airways and alveoli, and also between the alveoli and the pulmonary capillary blood.

In a typical normal adult at rest the normal pulmonary blood flow of about 5 l/min carries 11 mmol/min (250 ml/min) of oxygen from the lungs to the tissues and normal ventilation of about 6 l/min carries 9 mmol/min (200 ml/min) of carbon dioxide out of the body. The pressures of oxygen and carbon dioxide in the arterial blood are closely controlled. The normal range of Pao_2 is 11–13 kPa (83–98 mmHg) and of $Paco_2$ 4·8–6·0 kPa (36–45 mmHg). Observation of changes in these pressures in disease is of importance in assessing the nature and severity of any disturbance of lung function (p. 209).

Ventilation

The respiratory muscles, in ventilating the lungs, do mechanical work of two kinds, elastic and non-elastic. The first is performed against elastic forces in the lungs and chest wall which together tend to bring the chest to the position it occupies at the end of a normal expiration. Movement of the chest from this position of equilibrium involves the performance of elastic work and the storage of kinetic energy which is later available for non-elastic work during the return to the resting position. This second kind of work is largely expended in overcoming the resistance of the airways to the inspiratory and expiratory flow of air and to a smaller extent in displacing soft and inelastic tissues. Most of the resistance in normal subjects lies in the large central airways. The peripheral airways, though individually smaller in calibre, contribute less to total resistance because of their large combined cross-sectional area.

During quiet breathing inspiration is 'active' and expiration 'passive'. Inspiration against abnormal resistance (whether elastic or non-elastic) may bring accessory muscles such as the sternomastoids and scaleni into play; expiration, if forced or performed against abnormal resistance, is accomplished with the aid of the accessory muscles of expiration, chiefly those of the abdominal wall.

Elastic work is increased when the lungs are made more rigid (less compliant) by pulmonary oedema or fibrosis or when the chest wall is made more unyielding by ankylosing spondylitis or scleroderma. Rapid shallow breathing is often observed in these conditions. Non-elastic work is increased by rapid breathing and by conditions causing airflow obstruction such as asthma, chronic bronchitis, emphysema and tumours of major bronchi.

The metabolic cost of breathing is normally low: an increase in ventilation of 1 l/min raises oxygen uptake by about 45 μmol/min (1 ml/min) at most. In disease, this figure may rise to as much as 450 μmol (10 ml) oxygen per min per l/min increase in ventilation. Under such circumstances breathing accounts for an important fraction of metabolic oxygen uptake.

Not all of the inspired air takes part in gas exchange in the lungs. Some of each breath ventilates the conducting airways (down to the respiratory bronchioles), which constitute the 'anatomical' dead space; also because of maldistribution (see below) some of each breath is wasted in ventilating underperfused parts of the lungs. The proportion of wasted ventilation in each breath (physiological dead space:tidal volume ratio, Vd/Vt) is normally one fifth to one third, but may be much increased, sometimes to as much as two thirds, in disease. The volume which remains takes part in gas exchange and provides *alveolar ventilation*, which is normally about 5 l/min at rest. It follows that if the proportion of wasted ventilation is greater than normal a greater total ventilation is needed to achieve normal alveolar ventilation.

Normally, alveolar ventilation is closely matched to the excretion of carbon dioxide and this matching is reflected in a normal level of arterial P_{CO_2}. If alveolar ventilation is reduced in proportion to carbon dioxide excretion, the arterial P_{CO_2} must rise (hypercapnia), and if alveolar ventilation becomes excessive, the arterial P_{CO_2} will fall (hypocapnia). Indeed, the arterial P_{CO_2} reflects alveolar ventilation and the production of carbon dioxide just as the blood urea concentration reflects renal urea clearance and the metabolic production of urea.

Generalised alveolar underventilation is most commonly found as a late result of chronic bronchitis and emphysema. It also occurs if respiration is centrally depressed by narcotics, anaesthetics or intracranial disease. It may ensue when the respiratory muscles are paralysed or when gross deformity of the chest wall limits thoracic or diaphragmatic movement, as in kyphoscoliosis. Lowering of the arterial P_{O_2} (hypoxaemia) is an inevitable result of alveolar underventilation when air is breathed. Giving oxygen will correct this, but hypercapnia is corrected only when alveolar ventilation is improved.

Alveolar overventilation occurs in asthma of mild or moderate severity, in interstitial lung disease, in pulmonary vascular disease (e.g. pulmonary thromboembolic disease), in salicylate overdosage, as a result of upper brain stem lesions, or from anxiety or hysteria. It is also a prominent manifestation of metabolic acidosis (p. 100).

Control of breathing. Rhythmical discharges originating in the reticular substance of the brain stem provide the basis for co-ordinated respiratory movements; it is convenient to use the term 'respiratory centre' for the neurones involved in breathing, but the distribution and organisation of these neurones is highly complex. From the respiratory centre, impulses reach the spinal motor neurones by the recticulospinal tracts, in contrast to impulses mediating conscious changes in breathing, which travel via the corticospinal tracts. Normal breathing is modified by afferent impulses from many sources, which are best considered in two groups:

1. Those arising within the central nervous system and from receptors other than chemo-receptors ('neural stimuli').

2. Those arising from chemoreceptors sensitive to the composition of blood or cerebrospinal fluid ('chemical stimuli').

Afferent impulses of the first group mediate (a) the changes in rate and depth of breathing which may be consciously maintained for short periods, (b) the central neurogenic overventilation which occurs in certain lesions of the upper brain stem, (c) the respiratory depression associated with medullary compression and (d) the respiratory stimulation which originates in limb receptors, as in exercise. These impulses may also arise from receptors in muscles and joints in the chest wall, and from pulmonary receptors sensitive to stretch, bronchial irritation or pulmonary capillary distension. Pulmonary inflation and deflation (Hering-Breuer) reflexes are present in the newborn, but are weak in adults except under general anaesthesia.

The second group of afferent impulses arises in chemosensitive cells located in the carotid and aortic bodies (peripheral chemoreceptors) and intracranially (central chemoreceptors). In animals central chemosensitive areas are located on the ventrolateral surface of the medulla, but in man their situation is uncertain.

Ventilation is increased when the peripheral chemoreceptors are stimulated by arterial hypoxia; at rest, the stimulus is not strong unless arterial P_{O_2} is below 8 kPa (60 mmHg), and becomes powerful at about 4 kPa (30 mmHg). The peripheral chemoreceptors are also stimulated by an increase in the hydrogen ion activity of arterial blood. Central chemoreceptors are stimulated by an increase in the hydrogen ion

activity of cerebrospinal fluid (CSF). A rise in P_{CO_2} of the arterial blood is accompanied by increasing acidity of both blood and CSF and therefore stimulates both central and peripheral chemoreceptors. For this reason, inhalation of carbon dioxide is one of the strongest known respiratory stimulants. In the presence of mild or moderate hypoxia its effect is increased, but severe hypoxia acts as a central depressant. Pyrexia increases the sensitivity of the respiratory centre; all sedatives, particularly opiates, depress it. Salicylates in large doses stimulate it.

In some patients with chronic bronchitis the normal sensitivity to increased arterial P_{CO_2} is greatly reduced. In such patients chronic alveolar underventilation may occur and relief of the concurrent hypoxaemia may, by removing one of the remaining stimuli to breathing, be followed by worsening of the hypercapnia.

Distribution of Gas and Blood in the Lungs

Gas exchange in the lungs is inefficient unless alveolar ventilation is distributed uniformly to different parts of the lungs and is matched by uniform distribution of blood flow. The composition of blood leaving an individual alveolus depends on the composition of the mixed venous blood entering the pulmonary capillaries and the ratio between the ventilation of and blood flow around the alveolus. The possible values of this ventilation:perfusion ratio ($\dot{V}_A/\dot{Q}$) lie between infinity (ventilation but no perfusion) and zero (perfusion but no ventilation). Thus areas of lung with $\dot{V}_A/\dot{Q} = \infty$ behave as dead space, giving rise to wasted ventilation, while areas with $\dot{V}_A/\dot{Q} = 0$ behave as a physiological right-to-left shunt or venous admixture effect, giving rise to wasted perfusion.

The possible range of alveolar ventilation:perfusion ratios is so large that it has become conventional to treat the lungs as if they were made up of three compartments:

(a) a compartment normally ventilated and perfused,

(b) physiological dead space, contributed to by all alveoli whose $\dot{V}_A/\dot{Q}$ exceeds unity, and including the anatomical dead space.

(c) physiological shunt, contributed to by all alveoli with $\dot{V}_A/\dot{Q}$ less than unity, and including the small anatomical or 'true' right-to-left shunts through such pathways as bronchial-pulmonary venous anastomoses.

It follows that if the range of ventilation:perfusion ratios found in the lungs is wider than normal the physiological dead space and physiological shunt will be larger than normal and gas exchange will become less efficient.

Even in the normal lung, distribution of ventilation and perfusion is imperfect. In the erect posture, gravity affects distribution of both ventilation and blood flow, causing regional $\dot{V}_A/\dot{Q}$ to be increased at the apices and reduced at the bases of the lungs. In most forms of lung disease, distribution of ventilation and perfusion is further impaired, and it is easy to visualise how pathological mechanisms may have this effect. For example, distribution of ventilation may be impaired by

(a) bronchial or bronchiolar obstruction (tumour, secretions, mucosal oedema, bronchoconstriction),

(b) destruction of elastic tissue (as in emphysema),

(c) pulmonary collapse, consolidation, fibrosis or oedema,

(d) chest wall deformities.

Blood flow is reduced or abolished by pulmonary embolism or thrombosis or by obliteration of areas of the pulmonary capillary bed by necrosis or fibrosis.

The consequences of maldistribution are twofold. First, as has been explained above, an increase in physiological dead space means that a greater total ventilation is needed to achieve a given alveolar ventilation. Second, any increase in physiological shunt causes arterial hypoxaemia. Any tendency to hypercapnia due to perfusion of alveoli with low $\dot{V}_A/\dot{Q}$ ratios can be compensated for by overventilation of alveoli with high $\dot{V}_A/\dot{Q}$ ratios. This preserves a normal or low arterial P_{CO_2}, but the arterial hypoxaemia is little affected. Maldistribution, with areas of low $\dot{V}_A/\dot{Q}$ ratio, is therefore the most important single cause of hypoxaemia in disease, and is found in a wide variety of conditions. Fortunately, administration of oxygen raises the alveolar P_{O_2}, even in poorly ventilated alveoli, and corrects the hypoxaemia.

Diffusion of Gases in the Lungs

Oxygen and carbon dioxide move by molecular diffusion in the gas phase along the terminal airways and alveoli, and are also exchanged across the alveolar membrane by diffusion in the liquid phase from a site of higher to one of lower partial pressure. It might be expected that if the alveolar wall became thickened, as in interstitial lung disease, diffusion of gases, particularly of oxygen, would be impaired. However, most conditions which might be expected to have this effect can also give rise to maldistribution of ventilation and perfusion, and analysis suggests that this is usually the chief cause of hypoxaemia in these conditions.

If the area available for gas exchange is reduced (e.g. in emphysema) or if, because of maldistribution, the effective area is reduced, the ability of the lung to transfer gases will also diminish. Such a reduction may not be significant at rest, but may limit the amount of oxygen which can be taken up during exercise and may become a cause of hypoxaemia under these circumstances.

The overall ability of the lung to transfer gases can be readily measured by relating the uptake of carbon monoxide to the alveolar CO pressure when a low concentration of the gas is breathed. By this method, values for *gas transfer factor* or *diffusing capacity* of the lung are obtained. The former name is preferable, since 'diffusing capacity' carries the implication that diffusion itself is being measured, whereas in fact the measurement is affected by other factors, such as maldistribution.

COMMON MANIFESTATIONS OF RESPIRATORY DISEASE

Cough. This is the most frequent of all respiratory symptoms. It may be short, painful and half-suppressed, as when dry pleurisy accompanies pneumonia, loose and readily productive of sputum, as in bronchiectasis, or paroxysmal, ineffectual and exhausting, as in some cases of chronic bronchitis and asthma. In bronchial carcinoma it is usually an early symptom but may be a relatively late development in pulmonary tuberculosis. Generally it is worse at night or on waking.

Often it is aggravated by changes in temperature or humidity. The explosive character of a normal cough is lost when laryngeal paralysis is present ('bovine cough'). It is accompanied by stridor (p. 209) in whooping cough and in the presence of laryngeal or tracheal obstruction.

Sputum. Purulent sputum is due to bacterial infection in the respiratory tract and is typically seen in acute bronchitis, infective exacerbations of chronic bronchitis, bacterial pneumonia, bronchiectasis and lung abscess. In the last two conditions the sputum may be copious and is sometimes fetid. Mucoid sputum is due to over-secretion of bronchial mucus. It is frequently present in chronic bronchitis and bronchial asthma. In early cases of pulmonary tuberculosis the sputum is mucoid but in advanced cases it is usually purulent.

Haemoptysis. All grades of severity may occur, from slight streaking of sputum with blood to a massive haemorrhage. Although it is a common symptom in acute and chronic bronchitis, bleeding from the lower respiratory tract, however slight, must be regarded as of potentially serious significance demanding full investigation. Bronchial carcinoma, pulmonary infarction, bronchiectasis and pulmonary tuberculosis are its most important causes.

Chest Pain. There are four types of chest pain associated with respiratory disease:

1. Central retrosternal pain of a sore, 'scratchy' character made worse by coughing, usually caused by tracheitis.

2. Central chest discomfort caused by rapidly enlarging mediastinal tumours.

3. Unilateral chest pain, usually in the pectoral or axillary regions but sometimes in the back, of a sharp stabbing character, made worse by deep breathing and coughing, and caused by inflammation of the pleura or by a fractured rib.

4. Constant pain, unrelated to breathing, resulting from direct invasion of the chest wall by a malignant lung tumour, metastatic deposits in ribs or vertebral metastatic deposits compressing or invading intercostal nerve roots.

Pleural pain is thought to be due to stretching of the inflamed parietal pleura (the visceral pleura is insensitive to painful stimuli) and is maximal towards the end of inspiration. Patients with pleural pain try to minimise it by taking shallow breaths and by suppressing cough as much as possible.

The pain is referred to the area of skin supplied by the same spinal nerves as those supplying the inflamed area of pleura. Usually it is referred to the chest wall, but when the pleura lining the diaphragm is inflamed it may be referred to the cutaneous distribution of the supraclavicular nerves which have the same spinal roots (third and fourth cervical) as the phrenic nerve. Pain in the front and top of the shoulder is thus characteristic of diaphragmatic pleurisy. Pleural pain may also be referred to the anterior abdominal wall, where it may be difficult to distinguish from the pain of an acute abdominal emergency.

A *pleural rub*, which is a common physical sign in pleurisy, is due to the rubbing together of pleural surfaces roughened by fibrinous exudate. The effusion of fluid between the layers of the pleura diminishes pain by reducing the movement of the chest wall and abolishes the pleural rub by separating the pleural surfaces.

Dyspnoea. It has been said that breathing is the only involuntary act which is carried out by voluntary muscle, and this is normally so. Dyspnoea is a subjective sensation in which the effort of breathing reaches consciousness, usually under circumstances in which a normal person would not be aware of breathing at all. It should be distinguished from *hyperpnoea*, where the volume of ventilation is increased, but no abnormal sensation is felt, and *tachypnoea*, an excessive respiratory rate.

Dyspnoea occurs as a symptom in a wide variety of diseases, and no single theory can adequately explain why it occurs. In conditions where resistance to airflow is high, such as asthma or chronic bronchitis, the increased mechanical work needed to achieve a given volume of ventilation may account for it. A similar explanation may be given for dyspnoea in diseases causing lung stiffness, such as fibrosing alveolitis, with the added factor that the hypoxaemia which occurs readily during exercise in such diseases may still further increase the drive to breathe. This explanation is less satisfactory for the dyspnoea of heart disease, and still less so for the dyspnoea found in anaemia, where both the lungs and the arterial oxygen pressure are normal.

It has been suggested that the sensation arises from 'inappropriateness' between the amount of breathing which the patient feels is needed for a given task and the amount that in fact has to be produced — a feeling comparable to that experienced when picking up what seems to be an ordinary rubber ball and finding it is filled with lead. This throws some light on the nature of the sensation, but still leaves its cause obscure.

In mild heart or lung disease, dyspnoea is noticeable only on effort, and the presence of dyspnoea at rest is an indication that the disease is severe or advanced. In conditions such as chronic bronchitis, much of the respiratory reserve may have been lost before a sedentary patient complains of dyspnoea, but measurements of ventilatory capacity will confirm that severe airflow obstruction is already established. Complaints of dyspnoea should therefore be taken seriously, for although the symptom is commonly found in anxiety states, it also may occur early in diseases such as pulmonary thrombo-embolism or allergic alveolitis at a stage when abnormalities may not be apparent clinically or radiologically. Tests of pulmonary function and objective assessment of exercise capacity are then of value.

Wheeze. In all diseases causing airflow obstruction, particularly bronchial asthma, wheeze is usually a conspicuous symptom. It is a musical sound heard best during expiration, and is associated with numerous rhonchi on auscultation. *Stridor*, on the other hand, occurs when one of the major airways (larynx, trachea or main bronchus) is obstructed. It is a crowing sound heard best during inspiration, especially after coughing, and is associated with a persistent low-pitched rhonchus audible all over the chest.

Hypoxaemia is present if either the pressure or content of oxygen in arterial blood is reduced, and if severe enough may result in visible central cyanosis. The normal arterial Po_2 is over 12 kPa (90 mmHg) at the age of 20, and falls to around 11 kPa (82 mmHg) at 60. Above this age a further fall in Po_2 of up to 1·3 kPa (10 mmHg) may occur on recumbency because of closure of airways in the dependent regions of the lungs.

The most frequent and important cause of hypoxaemia in respiratory disease is the presence in the lungs of areas where the distribution of ventilation and perfusion is disturbed and where ventilation is low in relation to perfusion. Hypoxaemia also inevitably results from alveolar underventilation (because alveolar and arterial Pco_2 are increased) or if an atmosphere poor in oxygen is breathed, as at high altitudes. Impairment of diffusion across the alveolar wall may cause hypoxaemia during exercise, but is hardly ever an important factor at rest. The hypoxaemia due to all these causes is reversed by giving oxygen. Hypoxaemia due to congenital heart disease or vascular anomalies, with shunting of blood from the right to the left of the circulation past the lungs, cannot be entirely reversed by oxygen. Hypoxaemia also occurs if the oxygen capacity of the blood is reduced, as in anaemia or carbon monoxide poisoning.

Hypercapnia is present if the pressure of carbon dioxide in the arterial blood ($Paco_2$) is above the upper limit of normal of 6·0 kPa or 45 mmHg at rest, but values of up to 6.5 kPa (50 mmHg) are seldom of clinical importance. As has been explained, the finding of a raised $Paco_2$ implies that alveolar ventilation is inadequate in relation to the carbon dioxide production of the body; the causes of hypercapnia are therefore those of alveolar underventilation. Alveoli in which the ventilation:perfusion ratio is low also contribute to hypercapnia.

The finding of hypercapnia implies either that the normal sensitivity of the respiratory centre to carbon dioxide has been reduced, or that mechanical limitation or failure of neuromuscular transmission prevents a normally responsive centre from maintaining adequate alveolar ventilation.

Clinical features suggestive of hypercapnia include peripheral vasodilatation, with warm extremities and bounding pulses, sweating, muscle twitching, flapping tremor, headache, drowsiness, coma, retinal venous distension and, rarely, papilloedema. Unfortunately, none of these signs is specific and the diagnosis must be made by measurement of the pressure of carbon dioxide in arterial blood.

Hypercapnia has three consequences of clinical importance: (a) it aggravates hypoxaemia by lowering the pressure of oxygen in the alveolar gas,

(b) when acute, it increases the arterial hydrogen ion concentration (respiratory acidosis), although renal retention of bicarbonate tends to compensate for this over a period of hours or days (p. 98), and (c) when of a severe degree, it induces drowsiness, which may proceed to coma.

Respiratory failure is said to occur when the normal pressures of oxygen and carbon dioxide in the arterial blood are no longer maintained. For practical purposes, this means the finding of either a PaO_2 of less than 8 kPa (60 mmHg) or a $PaCO_2$ of more than 6.5 kPa (50 mmHg).

It follows that two varieties of respiratory failure can be recognised. In so-called Type I respiratory failure the $PaCO_2$ is normal or low, but PaO_2 is reduced. Type II respiratory failure, in which the $PaCO_2$ is elevated and the PaO_2 is reduced, is often termed 'ventilatory failure'. The mechanisms responsible for the hypoxaemia in each type have already been discussed (p. 209).

The causes of Type I respiratory failure are many, and include any of the pathological causes of maldistribution of ventilation and perfusion in the lungs (p. 207). Among the most important are bronchial asthma, pneumonia, pulmonary oedema, allergic and fibrosing alveolitis and pulmonary thromboembolism.

The most common pulmonary cause of Type II respiratory failure is chronic bronchitis, particularly when complicated by acute respiratory infection. Other causes include respiratory paralysis (p. 644), deformities of the chest such as severe kyphoscoliosis, and depression of the respiratory centre, particularly by narcotic or sedative drugs.

Adult respiratory distress syndrome (ARDS) is a severe form of Type I respiratory failure caused by non-cardiogenic pulmonary oedema. It is a grave and often fatal complication of shock following multiple injuries and fulminating viral or bacterial infections, particularly septicaemia.

Clubbing of the Fingers and Toes. The cause of clubbing, which is most readily recognised in the fingers, is not known but it is frequently found in patients with certain types of respiratory disease, notably bronchial carcinoma, chronic intrathoracic suppuration and fibrosing alveolitis. It does not occur in chronic bronchitis or emphysema unless there is accompanying pulmonary suppuration or if the patient has developed a tumour, nor in pulmonary tuberculosis except in advanced cases.

Clubbing also occurs in certain other conditions. It is usually present in infective endocarditis and cyanotic congenital heart disease, occasionally in Crohn's disease, malabsorption syndrome and cirrhosis of the liver, and rarely in healthy subjects as a familial trait. The earliest indication of finger clubbing is an abnormal degree of fluctuation at the bases of the nails. With more advanced clubbing there is, in addition, an increase in the curvature of the nails and bulbous swelling of the fingertips.

THE INVESTIGATION OF RESPIRATORY DISEASE

In most respiratory diseases a reasonably accurate diagnosis can be made from the history and physical examination alone, but in several important conditions, notably pulmonary tuberculosis and bronchial carcinoma, these methods are inadequate and the diagnosis can be confirmed or excluded only by more specialised procedures such as radiological, bacteriological or endoscopic examination.

The patient must always be asked about symptoms such as cough, sputum, haemoptysis, pain, breathlessness, wheeze and nasal discharge. Since some respiratory diseases are related to present or past occupational hazards (p. 265), contact with animals, particularly birds (pp. 225 and 249), or drug reactions (p. 248), a thorough enquiry must be made into these potential causes of respiratory illness.

Physical Examination

Before the chest itself is examined the temperature should be taken, and a note made of the rate and character of breathing, the type and severity of cough and the amount and character of any sputum. In addition, particular care must be taken to determine whether or not there is cyanosis, clubbing of the fingers or enlargement of the supraclavicular lymph nodes, these features being of special significance in respiratory disease.

The upper respiratory tract should be examined next, with particular regard to nasal discharge or obstruction, oral sepsis, and infection or enlargement of the tonsils. The presence of hoarseness or a 'bovine' cough would draw attention to the need for laryngoscopic examination (p. 251).

The chest wall should then be carefully inspected for soft tissue abnormalities such as cutaneous lesions, subcutaneous swellings (including lumps in the breast) and bulging or indrawing of intercostal spaces, and for skeletal abnormalities such as an increase in the anteroposterior diameter of the chest relative to its lateral diameter.

The position of the trachea and of the apex beat should be noted and the chest expansion measured. Chest wall movement, vocal fremitus and the percussion note should be compared in equivalent positions on the two sides. The terms used to describe the various types of percussion note are: hyperresonant, normal, impaired, dull and stony dull.

At auscultation, attention should be directed in turn to the breath sounds, added sounds and vocal resonance.

BREATH SOUNDS. The following terms are used: vesicular, vesicular with prolonged expiration, diminished vesicular, absent breath sounds, and high-pitched and low-pitched bronchial breath sounds.

ADDED SOUNDS. *Rhonchi* seem to be related to narrowing of the lumen of the bronchi caused by spasm of bronchial muscle, swelling of bronchial mucosa or tenacious mucus adherent to bronchial walls. Rhonchi may be high-pitched, medium-pitched or low-pitched, according to the size of the bronchi in which they originate.

Crepitations ('crackles') usually indicate the presence of secretions within alveoli, bronchi or pulmonary cavities. They may be fine, medium or coarse in quality, and may either disappear or become more numerous after coughing. Loud end-inspiratory crackles, unaltered by coughing, are a feature of interstitial lung disease (p. 265).

Pleural rub is a diagnostic sign of pleurisy. It is a grating or creaking sound, unaltered by coughing, audible during both inspiration and expiration.

VOCAL RESONANCE. The following terms are used: normal, increased, diminished or absent vocal resonance, aegophony and whispering pectoriloquy.

The Interpretation of Physical Signs. Certain groups of physical signs are typically associated with certain pathological changes in the lungs and pleura. Such changes are not necessarily specific for one particular disease. For example, consolidation may occur in pneumonia or tuberculosis, and fluid may be present in the pleural space in tuberculous pleurisy, empyema, malignant disease or cardiac failure. Each group of physical signs should therefore be correlated with the gross pathological lesion by which the signs are produced rather than with any specific disease, the diagnosis of which depends on an analysis of all the clinical and other evidence.

The physical signs of the more common lesions are shown on Table 8.1 (p. 212).

Special Methods of Investigation

Radiological Examination of the Chest. Many pulmonary diseases, including bronchial carcinoma and pulmonary tuberculosis, cannot be detected at an early stage without radiological examination of the chest. Facilities for this investigation are now readily available to most doctors, and it should always be undertaken whenever any serious form of intrathoracic disease is suspected. A lateral film may provide additional information about the nature and situation of a pulmonary, pleural or mediastinal abnormality.

Specialised techniques, such as bronchography, fluoroscopy, conventional tomography, computed tomography, radionuclide ventilation and perfusion scanning and pulmonary angiography may be of considerable diagnostic value in selected cases.

It may be very useful to obtain chest radiographs taken previously for comparison with a current film, since this may show whether a radiographic opacity is 'new' or progressive, and thus potentially serious, or 'old' and probably of no importance.

Some respiratory diseases, such as bronchial asthma and chronic bronchitis, and occasionally bronchial carcinoma, may not be associated with any radiographic abnormality, and a normal chest radiograph in these circumstances does not necessarily exclude serious intrathoracic disease.

Table 8.1 Summary of typical physical signs in the more common respiratory diseases

Pathological process	Movement of chest wall	Mediastinal displacement	Percussion note	Breath sounds	Vocal resonance	Accompaniments
Consolidation as in lobar pneumonia	Reduced on affected side	None	Dull	High-pitched bronchial	Increased (with aegophony) Whispering pectoriloquy	Fine crepitations early Coarse crepitations later
Collapse due to obstruction of major bronchus	Reduced on side affected	Towards lesion	Dull	Diminished or absent	Reduced or absent	None
Collapse due to peripheral bronchial obstruction	Reduced on side affected	Towards lesion	Dull	High-pitched bronchial	Increased (with aegophony) Whispering pectoriloquy	None early–coarse crepitations later
Localised fibrosis and/or bronchiectasis	Slightly reduced on side affected	Towards lesion	Impaired	Low-pitched bronchial	Increased	Coarse crepitations
Cavitation (usually associated with consolidation or fibrosis)	Slightly reduced on side affected	None, or towards lesion	Impaired	'Amphoric' bronchial	Increased Whispering pectoriloquy	Coarse crepitations
Pleural effusion Empyema	Reduced or absent (depending on size) on side affected	Towards opposite side	Stony dull	Diminished or absent (occasionally bronchial)	Reduced or absent (occasionally increased)	Pleural rub in some cases (above effusion)
Pneumothorax	Reduced or absent (depending on size) on side affected	Towards opposite side	Normal or hyper-resonant	Diminished or absent (occasionally faint bronchial)	Reduced or absent	Tinkling crepitations when fluid present
Bronchitis: Acute Chronic	Normal or symmetrically diminished	None	Normal	Vesicular with prolonged expiration	Normal	Rhonchi, usually with some coarse crepitations
Bronchial asthma	Symmetrically diminished	None	Normal	Vesicular with prolonged expiration	Normal or reduced	Rhonchi, mainly expiratory and high-pitched
Bronchopneumonia	Symmetrically diminished	None	May be impaired	Usually harsh vesicular with prolonged expiration	Normal	Rhonchi and coarse crepitations
Diffuse pulmonary emphysema	Symmetrically diminished	None	Normal	Diminished vesicular with prolonged expiration	Normal or reduced	Expiratory rhonchi
Interstitial lung disease	Symmetrically diminished	None	Normal	Harsh vesicular with prolonged expiration	Usually increased	End-inspiratory crackling crepitations uninfluenced by coughing

(After Macleod, J. (1979) *Clinical Examination*, 5th edn. Edinburgh: Churchill Livingstone.)

Microbiological and Cytological Examination. *Sputum* can be examined for bacteria, fungi and viruses. Microbiological examination seldom provides conclusive diagnostic information except when *Mycobacterium tuberculosis* is isolated. The findings in other circumstances must be interpreted in conjunction with the results of clinical and, if necessary, radiological examination. The demonstration of malignant cells in the sputum confirms a diagnosis of bronchial carcinoma. Sputum cytology may also identify excessive numbers of eosinophil leucocytes, as in asthma and bronchopulmonary eosinophilia.

Pleural Fluid. This should always be examined cytologically and bacteriologically. A special search should be made for *Myco. tuberculosis* if the fluid is serous and also for pyogenic organisms if it is purulent. The fluid should also be examined cytologically, particularly if malignant disease is suspected.

Blood Examination. Serological examination may be of value in the diagnosis of viral infections and allergic disorders.

Estimation of the total and differential leucocyte count may help to distinguish pyogenic infection from tuberculous or viral infection. An increase in the eosinophil count may occur for a variety of reasons (p. 248).

Skin Tests. The tuberculin test (p. 232) and Kveim test (p. 269) may be of value in the diagnosis of tuberculosis and sarcoidosis respectively. Skin sensitivity tests (p. 244) are useful in the investigation of allergic diseases.

Laryngoscopy and Bronchoscopy. The larynx is inspected either by means of a mirror placed in front of the uvula (indirect laryngoscopy) or through an illuminated telescopic tube (direct laryngoscopy).

The trachea and larger bronchi are inspected by a bronchoscope of either the rigid or the flexible fibreoptic type. Abnormal tissue can be removed for histological examination (bronchial biopsy), and bronchial brushings and washings can be taken for cytological and bacteriological examination. The range of vision with the rigid instrument extends to the origins of all segmental bronchi but the fibreoptic bronchoscope is more useful for the inspection and biopsy of lesions situated more peripherally, particularly in the upper lobes.

Biopsy. Histological examination of an enlarged lymph node removed from the neck or axilla, or cytological examination of a needle aspirate, may provide a diagnosis in conditions such as bronchial carcinoma, tuberculosis, lymphoma and sarcoidosis. A lymph node can also be obtained for histological examination from the mediastinum by the technique of *mediastinoscopy*.

In patients with pleural effusion it is possible to obtain a specimen of parietal pleura suitable for histological examination by means of Abrams' pleural biopsy 'punch'. This procedure is simple and safe and may be of considerable value in determining the cause of a pleural effusion. If it is unsuccessful, the pleural surfaces can be inspected with a thoracoscope inserted through an intercostal space, and if a pleural lesion is seen, a biopsy can be performed under telescopic vision.

When a diagnosis cannot be made in any other way it may be necessary to obtain a specimen of lung tissue for histological examination by needle biopsy through the chest wall, by transbronchial lung biopsy via a fibreoptic bronchoscope or by thoracotomy.

Tests of Pulmonary Function. Many of the procedures mentioned above are of great assistance in arriving at a pathological diagnosis, but investigations of a different type are necessary to determine the effects of disease on pulmonary function and to assess the response to therapy. Disturbances of the mechanical properties of the lungs, of ventilation, of control of breathing, of the distribution of ventilation and perfusion within the lungs and of diffusing capacity can all be measured (Fig. 8.2). Some of the tests require a high degree of skill and elaborate apparatus, but others are simple routine procedures which can be undertaken by any doctor without special training.

(a) ESTIMATION OF VENTILATORY CAPACITY. The patient is asked to take in as deep a breath as possible and then expel it as hard and as fast as possible. If the forced expiration is made into a recording spirometer of low resistance and low inertia, the *forced expiratory volume* in the standard time of 1 second (FEV_1) can be measured; if the forced expiration is continued till no more gas can be expelled, the *forced vital capacity* (FVC) is measured. The ratio of these two volumes may be expressed as a percentage (FEV/FVC%); normal people can expel between 65 and 80% of the FVC in 1 second, depending on age and sex.

In diseases which cause narrowing of the airways during expiration, such as asthma and chronic bronchitis, the FEV/FVC% is reduced, sometimes to 40% or less. This is due to a greater reduction in FEV than in FVC, and this type of ventilatory defect is called '*obstructive*'. In diseases such as interstitial lung disease or ankylosing spondylitis, which make the lungs or chest wall more rigid, FEV and FVC are reduced in the same proportion and FEV/FVC% is normal, as the airflow is relatively unaffected. This is called a '*restrictive*' ventilatory defect. Discovery of airflow obstruction is an indication to repeat the spirometric measurements after a bronchodilator drug has been given; reversibility of airflow obstruction is found in asthma and in some patients with chronic bronchitis.

During forced expiration, the *peak expiratory flow rate* (PEFR) can be measured by a device which is simpler and cheaper than a spirometer. PEFR is reduced in conditions causing airflow obstruction, and is a good indicator of the severity of the obstruction. The measurement has therefore become popular in clinical practice because of its speed and simplicity. PEFR is less affected by conditions causing a restrictive type of ventilatory defect, and is therefore of little value in diagnosing or assessing them.

Even if no apparatus other than a watch and stethoscope is available, forced expiration can still be used to assess ventilatory capacity. Normal people can empty their chests from full inspiration in 4 seconds or less. Prolongation of the *forced expiratory time* (FET) to more than 6 seconds indicates airflow obstruction and a reduction in FEV/FVC% to less than 50%. The endpoint of FET is detected by placing the chest-piece of a stethoscope over the trachea in the suprasternal notch.

(b) ANALYSIS OF ARTERIAL BLOOD. Apparatus for arterial blood-gas analysis is now available in most hospitals. Knowledge of the $Paco_2$ provides the answer to the question, 'Is the patient breathing enough?', and is of particular value in the management of Type II respiratory failure (p. 217). If the arterial hydrogen ion concentration (or pH) are known, it is often possible to deduce the type of disturbance of acid:base balance (p. 100) which may be present. Knowledge of the Pao_2 or arterial oxygen saturation allows accurate assessment of hypoxaemia and of the effects of oxygen therapy.

These simple measurements are thus of value in distinguishing between some types of respiratory disorder, as well as in providing an index of their severity. Serial measurements are valuable in following changes in pulmonary function, whether occurring spontaneously or in response to treatment.

THE TREATMENT OF RESPIRATORY DISEASE

Infection

The antimicrobial therapy of bacterial infection of the bronchi, lungs and pleura will be described in the sections on individual diseases. Bacteriological examination of sputum is seldom of much help in the clinical management of exacerbations of chronic bronchitis, but certain general principles are applicable to all other cases.

Before any treatment is started a specimen of sputum, a laryngeal swab (if there is no sputum) or a specimen of pleural fluid should be sent for bacteriological examination. In acute bacterial infection it is usually necessary to begin therapy before the results of bacteriological examination are available. The choice of antibiotic in these circumstances is based on clinical impressions of the nature and severity of the illness. If a clinical diagnosis of acute bronchitis, pneumonia or empyema is made and the patient is not seriously ill or if the acute infection is a complication of chronic bronchitis, asthma or bronchiectasis, ampicillin should be given initially. If the patient is gravely ill and there is any reason to suspect infection with *Staph. pyogenes*, an antibiotic to which that organism is unlikely to be resistant, e.g. flucloxacillin, must be added. As soon as the results of bacteriological examination and sensitivity tests are received, modifications in antibiotic therapy can be made, if necessary. Factors which interfere with the response to antibiotics must be corrected, e.g. an empyema must be aspirated or drained, and bronchiectatic cavities and lung abscesses must be kept empty by postural drainage.

The viruses which infect the respiratory tract are uninfluenced by chemotherapy, but secondary bacterial infection, which occurs in many cases, often requires treatment with an appropriate antimicrobial agent. Infection caused by small bacteria, such as coxiella, mycoplasma and chlamydia, usually responds to tetracycline.

The treatment of respiratory diseases caused by fungi is described on page 241.

Oxygen Therapy

Oxygen is present in the air at a concentration of 21% and at sea level the pressure of oxygen in inspired tracheal air is almost 20 kPa (150 mmHg). Arterial blood of normal haemoglobin concentration contains about 9 mmol oxygen per litre (20 ml/100 ml); at a Pao_2 of 13·5 kPa (100 mmHg) 135 μmol oxygen per litre (0·3 ml/100 ml) are dissolved in the plasma (i.e. a

---

Fig. 8.2 Relationships between structure and function of lungs and pulmonary function tests. The forced expirogram gives information about airway resistance and calibre and the maximal flow-volume loop supplements this with information about inspiratory resistance, airway collapsibility and behaviour of small peripheral airways. Vital capacity and lung volume measurements are influenced by tissue elasticity and airway resistance. Distribution of ventilation and blood flow may be assessed by blood gas analysis and by measurement of dead space and venous admixture. Overall gas exchange is assessed by arterial Po_2 and Pco_2 and by gas transfer factor.

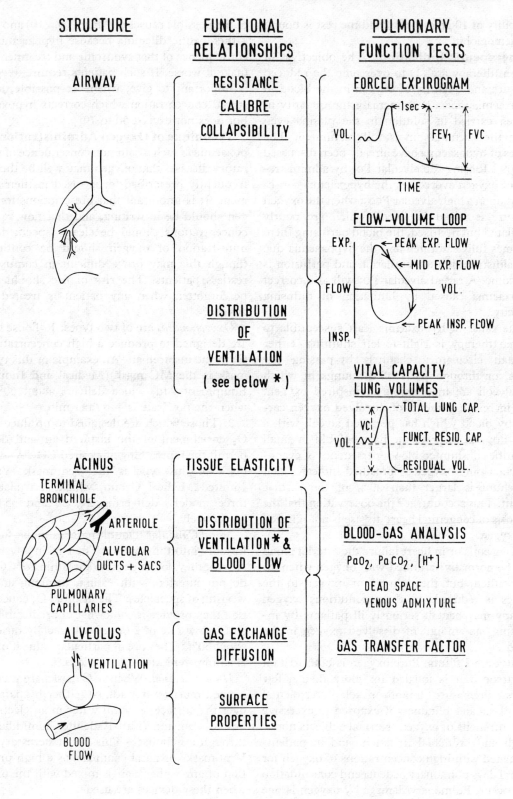

STRUCTURE

AIRWAY

ACINUS

TERMINAL
BRONCHIOLE

ARTERIOLE

ALVEOLAR
DUCTS + SACS

PULMONARY
CAPILLARIES

ALVEOLUS

VENTILATION

BLOOD
FLOW

FUNCTIONAL
RELATIONSHIPS

RESISTANCE
CALIBRE
COLLAPSIBILITY

DISTRIBUTION
OF
VENTILATION
(see below *)

TISSUE ELASTICITY

DISTRIBUTION OF
VENTILATION* &
BLOOD FLOW

GAS EXCHANGE
DIFFUSION

SURFACE
PROPERTIES

PULMONARY
FUNCTION TESTS

FORCED EXPIROGRAM

VOL.

1sec

FEV_1 FVC

TIME

FLOW-VOLUME LOOP

EXP.

PEAK EXP. FLOW
MID EXP. FLOW

FLOW

VOL.

INSP.

PEAK INSP. FLOW

VITAL CAPACITY
LUNG VOLUMES

TOTAL LUNG CAP.

VC

VOL.

FUNCT. RESID. CAP.

RESIDUAL VOL.

BLOOD-GAS ANALYSIS

PaO_2, $PaCO_2$, $[H^+]$

DEAD SPACE
VENOUS ADMIXTURE

GAS TRANSFER FACTOR

solubility of 10 μmol/l/kPa) and the rest is bound to haemoglobin.

Therapeutic Indications. The objectives of oxygen therapy are (1) to overcome the reduced pressure and quantity of oxygen in the blood in hypoxaemia, and (2) to increase the quantity of oxygen carried in solution in the plasma even when the haemoglobin is fully saturated. The causes of hypoxaemia have already been discussed (p. 209). Raising the alveolar Po_2 by administration of oxygen overcomes the hypoxaemia consequent upon a high alveolar Pco_2; when the oxygen pressure is raised in alveoli which are poorly ventilated but perfused, the blood perfusing them becomes fully saturated and the hypoxaemia due to maldistribution of ventilation and perfusion is overcome. A raised alveolar Po_2 will also correct hypoxaemia caused by limitation of diffusing capacity.

The cause of hypoxaemia least susceptible to oxygen therapy is right-to-left shunting, either through circulatory channels by-passing the lungs, or through parts of the lungs in which the alveoli are inaccessible to inspired oxygen. The increased amounts of dissolved oxygen carried by blood which has perfused alveoli with a high Po_2 can saturate the haemoglobin in small quantities of shunted blood; persistence of cyanosis when pure oxygen is breathed indicates that the shunt is larger than 20% of the cardiac output. This accounts for the observation that the cyanosis of congenital heart disease is not relieved by oxygen.

In anaemia or in heart failure the arterial blood may be normally saturated with oxygen when air is breathed, but the delivery of oxygen to the tissues is reduced. In these conditions oxygen therapy may benefit seriously ill patients by increasing the amount of dissolved oxygen in the blood.

Adverse Effects. Pure oxygen is both irritant and toxic if it is inhaled for more than a few hours. Premature infants develop retrolental fibroplasia and blindness if exposed to excessive concentrations of oxygen. Normal subjects notice cough and bronchial irritation, and in patients ventilated with high concentrations of oxygen for several days pulmonary oedema and consolidation may occur. Pulmonary damage by oxygen is one of the possible causes of ARDS (p. 210) and poses a therapeutic dilemma because hypoxaemia is a consequence of that syndrome and treatment may make it worse. If such patients require oxygen it is important to give, whenever possible, an inspired concentration which corrects hypoxaemia but does not exceed 60 to 70%.

Technique of Oxygen Administration. Hypoxaemia is such a common consequence of respiratory diseases that oxygen may well be the most frequently prescribed 'drug' used in their treatment. It is important that prescriptions for oxygen should be in writing, and that flow rates or concentrations should be clearly specified. Administration of oxygen should be continuous though this may prove difficult in confused or restless patients. The risk of fire should never be forgotten when any patient is treated with oxygen.

Oxygen masks are of two types: 1. Those which are designed to produce a high concentration of O_2 in the inspired air. An example of this type of mask is the MC mask (Medical and Industrial Equipment Ltd) which delivers about 60% O_2 when the flow rate is 4–6 l per min.

2. Those which are designed to produce slight O_2 enrichment of the inspired air and do not permit the rebreathing of expired CO_2. A suitable mask of this type is the Ventimask (Vickers Limited Medical Group) which is available in three models, delivering 24, 28 and 35% O_2 respectively.

Nasal Cannulae. Double nasal cannulae fit comfortably into the nostrils. Their main advantages are that they do not permit rebreathing of CO_2 and do not interfere with eating, drinking and the wearing of spectacles. The inspired O_2 concentration they provide is somewhat unpredictable, but an O_2 flow rate of 2 l/min. will usually raise it to about 30%. They are of particular value if oxygen is administered for long periods.

Humidification. When MC masks are used, the oxygen must be humidified, either by passing it over the surface of warm water in an electrically heated canister (East-Radcliffe humidifier) or through a nebuliser. This is not necessary with Ventimasks or nasal cannulae, as a high proportion of atmospheric air is mixed with the oxygen when these devices are used.

Treatment of Respiratory Failure

Acute Type I Respiratory Failure. Severe hypoxaemia associated with a normal or low $Paco_2$ can develop rapidly in many respiratory and cardiac disorders. Treatment is that of the underlying cause (e.g. pulmonary oedema, pneumonia, adult respiratory distress syndrome) and correction of the hypoxaemia by administration of oxygen in high concentration by oronasal mask. Young children may have to be treated in oxygen tents since few of them tolerate masks. Very ill patients may require artificial ventilation with oxygen-enriched air through a cuffed endotracheal tube.

Chronic Type I Respiratory Failure. Chronic hypoxaemia without carbon dioxide retention has many causes, mainly respiratory, which include fibrosing alveolitis and other types of interstitial lung disease (p. 264). Treatment is that of the underlying disorder, combined with high concentration oxygen therapy. Patients with chronic respiratory failure of this type are rarely treated with artificial ventilation, since the prognosis is generally poor and aggressive therapy is usually considered to be ethically unjustified.

Acute Type II Respiratory Failure. Acute Type II respiratory failure (asphyxia) may be produced by obstruction of the upper airways, severe acute asthma, major chest injuries, particularly those associated with tension pneumothorax, massive haemothorax or multiple rib fractures (flail chest), acute brain stem and cervical cord lesions resulting from trauma to the head and neck, arterial occlusion or viral infection, paralysis of respiratory muscles and poisoning with narcotic and other drugs.

Acute retention of carbon dioxide in this form of Type II respiratory failure, causes severe respiratory acidosis (p. 210). This may also supervene when carbon dioxide retention increases rapidly in patients with chronic Type II respiratory failure who develop a respiratory infection.

The treatment of the various causes of acute Type II respiratory failure is summarised in Table 8.2.

Chronic Type II Respiratory Failure. The most important cause of chronic retention of carbon dioxide (hypercapnia) and associated hypoxaemia is chronic bronchitis, but Type II respiratory failure also occurs preterminally in other progressive respiratory diseases. Chronic hypercapnia leads to renal conservation of bicarbonate which usually corrects the resultant respiratory acidosis. In these circumstances the arterial hydrogen ion concentration may be normal, but acidaemia recurs whenever a further reduction in alveolar ventilation again increases the degree of hypercapnia. High concentrations of oxygen can cause deterioration because they reduce the hypoxic drive to breathing in patients whose central (brain stem) response to carbon dioxide is diminished or absent.

Associated right ventricular failure is almost invariably made worse by hypoxaemia, which aggravates pulmonary hypertension.

Respiratory infection and retained bronchial secretions are the main factors responsible for exacerbations of Type II respiratory failure in patients with chronic lung disease. Efforts to encourage efficient expectoration, which may be difficult in patients made drowsy by carbon dioxide retention, must be pursued with the utmost vigour and appropriate antimicrobial therapy prescribed. If there is evidence of bronchospasm, bronchodilators and, if necessary, corticosteroids should be given in an attempt to reduce airflow obstruction. Analeptic drugs have a limited but useful place in drowsy and comatose patients. Nikethamide (2–4 ml of a 25% solution 1–2 hourly) or doxapram (infusions of up to 3 mg/minute) given intravenously for 24 hours, may successfully tide the patient over a period of hypoventilation during which time bronchopulmonary infection, bronchospasm and right ventricular failure can be treated, the last with a powerful diuretic. The main reason for giving analeptic drugs is to improve the level of consciousness so that effective expectoration can be encouraged. If these measures fail patients who were able to lead a fairly active life before the onset of the acute episode may be considered for artificial ventilation.

Mechanical Ventilation — Intermittent Positive-Pressure Ventilation (IPPV). Patients with both types of respiratory failure may have to be treated by IPPV through a cuffed endotracheal tube introduced through the mouth

Table 8.2 Treatment of acute Type II respiratory failure.

Cause	Treatment
1. *Upper airways obstruction* (a) Inhaled foreign body	Try to dislodge it by turning child upside down and forcibly compressing the thoracic cage or by Heimlich manoeuvre (p. 251) in adult. If ineffective, extract foreign body by laryngoscopy or bronchoscopy.
(b) Acute epiglottitis, laryngeal oedema, bilateral vocal cord paralysis	Treatment of cause. If medical treatment ineffective, tracheal intubation or tracheostomy.
2. *Severe acute asthma*	Medical treatment (p. 246). If not rapidly effective, tracheal intubation and intermittent positive-pressure ventilation.
3. *Chest injuries* (a) Tension pneumothorax	Pleural decompression by intercostal tube.
(b) Massive haemothorax	Drainage of blood through intercostal tube. Thoracotomy if necessary for evacuation of clot and ligation of bleeding points.
(c) Flail chest	Tracheal intubation and intermittent positive-pressure ventilation. Fixation of rib and sternal fractures.
4. *Brain stem and cervical cord lesions. Paralysis of respiratory muscles*	Tracheal intubation and intermittent positive-pressure ventilation. Treatment of cause where possible.
5. *Poisoning with narcotic and other drugs*	Measures to eliminate poison. Specific antidote (e.g. naloxone for opium alkaloids). Tracheal intubation and intermittent positive-pressure ventilation.

or nose under general anaesthesia. Positive end-expiratory pressure (PEEP) may be useful in some cases with Type I respiratory failure to correct ventilation-perfusion imbalance. Powerful ventilators delivering a fixed volume are required for the treatment of patients with Type II respiratory failure associated with airflow obstruction e.g. asthma and chronic bronchitis. Whenever IPPV is likely to be necessary for more than a few days, for example in patients with respiratory muscle paralysis, the patient should have a tracheostomy and the endotracheal tube should be replaced by a cuffed tracheostomy tube.

Endotracheal intubation and tracheostomy allow tracheo-bronchial suction to be performed as often as necessary to clear the airways of secretions. This can be done more efficiently by fibre-optic bronchoscopy which is of particular value if lobar collapse has occurred because of retained secretions.

Most adults require a ventilatory volume of about 10 l/min. to maintain a normal $Paco_2$ and sufficient oxygen is added to the 'inspired' air in order to achieve a satisfactory Pao_2. Attempts to discontinue ventilation can be started as soon as the underlying cause of respiratory failure has been successfully treated. It is usual for the patient to be allowed to breathe humidified air spontaneously through the tracheostomy tube for longer periods each day until assisted ventilation is no longer required. At this stage the tracheostomy tube can be removed, providing it is not still necessary to prevent aspiration of secretions into the trachea in patients who cannot swallow normally because of brain stem lesions.

Symptomatic Treatment in Respiratory Disease

Cough, when productive of sputum, should be encouraged and not suppressed. Those who are physically weak should be exhorted at regular intervals to clear their bronchi of secretion. Those with bronchiectasis or lung abscess should practise postural drainage, and those with tenacious sputum should be given hot drinks and inhalations of either steam or nebulised normal saline to help them to bring up sputum more easily. Cough, particularly during the night, may be a prominent symptom of bronchial asthma, and is relieved by treatment of that disease.

Unproductive, distressing cough should be suppressed, especially if sleep is disturbed. The two most effective preparations, suitable for use in bronchitis, pneumonia, bronchial carcinoma and pulmonary tuberculosis, are pholcodine and methadone.

Haemoptysis. A sedative may be given to allay anxiety, e.g. diazepam. Morphine, which depresses the cough reflex, may have the effect of allowing blood clot to accumulate in the bronchi and should not be prescribed. Haemoptysis nearly always stops spontaneously and reassurance to this effect lessens the strain of what, to patient and relatives, is a most alarming experience.

If the haemorrhage is very severe blood volume should be restored by transfusion and, if respiratory obstruction develops, the blood must be removed from the bronchi by aspiration through a bronchoscope. Control of the bleeding by surgical measures is occasionally required.

Airflow obstruction in bronchitis and asthma is treated by bronchodilators (p. 245) and in some cases by corticosteroids given by inhalation or as tablets (p. 246).

Chest Pain. For pleural pain mild analgesics, such as acetylsalicylic acid or codeine, may be adequate in most cases but a few patients may require pethidine, 50–100 mg by mouth or intramuscular injection, or even morphine, 10–15 mg i.m. Opiates must, however, be avoided in patients with poor respiratory function.

The pain of acute tracheitis usually responds to the application of heat to the front of the chest, combined with inhalations of steam medicated with benzoin (p. 222). Pain due to invasion of the chest wall by a malignant tumour, if not relieved by radiotherapy, usually demands a powerful analgesic such as pethidine or morphine, given by injection. In advanced cases these drugs may become ineffective and neurosurgical measures may be required for the relief of intractable pain.

INFECTIONS OF THE RESPIRATORY SYSTEM

Infections of the respiratory tract may be caused by viruses, bacteria and fungi. Viruses are frequently responsible for upper respiratory illnesses. Although viral infection is a relatively uncommon specific cause of pneumonia, it is often complicated by bacterial infection of the bronchi and lungs as, for example, in influenza. The bacteria most frequently responsible for respiratory infection, including pneumonia, are *Streptococcus pneumoniae*, often in association with *Haemophilus influenzae, Staphylococcus pyogenes* and various species of gram-negative bacilli. The so-called small bacteria, such as mycoplasma, coxiella and chlamydia, and also legionnella, are other, but much less common, causes of acute pneumonia. Pulmonary infection by *Mycobacterium tuberculosis*, atypical mycobacteria and fungi results in diseases of a more chronic type, which are described in separate sections of the chapter.

Upper Respiratory Tract Infections

The vast majority of these illnesses, of which acute coryza is by far the most common, are caused by viruses (Table 8.3). Immunity is short-lived, and specific for each virus. The average person can, therefore, expect to have at least two or three attacks of coryza every year. Other viral infections include pharyngoconjunctival fever, herpangina, acute laryngitis and acute laryngotracheobronchitis. Bacterial infection is the cause of acute tonsillitis, otitis media and epiglottitis.

Acute Coryza. The onset is usually sudden with a tickling sensation in the nose accompanied by sneezing. The throat often feels dry and sore, the head feels 'stuffed' and there is a profuse

Table 8.3 Upper respiratory tract infections caused by viruses. A classification of viruses is on page 727.

Aetiological agent	Clinical syndrome
*Adenoviruses	Acute coryza
	Pharyngoconjunctival fever
	Acute laryngitis
Coronaviruses	Acute coryza
Coxsackie viruses	Pharyngoconjunctival fever
	Herpangina
Echo viruses	Acute coryza
	Pharyngoconjunctival fever
*Influenza virus A, B, (C)	Epidemic influenza
	Acute laryngotracheobronchitis (croup)
*Parainfluenza virus 1–4	Acute coryza
	Acute laryngotracheobronchitis (croup)
*Respiratory syncytial (RS) virus	Acute coryza
	Acute laryngotracheobronchitis (croup)
Rhinoviruses	Acute coryza

*May also cause pneumonia

watery nasal discharge (rhinorrhoea). These symptoms last for 1 to 2 days, after which, with secondary infection, the secretion becomes thick and purulent, and impedes nasal breathing.

Coryza may be complicated by sinusitis when there is usually more systemic upset. Sinus infection is liable to become chronic, particularly in the maxillary sinuses, causing persistent purulent discharge from the front and back of the nose, often accompanied by nasal obstruction and headaches.

Other complications are infections of the lower respiratory tract, catarrh of the auditory tubes causing deafness, and otitis media causing fever and aural pain.

Frequent attacks of sneezing and watery rhinorrhoea, without systemic upset, suggest nasal allergy rather than viral infection.

Pharyngoconjunctival Fever. The pharyngeal syndrome, which is sometimes accompanied by conjunctivitis, occurs particularly amongst school children in spring and summer and in holiday camps. It may be caused by several viruses (Table 8.3), especially adenoviruses. Herpangina may occur in infections with Coxsackie A viruses.

Conjunctivitis may be the first symptom, but sore throat is the dominant feature and may be slight or severe. The pharynx, tonsils and ad-enoids become inflamed, and yellow exudate may be present. Cervical lymph nodes are enlarged and tender. The degree of constitutional symptoms — shivering, malaise, anorexia, headache and fever — is variable. In herpangina, typical vesicles, which may become punched-out ulcers, are present on the fauces. Acute streptococcal sore throat may be clinically indistinguishable from pharyngoconjunctival fever, but *Strep. pyogenes* will be isolated from such cases. Infectious mononucleosis (p. 519) may also be difficult to differentiate from the pharyngeal syndrome in the early stages. The possibility of diphtheria and of gonococcal infection should not be overlooked.

Acute Laryngitis. This usually occurs either as a complication of coryza or as a manifestation of one of the infectious fevers, for example, measles. The laryngeal mucous membrane is swollen, congested and coated with mucus.

The throat is dry and sore. The voice is at first hoarse and then reduced to a whisper. Speaking may be painful. There is an irritating non-productive cough, but the general upset is usually mild. In children the small laryngeal opening may be obstructed by oedema and viscid secretion, giving rise to stridor (croup).

Acute laryngitis usually clears up in a few days, but frequently recurring episodes may predispose to chronic laryngitis. Downward spread of the infection may cause tracheitis, bronchitis or even pneumonia.

Acute Laryngotracheobronchitis. This illness, which is particularly serious in very young children because of the small calibre of their airways, may be caused by several viruses (Table 8.3). Superinfection with bacteria, especially *Strep. pneumoniae* and *Staph. pyogenes*, may occur. The mucosa is intensely inflamed, the secretions are extremely tenacious and fibrinous casts of the bronchi may form.

The initial symptoms may be those of the common cold. These are followed by severe and sometimes violent cough which may be paroxysmal, accompanied by dyspnoea and stridor (croup), contraction of accessory muscles and indrawing of intercostal spaces. The child may be cyanosed, and asphyxia may occur if appropriate treatment is not given.

Acute Epiglottitis. This is a rare, but serious

disease of young children. Bacterial infection, almost always with *Haemophilus influenzae*, is the cause of this condition which presents with fever and sore throat. Stridor develops rapidly because of inflammatory swelling of the epiglottis and surrounding submucosa, and death may occur from asphyxia. Stridor and cough without hoarseness are features of acute epiglottitis which help to distinguish it from laryngeal causes of stridor. When this diagnosis is suspected, attempts to examine the throat using a tongue depressor or any instrument should be avoided since this may cause complete respiratory obstruction.

Investigation and Treatment of Upper Respiratory Tract Infections

Most patients with these infections recover rapidly and specific investigation is indicated only in the more severe cases. Viruses can be isolated from throat swabs, and viral infections may be identified by serological tests. Throat swabs may also be helpful if streptococcal sore throat is suspected, and examination of the blood will identify infectious mononucleosis. Radiographic examination may be required to confirm the presence of chronic sinus infection.

The spread of viral infections can be reduced by voluntary isolation of patients for 2–3 days during the early highly infectious stage. Excessive nasal secretions can be reduced by periodic use of decongestants either sprayed or dropped into the nose. Lozenges containing local anaesthetic, for example benzocaine, are helpful when the throat is painful. A mild analgesic such as aspirin or paracetamol, relieves systemic symptoms. Antibiotics are unnecessary except in the treatment of acute epiglottitis, streptococcal sore throat and bacterial complications of viral infection, such as acute sinusitis or otitis media. Ampicillin is normally the drug of choice in these conditions. In acute epiglottitis, however, either ampicillin in high dosage, or chloramphenicol, should be given intravenously.

Inhalations of steam are helpful in laryngitis. In acute laryngotracheobronchitis clearing of secretions is of utmost importance. Bronchoscopy, endotracheal intubation or tracheostomy may be required as life-saving measures in patients with severe respiratory obstruction. Oxygen therapy is necessary in some patients and adequate hydration should be maintained.

INFLUENZA

Influenza is a specific acute illness caused by a group of myxoviruses. It occurs in epidemics, and occasionally pandemics, often explosive in nature.

Aetiology. Three types of virus are described, A, B and C. At least four strains of influenza A, which is responsible for the pandemics, have been identified. The H3N2 strain (Hong Kong) has been implicated in most recent epidemics. Influenza B is usually associated with smaller and less virulent outbreaks. The C virus is found only rarely. The immunity which follows is type-specific and of relatively short duration. This causes problems in providing effective immunisation.

Clinical Features. The incubation period is 24 to 48 hours. The illness starts suddenly with malaise, headache, pain in the back and limbs, anorexia and sometimes nausea and vomiting. Pyrexia to 39°C remits for 2 to 3 days, with chills and shivering but seldom rigors. The face is flushed, conjunctivae suffused and fauces hyperaemic with prominent lymphoid follicles. The pulse is rapid. There is often leucopenia. There may be a harsh unproductive cough, without physical signs over the lungs.

The disease may spread rapidly throughout a household or institution. During epidemics, the diagnosis is usually easy. Most sporadic cases are identifiable only as respiratory virus infections unless the virus is isolated, or demonstrated by the fluorescent antibody technique, or if serological tests for specific antibodies are positive.

Course and Complications. In many cases, no further symptoms develop and recovery ensues within 3 to 5 days. The disease may, however, be complicated by tracheitis, bronchitis, bronchiolitis and bronchopneumonia. Secondary bacterial invasion by *Strep. pneumoniae*, *H. influenzae* and occasionally *Staph. pyogenes* causes these complications.

Toxic cardiomyopathy may cause sudden death, especially when there is pre-existing cardiac disease. Encephalitis and post-influenzal demyelinating encephalopathy are rare complications. Post-influenzal asthenia and depression are common, often marked, and may last for a week or two.

Treatment and Prevention. The patient should be kept in bed until the fever has subsided. A mild analgesic usually relieves the headache and backache. A linctus containing pholcodine or methadone may be used to suppress unproductive cough. The treatment of complications such as bronchitis and pneumonia is dealt with later.

Immunity is type-specific and if the antigenic constitution of a new strain can be detected early, a specific vaccine may give about 70% protection. Annual winter vaccination is recommended for patients suffering from chronic pulmonary, cardiac or renal disease.

ACUTE BRONCHITIS

Aetiology. This condition is an acute inflammation of the trachea and bronchi caused by pyogenic organisms such as *Strep. pneumoniae, H. influenzae* and, rarely, *Staph. pyogenes*. Infection by these organisms is a common sequel of coryza, influenza, measles and whooping-cough, and is particularly prone to develop in patients with chronic bronchitis.

Other factors predisposing to bacterial infection include cold, damp, foggy and dusty atmospheres and cigarette smoking.

Clinical Features. The first symptom is an irritating, unproductive cough accompanied by upper retrosternal discomfort or pain caused by tracheitis. When the bronchi become involved there is also a sensation of tightness in the chest, and dyspnoea with wheeze may be present. Respiratory distress may be particularly severe when acute bronchitis complicates chronic bronchitis and emphysema.

The sputum is at first scanty, mucoid, viscid and difficult to bring up, and occasionally may be streaked with blood. A day or two later it becomes mucopurulent and more copious. As the infection extends down the bronchial tree there may be a general febrile disturbance, with a temperature of 38–39°C and a neutrophil leucocytosis. In the vast majority of cases recovery takes place gradually over the next 4 to 8 days without the patient ever becoming seriously ill. Occasionally the dyspnoea and general symptoms increase in severity, cyanosis appears, and if the infection reaches the smaller bronchi and bronchioles ('bronchiolitis') the condition becomes indistinguishable from bronchopneumonia.

Tracheitis without bronchitis produces no abnormal physical signs. In bronchitis there is no impairment of chest wall movement or percussion note. The breath sounds are vesicular, or vesicular with prolonged expiration, and are accompanied by bilateral rhonchi and, occasionally, coarse crepitations.

The disease is usually mild and of short duration, the patient recovering within a few days if a suitable antibiotic is given. In severe cases it lasts longer, especially if bronchiolitis and bronchopneumonia develop.

Treatment. The patient should be confined to bed and oxytetracycline or ampicillin, 250–500 mg 4 times daily, given by mouth. Co-trimoxazole is equally effective in a dose of 2 tablets twice daily. In the early stages, when cough is painful and unproductive, the tough viscid secretion should be loosened by the inhalation 3 or 4 times a day of steam medicated with benzoin or menthol. A steam kettle or steam tent is more suitable for children. The cough should be controlled at night by pholcodine. If symptoms or signs of airflow obstruction are present a bronchodilator drug may be of some value. Oxygen is seldom required in uncomplicated acute bronchitis and antibacterial drugs may be unnecessary in mild cases.

THE PNEUMONIAS

Pneumonia is the term used to describe inflammation of the lung. There are many different kinds of pneumonia, some common, others rare. Aetiologically, they can be divided into the *primary pneumonias*, in which the disease is caused by a specific pathogenic organism, and the *secondary pneumonias*, in which some abnormality of the respiratory system predisposes to the invasion of the lung by organisms of relatively low virulence, and infection generally reaches the alveoli by aspiration from other parts of the respiratory tract.

In the secondary pneumonias, *H. influenzae*, some types of *Strep. pneumoniae* and certain of the bacteria forming the flora of the upper respiratory tract and mouth are the organisms most frequently cultured from the sputum.

In some types of primary and secondary pneumonia, prominent features are destruction of lung tissue by the inflammatory process, a high incidence of abscess formation and the subsequent development of pulmonary fibrosis and bronchiectasis. The term '*suppurative pneumonia*' has been applied to this group of cases and this condition merits separate description (p. 226).

THE PRIMARY PNEUMONIAS

Pneumococcal pneumonia, caused by *Strep. pneumoniae*, is the most common type of primary pneumonia. Other bacteria which may cause primary pneumonia include *Staph. pyogenes*, *Strep. pyogenes*, *Klebsiella pneumoniae*, *H. influenzae*, *Legionella pneumophila* and so-called small bacteria such as *Mycoplasma pneumoniae*, *Coxiella burnetii* and *Chlamydia psittaci* (psittacosis and ornithosis). Anaerobic organisms, including *Actinomyces israeli*, are rare causes of primary pneumonia. Primary viral pneumonia is most frequently due to influenza viruses in adults and to the respiratory syncytial virus in children.

Pneumococcal Pneumonia (Acute Lobar Pneumonia)

Pneumococcal pneumonia is characterised by homogeneous consolidation of one or more lobes or segments. The disease occurs at all ages but most frequently in early and middle adult life. The highest incidence is in winter. It is usually a sporadic disease, the mode of spread being by droplet infection.

Clinical Features. The onset is sudden, often with rigors, or with vomiting or a convulsion in children. The temperature rises in a few hours to 39–40°C. Malaise, loss of appetite, headache, and aching pains in the body and limbs accompany the pyrexia. Localised pain of pleural type develops at an early stage in the illness. It is generally referred to the chest wall but may on occasion be referred to the shoulder or to the abdominal wall.

There is a short, painful cough, dry at first but later productive of tenacious sputum which is often rust-coloured and occasionally frankly blood-stained. Respiration is rapid (30–40 per minute in adults, 50–60 in children), shallow and painful. The pulse is rapid, the skin is hot and dry, the face is flushed, and central cyanosis may be observed in severe cases. Herpes labialis is often present. A marked neutrophil leucocytosis is characteristic. *Strep. pneumoniae* can usually be isolated from the sputum, and a positive blood culture may be obtained.

Physical Signs in the Chest. In the first 24 to 48 hours of the illness, there is diminution of respiratory movement, slight impairment of the percussion note and often a pleural rub on the affected side. At a variable time after the onset, generally within 2 days, signs of consolidation appear (p. 212), the breath sounds being of the high-pitched bronchial type. When resolution begins, numerous coarse crepitations are heard, indicating liquefaction of the alveolar exudate. If a serous or purulent effusion develops, the physical signs of fluid in the pleural space are usually found, but often bronchial breath sounds persist and the presence of an effusion may be suspected only from stony dullness on percussion.

Radiological examination shows a homogeneous opacity localised to the affected lobe or segment, appearing within 12 to 18 hours of the onset of the illness. Radiological examination is particularly helpful when the diagnosis is in doubt or if a complication such as pleural effusion or empyema is suspected.

Course. Most cases respond promptly to chemotherapy and within a week the patient is well again. Delayed recovery suggests either that some complication such as empyema has developed or that the diagnosis is incorrect.

Other Types of Primary Pneumonia

Staphylococcal Pneumonia. Pneumonia due to *Staph. pyogenes* may occur either as a primary respiratory infection or as a blood-borne infection from a staphylococcal lesion elsewhere in the body, for example, osteomyelitis. The second condition is essentially one of pyaemic abscess formation in the lungs. Unless an empyema is produced by rupture of an abscess into the pleura, the pulmonary lesions may pass unnoticed, overshadowed by the severe general illness.

Primary staphylococcal pneumonia, although it occurs much less frequently than pneumococcal pneumonia, is a relatively common illness, especially as a complication of influenza. It may present as a lobar or segmental pneumonia, which may be difficult to distinguish clinically from a severe pneumococcal infection, or as a suppurative pneumonia (p. 226) with multiple lung abscesses which may persist as thin-walled cysts after the acute infection has subsided.

Culture of the sputum yields a growth of coagulase-positive staphylococci which are frequently resistant to benzylpenicillin, ampicillin, tetracycline and co-trimoxazole. At the present time, few-strains of staphylococci causing pneumonia are resistant to erythromycin, flucloxacillin, cephalosporins, gentamicin or sodium fusidate, but this relatively favourable situation may alter.

Klebsiella Pneumonia. Pneumonia due to *Kl. pneumoniae* is a rare disease with a high mortality. There is usually massive consolidation and excavation of one or more lobes, the upper lobes being most often involved, with profound systemic disturbance and the expectoration of large amounts of purulent sputum, sometimes chocolate-coloured. The diagnosis is made by the radiological appearances and the isolation of the causative organism from the sputum. It is usually sensitive to chloramphenicol, mezlocillin and cefotaxime.

Legionella pneumonia (legionnaires' disease) is caused by a bacillus which may be transmitted in water droplets from infected cisterns used to provide water for showers, particularly in warm climates. It is often a serious and occasionally a fatal illness, characterised by gastrointestinal symptoms, mental confusion, hyponatraemia and proteinuria as well as pneumonia. The organ is sensitive to erythromycin and rifampicin.

Actinomycosis. Formerly included amongst the fungal diseases, this is now regarded as a bacterial infection. It is caused by *A. israeli*, an anaerobic organism, which exists as a commensal in the mouth. When local defences are impaired, actinomycosis can cause cervicofacial, abdominal or, occasionally, pulmonary infection such as a widespread suppurative pneumonia (p. 226). Empyema, often bilateral and associated with persistent chest wall sinuses, may develop later, or occasionally *de novo*. The pus may contain 'sulphur granules'. Sinuses are also a feature of cervicofacial and abdominal infections.

Pneumonia caused by Viruses and Small Bacteria. A distinctive form of pneumonia may be produced by certain viruses, and also by small bacteria which exhibit a similar pathogenicity to lung tissue. The clinical picture differs from that of the bacterial pneumonias in that fever and toxaemia usually precede the respiratory symptoms by several days. Severe headache, malaise and anorexia are characteristic features in the early stages. The physical signs in the chest, if there are any, appear later and are seldom gross. The existence of a pulmonary lesion may not be recognised without a radiograph. The spleen may be palpable in the first week. The white blood count is generally normal and the pyrexia does not respond to penicillins. The diagnosis can often be confirmed by isolation of the causal organism or by serological tests.

The disease is usually self-limiting. The pyrexia subsides by lysis after 5 to 10 days, and complete recovery and radiographic resolution follow, the latter sometimes being slow. Very rarely, death takes place from widespread extension of the pneumonia or from viral encephalitis.

The *influenza, parainfluenza* and *measles* viruses rarely produce a specific pneumonia. The pneumonia caused by *chickenpox* virus, however, is usually characteristic. The radiograph shows numerous miliary nodular shadows which may eventually calcify. It occurs almost exclusively in adults. The *adenoviruses* cause occasional mild epidemics of specific pneumonia.

Respiratory syncytial virus is the most important respiratory pathogen of early childhood, especially in the first 2 months of life. This is because it causes bronchiolitis and pneumonia, and carries a risk of mortality. The infant is fevered, and cough, wheezy respiration and occasionally an erythematous rash are prominent features. The virus is not susceptible to any known therapy, and immunisation is ineffective.

Chlamydia psittaci causes psittacosis (ornithosis), a systemic illness contracted from infected birds. The pneumonia associated with it may be extensive, with severe toxaemia. Headache is a prominent early symptom.

Mycoplasma pneumoniae is a pleomorphic bacterium which is susceptible to tetracyclines though a few strains are sensitive only to erythromycin. Cold agglutinins (p. 513) can be demonstrated in a high proportion of cases. Antibodies can be detected, and haemagglutination and complement-fixation tests are available for diagnosis. Outbreaks of pneumonia caused by this organism are common in barracks and institutions. Most cases occur in children and young adults. Maculopapular rashes, haemolytic anaemia and meningoencephalitis occur rarely.

Coxiella (Rickettsia) burnetii is the organism responsible for *Q-fever*. Endocarditis may occur, as well as pneumonia, in this disease (p. 165).

Pneumonia due to Opportunistic Infections. Patients whose immunological defences have been compromised by disease, or by immunosuppressive, corticosteroid or prolonged antibiotic therapy, may develop pneumonia due to opportunist infections. The commonest causes are gram-negative bacilli (coliforms and *Ps. aeruginosa*), fungi (*Cryptococcus neoformans, Candida albicans* and *Aspergillus fumigatus*), viruses (cytomegaloviruses, herpes viruses) and protozoa (*Pneumocystis carinii*).

THE SECONDARY PNEUMONIAS

This group, sometimes described as 'nonspecific' or aspiration pneumonias, comprises a large number of different conditions, their common features being the absence of any specific pathogenic organism in the sputum and the existence of some abnormality of the respiratory system which predisposes to the invasion of the lung by organisms of relatively low virulence derived from the upper respiratory tract or from the mouth, for example, streptococci, certain types of pneumococci, *H. influenzae* and various species of anaerobic bacteria.

Infection may reach the lungs in various ways. Pus may be aspirated from an infected nasal sinus, or septic matter may be inhaled during tonsillectomy or dental extraction under general anaesthesia. Vomitus or the contents of a dilated oesophagus may enter the larynx during general anaesthesia, coma or even sleep. Infected secretion in the bronchi and pus from acute bronchitis, dilated bronchi or a lung abscess may also be carried into the alveoli by the air stream or by gravity.

Ineffective coughing caused by post-operative or post-traumatic thoracic or abdominal pain, by debility or immobility, or by laryngeal paralysis may also predispose to the development of secondary (aspiration) pneumonia.

Bronchial obstruction, partial or complete, as for example by a carcinoma, is another potential cause of secondary pneumonia, as it allows infection derived from the upper air passages to become established in the inadequately drained portion of lung beyond the obstruction.

Acute Bronchopneumonia

This type of aspiration pneumonia is invariably preceded by bronchial infection, which accounts for the widespread patchy distribution of the lesions. It occurs most frequently at the extremes of life, and may be described as 'hypostatic pneumonia' when it occurs in elderly or debilitated patients. In children, it is often a complication of measles or whooping cough, and in adults of acute bronchitis or influenza. It is particularly common in patients with chronic bronchitis.

Pathology. There is acute inflammation of the bronchi, especially the terminal bronchioles, which are filled with pus. Collapse and consolidation of the associated groups of alveoli follow. The lesions are distributed bilaterally in small patches which tend to become larger by confluence and are often more extensive in the lower lobes. The alveolar exudate consists of neutrophil leucocytes with a small amount of fibrin. There is interstitial oedema and cellular proliferation in the alveolar walls, and compensatory emphysema around the collapsed alveoli. Resolution of bronchopneumonia may be incomplete, and in such cases pulmonary fibrosis and bronchiectasis are common sequelae.

Clinical Features. After 2 or 3 days of acute bronchitis, as bronchopneumonia develops, the temperature rises to a higher level, the pulse and respiration rates increase, and dyspnoea and central cyanosis appear. There is generally a severe cough with purulent sputum. Pleural pain is relatively uncommon, in contrast to pneumococcal pneumonia.

During the early stages the physical signs are those of acute bronchitis but crepitations later become more numerous. In many cases, no signs of consolidation can be detected, until the lesions coalesce, when radiological examination shows mottled opacities in both lung fields, chiefly in the lower zones. A neutrophil leucocytosis is present.

Course and Complications. The disease is of more insidious onset and tends to run a more protracted course (up to 10 days) than pneumococcal pneumonia. Incomplete resolution may lead to bronchiectasis, but the number of patients developing this complication has fallen dramatically since antibiotics became available. The mortality is higher at the extremes of life, especially if the disease supervenes on chronic bronchitis and emphysema or any debilitating illness.

Prevention. The incidence of bronchopneumonia can be reduced by careful attention to apparently benign upper respiratory infections such as coryza and acute bronchitis, especially when they occur in children or elderly subjects and in patients with chronic bronchitis. Measures to prevent whooping cough and measles, and adequate treatment of those diseases, are also important in prophylaxis.

Benign Aspiration Pneumonia

This type of secondary pneumonia is due to the aspiration of infected secretion into the lungs during the course of an upper respiratory infection such as coryza or sinusitis. It is thus often associated with segmental pulmonary collapse. The organisms causing the pneumonia, being derived from the upper respiratory tract, are generally of low virulence and the degree of systemic disturbance is usually slight. In fact, the symptoms are often no more severe than would be expected with an uncomplicated upper respiratory infection and the existence of a pneumonia may be discovered only by radiological examination.

As a rule, however, the condition manifests itself by cough, purulent sputum, low-grade pyrexia and sometimes pleural pain, in association with a frank upper respiratory infection. Localised coarse crepitations are often the only abnormal physical finding. A neutrophil leucocytosis is usually present. The radiological lesions are typically unilateral, the characteristic appearance being a mottled opacity involving a single lobe or segment, which in some cases may be collapsed.

The condition is liable to be confused with viral pneumonia, but the coexistent upper respiratory infection and the minimal systemic upset are useful distinguishing features. Pulmonary tuberculosis may be erroneously diagnosed on the basis of a single radiograph. Re-examination 10 to 14 days later, following treatment with an antibiotic, will clarify the diagnosis as resolution is generally rapid in aspiration pneumonia.

Suppurative Pneumonia (Including Pulmonary Abscess)

Suppurative pneumonia is the term used to describe a form of pneumonic consolidation in which there is destruction of lung parenchyma by the inflammatory process. Although microabscess formation is a characteristic histological feature of suppurative pneumonia, it is usual to restrict the term 'pulmonary abscess' to lesions in which there is a fairly large localised collection of pus, or a cavity lined by chronic inflammatory tissue, from which pus has ruptured into a bronchus.

Suppurative pneumonia and pulmonary abscess may be produced by infection of previously healthy lung tissue with *Staph. pyogenes* or *Kl. pneumoniae*. These are, in effect, primary bacterial pneumonias associated with pulmonary suppuration. More frequently, suppurative pneumonia and pulmonary abscess are forms of secondary pneumonia. They may develop after the inhalation of septic material during operations on the nose, mouth or throat under general anaesthesia, or of vomitus during anaesthesia or coma.

In such circumstances gross oral sepsis may be an important predisposing factor. Bacterial infection of a pulmonary infarct or of a collapsed lobe, may also produce a suppurative pneumonia or a pulmonary abscess. The organisms isolated from the sputum may include *Strep. pneumoniae*, *Staph. pyogenes*, *Strep. pyogenes*, *H. influenzae*, and in a few cases, anaerobic bacteria. In some cases, however, no pathogens can be isolated, particularly when antibiotics have been given.

Clinical Features. These depend to a large extent on the pathogenesis of the lesion. The onset of the illness may be either insidious or acute, but cough with purulent sputum, usually large in amount, sometimes fetid and occasionally blood-stained, is present from an early stage. There is high, remittent pyrexia with shivering and sweating, and a neutrophil leucocytosis. Pleural pain is common and clubbing of the fingers may develop as early as 10 to 14 days after the onset of the illness. Progressive deterioration in general health with marked loss of weight ensues if the patient remains untreated. The rupture of a large abscess into a bronchus can be assumed when a large quantity of pus is suddenly expectorated. Such an incident is often preceded by blood-staining of the sputum and followed by remission of the pyrexia.

Physical signs in the chest also depend on the nature of the primary pathological process. Signs of consolidation (p. 212) are the most frequent; signs of cavitation are rarely found. A pleural rub is often present.

Radiological Examination. There is a homogeneous lobar or segmental opacity consistent with consolidation or collapse. A large, dense opacity, which may later cavitate and show a fluid level within it, is the characteristic finding when a frank pulmonary abscess is present.

Course and Prognosis. In most cases, there is a good response to antibacterial therapy (p. 229), and although residual fibrosis and bronchiectasis are common sequelae, these seldom give rise to serious morbidity. Empyema (p. 272) may complicate the acute phase of the disease.

Prevention. Every precaution should be taken during operations on the mouth, nose and throat to prevent the inhalation of blood, tonsillar fragments, etc. Oral sepsis should be eradicated, especially if a general anaesthetic is contemplated.

Investigation of Pneumonia

An attempt should always be made to establish a positive microbiological diagnosis, though this is not always possible, particularly if antibiotics have been given before specimens are submitted for examination. Direct smear examination of *sputum* by Gram and Ziehl-Neelsen stains may give an immediate indication of possible pathogens, and indicate what treatment should be prescribed. Culture (including anaerobic culture where indicated) and sensitivity testing should be carried out.

Where a microbiological diagnosis is essential, as in severely ill immunosuppressed patients, and a specimen of sputum cannot be obtained, an attempt should be made to aspirate secretions or washings from the trachea or bronchi either by bronchoscopy or by inserting a needle through the cricothyroid membrane. Transthoracic lung puncture has been advocated if the other techniques are unsuccessful, but carries the risk of producing a pneumothorax, which may have lethal consequences in dangerously ill patients.

Blood culture should be performed in patients with severe pneumonia, and may yield a positive result when sputum examination is negative, particularly in pneumococcal pneumonia. Pneumococcal antigen may also be detected in serum.

Serological tests may be helpful, specimens being examined at 10-day intervals for viral titres. A four-fold rise suggests recent infection. Nose and throat swabs, and post-nasal and bronchial aspirates, can be cultured for viruses or examined by immunofluorescence or electron microscopy.

The *total and differential white blood count* is often below $5 \cdot 0 \times 10^9/l$ in patients with viral infection, and a high neutrophil polymorph leucocytosis favours bacterial infection. The ESR is usually elevated, but is of no help in diagnosis.

Arterial blood gas studies are of vital importance in all patients who are seriously ill and in those with a previous history of chronic respiratory disease. It is impossible to make any rational decisions on oxygen therapy unless the Pao_2 and $Paco_2$ and the hydrogen ion concentration or pH of arterial blood are known.

Radiological examination is essential for confirmation of the diagnosis and for the early detection of complications such as pleural effusion and empyema. Follow-up radiological examination is important, because if a pneumonia fails to resolve, it may be secondary to bronchial obstruction by a carcinoma.

Transbronchial lung biopsy or *microscopical examination* of *bronchial brushings* or *washings* are the only means of confirming a diagnosis of *Pneumocystis carinii* pneumonia.

Complications of Pneumonia

Pulmonary: in most cases, the abnormal physical signs disappear within 2 weeks and the radiographic opacity within 4 weeks. Although resolution is occasionally delayed for longer periods, and may be incomplete, particularly in patients with suppurative pneumonia, this is always an indication for further investigation, including bronchoscopic examination. Bronchiectasis is a common complication of suppurative pneumonia.

Pleural: spread of the infection to the pleura may occur, with the development of a sterile pleural effusion or empyema. Staphylococcal lung abscess may be complicated by pyopneumothorax.

Cardiovascular: these are acute circulatory failure (due to bacteraemia), acute pericarditis and rarely endocarditis.

Neurological: meningism is not uncommon in children and lumbar puncture may be required to distinguish it from meningitis. Pneumococcal meningitis is rare. Mental confusion may be a prominent feature of legionnaires' disease.

Differential Diagnosis of Pneumonia

The following conditions may be difficult to distinguish from pneumonia:

Pulmonary infarction, in which pyrexia is less marked and is uninfluenced by antibiotics, frank haemoptysis is common, cough is inconspicuous and the source of an embolus can be identified in some cases.

Tuberculous pleurisy with effusion, in which the correct diagnosis can usually be suspected from the insidious onset, the virtual absence of cough and sputum, the physical signs of pleural effusion, the absence of leucocytosis, the failure of the pyrexia to respond to antibiotics, the radiological findings and the aspiration of serous fluid, in which lymphocytes predominate, from the pleural space.

Pulmonary tuberculosis, acute cases of which may simulate pneumonia. The patient is, however, seldom as acutely ill as in other specific pneumonias, it is uncommon for the respiratory rate to be markedly increased and the white blood count is seldom above $12.0 \times 10^9/l$. The diagnosis can usually be made by radiological examination, and the isolation of tubercle bacilli puts it beyond doubt.

Pulmonary oedema, which may be difficult to distinguish from pneumonia. If fever is present, pneumonia is the more likely diagnosis, but where there is any doubt, both an antibiotic and a diuretic should be given.

Inflammatory conditions below the diaphragm, such as cholecystitis, perforated duodenal ulcer, acute appendicitis, subphrenic abscess, generalised peritonitis, acute pancreatitis and hepatic amoebiasis, which may occasionally be mistaken for pneumonia. A carefully taken history is one of the most valuable means of determining the site and nature of the primary disease. A high temperature and a rapid respiration rate favour a diagnosis of pneumonia, whereas tenderness of the abdominal wall suggests that the primary lesion is below the diaphragm. Sometimes radiological examination of the chest is necessary before the presence of pneumonia can be confirmed or excluded.

Treatment of Pneumonia

Antimicrobial Therapy. The principles governing the specific treatment of bacterial infections of the respiratory tract have already been stated (p. 214). The appropriate therapy in relation to the various aetiological agents is shown in Table 8.4.

When a clinical diagnosis of pneumonia is made, provided the patient is not gravely ill, the initial treatment should consist of ampicillin, 500 mg four times daily, or co-trimoxazole, 2 tablets twice daily. Patients who are gravely ill and in whom a staphylococcal or a Gram-negative infection is suspected, should receive, in addition to ampicillin by intravenous injection, antibiotics to which the causative organism is unlikely to be resistant, for example, flucloxacillin, 250 mg 6-hourly by intravenous injection, and gentamicin, 2–5 mg/kg daily in divided doses 8-hourly by intramuscular or intravenous injection.

Table 8.4 Treatment of pneumonia with antimicrobial agents

Organism	Choice of drug
Streptococcus pneumoniae	benzylpenicillin, ampicillin
Haemophilus influenzae	ampicillin, co-trimoxazole
Staphylococcus pyogenes	benzylpenicillin *plus* flucloxacillin; gentamicin, cefuroxime, sodium fusidate.
Klebsiella pneumoniae	chloramphenicol, mezlocillin, cefotaxime
Proteus mirabilis	ampicillin, co-trimoxazole
Pseudomonas pyocyanea	ticarcillin, azlocillin, ceftazidine
Mycoplasma pneumoniae	oxytetracycline, erythromycin
Coxiella burnetii	oxytetracycline, erythromycin
Chlamydia psittaci	oxytetracycline, erythromycin
Legionella pneumophila	erythromycin, rifampicin
Anaerobes	benzylpenicillin, metronidazole, clindamycin

1. If *Strep. pneumoniae, Strep. pyogenes* or *H. influenzae* is isolated, or no pathogenic organisms are reported on culture, and the patient appears to be making satisfactory clinical progress, treatment with ampicillin or co-trimoxazole should be continued, but the dose of ampicillin can be reduced to 250 mg 6-hourly.

2. If *Staph. pyogenes* is isolated, treatment must be modified in accordance with the results of sensitivity tests. Resistance to penicillin may be due to the production of penicillinase, and such infections can usually be controlled by a combination of benzylpenicillin (600 mg b.d.) and flucloxacillin (250–500 mg 6-hourly) by intravenous or intramuscular injection. In other cases sodium fusidate (500 mg t.i.d.) by mouth, or gentamicin (80 mg) or cefuroxime (750 mg) 8-hourly by intramuscular or intravenous injection, may be indicated. There may be an advantage in combining two of these drugs.

3. If an anaerobic bacterial infection is suspected from fetor of the sputum, a combination of benzylpenicillin and metronidazole should be given.

4. If *Actinomyces israeli* is isolated, benzylpenicillin is given by intravenous infusion in a dose of 5 g daily.

5. If bacteriological examination is uninformative and there is no neutrophil leucocytosis in the blood, the pneumonia may be due to *Coxiella burnetii, Mycoplasma pneumoniae* or *Chlamydia psittaci*. In these circumstances, tetracycline, 500 mg four times daily is recommended. Erythromycin, 1 g four times daily should be given if infection with *Legionella pneumophila* is suspected. Pneumonia caused by viruses does not respond to antibiotic therapy.

6. If recovery is progressing satisfactorily, the isolation of an organism showing *in vitro* resistance to the antibiotic in use is not necessarily an indication for a change in treatment. If, however, the patient is not improving and is still febrile when such an organism is isolated, an appropriate change in antibiotic is imperative.

The impulse to substitute another antibiotic, where there is no bacteriological indication for doing so, should be resisted. The failure of patients to respond to treatment may be due to pleural infection, tuberculosis or bronchial obstruction by a tumour, and these conditions must be excluded before the antibiotic is changed.

7. No definite rule can be laid down for the duration of chemotherapy. In most cases of uncomplicated pneumococcal pneumonia, a 7-day course of treatment is usually adequate but this may have to be extended if the response to treatment is slow. In staphylococcal and klebsiella pneumonia, and in other forms of suppurative pneumonia, chemotherapy should be continued for a minimum of 2 weeks and should not be stopped until the causative organism has been eliminated from the sputum.

General Measures. The usual regimen of treatment for an acute infection should be instituted and attention paid to hydration, oral hygiene and care of the skin. If respiratory distress is marked the patient should be propped up comfortably with pillows or a backrest.

Cough, when distressing and unproductive, should be controlled by the measures described on page 219. When secretions are present in the bronchi the patient should be firmly encouraged to cough up sputum, even if the effort to do so causes pleural pain. In these circumstances an analgesic and the support of a nurse's hand on the painful side of the chest may relieve the distress of coughing. Postural drainage is of value if the sputum is difficult to bring up, particularly if it is copious, as in suppurative pneumonia, or when pneumonia complicates bronchiectasis. Skilled physiotherapy may be invaluable.

Pleural pain should be treated with analgesics (p. 219). It is, however, dangerous to prescribe morphine if even a mild degree of ventilatory insufficiency is present, and probably the safest policy is not to use this drug at all in the treatment of pneumonia.

Hypoxia demands oxygen therapy (p. 214).

Delirium, which in the early stages is caused mainly by the high temperature, and later by cerebral hypoxia, may have to be controlled by sedation. The safest drug to use is diazepam (5–10 mg i.m.).

Bacteraemic shock (p. 50) carries a high mortality and admission to an intensive therapy unit affords the best prospect of survival. The three most important therapeutic measures are (1) the administration of appropriate antibiotics in high dosage, (2) the maintenance of oxygenation, if necessary by tracheal intubation and intermittent positive-pressure ventilation, and (3) restoration of the depleted circulating blood volume by intravenous infusion of a 5% glucose solution, dextran or plasma, monitored by measurements of central venous pressure. Massive doses of intravenous hydrocortisone (3 g per day or more) have been advocated, but this treatment is of doubtful value.

Abscess Formation. Suppurative pneumonia is not in itself a reason for any departure from standard antibiotic policy. When an abscess cavity is present, however, it must be kept empty by regular postural drainage. Medical treatment is almost invariably successful and surgical measures nowadays are seldom required. In occasional instances, however, a large abscess may have to be drained externally or residual bronchiectasis resected.

TUBERCULOSIS

Although tuberculosis is a problem of rapidly diminishing proportions in Western Europe and North America, it remains, in the words of a WHO report: 'the most important specific communicable disease in the world'. As the disease decreases in frequency there is a tendency for tuberculosis to be overlooked.

Aetiology. Three types of mycobacteria are responsible for the disease in man: (1) *Myco. tuberculosis* (human type) — now the cause of almost all infections in man; (2) *Myco. bovis* — endemic in cattle, but now rarely responsible for disease in man, and (3) the *atypical* or *opportunistic* mycobacteria. The clinical importance of the last group of organisms lies in their ability to cause infection in cervical lymph nodes in children and, rarely, pulmonary disease in adults, when treatment may be a problem because the mycobacteria are primarily resistant to many drugs.

Entry of the tubercle bacillus into the body by the alimentary or respiratory tract is not necessarily followed by a clinical illness, the development of which is dependent on several other factors. Those of most practical importance are:

Age and Sex. In Europe and America, tuberculosis used to affect predominantly the young people in the community, especially females, but there has been a radical change in the age and sex incidence. Twenty years ago, 80% of notifications were of patients under 45 years of age, but nowadays 60% of patients are over that age, males predominating. This change is important in case-finding.

Natural Resistance. Susceptibility to tuberculosis is not inherited in the strict sense of the word, but the fact that certain races, and even certain regional groups, such as the inhabitants of the Western Isles of Scotland and of Ireland, are more prone to develop tuberculosis suggests that natural resistance varies from race to race and even from region to region. The natural resistance of a community tends to rise as the period of exposure to tuberculosis increases. Immigrants to Britain from Asia are more prone to have the disease than the indigenous population, and tend to have more florid types of the disease.

Standard of Living. The prevalence of tuberculosis diminishes as social and economic conditions improve. Poor housing with associated overcrowding increases the risk of massive infection or reinfection if one of the occupants suffers from infectious tuberculosis.

Conditions Affecting Individual Patients. Diabetes mellitus, gastrectomy and silicosis all predispose to the development of tuberculosis, as does treatment with corticosteroids or immunosuppressive drugs.

Pathology. The initial *'primary'* tuberculous

infection usually occurs in the lung but occasionally in the tonsil or in the alimentary tract, especially the ileocaecal region. The primary infection differs from later infections in that the primary focus in lung, tonsil or bowel is almost invariably accompanied by caseous lesions in the regional lymph nodes, i.e. in the mediastinal, cervical or mesenteric groups respectively.

In most people the primary infection and the associated lymph node lesions heal and calcify. In a few, healing, particularly in lymph nodes, is incomplete and surviving tubercle bacilli may under certain circumstances, such as a lowering of the general health or a disturbance of cell mediated immunity, be discharged into the blood stream. Such patients may in consequence develop tuberculous lesions elsewhere. The most common sites for 'haematogenous' lesions of this kind are the lungs, bones, joints and kidneys. Such lesions may develop months or even years after the primary infection.

The primary infection may in some cases fail to heal. A primary pulmonary lesion, particularly when it occurs during adolescence or early adult life, may lead to progressive pulmonary tuberculosis. A tuberculous mediastinal lymph node, in children especially, may compress a lobar or segmental bronchus (rarely a main bronchus) and produce pulmonary collapse. Occasionally the node may ulcerate through the bronchial wall and discharge caseous material into the lumen, with the production of acute tuberculous lesions in the related lobe or segment. Infection may also be carried by lymphatics from tuberculous mediastinal lymph nodes to the pleura or pericardium with the production of tuberculous pleurisy or pericarditis. Comparable complications may occur when the primary lesion is in the tonsil or gut, e.g. 'cold abscess' of the neck or tuberculous peritonitis.

Rarely, a caseous tuberculous focus either at the site of the primary infection or, more commonly, in an associated lymph node ruptures into a vein and produces acute dissemination of the disease throughout the body, a condition known as *acute miliary tuberculosis*. Tuberculous meningitis often complicates this condition.

Progressive pulmonary tuberculosis may develop directly from a primary lesion or it may occur later, following reactivation of an incompletely healed primary focus in the lung or as a result of haematogenous dissemination from an unhealed lymph node lesion. Alternatively it may be the result of reinfection from an outside source after the primary focus has healed completely.

All these forms of pulmonary tuberculosis, although differing in pathogenesis, have similar pathological features and can be grouped together under the term *postprimary pulmonary tuberculosis*. The characteristic pathological feature of this condition is the tuberculous cavity, which forms when the caseated and liquefied centre of a tuberculous pulmonary lesion is discharged into a bronchus. Extension of the infection to the pleura either by direct or lymphatic spread causes tuberculous pleurisy, which is sometimes accompanied by effusion and is occasionally followed by the development of a tuberculous empyema. Bloodborne dissemination to other organs is uncommon in postprimary pulmonary tuberculosis.

Clinical Features. There are two groups of clinical features in tuberculosis:

1. Those due to the systemic effects of the disease, which include lassitude and malaise, impairment of appetite, loss of weight, anaemia, sweating especially during sleep, tachycardia and pyrexia. The last is usually most marked in the late afternoon or evening and sometimes occurs only at these times. The absence of symptoms does not necessarily mean that the disease is inactive.

2. Those caused by the local effects of the tuberculous lesions, which are summarised below according to anatomical site:

Lungs and bronchi: cough, sputum, haemoptysis, dyspnoea.

Pleura: pleural pain, dyspnoea due to pleural effusion.

Larynx: hoarseness, with dysphagia at a later stage from involvement of pharynx.

Tongue: ulceration (rare).

Intestine: diarrhoea, malabsorption or intestinal obstruction.

Peritoneum: ascites, recurrent intestinal obstruction due to plastic peritonitis.

Pericardium: pericardial effusion, constrictive pericarditis later.

Kidneys and bladder: haematuria, increased frequency of micturition. These are relatively late developments, early renal lesions being symptomless.

Epididymis: painless craggy swelling, sinus formation later.

Fallopian tubes: salpingitis, tubal abscess, infertility.

Brain: tuberculoma with or without focal neurological signs.

Meninges: headache, neck stiffness.

Lymph nodes: enlargement of nodes, often with 'cold' abscess and sinus formation later.

Adrenal glands: Addison's disease.

Bones and joints: arthritis, osteomyelitis, 'cold' abscesses.

Skin: lupus vulgaris, erythema nodosum.

Eyes: phlyctenular keratoconjunctivitis, iridocyclitis, choroiditis.

In the sections which follow an account is given of those manifestations of tuberculosis which involve the lungs, namely primary pulmonary tuberculosis, acute miliary tuberculosis and post primary pulmonary tuberculosis. In some cases the pleura is also involved. For information regarding other manifestations of tuberculosis the reader should refer to appropriate sections of the book. The treatment and prevention of tuberculosis are dealt with on pages 236–240.

Primary Pulmonary Tuberculosis

The pathological features of this type of tuberculosis have been described on page 230. The primary infection usually occurs in childhood but is sometimes delayed until adult life. A history of contact with a case of active pulmonary tuberculosis is obtained in many instances.

Clinical Features. In the vast majority of patients the primary infection produces no symptoms or signs and passes unnoticed unless routine radiological examination of the chest happens to be carried out at the appropriate time or serial tuberculin tests show conversion from negative to positive.

In a few patients the primary infection produces a febrile illness. It is generally mild and

lasts for no more than 7 to 14 days, but it may be accompanied by other systemic features of tuberculous infection. It is unusual for gross focal symptoms or signs to develop in an uncomplicated case, but a slight dry cough is occasionally present. The leucocyte count is usually normal but the ESR is raised.

The primary infection may be accompanied by *erythema nodosum*. This condition is characterised by bluish-red, raised, tender cutaneous lesions on the shins and, less commonly, on the thighs, and is associated in some cases with pyrexia and polyarthralgia. Erythema nodosum may be the first clinical indication of a tuberculous infection. In such cases the tuberculin reaction (below) is always strongly positive and evidence of primary tuberculosis can usually be detected on the chest radiograph. Erythema nodosum may, however, be seen in conditions other than primary tuberculosis, e.g. sarcoidosis, streptococcal infections and drug reactions. It may also occur as an isolated phenomenon without apparent cause.

Occasionally the primary pulmonary infection pursues a progressive course (p. 231). Symptoms and signs due to its complications may appear either during the course of the initial illness or after a latent interval of weeks or months. Such complications include dry pleurisy or pleural effusion (p. 270), lobar or segmental collapse (p. 259), acute miliary tuberculosis (p. 233), tuberculous meningitis (p. 638), and postprimary pulmonary tuberculosis (p. 234).

Investigation. The three most valuable diagnostic investigations in primary pulmonary tuberculosis are:

1. *Radiological Examination of the Chest*. In children this usually shows unilateral enlargement of the hilar lymph nodes and demonstrates the primary intrapulmonary lesion if it is large enough to be visible radiologically. In adolescents and young adults the lymph node component of the primary complex is usually less conspicuous than in children and the pulmonary lesion more prominent. Complications such as pleural effusion, lobar or segmental collapse and acute pulmonary tuberculosis may be superimposed.

2. *Tuberculin Test*. With the Mantoux technique a solution of Old Tuberculin or purified protein derivative (PPD) tuberculin is injected

intradermally on the flexor aspect of the forearm. The test is regarded as positive if, 2 to 4 days after injection, there is a reaction consisting of a raised area of inflammatory oedema not less than 5 mm in diameter, with surrounding erythema. The test is regarded as negative if there is no reaction or if there is an immediate (non-specific) reaction which disappears completely within 48 hours.

The test should first be carried out with 1 tuberculin unit (TU) in 0·1 ml of normal saline. If there is no reaction it should be repeated with 10 TU in the same volume of saline. In order to obtain accurate results it is essential to use freshly prepared dilutions of tuberculin. Differential tuberculin testing with antigens prepared from other mycobacteria, e.g. PPD-A (*Myco. avium*) or PPD-Y (*Myco. kansasii*) is often a satisfactory method of distinguishing atypical mycobacterial infection from tuberculosis.

The younger the patient the greater is the diagnostic significance of a positive tuberculin test. A repeatedly negative test over a period of 6 weeks from the onset of symptoms practically rules out a diagnosis of tuberculosis except in the elderly, after acute exanthemata, in the later stages of miliary tuberculosis and tuberculous meningitis and in patients taking immunosuppressive drugs. The tuberculin test is almost invariably negative in patients with hilar and mediastinal lymph node enlargement caused by sarcoidosis.

Tuberculin testing is an essential part of the examination of the family contacts of cases of tuberculosis. Apart from its value as a diagnostic measure it indicates which of the contacts should be vaccinated with BCG. When large numbers are being tested, particularly children, a *multiple puncture technique*, which is quick and almost painless, is preferable to the Mantoux test. A disposable tine test unit should be used for this purpose. It has four prongs ('tines') 2 mm in length mounted on a disc and coated with Old Tuberculin. If firmly pressed on the skin of the forearm, it yields results as reliable as those obtained with the Heaf unit which, being difficult to sterilise, may carry some risk of transmitting hepatitis.

The test should be read after 3 days and the following four grades of positivity are recognised:

Grade   I: One or two faint papules
      II: Four discrete papules
      III: The area encircled by the papules is completely indurated.
      IV: Any reaction which is greater than III, including central necrosis.

Reaction in grades III and IV indicates infection with mammalian tubercle bacilli and a grade I reaction may indicate infection with atypical mycobacteria. The significance of a grade II reaction is uncertain.

3. *Bacteriological Examination*. Sputum is seldom available in cases of primary pulmonary tuberculosis, but tubercle bacilli can sometimes be isolated by culture of fasting gastric washings or of secretion obtained by swabbing the larynx. At least three specimens should be examined. The isolation of tubercle bacilli is absolute proof of the diagnosis, but a negative result does not exclude it.

Prognosis. Since primary pulmonary tuberculosis and its complications respond satisfactorily to antituberculosis chemotherapy (p. 236), which should be given in every case, the prognosis is excellent.

Miliary Tuberculosis

The pathogenesis of this condition has already been discussed. Hitherto it has occurred chiefly in children and young adults. With the changing age-structure of tuberculosis in many countries it is now affecting persons in older age groups in whom it takes the form of an insidious illness — the so-called 'cryptic' type — which is often difficult to diagnose. Before the introduction of chemotherapy the disease was invariably fatal but most patients now recover completely.

Clinical Features. The disease may start suddenly or may be preceded by a few weeks of vague ill-health. In children and young adults the systemic disturbance rapidly becomes profound. In particular there is high remittent or intermittent pyrexia with drenching sweats during sleep, marked tachycardia, loss of weight and usually progressive anaemia. Cough and dyspnoea are occasionally present. There may be no abnormal physical signs in the lungs, although widespread fine crepitations may be heard at later stages of the disease. The liver is often enlarged and the spleen may be palpable and sometimes tender. Choroidal tubercles may be visible on ophthalmoscopy but are rarely present in acute miliary disease affecting the elderly. Leucocytosis is usually absent or slight. If chemotherapy is not given the patient's condition deteriorates rapidly and death takes place from exhaustion or from tuberculous meningitis within weeks.

'Cryptic' miliary tuberculosis occurs in older age groups, particularly females. Lassitude and eventual exhaustion, loss of weight, and anaemia are common presenting features. Respiratory symptoms are rare, and the characteristic miliary shadows are absent. Choroidal tubercles are not observed in this form of the disease. A variety of specific blood disorders — neutropenia, pancytopenia and leukaemoid reaction — may be found. The clinical features are often so non-specific that the diagnosis is frequently made only at autopsy.

Investigation. The diagnosis of acute miliary tuberculosis can be made with confidence only when radiological examination of the chest shows the characteristic fine 'miliary' mottling symmetrically distributed throughout both lung fields or when choroidal tubercles are seen. These changes take a few weeks to develop but the diagnosis can often be suspected at an earlier stage by the symptoms, progressive clinical deterioration, persistent pyrexia and splenomegaly.

Bacteriological confirmation should be sought by culture of sputum, urine or bone-marrow. In difficult cases, liver biopsy may be diagnostic. Although the tuberculin reaction is usually positive, a negative result does not always exclude acute miliary tuberculosis, as tuberculin sensitivity is occasionally depressed in the later stages of the illness.

In patients suspected to have the cryptic form of miliary tuberculosis a therapeutic trial of chemotherapy with ethambutol and isoniazid (p. 237) is indicated; if the diagnosis is correct, clinical improvement is usually evident within 10 days.

Prognosis. Antituberculosis chemotherapy (p. 236) has reduced the mortality of miliary tuberculosis from 100% to less than 5%. The cause of death is often tuberculous meningitis, although many patients who develop this complication make a complete recovery, provided there has been no delay in starting treatment.

Postprimary Pulmonary Tuberculosis

Most of the morbidity and mortality from tuberculosis is caused by this form of the disease. Although in developing countries it is most prevalent in adolescence and early adult life, the majority of cases in Western Europe and North America now occur in middle-aged and elderly subjects, particularly males.

The lesions are most frequently situated in the upper lobes. Another common site is the apex of a lower lobe. The disease is often bilateral; usually it starts in one lung and spreads via the bronchi to the other. Less commonly it develops in both lungs at the same time. Occasionally, when the disease takes an acute form, a whole lobe may be consolidated.

Clinical Features. The onset of postprimary pulmonary tuberculosis is usually insidious, with the gradual development of general symptoms or of cough and sputum. Sometimes a dramatic incident such as haemoptysis, pleural pain or a spontaneous pneumothorax marks the onset of the disease, but the diagnosis is now frequently made by radiography before any symptoms have appeared.

The following respiratory symptoms may occur during the course of post-primary tuberculosis:

(a) Cough may be one of the earliest symptoms or may not be troublesome until a late stage. Its absence does not exclude a diagnosis of pulmonary tuberculosis.

(b) Sputum, like cough, may not become a prominent feature until the disease has reached an advanced stage. It is usually mucoid at first but later becomes purulent. It is rarely fetid.

(c) Haemoptysis, in the early stages, is due to the erosion of a small vessel in a caseating lesion and the bleeding is usually slight. In the late stages it can originate from a large vessel in the wall of a cavity and haemorrhage may be large, occasionally fatal.

(d) Dyspnoea on exertion is usually a late symptom, but may develop acutely when due to a spontaneous pneumothorax or to a rapidly developing pleural effusion.

(e) Pleural pain is usually due to dry pleurisy but occasionally to spontaneous pneumothorax.

At first, no abnormal physical signs may be

present, but despite this an extensive lesion may be visible radiologically. The earliest physical signs consist of a few medium or coarse crepitations, usually situated over one or other lung apex posteriorly. These crepitations may be present only after coughing.

As the disease advances the percussion note over the site of the lesion loses its normal resonance, there is a change in the character of the breath sounds, which may become bronchial, and numerous coarse crepitations appear. Ultimately, physical signs of consolidation, cavitation and fibrosis may develop (Table 8.1), and occasionally those of pleurisy, with or without effusion, or spontaneous pneumothorax.

Radiological Examination. This is of paramount importance for diagnosis in the early stages before physical signs appear and for assessment of the extent and progress of the disease.

The earliest radiological change is an ill-defined opacity or opacities, usually situated in one of the upper lobes. In more advanced cases opacities are larger and more widespread, and may be bilateral. Occasionally there is a dense, homogeneous shadow involving a whole lobe ('pneumonic tuberculosis'). An area or areas of translucency within the opacities indicates cavitation. Very large cavities may be visible in some cases. When the infection is controlled the opacities shrink, become more clearly defined, and may later show calcification. When fibrosis is marked the trachea and heart shadow are displaced towards the side of the lesion.

In any case of tuberculosis it is common for lesions at different stages of development to coexist. Thus in one area there may be cavitation, in a second evidence of fibrosis and in a third an opacity due to recent disease.

The presence of cavitation in an untreated case usually indicates that the disease is active. When cavitation is absent, however, it may sometimes be difficult to assess the activity of a tuberculous lesion from a single radiograph. Observation of the lesion over a period of time will be necessary in doubtful cases.

The radiological appearances of pleural effusion and pneumothorax, which may accompany those of pulmonary tuberculosis, are described on pages 270 and 275.

Diagnosis. The symptoms and signs suggesting a diagnosis of tuberculosis have already been stated. The grounds on which pulmonary tuberculosis should be suspected are: (1) unexplained cough persisting for more than three weeks; (2) haemoptysis; (3) pleural pain not associated with an acute illness; (4) spontaneous pneumothorax (although most cases are not caused by tuberculosis); (5) unexplained tiredness or loss of weight, even in the absence of respiratory symptoms.

The presence of any of these symptoms demands immediate radiological examination of the lungs and, if an abnormality is found, the examination of at least three specimens of sputum for tubercle bacilli. When bacilli are numerous, the diagnosis can readily be made by microscopical examination of sputum smears stained by the Ziehl-Neelsen method, but culture of sputum (or fasting gastric washings or laryngeal swabs, if no sputum can be obtained) is essential for the isolation of bacilli present in small numbers and for the detection of drug resistance (p. 238). Cultural methods are thus of great practical value and should be used in the examination of every specimen, if facilities permit.

In the vast majority of cases the diagnosis of pulmonary tuberculosis can be made with confidence by radiological examination of the chest, bacteriological examination of the sputum for tubercle bacilli, or a combination of the two. In some cases it is necessary to carry out further radiological examination after a course of treatment with an antibiotic, such as ampicillin, in order to exclude an acute inflammatory cause for an abnormal shadow.

Active pulmonary tuberculosis should be suspected if one or more of the following features is present:

1. Local or general symptoms, particularly haemoptysis or pleural pain
2. A radiological opacity known or suspected to be of recent development, or one which has increased in extent during a period of observation
3. Radiological evidence of cavitation

The isolation of tubercle bacilli from sputum, gastric washings or laryngeal swabs confirms that the disease is active and requires treatment.

Complications

Pleurisy with or without effusion (p. 269).

236 PRINCIPLES AND PRACTICE OF MEDICINE

Spontaneous pneumothorax may be due to rupture of a tuberculous lesion into the pleural space (p. 274).

Tuberculous empyema or pyopneumothorax (p. 275) may complicate spontaneous pneumothorax.

Tuberculous laryngitis usually occurs as a complication of advanced pulmonary disease.

Tuberculous enteritis is practically confined to advanced cases. It is due to the swallowing of heavily infected sputum.

Ischiorectal abscess and fistula-in-ano. The abscess forms as a result of tubercle bacilli passing through the rectal mucosa. Secondary pyogenic infection invariably occurs, and a fistula may form when the abscess is incised or if it ruptures spontaneously.

Dissemination of tuberculosis via the blood stream is very unusual in post-primary pulmonary tuberculosis, but may occur in advanced cases with the production of renal tuberculosis or tuberculous meningitis.

Respiratory failure (p. 210) and *right ventricular failure* (p. 255) are important late complications if extensive areas of lung tissue are destroyed by tuberculosis or were resected when surgery was the only effective treatment. Although the tuberculous infection itself can be controlled, the residual pulmonary damage it has caused may leave the patient seriously disabled by exertional dyspnoea.

Secondary infection of a healed cavity with fungi such as *Aspergillus fumigatus* may lead to the development of a mycetoma (p. 240). This can be a cause of haemoptysis, as can bronchiectasis in lung tissue severely damaged by tuberculous infection.

Prognosis. With the advent of effective chemotherapy there has been a remarkable decline in the mortality from pulmonary tuberculosis. Provided the tubercle bacilli are not initially drug-resistant and chemotherapy is used correctly, a fatal outcome is extremely uncommon, even if the disease has reached an advanced stage when it is first recognised.

The advent of new effective antituberculosis drugs has also improved the outlook for those patients whose bacilli are resistant to two or three drugs. The late complications of respiratory failure and secondary infection with pyogenic bacteria or fungi can be prevented if pulmonary tuberculosis is diagnosed at a reasonably early stage and is efficiently treated.

THE TREATMENT OF TUBERCULOSIS

General Principles

Antituberculosis chemotherapy is by far the most important measure in the treatment of all forms of tuberculosis and should be given to every patient with active disease.

Rest is unimportant except in a few specific circumstances. The current practice is to keep patients in bed only until acute symptoms have subsided. The majority of patients are ambulant throughout treatment, many of them remaining at work. Immobilisation is of course necessary in certain forms of skeletal tuberculosis.

Isolation of patients who are excreting tubercle bacilli and who are therefore potentially infectious has previously been an important principle. The observation made in Madras that the frequency of disease amongst contacts was no greater when the patient was treated at home than in a sanatorium has led to the adoption of a policy whereby the majority of patients, even those who are sputum-positive on smear examination, are treated wholly as out-patients. However, many authorities still prefer to isolate patients from contact with young children. Hospitalisation for an initial period of treatment, as distinct from isolation, may be recommended for patients who cannot be relied upon to take their drugs regularly and for those who present difficult therapeutic problems.

Surgical treatment such as pulmonary resection, nephrectomy or removal of superficial lymph nodes is now rarely required. However, an irreparably damaged kidney should be removed and drainage of an abscess from tuberculous lymph nodes or of an empyema may be necessary. Surgical treatment of tuberculosis of the spine may be essential to prevent paraplegia.

Chemotherapy

Effective treatment of tuberculosis demands not only a detailed knowledge of the drugs available but also of the most appropriate regimen for the individual patient.

In Britain, five drugs — rifampicin, isoniazid, ethambutol, streptomycin and pyrazinamide — are normally considered in the initial treatment of tuberculosis. Thiacetazone, which is cheap, is widely used in developing countries. Pyrazinamide is particularly useful in the treatment of tuberculous meningitis because it diffuses well into the cerebrospinal fluid. Apart from a few minor variations in dose and duration of treatment (see below and p. 238) the policy governing the use of antituberculosis drugs is the same for all forms of the disease.

The drugs should be used in the following once daily doses:

Rifampicin†	Children	10–20 mg/kg
	Adults weighing less than 50 kg and in the elderly	450 mg
	Adults weighing more than 50 kg	600 mg
Isoniazid	Children	3 mg/kg
	Adults	200–300 mg
	Intermittent regimen	15 mg/kg*
	Miliary/meningitis	10–12 mg/kg*
Ethambutol	Children and adults:	
	initial 8 weeks	25 mg/kg
	subsequently	15 mg/kg
	In renal failure	According to serum levels
Strepto-mycin sulphate	Children	30 mg/kg
	Adults under 40 years and weighing more than 45 kg	1 g
	Adults 40–60 years or weighing less than 45 kg	0·75 g
	Adults over 60 years or in patients with renal failure	According to serum levels
	Intermittent regimens	0·75–1 g
Pyrazin-amide	Children and adults:	35 mg/kg (max 2·5 g)

†Taken at least 30 minutes before breakfast
*Plus pyridoxine 10 mg to prevent peripheral neuropathy (p. 79)

ADVERSE EFFECTS. In choosing a suitable drug regimen for individual patients it is important to bear in mind those side-effects which are particularly liable to cause serious chronic disability, such as vestibular disturbance due to streptomycin and optic neuritis due to ethambutol. Streptomycin must be prescribed with caution in the middle aged and elderly, who find difficulty in compensating for vestibular disturbance. Even in the relatively low dose recommended for ethambutol, a few patients develop optic neuritis and some are left with a permanent visual defect. This potential hazard must be taken into consideration whenever ethambutol is prescribed, particularly in children. Patients should be instructed to test their own visual acuity daily.

Streptomycin and occasionally isoniazid, ethambutol and rifampicin may produce a hypersensitivity reaction, consisting of pyrexia and an erythematous skin eruption, which usually develops 2 to 4 weeks after treatment is started.

Rifampicin, which colours the urine orange-pink, is a potent liver enzyme inducer (p. 339) and should be used with appropriate caution when the following drugs are prescribed: oestrogens (e.g. oral contraceptives), warfarin, corticosteroids and digoxin. It should, if possible, be avoided in patients with liver disease.

The principal adverse effects of the most commonly prescribed drugs are:

Rifampicin: drug interaction (see above); hypersensitivity (occasionally, see above); hepatitis (rare); vasculitis (rare); fever, respiratory, cutaneous and abdominal syndromes (intermittent regimens only). Rifampicin should not be given again if the respiratory syndrome or vasculitis has occurred.

Isoniazid: hypersensitivity (occasionally, see above); polyneuropathy (rare); lack of mental concentration (rare).

Ethambutol: optic neuritis (see above); hypersensitivity (rare, see above).

Streptomycin: vestibular disturbance (see above); hypersensitivity (see above); deafness (rare).

Pyrazinamide: hepatitis; gout; hypersensitivity (rare).

REGIMENS. The following regimens are virtually 100% effective in the treatment of tuberculosis:

1. *Duration 9 months*

Initial Phase (2 months): ethambutol or streptomycin plus isoniazid plus rifampicin.

Continuation Phase (7 months): isoniazid plus rifampicin.

2. *Duration 6 months*

Initial Phase (2 months): ethambutol or streptomycin plus isoniazid plus rifampicin plus pyrazinamide.

Continuation Phase (4 months): isoniazid plus rifampicin.

Most advanced countries have adopted the 9-month regimen as standard treatment, but the high level of success of the 6-month regimen may lead to its increased use in future.

Any patient who cannot be trusted to take oral antituberculosis drugs regularly without supervision should be kept in hospital for the initial (two-month) phase of treatment. Thereafter, for 10 months, the following should be given at home twice weekly (at 3 and 4 day intervals): streptomycin sulphate, (1 g i.m.) and isoniazid, (15 mg/kg by mouth) with pyridoxine, (10 mg) to prevent peripheral neuropathy. This type of chemotherapy should be wholly supervised, the tablets being administered at the same time as the injections.

Inexpensive Treatment Regimens. In developing countries it will usually be impossible for economic reasons to adhere to ideal chemotherapeutic regimens. The following inexpensive forms of treatment are reasonably effective if administered for 12 months: (1) Streptomycin (1 g) by intramuscular injection *plus* isoniazid (15 mg/kg) by mouth with pyridoxine (10 mg) on 2 days per week. This is 90 to 95% effective: if daily treatment with standard dose of streptomycin and isoniazid can be afforded for the initial phase, the effectiveness of this regimen is nearly 100% in the absence of primary drug resistance. (2) Isoniazid (300 mg) *plus* thiacetazone (150 mg) given in a single daily dose by mouth is extremely cheap, and is about 80 to 95% effective.

RESPONSE TO TREATMENT. If the bacilli at the start of treatment are fully sensitive to the drugs in use it is most unusual, even in advanced cases, for cultures of sputum, gastric washings, laryngeal swabs or urine to remain positive for longer than 6 months. Where facilities for sensitivity testing do not exist, reliance must be placed on smear examination. Persistence of a positive sputum culture after 6 months' treatment suggests that drug resistance has occurred. Alternatively, failure may have been due to irregular treatment. A simple urine test for isoniazid metabolites can be used to assess the patient's cooperation in treatment.

DRUG-RESISTANT TUBERCLE BACILLI. The treatment of patients infected with drug-resistant tubercle bacilli presents a problem requiring specialised knowledge for its solution. Additional drugs available for the treatment of such cases are: Sodium aminosalicylate (PAS–5 g b.d. by mouth), ethionamide or prothionamide (0·75–1 g once daily by mouth), capreomycin (0·75–1 g once daily i.m.) and cycloserine (0·75–1 g once daily by mouth).

Corticosteroid Drugs

These agents suppress the cell-mediated reaction induced by the tubercle bacillus and by interfering with tissue defence mechanisms may promote a rapid dissemination of infection throughout the body. If, however, a corticosteroid drug is given in conjunction with effective antituberculosis chemotherapy, it may exert a favourable influence on the course of the disease by reducing the severity both of the local inflammatory reaction and of the associated systemic disturbance. In acute cases of pulmonary tuberculosis such treatment will rapidly relieve pyrexia and will often produce a dramatic improvement in the radiological appearances. The effect is temporary and ceases when the corticosteroid drug is withdrawn, but it may save the lives of patients with fulminating tuberculous infection by enabling them to survive until antituberculosis chemotherapy has had time to exert its influence. Prednisolone is given in a dose of 20 mg daily for about 3 months.

Corticosteroid drugs in combination with chemotherapy may also be of value in tuberculous pleural and pericardial effusion, tuberculous disease of intrathoracic or superficial lymph nodes, tuberculosis involving the eye and in tuberculous meningitis. Whenever there is evidence of ureteric obstruction in genitourinary tuberculosis, corticosteroids should be administered in addition to chemotherapy, for such treatment significantly reduces the need for surgery.

Symptomatic Treatment

Pleural pain due to dry pleurisy or spontaneous pneumothorax, *cough* and *haemoptysis* are treated as described on page 219. *Fever and sweating* usually subside soon after chemotherapy is started. When persistent and excessive they should be treated by repeated tepid sponging. *Hoarseness* is usually due to tuberculous laryngitis, which responds rapidly to specific chemotherapy provided the organism is not drug-resistant. Severe and continuous *diarrhoea* in a patient with pulmonary tuberculosis is usually due to tuberculous enteritis. In most cases it can be rapidly controlled by chemotherapy.

The Prevention of Tuberculosis

Mortality rates are no longer considered so important in the assessment of the success of control measures because of the very low rates now existing in some countries and the inaccuracy of certification in the many countries where tuberculosis remains a major problem. The frequency of tuberculous meningitis is, however, a crude yardstick of the progress being made towards eradication.

Notification rates are of limited value because of the adoption of varying standards, but the annual recording of the number of smear-positive patients with pulmonary tuberculosis is a useful indication of the efficiency of preventive measures.

Another useful parameter is the *tuberculin index*, i.e. the percentage of positive reactors to tuberculin at a standard age, e.g. 5 or 13 years. It is important to assess the possible influence of the prevalence of atypical myocobacteria in the community and of BCG vaccination policy on the tuberculin index. It is also useful to estimate periodically the percentage of patients who on initial diagnosis excrete drug-resistant tubercle bacilli.

The following control measures are important in the achievement of the goal of eradication of the disease.

Improvement in socio-economic conditions mainly in respect of adequate housing, ventilation and nutrition may still be the most important control measure of all.

Case-finding. Mass radiography is an expensive method of case-finding and should now be used in a selective manner concentrating on certain specific groups. The highest yield by far is from patients referred by general practitioners because of symptoms. Open access to chest radiography for general practitioners and minimum waiting time for patients are essential for success. Other important groups are persons in prisons, borstals and mental hospitals, elderly men, especially those in lodging houses, and immigrants from Asia.

Sputum-smear examination is an important and inexpensive method of case-finding in developing countries. The provision of a microscope and the training of a health worker in the examination of smears can be readily organised.

Contact examination achieves a high yield in case-finding. Efforts should be concentrated on the immediate examination of household contacts of sputum-smear positive patients especially amongst contacts under 25 years of age. Asian immigrants should have a chest radiograph annually for two years.

Chemotherapy. The proper use of modern highly-effective chemotherapy, by rendering patients non-infectious rapidly, makes a very important contribution to the control of the disease.

Isolation of patients is rarely considered necessary nowadays even in smear-positive patients except where very young children are at risk, provided the source case is being properly treated by chemotherapy.

BCG Vaccination. This is carried out by the administration of freeze-dried vaccine, reconstituted at the time of use, by the intradermal route (0·1 ml) injected at the junction of the upper and middle thirds of the upper arm. The multiple puncture method (40 needles) is less commonly used. Complications such as local abscess formation and enlargement of regional lymph nodes are very rare. BCG vaccine should not be given in the presence of immunodeficiency. The duration of protection is from 3 to 7 years. Vaccination reduces the incidence of pulmonary tuberculosis in young adults by 80% and minimises the risk of serious disseminated disease — miliary tuberculosis and tuberculous meningitis.

Policy in relation to BCG vaccination in a community depends upon the size of the problem locally. If the infection rate is very low (1% or less) vaccination is inappropriate on the grounds of cost and the fact that BCG interferes with the diagnostic value of the tuberculin test in such a situation. Where there are many positive tuberculin reactors, as occur in communities with low living standards, vaccination of the newborn is usually indicated. Where infection rates are falling to low levels, vaccination at puberty may be appropriate.

Chemoprophylaxis. The concept of administering chemotherapy to individuals in order to try to prevent the development of tuberculosis is adopted in different communities with varying degrees of enthusiasm. Chemoprophylaxis, using isoniazid (5 mg/kg by mouth) daily for 1 year, is indicated in: (a) non-BCG vaccinated tuberculin positive children under 3 years of age, as this is a vulnerable group in respect of miliary tuberculosis and tuberculous meningitis; (b) unvaccinated individuals who have recently become tuberculin-positive; (c) patients on immunosuppressive drugs.

Chemoprophylaxis may also be considered in: (a) tuberculin-positive adolescents with a high level of tuberculin sensitivity; (b) infants of highly infectious parents, when isoniazid-resistant BCG vaccine may be administered, isoniazid chemoprophylaxis being given for 6 weeks thereafter to prevent infection until vaccination exerts its protective effects.

Elimination of Bovine Infection. Although such infection is now extremely rare in Western countries constant vigilance will be required to ensure that it remains so.

RESPIRATORY DISEASES CAUSED BY FUNGI

Most fungi encountered by man are harmless saprophytes, but some species may in certain circumstances infect human tissue or promote damaging allergic reactions.

The term *mycosis* is applied to disease caused by fungal infection. Predisposing factors include metabolic disorders, such as diabetes mellitus, toxic states such as chronic alcoholism, diseases such as leukaemia and myelomatosis in which immunological responses are disturbed, treatment with corticosteroids and immunosuppressive drugs, and radiotherapy. Local factors, such as tissue damage by suppuration or necrosis and the elimination of the competitive influence of a normal bacterial flora by antibiotics, may also facilitate fungal infection.

Allergic reactions to fungi may cause bronchial asthma (*Aspergillus fumigatus* and *Cladosporium herbarum*), bronchopulmonary eosinophilia (*A. fumigatus*) or extrinsic allergic alveolitis (*Micropolyspora faeni, Thermoactinomyces vulgaris, Con-*

iosporium corticale and *A. clavatus*). These conditions are described in the following section on allergic diseases of the respiratory tract.

The diagnosis of fungal diseases is usually made by mycological examination of the sputum, supported by serological tests for precipitating antibodies, and in some instances by skin sensitivity tests.

Aspergillosis. This is the most common respiratory mycosis in Britain. Inhaled air-borne spores of *Aspergillus fumigatus* lodge and germinate in damaged pulmonary tissue. In some cases the fungal infection remains localised to the site of the original lesion, but, particularly in immunodeficient or immunosuppressed patients, it may spread rapidly, with the production of consolidation, necrosis and cavitation and grave systemic disturbance (*invasive pulmonary aspergillosis*).

When a pre-existing pulmonary cavity or cyst is infected by *A. fumigatus*, a large spherical mass of fungal mycelium may form within the cavity, producing on radiological examination a tumour-like opacity to which the term *mycetoma* or *aspergilloma* is applied. This type of lesion can readily be distinguished from a peripheral bronchial carcinoma by the presence of a crescent of air between the mycelial mass and the cavity wall. An aspergilloma often produces no specific symptoms, but may be responsible for recurrent severe haemoptysis.

Whenever a large amount of mycelium is present in a pulmonary cavity, or in any other lesion, precipitating antibodies can be detected in the serum by means of a gel diffusion test, using an antigen derived from *A. fumigatus*. This test is of considerable diagnostic value.

Candidiasis. Occasionally, in debilitated subjects oral thrush (p. 286) extends into the respiratory tract to involve the bronchi or lungs.

Other Pulmonary Mycoses. These, all of which are rare, include nocardiosis, cryptococcosis (p. 805), mucormycosis, blastomycosis (p. 805) and sporotrichosis (p. 803). Only the first three of these conditions have been encountered in Britain. In a somewhat different category are histoplasmosis (p. 803) and coccidioidomycosis (p. 804), which are endemic in certain areas of North America and Africa, and produce local or systemic granulomatous lesions resembling tuberculosis.

Treatment of the pulmonary mycoses is difficult and unsatisfactory. The administration of antibacterial drugs should be stopped, and antifungal agents substituted. Nystatin or natamycin by inhalation may control the more superficial respiratory mycoses involving the trachea and bronchi. For grave pulmonary infections amphotericin (p. 804), a potent but highly toxic antifungal agent may have to be given intravenously. Flucytosine and the antifungal imidazoles (p. 48) may be useful in the treatment of less severe infections. The effective dose of amphotericin, and thus its toxic effects on the kidney, can be reduced by combining it with flucytosine. Surgical treatment for a mycetoma may have to be considered if severe haemoptysis occurs.

ALLERGIC DISEASES

Many types of particle suspended in the atmosphere possess antigenic properties, and are capable of stimulating the production of specific antibody when inhaled. Further exposure to antigen of an individual 'sensitised' in this way may provoke an allergic reaction which causes pathological changes and disturbances of function in the tissue where the reaction occurs.

Three types of allergic response are concerned in the production of respiratory disease. The Type I or anaphylactic response (p. 24), mediated by immunoglobulin IgE, is associated with an immediate hypersensitivity reaction, the clinical manifestations of which include allergic rhinitis and bronchial asthma. The Type III or immune complex response, mediated by immunoglobulin IgG, is associated with a late hypersensitivity reaction which may contribute to the production of allergic alveolitis. Both Type I and Type III responses may be concerned in the production of some forms of bronchopulmonary eosinophilia, such as allergic aspergillosis. Type IV or tuberculin-type allergic responses, which are cell-mediated and do not involve circulating antibody, are usually associated with delayed hypersensitivity reactions in conditions such as tuberculosis, but may be involved in predominantly Type III reactions, such as allergic alveolitis.

Ingested antigens, or drugs such as aspirin and sulphasalazine, occasionally produce allergic respiratory disorders, such as bronchial asthma and bronchopulmonary eosinophilia, and auto-antigens may have a similar role in conditions such as polyarteritis nodosa and systemic lupus erythematosus.

In this chapter, allergic rhinitis, bronchial asthma, bronchopulmonary eosinophilia and allergic alveolitis will be described in some detail, but for a description of other forms of allergic disorder the reader should refer to Chapter 2.

ALLERGIC RHINITIS

This is a disorder in which there are episodes of nasal congestion, watery nasal discharge and sneezing. It may be *seasonal* or *perennial*.

Aetiology. Allergic rhinitis is due to an anaphylactic antigen-antibody reaction in the nasal mucosa (p. 24). The antigens concerned in the seasonal form of the disorder are pollens from grasses, flowers, weeds or trees. Grass pollen is responsible for *hay fever*, the most common type of seasonal allergic rhinitis in Britain, and this disorder is at its peak between May and July.

Perennial allergic rhinitis may be a specific reaction to antigens derived from house dust, fungal spores or animal dander, but similar symptoms can be caused by physical or chemical irritants, such as pungent odours or fumes, including strong perfumes, cold air and dry atmospheres. In this context the term 'allergic' is a misnomer.

Clinical Features. In the seasonal type there are frequent sudden attacks of sneezing, with profuse watery nasal discharge and nasal obstruction. These attacks last for a few hours, and are often accompanied by smarting and watering of the eyes and conjunctival injection. In the perennial type the symptoms are similar, but more continuous and generally less severe.

In seasonal allergic rhinitis, skin sensitivity tests with the relevant antigen are usually positive, and are thus of diagnostic value, but these tests are less useful in perennial rhinitis, and may all be negative.

Treatment. The following symptomatic measures, singly or in combination, are usually effective in both seasonal and perennial allergic rhinitis: (1) an antihistamine drug, such as terfenadine (60 mg b.d.). (2) a decongestant nasal spray, e.g. 1% ephedrine hydrochloride in saline. (3) sodium cromoglycate nasal spray, one metered dose of a 2% solution, into each nostril 6 times daily. (4) beclomethasone dipropionate nasal spray, one metered dose of 50 μg into each nostril 4 times daily.

Patients failing to respond to these measures may obtain symptomatic relief from intramuscular injections of 0·5–1 mg of tetracosactrin zinc, but this form of treatment should be reserved for those patients whose symptoms are very severe and interfere seriously with business and social activities.

Prevention. In the seasonal type an attempt should be made to reduce exposure to pollen, for example by avoiding country districts and keeping indoors as much as possible, with the windows closed, during the pollen season. Some patients with hay fever may benefit from pre-seasonal hyposensitisation (p. 245) with a grass pollen extract. The prevention of perennial rhinitis consists of avoiding, as far as possible, exposure to any identifiable aetiological factors. Specific hyposensitisation is probably of little value.

BRONCHIAL ASTHMA

Bronchial asthma is characterised by paroxysms of dyspnoea accompanied by wheezing, resulting from narrowing of the bronchial airways by muscle spasm, mucosal swelling or viscid secretion. The airflow obstruction causes mismatching of alveolar ventilation and perfusion and increases the work of breathing. Being more marked during expiration it also causes air to be 'trapped' in the lungs. The narrowed bronchi can no longer be effectively cleared of mucus by the act of coughing, and in patients with severe acute asthma many of the smaller bronchi become obstructed by inspissated and often very tenacious mucus. This is usually the most conspicuous finding at autopsy. The cause of death is progressive alveolar hypoventilation and severe arterial hypoxaemia, culminating in cardiac arrest.

Aetiology. Asthma in most cases starts either in childhood or in middle age. 'Early onset' asthma is slightly more common in males, and 'late onset' asthma in females.

'Early onset' asthma generally occurs in atopic individuals, i.e. those who readily form IgE antibodies to commonly encountered allergens (p. 241). Such individuals can be identified by skin sensitivity tests (p. 244), which produce positive reactions to a wide range of common allergens. They often suffer from other allergic disorders, such as allergic rhinitis and eczema, and a family history of these disorders and of 'early onset' asthma is common. It is unusual for a single allergen to be the sole cause of asthma, and clinical experience indicates that many different allergens are implicated in almost every case, although the importance of each of them may vary from time to time.

'Late onset' asthma generally occurs in nonatopic individuals, and it would appear that external allergens play no part in the production of this form of the disease, to which the term 'intrinsic asthma' is sometimes applied.

The allergens responsible for asthma in atopic individuals generally enter the bronchi with the inspired air, and are derived from organic material, such as pollen, mite-containing house dust, feathers, animal dander and fungal spores. Previous exposure to these agents will have stimulated the formation of reaginic antibody (the immunoglobulin IgE), and an anaphylactic antigen-antibody reaction in the bronchi may follow further exposure to specific allergen. This releases pharmacologically active substances, such as histamine, kinins and leukotrienes from mast cells which provoke bronchial constriction and an inflammatory reaction of allergic type in the bronchial mucosa. Much less frequently, similar effects may be produced by ingested allergens derived from certain foods, such as fish, eggs, milk, yeasts and wheat, which presumably reach the bronchi via the blood stream.

An immune complex allergic reaction may also be implicated in the pathogenesis of bronchial asthma, particularly where antigens derived from fungi, such as *A. fumigatus*, are implicated. Acute attacks of asthma may be caused by drugs such as aspirin and by exposure to chemical substances in the electronics, plastics and other industries (Tables 8.5 and 8.11).

Table 8.5 Allergens and other substances liable to provoke attacks of asthma.

Causative agent	Preventive measures	Efficacy
Pollens	Try to avoid exposure to flowering vegetation. Keep bedroom windows closed.	Low
Mites (e.g. *D. pteronyssinus*)	Vacuum-clean mattress daily. Shake out blankets daily. Dust bedroom thoroughly.	Doubtful
Animal dander	Avoid contact with dogs, cats, horses or other animals.	High
Feathers in pillows or quilts	Substitute latex foam pillows and terylene quilts.	High
Drugs (e.g. aspirin)	Avoid all preparations of relevant drugs.	High
Foods	Identify and eliminate from diet.	Low*
Industrial chemicals (e.g. diisocyanates, epoxy resins)	Avoid exposure to chemical, or change occupation.	High

*More effective in control of eczema

Asthma is often aggravated by non-specific factors, such as bronchial irritation caused by tobacco smoke, dust and acrid fumes, respiratory infection, and emotional stress. In children and young adults, usually atopic subjects, an attack of asthma may follow strenuous exertion (*exercise-induced asthma*) or exposure to cold air.

Clinical Features. Bronchial asthma may be either *episodic* or *chronic*, and although there is a good deal of overlap between these two syndromes, the distinction is clinically useful, particularly in terms of prognosis and management. In general, atopic individuals tend to develop episodic asthma, and non-atopic individuals chronic asthma.

In *episodic asthma* paroxysms of wheeze and dyspnoea occur at any hour of the day or night, are of sudden onset, and may be preceded by a feeling of tightness in the chest. Expiration is exhausting, while inspiration is short and gasping. The patient adopts an upright position, fixing the shoulder-girdle to assist the accessory muscles of expiration. Wheeze is chiefly expiratory and there is often an unproductive cough which aggravates the dyspnoea. In severe attacks there is tachycardia, pulsus paradoxus and central cyanosis.

The attack may end abruptly within an hour or two, sometimes with the coughing up of viscid sputum, or may persist for many hours or even for several days. The sputum, usually scanty, may contain numerous eosinophil leucocytes and, occasionally, gelatinous casts of small bronchi. In most cases there is an increase in the number of eosinophil leucocytes in the blood.

The term, *severe acute asthma*, has now replaced 'status asthmaticus' for the description of life-threatening attacks associated with extreme respiratory distress and arterial hypoxaemia.

In *chronic asthma* the paroxysmal character of the symptoms is usually less conspicuous, the chief clinical features being continuous wheeze and breathlessness on exertion. Cough and mucoid sputum, with recurrent episodes of frank respiratory infection, are common in this type of asthma, which may be difficult to distinguish from chronic bronchitis.

Physical Signs in the Chest. 1. During a paroxysm the chest is held near the position of full inspiration. The percussion note may be hyper-resonant. The breath sounds, which are obscured by numerous high pitched rhonchi, are vesicular in character with prolonged expiration. In very severe asthma airflow may be insufficient to produce rhonchi, and a 'silent chest' in such patients is an ominous sign.

2. Between paroxysms there are usually no abnormal physical signs except in patients with chronic asthma, who are seldom without rhonchi. Severe asthma starting in childhood may cause a 'pigeon chest' deformity.

Investigation. *Radiological Examination.* In an acute attack of asthma the lungs appear hyper-inflated. In long-standing cases the features of emphysema may be present, and the lateral view may demonstrate a 'pigeon chest' deformity. Occasionally, when a bronchus is obstructed by tenacious mucus, there is an opacity caused by lobar or segmental collapse.

Pulmonary Function Tests. Measurements of the forced expiratory volume in 1 second (FEV_1) and forced vital capacity (FVC) or of the peak expiratory flow rate (PEFR) provide a fairly reliable indication of the degree of airflow obstruction (p. 213), and can also be used to determine whether and to what extent it can be relieved by bronchodilator drugs or corticosteroids, or to confirm that it is provoked by exercise (Fig. 8.3) or hyperventilation. Such tests thus have an important place in the diagnosis and treatment of bronchial asthma. Frequent recordings of PEFR are useful in the assessment of those patients ('morning dippers') whose asthma shows marked diurnal variations in severity (Fig. 8.4). Measurements of arterial blood gas pressures (Pao_2 and $Paco_2$) are indispensable to the management of patients with severe acute asthma.

Skin Sensitivity Tests. A prick is made in the skin with a fine needle through a drop of an aqueous extract of the substance to be tested, and a positive reaction is indicated by the development of a wheal and flare, which begin to appear within a few minutes. Tests are usually performed with a group of common allergens known

Fig. 8.3 Exercise-induced asthma: serial recordings of forced expiratory volume in one second (FEV_1) in patient with bronchial asthma before, during and after 6 minutes of strenuous exercise. Note initial slight rise on completion of exercise, followed by sudden fall and gradual recovery.

to cause bronchial asthma. It is seldom possible with these tests to identify one particular allergen as the cause of asthma in an individual case, and their chief value is to distinguish atopic from non-atopic subjects.

Fig. 8.4 'Morning dipping': serial recordings of peak expiratory flow rate (PEFR) in patient with chronic asthma showing marked diurnal variations. Note sharp overnight fall and subsequent rise during the day.

Course and Prognosis. The prognosis of the individual attack is good, except in severe acute asthma where there is occasionally a fatal outcome, especially if treatment is inadequate or delayed. Spontaneous remission is fairly common in episodic asthma, particularly in children, but rare in chronic asthma, which often causes permanent pulmonary damage. Seasonal fluctuations occur in both types of asthma. Atopic subjects with episodic asthma are usually worse in the summer, when they are more heavily exposed to antigens, while chronic asthmatics are usually worse in the winter months because of their increased liability to infection.

Treatment. The following measures may be of value in the management of patients with bronchial asthma: (1) Reduction of exposure to relevant allergens. (2) Hyposensitisation, which may prevent damaging antigen-antibody reactions. (3) Drugs, such as sodium cromoglycate, which prevent release from mast cells in the bronchial wall of pharmacological mediators of bronchoconstriction. (4) Drugs, such as bronchodilators or corticosteroids, used to control or suppress clinical manifestations of asthma. (5) Measures to counter the effects of aggravating factors such as exercise, infection and emotional stress.

1. AVOIDANCE OF ALLERGENS. There are a few instances in which a single agent can be identified as the cause of attacks of asthma. These include grass pollens, mites, animal dander, drugs such as aspirin, a few industrial chemicals such as diisocyanates and certain articles of diet. The measures which can be taken to prevent or reduce exposure to these agents, and the degree of success likely to be achieved, are summarised in Table 8.5. In the vast majority of cases, however, asthmatic patients are sensitive to a wide range of allergens and attempts to avoid them all are impracticable.

2. HYPOSENSITISATION. This is the only specific measure available for the prevention of damaging antigen-antibody reactions. It involves the subcutaneous injection of initially very small, but gradually increasing, doses of extracts of allergens believed to be responsible for the patient's asthma. It may be of some value when only a single allergen, such as grass pollen or animal dander, is implicated but it is not devoid of the risk of producing an acute anaphylactic reaction. Hyposensitisation with a mixture of allergens is irrational and cannot be recommended. Although allergy to the house dust mite is widely believed to be an important cause of nocturnal asthma, the results of hyposensitisation with a 'mite vaccine' have proved to be disappointing.

3. PREVENTION OF THE RELEASE OF PHARMACOLOGICAL MEDIATORS OF BRONCHOCONSTRICTION. The only drug which has so far been shown to exert this effect is sodium cromoglycate administered by inhalation. It seems to be of particular value in children with extrinsic (atopic) asthma, and should be given a trial of 4 weeks' duration in all such patients. If it is found to be effective, regular inhalation of 20 mg in a dry powder by 'Spinhaler' or of 2–4 mg from a pressurised dispenser four times daily may completely prevent recurrence of asthma in this group of patients. It may also be of value in some cases of intrinsic (nonatopic) asthma.

A similar mode of action has been claimed for ketotifen by mouth, but that drug is less effective than sodium cromoglycate and has the serious disadvantage in some patients of causing drowsiness which may be a dangerous side-effect in patients driving cars or operating machinery.

4. DRUGS WHICH CONTROL OR SUPPRESS CLINICAL MANIFESTATIONS OF ASTHMA.

(i) *General Principles.* It is important to distinguish between bronchodilators, which have a direct and immediate effect on airflow obstruction, and corticosteroids, which relieve or prevent airflow obstruction indirectly by their less rapid anti-inflammatory action. Thus a corticosteroid aerosol cannot be expected to relieve an acute episode of asthma. On the other hand, if a patient with severe acute asthma does not respond rapidly to bronchodilator aerosols, systemic treatment with corticosteroids in high dosage by mouth or intravenously, is the only measure likely to be effective. In such a situation, there may be a delay of a few hours before a severe attack of asthma responds to corticosteroids and, during that period, intensive bronchodilator and oxygen therapy may be essential to the patient's survival.

There is considerable controversy about the relative efficacy of the various methods of administering bronchodilator drugs. In the case of selective β_2-adrenoceptor agonists, such as salbutamol, terbutaline or fenoterol, the inhalation of an aerosol has clear advantages over oral administration because it reduces airflow obstruction more rapidly. Since the effective dose is much lower, it is less liable to produce side-effects such as tremor and anxiety. When a patient fails to obtain the accustomed degree of relief from the inhalation of a bronchodilator aerosol, this means that the asthma is in a refractory phase, and that a more potent form of treatment, such as a course of prednisolone by mouth, is urgently required.

Methylxanthine derivatives, such as theophylline or aminophylline, can be given by intravenous injection, mouth or suppository. Intravenous aminophylline (375 mg) is often an effective form of treatment for severe acute asthma, although it is probably not superior to salbutamol (0·5 mg) administered by the same route. There has been a revival of interest in the oral methylxanthines since the introduction of sustained-release formulations. This is based chiefly on the claim that these preparations can maintain serum concentrations of theophylline at therapeutically effective but subtoxic levels. It is, however, still open to doubt whether oral methylxanthines, even when the dose is monitored by serum concentrations, have any real advantage in terms of efficacy and safety over the regular inhalation of β_2-adrenoceptor agonist aerosols, except possibly for the prevention of nocturnal wheeze.

(ii) *Episodic Asthma.* Where episodes of asthma are mild and infrequent, they can be controlled by inhalation of a bronchodilator aerosol, for example, 2 metered doses of salbutamol (200 µg) as required. When the episodes are more frequent, this should be supplemented by a regular prophylactic measure, such as sodium cromoglycate or a corticosteroid aerosol by inhalation. In general, sodium cromoglycate is more effective in atopic individuals, particularly children and corticosteroid aerosols in non-atopic individuals, particularly adults. Sodium cromoglycate has virtually no side-effects, but corticosteroid aerosols are apt to cause oropharyngeal candidiasis and a husky voice.

(iii) *Exercise-Induced Asthma.* This fairly common phenomenon, which occurs particularly in atopic children with episodic asthma, can often be prevented by regular treatment with sodium cromoglycate. If that fails, the inhalation of two metered doses of salbutamol (200 µg), a few minutes before the patient expects to undertake strenuous exertion, is usually effective.

(iv) *Chronic Asthma.* Some form of suppressive treatment is necessary in all patients with chronic asthma. Sodium cromoglycate is always worth a trial in such cases, but there is usually a better response to the regular inhalation of a corticosteroid aerosol — four metered doses of beclomethasone dipropionate (200 µg) or of betamethasone valerate (400 µg) twice daily. In severe cases, this may have to be supplemented by a small maintenance dose of prednisolone given by mouth (5–7·5 mg/day) and/or by occasional short courses of prednisolone in higher dosage (20 mg/day or more for a week).

There is some evidence that supplementary treatment with oral prednisolone may be required less frequently if the dose of inhaled corticosteroid aerosol is increased, in the case of beclomethasone dipropionate to 1000 or 1500 µg per day. The latter dose should, however, not be exceeded because systemic absorption of the drug may then cause impairment of pituitary-adrenal function. Most patients with chronic asthma also require to inhale a bronchodilator aerosol either regularly or periodically to control recurrences of wheeze. When regular treatment is needed, it is best given a few minutes before the inhalation of sodium cromoglycate or a corticosteroid aerosol to ensure that the largest possible amounts of these drugs enter the bronchi. Oral bronchodilator drugs are seldom as effective as aerosols in the treatment of chronic asthma, but slow-release oral preparations of β_2-adrenoceptor agonists and methylxanthines taken at bedtime may prevent nocturnal wheeze.

(v) *Severe Acute Asthma.* When an acute attack of asthma becomes severe and life-threatening, the patient will have ceased to show any response to bronchodilator aerosols and it is futile, and perhaps dangerous for hypoxic asthmatics, to persist with this form of treatment. All such patients should be admitted to hospital as quickly as possible and emergency admission schemes, which eliminate the delays inherent in normal hospital admission procedures, can do much to reduce the number of unnecessary deaths from severe acute asthma. It is equally important that, before the ambulance arrives, the general practitioner should start effective treatment (Table 8.6).

Table 8.6 Treatment of severe acute asthma in the home.

1. Administer oxygen from portable cylinder (preferably by MC mask).
2. Give bronchodilator intravenously: aminophylline (375 mg in 20 ml saline) *or* salbutamol (0·5 mg in 20 ml saline) *or* terbutaline (0·5 mg in 20 ml of saline). Alternatively, give salbutamol (5 mg) or terbutaline (10 mg) by inhalation
3. Give hydrocortisone sodium succinate 200 mg intravenously.
4. Arrange for emergency admission to hospital in ambulance equipped for oxygen therapy.
5. Give prednisolone 60 mg by mouth.

N.B. The above doses are for adults — those for children should be proportionately smaller.

Since all bronchodilator drugs may produce a significant increase in arterial hypoxaemia, which may have grave consequences in patients with severe acute asthma, it is strongly advisable for oxygen to be given from a portable cylinder before and after these drugs are administered. Oxygen therapy (35% by Ventimask) should be continued in the ambulance conveying the patient to hospital.

On arrival in hospital most patients respond to treatment with high doses of corticosteroid, supplemented by bronchodilator drugs administered by intravenous injection or infusion, or in the form of an aqueous aerosol delivered in oxygen from a nebuliser. Only occasionally is it necessary to employ major resuscitative measures, such as tracheal intubation, mechanical ventilation and bronchial lavage, because most patients nowadays are admitted before they have become desperately ill, and most of them have received adequate emergency treatment from their general practitioners.

Recently there has been an increase in the use of electric nebulisers for the self-administration of bronchodilators by patients in their homes, but those who are hypoxaemic and do not have access to oxygen may be at some risk from this form of treatment. Furthermore, overconfidence in its efficacy can lead to delay in seeking medical advice during an episode of severe asthma when prompt admission to hospital may be vital to survival. Doctors must, therefore, ensure that patients who are provided with nebulisers fully understand their potential dangers and how these can be avoided.

BRONCHOPULMONARY EOSINOPHILIA

This term is applied to a group of allergic disorders of different aetiology in which lesions of the bronchi and/or the lungs are associated with an increase in the number of eosinophil leucocytes in the blood. In some of these diseases the bronchi appear to be primarily affected, although there may be secondary effects on lung tissue, while in others the pathological changes are confined to the lungs. It is therefore appropriate to subdivide the syndrome into bronchial and pulmonary eosinophilia (Table 8.7).

Table 8.7 Bronchopulmonary eosinophilia.

Bronchial eosinophilia:	Bronchial asthma Eosinophilic bronchitis with bronchial obstruction (including allergic bronchial aspergillosis)

Pulmonary eosinophilia:	Helminthic eosinophilic pneumonia
	  localised
	  diffuse
	Fungal eosinophilic pneumonia
	Drug-induced eosinophilic pneumonia
	Cryptogenic eosinophilic pneumonia

Bronchial Eosinophilia

Although bronchial asthma could logically be included in this category, it is not customary to do so, and the term is normally restricted to patients with a severe allergic reaction in the bronchi which gives rise to the production of inspissated mucus heavily coated with eosinophils ('eosinophilic bronchitis'). These casts frequently obstruct bronchi and produce lobar or segmental collapse. In some cases, the allergic reaction extends into the collapsed lung tissue, but because lung biopsy is seldom indicated in patients with bronchopulmonary eosinophilia, the frequency of this complication is uncertain.

There is evidence that eosinophilic bronchitis

is the result of dual anaphylactic and immune complex antigen-antibody reactions (p. 241) in the bronchial wall, and that an antigen derived from the fungus, *Aspergillus fumigatus*, is often the causal agent. In many cases that fungus can be isolated from the sputum or from a bronchial cast, skin tests (immediate and late) with an *A. fumigatus* antigen are positive and precipitating antibodies can be detected in the serum. The term, *allergic bronchial aspergillosis* can be used to describe such cases. Occasionally all investigations are negative and a causal antigen cannot be identified.

Clinical Feature. Chronic asthma is the dominant clinical manifestation of bronchial eosinophilia, but at irregular intervals bronchi, usually in the upper lobes, are obstructed by casts, with the production of lobar or segmental collapse, which may cause a mild febrile illness. When these episodes recur over a period of years, as they usually do, they result in permanent damage to the bronchi and lungs. Cast formation first produces dilatation of the larger bronchi ('proximal bronchiectasis'), and at a later stage bacterial and possibly fungal infection in lung tissue distal to the bronchial obstruction causes extensive pulmonary fibrosis and bronchiectasis. These changes, together with the associated chronic asthma, which seldom responds well to treatment, eventually cause respiratory failure, pulmonary hypertension and right ventricular failure.

Investigation. In early cases, the diagnosis is made by observing recurrent transient radiographic opacities, usually of lobar or segmental distribution, in young adults (seldom children) with chronic asthma and an increased eosinophil count in the blood. Often the investigations already described will identify *A. fumigatus* as the cause of the allergic reaction. In advanced cases, however, chronic respiratory failure overshadows the earlier and more specific features, and radiological examination shows extensive bilateral fibrosis and bronchiectasis predominantly affecting the upper lobes.

Treatment. Initially, a short course of prednisolone (5 mg by mouth 6-hourly for a week), presumably by relieving airflow obstruction, may be followed by the expectoration of bronchial casts and clearing of the pulmonary opacities. If not, it may be necessary to extract the cast or casts by bronchoscopy in an attempt to avert permanent bronchopulmonary damage. Further cast formation can in some cases be prevented by a maintenance dose of prednisolone (5–10 mg per day), but in many cases this does not halt the development of progressive pulmonary fibrosis and bronchiectasis, particularly when bronchial eosinophilia is a manifestation of allergic aspergillosis.

Pulmonary Eosinophilia

As the term implies, this condition predominantly involves lung tissues although in a few cases it may be associated with chronic bronchial asthma. There is a cellular infiltrate, chiefly consisting of eosinophil leucocytes, in the alveoli and alveolar walls, to which the term, *eosinophilic pneumonia*, can suitably be applied. This may be localised or diffuse, and appears to be an immunological reaction in the lung to a variety of antigens (Table 8.8). In some cases eosinophilic pneumonia, which may be severe and extensive, develops in the absence of any identifiable cause. The term, *cryptogenic pulmonary eosinophilia*, is applied to this form of the disease, for which an autoimmune mechanism may be responsible.

Table 8.8 Some causes of pulmonary eosinophilia.

Helminths	*Ascaris lumbricoides* (localised eosinophilic pneumonia).
Microfilaria	(diffuse eosinophilic pneumonia).
Fungi	*Aspergillus fumigatus* (localised eosinophilic pneumonia).
Drugs	Nitrofurantoin, para-aminosalicyclic acid, sulphasalazine, imipramine, chlorpropamide, phenylbutazone, aspirin (localised or diffuse eosinophilic pneumonia).
Chemicals	Di-isocyanates (diffuse eosinophilic pneumonia)

Clinical Features. These vary widely in severity, depending on the aetiology and on the extent of pulmonary involvement. Many patients have only a trivial febrile illness, the nature of which would have passed unrecognised in the absence of radiological and haematological investigation. Others, particularly those in whom the illness is an allergic reaction to microfilariae (*tropical pulmonary eosinophilia*) (p. 799) or to drugs, may become gravely ill with high fever and severe dyspnoea, and a similar clinical picture may be observed in cryptogenic pulmonary eosinophilia. In most patients with a severe clinical illness, the absolute eosinophil count in the blood is high, often exceeding $5.0 \times 10^9/l$.

Investigation. Pulmonary eosinophilia should always be suspected in patients with unexplained radiographic opacities in the lungs, either localised or diffuse. It can readily be mistaken for pulmonary tuberculosis or bacterial pneumonia unless an eosinophil count is carried out. After the diagnosis is established, an attempt should always be made to discover the relevant aetiological factor, such as an intestinal helminth, filariasis or treatment with a drug or exposure to a chemical substance previously reported to have caused the disease. If all such causes are excluded, and tests for fungal allergy are negative, a diagnosis of cryptogenic pulmonary eosinophilia has to be accepted.

Treatment. If a cause is found or suspected it must be treated or removed. Helminthic intestinal infections should be eradicated and any drug likely to be responsible for the pulmonary eosinophilia should be withdrawn. When the condition is due to microfilariae the patient should be given diethylcarbamazine (p. 796) and rapid clinical and radiographic improvement will follow. Cryptogenic pulmonary eosinophilia usually responds dramatically to prednisolone (5 mg 6 hourly by mouth) but because it is apt to recur after corticosteroid therapy is withdrawn, a small maintenance dose may have to be continued for some months, or even for a few years.

EXTRINSIC ALLERGIC ALVEOLITIS

In this condition the inhalation of certain types of organic dust produces a diffuse allergic reaction in the walls of the alveoli and bronchioles. There is a cellular exudate consisting of polymorphs, lymphocytes and plasma cells, and small epithelioid granulomata may also be seen. These changes cause decreased pulmonary compliance and ventilation: perfusion maldistribution. They are presumably also responsible for the widespread crackling crepitations heard on auscultation, and for the diffuse micronodular shadowing seen on the chest radiograph.

Precipitating antibodies in the serum against the relevant antigens would seem to indicate that allergic alveolitis is an immune complex reaction, but the finding of small pulmonary granulomata suggests that cell-mediated hypersensitivity may also be implicated.

Some of the agents which produce extrinsic allergic alveolitis, the source of these agents, and the names applied to the resulting diseases are shown in Table 8.9. If patients with this disorder continue to be exposed to the relevant antigen for long periods, they may eventually develop permanent pulmonary damage with severe respiratory disability.

Table 8.9 Examples of extrinsic allergic alveolitis.

Agent	Source	Disease
Avian protein from pigeons and budgerigars	Pigeon loft or bird cage	Bird fancier's lung
Micropolyspora faeni	Mouldy hay	Farmer's lung
Thermophilic actinomycetes	Compost	Mushroom worker's lung
	Mouldy sugar cane fibre	Bagassosis
Aspergillus clavatus	Malting barley	Maltworker's lung
Coniosporium corticale	Bark of maple trees	Maple bark disease

Clinical Features. Extrinsic allergic alveolitis should be suspected when a person regularly exposed to a heavy concentration of organic dust complains, a few hours after re-exposure to the same dust, of malaise, pyrexia, dry cough and dyspnoea without wheeze, or insidiously develops similar symptoms after constant exposure to antigen, as in some cases of bird fancier's lung.

At this stage the patient may be febrile, cyanosed and dyspnoeic at rest, coarse crepitations (but no rhonchi) can be heard over both lungs and a chest radiograph may show diffuse micronodular shadowing. The FEV_1 and FVC are both reduced, but the FEV_1/FVC ratio is normal, indicating a restrictive ventilatory defect without airflow obstruction. The Pa_{O_2} is reduced, and the

$Paco_2$ is slightly subnormal as a result of overventilation. Gas transfer (p. 207) is impaired.

The diagnosis of extrinsic allergic alveolitis is confirmed serologically by a positive precipitin test and, if necessary, by a positive provocation test, in which the inhalation of an aerosol containing the relevant antigen is followed after 3 to 6 hours by pyrexia and a reduction in VC, often associated with a recurrence of symptoms.

Treatment. Mild forms of extrinsic allergic alveolitis rapidly subside when exposure to the antigen ceases. In acute cases a corticosteroid preparation should be given for 3 to 4 weeks, starting with 40–60 mg of prednisolone per day, and severely hypoxic patients may require oxygen in high concentration (60%). Most of these patients recover completely, but when there is a long history of exposure or subsequent re-exposure to the relevant antigen, the development of interstitial fibrosis causes permanent disability.

DISEASES OF THE LARYNX, TRACHEA AND BRONCHI

Acute infections have already been described (p. 220). Other common disorders of the larynx include chronic laryngitis, laryngeal tuberculosis (p. 231), laryngeal paralysis and laryngeal obstruction. Tumours of the larynx are relatively common, but for information on these conditions the reader should refer to a textbook of diseases of the ear, nose and throat.

Chronic Laryngitis

Chronic laryngitis occurs as a result of (i) repeated attacks of acute laryngitis, (ii) excessive use of the voice, especially in dusty atmospheres, e.g. in auctioneers, (iii) heavy tobacco smoking, (iv) mouth-breathing from nasal obstruction and (v) chronic infection of the nasal sinuses. The chief symptom is hoarseness and the voice may be lost. There is irritation of the throat and spasmodic cough. The disease pursues a chronic course frequently uninfluenced by treatment, and in long-standing cases the voice is often permanently impaired.

As chronic and progressive hoarseness may also be caused by tuberculosis and tumours of the larynx and by laryngeal paralysis, these conditions must be considered in the differential diagnosis if the hoarseness does not improve within a few weeks. In some cases a chest radiograph may bring to light unsuspected pulmonary tuberculosis or a bronchial carcinoma. If no such abnormality is found the patient should be referred to a specialist for laryngoscopic examination.

The voice must be rested completely. This is particularly important in the case of public speakers. Smoking should be prohibited. Some benefit may be obtained from frequent inhalations of medicated steam.

Laryngeal Paralysis

Aetiology. Laryngeal paralysis is due to interference with the motor nerve supply of the larynx and may be caused by lesions of the brain stem, e.g. bulbar paralysis, or of the vagus nerve or its recurrent laryngeal branch.

Interruption of the recurrent laryngeal nerve, or of the vagus trunk above the origin of that nerve, by tumour, aneurysm or trauma is the most common way in which laryngeal paralysis is produced. The paralysis is nearly always unilateral and, by reason of the intrathoracic course of the left recurrent laryngeal nerve, usually left-sided. Accidental division of one or both recurrent laryngeal nerves is one of the hazards of thyroidectomy.

Hoarseness or complete loss of voice (aphonia) may occur as a manifestation of hysteria.

Clinical Features. *Hoarseness* always accompanies laryngeal paralysis whatever its cause. Paralysis of organic origin is seldom reversible, but when only one vocal cord is affected the hoarseness may improve or even disappear after a few weeks as a result of a compensatory adjustment whereby the unparalysed cord crosses the midline and approximates with the paralysed cord on phonation.

'Bovine' cough, which is a characteristic feature of organic laryngeal paralysis, results from the loss of the explosive phase of normal coughing consequent upon the failure of the cords to close the glottis. The difficulty in bringing up sputum which some of these patients experience can be

explained on the same basis. A normal cough in patients with partial loss of voice or aphonia virtually excludes laryngeal paralysis.

Dyspnoea and *stridor* are occasionally present but are seldom severe except with bilateral laryngeal paralysis of organic origin.

Laryngoscopy is necessary to establish the diagnosis of laryngeal paralysis with certainty. The paralysed cord lies in the so-called 'cadaveric' position, midway between abduction and adduction. In hysteria only adduction of the cords, a voluntary movement, is affected.

Treatment. The cause of the laryngeal paralysis should be treated if that is possible. In unilateral paralysis the voice can be improved by the injection of teflon into the affected vocal cord. In bilateral organic paralysis, tracheal intubation, tracheostomy or a plastic operation on the larynx may be necessary. Psychiatric treatment is indicated for hysterical aphonia.

Laryngeal Obstruction

Aetiology. The laryngeal opening (glottis) may be obstructed by (1) inflammatory or allergic oedema or exudate, (2) spasm of the laryngeal muscles, (3) inhaled foreign body, (4) inhaled vomitus in an unconscious patient, (5) tumours of the larynx, (6) bilateral vocal cord paralysis and (7) fixation of both cords in advanced rheumatoid arthritis. Laryngeal obstruction is more liable to occur in children than in adults because of the smaller size of the glottis.

Clinical Features. Sudden complete laryngeal obstruction by a foreign body produces the clinical picture of acute asphyxia — violent but ineffective inspiratory efforts with indrawing of the intercostal spaces and the unsupported lower ribs, accompanied by deep cyanosis. Unrelieved, the condition progresses rapidly to coma, and death ensues within 5 to 10 minutes. When, as in most cases, the obstruction is incomplete at first, the main clinical features are progressive dyspnoea and cyanosis, stridor and indrawing of the intercostal spaces and lower ribs on both sides. The great danger in these cases is that the obstruction may at any time become complete and result in sudden death.

Treatment. Transient attacks of laryngeal obstruction due to exudate and spasm, which may occur with acute laryngitis in children (p. 220) and with whooping cough, are potentially dangerous but can usually be relieved by the inhalation of steam.

Laryngeal obstruction from all other causes carries a high mortality and demands prompt treatment. The following measures may have to be employed:

1. *The Relief of Obstruction by Mechanical Means.* When a foreign body is known to be the cause of the obstruction in children it can often be dislodged by turning the patient's head downwards and thumping the back vigorously. In adults this is often impossible, but sudden forceful compression of the upper abdomen (Heimlich manoeuvre) may be effective. In other circumstances the cause of the obstruction should be investigated by direct laryngoscopy, which may also permit the removal of an unsuspected foreign body or the insertion of a tube past the obstruction into the trachea. Tracheostomy must be performed without delay if these procedures fail to relieve the obstruction, but except in dire emergencies the operation should be performed in the operating theatre by a surgeon.

2. *Treatment of the Cause.* In cases of diphtheria, antitoxin should be administered and for other infections the appropriate antibiotic should be given. In angio-oedema the patient should receive adrenaline (0·5–1·0 ml of 1:1000 solution s.c.), chlorpheniramine maleate (10–20 mg i.v.) and hydrocortisone hemisuccinate (100 mg i.v.). These remedies take time to act and tracheostomy may be required in the intervening period.

Diseases of the Trachea

Acute tracheitis is a common complication of viral and bacterial infection of the upper respiratory tract (p. 219), and is usually associated with acute bronchitis (p. 222). Other primary disorders of the trachea are rare.

Tracheal Obstruction. Intrinsic benign and malignant tumours may produce tracheal obstruction, but external compression by enlarged mediastinal lymph nodes containing metastatic deposits from a bronchial carcinoma is a much more common cause. Rarely, the trachea may be compressed by an aneurysm of the aortic arch, or in children by tuberculous mediastinal lymph nodes. Tracheal stricture is an occasional complication of tracheostomy.

Stridor (p. 209) can be detected in every patient with severe tracheal obstruction. Endoscopic examination of the trachea should be undertaken without delay in these patients to determine the degree of obstruction and its nature.

Localised tumours of the trachea can be resected, but reconstruction of the resected segment may present complex technical problems. Radiotherapy or the administration of cytotoxic drugs may temporarily relieve compression by malignant lymph nodes. Tracheal strictures can sometimes be dilated, but may have to be resected.

Tracheo-oesophageal Fistula. This may be present in newborn infants as a congenital abnormality. In adults, it is usually due to malignant lesions in the mediastinum, such as carcinoma or lymphoma, eroding both the trachea and oesophagus, to produce a communication between them. Swallowed liquids enter the trachea and bronchi through the fistula, and provoke a 'spluttering' cough. Surgical closure of a congenital fistula, if undertaken promptly, is usually successful, but malignant fistulae are incurable, and death from overwhelming pulmonary infection rapidly supervenes.

CHRONIC OBSTRUCTIVE AIRWAYS DISEASE

Although chronic bronchitis and emphysema are pathologically distinct, they frequently co-exist, and it may then be difficult or impossible to determine the relative importance of each condition in the individual case. Generalised airflow obstruction is the dominant feature of both diseases In chronic bronchitis it is chiefly due to swelling of the bronchial mucosa and the accumulation of tenacious mucus within the air passages. In emphysema, on the other hand, the main factor in the production of airflow obstruction is extramural bronchial compression and collapse caused by overdistended alveoli in which air has been 'trapped' during expiration. This phenomenon is aggravated by chronic bronchitis and bronchopulmonary infection.

Chronic bronchitis and emphysema are often grouped together under the heading of 'chronic obstructive airways disease', and can be regarded as forming a spectrum, with 'pure' chronic bronchitis at one end and 'pure' emphysema at the other. For descriptive purposes, however, it is convenient to deal with them separately, with emphasis on their similarities and differences, and on the relationships which frequently exist between them.

Chronic Bronchitis

Aetiology. Chronic bronchitis is the name given to the clinical syndrome which many individuals develop in response to the long-continued action of various types of irritant on the bronchial mucosa. The most important of these is tobacco smoke, but they also include dust, smoke and fumes, occurring as specific occupational hazards or as part of a general atmospheric pollution in industrial cities and towns. Infection is sometimes a precipitating factor in the onset of chronic bronchitis, but its main role is in aggravating the established condition. Exposure to dampness, to sudden changes in temperature and to fog may also be responsible for exacerbations of chronic bronchitis.

The disorder occurs most commonly in middle and late adult life and more males are affected than females. It is much more common in smokers than in non-smokers, and in urban than in rural dwellers.

On culture of the sputum, *Strep. pneumoniae* and *H. influenzae* are isolated in most cases. These organisms become more numerous during acute exacerbations.

Pathology. In all cases there is overactivity of the mucus-secreting glands and goblet cells in the bronchi and bronchioles. The vast excess of mucus so produced coats the bronchial walls and clogs the bronchioles. Mucosal oedema further reduces the calibre of the air passages and as the degree of obstruction is greater during expiration air is 'trapped' in the alveoli. With the passage of time the alveoli become permanently over distended and there is extensive rupture of their walls. These changes, which constitute one form of 'emphysema', are also discussed on page 254.

Clinical Features. The disease usually starts with repeated attacks of 'winter cough', which show a steady increase in severity and duration with successive years, until cough is present all the year round. Wheeze, dyspnoea and tightness in the chest are common complaints, especially in the morning before the bronchial secretions are cleared, often with difficulty, by coughing. The sputum may be scanty, tenacious mucoid, and occasionally streaked with blood, or copious and watery. A frankly purulent sputum is indicative of bacterial infection, which supervenes from time to time in most cases of bronchitis.

Dyspnoea in chronic bronchitis is caused by airflow obstruction, and is aggravated by infection, excessive cigarette smoking and adverse atmospheric conditions.

Variable numbers of inspiratory and expiratory rhonchi, mainly low and medium pitched, are present in most cases of chronic bronchitis and there may also be some coarse crepitations. Physical signs attributable to emphysema may coexist.

Investigation. *Radiological Examination.* Chronic bronchitis produces no characteristic abnormality in the radiograph, but the features of emphysema (p. 255) may be prominent in some cases. Bronchography shows various irregularities of bronchial outline, calibre and branching, but is no longer a routine investigation in chronic bronchitis.

Pulmonary Function Tests. 1. The forced expiratory volume in 1 second (FEV_1) is reduced, and the ratio of FEV_1 to forced vital capacity (FVC) is also subnormal. In advanced cases the FEV_1 may be less than 1 l, and the FEV/FVC ratio may be as low as 30%. Such changes are common to all forms of obstructive airways disease.

2. With 'air trapping' and alveolar distension the residual volume of the lungs is increased at the expense of vital capacity.

3. As the distribution of ventilation and perfusion within the lungs becomes disturbed (p. 206), the Pao_2 falls below normal.

4. Impairment of carbon monoxide transfer occurs in a proportion of patients and marked reduction may provide an indication of the presence of emphysema.

5. In the later stages, when generalised alveolar underventilation supervenes, there is a further fall in Pao_2 and a sustained rise in $Paco_2$ (chronic Type II respiratory failure p. 210). Hypoxaemia becomes more severe during sleep, and some patients have periods of 'sleep apnoea' which cause profound falls in Pao_2. These may be factors in the production of pulmonary hypertension (p. 255).

Course and Prognosis. Chronic bronchitis is usually a progressive disease, punctuated by acute exacerbations and remissions, and eventually causing respiratory and cardiac failure. Some patients die within a few years of the onset of symptoms, while others survive for many years, with gradually diminishing respiratory reserve.

Treatment. 1. *Bronchial irritation* must be reduced to a minimum. If a smoker, the patient should be urged to give up the habit completely and permanently. Dusty and smoke-laden atmospheres should be avoided, which may involve a change of occupation.

2. *Respiratory infection* must be promptly controlled, as it aggravates dyspnoea and may precipitate ventilatory failure. The patient should be instructed to observe the colour of the sputum every morning, and, if it becomes purulent, should be given oxytetracycline or ampicillin in a dose of 250 mg four times daily or co-trimoxazole, 2 tablets twice daily, for 5 to 7 days. Intelligent patients can be provided with a stock of antibiotic tablets, and permitted to start a course of treatment on their own initiative when the need arises.

As the vast majority of bacterial infections in chronic bronchitis are caused by *Strep. pneumoniae* or *H. influenzae*, bacteriological examination of sputum is essential only when the response to standard treatment is unsatisfactory, and the sputum remains purulent. In that event a change of antibiotic, guided by the results of bacterial sensitivity tests, will be indicated. Continuous suppressive treatment with a tetracycline or ampicillin given throughout the winter or even throughout the year, is not advised, since it is apt to promote the emergence of a drug-resistant respiratory tract flora, and may merely add to the therapeutic problems.

3. *Symptomatic measures* may be required to control unproductive cough during the night, to enable sputum to be coughed up more easily and to relieve breathlessness and wheeze. Nocturnal unproductive cough will often be less troublesome if the patient sleeps in a heated bedroom, but pholcodine or methadone may be required to control it. A hot drink or the inhalation of steam helps to liquefy sputum and make it easier to bring up. So-called expectorant cough mixtures and drugs claimed to reduce sputum viscosity are of little or no value. Bronchodilators (p. 245) are much less effective in chronic bronchitis than in asthma, but are of value in those patients with demonstrable reversibility of airflow obstruction.

4. *Type II respiratory failure* must be promptly treated (p. 217).

Prevention. The abandonment of smoking is the most important preventive measure. The control of atmospheric pollution in urban areas and the increased use of measures to prevent the inhalation of dust by industrial workers will also help to reduce the prevalence of chronic bronchitis. Respiratory infection should be promptly and efficiently treated.

EMPHYSEMA

The word 'emphysema' means 'inflation' in the sense of unnatural distension with air, and this phenomenon, thus defined, can occur anywhere in the body. Air may, for example, enter the mediastinum (*mediastinal emphysema*) following the rupture of overdistended alveoli into the interstitial tissues of the lung in patients with severe bronchial asthma, or following rupture of the oesophagus. If a very large amount of air escapes rapidly into the mediastinum, it may produce cardiac tamponade (p. 187), but in most cases it tracks harmlessly upwards into the soft tissues of the neck, where it imparts a characteristic crackling sensation to the palpating fingers (*subcutaneous emphysema*). Penetrating wounds of the chest wall may also cause subcutaneous emphysema, and when a spontaneous pneumothorax is treated by pleural decompression with an intercostal tube (p. 275), widespread subcutaneous emphysema is an occasional complication, which is alarming but not serious.

Pulmonary Emphysema

The term 'pulmonary emphysema' covers a wide variety of pathological processes, ranging from overdistension of otherwise normal alveoli in conditions such as bronchial asthma, obstructive emphysema and compensatory emphysema to the widespread disruption of the alveolar walls which occurs in the more serious forms of pulmonary emphysema. There is a close association between the latter and chronic bronchitis, but the physical signs and radiological changes attributable to 'emphysema' may be more conspicuous in some cases of chronic bronchitis than in others.

In 'pure' emphysema generalised destruction of the alveolar walls ('panacinar' emphysema) is the dominant lesion. Where emphysema occurs along with a major component of chronic bronchitis, it is usually 'centrilobular' or 'centriacinar', and principally affects these alveoli which are most closely related to the respiratory bronchioles.

Although these two types of emphysema develop in different ways, factors such as bacterial infection, alveolar overdistension and distortion of the airways may eventually blur their distinctive features. The predominance of either chronic bronchitis or emphysema may, however, be sufficiently clear-cut to produce two separately identifiable syndromes. In the chronic bronchitis syndrome, ventilatory capacity is fairly well preserved, but severe hypoxia and hypercapnia, pulmonary hypertension and right ventricular failure occur at an early stage (the *'blue bloater'*). In the emphysema syndrome, on the other hand, grave impairment of ventilatory capacity and disabling exertional dyspnoea may antedate by many years the manifestations of respiratory and cardiac failure (the *'pink puffer'*). A mixed syndrome of chronic bronchitis and emphysema is, however, much more commonly seen than either of the two individual syndromes.

Emphysema in young adults may be associated with genetically determined α_1-antitrypsin deficiency (p. 344). It is believed that connective tissue in the lung is digested by proteolytic enzymes normally inhibited by α_1-antitrypsin, the serum concentration of which can be measured in most hospital laboratories.

Clinical Features. Most patients with pulmonary emphysema complain of exertional dyspnoea, but since other causes of airflow obstruction, such as chronic bronchitis and bronchial asthma, often co-exist, it is seldom possible to assess the contribution of emphysema *per se* to the production of this symptom. There is a progressive increase in respiratory disability, but the tempo of deterioration varies widely from one case to another. For example, in patients with a relatively minor component of chronic bronchitis, the exertional dyspnoea increases slowly over a period of several years, but the course of the disease tends to be more rapid where chronic bronchitis is a dominant feature.

The physical signs which may be observed in emphysema and other forms of chronic airflow obstruction are summarised in Table 8.1. Other clinical abnormalities include (1) a reduction in the length of the trachea palpable above the sternal notch, (2) tracheal descent with inspiration, (3) contraction of the sternomastoid and scalene muscles on inspiration, (4) excavation of the suprasternal and supraclavicular fossae during inspiration, (5) jugular venous filling during expiration, (6) indrawing of the costal margins during inspiration, and (7) an increase in the anteroposterior diameter of the chest relative to the lateral diameter.

Investigation. *Radiological Examination.* A diagnosis of emphysema can be made with reasonable confidence if the following abnormalities are present: (1) Unusually translucent lung fields, with loss of peripheral vascular markings. (2) Bullae (below). (3) A low flat diaphragm, which moves poorly on fluoroscopy (2 cm or less). (4) Prominence of the pulmonary hilar arterial shadows at both hila.

Abnormalities caused by pulmonary infection ('inflammatory shadowing') may also be present. In the late stages, when pulmonary hypertension and right ventricular failure supervene, there is enlargement of the main pulmonary artery, the right ventricle and the right atrium.

Pulmonary Function Tests. See page 253.

Complications. 1. *Type I and II Respiratory Failure* (p. 210). The latter may be associated with *secondary polycythaemia* as a consequence of prolonged severe hypoxaemia.

2. *Pulmonary Hypertension and Right Ventricular Failure.* The increase in pulmonary arterial pressure is due to vasoconstriction mediated by the effect of hypoxia on pulmonary arterioles and ultimately to destruction of the pulmonary vascular bed. As hypoxia is aggravated by any increase in the degree of airflow obstruction, bacterial infection in the respiratory tract, oedema of the bronchial mucosa, oversecretion of bronchial mucus and spasm of the bronchial muscles (which can all cause hypoxia) are liable to increase the pulmonary arterial pressure and precipitate right ventricular failure. Conversely, effective treatment of these causes of hypoxia, combined with oxygen therapy and diuretics, may relieve pulmonary hypertension and cardiac failure, at least for a time.

3. *Pulmonary bullae*, single or multiple, large or small, may develop in emphysematous lung tissue, regardless of the primary pathology. Bullae are inflated thin-walled spaces created by rupture of the alveolar walls. They are usually situated subpleurally, and are commonly found along the anterior borders of the lungs. A small bulla may rupture, causing spontaneous pneumothorax. In other circumstances bullae may increase progressively in size, and eventually become so large that they interfere seriously with pulmonary ventilation.

Treatment. There is no specific remedy for emphysema, but the patient may benefit considerably from the treatment of associated chronic bronchitis (p. 253), and of respiratory failure (p. 217), which is a common complication. Obesity must be prevented or corrected, as excess weight is an intolerable burden on the reduced cardiorespiratory reserve. The purpose of physiotherapy should be to induce relaxation of the cervical muscles and to show the patient how to exhale slowly and steadily through pursed lips. It should also be used to encourage expectoration. Regular mild exercise has also been shown to increase mobility, even in severely disabled patients. The surgical ablation of giant bullae, where this is feasible, may allow relatively normal lung tissue compressed by the bullae to re-expand

and may bring about a dramatic improvement in pulmonary function.

BRONCHIECTASIS

Aetiology and Pathogenesis. Bronchiectasis, which is the term used to describe abnormal dilatation of the bronchi, may be produced in different ways. In most cases bronchiectasis is secondary to severe bacterial infection, including tuberculosis, in the lungs. It is also a complication of bronchial eosinophilia (p. 247).

When pulmonary collapse follows obstruction of groups of small bronchi by secretion, the shrinkage of the affected portion of lung exerts outward traction on the walls of the medium-sized bronchi, which become dilated. Bronchiectasis arising in this way may be reversible if the obstructed bronchi can be cleared of secretion before the walls of the dilated bronchi are seriously damaged by infection.

Bronchiectasis may be due to bronchial distension resulting from the accumulation of pus beyond a lesion obstructing a major bronchus, such as a tuberculous hilar lymph node, an inhaled foreign body or a bronchial carcinoma. In cystic fibrosis (p. 308) recurrent infection and chronic obstruction by viscid mucus are both factors in causing bronchiectasis. Rarely, it may be the result of congenital dysfunction of the cilia, which is a feature of, for example, Kartagener's syndrome (bronchiectasis, sinusitis and transposition of the viscera).

Because of the many different causes of bronchiectasis no precise age incidence can be stated. When it occurs following acute pulmonary infections or secondary to obstruction of a bronchus by tuberculous lymph nodes (the two most common causes), the disease usually starts in childhood but may not produce severe symptoms until some years later.

Pathology. Although bronchiectasis may involve any part of the lungs, depending on the site of the primary pathological process, the lower lobes are more frequently affected than the upper and middle, but the more efficient drainage by gravity of the upper lobes renders bronchiectasis there less liable to produce serious symptoms than when it involves the lower lobes. The bronchiectatic cavities may be lined by granulation tissue, squamous epithelium or normal ciliated epithelium. There may also be inflammatory changes in the deeper layers of the bronchial walls and chronic inflammatory and fibrotic changes in the surrounding lung tissue.

Clinical Features. Three groups of clinical features occur in bronchiectasis:

1. *Those due to the accumulation of pus in the dilated bronchi* are chronic cough, usually worse in the mornings and often induced by changes in posture, and purulent sputum which in advanced cases is copious and sometimes fetid.

2. *Those due to inflammatory changes in the surrounding lung tissue and pleura.* Febrile episodes usually last for a few days but occasionally for weeks. Malaise, shivering and sleep sweating accompany the pyrexia; there is an increase in the amount of cough and sputum, a neutrophil leucocytosis is usually present and there may be radiological evidence of pneumonia. Dry pleurisy frequently accompanies the febrile episodes. Empyema is an occasional complication of bronchiectasis.

When chronic suppuration, either in the bronchi or in the lungs, is a marked feature it causes a decline in the patient's general health, with lassitude, anorexia, loss of weight, sleep sweating and clubbing of the fingers and toes. In many cases, however, symptoms are slight, consisting merely of recurrent episodes of cough and purulent sputum with no symptoms in the intervening periods and no deterioration in health.

3. *Haemoptysis* is caused by bleeding from thin-walled anastomotic vessels connecting the pulmonary and bronchial arteries, and situated in the walls of the dilated bronchi. It ranges in amount from blood-stained sputum to massive haemorrhage. It may be present in association with the first two groups of symptoms, but recurrent haemoptysis may also occur as an isolated symptom in the absence of cough and sputum ('dry' bronchiectasis).

Physical signs may be unilateral or bilateral and are usually basal. If the bronchiectatic cavities are dry and there is no lobar collapse, there may be no abnormal physical signs. If a large amount of secretion is present, numerous coarse crepitations are heard over the affected areas. When collapse is present the character of the physical signs depends on whether or not the proximal bronchi in the collapsed lobe are patent (Table 8.1).

Investigation. In ordinary radiographs the dilated bronchi themselves may not be visible, but changes may be produced by associated pulmonary inflammation or collapse. A diagnosis of bronchiectasis can be made with certainty only by bronchography.

Bacteriological examination of the sputum is necessary in every case to exclude tuberculosis and to identify other pathogenic bacteria.

Treatment. *Postural Drainage*. The purpose of this measure is to keep the dilated bronchi emptied of secretion. Efficiently performed it is of great value both in reducing the amount of cough and sputum and in preventing the 'toxaemia' caused by associated bronchopulmonary infection. In its simplest form, postural drainage consists of adopting a position in which the lobe to be drained is uppermost, so as to allow secretions in the dilated bronchi to gravitate towards the trachea, from which they can readily be cleared by vigorous coughing. The optimum duration and frequency of postural drainage depends on the amount of sputum, but 5 to 10 minutes once or twice daily is adequate in most cases.

Chemotherapy. The policy governing the use of antibiotics in bronchiectasis is the same as that in chronic bronchitis. Some patients, including those with cystic fibrosis, present difficult therapeutic problems arising from secondary infection with bacteria such as staphylococci and gram-negative bacilli, especially pseudomonas species.

Surgical Treatment. If surgical treatment is being considered, it is essential to obtain bronchograms demonstrating exactly the extent of the bronchiectasis. For this purpose the bronchi of all segments of both lungs must be outlined with a radio-opaque contrast medium. Pulmonary function should also be assessed.

The use of antibiotics has greatly reduced the need for surgical treatment. Unfortunately many of the cases in which medical treatment has been unsuccessful are also unsuitable for surgical treatment either because the bronchiectasis is too extensive or because most of the symptoms are due to coexisting chronic bronchitis. Emphysema of even moderate severity is a contraindication to surgical treatment, as the increase in exertional dyspnoea which inevitably results is more distressing to the patient than the symptoms of bronchiectasis. The most favourable cases for surgery are children and young adults in whom the bronchiectasis is confined to a single lobe or part of a lobe. Lobar or segmental resection in these patients is a highly satisfactory operation, carrying little risk.

Prevention. As bronchiectasis commonly starts in childhood following measles, whooping cough or a primary tuberculous infection, it is essential that these conditions receive adequate treatment. The early recognition and treatment of bronchial obstruction is particularly important in this respect.

Prognosis. With antibiotic therapy the prognosis, even in advanced cases, has greatly improved and the incidence of complications such as pneumonia, empyema, cerebral abscess and amyloidosis has fallen considerably.

BRONCHIAL OBSTRUCTION

Aetiology. The lesions most likely to obstruct a large bronchus are: (1) tumours, e.g. bronchial carcinoma or adenoma; (2) enlarged tracheobronchial lymph nodes, malignant or tuberculous; (3) inhaled foreign bodies; (4) bronchial casts or plugs, consisting of inspissated mucus or blood clot; (5) collections of mucus or mucopus retained in the bronchi as a result of ineffective expectoration.

Rare causes of bronchial obstruction include congenital bronchial atresia, fibrous bronchial stricture (often post-tuberculous), aortic aneurysm, giant left atrium and pericardial effusion.

Clinical Features. The manifestations of obstruction of a large bronchus depend on whether the obstruction is complete or partial, on secondary infection and on the effect on pulmonary function. The clinical features also vary with the cause of the obstruction.

1. COMPLETE OBSTRUCTION. When a large bronchus is completely obstructed, the air in the lung, lobe or segment it supplies is absorbed, the alveolar spaces close, and the affected portion of lung tissue becomes collapsed and solid. The percussion note over the collapsed lung or lobe is dull,

the breath sounds are absent or diminished, and radiological examination shows displacement of the trachea and/or heart shadow towards the side of the lesion, elevation of the diaphragm on the same side and a dense pulmonary opacity of characteristic size, shape and position.

If the collapse involves a smaller portion of lung (e.g. the right middle lobe or a bronchopulmonary segment), displacement of the mediastinum may not occur, and abnormal physical signs may be difficult to detect, but a characteristic radiographic opacity will be present.

The radiological features of pulmonary and lobar collapse are shown in Figures 8.5 and 8.6. Semisolid material, such as mucus, mucopus or blood clot, obstructing a large bronchus is apt to fragment, and portions of it may then be aspirated into the peripheral bronchi, leaving the larger bronchus clear. The absent or diminished breath sounds are then replaced by bronchial breath sounds, but the other clinical and radiological abnormalities do not change.

2. PARTIAL OBSTRUCTION. If a large bronchus is partially obstructed, a situation occasionally arises in which there is less resistance to air flow through the narrowed bronchus during inspiration than during expiration, when the obstruction may become temporarily complete. This differential between inspiratory and expiratory airflow, which is increased by coughing, results in overdistension of the lung, lobe or segment supplied by the partially obstructed bronchus (*obstructive emphysema*). The percussion note over such a

lesion is resonant or hyperresonant, and the breath sounds are diminished. A chest radiograph shows hypertranslucency of the affected part of lung, and on fluoroscopic examination the mediastinum can be seen to move towards the opposite side of the chest during expiration, because the volume of the affected lung then exceeds that of the contralateral lung.

3. SECONDARY INFECTION. Whenever a bronchus is narrowed, bacterial infection of the lung tissue it supplies is virtually inevitable, and this may occur even when the degree of obstruction is insufficient to cause pulmonary collapse. This explains why pneumonia may be the first clinical manifestation of bronchial carcinoma. The infection is usually of low virulence, but in some cases severe pulmonary suppuration may occur, with empyema as a further complication.

4. PULMONARY FUNCTION. Bronchial obstruction impairs pulmonary function, but this is unlikely to produce symptoms unless a main or lobar bronchus is involved, or if the patient's overall pulmonary function is so poor that obstruction of a smaller bronchus critically diminishes the respiratory reserve. Sudden occlusion of a main or lobar bronchus by mucus or mucopus occurring as a postoperative complication may cause severe dyspnoea and hypoxaemia.

5. CLINICAL FEATURES RELATED TO THE CAUSE OF THE OBSTRUCTION.

(i) *Tumours*. Bronchial obstruction by a carcinoma usually produces pulmonary collapse at an early stage and seldom causes obstructive emphy-

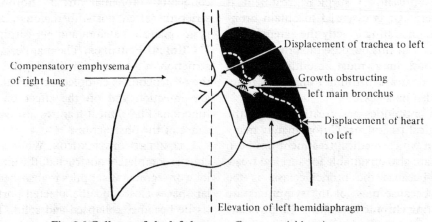

Compensatory emphysema of right lung

Displacement of trachea to left

Growth obstructing left main bronchus

Displacement of heart to left

Elevation of left hemidiaphragm

Fig. 8.5 Collapse of the left lung — effects on neighbouring structures.

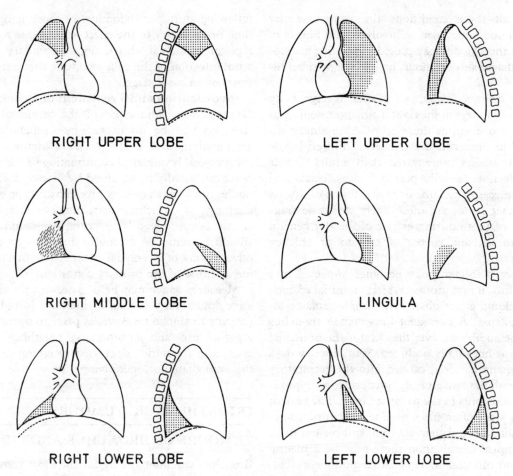

Fig. 8.6 Radiological features of lobar collapse caused by bronchial obstruction. The dotted line represents the normal position of the diaphragm.

sema. Pulmonary infection is common, and this may be complicated by empyema. The degree of exertional dyspnoea produced by a bronchial carcinoma is directly related to the size of the obstructed bronchus. The rate of growth of a bronchial adenoma is much less rapid than that of a carcinoma. Complete bronchial obstruction and pulmonary collapse are therefore later developments in the presence of an adenoma, and obstructive emphysema, caused by partial bronchial obstruction, may be observed during the intervening period.

(ii) *Enlarged Tracheobronchial Lymph Nodes.* By compressing or invading the bronchial wall, enlarged lymph nodes may produce the same clinical manifestations of bronchial obstruction as a tumour within the lumen, and in bronchial

carcinoma both types of lesion may co-exist. Bronchial obstruction by enlarged lymph nodes in Hodgkin's disease and other forms of lymphoma is less common than in bronchial carcinoma, presumably because these are less invasive types of tumour.

In some children with primary tuberculous infection, large caseous tracheobronchial lymph nodes may compress and erode lobar or segmental bronchi, occasionally even a main bronchus. Caseous material and granulation tissue from the lymph node may be extruded into the bronchial lumen and increase the degree of bronchial obstruction. Tuberculous infection may develop in the collapsed lobe or segment, and later complications include bronchial stricture and bronchiectasis.

In all these conditions the supraclavicular lymph nodes may also be involved, and biopsy of one of these nodes may provide a positive histological diagnosis of tumour, lymphoma or tuberculosis.

(iii) *Foreign Bodies*. An inhaled foreign body generally lodges in the right main, intermediate or lower bronchus, as these bronchi are almost directly in line with the trachea. Children inhale foreign bodies more often than adults. These include nuts (usually peanuts), peas, beans and small pieces of metallic or plastic toys. Adults, on the other hand, are more likely to inhale fragments of tooth during extractions under general anaesthesia, and pieces of mutton or chicken bone.

When a foreign body becomes impacted in a bronchus, it first produces, after an initial episode of choking, either obstructive emphysema or lobar collapse. A persistent low-pitched rhonchus may be audible all over the chest if the bronchial lumen is not totally occluded. Within a few days pathogenic bacteria, carried into the respiratory tract with the foreign body, give rise to a suppurative pneumonia in the collapsed lobe. The patient at this stage often has a high temperature, cough productive of purulent sputum, and pleural pain. On clinical examination there may be a pleural rub and physical signs of either pulmonary collapse or consolidation. Radiological examination shows either obstructive emphysema or collapse and/or pneumonic consolidation. It may also detect and locate a radio-opaque foreign body.

(iv) *Bronchial Casts or Plugs*. These may consist of either inspissated mucus or blood clot. Plugs of mucus may cause bronchial obstruction in patients with asthma or bronchial eosinophilia (p. 247). Secondary bacterial infection of the collapsed lung may occur, but is seldom severe. Bronchial obstruction by blood clot frequently follows severe haemoptysis, but as this complication is usually recognised and treated at an early stage, secondary bacterial infection of collapsed lung tissue seldom occurs.

(v) *Retained Secretions*. A main, lobar or segmental bronchus may be obstructed by retained mucus or mucopus when a patient is unable to cough effectively because of chest pain, muscular weakness or general debility. Pulmonary collapse following an upper abdominal or thoracic operation, or an injury to the chest wall, is due to this type of bronchial obstruction. Secondary bacterial infection of the collapsed lung tissue supervenes at an early stage.

Investigation and Treatment of Bronchial Obstruction. The cause of the bronchial obstruction can be discovered by bronchoscopic examination, and in the case of tumour and tuberculosis histological confirmation of the diagnosis can usually be obtained by biopsy. Foreign bodies can be extracted by bronchoscopy or bronchotomy. If bronchial casts, plugs or secretions cannot be dislodged by postural coughing, they should be removed through a bronchoscope. In other forms of bronchial obstruction the treatment is that of the primary condition.

Measures which may help to prevent postoperative pulmonary collapse include forbidding patients to smoke for 3 weeks prior to operation, vigorous pre- and postoperative breathing exercises, and regularly supervised coughing during the immediate postoperative period.

INTRATHORACIC TUMOURS

TUMOURS OF BRONCHUS AND LUNG

Bronchial carcinoma is by far the most common malignant pulmonary tumour. Benign tumours are rare. A primary carcinoma in any organ, but particularly in breast, kidney, uterus, ovary, testis, thyroid or in lung itself, may give rise to pulmonary metastatic deposits, as may an osteogenic or melanotic sarcoma.

Bronchial Carcinoma

Bronchial carcinoma accounts for more than 50% of all male deaths from malignant disease. It is four times more common in men than in women (although this ratio is now narrowing), and occurs most frequently between the ages of 50 and 75. Cigarette smoking is responsible for most cases of bronchial carcinoma, and the increased risk is directly proportional to the amount smoked and to the tar content of the cigarettes. For example, the death rate from the disease in heavy cigarette smokers is 40 times that in non-smokers. It is slightly higher in urban than in rural dwellers, presumably because of atmospheric pollution. There is also a higher incidence of bronchial carcinoma in asbestosis.

Pathology. The tumour, may be a squamous carcinoma (55%), a small cell carcinoma (25%) a large cell carcinoma (10%) or an adenocarcinoma (10%). It arises from bronchial epithelium or mucous glands and at an early stage may occlude the bronchial lumen. It also invades the deeper layers of the bronchial wall and the surrounding lung tissue. When the tumour obstructs a major bronchus it causes pulmonary collapse and infection (p. 257). A tumour arising from a peripheral bronchus may attain a very large size without producing a significant degree of collapse. Such a tumour, which is usually of the squamous type, may undergo central necrosis and cavitation.

The tumour may involve the pleura either directly or by lymphatic spread, causing a pleural effusion which is often blood-stained. It may also extend into the chest wall and cause severe pain by invading intercostal nerves or the brachial plexus. The tumour or its lymph node metastases may extend into the mediastinum, involving the phrenic and recurrent laryngeal nerves, the sympathetic trunk, the superior vena cava, the pericardium and myocardium, the trachea and the oesophagus.

Lymphatic spread may occur to the supraclavicular ('scalene') lymph nodes as well as to the mediastinal lymph nodes and pleura. Blood-borne metastases occur most commonly in liver, bone, brain, suprarenals, skin and kidneys. Even a small primary tumour may cause widespread metastatic deposits. A carcinoma of the small cell type has often spread beyond the lung by the time it is diagnosed.

Clinical Features. Cough is the most common early symptom. Sputum is purulent if there is secondary bacterial infection. Repeated slight haemoptysis is a common and characteristic feature. Dyspnoea may occur early when a lobe or lung is collapsed, or if there is a large pleural effusion, but in other circumstances is a late symptom unless the patient is coincidentally suffering from chronic bronchitis and emphysema. Pleural pain is a frequent symptom and may be due either to infective pleurisy or to malignant invasion of the pleura. Pain in the chest wall or in an upper limb with a nerve root distribution may be present if the tumour involves intercostal nerves or the brachial plexus. An apical bronchial carcinoma may cause Horner's syndrome (p. 615). The symptoms and signs which may occur if the tumour invades the mediastinum are described in the section on mediastinal tumours (p. 263).

Occasionally the presenting symptom is due to metastases, e.g. headache, fits or personality change, jaundice, bone pain, haematuria or skin nodules which may be tender. Lassitude, anorexia and loss of weight are late symptoms, usually indicative of extensive metastatic spread.

Clubbing of the fingers is often seen and a few patients present with the features of hypertrophic pulmonary osteoarthropathy. These are examples of non-metastatic extra-pulmonary manifestations of bronchial carcinoma; other paraneoplastic syndromes are listed in Table 8.10. Two of the endocrine syndromes, inappropriate ADH secretion (p. 427) and ectopic ACTH secretion (p. 445) are associated with small cell carcinoma, and a third, hypercalcaemia, usually with squamous carcinoma. The neurological syndromes (p. 668) may occur with any type of bronchial carcinoma, but perhaps more often with small cell tumours.

Table 8.10 Non-metastatic extra-pulmonary manifestations of bronchial carcinoma.

Endocrine	Inappropriate secretion of antidiuretic hormone (ADH)
	Ectopic ACTH secretion
	Hypercalcaemia
	Carcinoid syndrome
	Gynaecomastia
Neurological	Polyneuropathy
	Myelopathy
	Cerebellar degeneration
Other	Digital clubbing
	Hypertrophic pulmonary osteoarthropathy
	Nephrotic syndrome
	Myasthenia
	Polymyositis and dermatomyositis

Physical signs in the chest depend on the size of the tumour, but even more on the nature and extent of its secondary effects on lung and pleura. In the early stages a tumour may cause no abnormal physical signs. A tumour obstructing a large bronchus produces the physical signs of collapse or obstructive emphysema. Pulmonary infection beyond an obstructing tumour gives rise to pneumonia which is unusually slow to respond to treatment. A massive tumour may give rise to signs resembling those of a pleural effusion. Involvement of the pleura either by infection or by tumour may produce signs of dry pleurisy or of a pleural effusion.

Investigation. *Radiological Examination.* A bronchial carcinoma may produce (i) a dense, irregular, hilar opacity, (ii) a dense, fairly well circumscribed, peripheral pulmonary opacity, often large when first discovered, sometimes irregularly cavitated or (iii) an opacity consistent with collapse of a whole lung, a lobe or a segment which may be associated with a hilar opacity due to the tumour itself.

In some cases radiological examination may show a pleural effusion (usually due to malignant spread but occasionally to bacterial infection), broadening of the mediastinal shadow (due to lymph node metastases), osteolytic lesions of the ribs (indicating either direct invasion by tumour or blood-borne metastases) or unilateral diaphragmatic paralysis (indicating involvement of the phrenic nerve). A paralysed hemidiaphragm is usually raised and on fluoroscopic examination moves 'paradoxically' when the patient sniffs, i.e. it moves upwards instead of downwards.

Bronchoscopy. Inspection of the intrabronchial portion of the tumour and removal of tissue for histological examination is possible in over 70% of cases.

Other investigations, such as transbronchial or percutaneous lung biopsy, scalene node biopsy or mediastinoscopy may be required to confirm the diagnosis.

Cytological examination of sputum or bronchial brushings for malignant cells is a valuable diagnostic measure when practised by a pathologist with special expertise in this technique. Percutaneous needle aspiration biopsy is a useful method of obtaining a positive cytological diagnosis in peripheral tumours, and when metastatic spread has occurred to lymph nodes, skin or liver.

The stage of the tumour (p. 110) is defined from the information obtained from the foregoing procedures.

Treatment and Prognosis. Unless surgical treatment is practicable, the average period of survival, after the diagnosis is made, is less than a year. Resection of the lung (pneumonectomy) or, in some cases, of the lobe containing the tumour (lobectomy) offers the best prospect of survival. The operation can be performed only on the small number of cases (about 20%) in which the tumour is discovered at an early and relatively localised stage and pulmonary function is adequate. The tumour is liable to recur even after an apparently successful operation, and only 30% of such patients survive for more than 5 years. Early diagnosis provides slightly better results, but the prognosis depends to an even greater extent on the histological type of tumour and on the presence or absence of metastatic deposits in the hilar lymph nodes. The outlook is particularly unfavourable when the tumour is a small cell carcinoma.

Small tumours can occasionally be eradicated by radiotherapy, but this form of treatment is more often used to relieve distressing complications such as superior vena caval obstruction, recurrent haemoptysis and pain caused by chest wall invasion or by skeletal metastatic deposits. Obstruction of the trachea and main bronchi can also be relieved temporarily by radiotherapy, but as the latter may initially produce tumour swelling and a dangerous increase in the degree of obstruction, prednisolone should be given for 24–48 hours before treatment is started.

The treatment of small cell carcinoma with combinations of cytotoxic drugs can increase the median survival of patients with this highly malignant type of bronchial carcinoma from 3 months to over a year. This form of treatment is, however, still in the experimental stage and because of problems arising from the toxicity of the drugs it should for the present be undertaken only in specialised centres. It is of little value in the treatment of other histological types of bronchial carcinoma.

Bronchial Adenoma

This is an uncommon tumour occurring in a younger age group than carcinoma, and affecting females as often as males. Although classified as a benign tumour it possesses some of the properties of a malignant growth and may eventually give rise to metastases. There are two histological types of bronchial adenoma, the relatively more common carcinoid tumour and the rare cylindroma, or 'adenoid cystic carcinoma', which often arises at the tracheal bifurcation. A carcinoid tumour may secrete 5-hydroxytryptamine, and give rise to the carcinoid syndrome (p. 32). The usual primary pathological lesion is a small, vascular tumour within the bronchial lumen with a large encapsulated extrabronchial extension.

The clinical features, which may have a duration of several years, are recurrent haemoptysis, due to the vascularity of the tumour, recurrent pulmonary infection resulting from bronchial obstruction and, in rare cases, usually when metastatic spread has occurred, the carcinoid syndrome. The physical signs most frequently found are those of collapse. The diagnosis from bronchial carcinoma can be made only by bronchoscopy and histological examination of a portion of the tumour.

Treatment consists of resection of the pulmonary lobe or segment containing the tumour along with the bronchus from which it arises.

Secondary Tumours of the Lung

Blood-borne metastatic deposits in the lungs may be derived from malignant disease almost anywhere in the body. The usual sites of the primary tumour have already been stated (p. 260). The secondary deposits are usually multiple and bilateral. Haemoptysis occurs in a few cases but often there are no respiratory symptoms and the diagnosis is made by radiological examination.

Extensive infiltration of the pulmonary lymphatics by tumour may develop in patients with carcinoma of breast, stomach, pancreas or bronchus. This condition, *pulmonary lymphatic carcinomatosis*, causes severe and rapidly progressive dyspnoea.

TUMOURS OF THE MEDIASTINUM

Classification. *Tumours of the lymph nodes,* e.g. secondary carcinoma, usually from bronchus

or breast; lymphomas, including Hodgkin's disease; leukaemia.

Thymic tumours, e.g. benign or malignant thymoma.

Connective tissue tumours, e.g. fibroma, lipoma (benign); sarcoma (malignant).

Neural tumours, e.g. neurofibroma.

Developmental tumours and cysts, e.g. teratoma; dermoid, bronchogenic and pleuro-pericardial cysts.

Other lesions presenting as mediastinal tumours, e.g. aortic aneurysm, aneurysmal dilatation of left atrium, intrathoracic goitre, sarcoidosis involving lymph nodes.

Pathology and Clinical Features.

BENIGN TUMOURS AND CYSTS. The conditions in this category, which are all rare, include neural tumours, teratoma, developmental cysts and intrathoracic goitre. They may compress, but do not invade, vital structures. The diagnosis of benign tumour or cyst is usually made by chance, when radiological examination of the chest is undertaken for some other reason. If a tumour becomes very large it may cause dyspnoea by compression of lung tissue, or occasionally by narrowing the trachea. A benign tumour in the upper part of the thorax occasionally compresses the superior vena cava (p. 264). A dermoid cyst occasionally ruptures into a bronchus.

MALIGNANT TUMOURS. Included in this category are mediastinal lymph node metastases, lymphomas, leukaemia, malignant thymic tumours and mediastinal sarcoma. Aortic and innominate aneurysms have destructive features resembling those of malignant mediastinal tumours. All these conditions, except lymph node metastases, are uncommon.

The distinguishing feature of this group of tumours is their power to invade as well as to compress mediastinal structures, bronchi and lungs. As a result of this property even a small malignant tumour can produce symptoms, although as a rule the tumour has attained a considerable size before this happens. The structures which may be invaded or compressed and the symptoms and signs produced in each case are:

Trachea: dyspnoea, stridor, paroxysmal cough.

Main bronchus: pulmonary collapse, dyspnoea.

Oesophagus: dysphagia, oesophageal displacement or obstruction on barium swallow examination.

Phrenic nerve: diaphragmatic paralysis.

Left recurrent laryngeal nerve: paralysis of left vocal cord, hoarseness, bovine cough.

Sympathetic trunk: Horner's syndrome.

Superior vena cava: oedema and cyanosis of head and neck, and sometimes of upper limbs also, with distension of external jugular veins and dilated anastomotic veins on anterior chest wall and in axillary regions.

Pericardium: pericarditis, either dry with pericardial rub, or with effusion.

Investigation. *Radiological Examination.* A benign mediastinal tumour generally appears as a large, round, sharply circumscribed opacity, situated mainly in the mediastinum but often encroaching on one or both lung fields. A malignant mediastinal tumour seldom has a clearly defined margin and often presents as a general broadening of the mediastinal shadow. Fluoroscopic examination of the diaphragm and oesophagus should be undertaken in all suspected cases of mediastinal tumour.

As bronchial carcinoma is such a common primary cause of mediastinal tumour, *bronchoscopy* should be carried out in all cases. If enlarged mediastinal lymph nodes are suspected one of these can be removed for histological examination by the technique of *mediastinoscopy* (p. 213). In some cases, however, an exact diagnosis cannot be made without *surgical exploration* of the chest and removal of the tumour or a portion of it for histological examination.

Treatment. Benign mediastinal tumours should be removed surgically as soon as they are discovered because (a) they tend to produce symptoms sooner or later and (b) some of them, particularly cysts, may become infected while others, especially neural tumours, may become malignant. The operative mortality is low.

The treatment of lymphoma and leukaemia is described on pages 522 and 534 respectively. A malignant thymoma usually responds dramatically to radiotherapy. Lymph node metastases from bronchial carcinoma may respond well to radiotherapy or to cytotoxic chemotherapy, especially if the tumour is of the small cell type; complications such as superior vena caval and tracheal obstruction can often be relieved in this way.

PULMONARY FIBROSIS AND RELATED DISEASES

There are three main types of pulmonary fibrosis:

1. *Replacement fibrosis*, in which the fibrous tissue replaces lung parenchyma damaged by infection or by some other destructive process (e.g. infarction). Fibrosis of this type is a common feature of pulmonary tuberculosis and of all types of pulmonary suppuration (p. 226), and is often associated with bronchiectasis.

2. *Focal fibrosis*, which is a common manifestation of pneumoconiosis.

3. *Interstitial fibrosis*, which is the end-result of interstitial lung disease.

If pulmonary fibrosis is extensive, it will cause exertional dyspnoea and hypoxaemia, and this is more likely to be the case in focal and interstitial fibrosis than in replacement fibrosis. On the other hand, the physical signs and radiological changes will usually be more conspicuous in replacement fibrosis, which generally produces gross localised abnormalities.

INTERSTITIAL LUNG DISEASE

This term is applied to a group of pulmonary diseases which have the following features in common: (1) thickening of the alveolar walls by oedema, cellular exudate or fibrosis; (2) increased stiffness of the lungs (reduced compliance), associated with exertional dyspnoea; (3) maldistribution of pulmonary ventilation and perfusion, and a gas transfer defect leading to hypoxaemia, hyperventilation and hypocapnia.

Aetiology. Interstitial lung disease is caused by several different pathological processes, but these all give rise to similar symptoms, physical signs, radiological changes and disturbances of pulmonary function. They are thus worthy of collective consideration. Causes of interstitial lung disease are:

1. Chronic pulmonary oedema e.g. secondary to mitral valve disease (p. 158).

2. Extrinsic allergic alveolitis (p. 249).

3. Fibrosing alveolitis associated with the connective tissue disorders, or of unknown aetiology (cryptogenic fibrosing alveolitis).

4. Pulmonary damage following radiotherapy to the thorax.

5. Sarcoidosis (p. 268), asbestosis (p. 267), and idiopathic pulmonary haemosiderosis (see below).

Fibrosing Alveolitis

This condition exemplifies many of the typical features of interstitial lung disease. It may be a manifestation of one of the connective tissue disorders, such as rheumatoid disease, systemic lupus erythematosus or systemic sclerosis, or it may occur as an isolated pulmonary abnormality.

Progressive exertional dyspnoea is usually the presenting symptom, often accompanied by a persistent dry cough. In most cases there is gross clubbing of the fingers and toes. Chest expansion is poor, but hyperventilation is always a striking feature. Numerous bilateral crackling crepitations are audible on auscultation.

Radiologically, there are diffuse pulmonary opacities, the diaphragm is high and the lungs appear small. There is a restrictive ventilatory defect, with proportionate reduction of FEV_1 and vital capacity. The carbon monoxide transfer factor is low, and there is arterial hypoxaemia and hypocapnia. The diagnosis can usually be made with confidence from these findings, but should in doubtful cases be confirmed by lung biopsy. Serological tests for antinuclear and rheumatoid factors may be positive, even in cases without evidence of a connective tissue disorder.

The rate of progression of the pulmonary changes varies considerably, from death within a few months to survival with minimal symptoms for many years.

Treatment with corticosteroids is effective in perhaps 30% of the acute cases, but is of little or no value in the others, few of which survive for more than 5 years.

Honeycomb Lung. The radiological phenomenon of 'honeycomb lung' in which diffuse pulmonary shadowing is interspersed with small cystic translucencies, may be observed in some cases of interstitial lung disease, but it may also be a characteristic feature of certain rare diseases, such as histiocytosis X and tuberous sclerosis. Honeycomb lung, whatever its cause, is associated with an increased incidence of spontaneous pneumothorax, and eventually produces respiratory failure, pulmonary hypertension and right ventricular failure.

Idiopathic Pulmonary Haemosiderosis

This is a rare disease of unknown cause, in which spontaneous haemorrhage into the lungs causes recurrent episodes of pyrexia, haemoptysis and iron-deficiency anaemia. With every incident, red blood cells in large numbers are extravasated into the interstitial tissues of the lungs, where haemosiderin released from macrophages stimulates fibroblastic activity. If the patient survives the acute haemorrhagic episodes, the interstitial fibrosis may eventually cause respiratory failure and pulmonary hypertension. Pulmonary haemosiderosis may also be associated with acute glomerulonephritis (Goodpasture's syndrome, p. 358).

During the acute episodes, widespread coarse crepitations are present, and diffuse stippled shadowing, chiefly involving the mid-zones of both lung fields, is seen on the chest radiograph. In the later stages the clinical and radiographic abnormalities may be indistinguishable from those of fibrosing alveolitis.

OCCUPATIONAL LUNG DISEASES

In certain occupations the inhalation of dusts, fumes or other noxious substances may give rise to specific pathological changes in the lungs. The nature of each substance, the occupation in which the hazard occurs, the description of each disease and the pathological changes produced in the lungs are summarised in Table 8.11.

Since a diagnosis of occupational lung disease can easily be overlooked and the victims of it may be eligible for compensation, it is most important to take a detailed occupational history, past as well as present. It must also be emphasised that in many types of pneumoconiosis a long period of exposure to dust is required before radiological changes appear and these may precede symptoms by several years. Notes on diagnosis and claims

Table 8.11 Causes and effects of occupational lung disease.

Cause	Occupation	Description of disease	Pathological changes
Mineral dusts:			
Coal dust	Coal mining	Coal-worker's pneumoconiosis	Focal and interstitial fibrosis
Silica	Gold mining	Silicosis	Centrilobular emphysema
	Iron and steel industries		Progressive massive fibrosis
	Metal grinding		
	Stone dressing		
	Pottery		
Asbestos	Manufacture of fireproof and insulating materials	Asbestos-related disease	Asbestos bodies
			Interstitial fibrosis
	Shipbreaking		Bronchial carcinoma
			Pleural mesothelioma
Iron oxide	Arc welding	Siderosis	Mineral deposition only
Tin dioxide	Tin ore mining	Stannosis	
Beryllium	Aircraft and atomic energy industries	Berylliosis	Granulomata
			Interstitial fibrosis
Organic dusts:			
Cotton, flax or hemp dust	Textile industries	Byssinosis	Acute bronchiolitis
			Bronchoconstriction
Fungal spores from mouldy hay, straw or grain, mushroom compost, bagasse, etc.	Agriculture and related industries	Farmer's lung Maltworker's lung Mushroom worker's lung Bagassosis	Extrinsic allergic alveolitis
Gases and fumes:			
Irritant gases (ammonia, chlorine, phosgene, sulphur and nitrogen dioxide)	Various industries (accidental exposure)		Acute pulmonary oedema
Cadmium	Welding and electroplating		Chronic bronchitis and emphysema
Isocyanates, e.g. toluene di-isocyanate, diphenylmethane di-isocyanate, hexamethylene di-isocyanate	Manufacture of plastic foam, synthetic inks, paints and adhesives. Paint-spraying of vehicles in motor industry and car repair workshops		Bronchial asthma Eosinophilic pneumonia Alveolitis
Platinum salts	Platinum refining Laboratory work involving platinum compounds		Bronchial asthma
Acid anhydride and amine hardening agents (including epoxy resin curing agents)	Manufacture of epoxy resins Manufacture of adhesives Moulding of resins and plastics		Bronchial asthma
Rosin (colophony) used in soldering fluxes	Electronics industry		Bronchial asthma
Biological substances:			
Proteolytic enzymes, e.g. *Bacillus subtilis*, pancreatic extracts, papain	Detergent manufacturing Pharmaceutical industry Food processing		Bronchial asthma
Animal and insect excreta	Animal laboratories Farming Flour milling		Bronchial asthma
Grain dust contaminated by mites and fungal spores	Combine harvesting Handling of stored grain.		Bronchial asthma

for benefits in pneumoconiosis, occupational asthma and other related occupational diseases in Britain are contained in government pamphlets (p. 227). New industrial processes are constantly being introduced and it is necessary to remain alert to the possibility that they may be associated with new occupational lung diseases.

DISEASES CAUSED BY MINERAL DUSTS (PNEUMOCONIOSIS)

The dust particles, after inhalation, are conveyed by macrophages from the bronchial mucosa to minute foci of lymphoid tissue throughout the lungs. There the irritation produced by solution of the particles in tissue fluid may initiate widespread pulmonary fibrosis. The fibrogenic capacities of mineral dusts vary, silica being markedly fibrogenic whereas iron is almost inert. The most important types of pneumoconiosis are coal-worker's pneumoconiosis, silicosis and asbestosis.

Coal-worker's Pneumoconiosis

The disease results from prolonged inhalation of coal dust. For clinical purposes (and for certification) the condition is subdivided into simple pneumoconiosis and progressive massive fibrosis. It must be emphasised that for certification purposes in Britain the diagnosis rests at present on radiological, and not clinical, features.

Simple Coal-worker's Pneumoconiosis. This is categorised radiologically into 3 grades, depending on the size and extent of the nodulation present. It does not progress if the miner leaves the industry.

Progressive Massive Fibrosis. In this form of the disease, large dense masses, single or multiple, occur mainly in the upper lobes. These may be irregular in shape and may cavitate. This type of disease may be complicated by tuberculosis. It may be disabling, may shorten life expectancy and may progress even after the miner leaves the industry.

Cough and sputum due to associated chronic bronchitis are frequently present. The sputum may be black. Progressive breathlessness on exertion occurs in the later stages, and ventilatory and right ventricular failure supervene as terminal events. There may be no abnormal physical signs in the chest, but where present they are those of chronic obstructive airways disease.

Antinuclear factor is present in the serum of about 15% of patients with coal-worker's pneumoconiosis. Rheumatoid factor is present in some patients, as in *Caplan's syndrome*, in which rheumatoid arthritis coexists with rounded fibrotic nodules 0·5 to 5 cm in diameter, mainly in the periphery of the lung fields. This syndrome may also occur in other types of pneumoconiosis.

Silicosis

This disease is becoming much more rare as the standards of industrial hygiene improve. It is caused by the inhalation of fine free crystalline silicon dioxide (silica) dust or quartz particles. It occurs in the following occupations: mining of coal, tin, gold and other minerals; quarrying, mining and dressing of sandstone and granite; the pottery and ceramics industry; the manufacture of silica bricks and abrasive soaps; iron and steel industries; sand blasting, metal grinding and boiler scaling.

Silica is a very fibrogenic dust and causes the development of hard nodules which coalesce as the disease progresses. Tuberculosis may modify the silicotic process, and caseation and calcification may occur. The radiological features are similar to those seen in coal-worker's pneumoconiosis though the changes tend to be more marked in the upper zones. The hilar shadows may be enlarged and 'egg-shell' calcification in the hilar lymph nodes is a distinctive feature. The disease tends to progress even when exposure to dust ceases. The sufferer should therefore be removed from the offending environment as soon as possible.

Clinical features are similar to those described in coal-worker's pneumoconiosis.

Asbestos-related Diseases of the Lungs and Pleura

The main types of asbestos are chrysotile, which accounts for 90% of the world's production, and crocidolite (blue asbestos). Exposure occurs in the following occupations: mining and milling of the mineral; manufacturing processes involving asbestos; pipe lagging and spraying of limpet asbestos. Demolition workers, including those who may work alongside them, e.g. joiners, painters and electricians are also at risk.

Three forms of disease related to inhalation of asbestos are recognised — benign pleural plaques, progressive pulmonary fibrosis (pulmonary asbestosis) and malignant disease of pleura (mesothelioma).

Pleural plaques, which are often calcified, are best seen in the early stages on oblique films. They are most commonly found on the diaphragm and anterolaterally.

Pulmonary asbestosis is characterised by increasing shortness of breath on exertion and cough, by the presence of clubbing of the fingers and crackling crepitations at the bases and anterolaterally, and by typical radiological and physiological abnormalities.

The radiological abnormalities are usually confined to the lower two-thirds of the lung fields and consist of mottled shadows with some streaky opacities and sometimes 'honeycombing'. The cardiac silhouette becomes 'shaggy'.

The most important physiological abnormalities are a reduced carbon monoxide transfer factor (p. 207) and a restrictive ventilatory defect (p. 213). Respiratory and right ventricular failure eventually supervene. The incidence of bronchial carcinoma is much increased, about ten-fold, in persons suffering from asbestosis.

The diagnosis of pulmonary asbestosis is based on evidence of exposure, clubbing of fingers, characteristic crepitations, typical radiological features, and physiological abnormalities. Lung biopsy may be required to confirm the diagnosis, but is not without risk and should not be carried out solely for the purpose of allowing patients to claim benefits.

Mesothelioma of the pleura is usually linked with exposure, often relatively trivial, to blue asbestos. The patient frequently presents with chest pain. A pleural effusion, often blood stained, may develop, and cause breathlessness. In some cases the diagnosis can be confirmed histologically by pleural biopsy (p. 213), but tumour masses may later develop in the chest wall at the site of biopsy. Thoracotomy is seldom justified as a diagnostic procedure in patients with suspected mesothelioma. There is no effective treatment for this disease.

Treatment and Prevention of Pneumoconiosis

No specific treatment is available. In the later stages treatment is required for associated conditions such as chronic bronchitis and respiratory failure, pulmonary tuberculosis or malignant pleural effusion.

Improvement of standards of industrial hygiene are now enforced by law in many countries; such measures as wearing respirators, damping dust and efficient ventilation systems are already proving effective in a number of industries.

DISEASES CAUSED BY ORGANIC DUSTS

In *byssinosis* the initial lesion is an acute bronchiolitis, associated with symptoms and signs of generalised airflow obstruction which tend to be worse after week-end breaks, but eventually become continuous. There is no radiological abnormality. Recovery usually follows removal from exposure to the dust hazard.

All the other diseases caused by organic dusts are forms of asthma or extrinsic allergic alveolitis, described on pages 266 and 249.

SARCOIDOSIS

Sarcoidosis is a multisystem granulomatous disease. It is associated with imbalance between subsets of T lymphocytes and other disturbances of cell-mediated immunity, but the relationship between these phenomena and sarcoidosis has not so far been explained. Apart from absence of caseation and tubercle bacilli, the lesions are histologically similar to tuberculous follicles, but there is no convincing evidence to support the view that the disease is caused by any of the mycobacteria. Chronic beryllium poisoning produces a disease which mimics sarcoidosis both pathologically and clinically, but exposure to beryllium is extremely uncommon and such cases are rare. Histological changes resembling those of sarcoidosis are occasionally seen in individual organs, such as lymph nodes, in conditions such as carcinoma, and fungal infections, but these localised 'sarcoid reactions' are not associated with systemic sarcoidosis.

Pathology. The mediastinal and superficial lymph nodes, lungs, liver, spleen, skin, eyes, parotid glands and phalangeal bones are most frequently involved. The characteristic histological feature consists of non-caseating epithelioid follicles. These lesions usually resolve spontaneously but in some cases they stimulate the production of fibrous tissue, which may have grave effects on local structure and function. The disease is seldom fatal, and then only when it affects vital organs such as the lungs, the heart or the central nervous system. Calcium metabolism may be disturbed causing hypercalcaemia and, rarely, nephrocalcinosis and renal failure.

Clinical Features. Sarcoidosis may present in a subacute or a chronic form. *Subacute sarcoidosis* is usually a benign and self-limiting disorder, spontaneous resolution occurring within a year in most cases. One of its most common manifestations is bilateral and often symmetrical enlargement of the hilar lymph nodes. The paratracheal lymph nodes may also be involved. Erythema nodosum, pyrexia and polyarthritis (p. 572) may be present at the outset. Later, transient pulmonary changes may be seen on radiological examination in addition to the lymph node enlargement. Other cases of subacute sarcoidosis may present with bilateral parotid swelling or iritis. Neurological manifestations, which are uncommon, include arachnoiditis, cranial nerve lesions and polyneuropathy.

Chronic sarcoidosis is a more serious condition, which is less likely to resolve spontaneously and is more liable to cause permanent damage to the structures it involves. Chronic pulmonary sarcoidosis may lead to the development of interstitial fibrosis, pulmonary hypertension and cor pulmonale. The vital capacity and carbon monoxide transfer factor (p. 207) are the most useful indices of impairment of lung function in this form of the disease. Sarcoidosis may involve the myocardium and produce arrhythmias.

The commonest ocular lesion is bilateral chronic iritis which, if untreated, may cause blindness. Various types of skin lesion may be seen, such as cutaneous 'sarcoids' (reddish-brown papules) or lupus pernio (raised purple plaques, usually on the nose and cheeks, resembling chilblains). Cystic lesions may develop in the phalangeal bones of the hands or feet.

Investigation. In most cases skin sensitivity to tuberculin is depressed or absent, and the Mantoux reaction (p. 232) is therefore a useful 'screening' test, a strongly positive reaction to 1 TU virtually excluding sarcoidosis. Although the diagnosis can often be made with a fair measure of confidence from the clinical and radiological features and the tuberculin test, it should, if possible, be confirmed histologically by biopsy of a superficial lymph node or of a skin lesion, when these are present.

The Kveim test is also a useful diagnostic procedure, provided a potent antigen can be obtained from human sarcoid tissue. The antigen (0·1 ml) is injected intradermally and when the test is positive a small nodule develops about 4 weeks later, biopsy of which reveals typical sarcoid follicles.

Bronchoalveolar lavage (p. 276), gallium lung scanning and measurement of angiotensin-converting enzyme in the plasma may be of value in the diagnosis of pulmonary sarcoidosis, and in assessing its activity and response to treatment.

Treatment. As subacute sarcoidosis usually resolves spontaneously treatment is seldom required, but occasionally patients with persistent erythema nodosum, pyrexia, parotid swelling or iridocyclitis may have to be given oral corticosteroid therapy for a short period.

Patients with chronic sarcoidosis, particularly if it involves the lungs, eyes or other vital organs, are much more likely to require treatment with corticosteroids, which may have to be continued for several years. The dose should be kept to the minimum required to suppress the manifestations of the disease.

DISEASES OF THE PLEURA AND CHEST WALL

FIBRINOUS ('DRY') PLEURISY

This term is used to describe cases of pleurisy at the stage of fibrinous exudation when there is no significant degree of effusion. It is usually secondary to bacterial infection in the underlying lung, but may also occur in association with a viral infection (coxsackie B), which primarily involves the intercostal muscles and is known as 'Bornholm disease'. Dry pleurisy is a common feature of pulmonary infarction, and may be an early manifestation of pleural invasion by a pulmonary tumour or of pulmonary tuberculosis.

Clinical Features. The characteristic symptom of dry pleurisy is pleural pain. On examination, rib movement is restricted and the breath sounds may be diminished on the affected side. A pleural rub is present in many cases, particularly when the patient is asked to take a deep breath. It is not heard when the breath is held, except near the pericardium where a so-called pleuropericardial rub may be present. In the acute stage of dry pleurisy, respiration may be so painful that the limited range of movement of the chest wall may be insufficient to produce an audible rub.

The other clinical features depend on the nature of the lesion causing the pleurisy. Depending on the cause, complete clinical recovery may ensue or an effusion may develop, either serous or purulent.

Radiological examination must be performed in every case but a negative radiograph does not necessarily exclude a pulmonary cause for the pleurisy. A preceding history of a few days' cough, purulent sputum, and pyrexia is presumptive evidence of a pulmonary infection which may not have been severe enough to produce a radiographic abnormality or which may have resolved before the film was taken.

Treatment. The primary cause of the pleurisy must be treated. The symptomatic treatment of pleural pain is described on page 219.

PLEURAL EFFUSION

This term, by general consent, is applied only to serous effusions. The condition of purulent effusion or empyema is described on page 272. The passive transudation of fluid into the pleural cavity (*hydrothorax*) occurs in cardiac failure, nephrotic syndrome, advanced cirrhosis of the liver and severe malnutrition.

The most common causes of pleural effusion are pneumonia, tuberculosis, malignant disease and pulmonary infarction. Pleural effusion, often bilateral, may also be a manifestation of rheumatoid disease, systemic lupus erythematosus and lymphoma. Inflammatory lesions below the diaphragm, such as subphrenic abscess, amoebic liver abscess and pancreatitis, occasionally produce a pleural effusion. The cause of the majority of pleural effusions can be identified if a careful history is taken and comprehensive clinical examination performed.

Where the cause is obscure a lead may be given by enquiry regarding travel abroad, occupation (for example exposure to asbestos), contact with tuberculosis, or causes of thromboembolism (oral contraception; recent operation). Detailed investigations as described below may, however, be necessary.

Clinical Features. The symptoms and signs of dry pleurisy often precede the development of effusion, but the onset in other cases may be insidious with little or no pleural pain. Pyrexia occurs in most cases, whatever the primary cause, but is more severe in the presence of infection and more protracted when the infection is tuberculous. Dyspnoea is the only symptom related to the effusion itself. Its severity depends on the size of the effusion and the rate at which it accumulates. The physical signs in the chest are those of fluid in the pleural space (p. 212).

Investigation. *Radiological examination* shows a dense uniform opacity in the lower and lateral parts of the hemithorax shading off above and medially into translucent lung. Occasionally the fluid is localised below the lower lobe, the appearances simulating an elevated hemidiaphragm. When the effusion is loculated, for example, in an interlobar fissure, a localised opacity is seen.

Ultrasonography may be of value in detecting and localising an effusion.

Pleural Aspiration. Absolute proof that an effusion is present can be obtained only by the aspiration of fluid. A needle should be inserted through an intercostal space over the area of maximum dullness on percussion or, ideally, at the site of maximum radiological opacity as shown by postero-anterior and lateral films or by fluoroscopy. At least 50 ml of fluid should be withdrawn, 20 ml or more being placed in a sterile container for bacteriological examination, 20 ml in a citrated container for cytological examination and 10 ml in a chemically clean container for biochemical examination. Pleural biopsy (p. 213) is always indicated whenever a diagnostic aspiration of pleural fluid is performed.

The appearance of the fluid should be noted — straw coloured, blood stained, purulent or chylous. The protein content will give an indication as to whether the effusion is an exudate (>30 g/l) or a transudate (<30 g/l). The predominant cell type (polymorph, lymphocyte, red blood cell) gives useful information, and the fluid should be examined for malignant cells.

The glucose content is often measured, but is now considered to be unhelpful. There is a high amylase level in effusions secondary to acute pancreatitis and a high concentration of cholesterol in most chronic rheumatoid effusions. Microbiological investigation, including culture for *Myco. tuberculosis* should be performed where appropriate.

Other investigations may be required to determine the primary cause of a pleural effusion. Estimation of the total and differential leucocyte count in the peripheral blood, a tuberculin test, and examination of the sputum for tubercle bacilli should never be omitted. Radiological examination of the chest may disclose underlying pulmonary disease and indicate its nature. If the lung is obscured by a massive effusion, this examination should be repeated after a large volume of fluid has been aspirated. Other investigations which may help to determine the cause of a pleural effusion include bronchoscopy, biopsy of a scalene lymph node, thoracoscopy and serological tests for antinuclear and rheumatoid factors.

The main features of the more important causes of pleural effusion are shown in Table 8.12.

Treatment. Aspiration of pleural fluid may be necessary to relieve breathlessness caused by a large effusion. It is inadvisable to remove more than one litre on the first occasion, since pulmon-

Table 8.12 Pleural effusion: main causes and features.

	Appearance of fluid	Type of fluid	Predominant cells in fluid	Other diagnostic features
Tuberculous	Serous, usually amber coloured	Exudate	Lymphocytes	Positive tuberculin test. Isolation of *M. tuberculosis*. Positive pleural biopsy (80%).
Malignant disease	Serous, often blood-stained	Exudate	Serosal cells and lymphocytes. Often clumps of malignant cells	Positive pleural biopsy (40%). Evidence of malignant disease elsewhere.
*Cardiac failure	Serous, straw-coloured	Transudate	Few serosal cells	Other evidence of left heart failure. Response to diuretics.
*Pulmonary infarction	Serous or blood-stained	Exudate	Red blood cells Eosinophils	Contralateral evidence of infarction. Source of embolism. Factors predisposing to venous thrombosis.
*Rheumatoid disease	Serous Turbid if chronic	Exudate	Lymphocytes and serosal cells	Rheumatoid arthritis. Rheumatoid factor in serum. Cholesterol in chronic effusion.
*Systemic lupus erythematosus	Serous	Exudate	Lymphocytes and serosal cells. Occasionally LE cells	Other manifestations of SLE. ANF or anti-DNA in serum.
Obstruction of thoracic duct	Milky	Chyle	None	Chylomicrons

*Effusion often bilateral

ary oedema occasionally follows the aspiration of larger amounts. Even a careful operator may accidentally produce a pneumothorax and a radiograph of the chest should be taken after the procedure.

Treatment of the underlying cause, for example, heart failure, pneumonia, pulmonary embolism and subphrenic abscess, will often be followed by resolution of the effusion, but certain conditions require special measures.

Postpneumonic pleural effusion may require aspiration, as necessary, to ensure that an empyema has not developed and to prevent pleural thickening.

Tuberculous pleural effusion should always be treated with antituberculosis chemotherapy (p. 236). Aspiration is required initially if the effusion is large and causing dyspnoea, but the addition of prednisolone by mouth (20 mg/d for 6 weeks) will promote rapid absorption of the fluid and obviate the need for further aspiration. No restrictions need be placed on the activities of such patients.

Malignant effusions reaccumulate and to avoid the distress of repeated aspirations, an attempt should be made to obliterate the pleural space (pleurodesis) by injecting substances which produce an inflammatory reaction and extensive pleural adhesions. The agents most frequently used for this purpose are mustine hydrochloride, inactivated *Corynebacterium parvum* and tetracycline.

EMPYEMA THORACIS

This is the term used to describe the presence of pus in the pleural space. The pus may be as thin as serous fluid, or so thick that it is difficult to aspirate even through a wide-bore needle. Microscopically, neutrophil leucocytes are present in large numbers. The causative organism may or may not be isolated from the pus. An empyema may involve the whole pleural space ('total' empyema) or only part of it ('loculated' or 'encysted' empyema). It is almost invariably unilateral.

Aetiology. Empyema is always secondary to infection in a neighbouring structure, usually the lung. The principal infections liable to produce empyema are the bacterial pneumonias and tuberculosis. Other causes of empyema are infection of a haemothorax and rupture of a subphrenic abscess through the diaphragm. Empyema has become a relatively rare disease because pulmonary infection can now be so readily controlled by antibacterial therapy.

Pathology. Both layers of pleura are covered with a thick, shaggy, inflammatory exudate. In the course of time the exudate becomes converted into fibrous tissue which may encase the collapsed lung so rigidly that it cannot re-expand when the pus is removed by aspiration or by an external drainage operation. The pus in the pleural space is often under considerable pressure and if the condition is not adequately treated it may rupture into a bronchus, from which it is expectorated, or through an intercostal space with the formation of a subcutaneous abscess or sinus. When an empyema ruptures into a bronchus, a bronchopleural fistula is produced. This allows air to enter the pleural space, and a pyopneumothorax is formed.

The only way in which an empyema can heal is by apposition of the visceral and parietal layers of the pleura with obliteration of the empyema space by organisation of the intervening exudate. This cannot occur unless re-expansion of the collapsed lung is secured at an early stage by removal of all the pus from the pleural space. Re-expansion of the lung cannot take place if, through delay in treatment or inadequate drainage, the visceral pleura becomes grossly thickened and rigid, if the pleural layers are kept apart by air entering the pleura through a bronchopleural fistula, or if disease in the lung itself, such as bronchiectasis, bronchial carcinoma or pulmonary tuberculosis, renders it incapable of re-expansion. In all these circumstances an empyema tends to become chronic and healing may not take place without recourse to major thoracic surgery.

Clinical Features. Empyema should be suspected in patients with pulmonary infection if there is a recurrence of pyrexia which fails to respond or responds only partially to the continued administration of a suitable antibiotic. In other cases the illness produced by the primary infective lesion may be so slight that it passes unrecognised and the first definite clinical features are due to the empyema itself.

In the fully developed case two separate groups of clinical features are found:

Systemic features: (*a*) Pyrexia, usually high and remittent but sometimes slight. (*b*) Rigors, sweating, malaise, anorexia and loss of weight. (*c*) Neutrophil leucocytosis.

Local features: (*a*) Dyspnoea, when the empyema is large. (*b*) Pleural pain, usually confined to the initial stage of the illness. (*c*) Cough and purulent sputum, usually related to the primary lung disease, but occasionally caused by the rupture of an empyema into a bronchus. An empyema usually produces the typical signs of fluid in the pleural space (p. 212), but a small localised empyema, particularly when situated in an interlobar fissure, may produce no abnormal physical signs.

Investigation. *Radiological Examination.* The appearances are indistiguishable from those of serous pleural effusion (p. 270). When air is present in addition to pus (pyopneumothorax), a horizontal 'fluid level' marks the interface of liquid and air if the film is taken in the erect position.

Confirmation of the presence of an empyema depends on the *aspiration of pus*. A wide-bore needle should be inserted through an intercostal space over the area of maximal dullness on percussion. Whenever possible the position of the empyema should have previously been confirmed by posteroanterior and lateral radiographs.

Bacteriological examination of the pus may help to determine the cause of the empyema. In postpneumonic cases where intensive treatment with antibiotics has been given the pus is frequently sterile. The distinction between tuberculous and non-tuberculous cases can usually be made from the radiological changes in the lungs or by the isolation of tubercle bacilli from pus or sputum.

Treatment

NON-TUBERCULOUS EMPYEMA

1. *Acute.* When the patient is acutely ill, and the pus is thin in consistence:

(*a*) An intercostal tube should be inserted into the most dependent part of the empyema space and connected to a water seal drainage system (p. 275).

(*b*) An antibiotic to which the organism causing the empyema is sensitive should be given.

If treatment is started early enough, and the organisms are drug-sensitive, an empyema can often be aborted by these measures. If, however, the intercostal tube is not providing adequate drainage, which is apt to happen when the pus thickens and clots, a short segment of rib should be resected, the empyema cavity cleared of pus and clot, and a wide-bore tube inserted.

2. *Chronic.* If the diagnosis is made before any drainage procedure is carried out, it may be feasible to resect the empyema sac *in toto*, provided the patient is fairly fit and the underlying lung is healthy. If open drainage has been performed, and re-expansion of the lung is prevented by gross thickening of the visceral pleura, 'decortication' may be required. This procedure will allow the lung to re-expand and obliterate the pleural space. Few patients nowadays need to be left with a permanent pleural drain, but this may be unavoidable if the patient is unfit for major surgery.

TUBERCULOUS EMPYEMA. Antituberculosis chemotherapy (p. 236) should be started immediately, and the pus in the pleural space should be aspirated through a wide-bore needle until it ceases to reaccumulate. In many cases no other treatment is necessary, but surgery is occasionally required to ablate the residual space.

Prognosis. With early drainage and antibiotic therapy most patients with acute empyema quickly recover. Chronic empyema, on the other hand, causes general ill-health, recurrent episodes of pyrexia, clubbing of the fingers and, in severe cases, amyloid disease. It always requires surgical treatment. With specific chemotherapy tuberculous empyema is no longer a serious condition, but complete recovery may take some months.

SPONTANEOUS PNEUMOTHORAX

Aetiology. The two chief causes of spontaneous pneumothorax are: (1) rupture of a subpleural emphysematous bulla or of the pulmonary end of a pleural adhesion; (2) rupture of a subpleural tuberculous focus into the pleural space.

In Britain the first cause is very much more common. Active pulmonary tuberculosis is, in fact, responsible for very few cases of spontaneous pneumothorax, a finding which is in sharp contrast with the experience of 50 years ago. Other conditions such as staphylococcal lung abscess, pulmonary infarction and bronchial carcinoma may, in rare instances, give rise to spontaneous pneumothorax.

Pathology. There are three types of spontaneous pneumothorax (Fig. 8.7):

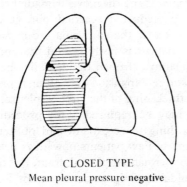

CLOSED TYPE
Mean pleural pressure negative

OPEN TYPE
Mean pleural pressure atmospheric

VALVULAR (TENSION) TYPE
Mean pleural pressure positive

Fig. 8.7 Types of spontaneous pneumothorax.

1. *Closed.* The communication between pleura and lung seals off as the lung collapses, and does not reopen. In this type of case the air is gradually absorbed and the lung re-expands.

2. *Open.* The communication is generally with a bronchus (bronchopleural fistula) and does not seal off when the lung collapses. The air pressure in the pleural space thus approximates to atmospheric pressure on both inspiration and expiration and the lung cannot re-expand. Moreover, the large bronchial communication facilitates the transmission of infection from the air passages into the pleural space and empyema is a common complication. The term 'open' is also applied to a pneumothorax resulting from a penetrating wound of the chest wall.

3. *Valvular.* The communication between pleura and lung persists but is small and acts as a one-way valve which allows air to enter the pleura during inspiration but prevents it from escaping during expiration. Very large amounts of air may be 'trapped' in the pleural space during bouts of coughing and the intrapleural pressure may rise to well above atmospheric level. This results not only in complete collapse of the underlying lung but also in mediastinal displacement towards the opposite side with compression of the opposite lung. This type of pneumothorax is usually referred to as 'tension pneumothorax'.

Clinical Features. The onset is usually sudden, with pain or a feeling of 'tightness' on the affected side of the chest, which may be aggravated by deep inspiration. The patient then becomes increasingly breathless and in severe cases central cyanosis may be present. The physical signs in the chest are those of air in the pleural space (p. 212). When the pneumothorax is small and localised there may be no abnormal signs, and the condition may be revealed only by radiological examination.

Closed Spontaneous Pneumothorax. Dyspnoea, which is seldom severe, gradually abates over the course of a few days. Progressive spontaneous absorption of the air takes place and re-expansion of the lung is complete between 2 and 4 weeks later, depending on the initial size of the pneumothorax. Pleural infection is uncommon in this type of pneumothorax.

Open spontaneous pneumothorax is usually due to the intrapleural rupture of a tuberculous cavity or a lung abscess. The onset is similar to that of the closed type, but the dyspnoea, although it is not rapidly progressive, does not improve and within a few days the appearance of pyrexia and systemic disturbance, accompanied by physical and radiological signs of air and fluid in the pleural space, indicate the development of a pyopneumothorax. In tuberculous cases acid-fast bacilli can be isolated from the pleural fluid.

Valvular pneumothorax ('tension pneumothorax') produces the most dramatic clinical picture of all. The dyspnoea is rapidly progressive from the start and is accompanied by central cyanosis. The patient may die from asphyxia within a few minutes, but usually the course of events is less rapid and medical attention can be obtained in time to avert a fatal outcome.

Recurrent spontaneous pneumothorax is not uncommon, especially in patients with emphysematous bullae. Subsequent incidents are usually on the same side as the first but may also occur on the opposite side.

Radiological examination shows the sharp edge of the collapsed lung, and between this and the chest wall there is complete translucency with no lung markings. The degree of pulmonary collapse varies from case to case. Radiographs also show the degree of mediastinal displacement, and give information regarding the presence or absence of pleural fluid and underlying pulmonary disease.

Treatment. 1. *Closed Spontaneous Pneumothorax.* When the pneumothorax is small and the patient is only slightly dyspnoeic no treatment is required but observation should be continued until re-expansion of the lung is complete. If, however, the pneumothorax is large and causing moderate or severe dyspnoea, it is essential to employ more active measures. Rapid and complete re-expansion of the lung can be obtained by inserting a catheter into the pleural cavity through an intercostal space and connecting it to a water-seal drainage system (Fig. 8.8) or a non-return (Heimlich) valve. The catheter is left in place for 5 or 6 days. This form of treatment considerably shortens the period of incapacity.

If a tuberculous aetiology is suspected, specific chemotherapy (p. 236) should be started immediately. If a pleural effusion develops, the fluid may be drained through the catheter by suitable posturing or aspirated with a needle and syringe.

2. *Open Spontaneous Pneumothorax.* There is a large bronchopleural fistula, and pleural infection rapidly supervenes. Such cases are seldom amenable to medical treatment and, whether tuberculous or non-tuberculous, should be referred to a thoracic surgeon for treatment of the resulting pyopneumothorax.

3. *Tension Pneumothorax.* This constitutes an acute medical emergency. An intercostal catheter should be inserted at once and connected to a water-seal drainage system, as shown in Figure 8.8. Symptomatic relief is immediate and dramatic. If suitable equipment for this procedure is not at hand a wide-bore plastic cannula should be used instead. This should be attached to a length of tubing, the end of which should be placed under water in a bottle or basin. Surgical treatment may be required for a persistent pneumothorax of this type.

Fig. 8.8 Treatment of spontaneous pneumothorax by pleural intubation and 'water-seal' decompression. The water-seal allows air to leave the pleural space but prevents it from re-entering. This reduces the intrapleural pressure and promotes re-expansion of the lung. The insert shows the position of the self-retaining (Malecot) catheter in the pleural space.

4. *Recurrent spontaneous pneumothorax*, unilateral or bilateral, is first treated by the introduction of an irritant substance, such as kaolin, into the pleural space. This procedure (artificial pleurodesis) produces an aseptic pleurisy, which results in

the formation of extensive adhesions between the parietal and visceral surfaces, and usually prevents further episodes of spontaneous pneumothorax. In a few cases thoracotomy and abrasion of the parietal pleura may be required to obliterate the pleural space.

DEFORMITIES OF THE CHEST WALL

An increase in the anteroposterior diameter of the chest relative to the lateral diameter is a common feature of emphysema, but only the most severe forms of this abnormality merit the description of 'barrel chest'. *Pectus carinatum* ('pigeon chest') is seen in patients who have suffered from chronic asthma since early childhood. *Pectus excavatum* ('funnel chest') is a condition in which the body of the sternum, often only its lower end, is curved backwards. The heart is displaced to the left, and may be compressed between the sternum and vertebral column, but only very rarely is this associated with disturbance of cardiac function. It may, however, restrict chest expansion and reduce the vital capacity. The impairment of cardiac or pulmonary function is seldom sufficiently severe to warrant surgical correction, but this may be indicated for cosmetic reasons.

Severe *thoracic kyphoscoliosis* restricts and distorts expansion of the chest wall which causes maldistribution of ventilation and blood flow in the lungs. Patients with this type of chest deformity may later develop Type II respiratory failure, pulmonary hypertension and right ventricular failure, and few survive beyond middle age. The tempo of deterioration is often accelerated by bacterial infection in the bronchi and lungs. The prognosis in these cases can be improved only by early surgical correction of the spinal deformity. Respiratory failure may also occur in ankylosing spondylitis, particularly if there is any interference with the function of the diaphragm.

PROSPECTS IN RESPIRATORY MEDICINE

Advances in immunology, immunopathology and immunopharmacology have already opened the way to a clearer understanding of the nature of certain respiratory diseases, notably bronchial asthma, bronchopulmonary eosinophilia and extrinsic allergic alveolitis, and may in time help to elucidate the pathogenesis of conditions such as cryptogenic fibrosing alveolitis, some types of occupational lung disease and even bronchial carcinoma. Cytological and biochemical examination of material obtained from the bronchi and lungs by bronchoalveolar lavage may also prove to be a useful diagnostic and research technique in many obscure forms of diffuse pulmonary disease. It may, for example, help to identify the type of interstitial lung disease and to gauge its activity. Immunology has a further contribution to make in the field of respiratory infection. Until recently research effort was concentrated mainly on the pathogenic properties of microorganisms, but with increasing awareness of the importance of the host reaction there is now a growing interest in methods of investigating the integrity of the various mechanisms, local and systemic, which protect the lungs against both acute and chronic infection by bacteria, viruses and fungi.

New non-invasive techniques are becoming available for the diagnosis of localised pulmonary lesions and of diseases which cause abnormalities of ventilation and perfusion, such as emphysema and pulmonary thromboembolism. These techniques, which include computed tomography and new methods of radionuclide scanning, are still in an early stage of development, but when fully exploited are certain to revolutionise the investigation of respiratory disease. On a more mundane level further improvement can be expected in the technique of bronchoscopy and of bronchial and pulmonary biopsy.

The empirical treatment of respiratory disease has recently seen many important advances, particularly in regard to antibiotics, bronchodilator drugs and corticosteroids. Efforts to discover drugs or other forms of treatment which can influence the basic causes of allergic and malignant disease and of chronic bronchopulmonary infection have so far met with only limited success, but this situation is bound to change when we have more precise knowledge of the pathogenesis of these diseases.

G.K. CROMPTON
I.W.B. GRANT
G.J.R. McHARDY

FURTHER READING:

Cotes J.E. (1979). *Lung Function: Assessment and Application in Medicine*, 4th edn. Oxford: Blackwell.

Crofton J.W. & Douglas A.C. (1981). *Respiratory Diseases*, 3rd edn. Oxford: Blackwell.

Grant I.W.B. (1983). Examination of the respiratory system. In: Macleod J (ed.) *Clinical Examination*, 6th edn. Edinburgh: Churchill Livingstone.

James D.G. & Studdy P.R. (1981). *A Colour Atlas of Respiratory Diseases*. London: Wolfe.

Parkes W.R. (1982). *Occupational Lung Disorders*, 2nd edn. London: Butterworths.

Ross J.D. & Horne N.W. (1983). *Modern Drug Treatment in Tuberculosis*, 6th edn. London: Chest, Heart and Stroke Association.

Department of Health and Social Security NI 226 (1979). *Pneumoconiosis and Related Occupational Diseases: Notes on Diagnosis and Claims for Industrial Injuries Scheme Benefits.* London: DHSS.

Department of Health and Social Security NI 238 (1982). *Clinical Notes on Occupational Asthma: a Disease Prescribed under the Industrial Injuries Scheme.* London: DHSS.

9. Diseases of the Alimentary Tract and Pancreas

PHYSIOLOGY OF THE ALIMENTARY TRACT

The alimentary tract is a coordinated structure with the function of ingesting and absorbing nutrients and excreting unabsorbed and waste products. It should not be regarded as a series of separate organs, since the role of each component is closely related to that of other parts of the tract. Its operation may be considered under the following headings:

(1) *Controlling and Coordinating Mechanisms*. The autonomic nervous system and hormones, including gastrin, secretin and cholecystokinin (pancreozymin), control and coordinate motility and secretion.

(2) *Motility*. The carefully controlled motility of the tract is responsible for the orderly progression of nutrients through the system so that the stage of digestion and absorption is appropriate to a given region of the tract.

(3) *Secretion*. The secretion of enzymes and detergents enables protein, carbohydrate and fat to be digested prior to absorption. The secretion of electrolytes provides the correct pH for each stage of digestion.

(4) *Absorption*. The absorptive system consists of specialised cells, together with the portal venous system and lymphatics.

(5) *Defence Mechanisms*. These are necessary to protect the mucosa from its own digestive enzymes and from the bacterial population to which it is exposed. These mechanisms include a rapid turnover of the epithelial cells, the production of mucus and a specialised immunological system.

1. The Controlling and Coordinating Mechanisms

The cells of the gastrointestinal tract are controlled by the transmission of chemical messengers which are aminoacids or their derivatives, amines or peptides. The transmission of the message is called neurocrine when it is across a synapse, paracrine when it is through an intercellular space, and endocrine when it is via the blood (p. 417). Many hormones and peptides have now been discovered, each being produced by a distinctive cell type in the gastrointestinal mucosa or pancreas. Peptide hormones or paracrine substances are released in response to food in the upper gastrointestinal tract, their function being to control the progression of nutrients by modifying nervous stimuli, and to stimulate or inhibit secretions at the appropriate time. It is now recognised that each event is influenced by a multitude of nervous and hormonal stimuli. For example, the secretion of acid by the stomach is produced mainly by vagal stimuli and the release of gastrin, but many other enteric hormones probably have smaller roles to play.

The smooth muscle, secretory cells and blood vessels of the gastrointestinal tract are supplied by the autonomic nervous system. Preganglionic parasympathetic fibres of the vagi synapse with the parasympathetic motor neurones of the enteric plexuses. Sympathetic fibres run in the splanchnic nerves to join the plexuses which are situated at different levels in the bowel wall — subserous, myenteric, submucosal and mucosal — each varying in density from organ to organ. In general, the parasympathetic system is excitatory and the sympathetic inhibitory.

A peptidergic system is now recognised as a large and important component of the autonomic nervous system. The nerves contain such substances as vasoactive intestinal peptide, substance P and encephalins, as well as substances like cholecystokinin which also act as hormones. The entire autonomic nervous system exerts an effect on the contraction of the smooth muscle cells and on the secretion of enzymes, electrolytes and hormones by the mucosa. It is influenced by sensory nerves in the mucosa and gut wall which respond to chemical stimuli and to stretch, by the enteric hormones and by the release of paracrine substances.

2. Motility

Apart from the striated muscle in the upper oesophagus, smooth muscle is responsible for the motility of the gastrointestinal tract. The smooth muscle produces 'slow waves' which are conducted over long distances. These do not result in contraction but they enable contractions in different areas to be coordinated.

Oesophagus. The upper oesophageal sphincter is formed by the striated cricopharyngeus muscle which exerts constant tone to keep the sphincter closed except during swallowing. Once the upper oesophageal sphincter relaxes, peristalsis sweeps along the length of the body of the oesophagus, but occasionally, even in the normal oesophagus, the contractions are not coordinated. In the disorder of diffuse spasm these uncoordinated contractions predominate. The lowest few centimetres of the oesophagus form the lower oesophageal sphincter. This has a high resting tension which prevents reflux of gastric contents into the oesophagus. Normally the sphincter relaxes when the peristaltic wave arrives but the characteristic feature in achalasia is that it fails to do so. The sphincter is controlled by nervous and hormonal mechanisms.

Stomach. The normal tonic contraction of the stomach is inhibited by the arrival of food probably by means of a centrally mediated vagal reflex. This is termed receptive relaxation so that a large increase in volume is accompanied by only a small rise in pressure within the lumen. The gastric slow wave controls the frequency and direction of antral peristalsis which is responsible for the thorough mixing of the gastric contents and their progressive emptying into the duodenum.

Several mechanisms exist to prevent the duodenum receiving more nutrient than it can deal with. Chemoreceptors for fat and acid and osmoreceptors in the duodenal mucosa control gastric emptying by means of local reflexes and the release of secretin, cholecystokinin and other enteric hormones. Approximately half of a semi-solid meal has left the stomach in about 30 minutes.

Small Intestine. Here the coordination is due to the slow wave in the longitudinal muscle fibres. It is the pacemaker which dictates the times at which any given segment of the gut can contract. The frequency of the slow wave in the duodenum is greater than in the ileum, thus enabling the proximal bowel to override more distal areas. By this means contractions are coordinated both to mix and propel the small bowel content so that all nutrients can be exposed to the absorptive cells. It is thought that the myenteric plexus and the enteric hormones determine the local response to the slow wave so that contraction may or may not occur depending on the state of affairs in the lumen at any one time.

Colon. Motility here is poorly understood. There is probably a slow wave but it is not known how it coordinates contractions. Observation of the colon suggests two main types of contraction occur which may be associated with two different functions. First, there is segmentation which consists of contraction rings forming and disappearing over long periods of time: these produce a slow mixing of faeces but no propulsion, thus facilitating the absorption of water and electrolytes. Second, propulsion occurs through 'mass movement,' a peristaltic wave which occurs several times a day. This action carries out the second function of the colon, namely the elimination of faeces.

All activity in the colon is increased after eating, and defaecation is more likely to occur post-prandially. The enteric hormones may be responsible for this activity. The main activity in the colon, segmentation, causes mixing only and is responsible for the resistance to flow along the lumen. In constipation, segmentation is increased and there is resistance to flow along the lumen whereas in diarrhoea there is a reduction in segmentation so that the semi-formed contents of the right colon have an unimpeded transit through the colon.

3. Secretion

The production of secretions for the digestion of nutrients is under nervous and hormonal control.

Gastric Secretion. In response to the sight or smell of food, the vagus stimulates acid and pepsin secretion by a direct effect on the parietal and peptic cells. It also initiates the release of gastrin from the antrum. More sustained output of this hormone is produced by a rise in pH and by ingested protein. Gastrin then enters the bloodstream and acts on the body of the stomach to produce acid and pepsin to digest the protein. It stimulates acid secretion through the release of histamine. Mechanisms are also required to turn off gastric secretion once digestion within the stomach is complete. These are largely the same as those which slow gastric emptying, i.e. the release of the enteric hormones, secretin and cholecystokinin, and also the presence of a low pH in the gastric antrum which inhibits the further release of gastrin.

Pancreatic Secretion, Bile and Intestinal Secretions. Acid, fat and hypertonic solutions in the duodenum release the hormones secretin and cholecystokinin from the duodenal mucosa into the bloodstream. Secretin stimulates the acinar cells of the pancreas to produce bicarbonate which neutralises the gastric acid and provides a neutral pH for the activity of the pancreatic enzymes, lipase, amylase and trypsin. These are produced in response to cholecystokinin, which also causes contraction of the gall bladder so that an adequate supply of bile acids reaches the intestine at a time when fat has to be digested. The enteric hormones are also responsible for the secretion, by the mucosa of the small intestine, of succus entericus which contains bicarbonate and additional enzymes.

4. The Absorptive System

The area for absorption in the small intestine is increased several hundredfold by the presence of villi and microvilli. The surface of the individual cell is formed of microvilli which possess a multitude of enzyme systems for the final stages of digestion of nutrients followed by their absorption. In coeliac disease and tropical sprue the surface area of the small intestine is reduced because of the atrophy or loss of villi, and malabsorption results.

Under normal circumstances nutrients are transported from the absorptive cell by the lymphatic system (e.g. fat and fat soluble vitamins) or by the portal venous system (e.g. amino acids and hexoses).

The absorptive system is discussed in more detail on page 310.

5. Defence Mechanisms

Cell Turnover. The epithelial cells of the gastrointestinal tract are constantly renewed so that, for example, the epithelial surface of the small intestine is replaced every 48 hours. The desquamated cells are digested and their products reabsorbed. In the intestine, cellular turnover has been shown to be slower than normal in germ-free animals and it can be argued that this turnover is to some extent a protective mechanism.

Production of Mucus. Mucus producing cells are present throughout the gastrointestinal tract and mucus has a protective function. In the stomach, the mucous layer on the surface of the epithelium contains bicarbonate ions which form part of the barrier to gastric acid.

Immunological System. The lamina propria of the stomach and intestines contains many lymphocytes and plasma cells. Some of these cells synthesise secretory IgA (p. 23) which is resistant to digestion by intestinal enzymes and has a role in protecting mucosal surfaces from bacterial invasion. It is thus of particular importance in the small intestine where bacterial colonisation is deleterious.

THE SYMPTOMS OF ALIMENTARY DISEASE

Pain is often the most important symptom of gastrointestinal disease. It must be analysed in relation to its main site, radiation, character, severity, duration, frequency, times of occurrence, aggravating and relieving factors and any associated phenomena. The characteristics of abdominal pain are often diagnostic, for example in peptic ulceration and acute appendicitis.

Loss of appetite (anorexia) may have a local cause such as carcinoma of the stomach but may also be a feature of any debilitating disease or of a psychological disturbance.

Waterbrash is the sudden filling of the mouth with saliva which is produced as a reflex response to a variety of symptoms from the upper gastrointestinal tract, e.g. peptic ulcer pain.

Vomiting may occur in diseases of the stomach or intestine, peritonitis, appendicitis, or cholecystitis. Numerous other conditions may also be responsible, for example meningitis, uraemia, migraine, drugs such as digoxin or morphine and, in the child, infection. The type, timing and related features of the vomiting are important diagnostically. Sudden vomiting without preceding nausea may be due to direct stimulation of the vomiting centre in the medulla and thus be an indication of intracranial disease. Vomiting in the morning may be due to pregnancy, alcoholism or anxiety. Vomiting of large quantities of food and secretions late in the day or night indicates gastric outlet obstruction. Vomiting which relieves pain is often due to a peptic ulcer. The complaint of persistent vomiting without loss of weight is nearly always indicative of a psychological disturbance.

Heartburn is a burning retrosternal sensation due to reflux oesophagitis.

Regurgitation is the appearance of previously swallowed food in the mouth without vomiting. It usually has an acid or bitter taste because of the presence of gastric juice or bile but not in patients with obstruction in the oesophagus.

Dysphagia, i.e. difficulty in swallowing, is discussed on page 287.

Flatulence is often due to excessive swallowing of air (aerophagy) which in turn may be due to anxiety. Under normal circumstances a small amount of air is swallowed with food, drink and saliva. Some of this gas may be expelled as a belch. The remainder passes into the intestine. Some will be absorbed but most, particularly the nitrogen, will be expelled per rectum. A plain radiograph of the abdomen shows that gas is normally present in the stomach and colon but that very little is seen in the small intestine.

Constipation and diarrhoea are sometimes difficult to define. In Britain fewer than 10% of people have less than one bowel motion per day and only 1% have a bowel movement less frequently than 3 times a week. These latter should be regarded as constipated. In addition, if the stool is hard and difficult to pass the patient should be regarded as constipated whatever the frequency of bowel movement. In contrast, less than 1% of the population have more than three bowel movements daily and this should be regarded as abnormal, particularly if the stool is not formed. When the stool is liquid or semiformed it must be regarded as abnormal whatever the frequency of bowel movement. The diet in Western countries is low in roughage; where a high residue diet is usual, more than three bowel movements daily may be normal. An explanation must be found for any change in bowel habit.

Loss of weight may be due to a reduced intake of food because of anorexia, nausea or vomiting, to malabsorption of nutrients or to the loss of protein from a diseased bowel as in ulcerative colitis. Carcinoma is the most important alimentary cause of loss of weight.

INVESTIGATION OF THE ALIMENTARY TRACT

In addition to systematic examination of the abdomen by inspection, palpation, percussion and auscultation and of the rectum by digital examination along the lines described in *Clinical Examination* (p. 333), further investigation is frequently required, notably radiological and endoscopic examinations.

Radiological Examination

Plain radiographs show the normal soft tissue shadows due to the liver, spleen and kidneys and also abnormal shadows. Gas in the intestine acts as a contrast medium so that the distribution of the bowel within the abdomen can be assessed. In obstruction there may be an excessive amount of gas and fluid in the bowel above the obstruction and films with the patient erect will demonstrate fluid levels. Finally, areas of opacification due to stones or to calcification in the liver, pancreas, cysts or blood vessels may provide important diagnostic information.

A chest radiograph will show the diaphragms. Free gas may be seen under the diaphragm and may indicate a perforation. Gas with a fluid level may be associated with a subphrenic abscess. Pulmonary lesions, from which pain may be referred to the abdomen, can also be identified.

Barium Studies. These will demonstrate a break in the continuity of the outline of the organ, abnormalities in the appearance of the mucosa and disorders of motility. Preparation of the patient for each examination should always be undertaken so that mucosal detail will not be obscured by contents. For studies of the upper gastrointestinal tract, the patient is fasted and for barium enema examination the colon should be cleared of faeces by means of laxatives and colonic lavage.

The Barium Swallow and Meal Examination. The oesophagus is studied whilst barium is being swallowed. This may demonstrate a disorder of motility, filling defect caused by tumours or varices, a stricture, a diverticulum or a hiatus hernia.

The mucosa of the stomach can be examined by using a small amount of barium together with the introduction of gas — a double contrast study. An ulcer is usually seen face on as a small collection of barium with radiating folds of mucosa. An ulcer may also appear as a projection beyond the normal outline while tumours cause filling defects. Small cancers can be detected by irregularity in the mucosal pattern. Observation of the motility of the stomach may indicate an inert area caused by infiltrating carcinoma. The duodenal cap is examined by studying its contours when it is completely filled with barium, and its mucosal pattern when it is distended with gas and the mucosa coated with barium.

The Follow-through Examination. When disease of the small intestine is suspected, barium is observed during its passage through the small intestine and radiographs are taken at intervals. The outline of the barium may indicate structural abnormalities such as diverticula or strictures. When there is malabsorption, excess secretions may cause the barium to clump and flocculate.

Barium Enema. This procedure is uncomfort-able and sometimes exhausting, particularly in the elderly or in those with cardiac disease in whom arrhythmia may be induced. Barium enema must always have been preceded by digital examination of the rectum and preferably also by sigmoidoscopy a few days earlier. Barium alone or, for double contrast examination, barium and air, is run into the bowel through a self-retaining catheter. Radiographs are taken with the colonic mucosa coated with barium and the lumen distended with air. In this way the colonic mucosa can be studied in detail and polyps or small tumours identified. In inflammatory bowel disease mucosal abnormalities are readily recognised. In some patients there will be a reflux of barium into the terminal ileum which can be outlined.

Cautionary Note. Exposure to X-rays in the early months of pregnancy may upset normal development of the fetus and be responsible for deformity or still birth. These risks apply not only to radiographic examination of the abdomen such as barium enema but also to procedures such as excretion urography and radiographs of the lumbar spine and pelvis. Inadvertent irradiation in the first few weeks of pregnancy can be avoided by restricting radiological examination of the lower abdomen in women at risk to the 10 days immediately following the onset of the last menstrual period — 'the 10 day rule'.

Computed tomography is used to depict intra-abdominal organs and masses. It may be of particular value in the detection of pancreatic cancer since the pancreas is inaccessible to most other radiographic techniques.

Imaging Studies

Ultrasonography. This non-invasive technique is of value in detecting cysts, particularly of the pancreas, and abscesses and can show the size of the pancreatic duct.

Radionuclide scanning is used for examining the liver and spleen (p. 345) and for detecting the approximate site of gastrointestinal haemorrhage.

Endoscopy

With fibreoptic instruments it is not difficult to examine the whole of the oesophagus, stomach, duodenum and colon. Two bundles of many thousands of fine glass fibres are contained in the instrument's shaft. One bundle carries light to the tip of the instrument in order to illuminate the organ being examined whilst the other can transmit an image back to the observer. The fibre bundles are flexible so that the whole shaft can be bent and easily passed into the upper gastrointestinal tract or colon. The shaft of the instrument also carries controls so that the tip of the instrument can be moved, and channels through which air or forceps can be passed to insufflate the organ or to take a biopsy from the mucosa. Endoscopic instruments can also be used for the therapeutic procedures which would otherwise require laparotomy such as removal of a polyp.

Rigid instruments are used to examine the rectum and lower pelvic colon (sigmoidoscope) and occasionally the oesophagus (oesophagoscope).

Upper Alimentary Tract. It is usual to carry out the procedure with the patient under sedation, often as an out-patient. After a 12-hour fast the pharynx is anaesthetised with a spray. The instrument is passed with the assistance of the patient in swallowing, and the procedure, whilst uncomfortable, should be no more so than any other intubation. Possible complications are perforation of the oesophagus or stomach whilst passing the instrument or during biopsy, and the inhalation of secretions; these are rare with flexible fibreoptic instruments.

Where possible, the oesophagus, stomach and duodenum are all inspected at the same examination (panendoscopy), because the presence of one lesion does not exclude another and double lesions are not uncommon, e.g. oesophagitis and duodenal ulcer. This is particularly important when endoscopy is carried out in patients with haematemesis or melaena, since there may be more than one source of bleeding.

Oesophagoscopy should be carried out when there is dysphagia or when barium examination suggests a tumour or stricture. Other indications include suspected oesophagitis, varices or a motility disorder. Therapeutic procedures that can be carried out include dilatation of a stricture and injection of sclerosing material into oesophageal varices to control bleeding.

Gastroscopy is always indicated when a gastric ulcer has been demonstrated on barium studies so that biopsies can be taken to exclude malignancy; subsequent healing of the ulcer should also be confirmed. Gastroscopy is nearly always necessary in the investigation of patients with symptoms after gastric surgery because the appearances are difficult to define radiologically. *Duodenoscopy* is indicated in duodenal ulceration.

Endoscopic Retrograde Cholangio-Pancreatography (ERCP) is a special application of fibreoptic endoscopy. At duodenoscopy the ampulla of Vater is cannulated with a fine bore catheter passed through the shaft of the instrument and radio-opaque dye is injected into the biliary and pancreatic ducts. The procedure is of great value in patients suspected of having pancreatic disease since distortion or obstruction of the ductal system may indicate a diagnosis of chronic pancreatitis or pancreatic carcinoma. Obstruction or distortion of the common bile duct by a stone or a tumour can also be demonstrated and stones can be removed.

Lower Alimentary Tract. *Proctoscopy and Sigmoidoscopy*. These are simple procedures which should always be carried out in patients with symptoms referable to the lower bowel or anus. Both terms are inaccurate since proctoscopy visualises the anal canal and only 2–3 cm of the rectum, and sigmoidoscopy examines the rectum and the lower few centimetres of the pelvic colon. It is usual to carry out the procedures without preparation but if the rectum contains faeces, then endoscopy is repeated after the bowel has been emptied. The examination is carried out with the patient in the knee-elbow position, or on the left side with the knees drawn up. Digital examination of the rectum should always precede endoscopy and the instruments should be warmed and well lubricated. Proctoscopy is used for the demonstration and injection of haemorrhoids. Sigmoidoscopy is necessary for the diagnosis of polyps, cancer of the rectum, ulcerative proctitis or colitis and Crohn's disease of the large bowel. Biopsy of the mucosa or lesion is also taken. Sigmoidoscopy is carried out under anaesthesia when there is a painful condition of the anus such as a fissure; it should be performed only with extreme care in fulminating ulcerative colitis because of the danger of perforation.

Colonoscopy. The fibreoptic colonoscope permits inspection of the colon to the splenic flexure. A longer instrument enables the whole colon to be examined but the procedure is time-consuming and occasionally difficult. With either method the bowel must be carefully prepared over several days, first with laxatives and then by lavage so that no faecal material remains. During colonoscopy it is possible to take a biopsy of suspicious lesions and polyps can be removed using a diathermy snare.

Other Investigations

Biopsy of lesions is an essential part of each endoscopic procedure but the small size of the specimen may make interpretation by the pathologist difficult.

Biopsy of the small intestine is indicated if malabsorption is suspected and is carried out by means of the Crosby capsule. After an overnight fast the capsule is passed into the jejunum attached to a stiff radio-opaque catheter and the biopsy is taken just distal to the duodeno-jejunal flexure. Suction via the catheter draws mucosa into a small port on the side of the instrument. The negative pressure which develops within the capsule also fires the knife which severs the mucosa. The intubation and biopsy are completed in about one hour. Bleeding occurs occasionally and for this reason biopsies should not be carried out unless the platelet count and prothrombin time are normal. Another rare complication is perforation of the intestine. The biopsy specimens are inspected under the dissecting microscope immediately after removal from the capsule prior to fixation and histological examination (p. 313).

Secretory Studies. *The Pentagastrin Test.* The acid output is measured in response to pentagastrin, a synthetic pentapeptide which exerts the biological effects of gastrin. Preparation consists of an overnight fast and H_2-receptor antagonist drugs must be stopped for at least 48 hours before the test. The fasting contents of the stomach are aspirated and their volume measured; then the secretions are collected continuously for one hour. This is termed the 'basal acid output'. Then pentagastrin is given subcuta-

neously and the secretions are collected for a further hour. The acid output in this hour is termed the 'maximum acid output'.

The pentagastrin test is helpful because: (a) a large volume of fasting juice indicates obstruction of the gastric outlet; (b) a very high basal acid output suggests that the patient has the Zollinger-Ellison syndrome (p. 300); (c) in patients with peptic ulcer it provides a preoperative base line; (d) achlorhydria can be demonstrated.

The insulin test is used after gastric surgery to indicate the completeness of vagotomy. The preparation and procedure are similar to those described above but the gastric stimulant is soluble insulin which is given intravenously. The resulting hypoglycaemia stimulates the vagal centres and gastric acid is secreted if the vagal innervation of the stomach has not been completely divided.

Pancreatic function tests are described on page 305.

Bacteriological Studies. The malabsorption syndrome may be due occasionally to bacterial colonisation of the small intestine. When this is suspected, secretion can be obtained for bacteriological studies by passing a fine sterile tube into the upper small intestine. A mercury bag attached to the tip of the tube ensures that the tube moves rapidly to the correct site. The patient should not be receiving antibiotics.

Motility Studies. Barium examination gives some indication of the motility of the oesophagus, stomach and small intestine. Cineradiography or videotape studies are useful in the analysis of dysphagia arising in the pharynx. Motility can be studied more accurately by measuring the pressure changes in the lumen of the organ but only in the case of the oesophagus is this manometry of diagnostic value. Fine open ended tubes are passed into the stomach and pressures are transmitted to transducers and measured at intervals whilst the tube is gradually withdrawn with the patient swallowing. The procedure may be of value in establishing the relationship between chest pain and abnormal oesophageal contractions, for the diagnosis of motility disorders of the oesophagus and in determining the position and competence of the lower oesophageal sphincter.

Examination of the Stool. In malabsorption

the stool may be pale and frothy; in the irritable bowel syndrome it may be like pellets or ribbon with or without mucus. In mild ulcerative disease of the colon there may be flecks of blood in the mucus. Inspection of the stool is sufficient to diagnose fresh bleeding from the lower alimentary tract while the loss of over 60 ml of blood from a site proximal to the ascending colon will produce a black tarry stool.

Tests for occult blood (e.g. Hemoccult) detect small amounts of blood in the stool and are performed for several successive days because bleeding from the gastrointestinal tract is often intermittent. Specimens obtained on the finger-stall at rectal examination can be readily examined.

Microscopic examination is of value particularly in distinguishing amoebic dysentery and other parasitic diseases.

PARENTERAL AND ENTERAL NUTRITION

When normal nutrition cannot be maintained, nutrients can be given intravenously (parenteral nutrition) or by nasogastric intubation (enteral nutrition). There are many possible indications for the use of parenteral nutrition including preparation for major surgery, postoperative care of patients who have undergone extensive intestinal resection and the management of prolonged ileus, enterocutaneous fistula, acute pancreatitis with complications, and severe inflammatory bowel disease. Some patients with these disorders can be managed by enteral feeding which has fewer complications and is more manageable and economical.

Protein-energy requirements are discussed on page 53.

Parenteral nutrition provides energy, nitrogen, water, electrolytes and vitamins. Energy is supplied in the form of 20–50% glucose solutions and 10–20% lipid emulsions; mixtures of individual crystalline amino acids provide the nitrogen. These are made up in a balanced solution containing the requirements of electrolytes, water and water soluble vitamins. Various commercial preparations are available for different requirements of protein and electrolytes. The solutions are hypertonic and hence they must be given via a central vein. Inadequate therapy can result in various metabolic complications and nutritional deficiencies, for example, of zinc (p. 63).

Enteral Nutrition. The diet may be polymeric, i.e. protein, fat and carbohydrate in high molecular weight form; this is used when the patient's digestive and absorptive capacity is normal but when there is difficulty in swallowing, e.g. after oesophageal surgery. Alternatively the diet may be monomeric, i.e. amino acids, oligo- and monosaccharides; these are used when digestion is impaired, e.g. after bowel resection, or when stimulation of digestive secretions is to be avoided. Enteral feeding is usually given as a constant infusion via a nasogastric or nasoenteric fine bore tube; gastrostomy or jejunostomy can also be used.

DISEASES OF THE MOUTH

The mouth acts as a receptacle in which food can be broken down into small particles during mastication. Into the mouth flows the saliva which is secreted in response to the act of chewing and to the sight, taste and smell of food. Saliva has several functions. It facilitates speech, moistens the food and lubricates the process of swallowing. By its solvent action on the foodstuffs, it enables tasting to take place. It also contains an enzyme ptyalin which is concerned in the digestion of polysaccharides to disaccharides.

Disorders of the Teeth

Mastication of food to a soft pulp is a prerequisite for good digestion. The teeth should be inspected to determine if they are healthy, present in adequate numbers and in correct apposition in the upper and lower jaws to allow efficient mastication. If dentures are worn it should be ascertained if they are comfortable and efficient. Bacteraemia may have its source in gingivitis or an apical abscess. It is particularly liable to occur after dental manipulation and may cause endocarditis in patients with valvular disease of the heart; for this reason such patients should always be given prophylactic antibiotics both before and after dental extraction (p. 166). All patients should be advised to consult a dentist regularly in order to conserve the teeth and to prevent or treat foci of infection in the mouth.

Stomatitis

The mouth harbours a population of commensal micro-organisms which normally is controlled by a reasonable standard of oral hygiene; if this is neglected the bacterial population may proliferate and cause gingivitis or stomatitis. This may also occur when resistance to the commensal population is lowered by disease especially in the compromised host (p. 37).

Stomatitis due to deficiency of nutritional factors may arise directly from an insufficient intake or indirectly as a result of impaired absorption of vitamins, especially niacin, riboflavin, folate, and cyanocobalamin. When the deficiency is acute and severe, the tongue is red, raw and painful. When the deficiency is chronic and less severe the tongue appears moist and unduly clean because of atrophy of the papillae. Angular stomatitis often accompanies glossitis, especially in the case of gross iron deficiency. In severe vitamin C deficiency the gums become swollen and spongy and bleed readily.

Ulcerative stomatitis (Vincent's infection) occurs mainly in adults with malnutrition and poor dental hygiene; it is not commonly seen nowadays in Britain. Ulcers with ragged necrotic margins occur especially on the gums, but may involve the palate, the lips, or the inner aspects of the cheeks; the ulcers are covered by a grey slough surrounded by an erythematous margin. A stained smear shows many spirochaetes and fusiform bacilli; these organisms are present in small numbers in the normal commensal population of the mouth and the condition may be regarded as an endogenous infection due to impairment of host resistance. The condition is infectious, so that the patient's food vessels and cutlery should be sterilised.

The acute phase responds to local treatment with metronidazole (200 mg t.i.d. for 4 d), or to penicillin. Necrosis of the gums may occur, so that when the acute phase has been controlled it is important that proper dental treatment is undertaken.

Candidiasis. The fungus *Candida albicans* (p. 802) is a normal commensal in the mouth but it may proliferate to cause thrush in babies, the aged and particularly in debilitated or compromised patients. Thrush is also common in those receiving prolonged treatment with oral antibiotics. White patches appear on the tongue and buccal mucosa and may enlarge and coalesce to form an easily detached membrane; there is little surrounding inflammation. In severe infection, the lower pharynx and oesophagus may be affected, causing dysphagia, or the fungus may spread to the lungs.

Thrush may be treated by gentian violet mouth wash three times a day for 4 days or by nystatin tablets (500 000 units) retained in the mouth for as long as possible, and given four times daily for at least 4 days.

Aphthous ulceration is a common recurrent condition characterised by painful superficial ulceration in the mouth. The lesion begins as an indurated erythematous area followed in a day or so by ulceration. The ulcers are often multiple and may recur over several weeks. The aetiology is unknown and the patient is usually healthy otherwise. Emotional stress may precipitate an attack, and in some women ulcers tend to recur in cyclical fashion during the premenstrual phase. Severe chronic aphthous ulceration may be found in association with Crohn's disease, ulcerative colitis, coeliac or Behçet's disease.

Treatment involves the avoidance of trauma from ill-fitting dentures and over-brushing. Hydrocortisone hemisuccinate lozenges (2·5 mg t.i.d.) may be effective in the early phase of lesions. Pain can be reduced with topical anaesthetics and secondary infection controlled with tetracycline mouth washes.

Other Forms of Stomatitis. An allergic reaction to chemicals in toothpaste, dentures, foodstuffs and many drugs, especially antibiotics, can cause stomatitis. A characteristic blue-black punctate line may be seen where the gum margins adjoin the teeth in lead poisoning. Skin diseases such as lichen planus, pemphigus and erythema multiforme involve the mouth, sometimes before being seen on the skin.

Diseases of the Tongue

In health the tongue is moist with only a slight white fur on the dorsum. The papillae are readily seen. Mouth breathing causes a dry tongue, but otherwise dryness of the tongue is an indication of dehydration. The tongue may be coated with a whitish-yellow fur in persons who smoke excessively but in general, the presence of fur on the tongue has little clinical significance.

Glossitis may be a prominent feature of stomatitis resulting from nutritional deficiency (p. 79). *Geographical tongue* is the name given to a chronic migrating superficial glossitis; it looks odd but has no clinical significance.

When the patient complains of a persistently painful tongue (*glossodynia*) which appears normal on inspection and, unlike true glossitis, is not exacerbated by hot liquids or vinegar, then the symptom is usually psychogenic. A bad taste in the mouth may be caused by local disease in the oropharynx, by some of the materials used in dental conservation and by some drugs; when these causes can be excluded the symptom is usually neurotic in origin. The complaint of an offensive breath (*halitosis*), when it cannot be confirmed by the physician, is usually due to psychoneurosis. The breath has characteristic odours in conditions such as liver failure or diabetic ketoacidosis and after the ingestion of alcohol or garlic. In these circumstances, the subject is either unaware of the smell or has become accustomed to it and does not complain.

Syphilis may occur as a primary chancre, in the secondary stage as 'mucous patches', or in the tertiary stage as painless gummatous ulcers.

Leukoplakia is a chronic affection characterised by the presence of white, firm, smooth patches beginning at the side of the tongue and later spreading over the dorsum. In the early stages the tongue is not painful but later the patches are split by fissures with resultant pain and tenderness. The importance of leukoplakia is that it may precede the development of carcinoma, and a biopsy of such lesions should always be undertaken.

Carcinoma of the mouth and tongue is often related to excessive consumption of tobacco and alcohol and poor oral hygiene. It must be con-sidered in all cases of chronic ulcer of the tongue; if any doubt exists biopsy should be carried out.

Diseases of the Salivary Glands

Excessive salivary secretion may be a response to irritation or inflammation in the mouth, e.g. oral sepsis. Dryness of the mouth (*xerostomia*) may be due to dehydration or may be caused by anticholinergic or antidepressant drugs; commonly it is due to anxiety. Xerostomia is one of the features of Sjögren's syndrome (p. 554).

Parotitis may be due to the virus of mumps or to bacterial infection of the gland. The latter tends to develop during severe febrile illnesses and after major abdominal operations if adequate attention is not given to oral hygiene and to the prevention of dehydration and infection. Its treatment consists of the parenteral administration of penicillin and surgical drainage if abscess formation has occurred.

Enlargement of the parotid glands may be found in sarcoidosis.

Salivary calculi occur occasionally in the submandibular gland or its duct. They cause pain and swelling brought on by eating. Infection of the gland is a complication. Stones in the duct can be felt in the floor of the mouth and can be removed by incision over the duct. Stones in the gland may require excision of the gland.

A 'mixed' salivary tumour is essentially of epithelial origin but may contain stromal elements. It presents as a slow, painless enlargement of one salivary gland. The tumour shows a variable degree of malignancy, depending on which it is treated either by excision or excision and radiotherapy.

DISEASES OF THE OESOPHAGUS

Dysphagia

Since the only function of the oesophagus is the transmission of food from mouth to stomach, most diseases of the oesophagus and its adjacent structures cause difficulty in swallowing (dysphagia).

Causes of Dysphagia. 1. PAINFUL DISEASES of the mouth and pharynx, e.g. stomatitis, tonsillitis, tuberculous laryngitis or retropharyngeal abscess, produce dysphagia, the cause of which is usually apparent.

2. NEUROMUSCULAR DISORDERS. Pharyngeal causes of dysphagia include bulbar and pseudo-bulbar paralysis and myasthenia gravis. Motility disorders of the oesophagus e.g. achalasia, diffuse spasm, Chagas' disease and systemic sclerosis also cause dysphagia.

3. EXTRINSIC COMPRESSION — goitre or a mediastinal mass, e.g. malignant lymph nodes or aneurysm of the aorta.

4. INTRINSIC DISEASE OF THE OESOPHAGUS

(a) *Congenital Abnormalities*. Atresia, the upper oesophagus ending blindly at about the level of the tracheal bifurcation, occurs occasionally requiring urgent surgery in the newborn.

(b) *Ulceration and Stricture*. Oesophagitis is most commonly due to reflux of gastric contents through a sphincter made incompetent by a sliding hiatus hernia. There is acid-pepsin digestion of the oesophageal mucosa immediately above the hernia, with ulceration, spasm and eventual stricture formation. More unusual causes of oesophagitis are herpes simplex infection, candidiasis which occurs in the immunocompromised and a variety of drugs which when given as tablets or capsules, lodge in the oesophagus particularly in the elderly, to cause local ulceration.

Oesophagitis and stricture are occasionally caused by the ingestion, accidental or otherwise, of corrosives such as bleach and caustic soda.

(c) *Sideropenic Dysphagia* (*Plummer-Vinson Syndrome*). This form of dysphagia is associated with iron deficiency anaemia, glossitis, and perhaps koilonychia and splenic enlargement. There is degeneration and atrophy of the epithelium of the tongue, pharynx, oesophagus and stomach. A fold of atrophic epithelial cells — the 'postcricoid web' — may be demonstrable radiographically or endoscopically. The dysphagia is to solids rather than to liquids, is intermittent, and may therefore mistakenly be thought to be hysterical. The dilatation associated with diagnostic endoscopy is often sufficient to relieve the dysphagia. Treatment is with iron.

(d) *Carcinoma* of the oesophagus or of the cardia of the stomach is the usual cause of dysphagia in elderly patients with no preceding history.

Investigation. The exclusion of malignant disease is essential in the investigation of any patient who complains of dysphagia. Barium swallow and oesophagoscopy are required. Where the disorder appears to be one of function rather than structure, as for example in achalasia or systemic sclerosis, then manometry (p. 284) can give additional information.

Oesophageal Hiatus Hernia and Reflux Oesophagitis

Several mechanisms operate to prevent reflux of food and fluid from the stomach into the lower oesophagus. The most important are the lower oesophageal sphincter situated just above the oesophago-gastric junction, the position of this sphincter below the diaphragm so that it is reinforced by intra-abdominal pressure, and the angle of entry of the oesophagus into the stomach. The latter two mechanisms are lost when the oesophagogastric junction 'slides' through the oesophageal hiatus in the diaphragm. This proximal displacement is usually sufficient to allow reflux although the lower oesophageal sphincter may remain operative. If reflux persists the continued exposure of the lower oesophageal mucosa to the effects of gastric juice or bile results in oesophagitis.

Hiatus hernia and reflux oesophagitis are most frequent in middle-aged and elderly women. An increase in intra-abdominal pressure, as a result of obesity, and hormonal changes in pregnancy promote their development in earlier years.

Clinical Features. Heartburn is the characteristic symptom of reflux oesophagitis. It is a deeply placed 'burning' pain, felt retro-sternally and brought on by bending, or by the exertion of lifting or straining with consequent increase in intra-abdominal pressure. It may also occur on lying down at night and keep the patient awake; relief is obtained by sitting up, or by taking food or alkali. No other pain produced in the alimentary tract is so closely linked to change of posture as that of reflux oesophagitis. Many patients with hiatus hernia have no symptoms as these are related to the presence of oesophagitis. Occasionally the latter is itself symptomless and it may present with severe iron deficiency anaemia due to blood loss.

Other complications are chronic ulcer of the oesophagus, stricture of the oesophagus and gastric ulcer in the herniated gastric mucosa.

The diagnosis of oesophagitis is made on the visual and biopsy findings at endoscopy. The presence of a hiatus hernia is shown by a barium meal (Fig. 9.1) and ulcer in the hiatus hernia can be revealed by endoscopy or barium studies.

Fig. 9.1 Hiatus hernia with an ulcer (arrow) in the herniated portion of the stomach. (Courtesy of Dr. G.M. Fraser).

Treatment. There are several practical dietary and postural measures which the patient can take to minimise reflux and these should be explained. Meals should be of small volume and fatty foods should be avoided as they tend to promote reflux and delay gastric emptying. Weight reduction is essential in obese subjects and may be all that is required to relieve symptoms. Stooping from the waist should be avoided as far as possible. To reduce reflux at night, the patient should sleep with the head of the bed elevated. Smoking reduces lower oesophageal sphincter pressure and should be stopped.

All medications consumed by the patient should be reviewed. Non steroidal anti-inflammatory drugs should be reduced or stopped if possible and the patient should be instructed to take all tablets with a large volume of water when sitting or standing in order to ensure complete swallowing.

Heartburn can be effectively relieved by antacids which, when symptoms are severe, should be taken one and three hours after meals, before sleep, and whenever heartburn occurs. The antiemetic metoclopramide (10 mg t.i.d.) may be helpful; it increases the contraction of the lower oesophageal sphincter and promotes emptying of the stomach. Cimetidine or ranitidine (p. 296) relieve symptoms and a prolonged course may induce healing of oesophagitis. Patients with strictures will require a liquid or semi-liquid diet, pending dilatation. Anaemia will usually respond to oral iron, but transfusion may be required if blood loss has been severe.

Surgery is indicated if severe symptoms persist despite adequate medical therapy. The aim of surgery is to return the lower oesophageal sphincter to the abdomen and to construct an additional valve mechanism. Most oesophageal strictures can be treated by dilatation at endoscopy followed by further dilatation as necessary. However, a small proportion cannot be helped in this way and surgical resection of the stricture is necessary.

Paraoesophageal Hernia

Here a knuckle of stomach 'rolls' alongside the oesophagus through the hiatus. The lower oesophageal sphincter remains below the diaphragm and competent even in the extreme cases when most of the stomach rotates to follow the herniated knuckle into the chest. There may be mild dysphagia; a large hernia in the posterior mediastinum may cause cardiac arrhythmias and breathlessness but often there are no symptoms and the hernia is found incidentally on chest radiography. Occasionally symptoms become acute because of obstruction, distension and even gangrene of the herniated portion of stomach and then surgery may be required urgently. In a few patients, and as a planned procedure, surgical repair of the hernia is indicated if the disability is severe.

Diverticulum of the Oesophagus

A traction diverticulum is most commonly situated in the anterior wall of the oesophagus just below the level of the tracheal bifurcation. It is due to chronic inflammation, usually tuberculous, in adjacent lymph nodes. By the time the diverticulum is discovered, often accidentally during barium swallow, the disease in the lymph nodes has healed. It is seldom that the diverticulum itself causes symptoms and surgical treatment is rarely necessary.

A pharyngeal pouch develops at the site of the inferior constrictor of the pharynx. Its late onset and the fact that dysphagia precedes the formation of the pouch suggests that the condition is the result of muscle incoordination. It begins as a posterior bulge of mucosa which enlarges to form a sac that extends downwards and to the left between oesophagus and cervical spine. The fully-formed pouch causes dysphagia due to forward displacement of the oesophagus. There is swelling and gurgling in the neck on swallowing. The patient may present with recurrent attacks of stridor, or inhalation of contents of the sac may lead to pneumonia.

The condition is seen almost exclusively in middle-aged subjects.

Treatment is surgical, a one-stage resection of the pouch with careful suture of its neck being carried out after preliminary cleansing and under antibiotic cover. The danger is leakage or contamination with consequent mediastinitis.

In Edinburgh, pharyngeal pouch is remembered as the affliction of Lord Jeffrey (1773–1850), a Scottish judge and wit who, in those days before surgery, emptied his pouch with a specially designed silver spoon.

Achalasia of the Cardia

Although apparently confined to the lower end where there is failure of the sphincter to relax, this is in fact a motility disorder of the whole oesophagus which shows progressive atony and dilatation. The cause is probably a failure of nerve conduction due to diminution in the number of ganglion cells. Chagas' disease (American trypanosomiasis, p. 780) produces similar changes. Achalasia is also known, less appropriately, as *cardiospasm*.

Clinical Features. Dysphagia may at first be intermittent but later is always present. It is caused both by solids and liquids and can be localised behind the lower end of the sternum. In the initial stages, the patient continues to eat a normal diet but food accumulates in the capacious non-contractile oesophagus. Later the retained

food cannot be expelled into the stomach and weight loss ensues. Inhalation of food and secretions may occur at night and cause recurrent pulmonary infection.

Investigation. A chest radiograph may be sufficient to show a dilated oesophageal outline, perhaps with a fluid level behind the heart shadow. A barium swallow shows the dilated atonic oesophagus coming to a smooth pointed termination (Fig. 9.2). There is absence of the usual gas shadow in the fundus of the stomach. While the appearances are typical, they are not diagnostic because they can be mimicked by a carcinoma at the lower end of the oesophagus or in the cardiac portion of the stomach. Treated or untreated, patients with achalasia have an increased liability to carcinoma of the oesophagus which makes initial endoscopy essential and periodic review after treatment desirable.

Fig. 9.2 Achalasia of cardia. (Courtesy of Dr. D.H. Cummack)

Oesophagoscopy should always be carried out. Usually cleansing of the oesophagus is required with mechanical removal of the larger retained food fragments, and this may involve repeated lavage, aspiration and oesophagoscopy. Once the oesophagus is clean it can be inspected and biopsies taken if necessary.

Motility studies (p. 284) are of value in establishing the diagnosis and in determining the severity of the lesion.

Treatment may be by dilatation or cardiomyotomy. In the first a hydrostatic or pneumatic bag is positioned at the level of the diaphragm. It is then distended forcibly so as to weaken the lower oesophageal sphincter. One or more dilatations may be required to bring about adequate swallowing.

Failure of hydrostatic dilatation or inability to introduce the dilator are indications for operation, which takes the form of cardiomyotomy (Heller's operation). Here the muscle at the lower end of the oesophagus, and for some distance above and below, is slit to expose but not to penetrate the mucosa. The operation is relatively effective and safe, even in the elderly, but either procedure may be complicated by reflux oesophagitis, or more occasionally by oesophageal perforation.

Diffuse Spasm of the Oesophagus

This condition may be caused by a disorder of the oesophageal nerve cells similar to that in achalasia. Often there is hypertrophy of the muscle wall of the oesophagus. Spasm of the oesophagus may also occur in patients with the irritable bowel syndrome (p. 332).

The main symptom is pain precipitated by eating or by emotional stress. The pain is retrosternal and there may be radiation to the back, neck or arms, thus making the differential diagnosis from coronary artery disease difficult. The pain may or may not be accompanied by dysphagia. The diagnosis is established by barium swallow which shows a hold-up of barium in the oesophagus due to multiple uncoordinated contractions. The appearance resembles a 'corkscrew'. Manometry shows strong uncoordinated contractions.

Treatment involves education in eating in a relaxed atmosphere with adequate mastication. Any emotional stress should receive attention. Nitroglycerine may relieve pain. Since most patients are over the age of 60, the physician has to persist with medical management but in the occasional younger patient, an extended cardiomyotomy may be required.

Carcinoma of the Oesophagus

There are wide geographical variations in the incidence of this tumour; it is very common around the Caspian Sea and some parts of Southern Africa (p. 105).

In Western communities, the average age of patients with carcinoma of the oesophagus is between 60 and 70 years, and there is a slight male predominance. The most frequent site is the lower third of the oesophagus; it is less common in the middle third and least common in the upper third. The lesion is usually ulcerative and it extends circumferentially and longitudinally in the wall of the oesophagus, often producing stenosis. Direct invasion of surrounding structures and involvement of related lymph nodes is common by the time of diagnosis. Squamous carcinoma is most frequent. Of the 10–20% of adenocarcinomas, most have invaded the lower oesophagus from the stomach; the remainder arise from oesophageal glands and from columnar epithelium in the lower oesophagus.

Clinical Features. Progressive dysphagia is typical. It starts with the 'sticking' of solid food, at first intermittently and then regularly and proceeds to difficulty with semisolids and eventually with liquids. There is discomfort, not amounting to pain, at the site of the obstruction which is usually well localised by the patient. The development of symptoms occupies some months so that by the time the patient first attends, weight loss is already a feature and there may be metastases in lymph nodes, liver and related structures in the mediastinum.

Investigation. Obstruction and an irregular narrowing of the oesophagus, seen at barium swallow, are highly suggestive of the diagnosis (Fig. 9.3). At the lower end it may not be possible to distinguish between carcinoma of the oesophagus and achalasia of the cardia. Oesophagitis and a benign stricture may also simulate carcinoma.

Oesophagoscopy and biopsy should always be carried out. Repeated biopsy may be required to obtain positive confirmation of the diagnosis, and this is particularly so when stricture formation prevents further insertion of the oesophagoscope or the biopsy forceps. In these circumstances, the passage of a brush through the narrowed area and examination of dislodged cells are of value.

Treatment. The choice lies between palliation and radical treatment. The chances of cure seldom exceed 10%. In squamous carcinoma,

Fig. 9.3 Carcinoma of the oesophagus. (Courtesy of Dr. G.M. Fraser).

particularly of the upper and middle thirds, high voltage radiotherapy is the treatment of choice in those centres possessing the necessary facilities. Otherwise, and with tumours of the lower third, oesophagogastrectomy offers the best hope. There is the possibility that a combined approach of surgery with preoperative radiotherapy may lead to enhanced survival.

Extensive tumours that are unsuitable for radical surgery or for intensive radiotherapy are treated palliatively, occasionally by bypass surgery, but more often by endoscopic insertion of a permanent tube into the oesophagus. This allows liquids to be taken and is effective in relieving the patient of that most distressing problem — the inability to swallow saliva.

Gastrostomy as a palliative measure offers no relief to the patient, fails to prolong survival and is therefore not advisable.

DISEASES OF THE STOMACH AND DUODENUM

PEPTIC ULCER

The term 'peptic ulcer' refers to an ulcer in the lower oesophagus, stomach or duodenum, in the jejunum after surgical anastomosis to the stomach, or rarely in the ileum adjacent to a Meckel's diverticulum. Ulcers in the stomach or duodenum may be acute or chronic; both penetrate the muscularis mucosae but the acute ulcer shows no evidence of fibrosis. Erosions do not penetrate the muscularis mucosae.

Although the incidence of peptic ulcer is decreasing in many Western communities, it still affects, at some time, approximately 10% of all adult males. The male to female ratio for duodenal ulcer varies from 4:1 to 2:1 in different communities whilst that for gastric ulcer is 2:1 or less. Variations in the incidence of gastric and duodenal ulcer occur between different countries and between different parts of the same country; the incidence of peptic ulcer is higher in Scotland than in Southern England due to a preponderance of duodenal ulcers in Scotland. Peptic ulcer is becoming more common in many developing countries. There is growing evidence that cigarette smoking prevents healing of gastric and duodenal ulcers and may be a factor contributing to their development.

Aetiology of Chronic Ulceration. HEREDITY. Patients with peptic ulcer often have a family history of the disease; this is particularly the case with duodenal ulcers which develop below the age of 20 years. Gastric and duodenal ulcers are inherited as separate disorders; thus, the relatives of gastric ulcer patients have three times the expected number of gastric ulcers but duodenal ulcer occurs with the same frequency amongst relatives as in the general population.

ACID-PEPSIN VERSUS MUCOSAL RESISTANCE. The immediate cause of peptic ulceration is digestion of the mucosa by acid and pepsin of the gastric juice, but the sequence of events leading to this is unknown. Digestion by acid and pepsin cannot be the only factor involved, since the normal stomach is obviously capable of resisting digestion by its own secretions. The concept of ulcer aetiology may be written as 'acid plus pepsin versus mucosal resistance'. Some factors which affect this balance can be identified.

Gastric Hypersecretion. Ulcers occur only in the presence of acid and pepsin; they are never found in achlorhydric patients such as those with pernicious anaemia. On the other hand, severe intractable peptic ulceration nearly always occurs in patients with the Zollinger-Ellison syndrome which is characterised by very high acid secretion. Acid secretion is more important in the aetiology of duodenal than gastric ulcer, because patients with duodenal ulcer, as a group, secrete more hydrochloric acid than normal individuals and duodenal ulcer heals when gastric hypersecretion is reduced by drugs or by vagotomy.

Mucosal Resistance. Several mechanisms protect the gastric mucosa from hydrogen ions secreted into the lumen of the stomach. The surface epithelial cells secrete bicarbonate which creates an alkaline milieu at the surface of the mucosa; this bicarbonate secretion is under the influence of mucosal prostaglandins. The tight junctions between the epithelial cells, and their surface lipoprotein layer provide a mechanical barrier. The normal turnover of epithelial cells and gastric mucus also has a protective function. Collectively, all these mechanisms can be described as the 'gastric mucosal barrier'. Its integrity is important in preventing gastric ulcer and some of the mechanisms may also operate in the duodenum.

Factors Reducing Mucosal Resistance. Several drugs, particularly those used in rheumatoid arthritis, will disrupt the gastric mucosal barrier. When aspirin is in solution at a pH below 3·5 it is undissociated and fat-soluble, so that it is absorbed through the lipoprotein membrane of the surface epithelial cells; during absorption it damages the membrane and the tight junctions. It also inhibits prostaglandin synthesis thus reducing bicarbonate secretion by the surface epithelial cells. Aspirin has been shown to be an important aetiological factor in gastric ulcer in Australia, and this may also be so in other countries where there is a high consumption of aspirin. There is also a relationship between aspirin ingestion and acute bleeding from the upper gastrointestinal tract.

Reflux of bile and intestinal secretions into the stomach occurs more frequently in patients with gastric ulcers than in normal individuals or patients with duodenal ulcer, due presumably to a poorly functioning pyloric sphincter. Bile damages the gastric mucosal barrier, predisposing the mucosa to ulceration. Chronic gastritis is more common in patients with gastric ulcer and it may be caused by damage from regurgitated bile and intestinal secretions.

Aetiology of Acute and Stress Ulcers. Many of the factors described above also contribute to the development of acute ulcers. Aspirin is particularly important. Acute peptic ulcers developing after head injury, burns, severe sepsis, surgery or trauma are termed stress ulcers. Gastric hyper-secretion is the usual cause of acute ulcer after head injury, while the reflux of duodenal contents and mucosal ischaemia may be responsible factors after burns or shock.

Pathology. Chronic gastric ulcer is nearly always single; 90% are situated on the lesser curve within the antrum or at the junction between body and antral mucosa. Chronic duodenal ulcer is usually situated in the first part of the duodenum just distal to the junction of pyloric and duodenal mucosa; 50% are on the anterior wall. More than one peptic ulcer is found in 10–15% of cases. Acute ulcers or erosions are frequently multiple, and are more widely distributed.

Clinical Features. A duodenal ulcer follows a chronic course for up to 20 years and whilst treatment with histamine H_2-receptor antagonist drugs may effect prompt healing, there is no evidence that the natural history of the ulcer is affected. The course of gastric ulcer is probably less chronic. While there are good grounds for believing that gastric and duodenal ulcers are different diseases it is convenient to describe the general features of 'peptic ulcer' as inclusive of both, noting differences where they occur.

Peptic ulcer may present in different ways. The commonest is chronic, episodic pain extending over months or years. However, the ulcer may come to attention as an acute episode with bleeding or perforation, with little or no previous history. Occasionally the patient presents with the symptoms of gastric outlet obstruction, having had negligible trouble previously.

Pain is the characteristic symptom of peptic ulcer, and it has three notable features — localisation to the epigastrium, relationship to food, and periodicity. Ulcer pain is typically referred to the epigastrium, in the midline or to the right; it is usually localised so that the patient can indicate the site with one finger, 'the pointing sign'. Occasionally ulcer pain is not clearly localised; it may be referred diffusely in the epigastrium, the lower chest or to the back in the interscapular region in the fifth to eighth thoracic segments. Pain referred to the interscapular area suggests duodenal or post-bulbar ulceration. The description of the pain is not especially helpful, although patients commonly describe it as gnawing or burning. Pain varies considerably in severity, and it is sometimes helpful to ask the patient to qualify the symptom as 'pain' or as 'discomfort' as a measure of its intensity.

Most patients recognise a relationship of the pain to food, although the relationship varies between patients, and in the same patient from time to time. Duodenal ulcer pain tends to occur between meal times, so that the patient may describe it as 'hunger' pain, which is characteristically relieved by food. A notable feature of duodenal ulcer is pain awakening the patient from sleep 2 to 3 hours after retiring. The pain of gastric ulcer occurs less regularly; it frequently occurs within an hour of eating, is less often relieved by food and it rarely occurs at night. Besides the characteristic relief obtained after eating, ulcer pain is almost invariably relieved by antacids or vomiting.

Ulcer pain is characteristically episodic occurring regularly each day for days or weeks at a time, then disappearing, to recur weeks or months later. Between attacks, the patient feels perfectly well, and may eat and drink with impunity. Bouts of pain may at first last only a day or so at a time, and occur only once or twice a year. As the natural history evolves, however, episodes begin to last longer and occur more frequently, so that in severe cases remissions of pain may be short lived and pain or discomfort becomes more or less

persistent. The cause for these relapses is difficult to establish. Seasonal factors may be operative, sometimes psychological stress may be blamed, sometimes dietary indiscretion, and sometimes alcoholic excess. Most commonly, no reason can be found for the relapse.

Pain is sometimes absent or so slight as to be dismissed by the patient. Such individuals may complain of other symptoms such as a feeling of 'distension' in the epigastrium or a poorly defined sense of unease after eating. Other complaints include episodic nausea and sometimes anorexia, as well as heartburn or waterbrash. Vomiting in ulcer patients almost always relieves pain and when it is persistent may result in weight loss. This helps to distinguish it from vomiting of psychological origin, in which weight is usually maintained. Persistent vomiting in an ulcer subject usually indicates some degree of gastric outflow obstruction, whether due to spasm or organic narrowing. In such patients, vomiting is usually copious, so that the patient is 'surprised' at the volume; the patient often recognises food eaten twelve or more hours previously. Although there is no constant change in bowel rhythm during an ulcer relapse, some patients are aware of constipation or diarrhoea when dyspepsia reappears.

Physical Signs. The only physical sign that may be present is 'the pointing sign' which, when accompanied by localised tenderness, is practically diagnostic of an ulcer. However, tenderness may be completely absent. In patients with gastric outlet obstruction, the stomach may be visibly distended, a succussion splash may be present, and gastric peristalsis may be seen.

Investigation. At double contrast barium meal the ulcer is seen *en face* as a small collection of barium with mucosal folds radiating to the edge of the crater (Figs 9.4 and 9.5). Even when an ulcer cannot be seen, deformity of the duodenal cap can be important evidence of duodenal ulcer disease. Endoscopy is preferred by most physicians particularly when the ulcer is gastric, because a biopsy can be carried out to exclude carcinoma. Endoscopy will also locate some duodenal ulcers which are difficult to detect radiologically. In addition it will diagnose *duodenitis*, a generalised inflammation of the first part of the duodenum. This may be regarded as a variant of

Fig. 9.4 Gastric ulcer. (Courtesy of Dr. G.M. Fraser).

Fig. 9.5 Duodenal ulcer. (Courtesy of Dr. G.M. Fraser).

duodenal ulcer disease in which no ulcer crater is present.

Treatment. While various measures are available to alleviate symptoms and heal the ulcer, there is no evidence that the long term course of the disease is affected.

DIET, INJURIOUS DRUGS, TOBACCO AND ALCOHOL. There is no evidence that dietary manipulation affects symptoms or ulcer healing, and strict diets should be avoided. It is particularly important that aspirin and other anti-inflammatory drugs are not used in peptic ulceration. Their injurious

action should be explained to the patient. There is evidence that stopping smoking accelerates the healing of gastric ulcers and it is likely that this also applies to duodenal ulcers. Patients should therefore be advised to give up cigarettes. Most patients cannot consume alcohol during exacerbations of ulcer disease because it aggravates their symptoms. It seems reasonable to encourage moderation in drinking habits in all patients with peptic ulceration.

DRUGS. *Antacids* provide symptomatic relief in peptic ulcer disease; in large doses, given for 4 to 6 weeks they will induce healing but side effects usually preclude this usage. Many preparations are available, varying in neutralising capacity, side effects, palatability and cost. Sodium bicarbonate is the quickest acting and is widely used for self-medication. However it is very readily absorbed with the risk of alkalosis, so that its use should be discouraged and it should not be prescribed. The majority of antacids are based on combinations of calcium, aluminium and magnesium salts, all of which may cause side-effects. Frequently calcium and aluminium cause constipation and magnesium causes diarrhoea. Calcium compounds may lead to hypercalcaemia if dosage is high and prolonged. Aluminium compounds block the absorption of phosphate and may cause phosphate depletion, an effect which is utilised in the management of renal failure. They may also bind other drugs whose absorption will be reduced if given at the same time as the antacid. Magnesium compounds may cause toxic hypermagnesaemia when renal function is impaired. Almost all antacids contain appreciable amounts of sodium which may exacerbate fluid retention in patients with cardiac or liver disease.

For relief of minor discomfort, antacid preparations in tablet form are convenient; they may be carried in the pocket and chewed or sucked whenever pain occurs. For relief of more severe pain during exacerbations, 15–30 ml of liquid antacid are usually required. To heal duodenal ulcer, it is necessary to give 30 ml of liquid antacid one and three hours after food and at bedtime. Patient acceptance of this form of therapy is low because of poor palatability and the frequent occurrence of constipation or diarrhoea.

Histamine H$_2$-receptor Antagonist Drugs. It has

long been known that the stimulating effect of histamine on gastric secretion could not be blocked by the standard antihistamines. This led to the idea that there might be a second type of histamine receptor situated on, or near, the parietal cells. The possibility of blocking this second type of receptor and so reducing gastric secretion led to the development of the histamine H_2-receptor antagonists which are the treatment of choice for all forms of peptic ulcer. Two of these drugs, cimetidine and ranitidine, are available and when given for 4 weeks will heal over 80% of duodenal ulcers and 70% of gastric ulcers. Cimetidine is used in a dose of 200 mg three times a day with meals and 400 mg at night, or alternatively, 400 mg with breakfast and 400 mg at night. Ranitidine is given in a dose of 150 mg with breakfast and 150 mg at night.

The use of cimetidine in large numbers of patients suggests that it is a very safe drug. Gynaecomastia occurs in a few patients; confusion in the elderly and diarrhoea are other occasional side effects. Cimetidine also impairs the metabolism of some drugs and this is particularly important in the case of warfarin and phenytoin. To date, ranitidine has the disadvantage of less exhaustive testing but appears not to cause any of the above side effects of cimetidine; however it may disturb liver function.

Treatment with either drug usually renders nearly all patients asymptomatic within a week of the commencement of therapy, and most are asymptomatic within 48 hours. Failure to relieve symptoms should lead to a reconsideration of the diagnosis. Most patients with peptic ulceration will have one or two exacerbations per year and each can be treated with a 4 week course of cimetidine or ranitidine. However, for those patients with more frequent relapses or who have contraindications to elective surgery, such as age, respiratory or cardiac disease, the number of further relapses can be reduced by giving maintenance therapy of ranitidine 150 mg at night for several years or permanently.

Other Drugs used for Healing Ulcers. It has been shown that carbenoxolone sodium accelerates the healing of both gastric and duodenal ulcers. However, because of its aldosterone-like effects, it may cause sodium retention with oedema, hypokalae-mia and hypertension, so that it should not be prescribed in elderly patients or when there is a history of cardiac failure. The usual dose is 50 mg four times daily for 6 to 8 weeks.

Colloidal bismuth, one tablet four times a day, results in the same healing rate of chronic gastric and duodenal ulcers as histamine H_2-receptor antagonists but the symptomatic response may not be so rapid.

SURGICAL TREATMENT. This has much to offer the patient with intractable peptic ulceration. It can relieve severe or persistent symptoms and prevent complications. While in many cases the assessment of the patient's disability is straightforward, in patients in whom anxiety or depression is present, the decision becomes difficult. Elective surgery should be considered in the following circumstances:

1. When the ulcer relapses promptly after several courses of cimetidine or ranitidine, or more rarely when the ulcer fails to heal at all, particularly when symptoms interfere with the enjoyment of life or reduce the capacity to work. The indications for surgery are strengthened if the ulcer has developed in adolescence or young adult life, if there is a strong family history, or if there has been a previous complication such as haemorrhage or perforation. Finally, some patients fail to comply with medical therapy or express reservations about prolonged therapy, both points being in favour of elective surgical treatment.

2. When there is an ulcer which has produced gastric outlet obstruction, or an hour-glass stomach because of fibrosis.

3. When there is a gastric ulcer the nature of which is uncertain or which has failed to heal in three months.

4. In a recurrent ulcer following previous gastric surgery.

There is no single, ideal operation suitable for all ulcers and all patients. For a gastric ulcer, the operation of choice is partial gastrectomy preferably with a Billroth I anastomosis, in which the ulcer itself and the ulcer-bearing area of the stomach is resected (Fig. 9.6). For duodenal ulcer the acid secretory capacity of the stomach may be reduced by vagotomy which eliminates nervous stimulation (Fig. 9.6). At truncal vagotomy the

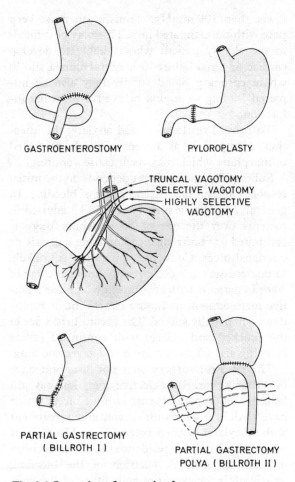

GASTROENTEROSTOMY   PYLOROPLASTY

TRUNCAL VAGOTOMY
SELECTIVE VAGOTOMY
HIGHLY SELECTIVE
VAGOTOMY

PARTIAL GASTRECTOMY
(BILLROTH I)

PARTIAL GASTRECTOMY
POLYA (BILLROTH II)

Fig. 9.6 Operations for peptic ulcer.

main nerves are divided and thereafter gastric emptying may be retarded so that a drainage operation such as pyloroplasty or gastroenterostomy has to be added. One of these procedures is also required in selective vagotomy in which vagal innervation to the small intestine, pancreas and biliary tree is preserved.

The aim of proximal (highly selective) vagotomy is to denervate only the acid-producing area of the stomach while leaving intact the vagal supply of the antrum and pylorus. Gastric emptying is thus not impaired and a drainage procedure is not required unless there is stenosis from ulcer scarring. The avoidance of a drainage procedure markedly reduces the incidence of post cibal syndromes and in particular dumping (p. 301). Vagotomy is preferred to partial gastrectomy be-

cause of the lesser mortality and lower incidence of long-term complications.

Complications of peptic ulcer are haemorrhage, perforation and gastric outlet obstruction. Ulcer-cancer is discussed on page 303.

Gastroduodenal Haemorrhage

Gastroduodenal haemorrhage is recognised by *haematemesis* (vomiting of blood) and/or *melaena* (passage of blood in the stools), and usually there are symptoms of hypovolaemia. Gastroduodenal haemorrhage carries a mortality that may reach 30% in elderly and shocked patients. A history of significant blood loss within the previous 48 hours should lead to immediate admission to hospital.

Aetiology. The common causes of bleeding are chronic gastric and duodenal ulcers (50%), erosions (15–30%), oesophageal varices (10%) and mucosal lacerations at the cardia due to vomiting (Mallory-Weiss syndrome — 7%). Less frequent causes are cancer of the stomach and other tumours such as leiomyoma, oesophagitis, stress ulcers and bleeding disorders.

Erosions are usually caused by the ingestion of aspirin either alone or in combination with alcohol or by corticosteroids or non-steroidal anti-inflammatory drugs (p. 558). In some patients the stomach shows petechiae, multiple erosions and areas of confluent mucosal bleeding; this appearance is called *acute haemorrhagic gastritis*. The usual presentation of stress ulcer, caused by burns or head injury, is with haematemesis and melaena.

Clinical Features. In severe bleeding from whatever cause, the patient complains of weakness, faintness, nausea, and sweating: these symptoms are followed by the vomiting of blood (*haematemesis*) or the passage of blood in the stools (*melaena*). Haematemesis and melaena occur together with a sudden large bleed whereas melaena alone indicates that bleeding is slower and less in amount. If blood remains in the stomach it becomes partially digested and appears brown and granular in the vomit or gastric aspirate, like 'coffee grounds'. Blood passing through the intestinal canal is also altered in appearance, so that the faeces become black and sticky, a 'tarry' stool. But in severe bleeding, transit may be so rapid that the blood in the rectum is bright red.

On examination, the patient may be shocked or restless and disorientated because of cerebral anoxia. These signs may be absent in the young patient in whom compensatory mechanisms are more effective.

The haemoglobin level will not alter until haemodilution occurs and this may not take place for some hours, nor be complete for some days. A reduced haematocrit on admission to hospital often indicates chronic bleeding prior to the acute episode. A raised urea with a normal serum creatinine indicates a blood loss of at least one litre. There is no simple laboratory procedure which will give a reliable estimate of the amount of blood loss until haemodilution is complete, so that in ordinary circumstances the assessment of the degree or rate of bleeding depends on clinical judgement. Serial recordings of the pulse rate and blood pressure give some indication, but for a more accurate assessment in patients who continue to bleed, measurement of central venous pressure is necessary. In patients with severe bleeding a record of urinary output by catheterisation is helpful.

Investigation. On admission there should be joint assessment by physician and surgeon and in large centres the management of gastroduodenal bleeding can with advantage be centralised in a single unit. The diagnosis and bleeding status should be established at the outset. Emergency endoscopy will show the source of the bleeding, whether it is continuing or whether it is likely to recur. Endoscopy is preferable to emergency barium studies in that it can demonstrate erosions and in the event of more than one lesion being present it can confirm which is bleeding.

The bleeding status is ascertained by passage of a nasogastric tube which should be aspirated at half hourly intervals and the quantity and type of aspirate recorded.

Treatment. Urgent treatment of hypovolaemic shock requires rapid and adequate blood replacement. Whole blood should be given as soon as it is available; until then, a colloidal solution such as dextran can be used. A blood transfusion is also indicated if the pulse rate is faster than 100 per minute or the systolic pressure

lower than 100 mmHg. Transfusion must keep pace with the estimated loss. This may be difficult in the elderly patient who is liable to develop cardiac or renal failure or cerebral anoxia and in whom coronary blood supply may also be impaired leading to angina or even myocardial infarction.

To control restlessness and anxiety, the injection of drugs such as diazepam is to be preferred to morphine which may itself cause vomiting.

Subsequent management depends on the initial response and on the site and cause of bleeding. In general, emergency surgery should be advised in patients over the age of 50 in whom there is continued or recurrent bleeding from a gastric or duodenal ulcer. Conversely operation is unlikely to be necessary in such patients under the age of 30 or in patients with erosions in whom conservative management, including cimetidine or ranitidine, will usually suffice. The greatest risks are in the shocked and elderly with continued severe bleeding and when operation is delayed too long.

The need for surgery does not disappear once the crisis is over. Early elective operation may still be indicated in patients with chronic ulcers which have bled, in those requiring continued treatment with salicylates or corticosteroids, and in patients whose occupation or residence makes supervision difficult. In general, excision of the bleeding gastric ulcer, or exposure and suture of the duodenal ulcer coupled in either case with vagotomy is safer than partial gastrectomy which should be reserved for the complicated case in expert hands.

Bleeding from oesophageal varices secondary to portal hypertension can be extremely severe and demands special measures for its management (p. 364).

Acute Perforation of a Peptic Ulcer

When free perforation occurs, the contents of the stomach escape into the peritoneal cavity. If perforation occurs without loss of contents, as in the accidental perforation of the empty stomach at gastroscopy, few symptoms are produced and the accident may even pass unnoticed. It follows that the symptoms of perforation are those of peritonitis, and they are in proportion to the extent of peritoneal soiling. Occasionally the symptoms of perforation appear and rapidly subside; presumably the perforation has then closed spontaneously, or more commonly the ulcer has perforated locally into an area confined by adhesions to adjacent structures. Perforation occurs more commonly in duodenal than in gastric ulcers, and usually in ulcers on the anterior wall. About one-quarter of all perforations occur in acute ulcers.

Clinical Features. Although perforation may be the first sign of ulcer, usually there is a history of recurrent epigastric pain. The most striking symptom is sudden, severe pain, the onset of which may be so incisive that the patient can time it to a minute. The pain is usually intense, and its distribution follows the spread of the gastric contents over the peritoneum. Thus, initially the pain may be referred to the upper abdomen, but very quickly it becomes generalised; shoulder tip pain may occur as a result of irritation of the diaphragm. The pain is accompanied by shallow respiration due to limitation of diaphragmatic movements and by shock. The abdomen is held immobile, and there is generalised board-like rigidity; intestinal sounds are absent, and liver dullness to percussion may decrease due to the presence of gas under the diaphragm. Vomiting is common. After some hours, the symptoms improve, though the abdominal rigidity remains. This period of improvement may deceive the clinician examining the patient for the first time; after this temporary improvement, manifestations of general peritonitis follow the initial peritoneal irritation and the patient's condition deteriorates.

A radiograph of the upper abdomen in the erect position may help to establish the diagnosis since free gas within the peritoneal cavity, if in sufficient amount, will show as a translucent crescent between the liver and diaphragm. Where doubt remains, an emergency Gastrografin meal may confirm that perforation has occurred.

Treatment and Prognosis. After initial treatment of the patient for shock, the acute perforation should be treated surgically either by simple closure, or occasionally in the case of perforation of a chronic ulcer by closure combined with vagotomy and drainage. More than half the patients who have a simple closure will eventually require a further elective operation for recurrence of ulcer symptoms, and for this reason some surgeons recommend a definitive procedure for the ulcer at the time of operation.

Acute perforation carries a mortality of about 5%. The outlook is poorest in elderly patients, when a large perforation results in extensive peritonitis or when operation is delayed.

Gastric Outlet Obstruction

An ulcer in the region of the pylorus may result in gastric outlet obstruction. This may be due to fibrous stricture or to oedema or spasm produced by the ulcer; frequently it is a combination of all three. Long-standing obstruction may lead to severe 'retention' gastritis, or even to secondary gastric ulcer.

In addition to chronic duodenal ulcer, or benign gastric ulcer at or near the pylorus, gastric outlet obstruction may be caused by carcinoma of the antrum and by a rare condition known as *adult hypertrophic pyloric stenosis*.

The syndrome of gastric outlet obstruction is loosely described as *'pyloric stenosis'*, even when the cause is chronic duodenal ulcer, and the stenosis is distal to the pylorus; thus in 'pyloric' obstruction due to duodenal stenosis, the pylorus itself may be seen radiologically to be greatly dilated.

Clinical Features. Symptoms of obstruction are usually preceded by a long history of duodenal ulceration. Without such symptoms, a patient with gastric outlet obstruction is likely to have a pyloric carcinoma. When there has been an ulcer, the symptoms change, so that vomiting becomes a prominent feature, and nausea replaces normal appetite. Vomiting produces such striking relief that a patient may start to eat immediately after the stomach has been emptied. If the obstruction progresses, the stomach dilates so that, eventually, surprisingly large amounts of gastric content may be vomited. Articles of food which have been eaten 24 hours or more previously may be recognised in the vomit. An earlier symptom is a sense of repletion soon after eating a relatively small amount of food. The loss of gastric contents results in water and electrolyte depletion. The blood urea may be raised because of dehydration. Alkalosis develops if large amounts of hydrochloric acid are lost, as occurs particularly in obstruction due to duodenal ulcer.

Physical examination shows evidence of wasting and dehydration, and there may be signs of tetany (p. 442). A succussion splash may be elicited four hours or more after the last meal or drink. In normal persons splashing occurs for less than an hour after meals because gastric emptying is rapid. Visible gastric peristalsis is diagnostic of gastric outlet obstruction and the abdomen should be inspected for its presence. If the patient takes a fluid diet with large amounts of milk, the signs of obstruction may be masked and nutrition may be well maintained.

Investigation. *Aspiration of the stomach contents* will confirm the diagnosis if the volume is in excess of 100 ml after fasting overnight or if the aspirate contains food residue, or is foul. However, a fine bore nasogastric tube may become blocked by debris; if in doubt a wide bore stomach tube should be used. If obstruction is suspected the stomach should be emptied prior to radiological examination.

The radiological signs are (1) an increase in the fasting residue of the stomach, (2) dilatation of the stomach with or without excessive peristalsis, (3) a lesion at or near the pylorus, and (4) delayed gastric emptying.

Endoscopy may demonstrate the cause of the obstruction and its degree.

Treatment. The stomach is washed out to remove all food debris and then aspirated 2 to 4 hourly for 3 to 4 days at which point, if the volume of aspirate has decreased, it may be possible to allow fluids by mouth. Dehydration and electrolyte disturbance must be corrected by intravenous fluids. In the first 24 hours 4 litres of isotonic saline are given and thereafter the daily requirement is based on the volume of aspirate together with other body losses. Potassium, 80 mmol/day, is given in the infusion. When obstruction is not severe a homogenised diet maybe prescribed. A multivitamin preparation should be given by injection to all but the mildest cases.

The majority of patients will be greatly improved by these methods; the volume of the gastric aspirate steadily declines, and the size of the stomach returns to near normal. It is then necessary to consider the timing of an operation; this should not be too long deferred. If obstruction persists, with no improvement after 5 to 7 days, nothing is gained by procrastination, and indeed the patient may deteriorate because of electrolyte imbalance. Relief of obstruction by conservative measures provides an opportunity to complete investigation and to render the patient as fit as possible for subsequent elective surgery.

Zollinger-Ellison Syndrome

This is a rare disorder in which severe peptic ulceration occurs due usually to an adenoma or hyperplasia of the islets of the pancreas secreting large amounts of gastrin which stimulates the parietal cells of the stomach excessively. The acid output may be so great that the 'acid tide' may reach the upper small intestine, reducing the luminal pH to 2 or less; at this pH, pancreatic lipase is inactivated and bile acids may be precipitated, causing diarrhoea and steatorrhoea. Excessive gastric secretion results in large volumes on aspiration under 'basal' conditions. Pentagastrin does not increase the secretory rate much above 'basal' values, since the stomach is already continuously secreting at or near maximal rates.

The ulcers are often multiple and severe and may occur in unusual sites such as the jejunum or the oesophagus. The history is usually short and bleeding and perforation are common. The syndrome may present in the form of severe recurrent ulceration following a standard operation for peptic ulcer, the underlying cause not having been recognised.

The diagnosis should be suspected in all patients with unusual or severe peptic ulceration, especially if the barium meal examination shows abnormally coarse gastric mucosal folds. It may be confirmed by finding very high levels of gastrin in the circulation.

Theoretically the condition should be cured by removing the pancreatic tumour, but this may not be possible because of its diffuse nature. In these circumstances it is necessary to eliminate, or very greatly reduce, acid secretion so that the ulcers may heal. In most patients continuous therapy with cimetidine or ranitidine is effective, but larger doses than those used to treat duodenal ulcer are required. In unresponsive patients, total gastrectomy is necessary.

Late Complications following Gastric Surgery

Although most operations carried out for the relief of peptic ulcer are successful, 10% of patients will develop complications months or years afterwards. Some of these, such as anaemia and nutritional impairment, develop insidiously, so that patients who have had an operation on the stomach should be reviewed at least once a year.

Recurrent ulcer, after surgery for duodenal ulcer, is usually due to insufficient reduction of the secretory capacity of the stomach because of incomplete vagotomy or inadequate gastrectomy. A jejunal ulcer develops just distal to the jejuno-gastric anastomosis, because the jejunal mucosa is more susceptible to acid-pepsin digestion than gastric or duodenal mucosa. About 15% of patients develop recurrent ulcer after highly selective vagotomy but the operation has the virtue of being free from the side effects associated with resection, truncal vagotomy or drainage procedures.

After months or years of freedom following the operation, ulcer pain recurs or the patient may present with melaena or severe anaemia without any dyspeptic symptoms. Occasionally perforation occurs. Rarely a jejunal ulcer penetrates the colon causing a *gastro-jejunal-colic fistula*; then there is bacterial contamination of the small bowel causing diarrhoea, malabsorption and wasting. The fistula can be demonstrated by barium enema.

Recurrent ulcer uncomplicated by perforation or fistula is best diagnosed by endoscopy which will also reveal the occasional ulcer due to an unabsorbed suture. This may be removed endoscopically. Recurrent ulcer can be treated by H_2-receptor antagonists but if medical therapy fails, a more radical surgical procedure may be necessary.

Biliary gastritis is the result of reflux of bile into the stomach through a drainage stoma. It may be symptomless and observed only on routine postoperative endoscopy. There may be epigastric discomfort, nausea, heartburn or vomiting of bile. Reduction in fluid intake, the eating of meals dry, avoidance of alcohol and stopping smoking may bring relief. Drugs are of little value

but some patients have symptoms due to delayed gastric emptying which are helped by metoclopramide (p. 289). Revisional surgery may be required if dietetic measures fail and especially when there is a mechanical cause for the reflux.

Post-cibal syndromes are mainly associated with gastrectomy and have become less frequent with the more general adoption of vagotomy.

1. *The Small Stomach Syndrome*. Discomfort and distension with meals leads to diminished intake and weight loss or failure to regain weight. High calorie small meals, with food supplements and, in some cases, revisional surgery are indicated.

2. *Dumping Syndrome*. After a meal and particularly after hot sweet foods, there is a feeling of intense drowsiness with weakness and nausea; there may also be flushing and palpitations. The syndrome usually disappears as the patient adapts and recognises the foods responsible. Occasionally further surgery may be necessary.

3. *Hypoglycaemia*. Rarely, one to two hours after a meal, the patient experiences attacks of weakness, tremor and faintness. The hypoglycaemia responsible for these symptoms can be relieved by glucose or barley sugar.

Diarrhoea may occur after any operation on the stomach, but especially after truncal vagotomy when most patients report some looseness of the stools. Moderate or severe diarrhoea occurs in about 10% and is characteristically episodic, several watery stools being passed daily for several days. A striking feature is the sense of urgency associated with the diarrhoea; defaecation may be precipitate, and the patient becomes worried because of the fear of soiling. Loperamide or codeine should be tried.

Mild steatorrhoea is common after all ulcer operations and does not require treatment, but if severe steatorrhoea occurs the cause (p. 311) should be identified so that appropriate treatment may be undertaken.

Anaemia is a common sequel to operations on the stomach, particularly partial gastrectomy, due to inadequate absorption of iron, or to recurrent minor blood loss from gastritis or oesophagitis. Its incidence increases in the first 10 years as the stores of iron are exhausted. The occurrence of anaemia is a measure of the adequacy of postoperative supervision, because it is preventable by and responds to the administration of iron. Megaloblastic anaemia may also occur (p. 503).

Nutritional Impairment and Osteomalacia. In a small proportion of patients there is some nutritional impairment following gastric surgery, and this increases with the extent of any resection. Severe weight loss is its most common manifestation. There may also be malabsorption with steatorrhoea and osteomalacia which may develop for the first time 15 to 20 years after partial gastrectomy, and may present as bone pain or as a pathological fracture. Treatment is described on page 70.

GASTRITIS

Gastritis signifies an acute or chronic inflammation of the stomach. Knowledge of the changes that occur in the gastric mucosa has been obtained by direct studies of the gastric mucosa in patients with gastrostomies, by gastroscopic observation and by histological examination of specimens removed at operation, biopsy or autopsy. There is poor agreement between these three approaches, so that the classification of gastritis is difficult. If histological specimens are examined, it is very rare to find a normal stomach completely free from any signs of inflammation. In this sense 'gastritis' is almost an invariable finding in adults. However, there are gross departures from this 'normal' state of affairs, even if they do not give rise to symptoms. For these reasons the condition is best defined in histological terms as acute or chronic gastritis.

Acute Gastritis

This is most commonly caused by the ingestion of aspirin, anti-inflammatory drugs and probably alcohol. It is also caused by the regurgitation of bile into the stomach, especially after gastric surgery. Macroscopically, there is engorgement of the mucosa with oedema and erosions or an acute haemorrhagic gastritis (p. 297). Microscopically there is loss of the surface epithelium, hyperaemia and some infiltration with inflammatory cells.

Acute gastritis may be asymptomatic. In some patients, there is anorexia, nausea, epigastric pain and heartburn. If gastritis persists, a slow loss of blood may lead to anaemia. The condition is diagnosed by the appearance of the mucosa at gastroscopy.

Drug consumption should be reviewed with a view to omitting or reducing drugs which are known to cause gastric mucosal damage. Alcohol should be avoided. The treatment of biliary gastritis is discussed on page 301.

Chronic Gastritis

The classification is histological; there are three stages which are progressive over many years. In *chronic superficial gastritis*, the mucosa is normal in thickness and there is patchy infiltration of lymphocytes and plasma cells. In *atrophic gastritis* there is a reduction of the specialised cells in the glands of the body and of mucous cells in the pyloric glands. There is epithelial metaplasia and an infiltrate of lymphocytes and plasma cells. In *gastric atrophy* the thickness of the mucosa is reduced, metaplasia is common but round cell infiltration is slight.

In pernicious anaemia and other autoimmune disorders, the chronic gastritis is due to an immunological process, and circulating antibodies to parietal cells and intrinsic factor are frequently found. Chronic gastritis is common in gastric ulcer, gastric cancer and after gastric surgery. In these instances, the gastritis is thought not to be immunological and circulating antibodies are absent.

The condition is asymptomatic; its importance lies in its association with the disorders noted above. The diagnosis may be suspected from the absence of mucosal folds at barium meal examination or from the gastroscopic appearances. However, the diagnosis is confirmed only by gastric biopsy. No treatment is known for stimulating the mucosa to regenerate.

CARCINOMA OF THE STOMACH

Carcinoma of the stomach is one of the commonest malignant tumours of the gastrointestinal tract, although its incidence varies considerably in different parts of the world — for example, the tumour is frequent in Japan and relatively uncommon in the USA: the incidence of gastric cancer in Japanese immigrants to America is much less than it is in Japan. Geographical variations have been attributed to environmental factors, such as trace elements in water, or differences in methods of food preparation. It has been suggested that nitrites, often used as preservatives in food can be converted to the carcinogens nitrosamines in the milieu of the stomach. Patients with pernicious anaemia have an increased risk of developing gastric cancer and this may extend to gastric atrophy from other causes.

Pathology. Almost 70% of all gastric cancers occur at the pylorus or in the antrum; the lesion does not spread to the duodenum. Such growths may produce symptoms of obstruction to the gastric outlet. Lesions of the body of the stomach often involve the greater curvature and produce a fungating ulcerating mass. Least common is a diffuse infiltrating lesion spreading throughout the body of the stomach and producing the so-called leather-bottle stomach. These are the descriptions of advanced cancer.

In the early stages, when the carcinoma is confined to the mucosa, the lesion may be represented only by a depressed area with obliteration or distortion of the mucosal folds, by irregular ulceration on an elevated base, or by a small polypoid lesion. Such changes can be seen and a biopsy taken during gastroscopy at a stage when the cancer is potentially curable by resection. The tumour is generally an adenocarcinoma and spreads by extension through the stomach wall, by lymphatic permeation and by embolism via the portal vein to the liver and thence to the systemic bloodstream.

Gastric carcinoma may present as a malignant ulcer, and whether it is then the result of malignant transformation of a benign ulcer is debatable. Most authorities believe that chronic peptic ulcer rarely becomes malignant, and that malignant ulcers, however long they have been present, have always been malignant. Whatever the truth of the matter the problem in the individual case is to decide whether a chronic gastric ulcer is benign or malignant.

Clinical Features. Loss of appetite, slight nausea and discomfort after meals occurring for the first time in middle age should always arouse suspicion. If the diagnosis is to be made early, then such patients require careful investigation. Unfortunately, the majority of patients have advanced gastric carcinoma before they seek advice. In some there have been no symptoms; in others symptoms have been present for 6 months or even a year. Dyspepsia, which is at first vague, becomes troublesome with increasing anorexia and nausea, discomfort or pain, vomiting and weight loss. There may be cachexia and pallor, a mass may be palpable or peristalsis visible. The abdomen may be distended by ascites from peritoneal metastases. Sometimes it is acanthosis nigricans (p. 109) or the presence of metastases in the liver, pelvis or scalene lymph nodes which first brings the patient to the physician.

Carcinoma of the stomach should always be considered as a cause of unexplained iron deficiency anaemia in the middle-aged person or as an uncommon cause of haematemesis or melaena. Tumours at the cardia may cause dysphagia, and tumours at the gastric outlet may cause vomiting. In the infiltrating type of tumour, diarrhoea may occur because of rapid emptying from the stomach.

Investigation. Early curable cancer is usually missed by a barium meal examination unless a double contrast study is carried out to show distortion of the mucosal pattern. The only method of establishing a positive diagnosis is by gastroscopy and biopsy of suspicious areas. These procedures are also necessary to distinguish malignant from benign gastric ulceration. The commonest appearance at barium meal is a filling defect in the antrum or body of the stomach (Fig. 9.7). In the rare diffuse infiltrating scirrhous carcinoma, the radiograph is that of a rigid tube through which the barium pours rapidly into the intestine. If dysphagia is the presenting symptom, a lesion in the cardia will probably be found, but symptomless lesions in this area can be very easily missed. Exfoliative cytology is sometimes used for diagnosis.

Treatment and Prognosis. The only curative treatment is gastrectomy, but it is usually only at laparotomy that the possibility of resection can be decided. About one-third of patients coming to operation are found to have tumours

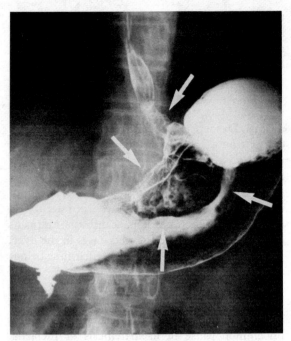

Fig. 9.7 Carcinoma of the stomach. (Courtesy of Dr. G.M. Fraser).

capable of removal; in the remainder it is possible to perform only a palliative procedure. This is worthwhile if pyloric obstruction is present, even if there are secondary deposits; such an operation relieves the distressing vomiting and gives the patient some comfort.

A total gastrectomy may be required for tumours involving the upper part of the stomach. Careful preoperative treatment is essential; this may require the restoration of fluid and electrolyte balance and the correction of anaemia. Every effort should be made to improve nutrition, if necessary by parenteral or enteral feeding (p. 285).

A small proportion of patients with cancer of the stomach obtain worth-while remission with cytotoxic drugs.

The prognosis in carcinoma of the stomach is very poor and has shown little improvement in the last 40 years. After an apparently successful resection, the 5 year survival rate is in the region of 20%. Pending an entirely new approach to the problem, the only means currently available by which the prognosis can be improved is the detection of gastric cancer when it is at a curable stage; this requires a vigorous approach to the problem of dyspepsia in the middle-aged, including careful radiological and endoscopic examination and the critical follow-up of doubtful abnormalities.

Malignant Ascites

Carcinoma of the stomach and other intra-abdominal tumours, including carcinoma of the colon and ovary, may be associated with the exudation of fluid into the peritoneal cavity. This follows the deposition of malignant cells on the peritoneal surface and is a sign of gross spread of the disease. The fluid is rich in protein and its sediment contains malignant cells which may be identifiable on microscopy.

Treatment is palliative. Relief of abdominal distension can be obtained by paracentesis, whilst instillation of an antimitotic agent such as methotrexate may slow the rate of reaccumulation.

DISEASES OF THE PANCREAS

The pancreas produces exocrine secretions which are important in digestion and also endocrine secretions concerned with the regulation of carbohydrate metabolism. The exocrine tissue, composed of acinar cells grouped in lobules and drained by a duct system, forms almost the entire mass of the gland. The exocrine secretion is discharged into the intestine through the pancreatic duct, which usually enters the duodenum together with the common bile duct at the sphincter of Oddi; in about 10% of individuals, however, the main outflow of the pancreatic juice reaches the duodenum by a separate duct.

The endocrine tissue is composed of specialised cells collected together in the small islets of Langerhans scattered throughout the gland, and accounts for only 1% of the mass of the pancreas. The endocrine secretions include insulin, which is produced by the beta cells of the islets, and glucagon from the alpha cells; both are discussed in the section on diabetes mellitus. The delta cell is one source of somatostatin (p. 419).

Pancreatic juice is an alkaline secretion (pH 7.5–8.5) which is isotonic with plasma, the main cations being sodium and potassium while the main anion is bicarbonate which is produced by the cells lining the duct system. The juice also contains enzymes which digest carbohydrate, fat and protein, the main ones being amylase, lipase and trypsin. These enzymes are synthesised by the serous cells of the pancreatic acini, and they are secreted in parallel concentrations; they all require an alkaline medium for optimal efficiency, so that theoretically digestion may be impaired if the bicarbonate content of the pancreatic juice is reduced.

Exocrine pancreatic secretion is stimulated partly through nervous and partly through hormonal mechanisms (p. 280), and a maximum flow is reached between 2 and 3 hours after a meal; in all, about 1 litre is secreted daily.

Investigation of the Pancreas

A plain radiograph may show evidence of duodeno-jejunal ileus in acute pancreatitis and calcification in chronic pancreatitis.

A barium meal will usually show stretching of the duodenal loop and upward displacement of the stomach when the head of the pancreas is enlarged by acute pancreatitis, cysts or tumours. Abnormalities of the mucosal folds of the duodenum, particularly on the medial wall, may be seen but these are best demonstrated by hypotonic duodenography.

The size, shape and position of the pancreas and the presence of tumours, cysts, oedema and dilated ducts can be shown by ultrasonography or by computed tomography. The former is more widely available and less expensive than CT scanning, but its value in the investigation of pancreatic disorders is greatly reduced if gas is present in overlying loops of bowel. CT scanning is more accurate in detecting pancreatic tumours especially in the tail of the gland. More specialised radiographic techniques include retrograde pancreatography of the duct system (ERCP p. 283).

Selective arteriography of the coeliac and superior mesenteric arteries can show distortion, compression, or abnormal distribution of vessels in relation to tumours. Radionuclide studies are now little used.

Tests of Exocrine Pancreatic Function. The exocrine function of the pancreas may be measured directly by passing a tube into the second part of the duodenum and collecting the secretory output of the gland in response to exogenous stimulation (secretin-cholecystokinin test) or endogenous stimulation by a meal (Lundh test).

In the secretin-cholecystokinin test the hormones are injected intravenously and pancreatic secretions are collected for 1 hour. Measurements are made of the volume of secretion and the concentration of bicarbonate and amylase or lipase. A special double lumened tube is used which allows gastric and pancreatic secretions to be collected separately to prevent neutralisation of pancreatic bicarbonate by gastric hydrochloric acid.

The Lundh test is simpler. A tube is passed into the duodenum and a liquid meal of fixed composition is given orally. The duodenal aspirate is collected by syphonage and the concentration of trypsin and amylase is recorded.

Both tests will detect the presence of pancreatic insufficiency, but usually give no information as to the cause; occasionally in patients with carcinoma of the pancreas the duodenal aspirate may be blood stained and malignant cells may be detected on cytological examination.

Fibreoptic duodenoscopy may allow the direct collection of pancreatic secretion for cytological examination. The value of all these tests is limited because of the technical difficulties involved and because early disease of the pancreas may not be detected.

Tests of Endocrine Pancreatic Function. A diabetic response to a glucose tolerance test in a patient with steatorrhoea suggests a pancreatic cause for the malabsorption of fat. When carcinoma of the pancreas is suspected, an abnormal glucose tolerance test is a frequent finding in a condition which is difficult to diagnose.

Acute Pancreatitis

This serious disorder is caused essentially by the digestion of the pancreas by its own enzymes. In the mildest cases the gland becomes swollen and oedematous; in more severe cases haemorrhagic necrosis occurs with the development of serious local and systemic complications. The disease is most common between the fourth and seventh decades, with an equal sex incidence.

Aetiology. In Britain about 50% of cases are associated with biliary disease and about 20% with alcoholism while in about 20% no cause can be identified. Alcoholism accounts for a much higher proportion in some countries, especially the USA and South Africa. Acute pancreatitis is a recognised complication of renal transplantation and may be caused also by drugs such as corticosteroids and oral contraceptives. It occurs occasionally after abdominal trauma or surgery and rarely in mumps, hyperparathyroidism, hyperlipidaemia or hypothermia.

The mechanisms which initiate the destruction of pancreatic tissue are not known. The frequent association with disease of the biliary tract led to the theory that obstruction of the sphincter of Oddi by a gallstone, oedema or spasm allows reflux of bile along the pancreatic duct, so activating the pancreatic enzymes and leading to autodigestion of the gland. Alcohol may cause pancreatitis by increasing the protein concentration in the pancreatic secretions; precipitation of the protein may then result in obstruction of the smaller ducts leading to pancreatitis. Obstruction from other causes, such as a tumour or stone may produce pancreatitis in the same way.

Clinical Features. The onset is sudden with severe pain in the epigastrium or right hypochondrium. It often occurs within 12 to 24 hours following the consumption of alcohol or a large meal. The pain is usually persistent and radiates most frequently through to the back, to either shoulder or to one of the iliac fossae before spreading to involve the whole abdomen. Nausea and vomiting are frequent. In severe cases profound shock soon supervenes and in addition to local complications such as ileus, systemic complications such as renal and respiratory failure may develop. In milder cases moderate fever occurs, and slight jaundice may develop, especially in cases with gallstones.

Despite the severity of the pain, there may be little or no guarding of the abdominal muscles at first. Later the upper abdomen becomes tender and rigid as peritoneal irritation increases and the initial shock passes off. The condition may simulate acute cholecystitis (with which it may coexist), and myocardial infarction. About one-third of cases are recognised for the first time at laparotomy, having been diagnosed as perforated peptic ulcer or acute appendicitis.

The swollen pancreas may cause obstruction to the duodenum or common bile duct. Bleeding may occur from inflamed or eroded areas of the stomach or duodenum.

Investigation. In the early stage of an acute case the serum amylase is elevated; this is short-lived because of rapid renal excretion. It follows that serum for amylase estimation must be taken immediately and that amylase measured in urine may provide the diagnosis when serum levels are normal (p. 820). A persistently raised serum amylase suggests the formation of a pseudocyst.

Biochemical findings may be helpful in the detection and monitoring of some complications. Hyperglycaemia is common in the first two days and hypocalcaemia may occur later because calcium is sequestered into the areas of fat necrosis which occur in severe pancreatitis.

A plain radiograph may show evidence of duodeno-jejunal ileus and absence of gas in the transverse colon. Ultrasonography, CT scanning or barium meal may demonstrate an enlarged pancreas.

Laparotomy is essential if diagnostic uncertainty persists.

Treatment. When the diagnosis of acute pancreatitis is made at laparotomy no direct surgical intervention should be attempted. Peritoneal lavage may be worthwhile and if there is definite evidence of associated biliary disease, the gallbladder may be drained. When the diagnosis can be established on clinical or biochemical evidence operation should be avoided unless complications develop. In about 10% of cases, acute pancreatitis is a catastrophic event, and death may ensue from acute circulatory, respiratory, or hepatorenal failure.

The immediate requirements are the energetic treatment of shock (p. 50) and of respiratory failure (p. 217) and the relief of pain. A central venous line may be necessary to monitor the need for fluid replacement, and to guard against overloading the circulation. Serial arterial oxygen pressures should be recorded because if respiratory failure becomes a major factor, endotracheal intubation and positive pressure assisted ventilation will be required (p. 217). The bladder should be catheterised so that urinary output can be measured. Intravenous saline, plasma, plasma expanders or whole blood may be required in large volumes as determined by the clinical response, urinary output and central venous pressure.

Ileus is almost inevitable in the acute phase and nasogastric suction will be required for decompression. Nasogastric suction has the additional benefit of suppressing pancreatic stimulation which may be further reduced by the intravenous administration of cimetidine.

Pain is best relieved by intravenous or intramuscular administrations of pethidine (100 mg) as required; morphine should be avoided because of its undesirable effect of causing spasm of the sphincter of Oddi.

Intravenous injections of calcium may be required if hypocalcaemia develops and blood sugar should be monitored regularly so that developing diabetes can be treated promptly.

There is no benefit from the administration of antibiotics in the acute phase; they are indicated if the necrotic pancreatic tissue becomes infected. Corticosteroids have no specific place in the treatment of acute pancreatitis and indeed may be a cause of it.

Prognosis depends upon the severity of the attack. Overall, the mortality is 10–20%. Patients with haemorrhagic pancreatitis have a mortality of over 50% whereas when there is only oedema of the pancreas, the mortality is less than 5%. Pancreatitis secondary to gallstones is unlikely to recur provided these are removed. Alcoholic pancreatitis will recur if alcohol consumption continues.

Chronic Pancreatitis

In the Western world the majority of cases of chronic pancreatitis occurs as a result of high alcohol consumption. It is possible that a small number result from cholelithiasis, but a causative relationship is difficult to establish because coincidental gallstones would be expected in a significant proportion of patients. It is rare for acute attacks of pancreatitis to proceed to chronic pancreatitis. In a few patients chronic pancreatitis may be caused by stenosis or disease of the sphincter of Oddi. In some parts of the tropics, chronic pancreatitis is common and malnutrition may be an aetiological factor.

On microscopy the pancreas shows fibrosis around the ducts and acinae which are gradually replaced. By contrast, there is preservation of the islets. The larger ducts are often irregular and dilated, and stones may be present in the lumen.

Clinical Features. The disease is most common in males between the ages of 35 and 45. Nearly all patients present with abdominal pain. Recurrent attacks occur at intervals of several weeks or months often within a few hours to two days of an alcoholic bout. In contrast to acute pancreatitis, the pain may begin gradually and persist for days or weeks. Pain is located in the epigastrium, right or left subcostal areas or around the umbilicus; characteristically it may radiate to the back between T10 and T12 and relief may be obtained by crouching forward or leaning forward over a chair.

Diabetes develops in about a fifth of patients and steatorrhoea in a third; occasionally one of these is the presenting feature. Both these complications are more likely when the pancreas is calcified. Jaundice may arise because of obstruction to the common bile duct and symptoms of duodenal obstruction due to the development of a pseudocyst. On examination there is often diffuse tenderness in the abdomen.

Investigation. In a small proportion of cases of chronic pancreatitis a plain radiograph of the abdomen shows calcification in the duct system or throughout the gland. Ultrasonography may show that the pancreas is abnormal. A barium meal or hypotonic duodenography may show deformity of the duodenal cap as a result of oedema, and flattening and rigidity of the medial wall of the duodenum. Pancreatic function tests (p. 305) may provide evidence of pancreatic insufficiency; the presence of steatorrhoea, or a diabetic glucose tolerance curve suggests that pancreatic insufficiency is severe. Estimation of serum amylase activity is of value only in an acute exacerbation.

Endoscopic retrograde pancreatography often

provides valuable evidence in favour of the diagnosis by showing stones and dilatation of the pancreatic ducts. This information is also helpful in planning surgical treatment.

Treatment. Pain is often severe and many patients require narcotics with the inevitable danger of addiction. When steatorrhoea is present, a diet containing over 2500 kcals per day is given, composed of carbohydrate and protein but only 40 g fat. Preparations of pancreatic extracts are given with and between meals to assist absorption; if they fail to bring about improvement, cimetidine or ranitidine given with meals will enhance their effect by preventing their inactivation by gastric acid. In diabetic patients, oral hypoglycaemic agents should be tried initially, but if these fail, insulin is usually required. It is imperative that the patient permanently abstains from drinking alcohol.

Surgery should be contemplated for the relief of intractable pain. Drainage of the pancreatic duct into the small bowel, removal of part or most of the pancreas, or sphincterotomy are the most usual procedures. The ultimate result is so dependent on the alcoholic's ability to stop drinking that operation is not worth while in the patient who cannot do so. The indication for surgery is stronger when cysts and the possibility of cancer of the pancreas are present. The best results are obtained in those patients who are shown to have stones in the bile ducts or stenosis of the ampulla of Vater. Correction of these abnormalities may relieve pain and result in recovery of pancreatic function.

Pancreatic Cysts

A pancreatic pseudocyst occurs as a complication of acute pancreatitis, chronic pancreatitis or trauma to the pancreas. A pseudocyst is a sac which contains fluid, pancreatic enzymes and blood. It usually occupies the lesser sac, displacing the stomach, and it may obstruct the duodenum. Most commonly the pseudocyst develops 3 to 4 weeks after the onset of acute pancreatitis. Epigastric pain, nausea and vomiting, weight loss, fever and jaundice are likely symptoms. On examination, a smooth, tender mass is felt in the upper abdomen in about half the cases.

There is a persistent leucocytosis and raised serum amylase activity. An abdominal radiograph shows a mass in the epigastrium and a barium meal or hypotonic duodenography confirms extrinsic pressure on the stomach, duodenum and small bowel. Ultrasonography will confirm the presence of a cyst in nearly all cases.

Pseudocysts which fail to resolve spontaneously within six weeks are treated surgically by drainage into the stomach or small intestine.

Intrapancreatic or retention cysts are usually small and multiple and are found in chronic pancreatitis. These cysts may cause abdominal pain but they are difficult to demonstrate except by retrograde pancreatography. Symptomatic cysts are treated surgically. Occasionally a cyst is secondary to carcinoma.

Cystic Fibrosis

This autosomal recessive disease is the major cause of pancreatic insufficiency and respiratory failure in childhood. Cystic fibrosis is characterised by generalised dysfunction of all exocrine glands, including those which secrete mucus. Blockage by viscid secretion causes cystic changes in the pancreas and also bronchiectasis.

Clinical Features. Frequently cystic fibrosis presents in infancy with repeated attacks of respiratory infection. Defective pancreatic enzymes give rise to impaired digestion and malabsorption of fat. The stools are bulky, foamy and foul-smelling. The child is often poorly nourished. Complications include intussusception and obstruction due to faecal masses.

Increasing numbers of patients are surviving to adulthood because of better treatment of respiratory infection. The respiratory problems become progressively more important in the adolescent and adult and determine the fate of the individual; by contrast malabsorption is less troublesome. There may be bronchiectasis, recurrent spontaneous pneumothorax, recurrent haemoptysis, pulmonary fibrosis and right ventricular failure. Sometimes there is cirrhosis leading to portal hypertension. Females with cystic fibrosis may become pregnant but males are nearly always infertile.

In the child, the diagnosis is established by the

finding of an increase in the concentration of sodium in the sweat (p. 819). The test is difficult to interpret after adolescence; the diagnosis is then made on the presence of chronic pulmonary disease, pancreatic insufficiency and a family history of cystic fibrosis.

Treatment. In the child, surgery may be required for a variety of complications. The replacement treatment for pancreatic insufficiency is very important to maintain adequate nutrition. The aims of treatment of respiratory disease are to control infection and to ensure adequate drainage of secretions by inhalation therapy, mucolytic agents, postural drainage and breathing exercises. In the adult these respiratory measures are of paramount importance.

Families with cystic fibrosis require long term support. Genetic advice should be made available to the parents (p. 17).

Carcinoma of the Pancreas

The incidence of carcinoma of the pancreas is increasing in many Western countries. It is more common in males than in females and it occurs most frequently between the ages of 55 and 70 years. Cigarette smoking and excessive coffee drinking may be aetiological factors. Most cancers are adenocarcinomas, commonly arising from the ducts but occasionally from the acinae; ductal carcinomas may be multicentric. Islet cell carcinoma (p. 310) and cystadenocarcinoma are rarer forms of cancer. Adenocarcinoma is of scirrhous nature and in two-thirds of cases it involves the head of the gland.

Clinical Features. Apart from carcinoma of the ampulla which may bleed into the duodenum, or cause jaundice at a relatively early stage, all cancers of the pancreas are advanced by the time they cause symptoms. Epigastric pain is common, but occasionally it may be absent throughout the course of the disease. The pain is variable in type but is characteristically dull and boring and radiates through to the back. It is often intensified by food and by lying supine, especially at night. It may be relieved by crouching forward. Vague dyspeptic symptoms are common and include anorexia, nausea, discomfort and sometimes vomiting. These symptoms may be the only manifestations until metastases occur.

Other clinical features depend largely on the site of the growth. In the majority of cases with involvement of the head of the pancreas, jaundice is the presenting feature and may be painless and progressive. A large firm liver eventually develops. An abdominal mass is present in one quarter of all patients and occasionally a distended gall bladder is palpable or ascites can be detected. Jaundice may not appear in cases where the lesion affects mainly the body and tail of the pancreas. The symptoms of diabetes mellitus or thrombophlebitis may occasionally be the presenting feature.

Carcinoma of the pancreas is a rapidly progressive emaciating disease especially in cases in which the head of the gland is involved, when death usually occurs within six months of the onset of obstructive jaundice.

Investigation. Pancreatic cancer may be suspected from the clinical features, a raised serum alkaline phosphatase and a diabetic glucose tolerance test. Diagnosis may be confirmed by ultrasonography or CT scanning; the latter is generally more accurate especially for lesions of the tail of the pancreas. A combination of angiography and ultrasonography or CT scanning may help to determine if resection is possible by demonstrating whether or not the portal vein is involved by tumour.

Barium meal or hypotonic duodenography usually provides supportive evidence when cancer is in the head of the pancreas. This may show distortion or displacement of the stomach or duodenum with possible invasion by tumour.

Duodenoscopy is important in detecting cancer of the ampulla; during this procedure, cannulation of the pancreatic duct may show stricture or obstruction of the duct and when jaundice is present, cannulation of the common bile duct may show the obstruction is within the pancreas. Occasionally malignant cells may be demonstrated in the pancreatic secretion (p. 305).

Treatment. Carcinoma of the ampulla can be treated by excision of the duodenum and head of the pancreas; the prognosis in such cases is better than for cancers elsewhere in the pancreas. Radical surgery is rarely possible for pancreatic cancer. Usually the aim is to relieve obstructive jaundice by implanting the common bile duct or gall bladder into the jejunum or to forestall duodenal obstruction by gastrojejunostomy. Less than 10% of patients with cancer of the pancreas survive for one year after diagnosis and only 2% survive for two years.

Islet-cell Tumours

A benign adenoma may arise rarely from the beta cells of the islets and produce hyperinsulinism with attacks of spontaneous hypoglycaemia (p. 473). Even more rare are tumours, usually malignant, from other islet cells which elaborate polypeptides, e.g. gastrin or allied substances, the secretion of which into the blood causes a variety of syndromes. The most common is the Zollinger-Ellison syndrome (p. 300).

DISEASES OF THE SMALL INTESTINE

MALABSORPTION

A number of disorders result in malabsorption of one or more of the essential nutrients, electrolytes, minerals or vitamins. Some or all of the following features may ensue: diarrhoea, abdominal pain and distension, loss of weight, anaemia, or other evidence of specific deficiency. However, some patients complain only of vague ill-health, and the diagnosis may not be made for many years.

The sequence followed in this section is first to review the basic processes of absorption and the means of testing them. Then the ways in which the processes of absorption can be deranged are discussed. Finally, the clinical presentation and treatment of malabsorption in general and then of specific disorders are described.

Tests of Absorption

Fat absorption takes place predominantly in the duodenum and upper jejunum. Dietary fat occurs largely in the form of insoluble long-chain triglycerides. These are emulsified mechanically in the stomach and by detergents (mainly bile acids) in the small intestine. Then pancreatic lipase hydrolyses the triglycerides to monoglyceride and fatty acids. Pancreatic bicarbonate is required to maintain the optimum pH for this hydrolysis and for the next step in fat absorption, the solubilisation of the monoglycerides and fatty acids by bile acids. This consists of their incorporation into micelles which orientate the fatty acid and monoglyceride in such a way that they can be presented to the intestinal mucosal cell for absorption (Fig. 10.2). Once in the absorptive cell, the monoglycerides and fatty acids are reformed (re-esterified) into triglycerides which are then coated with phospholipid and protein to form chylomicrons or converted into very low density lipoproteins. Both chylomicrons and very low density lipoproteins pass out of the cell to be transported by the lymphatic system into the blood (p. 336).

TEST OF FAT ABSORPTION. Fat excretion in the stool is measured over a 5-day period, whilst the patient is receiving a normal diet (which contains less than 100 g fat per day). The normal faecal fat excretion is less than 5 g per day (p. 819).

The fat-soluble vitamins A, D and K are absorbed in the same way as dietary fat and measurement of their absorption can be used as an indirect assessment of fat absorption. For example, the plasma vitamin A level can be measured after oral administration of retinol for two or three days.

Carbohydrate Absorption. Carbohydrate in the diet is in the form of starch (60%), lactose (10%) and sucrose (30%). These are digested to glucose, galactose and fructose. Glucose and galactose are absorbed into the cell by active transport mechanisms, the process requiring sodium ions and energy. The fructose molecule is too large to move across the cell membrane by simple diffusion and it is thought that it must be facilitated by a carrier.

TESTS OF CARBOHYDRATE ABSORPTION. *The glucose tolerance test* (p. 463) is sometimes used and the absence of a rise in blood sugar can indicate malabsorption, but there are so many variables that the test is difficult to interpret in the context of malabsorption.

In the *xylose absorption test*, 25 g of d-xylose are given orally after an overnight fast. Only a small proportion is metabolised within the body and

5–8 g should be excreted in the urine over the next 5 hours.

In the *lactose tolerance test*, 50 g of lactose are given orally and blood glucose levels are measured as in the glucose tolerance test. Normally this disaccharide is broken down by intestinal lactase to glucose and galactose which are absorbed so that blood glucose levels rise. If the enzyme lactase is deficient in the intestinal mucosa, there may be no rise in blood glucose and the patient may complain of colic and diarrhoea because the unabsorbed lactose acts as an osmotic agent in the gut.

Hydrogen Breath Test. This test is used to diagnose lactase deficiency. It has the advantage of not requiring blood samples and so is the preferred test in children. 50 g of lactose is given orally; lactose not absorbed in the small intestine passes into the colon where it is degraded by bacteria with the production of hydrogen. Hydrogen excretion in the breath is measured and this is proportional to the amount of lactose not absorbed by the small intestine.

Protein Absorption. Initial hydrolysis of dietary protein molecules is performed by gastric pepsin and pancreatic enzymes. Further hydrolysis of peptides takes place at the brush border and a mixture of peptides and amino acids is absorbed into the cell. A large amount of protein, other than dietary, enters the lumen of the gastrointestinal tract each day, derived from various secretions, desquamated cells and the exudation of plasma proteins. These are absorbed by the same mechanisms as dietary protein.

TESTS OF PROTEIN ABSORPTION. Measurement of the amount of nitrogen in the stool provides a very crude estimate of the above processes. Stools are collected for 3 to 5 days and no more than 2·5 g of nitrogen per day should be excreted.

An excessive loss of nitrogen in the stool can result from the loss of albumin and other plasma proteins into the lumen of the tract. This is termed *protein losing enteropathy* and it can be detected by labelling serum proteins with radioactive chromium and measuring radioactivity in the stool.

A low serum albumin level in the absence of hepatic or renal disease may indicate protein malabsorption or protein losing enteropathy.

Absorption of Other Substances. The Schilling test (p. 502) is used in investigating the absorption of vitamin B_{12}. The serum levels of folate, iron and calcium provide an index of the absorption of these substances.

Causes of Malabsorption

1. **Disorders of Intraluminal Digestion.** Here there is an insufficiency of a digestive enzyme or detergent within the lumen. The main feature is steatorrhea with deficiency of fat soluble vitamins. Since the intestinal mucosal cells are normal, there is no impairment of absorption of other substances less dependent on intraluminal digestion, e.g. carbohydrate, protein, vitamin B_{12}, folate and iron.

(a) DISTURBANCES OF GASTRIC FUNCTION. After gastric surgery it is possible for the correct enzymes, detergents and electrolytes to be delivered into the intestinal lumen and yet malabsorption may occur. This is because gastric emptying is no longer coordinated with the correct stage of digestion. For example, after gastroenterostomy or a Polya partial gastrectomy, bile and pancreatic juice may be delivered after food from the stomach has already passed down the efferent loop.

(b) PANCREATIC INSUFFICIENCY. A deficiency of pancreatic lipase causes malabsorption of fat, for example, in chronic pancreatitis, cystic fibrosis and carcinoma of the pancreas.

(c) DEFICIENCY OF BILE ACIDS. This may occur in two circumstances:

(i) *Interruption of the Enterohepatic Circulation of Bile Acids.* When there is disease, e.g. Crohn's, or resection of the terminal ileum, bile acids cannot be reabsorbed (p. 338) and are lost in the faeces. In the colon they prevent water and electrolyte absorption and stimulate their secretion; diarrhoea results. Synthesis by the liver cannot compensate for the loss of bile acids. There is therefore an inadequate concentration of bile acid in the upper jejunum and micelles cannot be formed.

(ii) *Colonisation of the Small Bowel by Bacteria.* The upper part of the small intestine is practically sterile under normal conditions. If a large number of bacteria are present (p. 314) bile acids are deconjugated, micelle formation becomes inefficient and steatorrhea results. Bacteria in the small intestine can also utilise vitamin B_{12} so that it is unavailable for absorption and anaemia ensues.

2. **Disorders of Transport in the Mucosal Cells.** In these disorders, the intraluminal digestive phase is normal, but the absorptive cells are not, because of:

(a) *Generalised mucosal damage* from coeliac disease, tropical sprue, giardiasis, Whipple's disease (p. 568) or extensive Crohn's disease. In these conditions, because the mucosa is damaged, it is usual to find widespread disturbances of absorption involving xylose, folate, vitamin B_{12}, iron, calcium and amino acids in addition to steatorrhoea.

(b) *Disorders with Histologically Normal Mucosa.* Here a specific substance is malabsorbed because of the absence of a particular enzyme. Thus there may be malabsorption of lactose because of an insufficiency of lactase in the mucosa. Another example is the malabsorption of vitamin B_{12} because of a lack of intrinsic factor in pernicious anaemia.

3. **Disorders of Transport from the Mucosal Cell.** These are rare and result from the blockage of the lymphatic system which is responsible for the transfer of chylomicrons from the absorptive cell to the systemic circulation. This may occur in abdominal lymphoma or tuberculosis or in the rare condition of primary lymphangiectasia involving the mesenteric lymphatic system.

Clinical Features and Investigation of Malabsorption

Clinical Features. The patient can present in various ways. In severe forms there may be general malnutrition, with loss of weight and energy and a slow deterioration in health or, in a child, a failure to grow and thrive. Abdominal distension is often a striking feature.

Steatorrhoea may be the presenting symptom. The patient complains of diarrhoea, with the passage of loose, pale, bulky and offensive stools which float on water. The patient may be anaemic due to a deficiency of iron, cyanocobalamin or of folate.

Haemorrhagic phenomena due to a deficiency

of vitamin K may be an occasional presenting feature. Hypocalcaemia may lead to tetany. The features of rickets or osteomalacia and various disorders due to deficiency of vitamins may be noted, such as sore tongue, angular stomatitis and dry, rough or cracked skin.

Hypoalbuminaemic oedema may occur. In other patients, malabsorption may be suspected because of gastric surgery or intestinal resection. In patients with mild malabsorption, there may be no diarrhoea and the condition may be diagnosed only after investigation for non-specific abdominal complaints or anaemia.

Investigation. The diagnosis may be suspected as a result of a barium follow-through examination in a patient with abdominal symptoms. The small intestine shows dilated loops with flocculation and segmentation of barium (Fig. 9.8).

Fig. 9.8 Malabsorption. Note dilated loops, segmentation and flocculation. (Courtesy of Dr. D.H. Cummack).

Malabsorption is confirmed by the tests of absorption which may also provide a clue as to the cause of the disorder. For example, malabsorption of several substances is likely when there is a generalised disorder of the absorptive cells.

Biopsy of the jejunum (p. 284) may show the villous atrophy of coeliac disease. Partial villous atrophy can occur in a variety of disorders, such as tropical sprue, Crohn's disease and in mild cases of coeliac disease. If the intestinal biopsy is normal, other investigations may be necessary to provide the diagnosis — for example, pancreatic function tests (p. 305) or the culture of intestinal aspirates for bacteria.

Treatment of Malabsorption

A gluten-free diet must be prescribed in coeliac disease. Pancreatic insufficiency is treated by pancreatic supplements (p. 308). Insufficiency of bile acids should not be treated with oral bile acids because these would pass into the colon, interfere with salt and water absorption, and so worsen the diarrhoea. The effect of the endogenous bile acids on the colon is counteracted by giving the binding agent cholestyramine in a dose of up to 12 g per day. In addition, a low fat diet should be given because cholestyramine will usually increase the faecal excretion of fat.

In severe forms of malabsorptive disease, it may be necessary to treat dehydration and electrolyte deficiency by intravenous infusions.

Replacement therapy is necessary for those patients with anaemia, bone disease or coagulation defects. Folic acid and iron supplements are given orally and vitamin B_{12} by a monthly injection. Vitamin D and calcium supplements may be required. Glossitis and cheilosis are indications for the administration of vitamin B complex.

THE PRINCIPAL DISORDERS CAUSING MALABSORPTION

These are coeliac disease, tropical sprue, lactose intolerance, bacterial colonisation of the small intestine and Crohn's disease.

Coeliac Disease

Coeliac disease is characterised by an abnormal mucosa in the small intestine, induced by a component of the gluten protein of wheat. Barley, rye and oats may also be injurious. It seems likely that local immunological responses to gluten are responsible.

Pathology. The mucosa of the normal small intestine has finger-like or leaf-like villi which can be seen with the dissecting microscope or on histological section. In coeliac disease the dissecting microscope appearance shows either (i) convolutions, like the surface of the cerebrum, which, when sectioned, appear as short wide villi, or (ii) a totally flat mucosa which is termed 'subtotal villous atrophy'. In addition, the height of the epithelial cells is reduced and there is an increase in the number of plasma cells in the lamina propria. All these histological features return towards normality during treatment with a gluten-free diet. In coeliac disease the mucosa at the duodeno-jejunal flexure is always abnormal and the abnormality extends distally for a variable distance.

Clinical features. Coeliac disease usually begins in the first 3 years of life. The child ceases to thrive and becomes fractious and irritable, the stools become voluminous and pale and, as the disorder progresses, growth is retarded, anaemia develops, and the abdomen becomes distended.

On the other hand, the disorder may manifest itself for the first time in adult life; the presenting symptoms range from those of a mild anaemia and listlessness of long duration, to a florid malabsorptive state developing rapidly over a period of weeks. The commonest features are diarrhoea, weight loss and anaemia, usually due to combined deficiency of folate and iron. There may be peripheral neuropathy and evidence of vitamin deficiency or hypoproteinaemia. Other features are finger clubbing, dermatitis herpetiformis, amenorrhoea and infertility.

Coeliac disease predisposes to the development of lymphoma of the small intestine; colicky abdominal pain and unexpected weight loss in a previously well-controlled patient should arouse suspicion.

Treatment. A gluten-free diet must be taken indefinitely. This requires the exclusion of wheat, rye, oats and barley, and imposes severe restrictions which must be fully explained to the patient. A booklet produced by the Coeliac Society (PO Box 181, London) containing diet sheet and recipes for gluten-free flour is of great value in this respect. Mineral and vitamin supplements are also given when indicated. If the patient deteriorates on a strictly supervised diet, corticosteroids may be tried; a diagnosis of lymphoma must also be considered.

Tropical Sprue (p. 719)

Lactose Intolerance

This disorder is being seen more often in Britain because Asian and African immigrants have insufficient lactase in the mucosa of the small intestine to digest the large amounts of lactose consumed in Britain. It may also be acquired, especially in children, as a temporary sequel to an infection of the bowel.

The patient complains of abdominal discomfort, colic and diarrhoea after the ingestion of milk or milk products. The diagnosis may be made by the lactose tolerance or hydrogen breath test (p. 311). The symptoms may be reproduced by the test and respond to the reduction of lactose in the diet.

Bacterial Colonisation of the Small Intestine

The effects of this proliferation have been discussed on page 311. The presentation is with steatorrhoea or anaemia due to vitamin B_{12} deficiency. Radiological investigation shows a lesion causing stasis in the intestine such as jejunal diverticula, a long afferent ('blind') loop after gastrectomy or gastroenterostomy, Crohn's disease, stricture formation or a fistula between colon and small intestine.

The Schilling test is abnormal (p. 502). The glycocholic acid breath test may be used for diagnosis; bacteria in the small intestine liberate ^{14}C glycine from the labelled glycocholic acid. The ^{14}C glycine is metabolised to $^{14}CO_2$ which is measured in the breath. The diagnosis is confirmed by the correction of steatorrhoea and vitamin B_{12} malabsorption by the administration of tetracycline.

Occasionally surgical correction of an abnormality may be required.

Crohn's Disease

This disease is characterised by localised areas of non-specific, granulomatous inflammation of the bowel. It was formerly termed regional ileitis or enteritis. However, the eponymous designation 'Crohn's disease' is preferable since the alimentary tract can be affected anywhere from the mouth to the anus, the sites most commonly involved being, in order of frequency, terminal ileum alone, terminal ileum and right side of colon, colon alone, ileum and jejunum. The term 'inflammatory bowel disease' comprises Crohn's disease and ulcerative colitis (p. 321).

Crohn's disease may occur at any age, but most commonly between the ages of 20 and 40; it affects both sexes equally. In its chronic form, it is a debilitating disease which often interferes profoundly with a patient's life requiring repeated admission to hospital for treatment.

Aetiology. The cause is unknown. No specific organism has been identified from the bowel content, the bowel wall or the regional lymph nodes. One of the histological characteristics of the disease is the presence of granulomas composed of collections of epithelioid and giant cells. These granulomas closely resemble those found both in tuberculosis and sarcoidosis. However caseation does not occur in Crohn's disease which is now accepted as being unrelated to either.

A current hypothesis is that Crohn's disease is the consequence of an abnormal immune response in the gut wall to an unidentified antigen. Crohn's disease, ankylosing spondylitis and ulcerative colitis all occur more commonly than might be expected amongst the families of patients with Crohn's disease, suggesting that all three diseases share a common but incomplete genetic basis.

Pathology. Although the disease may affect any part of the alimentary canal, the terminal ileum is most often involved. Macroscopically, the bowel is engorged and oedematous so that the lumen is markedly narrowed, sometimes enough to produce obstruction; the mucosa is oedematous, showing a 'cobble-stone' pattern with linear ulceration and fissuring. Characteristically, these changes are patchy; even when a relatively short segment of bowel is affected, it can be seen that the inflammatory process is interrupted by islands of normal mucosa occurring in the diseased area, the change from normal mucosa to the affected part being abrupt. The lesions may be discontinuous over a length of the bowel, a small lesion separated in this way from a major area of involvement being referred to as a 'skip' lesion. The affected lymph nodes are enlarged and the mesentery thickened.

Microscopically, inflammatory change involves all coats of the bowel wall. All grades of inflammation may be seen and characteristically there is oedema and hyperplasia of the lymphoid follicles. Granulomas are seen in about 50% of cases. Another feature is deep clefts or fissures opening on to the mucosal surface and sometimes passing through the entire thickness of the bowel wall. These clefts are responsible for the fistula formation which is such a characteristic feature of the disease. Fistulae may develop between adjacent loops of bowel or between affected segments of bowel and the bladder, uterus or vagina and may appear in the perineum.

Clinical features vary and depend in part on the site and extent of the bowel affected; many other diseases may be mimicked. Crohn's disease may present acutely with features indistinguishable from acute appendicitis. At laparotomy the terminal ileum is red and oedematous and provided the abdomen is closed without resection the prognosis is relatively good.

In the chronic form of the disease, pain is the commonest symptom and may be due either to peritoneal involvement, obstruction or both. Since the terminal ileum and right side of the colon are most commonly affected, this type of pain occurs most frequently in the right lower quadrant and it may be associated with local tenderness or guarding. A mass is palpable by abdominal and frequently by rectal examination. This consists of inflamed loops of bowel bound together, possibly including an abscess, and may be of any size. Colicky pain suggests obstruction, and may be associated with nausea and vomiting and excessive borborygmi. Indeed, recurrent episodes of colic due to attacks of subacute obstruction are a prominent feature in the life history of a patient with Crohn's disease; however, severe acute obstruction is uncommon.

Malabsorption occurs for a variety of reasons in Crohn's disease. The enterohepatic bile acid circulation may be interrupted by disease or resection of the ileum. Other areas of the small intestine may be involved, thus reducing the surface area for absorption. Strictures and fistula may lead to bacterial colonisation of the small intestine. The inflamed mucosa may cause a protein losing enteropathy.

Diarrhoea is frequent, but is rarely so marked as in ulcerative colitis. The stools may be formed or loose, and rarely contain frank blood, mucus or pus unless the colon is involved. In the latter case, the symptoms are indistinguishable from those of ulcerative colitis. A diagnostic feature, when present, is the occurrence of anal lesions such as oedematous skin tags or perianal abscesses and fistulas; they are more common when the colon is affected.

Weight loss is frequent and most patients have a low-grade fever and moderate anaemia. Clubbing of the fingers may be present. A number of other manifestations may occur, including enteropathic arthritis (p. 567), ankylosing spondylitis, iritis, aphthous stomatitis and erythema nodosum. Abnormal liver function tests are relatively common, while renal complications include hydronephrosis due to involvement of the right ureter in an inflammatory mass.

Investigation. Barium meal and follow-through examination may show alteration of the mucosal pattern, deep ulceration or the pathognomonic 'string sign' due to marked narrowing of a segment of affected bowel (Fig.9.9). In longstanding cases there may be stricture formation. The lesions tend to be discontinuous along the length of the bowel. A barium enema should be carried out since the disease may affect the small bowel and the colon simultaneously. In some patients there will be involvement of the colon segmentally or in its entirety. Crohn's disease of the colon can usually be differentiated from ulcerative colitis by the presence of shallow aphthoid or deep penetrating ulcers and discrete or eccentrically situated lesions.

Pus cells and red blood corpuscles may be found on microscopic examination of the faeces, but culture of the stool yields no specific organism. Moderate anaemia is usually present because

Fig. 9.9 Crohn's disease of the ileum with a fistula between the ileum and the bladder (arrow). (Courtesy of Dr. G.M. Fraser).

of blood loss, while protein loss from the inflamed, ulcerated mucosa may cause hypoproteinaemia. Vitamin B_{12} absorption is likely to be impaired if there is extensive disease of the terminal ileum, and this can be shown by an abnormal Schilling test (p. 502). The diagnosis may be confirmed either by rectal biopsy or by excision of perianal skin tags; a rectal biopsy will sometimes show the characteristic granulomatous lesions although the mucosa appears normal to the naked eye.

Sometimes no conclusive proof of Crohn's disease is obtained, and the diagnosis can only be presumptive; such patients should be kept under observation until the natural history of the illness declares itself.

Differential Diagnosis. The symptoms, signs and radiological findings are usually sufficient to suggest a lesion in the lower part of the small bowel. The other common diseases in this part of the intestinal tract are appendicitis or an appendix mass and carcinoma of the caecum. In the acute phase, it may be impossible to decide between these possibilities, so that a laparotomy may be necessary.

Ulcerative colitis is distinguished from Crohn's disease because it involves only the large bowel, whereas Crohn's disease may affect the alimentary tract from the mouth to the anus. The distinctive features of Crohn's disease are fistula and stricture formation, but when these are absent differentiation from ulcerative colitis may depend on demonstration of the extent and location of the disease and ultimately on biopsy. The possibility of carcinoma, either in association with or as a complication to Crohn's disease or ulcerative colitis, requires consideration.

Ileo-caecal tuberculosis may be indicated by the presence of tuberculosis elsewhere, for example, by the chest radiograph. A 'negative' tuberculin test is common in patients with Crohn's disease.

Caecal amoebiasis (p. 774) actinomycosis (p. 224) and lymphoma of the ileum or colon are rarer causes to be considered in the differential diagnosis.

Treatment. Crohn's disease is a chronic condition with remissions and relapses over many years. There is no known cure at present and treatment is largely a matter of managing particular problems as they arise and improving the general condition of the patient.

Dietary Measures. A low residue diet will reduce the frequency of intestinal colic.

Malabsorption with steatorrhoea may occur in patients with extensive involvement of the small intestine, contributing to weight loss and inanition. A low fat diet is then required and a course of oral antibiotics if bacterial colonisation of the upper intestine is suspected. Supplements of iron, folic acid, calcium, vitamins and electrolytes, especially potassium, may also be necessary. Hypoproteinaemia may require plasma or blood infusions in addition to a high protein diet.

An elemental diet is 'predigested' and absorbed high in the small intestine; it will relieve the symptoms of partial obstruction and restore nutrition. It is useful also in preoperative preparation, particularly for patients with external fistulas.

Drugs. Corticosteroids are beneficial when there is extensive active disease which is not improving with general medical measures. However they do not alter the long-term course of the disease. Prednisolone should be given in a dose of 40–60 mg daily in divided doses for 1 or 2 weeks depending on response, and the dose gradually reduced thereafter to 10–20 mg daily for 4 to 6 weeks and then withdrawn. Every effort should be made to stop the drug, but in the occasional case this may be difficult because of early relapse when the dose is reduced. In these circumstances, the effect of sulphasalazine (2–4 g daily) is worth a trial, much as it is used in ulcerative colitis (p. 325). Treatment with immunosuppressant drugs has been used with variable success in patients unresponsive to other forms of therapy.

Diarrhoea may be controlled with loperamide or codeine. When the terminal ileum is extensively diseased or has been resected, cholestyramine will reduce the diarrhoea due to the cathartic effect of the unabsorbed bile acids on the colon; hydroxocobalamin should be given to such patients for life since dietary vitamin B_{12} will not be absorbed.

Surgical Treatment. Although attacks of subacute obstruction can usually be managed conservatively by intestinal decompression and intravenous feeding (p. 285), operation may be necessary if attacks occur frequently. Surgery may also be required because of abscess or fistula formation. With localised disease, resection yields better results than bypass, but with extensive disease massive resection may result in malabsorption. Recurrence of the disease is always a danger, and therefore as much bowel as possible should be preserved. When the rectum and colon are extensively involved a total proctocolectomy as in ulcerative colitis may be the procedure of choice.

INTESTINAL OBSTRUCTION

Intestinal obstruction may be complete or incomplete, acute or chronic, intermittent or continuous. The most important point to decide is whether the obstruction is *simple* or associated with *strangulation*. The latter occurs when there is interference with the blood supply to the intestine, as when the bowel is trapped or twisted. Urgent relief is required if the dangers of gangrene, perforation and peritonitis are to be avoided.

Causes. Obstruction may be mechanical, when the lumen of the bowel is blocked, or paralytic, when there is inhibition of bowel motility. In general the former type will require surgical relief, while the latter may respond to conservative measures, but the distinction is not always clear cut. Sometimes the mechanically obstructed bowel becomes exhausted and non-contractile, or it perforates at the site of the obstruction or proximally, the resultant peritonitis being responsible for paralysis of the adjacent bowel loops.

Mechanical Obstruction. At all ages adhesions and hernias are common causes of obstruction. In childhood, intussusception is frequent, while in the elderly, volvulus, tumours of the large bowel and diverticular disease account for a large proportion of cases. Impaction of faeces in the rectum presents with spurious diarrhoea but can also cause intestinal obstruction in the aged or bedridden. In children in unhygienic surroundings a mass of round worms may be responsible (p. 791).

Paralytic obstruction (paralytic ileus) occurs temporarily after any abdominal operation and is a feature of shock, spinal injury and hypotension. Commonly it is due to peritonitis.

Clinical Features. *Pain.* In mechanical obstruction this is colicky and often originates at or about the site of the obstruction. Episodes of pain are accompanied by loud borborygmi. The advent of constant severe pain with tenderness is indicative of strangulation. Paralytic obstruction is associated with a dull constant pain in an abdomen which is ominously silent.

Vomiting. This is copious in high obstruction and may be late or absent in obstructions of the lower small bowel or large bowel. The effortless trickle of foul-smelling fluid from the corner of the mouth of the lethargic patient is seen in untreated paralytic ileus, whereas in mechanical obstruction vomiting is projectile and intermittent.

Distension. This may be absent or confined to some loops of the bowel which can be seen in the thin patient as ridges across the abdomen forming the so-called ladder pattern. Diffuse distension is late and may indicate chronic large bowel obstruction or paralytic ileus.

Bowel Movements. In complete obstruction neither faeces nor flatus is passed. In high obstructions, the bowels may move unaided or with enemas because of residual contents below the obstruction, while in large bowel obstruction, spurious diarrhoea may be due to a discharge of faecal-stained mucus.

Physical Examination. The diagnosis of obstruction and its cause can usually be made on physical examination alone. The hernial orifices should be palpated for the presence of a tender irreducible swelling. In fat patients particular care must be taken to check the femoral regions.

The presence of scars from previous abdominal operations is noted. Distension, particularly of individual loops, is significant. A distended caecum may be both seen and felt in thin patients and immediately points to a large bowel cause. Tenderness anywhere in the abdomen is suggestive of peritoneal irritation and bowel strangulation. A palpable mass is associated with large bowel tumours and diverticular disease. A transient mass, felt perhaps during bouts of colic, indicates intussusception. Classically bowel sounds are increased and tinkling in mechanical obstructions, but in advanced cases they are infrequent and auscultation must be prolonged to detect the occasional tinkle. In paralytic ileus, sounds are virtually absent.

Rectal examination usually reveals an empty ballooned rectum. In low obstructions there may be blood and mucus. Obstruction due to carcinoma of the rectum is rare.

In cases of doubt, and for confirmation of the diagnosis, serial measurements of abdominal girth will detect progressive abdominal distension.

Fluid and Electrolyte Changes. In obstruction of the upper small bowel, fluids and electrolytes are lost because of vomiting. When the obstruction is lower down, there is stagnation in the distended bowel loops, normal absorption from the gut is interrupted, and the body is deprived of fluid even in the absence of vomiting.

Biochemically, there is haemoconcentration with loss of water and electrolytes, particularly chloride, sodium and potassium. Elderly patients may develop secondary renal failure and this will add to the electrolyte imbalance. A vicious circle develops as increasing obstruction raises the tension in the bowel and further diminishes absorption; then increasing electrolyte imbalance interferes with intestinal peristalsis rendering the obstruction more complete. Recovery is heralded by diuresis, signifying return of peristalsis and reabsorption of fluid from the lumen of the bowel.

Radiological Examination. Plain radiographs, taken in the erect and supine positions, are most informative. The presence of fluid levels on the erect film, and of gas-distended loops on both films, indicate not only the diagnosis but also the site and probable cause of the obstruction (Fig. 9.10). Where the completeness of the obstruction is in doubt, serial films can be compared for any change in the gas patterns. If further localisation is necessary a small bowel barium follow through may be helpful.

Treatment. If intestinal obstruction is suspected, the opinion of a surgeon should be sought, even if non-operative measures are to be used.

The mainstays of treatment are decompression by gastrointestinal suction, the intravenous replacement of fluids and electrolytes, and operative relief of the obstruction. Urgent surgery is indicated for an irreducible hernia and where there is strangulation. In some countries, e.g. Uganda, volvulus of the sigmoid colon is a common cause of obstruction; it can be relieved by the passage of a rectal tube.

In cases of more gradual development where there is a possibility that the obstruction can be relieved even temporarily, and in paralytic ileus, conservative measures assume greatest importance. Passage of a nasogastric tube in an ill and nauseated patient requires skill and patience. Once in place, continuous suction with an electric pump, with periodic checks with a syringe to confirm that the tube is patent, will achieve upper intestinal decompression.

Intravenous infusion may require to be prolonged and biochemical estimations may be frequent, so that the veins should be treated with care. Where there has been blood loss, as in carcinoma of the bowel and diverticular disease, blood transfusion is required. Throughout conservative management, accurate fluid balance charts must be kept.

Fig. 9.10 Small bowel obstruction. Supine film on left showing dilated loops of small bowel. Erect film on right showing multiple fluid levels. (Courtesy of Dr. G.M. Fraser).

PERITONITIS

Peritonitis is the reaction of the peritoneum to an irritant. Usually this is infection, although sometimes the irritation is chemical, at least initially, as when bile or duodenal contents leak into the peritoneal cavity. Appendicitis is one of the commonest causes of peritonitis and *Esch. coli* is the organism usually responsible.

Infection or chemical irritation causes the peritoneum to become congested and oedematous. There is an exudation of fluid containing large quantities of leucocytes, protein and antibodies. Dilution and destruction of the irritant is accompanied by its localisation and by the formation of adhesions. Failure of these defence mechanisms is characterised by spread of the infection and by septicaemia and toxaemia. There is still a distressingly high mortality from generalised peritonitis.

Acute Peritonitis. In perforations, the onset is sudden, with severe abdominal pain, tenderness, rigidity and shock. The patient lies immobile, the respirations are short and grunting and the abdomen is retracted and motionless. These initial severe features then gradually decrease; the patient passes into a stage where he or she appears to have improved, and the diagnosis can be missed. Then, as paralytic ileus develops and fluid collects in the peritoneal cavity, there is increasing distension, the rigidity lessens, the tenderness remains and toxicity develops.

When peritonitis is secondary to inflammation of a viscus, such as appendicitis, the initial signs are those of the underlying disease, later to be replaced by the features of peritonitis. In advanced cases, only the history of onset remains to point to the probable cause.

Established peritonitis is treated by removal of the contaminating source when it is due to such conditions as appendicitis or perforation of the bowel or gall bladder. Anaerobic infection is controlled with metronidazole. Peritoneal toilet and lavage, intravenous replacement of fluids and electrolytes, and the treatment of the concomitant ileus by nasogastric suction are also required.

While the treatment of peritonitis is that of the cause, the ideal is its prevention. Thus acute appendicitis should be diagnosed before perforation and perforated peptic ulcer should be operated upon before the stage of chemical peritonitis is past.

General peritonitis may resolve completely, but often it localises to form an abscess at the primary site, in the subphrenic region or in the pelvis. Persistence of fever, or continued elevation of pulse rate, white blood count and ESR, should lead to efforts to locate such residual infections, for example by ultrasonography.

Pelvic abscess usually results from localisation of a general peritonitis and forms in the lowest part of the peritoneal cavity, in front of the rectum. The abscess may irritate the bladder causing frequency of micturition or involve the bowel causing diarrhoea with the passage of mucus and a feeling of incomplete emptying. It is evident on rectal or vaginal examination as a tender mass, which may discharge rectally or vaginally. Treatment with metronidazole is usually effective.

Subphrenic Abscess. Localisation of pus between diaphragm and liver on the right side or between the diaphragm and the liver, spleen and stomach on the left, is a complication of peritonitis most commonly due to perforation of the stomach, duodenum or gall bladder or to operation on these organs.

There are signs of persistent infection; there may be dullness at the base of the lung and tenderness and slight oedema over the lower ribs posteriorly. Diagnosis is aided by ultrasonography or a radiograph of the diaphragmatic region which may show elevation of the diaphragm, a fluid level below it or an effusion above it. Treatment is by drainage either at laparotomy or by insertion of a drain under ultrasound control.

Tuberculous peritonitis, although now rare in Britain, is still relatively common elsewhere, notably in tropical countries. It is secondary to a tuberculous focus in the abdomen, usually in a mesenteric lymph node and it is characterised by wasting, malaise and abdominal distension. Masses caused by matted omentum and loops of bowel may be palpable. The abdomen contains fluid rich in protein from which tubercle bacilli may be cultured. Diagnosis may also be made by biopsy of granulomas seen at laparotomy or laparoscopy.

In the adult, the condition may be confused with advanced malignant disease and an unnecessarily hopeless prognosis given. The response to antituberculous chemotherapy (p. 236) is good and often dramatic.

ACUTE APPENDICITIS

Acute appendicitis is more common in young people. Its rapid increase since the turn of the century is presumed to be connected with a change in diet and the adoption of a more sedentary existence. Acute appendicitis is usually obstructive, the lumen of the appendix being narrowed by swelling of lymphoid tissue in its wall, or by stricture from previous inflammation. Obstruction is made complete by impaction of a retained faecolith leading to gangrene, perforation and a local abscess or generalised peritonitis. In other cases an oedematous inflammatory appendix mass may ensue.

Clinical Features. The classical history is of the sudden onset of vague central abdominal pain followed in a few hours by shift of the pain to the right iliac fossa, where it becomes localised to McBurney's point, situated one-third of the distance along a line from the anterior superior iliac spine to the umbilicus. There is nausea and malaise. The breath is foul. There may be vomiting, but this is seldom severe and is often absent. The pulse rate is increased. In the early stages there is little elevation of temperature, so that rigors and a high fever make the diagnosis of appendicitis unlikely.

Locally there is tenderness and guarding in the right iliac fossa, progressing to rigidity as peritonitis develops. Rectal examination may disclose tenderness to the right.

The 'classical' history and findings account for less than 50% of cases. Because of variations in its anatomical position the inflamed appendix may simulate other diseases of the abdomen. The patient may present with diarrhoea or with urinary or gynaecological symptoms; acute cholecystitis or perforated peptic ulcer may also be mimicked.

In children and adolescents *non-specific mesenteric lymphadenitis* may resemble appendicitis. This condition is probably due to a virus. It is characterised by vague abdominal pain, slight fever and a doughy sensation on palpation. There is ill-defined tenderness in the right iliac fossa. The distinction from appendicitis may be difficult and if in doubt it is safer to operate; otherwise treatment is conservative, recovery taking place gradually over a few weeks.

In adults appendicitis may simulate other causes of a mass in the right iliac fossa (p. 316).

Treatment. The diseased appendix should be removed as early in the acute stage as possible. Attempts to temporise in the belief that mild forms of appendicitis can be distinguished from severe are dangerous, because the condition is notoriously deceptive. Even in the absence of obvious peritonitis, the acute case should have intraoperative antibiotic cover with rectal metronidazole and where there is obvious peritonitis systemic administration of ampicillin and metronidazole should be instituted.

A conservative policy is allowable only when a clearly defined appendix mass is present, without generalised abdominal signs. Once the mass has subsided, probably within 2 to 3 weeks, the appendix should be removed. Not all patients presenting with an appendix mass require antibiotics. Some need no more than rest, restriction of diet and the avoidance of purgatives. Others in whom there is more marked local tenderness, with low grade fever and malaise, benefit from ampicillin and metronidazole.

TUMOURS OF THE SMALL INTESTINE

Tumours of the small intestine are rare, although there is some evidence that lymphoma is more likely to develop in patients who have coeliac disease. Simple tumours such as polyps and leiomyomas may cause chronic anaemia or intussusception or may be found unexpectedly in the course of radiological investigation or laparotomy.

Carcinoid tumours arise from argentaffin cells. They are usually found in the appendix at appendicectomy and the prognosis is then excellent. When the primary is in the ileum, or elsewhere, for example in a bronchus, spread to the liver is common where metastases produce 5-hydroxytryptamine (serotonin) causing flushing, borborygmi, diarrhoea and, occasionally, fibrosis of the tricuspid or pulmonary valve. The diagnosis is made on the clinical features and confirmed by finding an excessive amount of 5-hydroxyindoleacetic acid in the urine.

Although long-term survival is possible, even with the systemic manifestations, the primary tumour and associated lymphatic and visceral metastases should be removed whenever possible with the aim of reducing the total volume of secreting tumour. Hepatic lobectomy can be considered when spread appears localised to one lobe.

DISEASES OF THE LARGE INTESTINE

The main functions of the large bowel are the removal of water from the intestinal contents, the storage of faeces and their evacuation at controlled intervals. Continence depends on training, on the function of a sphincter mechanism in the anal canal and on rectal sensation whereby the need to defaecate is appreciated.

The anal canal is sensitive to pain and touch, as is well demonstrated by the severe pain caused by fissures and inflamed piles. The rectum is insensitive to painful stimuli, so that the injection of a sclerosing agent for the treatment of haemorrhoids is painless. Rectal 'sensation' applies to an ability to appreciate distension and contraction.

In addition to clinical examination, including digital examination of the rectum, endoscopy (p. 283), stool examination (p. 284) and radiological investigation (p. 281) are all important aids to diagnosis.

Ulcerative Colitis

Apart from the bacillary and amoebic dysenteries and tuberculous enterocolitis, there are certain non-specific chronic inflammatory bowel diseases which are associated with ulceration of the colon.

One of these is Crohn's disease which may affect both the large and the small bowel; the other, commoner disease affecting the colon, is ulcerative colitis.

Aetiology. The aetiology of ulcerative colitis is not known. The disease may be due to an abnormal immune response, possibly to bacteria or to certain foods. In a few patients withdrawal of milk from the diet may improve the diarrhoea, suggesting perhaps that the condition is due to specific allergy to milk protein. However it seems much more likely that the improvement observed on milk withdrawal is due to a reduction in osmotic diarrhoea in patients who have developed secondary alactasia (p. 314).

A familial tendency is suggested by the increased incidence of the disease amongst relatives of patients and by the association between ulcerative colitis, ankylosing spondylitis and Crohn's disease (p. 314).

Some authorities believe that psychological disturbances are responsible and claim that patients with colitis have a particular personality structure characterised by traits such as undue dependence on others, extreme sensitivity to personal slight and obsessive tendencies. It seems probable, however, that these traits are largely due to the disease process itself, since they disappear or greatly improve during a remission; indeed, one of the most rewarding effects of successful treatment is the remarkable improvement that may occur in the psychological well-being of the patient. Moreover, similar psychological features occur in patients with severe long-standing diarrhoea due to specific causes such as dysentery; nevertheless the patient and the physician may relate the attack or exacerbation to a recent stressful event.

Pathology. The inflammatory process may be limited to the rectum, which is almost always involved (*proctitis*). The disease may also involve the distal colon (*distal colitis*) or the entire colon (*total colitis*). Whatever the extent of the disease, the inflammatory change is continuous throughout the affected part, in contrast to the patchy changes that occur in Crohn's disease of the colon.

In the early stages the mucosa is swollen and reddened, and punctate bleeding points may be seen. Thereafter, ulceration develops; the ulcers may be superficial or penetrate deeply, spreading longitudinally beneath the mucosa. In severe disease the mucosa may slough in parts to expose granulation tissue; the mucosa that remains becomes oedematous, hyperplastic and raised, giving the appearance of pseudo-polyposis. In *acute fulminant disease* the bowel, especially the transverse colon, may be greatly dilated (*toxic dilatation*) and the bowel wall becomes thin and may rupture. In long-standing disease, the colon is shortened and generally narrowed with a lack of haustrations.

Microscopically, in contrast to Crohn's disease, inflammation is confined to the mucosa. Initially there is congestion, oedema and intra-mucosal haemorrhage. The number of goblet cells is reduced and the lamina propria is infiltrated with lymphocytes and polymorphs; the latter also accumulate in the lumen of the crypts and are termed 'crypt abscesses'. These may progress to destruction of the mucosa which is replaced by granulation tissue. Finally, on healing, the mucosa has a reduced number of crypts.

Clinical Features. The disease occurs at all ages but most commonly between 20 and 40 years. The first attack is often the most severe and thereafter the disease is characterised by exacerbations and remissions although a minority of patients develop chronic symptoms. The clinical features and the management are largely determined by the extent to which the colon is involved, the severity of the inflammation and the duration of the disease.

The principal symptom is diarrhoea with loose bloody stools containing mucus and pus; defaecation is often accompanied by lower abdominal discomfort, although severe pain is uncommon. Tenesmus may occur because of proctitis. Tenderness may be present on palpation of the colon, especially in the left iliac fossa; when peritoneal irritation is present, it signifies that the serosa is involved in the inflammatory process.

In severe ulcerative colitis, there is exhausting diarrhoea and dehydration. *Toxic dilatation* represents the most serious form with tachycardia, a high swinging temperature and abdominal distension. Untreated, the patient dies as a result of colonic perforation.

In chronic ulcerative colitis the bowel is

permanently damaged as a result of fibrosis. The colon in such cases behaves as a rigid tube incapable of absorbing fluid properly or of acting as a faecal reservoir. There is no toxaemia, but the patient lives in chronic ill-health and with persistent diarrhoea.

When the disease is confined to the rectum, the symptoms may be trivial if the inflammation is mild and consist of loose motions and perhaps blood-streaking of the stool. However, a severe proctitis will cause tenesmus, and frequent small loose stools, together with bleeding per rectum, but systemic disturbance is absent. Paradoxically, in distal colitis, spasm may result in constipation, with retention of faeces in the proximal colon and small hard stools.

Relapse is often associated with emotional stress, intercurrent infection or the use of antibiotics. There is no special risk during pregnancy, when indeed it is usual for the disease to remit; in contrast there is a tendency for a severe relapse to occur early in the puerperium.

The patient is often anaemic and there may be leucocytosis and a raised ESR. In severe cases there are electrolyte disturbances and protein loss from the colon may lead to hypoalbuminaemia. Sometimes the liver function tests are abnormal. The stool should be cultured for pathogenic bacteria and a search of the mucus made for amoebae to exclude an infective cause for the colitis. Blood cultures are required if septicaemia is suspected.

Investigation. *Sigmoidoscopy* is essential in most cases; the mucosa appears engorged and hyperaemic and the normal vascular pattern is obliterated. In severe disease spontaneous bleeding will be seen; in less severe cases the mucosa appears intact, and bleeds only when it is gently rubbed, while in mild cases the only abnormality may be the absence of the normal vascular pattern. Rectal biopsy may be carried out to confirm the diagnosis and to exclude other causes of proctitis, such as Crohn's disease.

Radiological Examination. While sigmoidoscopy confirms the diagnosis of ulcerative colitis, a double contrast barium enema will demonstrate the severity and extent of the disease. The earliest radiological change is a granular appearance of the colonic mucosa. In more severe cases ulcera-

tion (Fig. 9.11) and pseudopolypi will be seen. In longstanding disease there may be shortening of the colon with narrowing of the lumen. Barium enema examination should not be performed in acute cases and where toxic dilatation is suspected because of the risk of perforation. In these, plain radiographs of the abdomen may allow a positive diagnosis to be made, since the colon will usually contain sufficient air to outline an abnormal mucosal pattern.

Fig. 9.11 Severe ulcerative colitis with deep ulcers and pseudopolyps affecting mainly the sigmoid colon. (Courtesy of Dr. G.M. Fraser).

Complications. *Toxic dilatation* and *perforation* have already been mentioned. *Stricture* may occur at any level in the colon or rectum; on the barium enema it is usually smooth, but is sometimes difficult to distinguish from carcinoma. *Carcinoma of the colon* develops more often in patients with long-standing ulcerative colitis than it does in the normal population, the risk being related to the duration, extent and age at onset of the disease. The risk increases greatly after the disease has been present for 10 years or more. It is greatest in patients with total colitis who develop the disease under the age of 20 years; in this group the risk of cancer of the colon is about 40 times greater than it is in a comparable normal population.

Extra-intestinal complications include enteropathic arthritis (p. 567), aphthous stomatitis, iritis and skin lesions such as erythema nodosum and, rarely but characteristically, pyoderma gangrenosum. Cholangitis and septicaemia may also occur. These complications are most common in advanced cases.

Differential Diagnosis. Ulcerative colitis has to be distinguished from other causes of inflammation of the colonic mucosa namely Crohn's disease (p. 314), amoebic colitis (p. 774), bacillary dysentery (p. 755), campylobacter infections (p. 753), and pseudomembranous colitis (p. 46). Colitis can also occur as a result of ischaemia (p. 330) and radiation therapy. Gonorrhoea is frequently overlooked as a cause of proctitis.

Treatment. Admission to hospital is required for patients with severe bowel symptoms, especially when there are general disturbances such as weight loss, anaemia, fever or tachycardia. Such patients may require intense supportive treatment until the disease remits or as a preparation for surgery. Parenteral nutrition through a central venous line allows correction of these deficiencies in the severely wasted patient and will do much to hasten recovery after operation. The measures should include correction of dehydration and electrolyte deficiencies, especially hypokalaemia, blood and plasma infusions to correct anaemia and hypoproteinaemia, and a high protein, low residue diet. Blood cultures should always be taken initially and be repeated throughout the course of the illness if fever persists. Gram-negative bacteria are the commonest organisms involved; if septicaemia is suspected parenteral administration of broad spectrum antibiotics is necessary. However, antibiotics have no special place in the primary management of ulcerative colitis; indeed a broad spectrum antibiotic may precipitate a relapse. Candidiasis of the mouth and upper pharynx is common, especially in ill patients on corticosteroids and must be treated (p. 286).

There is no satisfactory drug for controlling diarrhoea. Codeine phosphate or loperamide may be helpful but these drugs should be avoided in severely ill patients because they may precipitate an attack of toxic dilatation of the colon.

ANTI-INFLAMMATORY DRUGS. 1. *Corticosteroids.* Although there is no specific treatment for ulcerative colitis, the introduction of corticosteroids and corticotrophin has greatly improved the outlook.

(*a*) Local Treatment. When the disease is confined to the distal colon or the rectum, symptoms may be limited to moderate diarrhoea (three or four stools per day) with the passage of blood from time to time, while general health is maintained. Such patients may be treated by administration of corticosteroids as suppositories when there is local rectal involvement, or as self-administered enemas if the distal colon is involved. The preparations commonly used are prednisolone-21-phosphate or betamethasone, and both are available in disposable enema form. The patient is taught to administer the enema, twice daily, retaining the material for as long as possible; suppositories may be inserted twice or three times daily for the treatment of proctitis. Either form of treatment may be continued for several weeks, the duration being judged by the sigmoidoscopic appearances.

(*b*) Systemic Treatment. Prednisolone is given in doses of between 40–60 mg daily by mouth for 3 to 6 weeks depending on response. The usual contraindications to the use of these drugs must be observed (p. 453) and supplements of potassium salts should be given (p. 93). Used in this way, corticosteroids will induce remission in the majority of patients, the dose being reduced at weekly intervals as improvement takes place. Corticosteroids give rise to a sense of well-being and in addition improve appetite, so that the problem of persuading the patient to eat sufficient food is often solved; they are more effective in a first attack of ulcerative colitis, whereas corticotrophin may be more beneficial in the treatment of relapse. A long-acting form of corticotrophin (e.g. tetracosactrin zinc phosphate complex) should be used, and given in doses of the order of 1 mg daily by intramuscular or subcutaneous injection. This dosage is continued for a week after symptoms have remitted and it is then reduced at weekly intervals as in the case of corticosteroids. For convenience prednisolone may be substituted once the patient has responded adequately.

2. *Sulphasalazine* is split by bacteria in the colon into sulphapyridine and 5-aminosalicylic acid. The latter is probably the component responsible for reducing the chance of relapse of ulcerative colitis when corticosteroids have controlled the disease. It can also be used for mild or moderate attacks of colitis but is less effective than corticosteroids. The dose is 0·5–1 g q.i.d. with food for 1 to 2 years. Sulphasalazine can cause nausea, rashes, reversible sterility and occasionally blood dyscrasias, probably due to the sulphapyridine component.

3. *Other drugs.* Azathioprine (2·5 mg/kg) may be helpful in patients with chronic disease for whom surgery is inappropriate. Serious side effects may occur including suppression of the bone marrow with pancytopenia, so that patients must be carefully supervised.

Sodium cromoglycate given as a suppository or rectal enema is occasionally helpful in the management of proctitis or distal colitis; the drug may act on immunological mechanisms causing inflammation in the colon. There are no side effects.

SURGICAL TREATMENT. If the appropriate medical measures are carried out assiduously, the majority of patients with proctitis or moderately severe colitis will pass into remission. In severe forms of ulcerative colitis, where there is toxic dilatation of the colon or perforation and in the occasional patient with severe haemorrhage, emergency surgical treatment is required. In these urgent circumstances surgery is usually restricted to colectomy with ileostomy, the rectum and distal colon being removed at a later stage when the crisis is over.

Acute ulcerative colitis which fails to respond to medical treatment, or which relapses in spite of adequate treatment, is an indication for proctocolectomy. This is also indicated in chronic forms, where the disease burns out but leaves a permanently damaged bowel, perhaps with stricture formation. Long-standing disease, particularly when the onset has been in childhood, carries a risk of carcinoma and accordingly total bowel involvement, with activity extending over more than 10 years, should lead to serious consideration of surgery.

At all stages of the disease, the timing of and preparation for surgery are important and require a joint medical and surgical approach. In emergency situations, intensive pre-operative replacement of blood, fluid and electrolytes is needed and operation is performed as soon as the patient is fit to withstand surgery. In less urgent situations, the timing of surgery depends on the degree of improvement in the patient's general condition to be expected from preoperative medical measures. Shrewd judgement is required to choose the optimum time before the patient's condition deteriorates again.

Whenever possible, in addition to a full explanation of ileostomy and its management with a demonstration of the actual appliance to be used, the patient should have the opportunity before operation of meeting someone with an established ileostomy. Modern surgical techniques and the range of ileostomy appliances available make for easy management of the stoma and allow the patient to live an almost normal life with little restriction of physical activity. To be kept in touch with advances in techniques of ileostomy care, patients should join an ileostomy association or be enrolled in a stoma therapy clinic.

When the rectum is not grossly involved it may be preserved and ileo-rectal anastomosis performed. In selected cases ileo-anal anastomosis with formation of an ileal reservoir can be used. The risk of interference with sexual function is thus reduced and the need for a stoma avoided.

Prognosis. It is extremely difficult to give a prognosis in ulcerative colitis. The extent of involvement of the colon is an important consideration, the outlook being very much better, for example, if only the rectum is involved. The immediate death rate in patients with fulminating disease, however treated, is not less than 40%, and it is high also in patients developing an attack over the age of 60. In general, the overall mortality from ulcerative colitis is of the order of 10%, but this figure can be very greatly reduced when the patient is treated by those with special experience of the disease. Thus, the mortality from total proctocolectomy done during a remission by an experienced surgeon is about 2%, whereas mortality for proctocolectomy done as an emergency procedure is 10% in the best hands, and may be 20% or 30% in those with little experience of the disease. Attention has been drawn to the risk of carcinoma in long standing cases. Such patients should be kept under surveillance and preferably have periodic colonoscopic examinations to detect malignant changes.

Diverticular Disease

Though diverticula occur throughout the gastrointestinal tract, they are most common in the large bowel in middle-aged or elderly subjects. The presence of diverticula is known as *diverticulosis*; when they are inflamed the condition is known as *diverticulitis*. Such inflammation occurs almost exclusively in colonic diverticula. Because it is often difficult to separate the two conditions on clinical or radiological evidence, they are grouped together under the term '*diverticular disease*'.

Aetiology. In diverticulosis the muscular coat of the bowel is often greatly thickened, suggesting that the diverticula have formed as a result of increased intracolonic pressure. Manometric measurements support this view. It can be shown that pressure in the bowel is high and that there is an area of spasm or failure to relax at the pelvirectal junction. Epidemiological evidence suggests that dietary factors may be at least partly responsible. Diverticulosis is rare in areas of the world such as Africa and Asia where the usual diet is one of high residue; by contrast the incidence is increasing in Western countries where natural fibre (p. 80) is removed from the diet in the processes of food refining. Moreover there is evidence that intracolonic pressures vary with the bulk of the faecal residue, a high faecal residue being associated with a low intraluminal pressure and vice versa.

Diverticulosis occurs especially in middle-aged or elderly subjects and affects males and females equally.

Pathology. The pelvic colon is most commonly involved. Its muscle wall is thickened but the diverticula themselves are pouchings of the mucosa and have no muscle coat. It is not clear how they become inflamed. Radiological examination frequently shows the presence of a faecolith in a diverticulum, and it may be that faeces collect because of the inability of the diverticulum to contract. Faecal retention may then cause a local inflammatory reaction which may resolve spontaneously or progress to cause perforation, local abscess formation, fistula and peritonitis. When there are repeated attacks of diverticulitis, the bowel wall becomes progressively thickened with narrowing of the lumen leading eventually to obstruction.

Clinical Features. Pain or discomfort felt in the left iliac fossa is a common complaint and there may be associated local tenderness. Acute diverticulitis can give rise to severe pain, guarding and rigidity on the left side, the signs of peritonitis and obstruction being combined. Change of bowel habit, either of increasing constipation or constipation alternating with diarrhoea, is frequent. This is the most important symptom of distal colonic disease and can occur with any lesion. Before middle age, bowel habits are firmly established and a definite alteration usually betokens organic disease in the colon such as carcinoma or diverticulitis and always calls for investigation. Another presenting feature may be severe rectal bleeding.

In the chronic forms, there may be symptoms of subacute obstruction with increasing abdominal distension, borborygmi and colicky pain. Spread of inflammation to the bladder may cause urinary frequency and dysuria. Occasionally a fistula to the bladder gives rise to pneumaturia and faecal contamination of the urine.

On examination, the thickened tender colon may be palpable in the left iliac fossa. A mass may be present in those patients who have developed diverticulitis, with or without abscess.

Investigation. *Sigmoidoscopy* is necessary to exclude cancer of the rectum or pelvi-rectal junction. The principal indication for *colonoscopy* is to exclude colonic carcinoma, when the radiological appearances leave room for doubt. Colonoscopic examination may be difficult because of narrowing and rigidity of the bowel, but when the suspected abnormality can be seen and a biopsy carried out, a correct diagnosis is possible. Both diverticular disease and cancer may coexist or one may mimic the other to the extent that even at operation the true diagnosis is uncertain.

Radiological Examination. In diverticulosis, barium enema shows characteristic sacs along the contour of the gut (Fig. 9.12). After evacuation barium is frequently left behind in the diverticula which are clearly outlined. If diverticulitis is present, there will be narrowing, rigidity and lack of normal haustration of a segment of colon. Whether or not there are diverticula present, the main diagnostic difficulty is to distinguish the appearances from those of carcinoma and radiological differentiation may be impossible.

Fig. 9.12 Diverticular disease of the sigmoid colon. (Courtesy of Dr. G.M. Fraser).

Treatment. Asymptomatic diverticulosis is common, is often found accidentally and requires no treatment. A high fibre diet with vegetables, fruit, or bran is usually sufficient to relieve constipation. If not, a bulk laxative such as methylcellulose should be used in addition. Purgatives should be avoided.

During an attack of acute diverticulitis, bed rest, metronidazole or ampicillin, fluids intravenously and orally, or even cessation of feeding and nasogastric suction may be required. Most severe attacks subside spontaneously but a few require emergency surgery which will probably be confined to a temporary defunctioning proximal colostomy, to be followed later by local resection. An emergency partial colectomy may be required for acute bleeding.

Elective surgery is indicated, after recovery from an acute attack, in patients who develop obstructive features, who have complications such as fistula and in those in whom the possibility of carcinoma cannot be excluded. The treatment of choice is resection of the involved segment of pelvic colon with primary anastomosis.

A few patients fail to respond adequately to medical treatment and in some of these, resection of the most severely affected area of colon with end to end anastomosis is indicated.

Haemorrhage from the Lower Gastrointestinal Tract

The commonest source is haemorrhoids. Bleeding per rectum may also originate in the rectum itself, in the colon or terminal ileum. With bleeding from the proximal colon or ileum, the blood may appear as melaena. The usual causes are diverticular disease, cancer of the rectum or distal half of the colon and angiodysplasia in the mucosa of the bowel wall. Less common sources of bleeding are polyps, ulcerative colitis and ischaemic colitis.

Rectal examination and sigmoidoscopy will detect most rectal causes of bleeding.

If bleeding is proximal to the rectum, the patient is treated conservatively, as for upper gastrointestinal haemorrhage, and in most cases bleeding will stop. Thereafter barium enema and colonoscopy will detect most lesions. If bleeding continues, angiography of the superior and inferior mesenteric arteries can be performed to detect the site of bleeding and possibly treat it by embolisation through the arterial catheter. If bleeding fails to stop, the appropriate segment of the colon can be resected.

Carcinoma of the Colon and Rectum

In Britain, carcinoma of the large intestine is the most common malignant tumour of the alimentary tract. In contrast it is rare in Africa and Asia. The variation in incidence of the disease between different countries has led to speculation that dietary factors and differences in bacterial flora of the bowel may be of aetiological significance. Diseases known to be clearly associated with colonic carcinoma are long-standing ulcerative colitis and familial polyposis of the colon.

Pathology. In two-thirds of patients, cancer of the large bowel occurs in the left colon or rectum. Concomitant multiple tumours are present in 2% of cases. The risk of a second cancer may reach 10% in patients with adenomatous polyps. Macroscopically the tumour may be proliferative and fungating, ulcerative and infiltrating, polypoidal or encircling as a 'string' stricture. Perforation may occur at the site of the tumour, leading to peritonitis, localised abscess or a fistula.

Spread occurs directly in and through the bowel wall, by lymphatics and by the bloodstream through both portal and systemic circulations. Colonic carcinoma is capable of direct implantation on exposed surfaces, such as a suture line or area of trauma in the bowel. Metastases most commonly involve the liver.

Clinical Features. Symptoms vary depending on the site of the carcinoma. In tumours of the left colon, obstruction is early. Tumours of the right colon present with anaemia, cachexia and alteration of bowel habit, but obstruction is late because of the relatively fluid nature of the bowel contents. As a consequence left-sided tumours tend to be diagnosed earlier.

Change in bowel habit, anaemia, weight loss and sometimes excessive borborygmi, abdominal distension and colicky pains indicating subacute obstruction, all point to a large bowel tumour. Some, however, are relatively symptomless until the patient presents as an emergency with obstruction.

Carcinoma of the lower rectum will almost always cause early bleeding with mucus discharge; later there is tenesmus and a feeling of incomplete emptying of the bowel. Obstruction is a feature of tumours of the pelvirectal junction but not the rectum proper, which is capacious and distensible.

The findings on physical examination range from no obvious abnormality to the signs of advanced malignancy. The majority of rectal tumours can be palpated on digital examination. Fresh blood in the stool should always suggest the possibility of a tumour of the rectum or pelvic colon. Occult blood is found in the stool if an ulcerating lesion is present higher in the colon.

Investigation. *Endoscopy*. More than 50% of malignant tumours of the large bowel occur in a part accessible to direct inspection with the sigmoidoscope, i.e. the rectum and the lower pelvic colon and this procedure is mandatory. The whole or part of a growth may be seen and a biopsy carried out. Colonoscopic examination is valuable when a suspicious lesion is seen more proximally on the barium enema.

Radiological Examination. A barium enema will demonstrate advanced cancer as a filling defect or stricture (Fig. 9.13). For the demonstration of smaller, earlier tumours, careful preparation of the colon followed by a double contrast barium enema is necessary. A barium follow-through examination may be of value for tumours in the region of the caecum.

Fig. 9.13 **Carcinoma of the sigmoid colon** and a polyp in the transverse colon. (Courtesy of Dr. G.M. Fraser).

The *stage* of carcinoma of the rectum is defined by Dukes' classification (p. 110), and the role of CEA is discussed on page 107.

Treatment of choice is resection of the tumour as a one-stage procedure. If there is no colonic obstruction, or if it can be overcome by enemas, time should be spent in preparing the bowel by washouts and antibiotics. Anaemia should be corrected by preoperative transfusion.

Carcinoma of the rectum may require total removal of the rectum with permanent colostomy and for this the patient requires pre-operative introduction to colostomy and its management. However advances in suture techniques allow preservation of continuity in many more patients by means of a colo-rectal or colo-anal anastomosis. Success depends on early diagnosis and operation before spread has occurred and before obstruction renders the surgeon's task more complicated. The possibility of carcinoma of the colon must be considered when anyone of middle age presents with rectal bleeding, change of bowel habit or iron-deficiency anaemia.

Benign Tumours of the Large Intestine

Only polyps are found with any frequency. These tumours may be single or multiple and are most commonly found in the left side of the colon. They are sessile or pedunculated; in the latter case the stalk may allow the polyp to move up and down the lumen of the bowel. These tumours may be found incidentally at operation or on barium enema (Fig. 9.13), or they may cause bleeding, discharge of mucus, or intussusception. Occasionally, because of its mobility, a polyp may prolapse through the anus to appear as a red, cherry-like mass.

Although they are primarily benign, polyps of the colon may become carcinomatous. In general polyps of more than 1 cm in diameter are probably malignant. The malignant change may not extend into the stalk, so that removal of the polyp and stalk at colonoscopy may suffice. The stalk as well as the polyp itself should then be examined histologically. Colonoscopy should be repeated after 2 years to exclude recurrence.

Multiple Polyposis

In this condition, transmitted by autosomal dominant inheritance, there may be thousands of small polyps diffusely scattered over the mucosal surface of the colon and rectum. They appear at adolescence and become malignant in about 15 years, the patient often dying from carcinomatosis before the age of 40. The disease can be recognised by radiological or endoscopic examination from adolescence onwards of members of affected families. Prevention of carcinoma means removal of the colon and rectum with permanent ileostomy, although symptomless members of the family may find ileorectal anastomosis with diathermy removal of rectal polyps and periodic surveillance more acceptable.

Megacolon

Megacolon is a condition characterised by dilatation of the colon and obstinate constipation. The disease may be separated into two groups, congenital (Hirschsprung's disease) and acquired megacolon.

Hirschsprung's Disease. The cause is a congenital absence of the myenteric nerve plexus in the wall of the pelvic colon and upper rectum. Occasionally the defect extends proximally. Boys are more often affected than girls and symptoms of colonic obstruction (constipation, abdominal distension and vomiting) date from birth. Symptoms may be intermittent, but even between attacks there is persistent abdominal swelling. The rectum is empty on digital examination.

Radiological examination with small amounts of barium shows a small rectum, a narrow segment above and then wide dilatation of the colon full of retained faeces. The diagnosis can be confirmed by a rectal biopsy of sufficient thickness to include muscle of the bowel wall in which the ganglion cells are situated.

Treatment is by excision of the abnormal segment of colon and rectum.

Acquired Megacolon. In this group of cases, there is no defined aetiology and no particular age-group. Some are examples of a milder, short segment form of Hirschsprung's disease. Others are associated with cretinism. In Chagas' disease (p. 780) autonomic ganglia in the lower colon are destroyed by a trypanosome.

Radiologically, acquired megacolon usually shows no narrowed segment, the dilatation instead extending down to the anus. The rectum is full of faeces.

Most cases can be managed conservatively, by treatment of the cause where identifiable, by high residue diets, laxatives and perhaps saline enemas. In a few patients colonic resection has been used as a last resort in the relief of obstinate constipation.

Incontinence of Faeces

Incontinence is most common in elderly, debilitated or demented patients in whom the appreciation of rectal distension is diminished and the sphincteric and pelvic floor muscles are weakened. It may also be due to faecal impaction with overflow incontinence of soft faeces and require manual or instrumental disimpaction followed by the use of laxatives to prevent recurrence.

Incontinence also occurs when the sphincters and the supporting muscles are injured, for example by obstetric tear; various operative procedures are available for their repair. The sphincter mechanisms can be damaged by cancer, Crohn's disease or third degree haemorrhoids or their neurological control may be impaired by spina bifida or trauma to the lumbar spine.

There can be incontinence of faeces even when anal function is normal as in the presence of severe diarrhoea or in behavioural disturbances in children. In both instances treatment must be directed at the primary cause.

DISEASES OF THE ALIMENTARY TRACT

Any or several components of the alimentary tract may be involved by infection, ischaemia or psychogenic disorders.

Infections of the Alimentary Tract

Infections of the mouth due to thrush and other organisms are discussed on page 286 and gastroenteritis caused by bacterial food poisoning on page 753. Acute gastroenteritis may be caused by viruses such as rotavirus. Usually identification of the viral nature of the infection is not possible and diagnosis is presumptive on epidemiological grounds when no bacterial cause has been demonstrated.

The small intestine is involved in typhoid and paratyphoid fevers (p. 751), cholera (p. 755), staphylococcal enterocolitis (p. 743), tuberculosis (p. 230), giardiasis (p. 775), strongyloidiasis (p. 793) and ancylostomiasis (p. 793).

The principal infections involving the large intestine are bacillary dysentery (p. 755), amoebic dysentery (p. 773), antibiotic-associated pseudomembraneous colitis (p. 46) and schistosomiasis (p. 782). Some organisms, e.g. *Yersinia enterocolitica*, may infect both small and large intestines.

Rehydration together with oral glucose and electrolytes can be life-saving in the acute diarrhoeal illnesses which are a major cause of death in infants and children in the Tropics (p. 718).

Bacterial resistance to antimicrobial agents is readily induced by their indiscriminate use in infections of the gut, many of which are not of bacterial origin. When antimicrobial therapy is indicated by the presence of systemic upset, local knowledge of sensitivity is important as resistance may have been acquired to one or more of the agents commonly used in that area.

Abdominal infections complicating surgical or gynaecological operations and diverticulitis are commonly caused by *Bacteroides fragilis* and respond to metronidazole. Alternative therapy is provided by clindamycin or cefoxitin.

Travellers' Diarrhoea. A short attack of diarrhoea commonly affects travellers, especially in developing countries. The attack is usually acute, with watery stools and sometimes vomiting. It lasts 2 to 5 days and is self-limiting. Enterotoxigenic *Esch. coli* has been implicated in about 50% of cases and shigella in up to 20%. Other organisms, e.g. campylobacter or rotaviruses, may be involved but often the cause cannot be identified. In mild cases symptoms can be controlled by one of the synthetic narcotic analogues, loperamide or diphenoxylate. Severer cases should be treated early with co-trimoxazole or trimethoprim.

Persistence of diarrhoea after travel is a feature of giardiasis (p. 775) and amoebiasis (p. 773).

Ischaemia of the Alimentary Tract

The intestines are supplied by the coeliac, superior mesenteric and inferior mesenteric arteries. Of these, the superior mesenteric, which supplies the mid-gut, has poor collateral support from the other two arteries. It follows that intestinal ischaemia is usually due to sudden or slow occlusion of the superior mesenteric artery. However, it may also arise from obstruction to the venous outflow from the intestine, or from a reduction in blood flow due to shock or cardiac failure, without evidence of obstruction to the arterial or venous supply. The usual causes of blockage of the superior mesenteric artery are atheroma, thrombosis due to blood diseases, and embolism. Most cases of intestinal ischaemia occur in the elderly and in those with cardiac failure or arrhythmias.

Acute Intestinal Failure. This term is used to describe the consequences of acute obstruction of the superior mesenteric artery. A variable length of the small intestine undergoes necrosis of the superficial epithelium and over several hours this progresses to gangrene. The patient has abdominal pain, vomiting, watery and later bloody diarrhoea. Signs of peritonitis and hypovolaemic shock develop. There is marked leucocytosis. Early laparotomy is essential as most patients will die unless the affected bowel is resected. Occasionally, embolectomy or thrombectomy can restore the circulation and allow recovery.

Chronic Intestinal Ischaemia. This occurs when there is a gradual reduction of blood flow in the superior mesenteric artery with resulting impairment of the normal postprandial increase in blood flow to the small bowel. There is abdominal pain ('abdominal angina') some 30 minutes after each meal so that the patient is afraid to eat and loses weight. The condition is rare.

Ischaemia of the Large Intestine. Occlusion of the inferior mesenteric artery leads to ischaemia of the left colon, especially when blood flow in the superior mesenteric artery is also reduced. The disorder is termed *ischaemic colitis*. The patient presents with abdominal pain and bloody diarrhoea and the diagnosis is made by barium enema examination which shows oedema of the mucosa of the affected segment of colon. In contrast to ischaemia of the small intestine, the condition is usually transient, but in some patients it may proceed to gangrene or to stricture usually situated at the splenic flexure.

Psychogenic Disorders

Psychogenic Dyspepsia. Gastric secretion, motility of the alimentary tract and blood flow are influenced by emotion. Commonly psychological factors cause oesophageal and gastrointestinal disorders some of which mimic organic disease.

Patients under stress, or with an anxiety neurosis, may develop a wide range of symptoms such as dry mouth, a sensation of a lump in the throat, anorexia, nausea, vomiting, aerophagy with belching, abdominal discomfort and pain, diarrhoea or constipation. Patients with depressive illness may have anorexia, a bad taste in the mouth and constipation. It should not be forgotten that such patients may also have an organic lesion in the gastrointestinal tract.

A careful history will usually identify complaints of psychological origin; for example, pain of this type may have no discernible pattern with no clear time or food relationships and the patient often has difficulty in describing it. Pain which is diffuse, continuous, lacking in periodicity or present for months or even years is probably psychogenic. The more bizarre the description, the less likely is the symptom to be organic in origin. The history should also elicit features indicative of a psychological disturbance.

Physical examination may reveal a manifestation of anxiety such as inappropriate sweating or tachycardia. If abdominal tenderness is elicited, this is often quite disproportionate both to the patient's physical well-being and to the complaint. Further investigation is often necessary but must be selected with discrimination in relation to the individual problem.

The psychological origin of the symptoms should be sought and explained. Frequently, patients with psychogenic dyspepsia recognise that they have a 'weak stomach' which bears the brunt of recurrent stress, but they come to a doctor for reassurance from time to time. Some are helped by small doses of antacids or the anticholinergic dicyclomine 10–20 mg with meals; this may be a placebo response.

Globus hystericus describes the sensation of a lump in the throat which is independent of swallowing and indeed may be relieved by swallowing food or drink. The symptom occurs most frequently in tense, anxious individuals, but before accepting a psychogenic basis it is necessary to exclude organic disease by a barium swallow and if necessary by endoscopy.

Psychogenic vomiting is not an uncommon manifestation of anxiety neurosis. It occurs usually on wakening, or immediately after breakfast;

only rarely does it occur later in the day. It is probably a reaction to awakening and facing up to the worries of everyday life; in the young it can be due to school phobia. There may be retching alone or the vomiting of gastric secretions or food. Although psychogenic vomiting may occur regularly over long periods, there is little or no weight loss and this is of value in distinguishing it from vomiting due to organic disease of the alimentary tract. Early morning vomiting also occurs in pregnancy, alcohol abuse and depression.

It is essential in all cases to assess and, if possible, alleviate the underlying psychological disturbance. Tranquillisers and antiemetic drugs have only a secondary place.

The Irritable Bowel Syndrome

One of the commonest disorders of the alimentary tract is that of long-standing dysfunction associated with abdominal pain for which no organic cause can be found. Bowel habit is disturbed by diarrhoea or constipation occurring alone, or alternating. Some forms of this irritable bowel syndrome are also known as *spastic colon* and *idiopathic* or *nervous diarrhoea*.

Manometric studies from the distal colon have shown various patterns. When constipation and pain are the predominant symptoms, intraluminal pressure is usually increased and there is an increased frequency of pressure waves, whereas motor activity is often reduced in patients with painless diarrhoea. These changes are not constant so that motility studies are of no value for diagnostic purposes.

Although the aetiology of the irritable bowel syndrome is uncertain, psychological disturbances, especially anxiety, are frequent; patients are often tense, conscientious individuals who worry excessively about family or financial affairs. Some relate the onset of their symptoms to an attack of infective diarrhoea; in others certain foods may precipitate symptoms.

Clinical Features. The syndrome is most frequent in women between the ages of 20 and 40 years. The commonest symptom is pain referred to the left or right iliac fossa or the hypogastrium, sometimes flitting from site to site. Pain often occurs in attacks usually relieved by defecation and sometimes provoked by food, and may be severe. Bowel habit is variable. Almost all patients notice pellet like or ribbon like stools with or without mucus at some time. Diarrhoea may be painless and characteristically occurs in the morning, and almost never at night; defecation after meals may be precipitate due to an exaggerated gastrocolic reflex.

Other symptoms include bloating or abdominal distension, a sensation of incomplete emptying of the rectum, excessive flatus and audible borborygmi. Nausea, anorexia, headache and tiredness may also occur.

The patient may seem anxious but is otherwise well. The descending colon may be palpable and tender. Rectal examination is normal.

Investigation. Although the diagnosis is usually suggested by the history alone, organic bowel disease has to be excluded, especially in patient developing symptoms for the first time over the age of 40 years. Sigmoidoscopy is essential to exclude an organic lesion of the distal colon. The mucosa appears normal in the irritable bowel syndrome but the colon may show marked motor activity, contracting and relaxing quite unlike the normal inert bowel. Barium enema examination is necessary principally to exclude organic disease; there are no diagnostic radiological features. In patients whose principal complaint is painless diarrhoea, the possibility of lactose intolerance, hyperthyroidism or alcohol excess should not be overlooked.

Treatment. The patient must first be reassured on the basis of the normal findings on examination and investigation, as anxiety may precipitate or aggravate the condition and there is sometimes an underlying fear of cancer. In patients with persistent or troublesome symptoms, measures designed to modify the intestinal dysmotility are required. For constipation and pain, the patient should be encouraged to increase the roughage content of the diet and one of the hydrophilic colloids should be prescribed in a dose sufficient to ensure a normal bowel movement. It is important that the patient should stop laxatives.

Pain and diarrhoea may be relieved by an anticholinergic drug such as dicyclomine or an antispasmodic such as mebeverine hydrochloride thrice daily. For patients with painless diarrhoea, improvement is commonly obtained with some dietary restriction, particularly the avoidance of fresh fruits and salads. Codeine phosphate and loperamide are useful drugs which act quickly and can be carried by the patient to use in emergency or they can be taken before any event which is known to precipitate diarrhoea.

In all patients the psychological component of the syndrome should be explained

PROSPECTS IN ALIMENTARY DISEASE

The accurate diagnosis of most gastrointestinal diseases is now possible due to the development of sophisticated endoscopic and radiological procedures. This precision is being still further improved by developments in ultrasonography, computed scanning and nuclear magnetic resonance. All these techniques are being used increasingly to effect therapy. Thus imaging and radiographic techniques are used to control gastrointestinal bleeding and to localise, accurately, masses, abscesses and cysts which can then be biopsied or aspirated. Endoscopic procedures are being used in many different ways, for example for the removal of stones from the common bile duct and to carry out the coagulation of bleeding points. There is no doubt that advances along these lines will continue.

The ability to treat most cases of peptic ulceration with H_2-receptor antagonists and the success of highly selective vagotomy in those who require surgery, has led to more satisfactory management of the majority of such patients. There remains the significant problem of those who develop ulcers or bleeding from erosions as a result of consuming aspirin or other anti-inflammatory drugs. It is likely that an increased understanding of the components of the gastric mucosal 'barrier' and the development of drugs to strengthen it, for example the prostaglandins, will avoid these complications. The mechanisms which protect the epithelium of the entire gastrointestinal tract are also under study; this may provide new insights into diffuse conditions such as Crohn's disease, and ulcerative colitis.

Functional gastrointestinal disease remains a significant cause of illness. Our understanding of the mechanisms involved is rudimentary. The development of research into motility of the alimentary tract and the increased awareness of the large number of interacting gastrointestinal hormones and paracrine substances may eventually provide therapeutic benefits.

In some directions the surgical treatment of gastrointestinal disorders will continue to contract with the increasing efficiency and availability of medical, radiological and endoscopic alternatives. On the other hand sphincter sparing operations and other technical improvements will continue. Now that microvascular surgery and organ transplantation are established in other fields similar advances in the management of pancreatic and gut failure can be anticipated. Whilst these advances in technique offer more acceptable operations, the problem of gastrointestinal cancer remains; the utilisation of chemotherapy is in its infancy and the main hope still lies in the identification of carcinogens and their elimination from the diet and environment.

G.P. CREAN
D.J.C. SHEARMAN
W.P. SMALL

FURTHER READING:

Clinics in Gastroenterology. London: W.B. Saunders. A series of specialist volumes consisting of three numbers annually and each dealing with a specific disorder of the alimentary tract. Recommended for selective reading and as a reference library to current practice.

Macleod, J. (1983) Examination of the alimentary system. In *Clinical Examination*, 6th edn. Edinburgh: Churchill Livingstone. Complementary to this chapter and designed to be read in conjunction with it.

Shearman, D.J.C. & Finlayson, N.D.C. (1982) *Diseases of the Gastrointestinal Tract and Liver*. Edinburgh: Churchill Livingstone. A new textbook primarily for clinicians.

Sleisenger, M.H. & Fordtran, J.S. (1978) *Gastrointestinal Disease*, 2nd edn. London: W.B. Saunders. The most complete reference text presently available. Contains extensive bibliographies to each chapter.

10. Diseases of the Liver and Biliary Tract

THE LIVER

ANATOMY

The liver is the largest organ in the body, weighing 1200–1500 g. It has right and left lobes separated by the falciform ligament anteriorly, the fissure of the ligamentum teres inferiorly and the fissure of the ligamentum venosum posteriorly. The right lobe is the larger; it contains the quadrate lobe on the anteromedial part of the inferior surface and the caudate lobe on the medial part of the posterior surface. The left lobe is relatively larger in infancy and contributes to the protuberant abdomen at that age.

The liver has an arterial and a venous blood supply and total blood flow is normally about 1500 ml/min. The arterial supply is by the hepatic artery, a branch of the coeliac axis, which enters the liver in the porta hepatis and is distributed throughout the liver via the portal tracts. Its precise terminal distribution is uncertain, but most of its blood enters the sinusoids directly. In man, the hepatic artery supplies about 35% of the total liver blood flow and about 50% of its total oxygen supply. The portal vein drains the blood from the alimentary tract, spleen, pancreas and gall bladder. It also enters the liver in the porta hepatis, is distributed throughout the liver via the portal tracts and empties its blood into the sinusoids. The oxygen content of portal blood varies and is lowest during digestion. Autoregulation of blood flow by the hepatic artery compensates for variations of portal blood flow and ensures that total liver blood flow remains constant.

Histologically, the liver is divided into lobules based on a central vein and peripheral portal tracts with regular radiating sinusoids separated by plates of liver cells (hepatocytes). The central veins are tributaries of the hepatic veins which drain to the inferior vena cava; the portal tracts contain branches of the hepatic artery, the portal vein, lymphatics and the bile ducts; the sinusoids are capillaries which are lined by endothelial and phagocytic (Kupffer) cells and which receive blood separately from the hepatic arterial and portal venous systems and convey it to the central veins; the hepatocytes (Fig. 10.1) are arranged in single-cell plates which lie between and separate the sinusoids from one another. Between the hepatocytes and the sinusoidal cells is the space of Disse which contains fluid draining to the lymphatics in the portal tracts. The space of Disse also contains unique stellate (Ito) cells responsible for the storage of vitamin A. Individual hepatocytes either line the space of Disse or abut on other liver cells; electron microscopically, the part of the membrane lining the space of Disse has irregular microvilli, while a part of the membrane adjacent to other liver cells helps to form the lining of the bile canaliculi, and here regular microvilli project into the canalicular lumen. These bile canaliculi form networks between the hepatocytes and convey bile towards the terminal bile ducts which link the intralobular bile canaliculi to the larger interlobular bile ducts in the portal tracts (Fig. 10.1).

The electron microscopic features of the liver are complex and so far this technique has not proved of great clinical value. However, increasing knowledge is beginning to focus attention on the intracellular sites at which damage occurs in different forms of hepatocyte injury. Direct toxic injury (alcohol, drugs, pregnancy, Wilson's

Fig. 10.1 The hepatocyte and its main related structures. The hepatocyte has a prominent nucleus and nucleolus [N] and electron microscopy shows its cytoplasm to be rich in organelles such as mitochondria [M], endoplasmic reticulum [R], lysosomes [L] and Golgi apparatus [G], responsible for complex metabolic processes. The sinusoids (capillaries) are heavily fenestrated, and are therefore highly permeable. The inset shows a lobule with plates of hepatocytes and their relationship to the central vein [CV], bile ducts [BD] and portal tracts [PT].

disease, Reye's syndrome) principally damages mitochondria and causes centrilobular necrosis and fatty change; immunological damage (chronic active hepatitis, primary biliary cirrhosis, drugs) affects cell and canalicular membranes, and cholestatic injury (drugs) affects the bile secretory mechanism.

Clinical Aspects. The upper border of the liver extends from the fifth rib medial to the right midclavicular line to the sixth rib in the left midclavicular line. Its lower margin crosses the epigastrium midway between the xiphisternum and the umbilicus. As the liver descends 1–3 cm in inspiration, it can normally be palpated in adults below the right costal margin during deep inspiration. Heavy percussion from above and light percussion from below in the right midclavi-

cular line helps to determine liver size; percussion is of greatest value in revealing a small liver. Auscultation over the liver may reveal a rub due to perihepatitis, a venous hum between the xiphisternum and umbilicus due to collateral vessels in portal hypertension, or, rarely, an arterial bruit due to hepatocellular carcinoma or acute alcoholic hepatitis.

PHYSIOLOGY

Liver cells carry out a wide variety of metabolic functions facilitated by the rich blood supply derived from the gut as well as the systemic circulation, and by the intimate contact between hepatocytes and blood due to the highly permeable sinusoidal lining. All hepatocytes appear capable of performing the many functions of the liver.

Carbohydrate Metabolism. The liver is central to the maintenance of the blood glucose concentration which remains remarkably constant thus ensuring a steady supply of carbohydrate to extrahepatic tissues. During fasting, glucose derived from glycogen (glycogenolysis) or from newly synthesised glucose (gluconeogenesis) is added to the blood. Three quarters is derived initially from glycogenolysis, but glycogen reserves (70–80 g) become exhausted within 24 hours of fasting and gluconeogenesis becomes steadily more important. Precursors for gluconeogenesis include lactate, pyruvate, glucogenic amino acids and glycerol. Lactate derived from extrahepatic tissues is most important quantitatively, but lactate is itself derived from glucose and as fasting continues amino acids, especially alanine, become steadily more important precursors. After feeding, insulin stimulates the hepatic uptake of a half or more of the glucose absorbed, and it is stored as glycogen or used to produce glycerol and fatty acids thus avoiding marked hyperglycaemia. Fructose and galactose in dietary carbohydrate can also be used for glycogen synthesis.

Protein Metabolism. Dietary proteins enter the portal vein as amino acids and most are taken up by the liver except for the branched chain amino acids which are metabolised by the muscles. The liver utilises amino acids for endogenous hepatic protein and plasma protein synthesis and for the production of urea; a substantial proportion of the amino acids is released into the blood for the use of other tissues. During fasting, amino acids, including those reaching the liver from extrahepatic tissues, are used more for gluconeogenesis while endogenous protein synthesis, urea production and amino acid release to the blood are suppressed. Plasma protein synthesis, by contrast, varies little in relation to food intake and is a major function of the liver cells. Indeed, all the plasma albumin and most of its globulins, other than the gammaglobulins, are produced there.

Globulins made in the liver, often exclusively, include coagulation factors I (fibrinogen), II (prothrombin), V, VII, IX and X, many of the components of the complement system, transport proteins such as transferrin and haptoglobin and proteins with no certain physiological function such as caeruloplasmin, α-fetoprotein, α_2-macroglobulin and α_1-antitrypsin. The result of this extensive synthetic activity is that the electrophoretic pattern of the plasma proteins is largely determined by liver function.

Lipid Metabolism. Dietary fat is largely triglyceride, and it enters the body in chylomicrons (Fig. 10.2). Triglyceride is removed from the chylomicrons by lipoprotein lipase in the blood; the triglyceride is taken up by many tissues and the chylomicron remnants are removed by the liver. Triglyceride taken up by the liver is broken down to 2-carbon fragments which may be used in many metabolic processes. Free (non-esterified) fatty acids, liberated from the fat stores into the blood, are also taken up by the liver and used similarly.

Among these processes is the synthesis of new lipid molecules — triglyceride, phospholipid and cholesterol — which are combined with specific apoproteins to form lipoproteins which are released into the blood. These include very low density (pre β) lipoproteins (VLDL) and high density (α) lipoproteins (HDL). VLDL are converted by lipoprotein lipase in the blood to low density (β) lipoproteins (LDL) which transport triglyceride to muscles and other tissues as a source of energy or to the fat depots for storage. The functions of HDL are uncertain, but they may be important in cholesterol transport. The liver synthesises more cholesterol than any other organ and this can be incorporated into lipoproteins, converted into bile acids or excreted into the bile. In biliary obstruction of any severity the serum lipid concentration increases, largely due to the formation of an abnormal lipoprotein known as lipoprotein X.

Bilirubin is produced from the ferroporphyrin, haem, after removal of its iron component. Most (80%) is derived from haemoglobin breakdown by Kuppfer cells in the liver and other macrophages in the spleen and bone marrow, the rest being formed by catabolism of other haemcontaining proteins, particularly enzymes (e.g. cytochromes, peroxidases, and catalase) and myoglobin. This bilirubin is unconjugated and is not

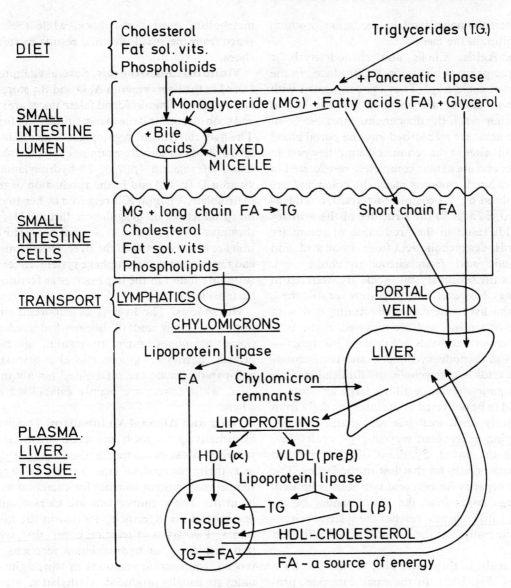

Fig. 10.2 Outline of fat metabolism See text pages 310 and 336.

water soluble; it is bound to albumin in the plasma and does not pass into the urine. It is taken up by the hepatocytes, conjugated with glucuronic acid and excreted into the bile. Bilirubin diglucuronide is formed in the microsomes by the enzyme glucuronyl transferase and is water soluble. It is excreted into the bile where it constitutes 80% of the bilirubin. The remaining 20% is bilirubin monoglucuronide, and its origin is uncertain. It is excreted into bile by active transport.

Conjugated bilirubin is not absorbed in the small intestine. Bacteria in the terminal ileum and colon, however, reduce it to a group of colourless chromogens. Most of these (stercobilinogen) are excreted in the stool (100–200 mg/day). Some are absorbed from the gut and pass to the liver where most are re-excreted in the bile; a small amount (4 mg/day) passes through the liver and is excreted in the urine where it is known as urobilinogen. Urobilinogen and its oxidation product urobilin in the urine are identical, respectively, with stercobilinogen and its oxidation product, stercobilin, in the faeces.

Bile Acids. Cholic and chenodeoxycholic acids, the primary bile acids, are produced in the liver from cholesterol. They are conjugated with glycine or taurine and secreted into the bile in which they reach the duodenum. Most (95%) of the bile acids are reabsorbed into the portal blood at specific sites in the terminal ileum; they pass to the liver and are almost completely re-excreted in the bile. Small amounts reach the colon and are metabolised by the colonic bacteria. Deconjugation and changes in the structure of the primary bile acids result in the production of secondary bile acids, deoxycholic acid from cholic acid, and lithocholic acid from chenodeoxycholic acid. Most of the secondary bile acids are excreted in the faeces. However, small amounts are absorbed, reach the liver where they are conjugated with glycine or taurine, and are excreted in the bile. Bile, therefore, contains two primary bile acids — cholic and chenodeoxycholic — and two secondary bile acids — deoxycholic and lithocholic. This *enterohepatic circulation* allows large amounts of bile acid to be delivered to the intestine daily from a relatively small total bile acid pool (6 mmols; 3 g) owing to frequent recycling (10 cycles/day) through the bowel. Synthesis of new bile acid compensates only for that lost in the faeces. The hepatic capacity for bile acid synthesis is limited, and large losses from the bowel cannot be replaced. Little bile acid reaches the systemic circulation normally, but the amount increases in liver disease.

Bile acids, as they enter bile, combine to form micelles (Fig. 10.2). In the small intestine, provided the bile acid concentration remains sufficient to maintain the micellar state, this greatly increases the efficiency of fat absorption. Insufficiency of bile acids results in poor absorption of dietary fat and fat-soluble vitamins, notably vitamins D and K. Such deficiency may result from impaired synthesis in chronic liver disease, biliary obstruction, small intestinal overgrowth of bacteria capable of deconjugating and dehydroxylating bile acids, and loss of bile acids into the colon in disease of the terminal ileum or after its resection. In this last instance, the bile acids interfere with colonic water and electrolyte metabolism causing diarrhoea, while their absence from the small intestine results in steatorrhoea.

Vitamins and Minerals. Several vitamins are stored in the liver; vitamin A, D and B_{12} stores are large whereas vitamin K and folate stores are small and soon disappear if the dietary intake is deficient. The liver can convert tryptophan to nicotinic acid (p. 76), and can activate vitamins as by phosphorylation of thiamin (p. 73), 25-hydroxylation of vitamin D (p. 66) and in the production of tetrahydrofolate. Vitamin K is required by hepatocytes for production of coagulation factors II (prothrombin), VII, IX and X. Normal tissue stores of iron are divided between the liver, striated muscle and the monocyte–macrophage system. Liver iron stores are found in the hepatocytes as ferritin and haemosiderin.

Hormones. The liver is an important site of hormone action and of hormone degradation. Some hormones such as insulin, glucagon, growth hormone, glucocorticoids, oestrogens, and parathormone are catabolised mainly in the liver, while others are mainly catabolised elsewhere.

Drug and Alcohol Metabolism. The liver is quantitatively the most important organ for this function. Most drugs metabolised are fat-soluble and their conversion into water-soluble substances makes them suitable for excretion in bile or urine. These conversions are carried out by enzymes of low specificity located in the microsomes. Two types of reaction occur; first, oxidation, reduction, or hydroxylation reactions, and second, conjugation reactions in which glucuronides are usually produced. Methylation, acetylation, sulphation and amino-acid conjugation may also occur.

The pharmacological results of drug metabolism vary. Barbiturates undergo oxidation with loss of activity; cyclophosphamide is metabolised from an inactive substance to an active alkylating agent; phenylbutazone is oxidised to another active agent, oxyphenbutazone; and codeine is converted in part to morphine. Conjugation, as occurs with salicylates, paracetamol and morphine, almost always causes loss of activity. Acetylation of sulphonamides makes them less soluble and therefore potentially more harmful from crystallisation in the urinary tract. When two drugs are metabolised by the same microsomal enzymes, each retards the metabolism of the other, leading to prolongation of drug action and the danger of overdosage. This is an example of one mechanism causing an undesirable drug interaction in therapy.

The action of many drugs is determined largely by their speed of metabolism in the microsomal enzyme system, the activity of which may be altered by dietary and hormonal factors. In particular, microsomal enzyme activity may be greatly increased by certain drugs they themselves metabolise, an effect referred to as *enzyme induction*, due to an increase in enzyme protein which disappears when the drug is withdrawn. Drugs producing this effect — 'inducing agents' — are many and include barbiturates, phenylbutazone and phenytoin. Enzyme induction has important therapeutic consequences, for an enzyme inducer such as a barbiturate may increase the required dose of another drug, such as warfarin; if only the inducing drug is then stopped, bleeding from overdosage of the anticoagulant may occur.

The liver metabolises about 90% of alcohol (ethanol) ingested, the rest being excreted by the lungs and kidneys. It is oxidised via acetaldehyde to acetate with the eventual formation of carbon dioxide. These reactions are carried out mainly by alcohol dehydrogenase, a mitochondrial enzyme, and the microsomal ethanol oxidising system. The last, like other microsomal enzyme systems such as γGT (p. 341) may be induced by drugs, including alcohol itself, and this may in part account for increased alcohol tolerance in drinkers and for their resistance to the action of microsomally metabolised drugs. Conversely, the effects of alcohol may be enhanced when a microsomally metabolised drug such as chlormethiazole is taken concomitantly; this is a very important example of drug interaction.

In liver disease, drug metabolism may be impaired, and care is needed to avoid overdosage, particularly with sedative drugs. The extent to which individual drugs are affected is very variable and cannot be predicted. Special care should, therefore, be taken whenever hepatic damage is present, particularly where there is evidence of severe liver damage, such as jaundice, ascites, encephalopathy, hypoalbuminaemia or a prolonged prothrombin time.

Function of the Monocyte-macrophage System. Approximately 20% of the hepatic cell mass is composed of monocytes and macrophages, including the Kupffer cells. These cells destroy effete erythrocytes and remove bacteria from the blood. The Kupffer cells also have important but poorly understood immunological functions. Antigens from the gut normally gain repeated access to the body. They are carried in the portal blood to the liver where the Kupffer cells phagocytose them and prevent their eliciting immunological responses. Kupffer cells are also very efficient at removing immune complexes from the blood. The liver, therefore, is able to prevent undesirable immunological reactions.

THE INVESTIGATION OF LIVER DISEASE

Liver Function Tests

The term 'liver function tests' refers to a group of biochemical investigations useful in confirming that the liver is diseased, in indicating whether hepatic cells (parenchymal liver disease) or the biliary tree (obstructive or cholestatic liver disease) is primarily involved, in giving an indication of the extent of liver damage and in assessing progress. The term is misleading in that many of the investigations do not measure liver functions and most liver functions are not tested in clinical practice; however, the term has become generally accepted. Liver function tests are variably abnormal in patients with liver disease and therefore a group of tests is usually done. It is important to realise that there are no patterns of abnormality indicative of specific diagnoses and that normality of all the commonly used tests does not prove that the liver is normal.

Bilirubin. Almost all the bilirubin normally present in the blood is unconjugated. Unconjugated hyperbilirubinaemia without any abnormality of other liver function tests may result from increased bilirubin production, as in haemolysis or ineffective erythropoiesis or from inability to transport bilirubin across the liver, as in Gilbert's syndrome. Except in the newborn, the hyperbilirubinaemia rarely exceeds 100 μmol/l (6 mg/dl), and there is no bilirubin in the urine. Conjugated hyperbilirubinaemia without any abnormality of other liver function tests, as in the rare Dubin-Johnson syndrome, is accompanied by bilirubinuria but is uncommon.

Estimates of unconjugated and conjugated bilirubin in the blood are hardly ever necessary, and cannot be done accurately when the total serum bilirubin is less than 70 μmol/l (4 mg/dl) using generally available methods. Hyperbilirubinaemia in hepatobiliary disease is predominantly conjugated, bilirubinuria is present, and other tests of liver function are almost always abnormal. The serum bilirubin in parenchymal liver disease varies widely depending on the severity of the disease and its activity. It gives an accurate measure of the depth of jaundice and repeated estimations may be useful in following the progress of disease. Very high concentrations of bilirubin occur most frequently in biliary tract obstruction, with sustained high levels where this is due to malignant disease and more fluctuating levels where obstruction is caused by gallstones.

Simple, sensitive, inexpensive dipstick tests for bilirubin in the urine are available and useful. Unconjugated bilirubin is bound to albumin in the blood and does not pass into the urine and conjugated bilirubin is not detectable in the urine of normal persons. Consequently, bilirubinuria implies a conjugated hyperbilirubinaemia and points to hepatobiliary disease. Conversely, absence of bilirubinuria in a jaundiced patient suggests haemolysis, ineffective erythropoiesis or a congenital non-haemolytic hyperbilirubinaemia such as Gilbert's syndrome.

Urobilinogen. A simple dip stick test is available to detect excessive urobilinogenuria. There is normally a diurnal variation in the urinary output of urobilinogen, maximal excretion occurring in the afternoon when tests are best performed. Since it is readily oxidised to urobilin on exposure to air at room temperature, only fresh urine samples should be used. Excess urinary urobilinogen occurs in haemolytic diseases owing to increased bilirubin excretion leading to increased urobilinogen formation; in these patients bilirubinuria is not present. Any cause of hepatic parenchymal dysfunction — viral hepatitis, cir-

rhosis, malignancy, partial biliary obstruction, pyrexia or cardiac failure — will reduce the biliary re-excretion of urobilinogen and increase its excretion in the urine; bilirubinuria may or may not be present. In cholestatic jaundice, absence of urinary urobilinogen for over a week indicates complete biliary obstruction.

Enzymes. Liver cells contain many enzymes which may be released into the blood in various pathological processes. Measurement of the activity of these enzymes in the blood may give evidence of hepatocellular disease and of its general nature. In practice, maximum information may be obtained by measuring the activity of relatively few enzymes. It must be remembered in interpreting the results of these tests that none of the enzymes usually measured is specific to the liver and alternative sources should be considered, particularly where abnormalities have been found incidentally in patients with minimal or no clinical evidence of liver disease.

Aminotransferases. The two important enzymes in this group are aspartate aminotransferase, AST (fomerly known as glutamic oxaloacetic transaminase, GOT) and alanine aminotransferase, ALT (glutamic pyruvic transaminase, GPT); both are present in the cytosol of the hepatocytes, the former also being found in the mitochondria. Normal serum contains low enzyme activity the source of which is unknown. Irrespective of the cause, whenever liver cells are damaged or killed the enzymes are liberated into the blood; this is therefore a test of the integrity of the liver cells. The highest activities are caused by any form of acute liver damage.

In viral hepatitis there is generally increased activity even in the prodromal phase and maximal levels of 10 to 100 times the normal value are usually reached in the jaundiced phase after which activity falls rapidly. Equally high activity occurs in acute hepatitis due to drugs, in acute circulatory failure and in exacerbations of chronic active hepatitis. Most patients (80%) with infectious mononucleosis or cytomegaloviral infection also have an acute hepatitis with serum transferase activity raised 2 to 10 times but few develop jaundice. Serum aminotransferase activity rarely rises more than five-fold in acute alcoholic hepatitis. Patients with cirrhosis usually show only modest elevations of serum transferase. In obstructive jaundice, activity may rise up to five-fold but rarely more unless cholangitis is present.

Increased serum aminotransferase activity is a very sensitive index of hepatic damage. Neither enzyme is specific to the liver, but as alanine aminotransferase is found there in much higher concentration than in other organs, increases in its activity indicate more specifically that hepatic damage is present. These enzymes are of principal value in the diagnosis of acute hepatitis and in differentiating hepatocellular from obstructive jaundice. They are of no prognostic value in either acute or chronic liver disease.

Alkaline Phosphatase. This enzyme occurs in almost all tissues; in liver cells it is situated principally in the canalicular and sinusoidal membranes. Normal serum contains alkaline phosphatase activity derived mainly from bone and liver, and to a lesser extent intestine; in pregnancy additional activity of placental origin is found. When hepatocytes are damaged, relatively little alkaline phosphatase is liberated into the blood, most probably coming from cells which are killed. In hepatocellular disease, either acute or chronic, alkaline phosphatase does not usually rise more than two and a half fold. When the biliary tract is obstructed at any level, new alkaline phosphatase is synthesised in the hepatocyte membrane much of which escapes into the blood. A greatly increased blood alkaline phosphatase activity is, therefore, the main indicator of biliary obstruction though it does not give any information regarding the site of that obstruction. The alkaline phosphatase activity has no prognostic significance in liver disease.

Sometimes a raised blood alkaline phosphatase activity may be found incidentally and may be the sole abnormality. Hepatobiliary disease may be present, but it is important to ensure that the alkaline phosphatase does not have an extrahepatic origin before investigating the liver further. This may be done by electrophoretic separation of the isoenzymes of alkaline phosphase or by finding abnormal activities of enzymes more specific for the liver such as γ-glutamyl transferase or 5' nucleotidase. Bone is the main alternative origin of a raised serum alkaline phosphatase; it results from increased osteoblastic activity, such

as occurs in adolescents when it may increase up to two and a half fold, in Paget's disease, rickets, hyperparathyroidism, and in metastatic tumour in bone. Myelomatosis, though affecting bone extensively, is not associated with much bone repair, and the blood alkaline phosphatase is not usually raised. During the third trimester of pregnancy, alkaline phosphatase of placental origin may increase the serum activity up to two and a half fold.

Gamma-glutamyl Transferase (γ-GT). This is a microsomal enzyme which is distributed widely in body tissues. Increased serum γ-GT activity is a sensitive index of liver abnormality. The highest activities occur in biliary obstruction, but marked increases also occur in acute parenchymal damage from any cause. In practice, γ-GT measurements give little information in patients with liver disease beyond that provided by transferase and alkaline phosphatase measurements. Serum γ-GT activity is also increased by microsomal enzyme inducing agents (p. 339) such as alcohol and various drugs. Increased γ-GT activity can therefore be used to detect and follow alcohol abuse in patients with little or no other abnormality of liver function provided they are not taking such drugs.

Plasma Proteins. *Albumin* is synthesised solely in the liver. In chronic liver disease, especially cirrhosis, the serum albumin concentration is frequently low. Impaired albumin synthesis can be the cause, but this is not invariably so and other factors such as malnutrition, fever and the dilutional effect of fluid retention with ascites may be important. Low serum albumin concentrations in general detect patients with more severe liver damage, and a falling concentration is a bad prognostic sign. Serum albumin has a long half-life (20–26 days) and consequently changes in concentration occur slowly. Thus, even in severe acute hepatitis, the serum albumin remains normal unless the illness continues for many weeks.

Globulins. It is characteristic of chronic liver disease that hyperglobulinaemia occurs in addition to hypoalbuminaemia; it may be found irrespective of changes in the serum albumin concentration in prolonged viral hepatitis or chronic active hepatitis. Once established, hyperglobulinaemia tends to persist in most patients with cirrhosis. It represents a reaction of the monocyte–macrophage system in general and does not directly reflect liver cell damage.

The causes of hyperglobulinaemia are not fully understood; increases in gammaglobulins are prominent and probably reflect an increased activity of the immune system, to which many factors may contribute. In those with hypoalbuminaemia it may represent a response to a reduced colloid osmotic pressure in the plasma. Individual immunoglobulins are variably increased, IgG mainly in chronic active hepatitis and cryptogenic cirrhosis, IgA mainly in alcoholic liver disease and IgM in primary biliary cirrhosis. Variations, however, are so frequent that Ig measurements are not of much diagnostic value.

Plasma Protein Electrophoresis. Various changes occur in the electrophoretic pattern of the plasma proteins in cirrhosis. The commonest are a decreased albumin and an increased gammaglobulin peak. There is some relation between certain electrophoretic patterns and particular forms of liver disease, but this is not precise enough to be of great diagnostic value. Monoclonal gammopathy occurs rarely but does not have any clear diagnostic or prognostic implication.

Coagulation Factors. Severe liver damage impairs the production of several coagulation factors. This is most readily detected by the one stage prothrombin time which depends, among other things, on coagulation factors II, VII and X of liver origin. As the plasma concentration of any one of these factors has to fall to less than 30% of normal before the prothrombin time becomes abnormal, prolongation in chronic liver disease indicates severe liver dysfunction. Furthermore, as the normal plasma half-life of these factors is short (5–72 hours), prothrombin time changes occur relatively quickly after liver damage and abnormalities are found in severe acute hepatitis. Indeed, in acute hepatitis, such as viral hepatitis, the prothrombin time is a most valuable prognostic guide; an abnormal value indicates severe damage and an increasing prothrombin time indicates a progressively worse prognosis.

Vitamin K is required for coagulation factor production by the liver, and deficiency of this should be corrected by giving vitamin K_1 10 mg i.v. This is particularly important in patients with biliary obstruction in whom vitamin K is poorly absorbed.

Bromsulphthalein (BSP) Clearance. Estimation of BSP clearance from the blood is a sensitive test for hepatic dysfunction. However, the test is invalid in jaundiced patients, gives misleading results in elderly, febrile or hypoalbuminaemic patients and serious sensitivity reactions to BSP occur occasionally. These factors and the high sensitivity of enzymic tests for hepatic abnormality have led to the virtual abandonment of the BSP test. It remains of value in the diagnosis of the Dubin-Johnson syndrome (p. 000); blood concentrations of BSP are measured 45 min and 120 min after injection and a higher value at 120 min confirms the diagnosis.

Reference Values Tables 21.3 and 21.4 (p. 817).

Other Investigations of Liver Disease

Hepatitis A Virus Antigens and Antibodies. The hepatitis A antigen (HAAg) is located on a particle thought to be the hepatitis A virus (p. 349). It is excreted in the stools during the last two weeks of the incubation period, and disappears soon after onset of the clinical illness. It is not found in the blood. Antibody to the hepatitis A virus (anti-HAV) appears at or soon after the onset of symptoms and is more important in diagnosis. The mere presence of the antibody is not enough for diagnosis, as hepatitis A viral infection is common in all communities and antibody to it persists for years after infection. A rising antibody titre, or antibody of the immunoglobulin M type which defines a primary immune response, is diagnostic of recent infection. Anti-HAV measurements can be used in studies of the prevalence of hepatitis A viral infection.

Hepatitis B Virus Antigens and Antibodies. The hepatitis B virus (p. 351) contains several antigens to which infected persons can make immune responses. These antigens and their antibodies are important in identifying hepatitis B virus infection (Fig. 10.3). The hepatitis B surface antigen (HBsAg) is located in the capsular material of the virus; it can be identified by sensitive haemagglutination and radioimmunoassay methods and is a reliable marker of hepatitis B virus infection. It appears in the blood late in the incubation period or in the prodromal phase of acute type B hepatitis; it may be present for only a few days, disappearing even before jaundice has developed, but usually lasts for 3–4 weeks or may persist up to 3 months. It should therefore be sought as soon as possible in acute hepatitis. Antibody to HBsAg (anti-HBs) usually appears after about 3 months and persists for many years or perhaps permanently. The presence of anti-HBs implies only that infection has occurred at some time; seroconversion alone indicates recent infection.

The hepatitis B core antigen (HBcAg) is located in the central part of the virus and is not found in the blood. However, antibody to the core antigen (anti-HBc) appears early in the illness, rapidly reaches a high titre, and then subsides gradually. This antibody is considered to be an index of infection and of viral replication and occasionally it can reveal hepatitis B virus infection when the HBsAg has disappeared and before anti-HBs has developed (Fig. 10.3). The central part of the virus contains another antigen, the hepatitis Be antigen (HBeAg), which appears only transiently at the outset of the illness and is followed by the production of antibody (anti-HBe).

About 5% of patients become chronic carriers of the hepatitis B virus after acute type B hepatitis, and they continue indefinitely with HBsAg and anti-HBc in the blood. In some cases the HBeAg is also present (p. 352). Some healthy persons and a variable proportion of patients with chronic hepatitis (p. 357), cirrhosis (p. 360), or hepatocellular carcinoma (p. 368) are also chronic carriers of the virus. Any chronic virus carrier can transmit hepatitis, and the risk is greatest for those with chronic liver disease or with the HBeAg, in the blood. The risk of transmitting infection is low for healthy carriers who have anti-HBe and close bodily contact or direct inoculation of infected blood or other body fluids is generally required.

Hepatitis B antigens and their antibodies can be used to study the epidemiology of hepatitis B virus infection.

Other Viruses. Cytomegalovirus and the Epstein Barr virus (infectious mononucleosis) are occasional causes of acute hepatitis and infection can be detected by serological tests. There are no tests for non-A, non-B hepatitis virus infection.

Autoantibodies. Three autoantibodies in the blood are important in liver disease; antinuclear antibody, smooth muscle antibody and antimitochondrial antibody. None is specific to liver disease; antinuclear and antimitochondrial antibodies occur in connective tissue diseases and in autoimmune diseases, including various thyroid disorders and pernicious anaemia, while smooth muscle antibody has been reported in infectious mononucleosis and in a variety of malignant diseases. In liver disease, smooth muscle antibody, and to a lesser extent antinuclear antibody, may occur transiently and at low titre in acute viral hepatitis. The autoantibodies are, however, more important in chronic liver disease where they are often present for long periods of time and at relatively high titres. They are found particularly in chronic active hepatitis, cryptogenic cirrhosis and primary biliary cirrhosis. In a patient with chronic liver disease, autoantibodies indicate the likelihood of one or other of these disorders, the differential diagnosis being made on other clinical and laboratory evidence. In a patient with

Fig. 10.3 Serological response to hepatitis B virus.

cholestasis, the antimitochondrial antibody is of particular value in indicating that primary biliary cirrhosis is present. Antimitochondrial antibody occurs in primary biliary cirrhosis in 95% of cases and in less than 1% of patients with obstruction of the large biliary ducts. An antimicrosomal antibody has also been described which may become important in certain forms of chronic active hepatitis. None of the autoantibodies damages liver tissue, and they are therefore unlikely to have aetiological importance.

Alpha-fetoprotein is made mainly by the fetal liver, production falling to low levels after birth. The reappearance of substantial serum concentrations in adult life is almost always due to a hepatocellular carcinoma, though rarely it may be associated with other tumours, for example of the testis (p. 107). Such substantial serum concentrations can be detected by electrophoresis in a quarter to a third of patients with hepatocellular carcinoma in Europe and North America, and in up to three quarters of those in Africa and Asia. Lesser serum concentrations, detectable by radioimmunoassay, occur in 90% of all patients, but sometimes too in acute viral hepatitis and in chronic liver disease, particularly chronic active hepatitis. Increasing concentrations in chronic liver disease suggest hepatocellular carcinoma. Increased concentrations in the blood and amniotic fluid in pregnancy are associated with defects of the neural tube in the fetus.

Caeruloplasmin is a copper-containing globulin produced by the liver. It is important in the diagnosis of Wilson's disease in which serum concentrations are low or undetectable. Low levels may also occur in fulminant hepatic failure and in other advanced and severe chronic liver diseases, as well as in protein-losing enteropathy and malabsorption.

Serum Iron and Ferritin. The serum iron concentration and the saturation of the serum iron-binding capacity are usually high when the body iron stores are increased. A high serum iron and a highly saturated iron-binding capacity in chronic liver disease suggests haemochromatosis but is not sufficient for a diagnosis as similar results occur in chronic alcoholic liver disease. The serum ferritin concentration reflects the total body iron more closely and is increased greatly in haemochromatosis. It is also the best single indication of iron overload in the asymptomatic relatives of patients. These tests can be used to follow the effects of venesection therapy. Haemochromatosis is excluded when they are all normal.

Alpha$_1$-antitrypsin deficiency, detectable by absence of the α_1 peak on serum protein electrophoresis, is a well-established cause of liver disease in infancy and childhood. Rarely, it can cause cirrhosis or emphysema (p. 254) in adults, and occasionally both diseases occur together.

Investigative Procedures in Liver Disease

Liver biopsy is a relatively safe procedure in the hands of an experienced clinician. It is carried out with a special needle, usually through an intercostal space, using local analgesia. It requires a co-operative patient who will stop breathing when the biopsy is actually taken. The haemostatic mechanisms must be intact as indicated by the prothrombin time and platelet count. After the procedure, the patient remains in bed for 24 hours, regular pulse and blood pressure measurements must be recorded and blood for transfusion (2 units) should be available. The main complications are abdominal and/or shoulder pain, bleeding and, rarely, biliary peritonitis which usually occurs when there is obstruction of a large bile duct. Liver biopsy should never be done lightly as the mortality rate is about 0.1%.

Biopsy yields only a small sample of liver and consequently the best results are obtained in patients with diffuse liver disease. The procedure is essential in the diagnosis of chronic hepatitis and in separating its persistent and aggressive forms. It is also important in establishing a diagnosis of cirrhosis in which it may indicate a cause such as alcohol abuse or haemochromatosis. In cholestasis it may suggest obstruction of a large bile duct or give evidence of a disease of the smaller bile ducts or liver cells such as primary biliary cirrhosis. Other investigations are now preferred initially in obstructive jaundice (p. 345). Biopsy is not usually required in acute hepatitis in which the diagnosis can normally be made on other grounds; it may be needed, however, in atypical cases. Localised disease, particularly malignancy, is less accurately diagnosed unless the site of disease is first identified by some other method. Operative liver biopsy may sometimes be valuable, as in the staging of lymphoma.

Laparoscopy can be performed under local analgesia or general anaesthesia and involves the creation of a pneumoperitoneum. The laparoscope provides an excellent view of the anterior and superior surfaces of the liver as well as some of its inferior aspect and the gall bladder. The spleen, the prominent blood vessels of portal hypertension and evidence of peritoneal disease may also be seen. Biopsies can be taken directly from diseased areas which is valuable in focal disorders, especially malignant disease. The main contraindications are haemostatic abnormalities, marked ascites and previous surgery which may have caused adhesions.

Imaging. Radionuclides, ultrasound, computed tomography or nuclear magnetic resonance can be used for imaging of the liver and biliary tract. *Radionuclide imaging* is the simplest and is usually performed with technetium (^{99m}Tc) sulphur colloid which is taken up by the monocyte–macrophage system. Its greatest application is in the detection of focal hepatic disease, though lesions have to exceed 2–4 cm in diameter to be seen. Patchy uptake of ^{99m}Tc sulphur colloid by the liver and increased uptake by the spleen and bone marrow are most characteristic of cirrhosis with portal hypertension. Radionuclide imaging should be used primarily to localise liver disease prior to biopsy and should not be used on its own to make a definitive diagnosis.

Ultrasonography requires a skilled operator. It is most useful in identifying dilatation of the extrahepatic and intrahepatic bile ducts in jaundiced patients and in detecting gallstones. It is similar to radionuclide imaging in detecting focal hepatic disease and can usually differentiate between tumours and abscesses or cysts. The portal vein can be identified.

Computed tomography has indications similar to those of ultrasound. The value of *nuclear magnetic resonance* remains to be determined.

Radiological Investigation. Specialised radiological techniques may be useful in investigating the liver. Angiography can define the site and nature of localised lesions and is valuable in planning hepatic surgery. Splenoportography,

mesenteric angiography and transhepatic or perumbilical portography can all be used to investigate the portal venous system in portal hypertension prior to the surgical creation of portasystemic shunts. The portal venous pressure can be measured at splenoportography or direct portography and by catheterising the hepatic veins, as the wedged hepatic venous pressure closely reflects the portal venous pressure in cirrhosis. Hepatic venography can be used to identify hepatic venous obstruction.

Paracentesis. Analysis of ascites may give useful information. In cirrhosis, the fluid is clear, the protein content usually below 30 g/l, and in the absence of infection there are less than 250 cells/cu.mm. Blood-stained ascites is usually due to malignant disease. Ascitic protein concentrations above 30 g/l occur in peritoneal infection, especially tuberculosis, peritoneal tumour, hepatic venous obstruction and ascites associated with pancreatic disease. Amylase activity is high in ascites caused by pancreatitis. Infections, such as spontaneous bacterial peritonitis (p. 319) or tuberculosis, can be identified by bacteriological examination and malignancy by cytology.

JAUNDICE

Jaundice is a clinical term referring to the yellow appearance of the skin and mucous membranes resulting from an increased bilirubin concentration in the body fluids. It is detectable when the serum bilirubin concentration exceeds 50 μmol/l (3 mg/dl); less marked hyperbilirubinaemia is called 'latent' jaundice. Internal tissues and body fluids are coloured yellow but not the brain as bilirubin does not cross the blood-brain barrier other than in the immediate neonatal period. Pathological mechanisms giving rise to jaundice fall into three groups: haemolytic, hepatocellular and cholestatic or obstructive.

Haemolytic Jaundice

This results from an increased rate of destruction of red blood cells causing the production of more bilirubin. As a healthy liver can excrete a bilirubin load six times greater than normal before unconjugated bilirubin accumulates in the plasma, jaundice due to haemolysis is usually mild. Exceptions to this occur in the newborn when the hepatic bilirubin transport mechanism is immature and in patients with liver disease. Haemolysis may be due to intrinsic defects of the red blood cell or to various extracorpuscular factors (p. 506).

Jaundice in haemolytic anaemia is usually mild. The serum bilirubin is usually less than 100 μmol/l (6 mg/dl), and as it is dominantly unconjugated there is no bilirubinuria. Increased bilirubin excretion leads to increased stercobilinogen and stercobilin in the stools which are therefore not pale, and to increased urobilinogen in the urine as more of this substance is absorbed from the gut. The urine rapidly becomes deep yellow on standing due to urobilin formation, and in the absence of biliary obstruction the stools are dark in colour. Pallor due to anaemia and splenomegaly due to excessive reticuloendothelial activity are usually present. Investigations show anaemia and reticulocytosis, and liver function tests other than the serum bilirubin are normal.

Hepatocellular Jaundice

Hepatocellular jaundice results from inability of the liver to transport bilirubin into the bile as a result of liver cell damage. Bilirubin transport across the hepatocytes may be impaired at any point between uptake of unconjugated bilirubin into the cells and transport of conjugated bilirubin into the canaliculi. In addition, swelling of cells and oedema resulting from the disease itself may cause obstruction of the intrahepatic biliary tree. In hepatocellular jaundice the concentrations in the blood of both unconjugated and conjugated bilirubin increase, perhaps because of the variable way in which bilirubin transport is disturbed.

Acute parenchymal liver diseases, usually due to the hepatitis viruses (p. 349) or to toxins, usually drugs or alcohol (p. 349), are common causes. Immature bilirubin transport mechanisms in the newborn, especially in prematurity, and congenital defects in bilirubin transport (p. 347) are very specific metabolic defects in the liver cell causing jaundice. Chronic hepatitis and cirrhosis can also cause hepatocellular jaundice.

The clinical features vary depending on the underlying diseases. Jaundice ranges from mild to very severe.

Cholestatic Jaundice

Cholestasis is a failure of bile flow, and its cause may lie anywhere between the hepatocyte and the duodenum. Jaundice becomes progressively severe in unrelieved cholestasis because conjugated bilirubin is unable to enter the bile canaliculi and also because there is a failure of clearance of unconjugated bilirubin arriving at the liver cell.

Aetiology. Causes of cholestatic jaundice are classified according to their site in the biliary tree. They can be situated in the large bile ducts, where they may be amenable to surgical treatment, or in the smaller intrahepatic bile ducts.

Large Duct Obstruction. The most common causes are impaction of a gallstone in the common bile duct and carcinoma of the head of the pancreas. Other causes include carcinomas of the papilla of Vater or bile duct, strictures of the bile duct, usually the result of previous surgery, metastatic tumours impinging on the bile ducts, sclerosing cholangitis and, very rarely, involvement of the common bile duct by a duodenal ulcer.

Small Duct Obstruction. Widespread small duct obstruction is required to produce cholestatic jaundice. Drugs and alcohol are important causes which may exert their effects either on the liver cells or on the bile ducts. Other conditions causing obstruction are often primary diseases of the liver cells which also involve the small bile ducts, particularly the biliary canaliculi whose walls are formed by the hepatocytes, and such conditions include the cholestatic episodes which may occur in viral hepatitis, chronic active hepatitis, cirrhosis and the cholestasis of pregnancy. Cholestasis, sometimes with deep jaundice, may also occur for unknown reasons following surgery, in severe bacterial infections and in Hodgkin's lymphoma. Diseases involving the smaller interlobular ducts and the ductules include primary biliary cirrhosis and the pericholangitis of ulcerative colitis. Widespread secondary carcinoma in the liver sometimes produces cholestatic jaundice.

Clinical Features. Apart from the manifestations of the causative disease, there is jaundice which, if prolonged and severe, may give the skin a greenish appearance. The stools are pale or clay-coloured due to deficiency of bilirubin and to steatorrhoea and the urine is dark due to the renal excretion of conjugated bilirubin. Some patients have generalised pruritus, anorexia, or a metallic taste in the mouth. Upper abdominal pain occurs particularly in large duct obstruction by a gall-stone or pancreatic carcinoma.

Fever, sometimes with rigors, suggests cholangitis, which occurs most often with gallstone obstruction. A palpable gall bladder strongly suggests large-duct obstruction by a carcinoma, usually of the pancreas. The absence of this does not exclude a neoplasm. A very large and irregular liver indicates hepatic neoplasm. In prolonged obstructive jaundice, xanthomatous skin lesions, especially on the upper eyelids, occasionally appear as well as features due to secondary intestinal malabsorption; these latter include weight loss, a haemorrhagic tendency (vitamin K deficiency) and pain due to bone disease (calcium and vitamin D deficiency). In long-standing cases, clinical and biochemical evidence of hepatocellular failure occurs.

Congenital Non-haemolytic Hyperbilirubinaemia

With the exception of Gilbert's syndrome, the congenital abnormalities of bilirubin transport are very rare. In adults they all have an excellent prognosis, need no treatment and are clinically important only because they may be mistaken for more serious liver disease.

Gilbert's Syndrome. This common benign condition is usually first recognised in adolescents or young adults. It probably has a varied aetiology, and in some cases is inherited as an autosomal dominant. Gilbert's syndrome generally presents as mild jaundice, occasionally following viral hepatitis from which there has been an otherwise complete recovery, or is found incidentally. Many patients have no symptoms; others suffer episodes of malaise, anorexia and upper abdominal pain, the last occasionally severe, with increases in the jaundice. These episodes may be related to infection, fatigue or fasting.

Apart from mild jaundice, examination is normal. Investigations show unconjugated hyper-bilirubinaemia, generally below 100 μmol/l (6 mg/dl), with no abnormality of other liver function tests. No bilirubin is found in the urine. The peripheral blood count, reticulocyte count and the serum haptoglobin concentration are normal, giving no evidence of overt haemolysis. Liver biopsy is normal; in the absence of a history suggesting liver disease, a biopsy is not necessary.

The main cause of the unconjugated hyperbilirubinaemia is a deficiency of glucuronyl transferase; in some cases uptake of unconjugated bilirubin from the plasma may also be impaired. Glucuronyl transferase activity may be increased by phenobarbitone (60 mg b.d.) which can be used to diminish jaundice and to ameliorate other symptoms.

Crigler-Najjar Syndrome. In the Crigler-Najjar syndrome (type I), there is complete absence of glucuronyl transferase from the liver. It causes severe unconjugated hyperbilirubinaemia and kernicterus in the newborn leading to early death, though a few patients have survived to adulthood. This autosomal-recessive condition is very rare. A milder form (type II), due to partial deficiency of the enzyme, also occurs. Jaundice is less severe, kernicterus is rare and most survive to adult life. This condition is autosomal-dominant and is also very rare.

Dubin-Johnson Syndrome. This very rare autosomal recessive condition is caused by a reduced ability to transport organic anions, such as bilirubin glucuronide, into the biliary canaliculi. It causes malaise and variable mild jaundice. The hyperbilirubinaemia is of the conjugated type and bilirubin is found in the urine.

Other organic anions which are poorly transported include BSP (p. 342), which can be used to diagnose the condition, and the contrast agents for biliary radiology so that the gall bladder, though normal, is frequently visualised poorly or not at all on cholecystography. Liver biopsy shows a characteristic dark pigment in the centrilobular hepatocytes. The prognosis is excellent.

Rotor Syndrome. This very rare condition causes mild jaundice, due to conjugated hyperbilirubinaemia, and bilirubinuria. The liver is normal histologically and BSP clearance is unimpaired. It is probably caused by poor uptake and storage of bilirubin by the liver cells. The prognosis is excellent.

Effect of Drugs on Bilirubin Metabolism

Numerous drugs and chemicals affect biluribin metabolism. In normal adults, drugs interfering with bilirubin disposal produce only mild hyper-bilirubinaemia, sometimes without jaundice, but more marked jaundice may occur where the ability to metabolise bilirubin is impaired. This occurs in the newborn, where hyperbilirubinaemia may become sufficient to cause kernicterus (p. 651), in those with congenital nonhaemolytic hyperbilirubinaemia and in patients with chronic liver diseases such as cirrhosis. Hyperbilirubinaemia disappears readily when the drug is stopped.

The main sites at which drugs may interfere with bilirubin metabolism are shown in Table 10.1. Sulphonamides and salicylates displace unconjugated bilirubin from the binding sites on serum albumin; given to a newborn child with haemolytic disease or to the mother in late pregnancy, they may precipitate the development of kernicterus without increasing the serum bilirubin. Drugs which raise the serum bilirubin may increase either its unconjugated or conjugated forms depending on whether they act prior to or at the stage of conjugation or thereafter. Unconjugated hyperbilirubinaemia occurs when drugs produce haemolysis, impair transport from the plasma to the conjugating site or reduce conjugation itself. Conjugated hyperbilirubinaemia occurs when transport of conjugated bilirubin into the biliary canaliculus is impaired; drugs which do this also reduce BSP transport and increase BSP retention in the blood. Inducing agents, such as phenobarbitone, can increase the capacity of the liver to conjugate bilirubin so that patients on long-term treatment with such agents, e.g. epileptics, tend to have low serum bilirubin concentrations.

Oral Contraceptives. These agents usually contain an oestrogen capable of causing cholestasis and a progestogen. Occasionally they cause jaundice, almost always within the first three cycles. The serum bilirubin often exceeds 170 μmol/l (10 mg/dl) and the alkaline phosphatase activity is high indicating cholestasis. The reaction is a complex one, however, as the serum aminotransferase activity is also moderately increased and liver biopsy shows some hepatocellular damage in addition to cholestasis. Those who develop jaundice due to oral contraceptives frequently also develop cholestasis of pregnancy and both conditions may reflect an unusual hepatic reaction to a steroid agent. This may have a genetic basis as both conditions show a similar geographic distribution.

ACUTE PARENCHYMAL DISEASE OF THE LIVER

Aetiology. In acute parenchymal liver disease (acute hepatitis) there is a sudden episode of widespread damage in which variable numbers of hepatocytes undergo necrosis. These episodes are due largely to infective or toxic agents.

Table 10.1 Effects of drugs on bilirubin metabolism. Sites of action of some drugs *reducing* the plasma protein binding of bilirubin or its uptake, transport, conjugation or excretion by hepatocytes

Site of action			
Plasma	Hepatocyte		
Protein binding	*Uptake and transport*	*Conjugation**	*Excretion into canaliculus*
Sulphonamides Salicylates	Rifampicin Filix mas Cholecystographic media	Novobiocin	Sulphadiazine Oral contraceptives Methyltestosterone Anabolic steroids (C–17α alkyl substituted testosterones)
Unconjugated bilirubin		Conjugated bilirubin	

*Phenobarbitone *increases* conjugation of bilirubin.

INFECTIONS. The most important infective causes are the hepatitis A and B viruses and the non A, non B viruses. Cytomegalovirus, Epstein-Barr virus and yellow fever virus occasionally cause clinically apparent acute hepatitis. Other viruses, however, have been implicated only rarely. Less frequently non-viral agents such as *Leptospira icterohaemorrhagiae* (Weil's disease), *Toxoplasma gondii* (toxoplasmosis) and *Coxiella burneti* (Q fever) may cause acute hepatitis. Impaired hepatic function can also occur in severe extrahepatic infections, especially with septicaemia, but this is not due to infective agents reaching the liver.

TOXIC SUBSTANCES. Most substances causing acute hepatitis are drugs. How often an individual drug is responsible depends on the frequency with which it is used and in what proportion of cases hepatic damage occurs. Usually, liver damage caused by drugs is due to idiosyncratic reactions (i.e. not related to the dose of the drug and occurring in only a few individuals). Among the drugs more commonly responsible are: chlorpromazine and other phenothiazines, phenelzine and other monoamine oxidase inhibitors, imipramine, amitriptyline, erythromycin, isoniazid, rifampicin (and occasionally other antituberculous drugs), halothane, methyldopa, phenylbutazone, indomethacin, chlorpropamide and thiouracil. Liver damage due to drugs is reported increasingly, and any drug should be suspected. A few drugs cause liver damage in all people in a dose-related manner. These include tetracycline, especially in pregnancy or in those with renal dysfunction, and paracetamol which is often used in self-poisoning.

Potent liver poisons include carbon tetrachloride and yellow phosphorus. Where there are strict rules regarding their use, damage due to these agents is rare. Occasionally severe liver damage occurs from eating poisonous fungi (*Amanita phalloides*). Alcohol is by far the most important liver toxin; in addition to chronic liver damage it may produce acute alcoholic hepatitis.

CIRCULATORY DISTURBANCES. Acute hepatic damage, sometimes sufficient to cause jaundice, may be caused by any form of shock or by right ventricular failure particularly when it is severe or develops rapidly.

Pathology. Viral and most drug-induced hepatitis show similar lesions. Cell damage throughout the liver is the dominant abnormality, particularly in centrilobular areas, though individual lobules are variably affected. Damaged hepatocytes have a swollen granular appearance, while dead ones become shrunken and deeply stained, sometimes losing their nuclei to form eosinophilic Councilman bodies; these bodies, originally described in yellow fever, suggest acute hepatitis. The lobules may be infiltrated with mononuclear cells. Polymorphonuclear leucocytes and fatty change are not seen. The portal tracts are enlarged with a predominantly mononuclear cell infiltrate.

More severe damage is accompanied by collapse of the reticulin framework, particularly between the central veins and portal tracts which become linked to one another; this is known as bridging or subacute hepatic necrosis. Very severe damage results in destruction of whole lobules (massive necrosis) and is the lesion underlying fulminant hepatic failure. Cholestasis is occasionally very prominent.

Circulatory disturbances cause centrilobular congestion and necrosis.

In some patients, the main histological abnormality is fatty change. This occurs in damage due to carbon tetrachloride, tetracycline and a number of other direct toxins.

Rarely, severe fatty degeneration of the liver may be encountered in pregnancy or in Reye's syndrome in children following a viral infection.

VIRAL HEPATITIS

Viral hepatitis is almost always caused by one or other of the hepatitis viruses. They give rise to illnesses which are similar in their clinical and pathological features and which are frequently anicteric or asymptomatic.

Acute Type A Hepatitis

Aetiology and Pathology. Type A hepatitis is due to a virus which can now be cultured though currently this is done only for research purposes. It may belong to the picornavirus group of enteroviruses (p. 727). It is highly infectious and is usually spread by human faeces entering the body via the oral route directly or indirectly. Infected persons excrete viruses in the faeces for about 2 weeks before the onset of the illness and for 5 to 7 days thereafter. Children are most commonly affected and conditions of overcrowding and poor sanitation facilitate spread. In occasional outbreaks, water, milk and shellfish have been the vehicles of transmission. Though faeces is the usual source, other body constituents may also spread disease; the hepatitis may, for example, be spread by blood transfusion. Homosexual activity, especially in men, can also transmit the infection. The sources in the community appear to be persons incubating or suffering from the disease; a carrier state, analogous to that for hepatitis B virus, has not been identified. The incubation period of type A hepatitis is about a month.

The disease is generalised with involvement of the gastrointestinal tract, heart, pancreas, spleen, etc., but the main lesion is in the liver (see above).

Clinical Features. In the case of average severity, prodromal symptoms precede the development of jaundice by a few days to 2 weeks. They are the usual manifestations of an acute infectious disease, and include chills, headache and malaise. Gastrointestinal symptoms may be prominent; anorexia and distaste for cigarettes are common and early complaints, and nausea, vomiting and diarrhoea may follow. A steady upper abdominal pain occurs as a result of stretching of the peritoneum over the liver as the organ enlarges; the pain is severe in some patients. Initially physical signs are scanty; the liver is usually tender, though not readily palpable, enlarged cervical lymph nodes may be found and splenomegaly may occur, particularly in children.

Dark urine and a yellow tint to the sclerae herald the onset of jaundice. As obstruction to the biliary canaliculi develops, the jaundice deepens, the stools become paler, the urine darker and the liver more easily palpable. At this time the appetite often improves and gastrointestinal symptoms diminish in intensity. Thereafter the jaundice usually recedes, the stools and urine regain their normal colour, the liver enlargement regresses and, in the course of 3 to 6 weeks, the great majority of cases gradually recover.

Milder cases occur or the disease may run an anicteric course which is recognised by the association of vague gastrointestinal complaints or malaise with bilirubinuria and biochemical evidence of hepatic dysfunction.

Investigation. A serum aminotransferase activity exceeding 400 units/l, even before jaundice develops, is the most striking abnormality. The serum bilirubin reflects the degree of jaundice, the alkaline phosphatase activity rarely exceeds 250 units/l (30 K.A. units/dl) unless marked cholestasis develops and the albumin concentration is normal. The prothrombin time is increased in severe cases and in these circumstances is a good guide to prognosis. Bilirubinuria is an early finding, occurring in the prodromal phase and usually continuing into the convalescent period. Urobilinogenuria appears just before jaundice, disappears at the height of the jaundice owing to intrahepatic cholestasis and reappears early in convalescence as a sign of recovery. Mild proteinuria may be present. The white cell count is normal or low in uncomplicated cases, sometimes with a relative lymphocytosis; this is of some value in differentiation from Weil's disease (p. 762). Measurement of anti-HAV allows a specific diagnosis to be made (p. 342).

Differential diagnosis is discussed on page 354.

Course and Prognosis. Almost all patients make a full recovery. During convalescence 5–15% relapse with a return of symptoms and signs; these cases of *relapsing hepatitis* almost always subside spontaneously. More frequently, the serum aminotransferase activity increases without any return of clinical illness; these asymptomatic 'biochemical' relapses also subside spontaneously. Either from the onset or during the course of the illness, more severe jaundice of a clinically and biochemically obstructive type may develop and it may follow a prolonged course. Liver biopsy shows the features of hepatitis with prominent cholestasis and no evidence of chronic liver damage. This clinical syndrome is known as *cholestatic viral hepatitis* and, though it may continue for many months, the prognosis is good.

Following clinical and biochemical recovery, debility for 2 to 3 months is common. Sometimes, particularly in anxious patients, there may be prolonged malaise, anorexia, nausea and right hypochondrial discomfort without clinical, biochemical or histological evidence of liver disease. This syndrome, which may be exacerbated by too frequent clinical and biochemical assessment, is known as the *posthepatitis syndrome*; it is not due to liver disease and should be treated by reassurance.

Death from acute type A hepatitis is uncommon. In young adults, the mortality is around 0.2%. With increasing age, however, the frequency of severe episodes and death increases so that over the age of 60 years mortality reaches about 3%. Evidence regarding mortality during pregnancy is conflicting; most reports suggesting an increased mortality are derived from countries in which the standard of living is low. In Europe and North America the mortality in pregnant women is probably not increased. Those who die of the acute illness do so after developing *fulminant hepatic failure* (p. 353). Rarely, *aplastic anaemia* may occur several months after recovery from viral hepatitis. Prolonged carriage of the virus and the development of chronic liver disease are not features of hepatitis A infection.

Treatment and Prevention. There is no specific therapy; general measures applicable to all forms of acute hepatitis are discussed on page 355. Although for many years patients have been treated in general medical wards without cross-infection occurring, indicating that isolation is not essential, precautions for preventing the spread of enteric infections are advisable.

The most effective prophylactic measures are to improve social conditions, particularly overcrowded and unhygienic situations. In sporadic cases, prevention of disease in contacts cannot be achieved as the patient is infectious during the incubation and prodromal stages. However, once the disease is recognised, contacts may be protected by immune serum globulin (0.04–0.06 ml/kg i.m.), especially those at particular risk such as close contacts, the elderly, those with other major disease and perhaps pregnant women. Persons travelling to endemic areas may be protected by immune serum globulin for about 3 months. The protective effect of immune serum globulin is attributed to its anti-HAV content.

A vaccine against type A hepatitis virus is not available.

Acute Type B Hepatitis

Aetiology and Pathology. Type B hepatitis is due to a virus which cannot yet be grown but which can be transmitted to certain primates, such as the chimpanzee, in which it can replicate. The virus and an excess of its capsular material circulate in the blood where it can be identified (p. 342). The classification of the virus remains uncertain, but its core contains DNA and has DNA polymerase activity. Blood and certain blood products are the main sources of infection. Coagulation factor concentrates which are manufactured from a plasma pool and cannot be sterilised are a particular hazard and account for the high incidence of hepatitis in haemophilia. Only blood products subjected to pasteurisation (albumin solutions, γ-globulin fraction) can be regarded as largely free of risk. Spread may follow transfusion of infected blood or blood products or injections with contaminated needles, a mode of spread most common among parenteral ('mainline') drug abusers who share needles. Tattooing or acupuncture may also spread this disease as needles are reused frequently.

The ability to identify the hepatitis B virus has led to the realisation that it may cause sporadic infections which cannot be attributed to parenteral modes of spread. Infected serum can transmit disease orally and the discovery of the HBsAg in body fluids, such as saliva, urine, semen and vaginal secretions, suggests many alternative modes of spread. Close personal contact seems necessary for spread and sexual intercourse, especially in male homosexuals, seems an important route of transmission. Finally, the virus may be spread from mother to child; transmission at or soon after birth seems more likely than transplacental spread. Humans are the only source of the hepatitis B virus; in addition to those incubating or suffering from the disease, some asymptomatic individuals carry the virus in the blood over long periods, perhaps for life. The incubation period of type B hepatitis is about 3 months. A negative test for the HBsAg in the blood does not exclude type B hepatitis (p. 342).

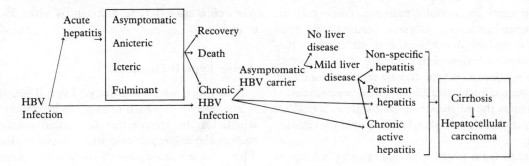

Fig. 10.4 HBV infection. Range of possible clinical effects.

The pathology is as for type A hepatitis (p. 349).

Clinical Features. The clinical features are similar to, but usually more severe than those of type A hepatitis. Transient rashes, including urticaria, may occur and arthralgia or arthritis is common. Though these can occur in type A hepatitis, they are much more suggestive of type B hepatitis. The latter tends to be a more severe disease than type A. The mortality depends on the virulence of the virus, the age of the patient and any underlying disease: In about 5% of cases chronic hepatitis B carriage follows the acute episode.

Chronic Asymptomatic Carriers. Some individuals with no history of acute hepatitis and lacking clinical evidence of liver disease are chronic carriers of the hepatitis B virus. They all have the HBsAg and anti-HBc in the blood, and some also have the HBeAg (p. 343) and DNA polymerase activity (p. 351). The frequency of chronic carriers in northern Europe and in North America is about 0·1%, but higher frequencies (1–15%) are found in Mediterranean countries, in Africa, and in Asia. Most asymptomatic chronic carriers have normal liver function tests and need not undergo liver biopsy as significant histological abnormalities are uncommon. Persistent biochemical abnormalities are more common in those with the HBeAg or DNA polymerase in the blood, and liver biopsy should be considered.

The prognosis for chronic asymptomatic carriers is uncertain, but the virus can be carried for many years without severe chronic liver disease occurring. Some develop chronic hepatitis and cirrhosis and there is an increased risk of hepatocellular carcinoma (Fig. 10.4). Close body contact and the body fluids of these individuals can transmit infection, particularly when the HBeAg, DNA polymerase activity, or liver disease are present, and precautions are therefore needed when they undergo medical or dental treatment.

Patients with impaired immune responses are very liable to become chronic carriers; this occurs particularly in Hodgkin's disease and other lymphomas, in those on immunosuppressive drugs, in patients on long-term dialysis, and in institutionalised patients with Down's syndrome.

Treatment and Prevention. No specific treatment is available. Supportive therapy is described on page 355.

Post-transfusion type B hepatitis can be largely prevented by scrupulous blood transfusion technique, by using volunteer donors and excluding those with a history of jaundice and by screening all blood for the HBsAg, using highly sensitive methods. Non-A, Non-B hepatitis viruses are now the cause of most cases of post-transfusion hepatitis, though type B virus hepatitis still occurs occasionally. Hepatitis caused by plasma can be virtually eliminated by limiting plasma pool sizes to 10 donors, but this cannot be done for the production of coagulation factor concentrates which carry a relatively high risk of hepatitis. Sterile needles and syringes should always be used and if disposable equipment is not available these should be autoclaved for 20 minutes at 120°C. Thorough washing followed by boiling in water for 20 minutes is an acceptable emergency procedure. Strict precautions should be observed by all persons involved in handling human blood.

Type B hepatitis can be prevented or minimised by the intramuscular injection of hyperimmune serum globulin prepared from blood containing anti-HBs. Where available, it should be given to persons without HBsAg in their blood within 24 hours, or at the most a week, of exposure to infected blood in circumstances likely to cause infection; these include accidental needle puncture, gross personal contamination with infected blood or exposure to infected blood in the presence of cuts and grazes.

A hepatitis B vaccine capable of producing active immunisation in all but about 5% of normal individuals has become available. This American vaccine is made by purifying HBsAg from the plasma of chronic hepatitis B virus carriers in such a way as to exclude the hepatitis B virus itself. The vaccine gives a high degree of protection and has proved safe so far, but it is expensive and supplies are limited. Its use can be considered in those at special risk of infection who are not already immune as evidenced by anti-HBs in the blood. Such persons include patients with haemophilia and those needing multiple blood transfusion, drug addicts, homosexuals, spouses of chronic hepatitis B virus carriers, and patients on long-term renal dialysis. Medical staff can also be considered where there is special risk. This includes particularly dentists and medical and nursing staff in emergency rooms, intensive care areas and renal, liver and oncology units. Laboratory staff are protected best by stringent technical precautions in handling blood products. The vaccine is ineffective in those already infected by the hepatitis B virus.

Non-A, Non-B Hepatitis

The existence of non-A, non-B hepatitis was recognised once infection with the hepatitis A and B viruses could be excluded by specific serological methods. The responsible agent or agents cannot yet be identified, but they can transmit infection in humans and confer specific immunity. Non-A, non-B hepatitis is diagnosed by excluding hepatitis A and B, cytomegaloviral, and Epstein-Barr viral infections. It may cause about a quarter of sporadic cases of acute viral hepatitis and it is known to cause 90% or more of post transfusion hepatitis in North America and Europe.

Long and short incubation forms of the disease occur, the clinical features are similar to those of type A and type B hepatitis and a chronic carrier state can follow infection. Immune serum globulin, useful in type A hepatitis, may also prevent or ameliorate non-A, non-B hepatitis the contribution of which to the production of chronic liver disease is not yet known.

Fulminant Hepatic Failure

Fulminant hepatic failure is a rare syndrome in which hepatic encephalopathy, characterised by mental changes progressing from confusion to stupor and coma, results from sudden severe impairment of hepatic function. The syndrome is defined further as occurring within 8 weeks of onset of the precipitating illness, in the absence of evidence of pre-existing liver disease, to distinguish it from those instances in which hepatic encephalopathy represents a deterioration in chronic liver disease.

Aetiology and Pathology. Acute viral hepatitis is the commonest cause, drugs (p. 349) being the next most frequent. Rarely, it occurs in pregnancy, in Wilson's disease, following shock or from poisons such as carbon tetrachloride. Reye's syndrome (p. 349) causes fulminant hepatic failure in children and adolescence.

Extensive parenchymal necrosis is the most obvious lesion (p. 349). In fatal cases, less than 30% of the liver cells appear viable histologically and often few such cells are seen. Severe fatty degeneration is characteristic of such causes of this syndrome as tetracycline, pregnancy and Reye's syndrome.

Clinical Features. Cerebral disturbance (encephalopathy) is the cardinal manifestation of fulminant hepatic failure. Its cause is unknown, but it is thought to be due to toxic substances, including ammonia, nitrogenous compounds which may act as false neurotransmitters and fatty acids. The earliest features are reduced alertness and poor concentration progressing through behaviour abnormalities including restlessness, aggressive outbursts and mania, to drowsiness and coma. Confusion, disorientation, inversion of sleep rhythm, slurred speech, yawning, hiccoughing and, in the late stages, convulsions may occur. More general symptoms include weakness, nausea, and vomiting. Right hypochondrial pain is only an occasional feature.

Examination shows jaundice which develops rapidly and is usually deep in fatal cases though, rarely, death may occur before it develops. Fetor hepaticus, a sweet musty odour to the breath, may be present and is said to be due to methyl mercaptan. A flapping 'hepatic' tremor of the extended hands is characteristic. The liver may be enlarged initially, but later becomes impalpable. Hepatic dullness on percussion may disappear indicating much shrinkage and a bad prognosis. Splenomegaly is uncommon and never prominent. Ascites and oedema occur in a few patients surviving a week or more. Purpura and overt bleeding such as melaena reflect severe haemostatic disturbance. Neurological examination may show pupillary abnormalities, chorea, muscle spasticity and extensor plantar responses. Other features include fever, sweating, hypotension, tachycardia, hyperventilation and renal failure.

Investigation. The serum bilirubin reflects the degree of jaundice. Initially, serum aminotransferase activity is high, as in acute viral hepatitis, but with progression of damage activity falls; this investigation has diagnostic but not prognostic significance. Alkaline phosphatase activity is variable. Serum albumin concentration remains normal unless the course is prolonged. Increased serum and urine amino acids are characteristic but are not generally measured. The prothrombin time rapidly becomes prolonged as coagulation factor synthesis fails; this is the laboratory test of greatest prognostic value, a progressive and marked prolongation being a very bad sign. White blood cell counts vary, leucocytosis occurring even in the absence of infection. The urine contains protein, bilirubin and urobilinogen.

Liver biopsy is contraindicated because of the severe haemostatic deficiency and because it rarely gives information required for management. Viral causes are sought serologically (p. 342). Wilson's disease (p. 366) should always be considered in patients under 30 years old.

Course and Progress. The progress of fulminant hepatic failure is closely related to the encephalopathy. When only minor signs are present and drowsiness is not prominent some two-thirds of patients survive. Once the patient is comatose only 10 to 20% survive. The prognosis is worse with increasing age and, perhaps, when due to certain agents such as halothane. In fatal cases, death usually occurs within a week. Life-threatening complications, some amenable to conservative therapy, may arise in the course of the illness. These include profound hypoglycaemia, cerebral oedema, respiratory failure, hypothermia, bacterial infections, bleeding due to coagulation disorders, pancreatitis and renal failure with severe oliguria. Electrolyte disturbances, particularly hyponatraemia, hypokalaemia and alkalosis, may also occur. The great majority of those who recover from fulminant hepatic failure regain normal hepatic structure and function.

Treatment. There is no specific therapy. Supportive measures are described on page 355.

Differential Diagnosis of Acute Parenchymal Disease of the Liver

Most patients with acute parenchymal liver disease are suffering from viral hepatitis. This diagnosis depends on the clinical features described above, a history of contact with a jaundiced person or of transfusion, or damage to the skin when handling blood within an appropriate incubation period, the results of liver function tests, and serological tests for the A and B hepatitis viruses. The possibility of drug-induced hepatitis should always be considered, the diagnosis depending on exposure to the drug within 2 weeks of the onset of symptoms with no other detectable cause for the illness.

In the pre-icteric phase there may be confusion with other acute generalised infections, acute abdominal emergencies when pain is present, or gastroenteritis. Especially in young persons, there may be confusion with *infectious mononucleosis* in which sore throat, lymphadenopathy and splenomegaly are prominent, atypical blood lymphocytosis is present, and the Paul-Bunnell test generally positive; in this disease abnormal liver function tests are common and jaundice may occur. *Cytomegalovirus infection* should be considered in those with poor immune responses who have received blood transfusion; a specific antibody response occurs, virus may be isolated from the urine, and giant cells and intranuclear inclusions found on liver biopsy.

Weil's disease (p. 762) may cause severe jaundice. In contrast to viral hepatitis, there is a polymorphonuclear leucocytosis and protein, blood and casts are found in the urine. The diagnosis is made by demonstrating a rise in specific antibodies, and leptospires may be isolated from the blood or urine.

A most difficult problem is to differentiate jaundice due to viral hepatitis from that due to *large-duct biliary obstruction* usually caused by a stone or a neoplasm. This is particularly so when an episode of viral hepatitis becomes prolonged and obstructive features develop. Clinically, a patient over 40 years old, previous attacks of abdominal pain, the gradual onset of fluctuant or progressive jaundice, marked pruritus, weight loss and right upper quadrant abdominal pain or a palpable gall-bladder indicate a large duct obstruction. Leucocytosis or a positive test for blood in the stool also suggest large-duct obstruction. Liver function tests are of greatest value at an early stage; in viral hepatitis serum alkaline phosphatase does not usually exceed 250 units/l (30 KA units/dl) and serum aminotransferase activity almost always exceeds 400 units/l, while in biliary obstruction the reverse usually obtains. This laboratory differentiation becomes less clear as the disease progresses, however, and in biliary obstruction cholangitis may increase serum aminotransferase activity. A plain radiograph of the abdomen may show gallstones, though only 10% of these are radio-opaque. Ultrasonography is of greatest value in revealing dilated bile ducts caused by large bile duct obstruction and by showing gallstones. Oral cholecystography and intravenous cholangiography are of no value in these jaundiced patients; the biliary tract may be demonstrated by either transhepatic cholangiography or endoscopic retrograde cholangiopancreatography (p. 283). Liver biopsy may also be useful in revealing hepatitis or features of bile-duct obstruction. The HBsAg and the antimitochondrial antibody must always be sought. Where viral hepatitis is a possibility, laparotomy should be avoided as such patients withstand anaesthesia and surgery poorly.

Treatment of Acute Parenchymal Disease of the Liver

Aetiological Factors. In most cases nothing can be done to eliminate the cause of the disease. It is important to detect drug-induced acute hepatitis so that the drug may be stopped and the patient warned to avoid its use in future. Penicillin, given early, is effective in Weil's disease (p. 762).

Bed Rest When symptoms are marked, bed rest should be advised, the patient rising to the toilet if desired. Thereafter, the younger patient may be up and about taking care only to avoid exhaustion. For those in whom the risks of hepatitis may be greater, bed rest should be empirically prolonged until symptoms and signs have disappeared and liver function tests have returned substantially towards normal. These patients include those over 50 years, the pregnant, and those with other major disease.

Diet. A good general diet containing some 3000 kcal daily is desirable. Initially, owing to anorexia and nausea, this is usually not tolerated, in which case a light diet supplemented by fruit drinks and glucose is usually acceptable. The content of the diet should be dictated largely by the patient's wishes; however, a good protein intake should be encouraged. If vomiting is severe, intravenous fluid and glucose may be required for a few days.

Drugs. Corticosteroids have been advocated in viral hepatitis. Current evidence, however, is that they do not aid recovery and that they may cause serious side-effects. In general, therefore, they should not be used. On the other hand, in patients with marked malaise, anorexia or vomiting they may cause rapid regression of symptoms with return of appetite. In this small group of patients, prednisolone may be given provided the HBsAg test is negative as there is some evidence that corticosteroids may lead to chronic HBs antigenaemia. The dose is reduced rapidly from 20 mg daily as symptoms remit. Drugs metabolised in the liver should be avoided where possible, a principle applying especially to sedative and hypnotic agents. Alcohol must be avoided during the illness and should not be taken in the ensuing 6 months. Oral contraceptives may be resumed after clinical and biochemical recovery.

Fulminant Hepatic Failure. There is no specific treatment but certain measures should be instituted as soon as possible once cerebral changes occur. The patient's life is sustained in the hope that hepatic regeneration will take place spontaneously. There should be close observation so that steps may be taken quickly to correct complications as they occur. The development of encephalopathy greatly alters management.

Encephalopathy is treated by withdrawing all nitrogen intake, by reducing the nitrogen-producing colonic flora with neomycin, (1 g orally 6 hourly) and by increasing faecal output with lactulose (p. 364). If tests for stool blood are positive the colon should be washed out. Electroencephalography may be used to follow the course of the encephalopathy. Sedative drugs must be used with very great care, restlessness and excitement being best controlled, if necessary, with diazepam 5 mg intravenously.

Cerebral oedema is a frequent cause of death and is difficult to diagnose as it often develops rapidly and rarely causes papilloedema. It can present as a sudden respiratory arrest. Unequal or abnormally reacting pupils, local or general myoclonus or focal fits, increasing hyperventilation, decerebrate posturing, fixed dilated pupils and continuing spontaneous respiration all point to cerebral oedema and the appearance of any one indicates the need for treatment. Mannitol 20% (1 g/kg body weight) should be infused intravenously rapidly, and the dose repeated if the clinical signs are not reversed. Most patients need two doses (range 1–4) for any one episode of cerebral oedema. Dexamethasone is of no value.

Nutrition. Calories are provided as glucose 300 g daily either orally, if necessary by nasogastric tube, or into a large central vein as a 10–20% solution (0·6–1·2 mol/*l*). Fluid and electrolyte therapy depends on maintenance of accurate fluid balance records and on daily measurements of serum urea, sodium, potassium and bicarbonate. Saline must be used cautiously to avoid sodium overload, and potassium deficiency, which occurs readily, should be corrected. The blood glucose should be measured 4 hourly in the severe phase as potentially fatal hypoglycaemia often occurs; its treatment may require large amounts of glucose. Estimations can be made simply by using dip-stick tests, but some checks by a laboratory method should also be made.

Haemorrhage. As these patients have poor vasomotor control, early detection of bleeding and rapid correction of blood volume by transfusion are required. This is facilitated by regular recordings of pulse, blood pressure, hourly urine output and if possible central venous pressure. Impaired haemostasis leads to bleeding, particularly from the gastrointestinal tract. Intramuscular injections are best avoided. The development of a bleeding tendency is detected by regular haemoglobin, platelet count, prothrombin time and faecal occult blood measurements. Treatment is discussed on page 546. Cimetidine (30 mg i.v. hourly) or ranitidine (25 mg/h/i.v. for 2 hours every 6–8 hours) should be given to prevent gastrointestinal bleeding.

Infection is common and serious. As fever and leucocytosis may result solely from the liver disease itself, they are no guide and regular blood, urine, and throat cultures and chest radiographs should be carried out. Prophylactic antibiotics should not be used; if infection is strongly suspected they may be given once specimens have been taken for culture. Suitable regimens are gentamicin and clindamycin or cefuroxime.

Other Measures. A close watch on the respiration is needed as initial hyperpnoea may rapidly become apnoea, requiring tracheostomy and assisted ventilation. Renal failure, revealed by a rising blood urea, may eventually require dialysis. The temperature must be measured 4 hourly as hypothermia can follow central loss of temperature control.

Fulminant hepatic failure requires intensive patient care, access to varied specialised help, and a hospital with great technical resources. Many special treatments have been tried. None is of proven value and some involve the risk of infecting staff; they include exchange transfusion, plasmapheresis, haemodialysis, and extracorporeal circulation of the patient's blood through various animal livers, isolated or *in situ*, or through coated-charcoal columns. Corticosteroids, or gammaglobulin containing anti-HBs in HBsAg positive cases are of no value.

CHRONIC PARENCHYMAL DISEASE OF THE LIVER

There are two main forms of chronic parenchymal liver disease: (1) chronic hepatitis, which comprises chronic persistent hepatitis and chronic active hepatitis, and (2) cirrhosis.

Aetiology. There are many causes of chronic hepatitis and cirrhosis. In Britain, cirrhosis is usually associated with alcohol abuse, chronic active hepatitis or primary biliary cirrhosis. No cause can be found in 30% of cases. Haemochromatosis accounts for about 5% of patients and all other causes are rare.

Alcohol. The mechanism whereby alcohol damages the liver is unknown; it is now, however, accepted as a direct liver toxin in man and in other primates. The production of cirrhosis requires a prolonged intake of alcohol of about 80 g or more daily for 5 to 15 years. Women may be at greater risk of liver damage than men, and a daily alcohol intake may be more likely to cause cirrhosis than episodic drinking.

Infection. Rarely, patients can develop cirrhosis over a few months or years after viral hepatitis. In some patients with chronic hepatitis or cirrhosis, the proportion showing marked geographic variation (0–30%), the HBsAg is found persistently in the blood and in such cases the hepatitis B virus is presumably the causative agent. The non-A, non-B viruses can cause chronic infection and are likely causes of chronic liver disease. The hepatitis A virus does not cause chronic liver disease.

Metabolic Disorders. These include excess hepatic deposition of iron in haemochromatosis and of copper in Wilson's disease. Most other metabolic conditions involving the liver manifest themselves first in childhood, e.g. glycogen storage disease, fibrocystic disease and α_1-antitrypsin deficiency.

Drugs. Chronic hepatitis and cirrhosis have been reported in patients on long-term treatment with methotrexate or methyldopa. Other drugs (e.g. phenylbutazone, sulphonamide) have been cited occasionally.

Cholestasis. Prolonged obstruction anywhere in the biliary tree may cause cirrhosis. In primary biliary cirrhosis, obstruction results from damage to interlobular bile ducts. Cirrhosis from large-duct obstruction may occur with biliary strictures or in sclerosing cholangitis. Neoplastic lesions do not cause cirrhosis as survival is short.

Congestion. Prolonged hepatic congestion can eventually cause cirrhosis. This is rare, as death usually occurs before cirrhosis develops. Congestion may be due to hepatic venous outflow obstruction, as in the Budd-Chiari syndrome (p. 367) or chronic heart failure.

Immunological Factors. Some patients with chronic liver disease of unknown cause have abnormal serum antibodies (p. 342). Though the autoantibodies themselves are not cytotoxic, their presence has suggested that liver damage may be produced by abnormal immune mechanisms. Currently, the possibility that sensitised lymphocytes may do this is being investigated; lymphocytes from patients with chronic liver disease have been shown to react to antigens in liver and bile and to be capable of damaging liver cells *in vitro*. The importance of these reactions in chronic liver disease, however, remains to be established. Immune reactions are also likely to be important in chronic liver disease caused by the hepatitis B virus.

Malnutrition. This often occurs secondarily in patients with cirrhosis, but it is unlikely that it is primarily responsible for cirrhosis. Permanent liver damage does not follow marasmus or kwashiorkor.

Cryptogenic Cirrhosis. In this heterogeneous group, no cause can be found.

Pathology. 1. CHRONIC HEPATITIS. Two types of chronic hepatitis are recognised histologically. Their names — persistent hepatitis and aggressive hepatitis — are easily confused with the clinical syndromes they underlie — chronic persistent hepatitis and chronic active hepatitis; this should be avoided.

In *persistent hepatitis* the essential feature is an infiltration of chronic inflammatory cells confined to the portal tracts which may be expanded or show short fibrous septa extending into the parenchyma. Changes in the hepatocytes are absent or slight; there may be small foci of liver cell necrosis with inflammatory cell infiltration (spotty necrosis) and sometimes the residual changes of viral hepatitis. Lobular architecture is normal and cirrhosis only rarely develops.

In *aggressive hepatitis*, the histological process underlying the clinical condition chronic active hepatitis, both the portal tracts and the parenchyma are involved, lobular architecture is distorted and cirrhosis often develops. The portal tract infiltration of mononuclear cells extends irregularly into the surrounding parenchyma so that swollen liver cells become isolated in the inflammatory cell infiltrate. This process of hepatocyte destruction is called 'piecemeal necrosis' and it leads to septum formation linking portal tracts and central veins. The ensuing disruption of lobular architecture is accompanied by the development of regenerative nodules and then by cirrhosis. Changes in the rest of the parenchyma are variable and resemble those of persistent hepatitis. These changes do not occur diffusely and may be more advanced in some areas than others, a point to be considered in interpreting biopsies.

2. CIRRHOSIS. In cirrhosis, widespread death of liver cells resulting from many causes is accompanied and followed by progressive fibrosis, regenerative (nodular) hyperplasia of surviving hepatocytes, and distortion of liver architecture resulting in portal-systemic vascular shunts. The whole liver is involved, though not necessarily every lobule. Cirrhotic livers have an infinitely variable appearance limiting the usefulness of anatomical classifications. Currently, a simple classification into micronodular, macronodular and mixed cirrhosis is used.

Micronodular cirrhosis is characterised by regular connective tissue septa, regenerative nodules approximating in size to the original lobules (1 mm in diameter) and involvement of every lobule. This form, also called portal, septal, nutritional, monolobular, or Laënnec's cirrhosis, is characteristic but not pathognomonic of the parenchymal damage induced by alcohol.

In *macronodular cirrhosis* the connective tissue septa vary in thickness and the nodules show marked differences in size, the larger ones containing histologically normal lobules. This form is also called posthepatitic or postnecrotic cirrhosis.

Mixed cirrhosis shows features of both micro-

nodular and macronodular cirrhosis. None of these types of cirrhosis is static; micronodular cirrhosis may, for example, develop into a macronodular stage.

1. CHRONIC HEPATITIS

It is important not to confuse gradually resolving acute hepatitis with chronic hepatitis. As there is no certain way to avoid this by clinical assessment or investigation, including biopsy, a diagnosis of chronic hepatitis should only be made firmly once liver disease has been present on clinical or other grounds for at least 6 months.

Chronic Persistent Hepatitis

Aetiology is discussed on page 357; pathology (persistent hepatitis) on page 357. Symptoms are mild and comprise fatigue, poor appetite, fatty food intolerance and upper abdominal discomfort, especially over the liver. The condition may be asymptomatic and revealed by biochemical tests done for other reasons. There may or may not be a history of acute hepatitis. Examination may show slight hepatomegaly, but is often normal. There are no features of chronic liver disease.

Serum bilirubin is normal or slightly raised, serum aminotransferase is raised up to fivefold and alkaline phosphatase is generally normal. Serum albumin and globulin are normal. The HBsAg may be present but autoantibodies are not found. Liver biopsy shows persistent hepatitis.

Differentiation should be made from the posthepatitis syndrome (p. 351) and Gilbert's syndrome (p. 347), as well as from the pericholangitis associated with Crohn's disease and ulcerative colitis (p. 321). The prognosis is usually excellent, the patient should be reassured and no treatment is required. Rarely, progression to chronic active hepatitis or cirrhosis may occur.

Chronic Active Hepatitis

Aetiology is discussed on page 357; pathology (aggressive hepatitis) on page 357.

Clinical Features. Chronic active hepatitis (CAH) is a more severe disease than chronic persistent hepatitis, but recently less severe forms of the disease have become increasingly recognised. No clinical classification has yet proved satisfactory, but patients with CAH associated with chronic hepatitis B virus infection on the whole have less florid signs of disease. CAH associated with hepatitis B virus infection occurs most often in males over 30 years of age and comes to attention when an episode of acute viral hepatitis fails to resolve, with the features of cirrhosis, or even incidentally in an asymptomatic individual. Examination often reveals little of note; hepatomegaly is the most common abnormality, jaundice is slight or absent and fewer than a third of patients have spider telangiectasia or splenomegaly. Systemic features other than arthralgia are uncommon.

CAH not associated with hepatitis B virus infection is usually a more florid disease though it too shows a wide range of severity. It occurs predominantly in females in the second and third decades. The onset is usually insidious with fatigue, anorexia and jaundice. Other features include fever, arthralgia, epistaxis and ready bruising. Amenorrhoea is the rule. In about a quarter of cases the onset is acute, resembling viral hepatitis which, however, does not resolve normally. On examination, the general health appears good; jaundice is mild to moderate or occasionally absent. Signs of chronic liver disease, especially spider telangiectasia and hepatosplenomegaly, are almost always present. Sometimes a 'Cushingoid' face with acne, hirsutism and pink cutaneous striae, especially on the thighs and abdomen, are present. Bruises may be seen.

Though liver disease usually dominates the clinical syndrome, many associated conditions occur in chronic active hepatitis emphasising its essentially systemic nature. These include migrating polyarthritis of large joints, a variety of rashes, most nonspecific but including inflammatory papules and urticaria, lymphadenopathy, thyroid disorders such as Hashimoto's thyroiditis, thyrotoxicosis and myxoedema, Coombs'-positive haemolytic anaemia, pleurisy, transient pulmonary infiltration, ulcerative colitis and glomerulonephritis. Some patients have Sjögren's syndrome (p. 554).

Investigation. Liver function tests vary; the activity of the disease is indicated by the serum aminotransferase activity, and the severity of liver damage is reflected in the serum albumin concentration and the prothrombin time. Abnormalities are often relatively mild at presentation in CAH associated with hepatitis B virus infection, but in the other forms of CAH, aminotransferase activity in relapse is usually more than ten times increased and hypoalbuminaemia and marked hyperglobulinaemia are common. The serum bilirubin reflects the degree of jaundice but usually does not exceed 100 μmol/l (6 mg/dl). The serum alkaline phosphatase activity reflects the degree of intrahepatic cholestasis. The HBsAg is found in patients with hepatitis B infection. Autoantibodies are often found in patients without hepatitis B infection; antinuclear antibodies are found in half the patients, smooth muscle antibodies in two thirds and antimitochondrial antibodies in a quarter.

Diagnosis and Prognosis. Differentiation from acute viral hepatitis can be impossible when CAH presents with an acute exacerbation. An acute hepatitis showing unremitting activity (aminotransferase increased at least tenfold, or increased at least fivefold with serum gammaglobulin increased at least twice) for 10 weeks is likely to be due to CAH, but in all cases the diagnosis should not be considered certain until a biopsy done at least 6 months after the onset is examined. Drugs should always be sought as a cause and Wilson's disease must be excluded (p. 366). Where ulcerative colitis coexists, cholestatic features suggest pericholangitis or sclerosing cholangitis rather than chronic active hepatitis. Difficulty in differentiation from persistent hepatitis usually occurs where the liver biopsy does not confirm the clinical diagnosis and in these cases a further biopsy is needed.

Most patients eventually progress to cirrhosis with the development of portal hypertension (p. 360), ascites (p. 360) and encephalopathy (p. 361). The course of CAH associated with autoantibodies is marked by exacerbations and remissions, and about half the patients die of liver failure within 5 years if no treatment is given. CAH due to hepatitis B virus infection progresses more slowly and usually without exacerbations.

Treatment. Corticosteroids are life-saving in

CAH not caused by hepatitis B virus infection, especially in the early stages, reducing activity and improving hepatocellular function. Initially, prednisolone 30 mg/day is given orally and the dose reduced gradually as the patient and liver function tests improve. Treatment for at least a year is needed, when gradual withdrawal of prednisolone may be tried. Relapse is frequent and prolonged maintenance therapy (10–15 mg/day) is often required. Where severe corticosteroid side-effects occur, azathioprine 50–100 mg/day orally may be given and the prednisolone reduced by half. Ascites, encephalopathy and portal hypertension are treated (p. 363). Corticosteroids do not seem to be of any value in CAH due to hepatitis B virus infection.

2. CIRRHOSIS OF THE LIVER

Aetiology is discussed on page 357 and pathology on page 357.

Clinical Features. These vary greatly and may include any combination of the manifestations described below. None is specifically related to particular causes of cirrhosis, though florid spider telangiectasia, gynaecomastia and parotid enlargement are more common in alcohol-associated cirrhosis. Autopsy experience shows that cirrhosis may be entirely asymptomatic, and in life it may be found incidentally at surgery or with minimal features such as isolated hepatomegaly. Enlargement of the liver tends to be more common in the early stages of the disease, disappearing as hepatocyte destruction and fibrosis reduce liver size. The patient may complain of weakness, fatigue or weight loss. Non-specific digestive symptoms such as anorexia, nausea, vomiting and upper abdominal discomfort may occur as does gaseous abdominal distension. Otherwise, clinical features are due mainly to portal hypertension and/or hepatic insufficiency.

Portal Hypertension. This results from destruction and distortion of the hepatic vasculature leading to obstruction of blood flow. In addition, there may be transmission of arterial pressure to the portal venous system. Cirrhosis is the commonest but not the only cause of portal hypertension; obstruction of the portal vein, e.g. from thrombosis, may have the same effect (p. 367).

Splenomegaly is caused mainly by portal hypertension and is its cardinal sign. The splenomegaly is seldom marked in adults, the tip rarely reaching more than 5 cm below the costal margin. In childhood and adolescence it may be much more marked. When the spleen is not enlarged clinically or radiographically, portal hypertension is unlikely.

Haematological Changes. Moderate leucopenia and thrombocytopenia frequently occur with splenomegaly and are attributed to hypersplenism (p. 538). Anaemia may occur and when hypochromic is usually due to blood loss from the gut. Macrocytes and target cells are common; though the marrow is usually normoblastic, megaloblastic anaemia sometimes occurs. Megaloblastic changes are usually due to nutritional folate deficiency; vitamin B_{12} deficiency is rare.

Collateral Circulation. This occurs where there are portal-systemic communications. These are in the distal oesophagus and proximal stomach, in the anus and distal rectum, in the falciform ligament and between the colonic, omental, splenic and retroperitoneal veins. Collateral vessels may be seen on the anterior abdominal wall and rarely they radiate prominently from the umbilicus ('caput medusae'). A venous hum can occasionally be heard over a large umbilical collateral vessel. The most important collateral vessels are in the oesophagus and stomach (oesophagogastric varices) as they can cause bleeding which may be severe and acute, or occult and chronic. Bleeding may occur from varices elsewhere in the gut but this is very rare. The presence of oesophagogastric varices establishes a diagnosis of portal hypertension. Special radiological procedures can demonstrate the patency of the splenic and portal veins, assess the extent of collateral circulation and allow the portal pressure to be measured (p. 345).

Ascites. Ascites in cirrhosis is due to a combination of liver failure and portal hypertension. Liver failure leads to salt and water retention by decreasing renal blood flow which produces both a reduced glomerular filtration rate with excessive tubular resorption of water and sodium, and an increased renal release of renin leading to secondary hyperaldosteronism. Failure of the liver to metabolise aldosterone intensifies the secondary aldosteronism and failure to metabolise vasopressin reduces renal water clearance. Hypoalbuminaemia lowers the colloid oncotic pressure of the plasma, encourages the formation of oedema and may contribute to a poor renal blood flow. Portal hypertension and lymphatic obstruction in the liver predispose to the localisation of fluid in the abdomen.

Jaundice. This is mainly due to failure of bilirubin metabolism. Intrahepatic cholestasis may also be a contributing factor. In cirrhosis jaundice is generally mild or absent. Increasing jaundice implies progressing liver failure.

Circulatory Changes. In cirrhosis the circulation tends to be hyperdynamic with increased peripheral blood flow and reduced visceral blood flow especially to the kidneys. The cause for this is unknown. Increased peripheral blood flow is indicated by palmar erythema. Arteriolar changes result in cutaneous *spider telangiectases*; these lesions comprise a central arteriole, which may raise the skin surface, from which small vessels radiate. They are usually confined to the area above the nipples and occur especially on the face, necklace area, forearms and dorsum of the hands. At an early stage they may appear as white spots on cooling the skin.

Reduced arterial oxygen saturation is frequent and central cyanosis may occur; this is probably due to the development of pulmonary venoarterial shunts and similar shunts may predispose to the development of clubbing of the fingers.

Endocrine Abnormalities. Gynaecomastia, sometimes unilateral, may occur. It can result from the liver disease or may be induced by spironolactone therapy. Loss of libido occurs in both sexes; there is impotence and testicular atrophy in men and breast atrophy and irregular menses or amenorrhoea in premenopausal women.

Haemorrhagic Tendency. This is found in advanced liver failure and is due largely to underproduction of coagulation factors (p. 539). Thrombocytopenia may also occur particularly when splenomegaly is present. It is seldom sufficient to cause spontaneous bleeding but may aggravate bleeding from other causes such as varices. Serum fibrinogen concentration is not reduced until the terminal stages, though occasionally fibrinolysis may be significant. Bruis-

ing, purpura, epistaxis, menorrhagia or gastrointestinal bleeding can all occur.

Skin Pigmentation. Generalised hyperpigmentation due to increased melanin deposition occurs in a minority; haemochromatosis must then be excluded.

Dupuytren's Contracture. Various studies have suggested that there is an increased incidence of Dupuytren's contracture in patients with cirrhosis but the statistical evidence for this is poor.

Fever. About a third of cirrhotic patients have a low-grade fever not due to infection.

Hepatic (Portal-systemic) Encephalopathy. The mental and neurological features described in fulminant hepatic failure (p. 353) occur in cirrhosis in a more chronic and intermittent fashion. This complication sometimes overshadows the liver disease and leads to a diagnosis of primary mental disorder. Rarely, irreversible central nervous system changes occur with paraplegia, parkinsonism, epileptic fits and dementia.

In addition to liver failure, the collateral venous circulation in cirrhosis bypasses the liver and allows nitrogenous substances from the gut to reach the systemic circulation thereby increasing the tendency to encephalopathy. Where anastomoses are extensive, encephalopathy may even occur despite relatively good liver function; this is rare in cirrhosis alone, but may be seen following a surgical portal-systemic shunt.

A number of factors precipitate hepatic encephalopathy in the cirrhotic patient including sedatives, a high protein diet, infection, trauma including surgery, gastrointestinal bleeding, hypokalaemia and constipation.

Renal Failure. Renal failure consequent on liver failure can occur in cirrhosis. The kidneys themselves are intrinsically normal, and renal failure is thought to result from a diminished renal flood flow. The condition is called functional renal failure of cirrhosis or the *hepatorenal syndrome*. It occurs in advanced cirrhosis, usually with ascites, and uraemia is characterised by the absence of proteinuria or abnormal urinary sediment, a urine sodium less than 10 mmol/day and a urine/plasma osmolality ratio greater than 1·5. The prognosis is very poor.

Investigation. The serum bilirubin may be normal; increases are very variable. Bilirubinuria may or may not be present, but excessive urobilinogenuria is usual. Serum aminotransferase activity is usually slightly increased by up to three-fold and serum alkaline phosphatase is raised similarly. All these tests may be normal and they are of no prognostic value. The serum albumin is reduced and the prothrombin time remains prolonged in spite of parenteral vitamin K in those with poor liver function; these tests, especially sequential results, are of considerable value as deteriorating levels indicate a poor outlook. The serum globulin is raised. BSP retention is almost always increased, though falsely normal values may occur in hypoalbuminaemia. Autoantibodies or the HBsAg may be found.

Differential Diagnosis. Alternative diagnoses to be considered depend on how the patient presents, for example with haematemesis (p. 360) or ascites (p. 360). In those with hepatomegaly, secondary carcinoma should be especially considered where enlargement is gross, irregular and hard and where the spleen is not palpable. The site of the primary tumour may be found. A primary liver tumour is also possible (p. 368). Cardiac failure, tricuspid valve disease and constrictive pericarditis should be sought especially where the liver is large, smooth and tender. Rarer causes of hepatomegaly include lymphoma, leukaemia, amyloidosis, sarcoidosis, abscess and hydatid cyst. In the tropics, kala azar, malaria or schistosomiasis may be present. Finally, a cause for cirrhosis must be sought, especially one which is treatable, such as haemochromatosis or Wilson's disease.

Prognosis. Although cirrhosis is a progressive disease, the rate of progression varies and the outlook is related to many factors. The prognosis is better where the cause of cirrhosis can be corrected, as in alcohol abuse, haemochromatosis and Wilson's disease. Worsening liver function evidenced by jaundice or ascites indicates a poor prognosis unless a treatable cause such as bleeding or infection is present. Encephalopathy not associated with an extensive collateral circulation is a poor prognostic sign and, as with ascites, a poor response to therapy is ominous. Acute bleeding from oesophageal varices is fatal in about 50% of cases. Marked hypoalbuminaemia (below 25 g/l), hyponatraemia (below 120 mmol/l) not due to diuretic therapy and a prolonged prothrombin time are bad prognostic signs. The course of cirrhosis is uncertain as unforeseen complications such as severe infection or hepatocellular carcinoma may lead to death.

Treatment is discussed on page 363.

BILIARY CIRRHOSIS

Biliary cirrhosis results from prolonged obstruction anywhere between the small interlobular bile ducts and the papilla of Vater.

Primary Biliary Cirrhosis. This disease affects predominantly women, usually in middle age. It was previously considered rare, but is now recognised as relatively common, affecting about 1 in 40 000 in Britain. A chronic granulomatous inflammation of unknown cause destroys the interlobular bile ducts in the liver with the eventual development of cirrhosis. Immune complexes are found in the blood but their importance in producing liver damage is unknown. Pruritus is the commonest initial complaint and may precede jaundice by months or even years. When the patient is jaundiced, pruritus is almost always present. Although there may be upper abdominal discomfort, the abdominal pain, fever and rigors of large bile-duct obstruction do not occur. Diarrhoea resulting from malabsorption of fat, and pain and tingling in the hands and feet due to lipid infiltration of peripheral nerves occasionally occur. Bone pain or fractures due to osteomalacia from malabsorption or osteoporosis are often prominent later.

Initially patients are well-nourished, but considerable weight loss can occur as the disease progresses. Scratch marks may be found. Jaundice is only prominent late in the disease when the patient may become a bottle-green colour. Xanthomatous deposits occur in a minority especially around the eyes, in the hand creases and over the elbows, knees and buttocks. Hepatomegaly is virtually constant. Splenomegaly occurs later as portal hypertension develops. The disease generally lasts 5 to 10 years terminating in liver failure or alimentary bleeding.

The diagnosis is based on the clinical picture, on liver function tests showing cholestasis, especially a very high serum alkaline phosphatase activity greater than 250 units/l (30 KA units/dl), and on a positive antimitochondrial antibody test. It is confirmed by liver biopsy and by the absence of dilated bile ducts on ultrasonography.

No specific therapy is available. Azathioprine is of no value and corticosteroids are contraindicated as they exacerbate or precipitate bone disease. Penicillamine has been used with contradictory results, and as it causes serious side-effects in up to a third of patients it cannot be recommended. Palliative measures, e.g. for pruritus, are described on page 365.

Secondary Biliary Cirrhosis. This develops after prolonged large duct biliary obstruction due to gallstones, bile duct strictures and, occasionally, sclerosing cholangitis (p. 365). There is chronic cholestasis with episodes of ascending cholangitis or even liver abscess manifested by upper abdominal pain, tender hepatomegaly, fever, rigors, leucocytosis and sometimes a positive blood culture or septicaemic shock. Finger clubbing is common and xanthomas and bone pain may develop. Cirrhosis, ascites and portal hypertension are late features.

Treatment of Hepatic Cirrhosis

Although no treatment can reverse cirrhosis or even ensure that no further progression occurs, medical therapy can promote improved general health and alleviate symptoms. The main problems are to detect treatable causes, to correct malnutrition, to control fluid retention, encephalopathy and alimentary bleeding and to manage chronic cholestasis. There is no satisfactory treatment for the hepatorenal syndrome.

Aetiological Factors. Treatable conditions such as alcohol abuse, drug ingestion, haemochromatosis and Wilson's disease should always be sought. Relief of biliary obstruction will prevent biliary cirrhosis.

Nutrition. In the absence of encephalopathy or ascites, a high energy (3000 kcal/day), protein-rich (80–100 g/day) diet should be advised. Where cholestasis is not a feature, fat intake need not be restricted. Alcohol must be forbidden. When a good diet is taken, vitamins and other supplements are not required.

Ascites. Treatment of ascites and oedema may relieve symptoms but does not improve the prognosis and, if over vigorous, may lead to fatal renal failure. Sources of excessive sodium intake should be sought and corrected first. These may be very salty foods, sodium-containing drugs such as certain antacids (sodium bicarbonate, magnesium trisilicate mixture, and magnesium carbonate mixture) alginates, salicylates, and effervescent calcium, or sodium-retaining drugs such as carbenoxolone, nonsteroidal anti-inflammatory agents and steroid hormones. Thereafter, in milder cases salt restriction alone may be sufficient; by using salt in cooking while avoiding salt at table, especially salty foods such as soups, ham and bacon, daily salt intake may be reduced to about 2 g of sodium chloride daily (40 mmol of sodium).

More severe ascites requires diuretics. Initially, a potassium sparing drug such as spironolactone (100–200 mg/d) or triamterene (100–200 mg/d) should be used. Additional diuresis may be obtained from a medium potency diuretic such as bendrofluazide. Potassium supplements may not be necessary with this drug combination but hypokalaemia should be avoided as it may precipitate or worsen encephalopathy.

Patients with marked ascites should be admitted to hospital. They generally have more severe liver dysfunction and require more vigorous therapy to which they are apt to react adversely. Bed rest, restriction of water intake to 1 l/d, restriction of salt to 22 mmol of sodium daily (1 g salt) and potassium supplements may induce diuresis. If this does not occur within 4 days spironolactone or triamterene should be added and potassium intake reduced. Only when this has failed should high potency diuretics such as frusemide (40–160 mg) be used. Treatment should aim to produce a weight loss of 0·5–1 kg/d, and regular checks should be made of the blood urea and electrolyte concentrations.

Occasionally patients do not respond to treatment; many are continuing to take salt and this should be checked. The temptation to remove fluid by paracentesis must be resisted as patients tolerate this very badly; up to 5 l may be removed over an hour without great risk to relieve respiratory distress caused by gross ascites. Ascites unrelieved by medical therapy can often be helped by a LeVeen shunt which carries ascites directly to the central veins. Intravenous reinfusion of ultrafiltered ascites or intravenous infusions of salt-poor albumin (25 g) over 3 hours with frusemide (40–80 mg i.v.) may also initiate diuresis in resistant cases. In special centres a Rhodiascit machine to ultrafilter ascites and return its colloid to the patient can be used.

Hepatic Encephalopathy. Episodes of encephalopathy develop in many patients with cirrhosis and are usually readily reversed until the terminal stages occur. The principles of treatment are as in fulminant hepatic failure (p. 356). All dietary protein is stopped or reduced below 20 g/d, and glucose (300 g/d) is given orally or parenterally.

Lactulose (15–30 ml t.i.d.) is given to produce two stools daily. Lactulose is a disaccharide which reaches the colon intact and is then split by colonic bacteria. It produces an osmotic laxative effect, reduces the pH of the colonic content thereby limiting colonic ammonia absorption and promotes the incorporation of nitrogen into bacteria. If the effect of lactulose is disappointing then neomycin may be added in a dose of 4–6 g/day. Neomycin, which acts by reducing bowel flora, is also used as an alternative to lactulose if diarrhoea becomes troublesome. Although neomycin is poorly absorbed a careful watch should be kept for ototoxic effects from long-term use especially if there is any uraemia.

As encephalopathy improves, dietary protein is increased by 10–20 g/d on alternate days to an intake of 40–60 g/d which is usually the limit in these cirrhotic patients. Levodopa (500 mg/d) and bromocriptine (1–5 mg/d) have been advocated for those who fail to improve adequately.

Variceal Bleeding. Acute bleeding from oesophagogastric varices is frequently severe. Blood transfusion is required, and every effort should be made to avoid hypotension which reduces liver blood flow and can produce significant liver damage. Measures to stop the bleeding include the reduction of portal venous pressure and portal blood flow, the local application of pressure to the varices, embolisation of vessels feeding the varices, operations on the varices themselves and portal-systemic shunt operations.

REDUCTION OF PORTAL VENOUS PRESSURE. *Vasopressin* helps to arrest bleeding by constricting the splanchnic arterioles and thereby reducing portal pressure and blood flow. It can be given intravenously in a dose of 20 units in 200 ml of 5% glucose over 20 minutes, and this may need to be repeated 3–4 times at hourly intervals as the drug is destroyed rapidly. Abdominal colic, evacuation of the bowels and facial pallor from general arteriolar constriction indicate that vasopressin is active, and absence of these suggests an inert preparation. Vasoconstriction can cause angina, arrhythmia and even myocardial infarction and vasopressin should not therefore be used in patients with ischaemic heart disease. Vasopressin can also be given by intravenous infusion 0·4 unit/minute until bleeding stops or for 24 hours and then 0·2 unit/minute for a further 24 hours. Cessation of bleeding is judged from nasogastric aspiration and from the pulse and blood pressure.

Glypressin (triglycyl lysine vasopressin) is a suitable alternative to vasopressin with certain advantages. Glypressin itself is not active, but vasopressin is released from it over several hours in amounts sufficient to reduce the portal pressure without producing systemic, including cardiac, effects. It is given in a dose of 2 mg intravenously every 6 hours until bleeding stops and then 1 mg every 6 hours for a further 24 hours. Cessation of bleeding is judged from nasogastric aspiration, pulse and blood pressure.

Propranolol has been advocated as a medical means for reducing portal venous pressure and preventing variceal bleeding but its efficacy remains to be proved fully.

LOCAL MEASURES. When initial bleeding has been controlled, its source should be determined by *endoscopy* as about a quarter of patients with varices are bleeding from some other lesion, especially acute gastric erosions. Persistent or recurrent bleeding from varices should then be controlled by a *Sengstaken tube*. This possesses two inflatable balloons which exert pressure in the lower oesophagus and gastric fundus. A useful modification, the *Minnesota tube*, allows secretions to be aspirated from the upper oesophagus when the balloons are inflated.

Transhepatic Embolisation. Persistent or recurrent bleeding can also be controlled by passing a catheter through the liver into the portal vein and obliterating the collateral vessels by injecting sclerosing material. Recurrent bleeding following treatment with a Sengstaken tube and/or transhepatic embolisation of the varices requires injection of the varices or surgery.

SURGERY and SCLEROTHERAPY. Surgical treatment is best restricted to an oesophageal transection of the varices which can now be done relatively easily with a stapling gun, though this technique does carry some risk of subsequent oesophageal stenosis. Emergency portal-systemic shunt surgery carries a mortality of 50% or more and is rarely practicable.

Recurrent variceal bleeding is the rule rather than the exception in patients who have had bleeding from oesophageal varices, and in the past *portal-systemic shunt surgery* was recommended widely for these patients as it effectively reduces recurrent bleeding. There has, however, been increasing dissatisfaction with this treatment as the operations do not prolong life and often cause troublesome hepatic encephalopathy perhaps because the shunts used previously (portacaval, splenorenal and mesocaval) divert all the portal blood away from the liver. In contrast the relative ease of endoscopy with fibreoptic instruments has led to a resurgence of interest in *injection sclerotherapy* for varices. Varices are injected with a sclerosing agent as soon as practicable after bleeding is controlled, and injections are repeated every 1–2 weeks thereafter until the varices are obliterated. Regular follow-up is then necessary to allow treatment of any recurrence of varices. The treatment is not free of risk as injections can cause ulceration and stricture formation, but, in general, morbidity is low; even those with poor liver function can be treated and recurrent bleeding is largely prevented.

Portal-systemic shunt surgery may still be preferred for some patients, and if possible a selective shunt, such as the distal splenorenal (Warren) shunt, which decompresses the varices while preserving much of the portal blood flow to the liver should be done as encephalopathy ensues much less frequently. Shunts should be considered only for those under 60 years of age with good liver function evidenced by good general health, no ascites or evidence of encephalopathy, serum bilirubin less than 35 μmol/l (2·0 mg/dl),

and serum albumin over 35 g/l. There is no place for the prophylactic use of shunt operations in patients with varices who have not bled.

Chronic Cholestasis. Where this is associated with irremediable large duct biliary obstruction, episodes of cholangitis require antibiotics. Such treatment should be reserved for exacerbations and not given continuously.

Pruritus, believed to be due to bile acids, is the main symptom demanding relief. This is best achieved with the anion-binding resin cholestyramine, which reduces the bile acids in the body by binding them in the intestine and increasing their excretion in the stool. A dose of 4–16 g/day orally is used. The powder is mixed in orange juice and the main dose (8 g) is taken with breakfast when maximal duodenal bile acid concentrations occur. Cholestyramine may bind other drugs in the gut (e.g. anticoagulants); the latter should therefore be taken one hour before the binding agent.

Anion-binding resins are not helpful in complete biliary obstruction; then methyltestosterone (25 mg sublingually daily) or, for women, norethandrolone (10 mg orally thrice daily) is usually effective. These drugs, however, increase cholestasis at the canalicular membrane and jaundice invariably worsens. Anion-binding resins and the androgens usually relieve pruritus within a week.

Steatorrhoea. Prolonged cholestasis is associated with steatorrhoea and malabsorption of fatsoluble vitamins and calcium. Steatorrhoea can be reduced by limiting fat intake to 40 g/day. Medium chain triglyceride supplements can be used to augment calorie intake. Monthly injections of vitamin K_1 (10 mg), vitamin D (calciferol 2·5 mg; alfacalcidol 1 μg/d orally) and calcium supplements should also be given, the last as effervescent calcium gluconate (2–4 g/day). This preparation, however, contains much sodium and, where there is fluid retention, calcium gluconate alone should be used.

MISCELLANEOUS DISEASES OF THE LIVER

Primary Haemochromatosis. This is an uncommon disease in which excessive iron absorption over years leads to a gross increase in total body iron from the normal level of 4 g to 20–60 g. It is caused by a genetic defect associated with the histocompatibility antigen HLA-A3. Iron is deposited widely: the important organs involved are the liver, pancreas, endocrine glands and heart. In the liver, iron deposition occurs first in the peripheral hepatocytes extending later to all hepatocytes. The gradual development of fibrous septa leads to the formation of irregular nodules and finally regeneration results in macronodular cirrhosis.

Clinical features generally occur in men aged over 45 years, menstruation and pregnancy providing protective mechanisms in women in whom the disease is ten times less common. There may be manifestations of hepatic cirrhosis, diabetes mellitus or heart failure. Leaden-grey skin pigmentation due to excess melanin and iron occurs especially in exposed parts, axillae, groins and genitalia, hence the term 'bronzed diabetes'. Impotence, loss of libido and testicular atrophy are also common.

The serum iron concentration is increased and the serum iron binding capacity is usually over 70% saturated. The serum ferritin is also high (p. 344). The diagnosis is confirmed by liver biopsy.

Haemochromatosis must be distinguished from other forms of cirrhosis, especially that due to alcohol in which there may be excess liver iron. Differentiation must also be made from other causes of excess body iron discussed below.

Treatment is by weekly venesection of 500 ml (250 mg iron) until the serum iron is normal; this may take 2 years or more. Thereafter, venesection is done to keep the serum iron normal. Other therapy includes that for cirrhosis and diabetes mellitus.

Secondary Haemochromatosis. Many conditions are associated with widespread secondary siderosis. Though they may cause features similar to haemochromatosis, these are rare and the history suggests the true diagnosis. Primary conditions include chronic haemolytic disorders, sideroblastic anaemia (p. 499), multiple blood transfusion (generally over 150 l) and dietary iron overload (p. 62). Marked hepatic siderosis may also occur in alcoholic cirrhosis.

Wilson's disease (hepato-lenticular degeneration) is a rare but important autosomal recessive condition caused by an abnormality of copper metabolism. Normally, dietary copper is absorbed from the stomach and proximal small intestine, and is rapidly taken up into the liver where it is stored, and incorporated into caeruloplasmin which is secreted into the blood. The functions of caeruloplasmin are unknown. The accumulation of excessive copper in the body is prevented by its excretion, and the most important route is via the bile. The precise nature of the biliary chemical defect in Wilson's disease is unknown, but it results in a failure of copper excretion leading to its accumulation in the body. There is almost always a failure of synthesis of caeruloplasmin also, though occasional patients with Wilson's disease have a normal plasma caeruloplasmin concentration. The amount of copper in the body at birth in Wilson's disease is normal but thereafter it increases steadily; the organs most affected by this are the liver, the basal ganglia of the brain and the eyes.

The clinical features usually arise between the ages of 5 and 30 years. Hepatic disease occurs predominantly in childhood and early adolescence while neurological damage causes basal ganglion syndromes (p. 651) in later adolescence. These manifestations can occur alone or simultaneously. Most patients presenting with Wilson's disease have Kayser-Fleischer rings, though these may be detectable only by slit-lamp examination; they are the most important single clinical pointer to the diagnosis. Kayser-Fleischer rings are characterised by a greenish-brown discolouration of the corneal margin appearing first at the upper periphery. They eventually disappear when treatment is given. Other manifestations include haemolysis, renal tubular damage and osteoporosis, but these are virtually never presenting features.

The clinical features of liver damage are not specific. Episodes of acute hepatitis can occur, especially in children, and may progress to fulminant hepatic failure. Chronic persistent hepatitis and chronic active hepatitis can also develop, and eventually cirrhosis with liver failure and portal hypertension.

Any patient under 35 years of age with recurrent hepatitis, chronic hepatitis or cirrhosis of unknown cause should be investigated for Wilson's disease. A family history of hepatic or neurological disease and Kayser-Fleischer rings are the most important clinical clues to the diagnosis, and a low serum caeruloplasmin concentration is the best single laboratory test. However, any cause of liver failure can lead to a low serum caeruloplasmin and occasionally the serum caeruloplasmin is normal in Wilson's disease. Other features of a disordered copper metabolism should therefore be sought; these include a low serum copper concentration, a high urine copper excretion (p. 820) and a very high hepatic copper content (p. 819). Rarely, it may be necessary to demonstrate failure of the liver to incorporate radioactive copper into caeruloplasmin.

The copper-binding agent penicillamine is the drug of choice in Wilson's disease. The dose given must be sufficient to produce cupriuresis and most patients require 1·5 g/day (range 1–4 g). The dose can be reduced once the disease is in remission, but treatment must continue for life and care taken to see that reaccumulation of copper does not occur. Young women should continue to take the drug during pregnancy as it does not seem to be teratogenic. Serious toxic effects of penicillamine (p. 560) are fortunately rare in Wilson's disease. If they do occur triethylene tetramine dihydrochloride is the next drug of choice.

The prognosis of Wilson's disease is excellent provided treatment is started before irreversible damage is done, and the long-term complication of hepatocellular carcinoma does not occur as it does in haemochromatosis. Siblings of patients with Wilson's disease should also be investigated and treatment should be given to any who have the disease even if it is asymptomatic.

Non-cirrhotic Portal Hypertension. Portal hypertension is virtually always due to obstruction to the portal blood flow somewhere in the portal venous system. The obstruction may be outside the liver (extrahepatic presinusoidal) in the portal or splenic vein where the result is the development of collateral vessels bypassing the obstruction as well as portal hypertension. Umbilical infection in the neonatal period is believed to be an important cause but other conditions leading to thrombosis include polycythaemia

vera, malignant invasion from adjacent organs and pancreatitis.

Obstruction in the portal tract (intrahepatic presinusoidal) may also be responsible and causes include schistosomiasis, congenital hepatic fibrosis, myeloproliferative disease, exposure to arsenic or vinyl chloride and primary biliary cirrhosis. Mixed intrahepatic obstruction is usually caused by cirrhosis but other causes include the Budd-Chiari syndrome and polycystic disease of the liver.

Cirrhosis is the commonest cause of portal hypertension in Europe and North America, but schistosomiasis is the commonest cause worldwide. Portal hypertension due to increased portal blood flow is exceptionally rare.

Hepatic venous outflow obstruction is an uncommon condition. It can occur in the larger hepatic veins (*Budd-Chiari syndrome*) and obstruction may be due to thrombosis, especially in polycythaemia vera and in women taking oral contraceptives, to invasion by tumours of the liver, kidney, or adrenal, or to congenital venous webs. In up to three-quarters of patients no cause can be found for the obstruction. The same syndrome may also develop in constrictive pericarditis or right ventricular failure. Obstruction may also follow damage to the central hepatic veins in *veno-occlusive disease*, occurring especially in children in Jamaica due to ingestion of toxic alkaloids in 'bush tea' infused from plants.

The condition generally develops fairly rapidly with abdominal pain, tender hepatomegaly and ascites. Liver biopsy shows severe centrilobular congestion. Hepatic venous obstruction is demonstrated angiographically. Mild cases can recover completely but severer cases often die rapidly or go on to develop cirrhosis.

Congenital hepatic fibrosis is a rare condition in which broad fibrous bands are found in the liver. Most patients have associated polycystic renal disease. Many die in early childhood of renal failure. Those who survive often develop gastrointestinal bleeding due to portal hypertension, usually presenting between 5 and 30 years of age.

The Liver in Protozoal and Helminthic Infections. Protozoal infections associated with liver changes include malaria, trypanosomiasis, visceral leishmaniasis, toxoplasmosis and amoebiasis; the last is the most important as it causes liver abscesses which respond promptly to treatment (p. 773). In some cases of persistent malarial infection gross splenomegaly and portal hypertension develop (p. 771).

Schistosomiasis is the most significant helminthic infection as it may cause portal hypertension (p. 784). Echinococcosis, giving rise to hydatid liver cysts (p. 789), is the next most important. Rarely the roundworm, *Ascaris lumbricoides* (p. 791), may obstruct the common bile duct, and liver flukes (p. 789) may cause inflammation and adenocarcinoma of the bile ducts.

Cysts. Solitary cysts are rare, probably congenital, vary greatly in size and occur more frequently in the right lobe.

Polycystic disease is characterised by many cysts of variable size; half the patients have associated polycystic disease of the kidneys (p. 405). Cysts may be found elsewhere as in the pancreas and lungs. Some patients have cerebrovascular aneurysms.

Hepatic cysts are usually found incidentally. Occasionally a large cyst may cause upper abdominal pain, nausea, vomiting and a palpable mass. Complications are rare and include obstructive jaundice, torsion, bleeding and rupture. Portal hypertension may occur in the polycystic form. Liver function tests are usually normal. Cysts show as rounded filling defects on radionuclide liver scans.

TUMOURS OF THE LIVER

Primary Malignant Tumours. *Hepatocellular carcinoma (hepatoma)* is the principal primary liver tumour. Its incidence shows great geographic variation, being common in Africa and S.E. Asia but rare in temperate climates. It occurs predominantly in males, and in 80% of cases cirrhosis is present. Cirrhosis may be of any type, but hepatocellular carcinoma appears most commonly in haemochromatosis and alcoholic cirrhosis, dominantly male diseases, and rarely in primary biliary cirrhosis, which mainly affects women. Other aetiological factors include chronic hepatitis B viral infection, ingestion of aflatoxin-contaminated foods in tropical countries (p. 720) and exposure to toxins such as thorotrast and arsenic. These last toxins usually produce angiosarcomas but they may also cause hepatocellular carcinomas. Oestrogens and androgens may cause adenomas or rarely hepatocellular carcinomas.

Macroscopically, the tumour may be a single mass or there may be multiple tumour nodules. Microscopically, the tumour is made up of trabeculae of well-differentiated cells resembling hepatocytes. Bile secretion by tumour cells may be seen and is diagnostic.

Deterioration in a patient with cirrhosis should always lead to suspicion of hepatocellular carcinoma, the clinical features of which include weakness, anorexia, weight-loss, fever, abdominal pain, abdominal mass and ascites. Hepatocellular carcinomas are vascular so that a bruit may be heard over the liver or intra-abdominal bleeding may occur. Metabolic abnormalities are recognised increasingly and include polycythaemia, hypercalcaemia, hypoglycaemia and porphyria cutanea tarda.

The detection of high concentrations of α-fetoprotein (p. 344) in the blood is virtually diagnostic. A liver scan almost always reveals a filling defect(s) and the diagnosis may be confirmed by liver biopsy. Surgical removal requires a tumour confined to one lobe in the absence of cirrhosis and is rarely feasible; the possibility should always, however, be considered. Doxorubicin (p. 528) can provide useful palliative therapy.

Other primary tumours are rare; they include haemangioendothelial sarcomas and adenomas. Cholangiocarcinoma is described on page 374.

Secondary malignant tumours are common and usually originate from carcinomas in the bronchus, breast, abdomen or pelvis. They may be single or multiple. Peritoneal dissemination frequently results in ascites.

Symptoms of the primary neoplasm are absent in about half the cases. Hepatomegaly may suggest cirrhosis, but splenomegaly is rare. There is usually rapid liver enlargement with fever, weight loss and jaundice. A raised alkaline phosphatase activity is the commonest abnormality but the liver function tests may be normal. Ascitic fluid has a high protein content, may be blood-stained and cytology may reveal malignant cells. Diagnosis can be made by needle biopsy in the area of a filling defect on liver scan or at laparoscopy.

Benign Tumours. Hepatic adenomas are rare vascular tumours which may present as an abdominal mass or with abdominal pain or intraperitoneal bleeding. They are more common in women and may be caused by oral contraceptives.

THE GALL BLADDER AND BILE DUCTS

ANATOMY AND PHYSIOLOGY

The junction of interlobular bile ducts leads to the formation of the right and left hepatic ducts which exit from the liver in the porta hepatis. These join immediately to form the common hepatic duct which, with the common hepatic artery and portal vein, lies in the free edge of the lesser omentum. The common hepatic and cystic ducts join to form the common bile duct which varies in length (2–9 cm) depending on where the junction occurs. The common bile duct, passing towards the duodenum, is usually divided into supraduodenal, retroduodenal, intrapancreatic and intraduodenal portions; it is, however, more useful to separate it into a thin-walled, wide-lumened proximal part up to 10 mm in diameter radiologically, and a thick-walled, narrow-lumened distal part 1–3 cm in length which may taper to a thread radiologically. The thick-walled part starts just outside the duodenal wall; it may be seen radiologically as a notch and is formed by the muscular choledochal sphincter (sphincter of Oddi). The common bile and pancreatic ducts usually fuse in the duodenal submucosa to enter the second part of the duodenum at the apex of the papilla of Vater.

The gall bladder is a pear-shaped sac of about 50 ml capacity situated under the right hepatic lobe. Its fundus lies close to the tip of the right ninth costal cartilage, its body and neck passing posterosuperiorly into the cystic duct which runs in a series of S-bends to join the common hepatic duct. Congenital abnormalities of the biliary system are rare; a folded gall bladder fundus ('phrygian cap') may be seen radiologically and biliary atresia or a choledochal cyst may occur.

The liver secretes bile continuously, producing 1–2 litres daily at a pressure of 15–25 cm of water. As the resting pressure in the common bile duct is somewhat higher than that in the gall bladder, bile enters the latter where it is concentrated about 10-fold by water and electrolyte absorption. The intraluminal pressure in the common bile duct is probably maintained by the choledochal sphincter. Bile duct pressures above 30 cm of water inhibit bile secretion. Reflux of bile into the pancreatic duct often occurs normally.

The gall bladder receives an autonomic nerve supply, mainly from the vagus; acetylcholine causes contraction of gall-bladder muscle and it is likely that vagal innervation controls gall-bladder tone while the sympathetic nerve supply has little or no effect. Gall bladder contraction is due mainly to cholecystokinin secreted by the duodenal mucosa in response to food (p. 280). The choledochal sphincter normally opens and closes rhythmically; cholecystokinin and glyceryl trinitrate cause it to relax, while secretin and the analgesic drugs morphine, pethidine and pentazocine cause contraction. Of the analgesic drugs, pentazocine causes least sphincteric contraction. Acetylcholine has variable effects. Peristalsis does not occur in the common bile duct.

INVESTIGATION

Radiological Investigation. *A plain radiograph* may show stones in the gall bladder or bile ducts, the soft tissue mass of an inflamed gall bladder, gas in the biliary tree due to a fistula into the intestine or pancreatic calcification. Only 10% of gallstones are radio-opaque.

Cholecystography. An iodine-containing compound is used which is absorbed from the gut, excreted into the bile and concentrated in the gall bladder so that it becomes radio-opaque; it is given the night before the investigation. The normal gall bladder shows as a homogeneous ovoid opacity. Non-opaque gallstones may show as 'filling defects' within the opaque area; much less commonly a tumour may do the same. Failure of the gall bladder to opacify is a frequent finding in gall bladder disease (non-functioning gall bladder). However, failure to take, or vomiting of, the tablets, pyloric stenosis, diarrhoea, occasionally intestinal malabsorption, poor liver function or a serum bilirubin above 35 μmol/l (2 mg/100 ml) can produce the same result. In addition, for unknown reasons, a normal gall bladder may fail to opacify in up to 20% of cases; for this reason the test should then be repeated, doses of the contrast medium being given on each of the 2 days prior to the test. If the gall bladder still fails to opacify, it is virtually certain to be diseased.

Intravenous cholangiography. Iodipamide methylglucamine (Biligrafin) given intravenously is excreted by the liver into bile. Provided liver function is good and the serum bilirubin not above 35 μmol/l the main biliary ducts and the gall bladder will be shown. This investigation may be used in those who have had a cholecystectomy. The extent of opacification of the biliary tree is much less than that achieved by cholecystography so that gallstones cannot be excluded confidently by this method. Furthermore side effects due to Biligrafin are fairly frequent; these can be reduced by infusing it slowly over an hour.

Percutaneous transhepatic cholangiography is of value in patients with obstructive jaundice and it may be done if the prothrombin time and platelet count are satisfactory. Under local analgesia, a narrow bore (Okuda) needle is passed into the liver and contrast material is injected under radiological control until a bile duct is entered. Where there is large-duct obstruction, the dilated biliary tree is usually entered readily allowing a demonstration of the site and often the nature of the obstruction. Less frequently the biliary tree is shown to be normal. Failure to enter the biliary tree cannot be taken to exclude fully a large duct obstruction. While narrow-bore needles have reduced the risk of biliary leakage and peritonitis, facilities for surgery should be available.

Operative Cholangiography. During operations on the biliary tract, the biliary tree should always be defined by injecting contrast material, either via the cystic duct or directly into the common bile duct.

Endoscopic Retrograde Cholangiopancreatography. (ERCP, p. 283).

Ultrasonography is the best method for the initial investigation of jaundice as it is capable of demonstrating dilatation of the biliary tree due to mechanical obstruction (p. 345). It can detect gallstones, and is particularly valuable for this purpose in pregnancy. Ultrasonography can also show the size of the gall bladder and the thickness of its wall. Results are much less satisfactory in obese patients.

Cholescintigraphy is a safe means of demonstrating biliary excretion and can be used to detect bile duct obstruction and cholecystitis.

GALLSTONES

Gallstone formation is the commonest disorder of the biliary tract. Indeed, gall bladder disease in its absence is a rarity.

Epidemiology and Pathology. The prevalence of gallstones is not known as in most instances they are asymptomatic; they are common in North America, Europe and Australia, but less frequent in India and the Far East, and rare in African blacks. The incidence of gallstones rises with age. In those less than 40 years there is a 3:1 female preponderance whereas in the elderly the sex ratio is about equal. In prosperous countries the incidence of symptomatic gallstones seems to be increasing and occurring at an earlier age.

In the past, gallstones have been classified by their macroscopic appearance into metabolic, inflammatory and mixed types. Biochemical analysis, however, has shown this to be misleading. In countries where gallstones are common, cholesterol is the most usual and frequently the major component irrespective of appearance. It is found in over three-quarters of gallstones accounting for 10–98% of their content. Some gallstones are composed almost wholly of calcium salts of bilirubin. The latter are commonest where there has been prolonged overproduction of bilirubin due to haemolysis; very little is known about the formation of calcium stones. Only the development of stones containing cholesterol will be considered here.

Aetiology. Current evidence suggests strongly that cholesterol gallstone formation is due mainly to physico-chemical changes in bile predisposing to cholesterol precipitation. Cholesterol, which is insoluble in water, is held in solution in bile by its association with bile acids and phospholipid in the form of mixed micelles (p. 310). In gallstone disease, the liver produces bile containing reduced amounts of bile acid and phospholipid relative to cholesterol with which the bile therefore becomes saturated or even supersaturated. Such bile is termed lithogenic. These changes precede gallstone formation and seem to be due mainly to a reduction in the size of the bile acid pool associated with reduced bile acid secretion into the bile. In a few patients there is also an increased secretion of cholesterol into bile. Although the liver produces the abnormal bile, the gall bladder is important in gallstone formation as it provides a site for cholesterol precipitation and a reservoir for gallstone growth. Infection and inflammation in the gall bladder may enhance the tendency to form stones.

Certain conditions predispose to gallstone formation. Disease or loss of the terminal ileum and long-term cholestyramine therapy leads to loss of bile acids in the faeces; cirrhosis reduces the secretion and pool of bile acids. Diets to lower serum cholesterol and the long-term use of oral contraceptives also increase the frequency of gallstones.

Clinical Features. Gallstones usually manifest themselves as recurrent biliary colic (p. 372) or as acute cholecystitis (p. 372). Biliary colic is not associated with fever or leucocytosis; severe pain lasts for about an hour and may be followed by upper abdominal soreness for a few days.

Some patients with gallstones complain of nonspecific symptoms such as eructations, nausea, vomiting and upper abdominal discomfort mainly in the epigastrium or right hypochondrium. These may be precipitated by fatty foods. However, while such symptoms do occur in chronic cholecystitis and can be relieved by cholecystectomy, they also occur frequently in patients with other organic and functional bowel disease. Hence, when a patient complains only of dyspeptic symptoms, other bowel diseases must be excluded carefully before they are attributed to the gall bladder.

Sometimes a gallstone passes into the common bile duct and causes obstructive jaundice. Upper abdominal pain is present in three quarters of these patients and there is frequently a history of biliary colic. Biliary infection causes fever in one third of cases; ascending cholangitis may then be severe, giving rise to liver abscesses or to septicaemia with shock. Obstruction is not usually complete so that the faeces remain pigmented and both bilirubin and excess urobilinogen are present in the urine. Occasionally, a gallstone may obstruct the common bile duct in the absence of abdominal pain or fever suggesting a pancreatic or biliary neoplasm. Alternatively, it may be associated with an attack of acute pancreatitis (p. 305).

Rarely, a larger gallstone which has reached the intestinal tract, usually via a cholecystenteric fistula, may cause intestinal obstruction. This usually occurs in elderly patients. The clinical features are those of small intestinal obstruction with or without a history of biliary colic; the obstruction is usually in the terminal ileum. Abdominal radiographs show small intestinal obstruction, perhaps the gallstone and possibly gas in the biliary tree.

Investigation. The results of liver function tests and of urine tests for bilirubin and urobilinogen will depend on the degree of obstruction to the common bile duct. Abdominal radiographs occasionally show gallstones. Cholecystography will show either gallstones or a non-functioning gall bladder. Ultrasonography should be used when cholecystography fails to show gallstones in a patient with suggestive symptoms. Ultrasonography usually shows dilated bile ducts where stones are causing jaundice, and transhepatic or retrograde cholangiography may then be needed.

Treatment. The most satisfactory treatment is cholecystectomy with the removal of any stones elsewhere in the biliary tract. Stones lodged in the common bile duct can be remove via a sphincterotomy carried out at endoscopy; this is a very important consideration in the management of elderly and infirm patients. The medical dissolution of gallstones is expensive and effective only with small radiolucent cholesterol stones in a gall bladder which functions on cholestography. The success rate is not impressive (less than 30%); it takes 6 months to 2 years to dissolve stones, and long-term prophylaxis thereafter is probably required. This form of treatment may however have a role when surgery is inadvisable or refused. Ursodeoxycholic acid may come to be preferred to chenodeoxycholic acid in that it causes less diarrhoea and less disturbance of liver function tests. It is given initially in a dose of 8–10 mg/kg.

Because of the need to follow patients radiographically, treatment should be supervised at hospitals.

A frequent problem results from the incidental finding of asymptomatic gallstones. Follow-up of persons with these shows a high incidence of subsequent symptoms, sometimes with the development of serious complications, especially in older patients. Whether or not cholecystectomy should be carried out remains controversial, but it should be considered only in those with no contraindication to surgery.

ACUTE CHOLECYSTITIS

Aetiology and Pathology. Acute cholecystitis is almost always associated with obstruction of the gall bladder neck or cystic duct by a gallstone. Occasionally, obstruction may be by mucus or rarely by a neoplasm. Initially, the inflammation is sterile being perhaps due to chemical irritation from an increasing concentration of the bile in the gall bladder. Later, enteric organisms, especially *Esch. coli* and *Strep. faecalis*, reach the gall bladder by unknown routes and secondary infection occurs. Culture of gall bladder contents within 24 hours of the onset of symptoms yields organisms in 30% of cases, whereas after 72 hours organisms are obtained in about 80%. Acute cholecystitis in the absence of stones is rare; it may develop in typhoid and paratyphoid fever during bacteraemia, or after major trauma, burns or surgery.

All degrees of inflammation occur from mild congestion to gross swelling and tenseness of the gall bladder with ulceration of its wall. Occasionally, perforation takes place or the gall bladder may become distended with pus (empyema). Prolonged obstruction of the cystic duct may also lead to distension of the gall bladder by mucus (mucocele); the patient may experience right upper abdominal discomfort and the gall bladder may be palpable. Rarely, gas forms in the wall (emphysematous cholecystitis), a condition more frequent in males and in diabetes mellitus.

Clinical Features. The disease occurs at any age. The time-honoured factors — fair, fat, fertile, and 40 to 50 years old — are only partly true. The disease is seen increasingly in persons aged under 40 years. The cardinal feature is upper abdominal pain mainly in the epigastrium and right hypochondrium. It is commonly severe, causing restlessness, pallor, sweating and vomiting. Its onset is sudden and it increases quickly to its maximum intensity. The pain usually remains intense for up to an hour, though it may persist for many hours unless relief is obtained from powerful analgesics. Although called '*biliary colic*' it rarely comes in waves like intestinal colic. There may be a history of previous similar pain.

Examination shows right hypochondrial tenderness and rigidity, worse on inspiration (Murphy's sign). Occasionally the gall bladder is palpable. Fever is present and rigors may occur. Jaundice is seen in a minority and is usually slight; it suggests obstruction of the common duct.

Conservative therapy is followed by recovery in 80–90% of cases though recurrences are common. Sometimes there is deterioration due to the development of empyema, perforation and peritonitis or ascending cholangitis. In these cases increasing abdominal pain and rigidity, high fever, tachycardia and hypotension occur.

Investigation. A plain radiograph of the abdomen may show gallstones. Cholecystography should not be done as it fails to reveal the gall bladder and ultrasonography usually shows gallstones. Intravenous cholangiography or cholescintigraphy may show the common bile duct but not the gall bladder implying cystic duct obstruction. The serum amylase may be slightly raised and a moderate leucocytosis is common. Bilirubinuria may or may not be present.

Differential diagnosis has to be made from other causes of severe upper abdominal pain. These are mainly perforated peptic ulcer, acute pancreatitis, appendicitis (especially retrocaecal) and intestinal obstruction. Myocardial infarction should always be considered. Investigations useful in this differentiation are the raised serum amylase in acute pancreatitis, chest and abdominal radiographs, and an electrocardiogram. Occasionally there may be confusion with renal colic, herpes zoster, epidemic myalgia, pleurisy and acute intermittent porphyria.

Treatment. Initially, conservative therapy is usual. This consists of bed rest, relief of pain, maintenance of fluid balance and chemotherapy.

Severe pain is relieved best by morphine 10–20 mg intramuscularly. Increased tone of the choledochal sphincter due to this drug may be minimised by atropine 0·6 mg intramuscularly. Less severe pain can be relieved by pethidine 100 mg or pentazocine 30 mg intramuscularly. Effective relief of pain may require repeated doses of analgesic every 2–3 hours. Provided persistent vomiting is not present, oral fluids can be given. Nasogastric aspiration is required only when there is persistent vomiting, in which case fluid must be given by the intravenous route. Co-trimoxazole or an antibiotic is usually prescribed.

The development of complications, most common in the elderly, is an indication for surgery. However, over 90% of patients recover. The finding of stones, a non-functioning gall bladder or a mucocele should lead to cholecystectomy within 2–3 months.

Early operation has been advocated for acute cholecystitis. Therapy is begun as above, ultrasonography is carried out as soon as possible and operation done within a week of the onset of the illness. It is emphasised that this is not an emergency operation. The results of such therapy are similar to those of conservative treatment. It does, however, require only the one hospital admission, and it obviates the possibility of recurrent attacks.

Postcholecystectomy Syndrome. Where cholecystectomy is carried out for gallstones, at least 70% of patients get complete relief of symptoms. When symptoms persist or biliary colic recurs, radiological examination of the biliary tree for gallstones or unrecognised neoplasia should be carried out. Endoscopic retrograde cholangiopancreatography is specially valuable. In some patients, neither this nor investigation for other diseases such as peptic ulcer or pancreatitis shows any abnormality. The patients are then often considered to suffer from a functional abnormality of the biliary tree — 'biliary dyskinesia'. There is, however, no good evidence for such a condition and these patients should not be treated by procedures such as sphincterotomy or choledochoduodenostomy. Antacids, simple analgesics, sedatives, avoidance of foods clearly followed by symptoms and reassurance should be tried.

MISCELLANEOUS DISEASES OF THE GALL BLADDER AND BILIARY TRACT

Non-calculous cholecystitis is rare. It may occur in typhoid fever, in polyarteritis nodosa, as emphysematous cholecystitis due to *Cl. welchii* in diabetes mellitus and in those on corticosteroid therapy. It may follow trauma or surgery and can complicate septicaemia.

Cholesterolosis of the Gall Bladder. In this condition lipid deposits in the submucosa and epithelium appear as multiple yellow spots on the pink mucosa. The changes are restricted to the gall bladder, symptoms are due to associated gallstones and the condition is recognised only at operation.

Adenomyomatosis of the Gall Bladder. In adenomyomatosis there is hyperplasia of all elements in the gall bladder wall. This is usually localised to the fundus where it shows as a filling defect on cholecystography. It may also be generalised in which case cholecystography shows a distorted gall bladder possibly with intramural contrast medium in Rokitansky-Aschoff sinuses. Frequently there are associated gallstones. Although in most cases there are no symptoms, recurrent biliary colic sometimes occurs. In symptomatic cases, treatment is by cholecystectomy though where there are no gallstones operation should not be done before excluding other diseases, especially peptic ulcer and pancreatitis. Cholecystectomy should be carried out if it is thought that the filling defect might be a neoplasm.

Sclerosing Cholangitis. In this condition there is fibrotic obliteration of the large bile duct system. It may be primary, associated with ulcerative colitis or retroperitoneal fibrosis, or secondary to cholelithiasis or biliary surgery. There is gradually progressive cholestasis and abdominal pain punctuated by episodes of cholangitis. Secondary biliary cirrhosis (p. 363) may occur. The diagnosis can be made at ERCP when material for cytology can be obtained or by biopsy of the bile ducts at laparotomy.

Choledochal Cyst. This cystic dilatation occurs in the common bile duct. It almost always presents by the age of 30 years with episodes of jaundice or abdominal pain. A mass is sometimes palpable in the right hypochondrium. Treatment is surgical, usually by drainage of the cyst or, rarely, excision.

Tumours of the Gall Bladder and Bile Ducts

Benign tumours of the gall bladder are uncommon and usually found incidentally at operation or autopsy. Cholesterol polyps, sometimes associated with cholesterolosis of the gall bladder, papillomas and adenomas are the main types.

Carcinoma of the gall bladder is an uncommon tumour occurring more often in women and hardly ever under the age of 50 years. It usually is in the fundus or neck of the gall bladder and some 90% are adenocarcinomas. The remainder are anaplastic or, rarely, squamous tumours. Gallstones are usually also present and these are often held to be important in the aetiology of the tumour.

Clinically, there is frequently a history of repeated attacks of biliary colic and cholecystitis followed by general deterioration in health, weight loss and constant right upper quadrant abdominal pain. The gall bladder or a mass is palpable in the right hyponchondrium in half the patients. Jaundice is also present in half the patients and is occasionally an early feature in tumours of the gall bladder neck.

Liver function tests most frequently show cholestasis. Gall bladder calcification (porcelain gall bladder), detectable on an abdominal radiograph, is strongly associated with cancer. Cholecystography may show a filling defect in the gall bladder but frequently jaundice prevents the procedure or a non-functioning gall bladder is found. Endoscopic retrograde or percutaneous transhepatic cholangiography may be helpful but frequently the diagnosis is made only at laparotomy.

In the majority of patients, the tumour is inoperable and survival is short.

Benign tumours of the bile ducts are extremely rare. Almost all are either papillomas or adenomas. They may cause biliary obstruction and generally are diagnosed only at operation.

Cholangiocarcinoma is an uncommon tumour arising anywhere in the biliary tree from the small intrahepatic bile ducts to the papilla of Vater. It is not associated with cirrhosis. Virtually all the tumours are adenocarcinomas of varying degrees of differentiation and often with a marked connective tissue stroma.

Clinically, obstructive jaundice is the usual presenting feature though this may be delayed where the tumour involves only the right or left hepatic duct or an intrahepatic radical. Half the patients have upper abdominal pain and weight loss. Intrahepatic tumours are diagnosed as described for hepatocellular carcinoma (p. 368) with the exception that alphafetoprotein is hardly ever found. Transhepatic or retrograde cholangiography are the best methods for diagnosing large duct tumours preoperatively. Tumours above the junction of the hepatic ducts are often missed at operation despite operative cholangiography which may not show the intrahepatic ducts.

It is rarely possible to remove the tumour surgically, but a bypass procedure to relieve itching is worthwhile as these tumours often grow only slowly. Relief of biliary obstruction by passing a drainage tube through the tumour by a transhepatic or perendoscopic retrograde route is much less onerous for these patients who are often elderly.

PROSPECTS IN HEPATOBILIARY DISEASE

The last 15 years has seen the development of serological means for identifying the hepatitis A and B viruses, and in the case of the hepatitis B virus serological methods can identify chronic virus carriers who are relatively highly infectious and who are at greater risk of developing chronic liver disease. Methods are now needed for identifying the non-A, non-B viruses, especially as they can cause chronic infection and may therefore cause chronic liver disease. Several serological methods are being developed to identify these viruses, and, though none are currently generally accepted, several show considerable promise.

The production of an effective vaccine against hepatitis B virus infection has been an important advance. This vaccine could have a major impact on reducing chronic viral infection, chronic liver disease and hepatocellular carcinoma especially in countries where chronic hepatitis B virus infection is common as in Asia. It should not be seen as a substitute for improving poor social conditions predisposing to spread of the virus. Production of vaccine is limited as the starting material is plasma from chronic carriers of the hepatitis B virus, which is in any case undesirable though elaborate precautions in production have led to a vaccine which has so far proved very safe. Current research aims to produce viral components synthetically which should eventually allow the production of large amounts of a much less costly vaccine; this is likely to be a long-term rather than a short-term prospect.

The most significant advance in the management of viral hepatitis would be the development of effective antiviral therapy. Many agents have been tried, especially in chronic hepatitis B virus infection, but none has proved effective.

In chronic liver disease, prevention must be the long term objective. Much will depend on how society faces the problem of alcohol abuse. Where disturbance of immunity seems to be an aetiological factor, recent observations indicate that the T lymphocyte has a significant role and advances in this area may lead to more rational therapy.

The development of a liver support system for the management of patients with liver failure has, as yet, met with only limited success. Difficulties include perfecting such materials as polymer-coated charcoal capable of adsorbing substances toxic to the liver. Progress in this field is urgently required if we are to reduce the very high mortality in acute liver necrosis and also to facilitate liver transplantation. The latter is now techni-cally feasible and there is steady progress in overcoming the immunity problems of organ transplantation and rejection. The use of cyclo-sporin for immunosuppression has improved the outlook in renal transplantation, but its value in liver transplantation remains to be proved.

Great advances have been made in understanding the pathogenesis of gallstones and perhaps these will lead to preventive measures in the future. Endoscopic retrograde cholangiography is an established diagnostic procedure, and the coming years will see an increasing use of endoscopic techniques for removing stones from the biliary tree and for improving its drainage (e.g. papillotomy). The place of computed tomography and nuclear magnetic resonance in hepatobiliary disease needs to be defined.

N.D.C. FINLAYSON
JOHN RICHMOND

FURTHER READING:

Popper, H. & Schaffner, F. (eds.) *Progress in Liver Diseases*. Vol. IV (1972), Vol. V (1976), Vol. VI (1979) and Vol VII (1982). New York: Grune & Stratton.

Schiff, L. (ed.) 1982 *Diseases of the Liver*, 5th edn. Philadelphia and Co (Harper and Row): Lippincott. A very comprehensive reference book.

Shearman, D.J.C. & Finlayson, N.D.C. (1982) *Diseases of the Gastrointestinal Tract and Liver*. Edinburgh: Churchill Livingstone. A textbook primarily for clinicians.

Sherlock, S. (1981) *Diseases of the Liver and Biliary System*, 6th edn. Oxford: Blackwell Scientific Publications. The standard textbook for reference purposes.

Wright, R., Alberti, K.G.M.M., Karran, S., Millward-Sadler, G.H. (eds) (1979) *Liver and Biliary Disease*. Philadelphia: W.B. Saunders. A very comprehensive reference book.

11. Diseases of the Kidneys and Genito-urinary System

ANATOMY AND PHYSIOLOGY

The kidneys are each composed of approximately one million nephrons, the basic structure of one of which is illustrated in Figure 11.1.

The blood supply of the kidneys is relatively large and amounts to about one-quarter of the cardiac output at rest, i.e. 1300 ml per minute. The afferent arterioles which give rise to the glomerular capillaries arise from branches of the renal artery. Emerging from the glomeruli the capillaries unite to form the efferent arterioles which then supply blood to the proximal and distal convoluted tubules surrounding the glomeruli. The medulla is supplied by arterioles which arise from those glomeruli situated in the deeper regions of the cortex.

For a short distance the afferent arterioles and distal convoluted tubules are in contact. At this point the tubular cells become tall and columnar in character, forming the macula densa and the wall of the arteriole is thickened by cells which contain large secretory granules. These structures together constitute the *juxtaglomerular apparatus* which is intimately concerned in the regulation of the volume of the extracellular fluids and blood pressure (p. 379).

The hydrostatic pressure of about 45 mmHg within the glomerular capillaries results in the filtration of fluid from the plasma into Bowman's capsule. This fluid is identical in its composition with plasma except that it normally contains no fat and very little protein. The filtrate thus formed then flows through the various parts of the tubule and is modified according to the needs of the body by tubular secretion and by the selective reabsorption of its constitutents.

Functions of the Kidneys

In health the volume and composition of the body fluids vary within narrow limits. The kidneys are largely responsible for maintaining this constancy and the excretion of the waste products of metabolism represents merely one aspect of this task. The various renal functions are conveniently considered under the following headings and some are shown diagrammatically in Figure 11.1.

Regulation of the Water Content of the Body. About two-thirds of the water filtered by the glomerulus is reabsorbed iso-osmotically by the proximal tubules. The remaining water passes through the distal tubules and collecting ducts where its reabsorption is regulated by vasopressin, the antidiuretic hormone of the posterior pituitary. In the presence of vasopressin the distal convoluted tubules become permeable to water which is then passively reabsorbed in response to the high concentration of sodium chloride and urea which exists in the medullary interstitium. The urine then becomes concentrated. In the absence of vasopressin the distal nephron is impermeable to water. In these circumstances a dilute urine is formed by the tubular reabsorption of sodium and chloride without water. Disorders of the water-regulating mechanism which result in oliguria or polyuria are described on pages 380 and 426.

Regulation of the Electrolyte Content of the Body. The electrolyte content is kept remarkably constant as a result of selective reabsorption and secretion by the renal tubules. A large part of the sodium, chloride and probably all the potassium, which are freely filtered by the glomeruli, are actively reabsorbed in the proximal

Fig. 11.1 Some of the events concerned in urine formation. In the proximal convoluted tubule about two-thirds of the filtered sodium, chloride, potassium and water are reabsorbed. The greater part of the filtered bicarbonate is also reabsorbed here by a process which involves the secretion of hydrogen ions. Sodium and chloride are reabsorbed without water in the ascending limb of the loop of Henle; the loops function as counter-current multipliers and are largely responsible for the hyperosmolality of the medullary interstitium. In the distal convoluted tubule and collecting duct, potassium is transported into the cells and diffuses into the lumen in response to an electrochemical gradient. Hydrogen ions and ammonia are also secreted there and water is passively reabsorbed in the presence of antidiuretic hormone.

convoluted tubules and pars recta. The remainder of the sodium passes into the distal tubules and collecting ducts where its reabsorption appears to be under the influence of hormones of the adrenal cortex, especially aldosterone. With reduced secretion of these hormones, excessive quantities of sodium and chloride ions are lost in the urine, whereas with the administration of corticosteroids, sodium retention occurs.

Urinary potassium is largely derived from potassium which diffuses into the tubular lumen from the distal tubular cells, in response to the electrochemical gradient. The chemical gradient is created by the active transport of potassium from the peritubular fluid into the cells and an intraluminal potential which is negative with respect to the peritubular fluid favours the diffusion of potassium into the lumen.

The dual actions of the adrenocortical hormones and of the antidiuretic hormone on the renal tubules play an important role in determining the total volume of water and the electrolyte content of the body. The rate of secretion of vasopressin is determined mainly by changes in

Fig. 11.2 Maintenance of the normal acid-base equilibrium of the blood. Carbonic acid is generated within the renal tubular cells from CO_2 and H_2O released within the tubular lumen. The hydrogen ions of this acid are then actively secreted into the tubular lumen in exchange for filtered sodium which is then reabsorbed into the blood. The bicarbonate ions liberated from the carbonic acid are absorbed with the sodium into the blood; this restores the concentration of plasma bicarbonate to normal and also regenerates other buffers which have been titrated by the invading acids.

Some of the hydrogen ions are buffered in the urine by disodium hydrogen phosphate to form dihydrogen sodium phosphate and in the distal tubules by ammonia to form ammonium ions. Anions of the inorganic and organic acids are excreted in the urine largely as ammonium salts.

osmolality of the blood; aldosterone secretion is influenced *inter alia* by changes in the composition of the fluid in the region of the macula densa and the renal perfusion pressure. These stimuli influence the rate of secretion of renin by the juxtaglomerular apparatus. It has also been shown that proximal tubular reabsorption of water and salt is influenced by the volume of the blood and the extracellular fluid. How this control is mediated is unknown but the activity of a natriuretic hormone has been postulated.

Maintenance of the Normal Acid-base Equilibrium of the Blood. The ability of the kidney to reabsorb sodium and regulate urinary acidification and secrete ammonia is essential to normal acid-base balance. The importance of preserving an adequate concentration of bicarbonate in the plasma is referred to on page 98. This is achieved by three mechanisms:

1. All filtered bicarbonate is reabsorbed up to a threshold of a plasma concentration of about 25 mmol/l. When the plasma concentration rises above this level, reabsorption becomes incomplete and the excess is eliminated in the urine. This mechanism thus maintains the plasma bicarbonate buffer system (p. 99).

2. The kidneys regenerate bicarbonate and restore its concentration in the plasma when reduced by metabolic acids. This is achieved by actively secreting hydrogen ions into the tubular urine, where they are buffered largely by disodium hydrogen phosphate (Fig. 11.2).

3. Ammonia formed within the distal tubular cells diffuses into the tubular lumen where it accepts more of the hydrogen ions to form ammonium ions.

The degree to which these mechanisms operate is adjusted in accordance with the nature of the food ingested and the amount of endogenous acid production. In health, on a normal diet,

40–80 mmol of acid are excreted daily into the urine. When a diet consisting mainly of fruit and vegetables is taken, disodium hydrogen phosphate and bicarbonate are excreted in the urine and tubular secretion of hydrogen and ammonium ions is suppressed.

Retention of other Substances vital to Body Economy, e.g. Glucose, Amino Acids, Phosphate, Bicarbonate, Proteins. Glucose is normally reabsorbed so completely by the proximal tubules that none can be detected in the urine by clinical tests. *Renal glycosuria* is a genetically determined benign defect of tubular reabsorption in which glucose appears in the urine in the presence of normal blood glucose levels. More rarely other *congenital or acquired abnormalities of tubular transport* result in abnormal loss in the urine of amino acids, phosphate, sodium, potassium, calcium and water. These defects may occur singly or in combination. Examples are cystinuria, familial hypophosphataemia, nephrogenic diabetes insipidus and the Fanconi syndrome, a disease which usually does not present until the third decade of life.

In health the great bulk of the bicarbonate filtered by the glomeruli is removed from the urine by tubular reabsorption, and this becomes complete when the urine is acid. *Renal tubular acidosis* is a defect in the power either to reabsorb bicarbonate (proximal RTA) or to acidify the urine (distal RTA) which then usually contains significant amounts of bicarbonate in the face of metabolic acidosis. Such defects may be acquired as a result of renal disease such as pyelonephritis; they also occur as a consequence of myelomatosis, hyperparathyroidism and Wilson's disease. Idiopathic renal tubular acidosis is a rare, inherited form. All types are apt to lead to osteomalacia, nephrocalcinosis and hypokalaemia.

In health only a small amount of protein $(0.2 \text{ g}/l)$ reaches the fluid in Bowman's capsule. The volume of glomerular filtrate, however, is so great that if this small amount were not reabsorbed, more than 3 g of protein rather than the normal 50 mg would be excreted in the urine in 24 hours.

Excretion of Waste Metabolic Products, Toxic Substances and Drugs. The end-products of metabolism, especially those of protein, include urea, uric acid, creatinine, phosphates and sulphates, and are excreted in the urine.

Hormonal and Metabolic Functions. The juxtaglomerular apparatus within the kidneys is believed to secrete renin, which converts angiotensin I in the blood to angiotensin II. This substance increases the rate of aldosterone secretion by the adrenal cortex and also causes vasoconstriction. This may be the sequence of events by which renal ischaemia produces hypertension.

The kidney is the main source of erythropoietin necessary for normal erythropoiesis (p. 490) and it is also responsible for the formation of 1,25 dihydroxycholecalciferol (p. 66). Two prostaglandins (PGE_2 and PGI_2) are also produced within the kidney. Both are powerful vasodilators; PGI_2 is probably a mediator in renin release. Both may be concerned in the control of the renal circulation.

INVESTIGATION OF RENAL DISEASE

In the majority of patients suffering from renal disease, symptoms and signs are not referred to the anatomical site of the kidneys. This is due to the fact that clinical features of renal disease most frequently arise from abnormalities in the chemical composition of the body or from hypertension, anaemia or metabolic bone disease. Their true origin therefore may be suspected only after the detection of urinary abnormalities and the importance of a routine examination of the urine cannot be overemphasised.

The tests which may be of value include the determination of the volume of urine passed in 24 hours, the detection of the presence of abnormal urinary constituents and bacteriological examination. Under certain standardised conditions the determination of the specific gravity or osmolality and pH of urine is of value. Chemical examination of the blood is mandatory and in addition it may be necessary to obtain further information by tests of glomerular and tubular function.

The urethra and bladder can be inspected by urethroscopy and cystoscopy and catheterisation of the ureters can provide samples of urine from each kidney.

Radiological examination includes a plain radiograph of the abdomen, excretion urography (intravenous pyelography), retrograde pyelography and renal angiography. Further information can be obtained by ultrasonic, radioisotope and computed scanning, and by renal biopsy.

Examination of the Urine

Urinary Volume. In health and in temperate climates the volume of urine excreted usually lies within the range of 800–2500 ml per 24 hours. There is a limit to the power of the kidneys to concentrate urine and on a normal diet a minimum volume of 500 ml is required to excrete the solid urinary constituents which consist mainly of urea and electrolytes. Less solute has to be excreted when a diet rich in carbohydrate and fat and low in protein and salt is eaten, and as little as 250 ml of urine per 24 hours is sufficient in these circumstances.

Oliguria is the production of insufficient urine to enable solute to be excreted in adequate amounts and the *milieu intérieur* of the body to be preserved. If the concentrating power of the kidneys is seriously reduced or if the solute to be excreted in the urine is increased above the normal, as occurs, for example, in severe infections or after traumatic injury, a daily output of as much as 2–3 litres of urine may be insufficient. Oliguria develops in conditions associated with a reduction in renal blood flow and rate of glomerular filtration, e.g. diseases giving rise to water and salt depletion, hypotension, cardiac failure, acute glomerulonephritis, and other organic diseases of the kidneys. In these circumstances urine flow sometimes ceases completely and *anuria* develops. Anuria from this cause should be distinguished from urinary retention. In the latter case distension of the bladder will be found on examination of the abdomen confirmed if necessary by catheterisation.

Polyuria denotes a persistent increase in urinary output. It must be distinguished from frequency of micturition, which may be defined as the frequent passage of small quantities of urine without an increase in the total volume.

There are two basic mechanisms which give rise to polyuria. It may be due (i) to the excretion of an abnormally large amount of solute which interferes with reabsorption of water in the nephron, or (ii) to a reduction in the ability of the kidney to concentrate urine so that an increased volume of water is needed to eliminate a given amount of solute. The second defect may arise because of lack of circulating vasopressin or insensitivity of the concentrating mechanism within the kidney to its action. Polyuria occurs in the following clinical circumstances:

1. Diabetes mellitus in which an osmotic diuresis occurs because of glycosuria due to hyperglycaemia.

2. Renal disease with uraemia in which the elevated concentration of urea in the blood acts as the osmotic diuretic.

3. Conditions in which there is decreased responsiveness of the distal nephron to vasopressin, e.g. in some cases of chronic renal disease, (amyloidosis, myelomatosis, some patients with chronic obstructive nephropathy or chronic pyelonephritis), during the recovery phase of acute renal failure, in hypercalcaemia, in potassium depletion and in inherited nephrogenic diabetes insipidus.

4. Drugs which may induce unresponsiveness to vasopressin; these include lithium carbonate and amphotericin.

5. Diabetes insipidus of neurohypophyseal origin in which there is diminished secretion of vasopressin.

6. Inhibition of vasopressin secretion due to excessive drinking of fluid either from choice or from psychiatric causes, i.e. compulsive polydipsia or as a result of a lesion of the hypothalamus.

7. The elimination of oedema, e.g. in recovery from heart failure or the nephrotic syndrome.

Specific gravity of urine is a measure of the quantity of solids in solution and is an approximate measure of osmolality. In health, urea and sodium chloride are the main solutes contributing to the specific gravity of urine. In diabetes mellitus, on the other hand, the quantity of glucose in the urine may far outweigh the total of all the other solutes present; water containing 1% glucose has a specific gravity of 1·004, while, in the case of proteinuria, 4 g protein per litre, which gives a strong reaction with dipstix, raises the specific gravity by only 0·001. The specific gravity of urine varies with the nature and quantity of food eaten as well as with the amount of water or other fluid consumed.

The maximal capacity of the kidneys to concentrate urine may be determined after either depriving the patient of fluid or after giving vasopressin, but if a random or prebreakfast sample of urine is found to have a specific gravity of 1·020 or more there is clearly no need to carry out these tests.

Reaction of the Urine and Acid Excretion. In health urinary pH ranges from about 4·3 to 8·0. A very high pH (over 8·0) nearly always indicates urinary tract infection with an organism which forms ammonia from urea. In certain circumstances the ability of the renal tubules to excrete hydrogen ions is depressed. This may be due to failure to form a very acid urine or the inability to secrete a sufficient quantity of the buffer base ammonia. Failure to reduce the pH of the urine to less than 5·3 following oral administration of ammonium chloride is characteristic of both proximal and distal renal tubular acidosis either of which can occur as an inherited or acquired defect. Distinction between the two forms of the disorder requires more elaborate investigation. In chronic renal failure the ability to form urine of pH less than 5·3 is commonly retained but excretion of the ammonium ion is reduced and this defect can be demonstrated after administration of ammonium chloride.

Abnormal Constituents of Urine Detectable by Routine Examination. PROTEIN in the urine, detectable by dipstix or salicylsulphonic acid almost invariably indicates the presence of disease of the kidneys. Its magnitude bears little relation to the overall level of renal function. Significant proteinuria does not occur in disease of the lower urinary tract, though a small amount can be detected in severe urinary tract infection or in obvious haematuria. Small amounts of protein are usually found in the urine in chronic renal disease, in the course of febrile illness and in heart failure. Larger amounts of protein (e.g. 3 g/day or more) are found in the nephrotic syndrome and invariably indicate glomerular disease.

The great bulk of the urinary protein is albumin and larger molecular weight plasma proteins are present in only small amounts. The pattern of proteinuria can be determined and an index of selectivity assessed. *A highly selective proteinuria* is one in which the larger molecular weight proteins are virtually absent, while a *non-selective* *proteinuria* is one which the larger proteins are found in significant amounts. The degree of selectivity is an indication of the amount of glomerular damage and is of help in predicting the response to be expected to the administration of corticosteroids.

Postural (Orthostatic) Proteinuria. In a number of apparently healthy children and adolescents, and less commonly in adults, protein is excreted in the urine in variable but usually small amounts without associated disease of the kidneys. The urine formed while these individuals are recumbent at night is free from protein so that examination of the first specimen voided immediately on rising in the morning is normal. On the other hand urine formed while the individual follows the usual daytime activities or following vigorous exercise is found to contain protein. Tests of renal function show no abnormality and further investigations are not justified. It should be remembered that postural proteinuria sometimes occurs in the presence of organic renal disease.

BLOOD is found in the urine in a wide variety of clinical conditions; haematuria commonly indicates serious disease of the urinary tract and the cause must always be sought without delay. The appearance of the urine varies with the amount of blood and is normal to the naked eye when only traces are present. When larger amounts of blood are present the urine may be smoky in appearance, bright red or reddish-brown. The brown discolouration is due to the formation of acid haematin from haemoglobin.

Red blood cells are found in varying number in the urine in acute glomerulonephritis, infective endocarditis, malignant hypertension, polyarteritis nodosa or systemic lupus erythematosus affecting the kidney, renal tuberculosis, congenital cystic disease, haemorrhagic disease, renal infarction and trauma to the kidneys. Red cells occur in the urine also in inflammation and tumours of the kidney and of the urinary tract, in benign hyperplasia and carcinoma of the prostate, and in the presence of urinary calculi. Red cells are absent, or very scanty, in minimal lesion and membranous glomerulonephritis and in most cases of the nephrotic syndrome due to other causes.

Many of these conditions can be diagnosed by the presence of characteristic symptoms and signs in addition to haematuria. When haematuria is the sole or presenting symptom the cause is most likely to be renal carcinoma, papilloma of the bladder, benign prostatic hypertrophy or, in some localities, schistosomiasis (p. 782).

When blood appears only at the beginning of micturition, the rest of the urine voided being clear, the source of bleeding is distal to the bladder. When blood is uniformly mixed with the urine, it may have come from any part of the urinary tract other than the urethra. Renal colic accompanying haematuria indicates that the bleeding is renal or ureteric in origin.

Haematuria may be mimicked by other rarer causes of discolouration of the urine:

1. *Haemoglobinuria*, which accompanies various intravascular haemolytic disorders (p. 505) and occasionally in normal people after strenuous exercise. The urine gives the chemical tests for haemoglobin, but no red cells are present on microscopic examination of the centrifuged deposit of a fresh sample of urine.

2. *Acute intermittent porphyria* in which large amounts of porphobilinogen are excreted in the urine. Fresh urine from such cases may appear normal, but on standing for some hours a dark red colour may develop. The presence of porphobilinogen may be suspected from the red colour produced by the addition of Ehrlich's aldehyde reagent. In contrast to that produced by urobilinogen, this colour is not extracted by chloroform.

3. *Beetroot, senna, dyes* used to colour sweets and *phenolphthalein* used in proprietary purgatives. These are rarer mimics of haematuria.

PUS CELLS AND BACTERIA. Pus cells may be found in the urine in inflammation of any part of the urinary tract. The urine should always be examined under the microscope and cultured when urinary tract infection is suspected. In obtaining the specimen for culture it is best to avoid catheterisation. A midstream specimen should be obtained from both male and female patients, and a culture should be made of this within 2 hours (p. 396).

CASTS are cylindrical structures of microscopic size which are found in the urinary deposit. They are formed in the renal tubules by the coagulation of protein. Red blood corpuscles or epithelial cells may be impressed upon this matrix, producing blood and epithelial casts respectively; such casts are found in the early stages of acute glomerulonephritis and other diseases in which there is glomerular inflammation. Granular casts are formed by degeneration of the impressed cells. Epithelial and granular cases are indicative of inflammation and degeneration of the renal tubules. Hyaline casts are formed by coagulated protein without the addition of cellular elements and are found in chronic glomerulonephritis and occasionally in small numbers in normal urine, especially after vigorous exercise.

OTHER ABNORMALITIES. Glycosuria (p. 463); biliuria and urobilinogenuria (p. 340).

REFERENCE VALUES FOR URINE Table 21.6 (p. 820).

Chemical Analysis of the Blood

With progressive impairment of renal function the composition of the body fluids becomes abnormal. These abnormalities may be detected by blood analyses. The products of metabolism which in health are excreted in the urine are retained in the blood, and the concentration of urea, creatinine and the anions such as phosphate and sulphate increases. Determination of the concentration of blood urea gives a useful indication of the degree of renal failure, but it should be remembered that it does not rise above the accepted normal maximum until renal function is reduced by at least 50%.

The diminishing capacity of the kidneys to excrete hydrogen ions results in their accumulation in the blood, and the severity of the consequent metabolic acidosis may be estimated by measurement of arterial pH and the concentration of plasma bicarbonate. Estimation of plasma sodium, potassium, calcium and protein concentrations is of value in certain circumstances.

REFERENCE VALUES for biochemical constituents of the blood, in SI and equivalent units, are given in Table 21.3 on page 817.

Renal Clearance. The ability of the glomeruli to perform their function is best studied by the measurement of renal clearance where clearance $C = UV \div P$, U and P being the urinary and plasma concentration of any given substance and V the minute volume of urine. If a substance in the plasma passes freely through the glomerular filter and is neither absorbed nor excreted by the tubules, the quantity excreted in the urine (UV) is identical with the amount filtered by the glomeruli; the clearance of such a substance therefore equals the rate of glomerular filtration (GFR). The polysaccharide, inulin, appears to be excreted in this way and its clearance is used to estimate GFR, which for the average adult is about 120 ml/min. In clinical practice the clearance of creatinine, which approximates to that of inulin, is usually carried out by collecting all the urine passed in a 24 hour period and withdrawing one sample of blood during the day of collection.

Radiological and Imaging Investigation

A *plain radiograph* of the abdomen should always be taken before proceeding to excretion urography. Its main purpose is to reveal radio-opaque calculi or other areas of calcification such as nephrocalcinosis. Calculi are easily missed, especially if they are less than 1 cm in diameter as they are easily obscured by bowel shadows, or overlie bone. The plain film may also demonstrate the renal outline and so give an indication of renal size, though this is often better visualised during excretion urography.

Excretion urography is carried out by the intravenous injection of an organic iodine-containing compound, about one third of which is excreted largely by glomerular filtration within the first hour. Following the injection, films are taken at timed intervals. There is first an increase in the radiographic density of the renal substance (nephrogram), as the contrast medium enters the renal tubules. In the adult, healthy kidneys usually measure 11–14 cm in length and differ from each other by less than 2 cm; they are usually smooth in outline, but the nephrogram may reveal scars of pyelonephritis, often in association with a calyceal abnormality, or reveal localised masses or tumours; sometimes fetal lobulation, a normal variation, is seen. In diffuse renal disease with reduced function the nephrogram is faint and the kidneys may appear small. An increase in opacification occurs on the affected side in renal artery stenosis.

Normally within a few minutes the contrast medium begins to be excreted into the calyceal system, pelvis and ureters, which are best seen within the first 20 minutes, and may outline anatomical abnormalities there. Usually each kidney is seen to possess 2–4 major calyces, each of which possesses 3–4 minor calyces moulded around a renal papilla, and giving a concave or cup-like opacification. Clubbed calyces and slow excretion are commonly found in chronic urinary obstruction. When obstruction is severe there is often distension of the pelvis and thinning of the renal cortex and calyceal opacification is then often absent (negative pyelogram). Calyceal abnormalities may also suggest papillary necrosis, renal tuberculosis or atrophic pyelonephritis. In renal tuberculosis calcification and cavitation are common. Pools or streaks of contrast medium within the pyramids without calyceal deformity suggest medullary sponge kidney. Polycystic disease causes bilateral renal enlargement and the calyceal structure is stretched and spidery.

Retrograde urography or pyelography is mainly used to investigate lesions of the ureter and to define the cause of obstruction. Contrast medium is injected under screening control into the ureteric orifice during cystoscopy; alternatively, a catheter can be introduced into the lower part of the ureters and the injection carried out later. Occasionally when retrograde pyelography is unsatisfactory or impossible, or a ureteric obstruction involves only the upper urinary tracts, percutaneous (antegrade) pyelography is carried out.

A micturating cystogram is of importance in the investigation of urinary infection in childhood, but because of risk to the gonads of radiation, it should be carried out only in those who show a urographic abnormality and are under the age of three years. It may also reveal abnormalities of the bladder outflow tract.

Renal arteriography is less often required than formerly, but may be helpful in identifying the nature of a renal mass detected by ultrasound examination and in revealing renal artery stenosis or intrarenal microaneurysms as occurs in polyarteritis nodosa.

Ultrasonography of the kidneys is complementary to other methods of investigation, but is most useful in assessing renal size and in distinguishing solid renal tumours from cystic lesions and hydronephrosis. Polycystic kidney disease is readily diagnosed by ultrasonography which has replaced excretion urography as a screening test for this condition.

Computed tomography is particularly helpful in the diagnosis of masses in the kidneys and retro-peritoneal tissues, and in defining the spread of bladder and prostatic tumours. Its use should be reserved for cases in which simpler methods fail to clarify the problem.

Radionuclide studies involve the injection of radioactive compounds which are concentrated and excreted by the kidney; the gamma radiation emitted is detected and the change in radioactivity with time is recorded by a gamma scintillation camera. The application of these techniques is of value in estimating the relative blood flow to the kidneys, in defining their size, shape, position and function, in the detection of tumours or abscesses and in estimating the effect of urinary tract obstruction on kidney function.

Renal Biopsy

The technique of renal biopsy has greatly increased understanding of renal disease and in particular, knowledge of glomerulonephritis. Tissue obtained can be examined by light and electron microscopy; immunoglobulins, complement and fibrin can be identified by the use of immunofluorescence microscopy. Biopsy is especially useful in diagnosis in patients with proteinuria of unknown origin, in unexplained renal failure when the kidneys are of normal size, in suspected systemic disease associated with abnormal urinary constituents and in haematuria in which lesions of the lower urinary tract have been excluded. In experienced hands it is a safe procedure, but should be carried out only in patients possessing two kidneys and after the exclusion of any bleeding disorder by an appropriate coagulation screen. Hypertension, if present, should be under control.

GLOMERULONEPHRITIS

The term 'glomerulonephritis' is used to describe a bilateral disease of the kidneys which usually affects all the glomeruli. In practice, cases can usually be placed in one of three histologically defined categories which are described below under the headings of (1) *proliferative glomerulonephritis*, (2) *minimal lesion glomerulonephritis*, and (3) *membranous glomerulonephritis*. Within the proliferative group there are, in addition to the acute diffuse type, several variants. The most important of these are IgA nephropathy, crescentic glomerulonephritis, mesangiocapillary glomerulonephritis and focal or segmental glomerulonephritis.

These histological appearances reflect the different ways in which the glomerulus reacts to injury and to some extent they influence the presenting clinical features. In the early stages of these disorders the histological pictures are dis-

Table 11.1 Glomerulonephritis (GN)

Histological type	Common presenting feature	Prognosis
1. *Proliferative*		
(i) Acute diffuse GN	Acute nephritic syndrome	Resolution in majority of children; Prognosis less good in adults
(ii) IgA Nephropathy	Recurrent haematuria	Usually a benign course; A minority develop renal failure
(iii) Crescentic GN	Acute nephritic syndrome	Rapid development of renal failure
(iv) Mesangiocapillary GN	Nephrotic syndrome	Slow development of renal failure
(v) Focal or segmental GN	Asymptomatic proteinuria; haematuria	Good. Small minority develop renal failure
2. *Minimal lesion GN*	Nephrotic syndrome; asymptomatic proteinuria	Reversible with corticosteroids or cyclophosphamide
3. *Membranous GN*	Asymptomatic proteinuria; nephrotic syndrome	20% spontaneous resolution 80% slow development renal failure

tinctive. In cases of proliferative glomerulonephritis which fail to recover completely, and in the later stages of membranous glomerulonephritis, the histological features become less clearly distinguishable. The fact that hypertension may accompany some stage of these diseases complicates the pathology still further by the changes due to arteriolosclerosis.

The severity and extent of the glomerular injury also influences the clinical manifestations of the disease and the prognosis. No single histological type is invariably associated with any specific clinical presentation but Table 11.1 indicates the most common presentation for each variant and indicates the most likely prognosis.

Proliferative Glomerulonephritis

This condition is characterised by an inflammatory reaction of the glomeruli of both kidneys which typically affects all glomeruli diffusely. In a small number of cases, the proliferative cellular response is confined to a limited number of glomeruli, the others being normal (*focal or segmental glomerulonephritis*). When the disease appears abruptly, the terms *acute (diffuse) glomerulonephritis* or *acute nephritis* are often applied.

Aetiology. The great majority of cases of proliferative glomerulonephritis is due to the deposition of immune complexes in the capillary wall of the glomerulus. The classical disorder follows infection with certain strains of β-haemolytic streptococci, causing acute tonsillitis, scarlet fever or upper respiratory infection. In developing countries streptococcal infection of wounds or skin are more often responsible but streptococcal infection anywhere may be the cause. Some viruses (e.g. varicella and EB) may also cause proliferative glomerulonephritis and a similar reaction can rarely follow infection with organisms as different as staphylococci, pneumococci, *Mycobacterium leprae*, *Plasmodium malariae* and schistosomiasis. It may also occur as a complication of infective endocarditis.

Glomerular disease caused by immune complexes is also found in systemic lupus erythematosus (antibody to DNA) and polyarteritis, in the course of some tumours and lymphomas which induce circulating antibodies and as a con-

sequence of an immunological reaction to drugs. However, in many patients and in the majority of cases that occur in Britain, there is no clue to the nature of the antigen.

Pathology. The commonest lesion is a diffuse reaction of the glomerular capillaries with variable swelling of the endothelial cells, proliferation of the mesangial cells and accumulation of polymorphonuclear leucocytes in the tuft and the glomerular space (Fig. 11.3). Within the first few weeks of the illness EM examination shows characteristic deposits of antigen-antibody complexes on the basement membrane; these are associated with a granular appearance on immunofluorescence for IgG and C3. In *IgA nephropathy* immunofluorescent studies show a great predominance of IgA antibodies in the glomerular capillary mesangium (Fig. 11.4).

There may be proliferation of the outer layers of Bowman's capsule to form minor or segmental epithelial crescents. In many cases the changes resolve with clinical recovery and the kidney returns to normal.

In persistent and in rapidly progressive cases the epithelial crescents, which arise as a result of the presence of red blood cells, fibrin and inflammatory exudate in Bowman's space, increase in size and compress the glomeruli interfering with their function. This is the variant known as *crescentic glomerulonephritis* (Fig. 11.4).

In crescentic glomerulonephritis progressive fibrosis of crescents and glomeruli occurs and the glomerular capillaries gradually become obstructed, resulting in secondary degeneration in the tubules. Ultimately many nephrons may be replaced by fibrous tissue, leading to small contracted kidneys. It appears likely that the immune complexes activate both the coagulation and the complement systems. The degree of intravascular glomerular thrombosis partly determines the rapidity of the deterioration and possibly also whether the condition resolves. This component of the disorder may be assessed by estimation of the degradation products of fibrinogen and fibrin (FDP) in the urine.

Goodpasture's syndrome is a rare form of glomerulonephritis associated with haemoptysis. It develops as a consequence of the formation of IgG antibodies to glomerular basement membrane which then 'home' onto this membrane and are deposited in a linear fashion along it.

Another factor influencing the histological picture and the outcome is the way in which the mesangial cells react and fulfil their phagocytic role. In some cases proliferation of the mesangial cells is so marked that they project into the glomerular capillaries and seriously interfere with their function. They also send extensions of mesangial cell cytoplasm between the endothelial cells and the basement membrane giving a lobular appearance. This variant is called *mesangiocapillary glomerulonephritis*; one type is characterised by large subendothelial deposits and a second by dense deposits throughout the basement membrane (Fig. 11.4).

The activation of complement in acute streptococcal glomerulonephritis is reflected in a transient fall in the C3 component of complement (p. 23) during the illness. In many cases of mesangiocapillary glomerulonephritis there is a persistent reduction of serum complement which antedates the disease. This abnormality, which is possibly genetically determined, may increase the susceptibility of the host to circulating immune complexes.

Clinical Features. Acute glomerulonephritis occurs most commonly in childhood and adolescence but may develop at any age. When it follows streptococcal infection a latent period is usual, the features of glomerulonephritis developing 1 to 3 weeks after the infection has subsided. The infection itself may be slight and may even pass unnoticed, and there is no relationship between its severity and the probability of the development of the disease.

In children the onset of the acute nephritic syndrome is usually abrupt, a striking feature being swelling of the face which is part of a generalised oedema caused by fluid retention. It is most marked around the eyes because the skin is more loosely attached to the subcutaneous tissues here and because the patient can usually lie flat. Oedema may be detected around the ankles if the patient is ambulant. Breathlessness due to pulmonary oedema may be present and in severe cases pleural effusions develop. Occasionally there is discomfort in the renal angles or upper abdomen. Epistaxis may occur. In acute cases there may be malaise, fever, anorexia, vomiting and headache. In most cases there is a moderate rise in blood pressure. In a few hypertensive encephalopathy occurs.

In adults, a history of acute streptococcal or other infection is less commonly obtained and the onset is subacute or insidious with progressive tiredness and slowly developing oedema of the lower limbs. Asymptomatic cases may be discovered after routine examination of the urine.

Urine. The daily output is usually reduced in volume due to a fall in the rate of glomerular filtration and increased tubular reabsorption of salt and water. Anuria may occur in very severe cases. The urine may appear red or smoky owing to the presence of blood and is usually concentrated. Proteinuria is of moderate degree, seldom exceeding 4 g daily, but the amount present is out of proportion to the haematuria. Microscopic examination of the urinary deposit reveals erythrocytes, some leucocytes, and red blood cell, epithelial and granular casts.

Renal function tests. In the early stages concentrating power is usually unimpaired, and the specific gravity of the urine is high. The rate of glomerular filtration may be transiently reduced and the concentration of urea in the blood raised. A moderate degree of acidosis is usual. When recovery occurs the filtration rate rises and the blood urea concentration falls to normal.

Course and Prognosis. Complete recovery

Fig. 11.3 Glomerulonephritis (GN). A composite diagram in which the normal capillary wall is contrasted with the pathological changes found in proliferative, minimal lesion and membranous GN [L = capillary lumen; M = mesangium; Mn = mesangial nucleus; Mm = mesangial matrix column]. (Courtesy of Department of Pathology, University of Edinburgh).

Fig. 11.4 Glomerulonephritis (GN). A composite diagram showing a section of Bowman's capsule, the walls of 4 capillaries and the related mesangium to illustrate the pathological changes found in IgA nephropathy, crescentic and mesangiocapillary GN. [L = capillary lumen; M = mesangium; Mn = mesangial nucleus; Mm = mesangial matrix column]. (Courtesy of Department of Pathology, University of Edinburgh).

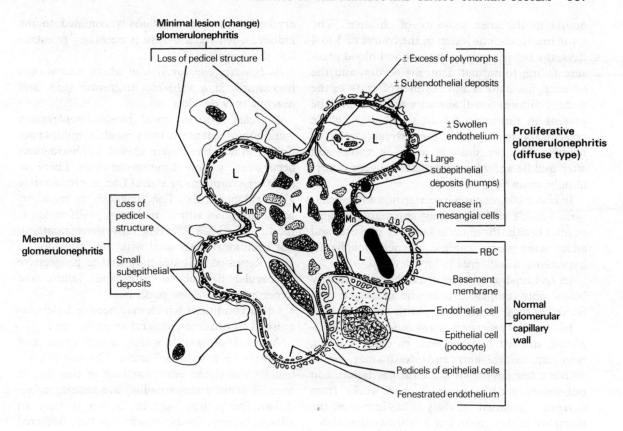

**Minimal lesion (change)
glomerulonephritis**

Loss of pedicel structure

± Excess of polymorphs

± Subendothelial deposits

± Swollen
endothelium

**Proliferative
glomerulonephritis
(diffuse type)**

± Large
subepithelial
deposits (humps)

Increase in
mesangial cells

Loss of
pedicel
structure

**Membranous
glomerulonephritis**

Small
subepithelial
deposits

RBC

Basement
membrane

**Normal
glomerular
capillary
wall**

Endothelial cell

Epithelial cell
(podocyte)

Pedicels of epithelial cells

Fenestrated endothelium

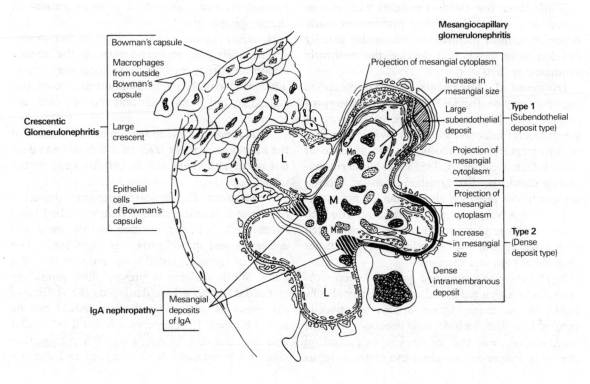

**Mesangiocapillary
glomerulonephritis**

Bowman's capsule

Macrophages
from outside
Bowman's
capsule

Projection of mesangial cytoplasm

Increase in
mesangial size

**Crescentic
Glomerulonephritis**

Large
crescent

Large
subendothelial
deposit

Type 1
(Subendothelial
deposit type)

Projection of
mesangial
cytoplasm

Epithelial
cells
of Bowman's
capsule

Projection of
mesangial
cytoplasm

Increase
in mesangial
size

Type 2
(Dense
deposit type)

Dense
intramembranous
deposit

Mesangial
deposits
of IgA

IgA nephropathy

occurs in the great majority of children. The acute manifestations lessen in the course of 3 to 4 days, the temperature, pulse rate and blood pressure falling to normal. Diuresis occurs, and the oedema, haematuria and number of casts in the urine diminish. Small amounts of blood may be present in the urine for 10 to 14 days, while proteinuria may persist for several weeks or months. The prognosis is worse in adults and after middle age when complete recovery occurs in only about 50% of cases.

In about 10% of cases hypertension and haematuria subside and the patient apparently regains normal health. Proteinuria however persists, and after many years chronic glomerulonephritis, hypertension and renal failure develop.

In *IgA nephropathy*, recurrent haematuria may be the only complaint. It can be associated with recurrent focal glomerulonephritis (see below).

In rapidly *progressive crescentic glomerulonephritis*, marked hypertension, extreme oliguria, recurrent convulsions and death may occur within a few days from acute cardiac failure and pulmonary oedema or in 2 or 3 weeks from uraemia. Treatment by dialysis has improved the mortality in this group but it still remains high.

While about one-third of patients with *mesangiocapillary glomerulonephritis* present an acute nephritic clinical picture, the remainder usually develop more slowly and develop the nephrotic syndrome (p. 390).

Differential Diagnosis. Poststreptococcal nephritis may be diagnosed if haemolytic streptococci can be isolated or if there is evidence of streptococcal infection as shown by a rising titre of antistreptolysin antibody. In the absence of other infective causes (p. 385) acute glomerulonephritis should be distinguished from the following conditions in which glomerular lesions occur:

1. *Henoch-Schönlein purpura* (p. 569) in which focal or diffuse glomerulonephritis is associated with purpura and swollen joints and sometimes abdominal pain and melaena.

2. *Polyarteritis nodosa and systemic lupus erythematosus* in which red blood cell casts may also be found in the urine. Other organs are usually involved in the pathological process, and the diagnosis of these two diseases is suspected on this basis. Polyarteritis nodosa and systemic lupus

erythematosus are occasionally confined to the kidney, when renal biopsy is necessary to establish the diagnosis.

3. *Infective endocarditis*, in which microscopic haematuria is a valuable diagnostic sign, and uraemia may develop.

4. *Acute recurrent focal glomerulonephritis*, a condition of unknown but probably multiple aetiology in which recurrent episodes of haematuria occur over a period of months or years. There are no other symptoms or signs of acute proliferative glomerulonephritis. The diagnosis is made by renal biopsy in which mesangial proliferation is found sometimes affecting only some glomeruli but commonly associated with the deposition of IgA. Repeated episodes may lead to progressive glomerular destruction with renal failure and hypertension in a few patients.

Other conditions which may need to be distinguished from acute glomerulonephritis are:

A. *Angio-oedema*, in which sudden swelling of the eyelids is a frequent feature. This condition is usually associated with swelling of the lips or tongue; urinary abnormalities are absent. In addition, the patient may be known to have an allergic history, similar attacks may have occurred previously, and eosinophilia is often present in the peripheral blood.

B. *Acute pyelonephritis*, in which oedema is absent while pain and tenderness in the lumbar region and frequency of micturition may occur. The urine contains micro-organisms, more pus cells than red blood cells and red cell casts are absent.

C. *Haematuria due to tuberculosis or tumours* of the kidney or urinary tract in which oedema does not occur and there are no cellular casts in the urine.

Treatment. Patients suffering from the acute nephritic syndrome should remain in bed until haematuria, hypertension and oedema have disappeared and proteinuria has decreased. The intake of protein should be reduced to 40 g daily. While oedema is present fluid should be restricted to half a litre daily plus the volume of the previous day's output. Salt should not be added to food. If oedema is severe a low salt diet and diuretics may be necessary. When hypertension and haematuria have subsided and diuresis has occurred the protein and salt content of the diet can be increased.

In the occasional rare case of severe nephritis with anuria or extreme oliguria the regime described on page 401 should be adopted.

Streptococcal infection should be treated with penicillin. Removal of infected tonsils or other septic foci should be delayed until convalescence is advanced, as operation may be followed by an exacerbation, especially if carried out during the acute stage. However, in a few cases with persistence or repeated recurrence of symptoms and signs, these features may disappear only after the removal of a focus of chronic infection, e.g. an abscess at the root of a tooth. In the event of operative treatment being needed, benzylpenicillin should be given on the day of operation and for 3 days after it. When the condition is associated with other infections appropriate antimicrobial treatment should be given.

Hypertension does not require treatment in the majority of cases but hypertensive encephalopathy should be treated as described on page 183. Attempts to influence the course of the disease by the use of corticosteroids or immunosuppressive drugs have not been successful. Plasma exchange has been used to remove antibasement membrane antibodies in Goodpasture's syndrome.

Minimal Lesion Glomerulonephritis and Membranous Glomerulonephritis

These conditions are associated with a marked increase in the permeability of the glomerular basement membrane. This leads to proteinuria which is often so severe that the nephrotic syndrome with hypoproteinaemia and oedema develop. The two conditions are described together because, although they tend to affect different age groups, their clinical presentation is similar.

Aetiology and Pathology. In membranous glomerulonephritis the histological appearances consist of a loss of pedicel (foot process) structure and thickening of the glomerular basement membrane associated with subepithelial deposition of IgG (Fig. 11.3). As the disease progresses the thickening becomes more severe and the glomerular tufts are converted into structureless hyaline tissue. Immunofluorescent studies show that

while immunoglobulins are deposited in the basement membrane, there is little or none of the endothelial or mesangial cell proliferation so characteristic of proliferative glomerulonephritis.

These findings taken together with experimental studies suggest that membranous glomerulonephritis is the result of antigen-antibody complexes sufficiently small to pass through most of the thickness of the glomerular basement membrane and become deposited on its external subepithelial aspect. While this could explain the lack of mesangial cell proliferation, the possibility of glomerular injury from other mechanisms cannot be excluded and the nature of the antigen or antigens is unknown in the vast majority of cases.

Antibodies to type B hepatitis are occasionally associated with membranous glomerulonephritis and the condition occasionally occurs in response to the presence of solid tumours and lymphomas. Membranous glomerulonephritis is also strongly associated with HLA-DR3.

In minimal lesion glomerulonephritis, the glomeruli show no lesion when examined by light microscopy. However, abnormalities of glomerular structure involving the pedicels of the epithelial cells are revealed by the electron microscope (Fig. 11.3). The evidence suggests that this condition does not progress to glomerular destruction as is usually the case with membranous glomerulonephritis, and there is no evidence that the condition is due to the deposition of immune complexes. Minimal lesion glomerulonephritis may rarely follow exposure to pollen and this suggests an anaphylactic immune response (p. 24); however there is no immunofluorescent or other evidence to implicate IgE in the disease process.

Clinical Features. Minimal lesion glomerulonephritis occurs predominantly in children and young adults while membranous glomerulonephritis mainly affects those over 30 years of age. Both diseases are insidious in onset. If the proteinuria is slight they may persist without symptoms and remain undetected for months or years. When proteinuria increases in severity, oedema occurs and it is in this way that attention may be drawn to the presence of disease. The oedema is generalised, involving first the subcutaneous tissue and later the serous sacs and lungs. The face presents a pale and puffy appearance. The general health may remain good for some considerable time but eventually becomes progressively impaired, with increased liability to infection of the oedematous tissues or the serous cavities. Protein malnutrition with striae in the skin and osteoporosis may occur.

The urine contains protein in moderate amounts though as much as 30 g may be excreted daily by occasional patients. Granular and hyaline casts are seen on microscopic examination, red cells being scanty or absent.

At first chemical examination of the blood shows little or no increase in urea. Plasma cholesterol is slightly raised and the plasma and ascitic fluid may look milky due to an increase in fat and β-lipoproteins. Total plasma proteins are greatly reduced e.g. to 30–40 g/l. There are quantitative changes in the various globulin fractions, but the chief reduction affects albumin. Proteins of larger molecular weight, e.g. α_2-macroglobulin, do not so readily pass the glomerular barrier and are retained in the blood and hence are increased relative to the other plasma proteins. The resulting fall of colloid osmotic pressure of the plasma is mainly responsible for the massive oedema which is the prominent clinical feature. The ensuing oligaemia stimulates the secretion of aldosterone which promotes further sodium and water retention and sometimes potassium loss.

In the early stage of the disease renal function tests reveal no impairment of glomerular filtration rate or of the ability to concentrate urine.

Course and Prognosis. Prior to the use of effective diuretics, antibiotics and corticosteroids, the oedema persisted in the majority of cases for months or years, with occasional spontaneous but temporary remissions. Most patients died either from intercurrent infection in the oedematous phase or from renal failure. There is now ample evidence that in patients with minimal lesion glomerulonephritis, corticosteroids and immunosuppressive treatment causes the proteinuria to subside and the condition to resolve in the great majority of cases. In membranous glomerulonephritis, however, the prognosis is less favourable. Arterial hypertension and hypertensive retinopathy develop and progressive renal destruction ultimately reduces the rate of glomerular filtration

in most cases. Proteinuria diminishes, and consequently the plasma proteins rise and oedema becomes less. There is gradual impairment of renal function as the disease progresses to chronic glomerulonephritis with uraemia (p. 391). In a minority of cases, however, slow resolution of the glomerular lesion occurs and patients may recover completely.

Differential Diagnosis of the Nephrotic Syndrome. The term 'nephrotic syndrome' is used to describe the clinical state of hypoproteinaemic oedema associated with marked proteinuria irrespective of its aetiology. *Minimal lesion glomerulonephritis* is the most common cause of the nephrotic syndrome in children and is responsible for about 20% of cases in the adult. *Membranous glomerulonephritis* is more common in adults; both must be distinguished from other renal disorders which give rise to a similar clinical picture. Sometimes the aetiology of the nephrotic syndrome is obvious from the presence of other clinical features of the causative disease. In most patients it is necessary to carry out a renal biopsy in order to make the diagnosis.

The various forms of *proliferative glomerulonephritis* are occasionally associated with marked proteinuria and massive oedema. In some patients the clinical history and the course of the disease are sufficient to make this diagnosis clear, but in many the true nature of the syndrome is detected only after renal biopsy. Mesangiocapillary glomerulonephritis is often then found to be responsible (p. 388).

Amyloidosis is an uncommon cause of the nephrotic syndrome. This is a multisystem disease which may be generalised or localised. When the kidney is involved, extracellular deposits of fibrils and protein damage glomerular capillaries and cause marked proteinuria. The diagnosis of amyloidosis can be established by renal biopsy. A search should then be made for the presence of an underlying disorder such as rheumatoid arthritis, chronic suppuration, lepromatous leprosy or multiple myeloma.

Renal vein thrombosis is a rare cause of the nephrotic syndrome. It should be suspected when proteinuria occurs in a patient with evidence of deep venous thrombosis in the lower limbs or if an illness is complicated by pain in the loins and the subsequent development of the nephrotic syndrome. Renal vein thrombosis may occasionally accompany membranous glomerulonephritis.

Other causes of the nephrotic syndrome with individual distinguishing features are diabetic nephropathy, drugs (e.g. penicillamine and gold), systemic lupus erythematosus, polyarteritis nodosa, tumours and *P. malariae* infection in children in parts of Africa.

The nephrotic syndrome must also be distinguished from:

Cardiac failure with severe oedema, in which dyspnoea is present, the venous pressure is increased, signs of underlying cardiac disease are present, oedema is usually absent from the face, and proteinuria is less severe.

Hypoproteinaemic oedema, due to causes other than loss of protein in the urine, namely impairment of intake, digestion, absorption or synthesis of protein and in protein-losing enteropathy.

Treatment is directed at relief of oedema and control of proteinuria. As long as the blood urea is not elevated, a liberal intake of protein is desirable in an attempt to make good the urinary loss of protein. At least 90–100 g protein should be given daily. This may be supplemented with proprietary salt-free protein concentrates.

Salt intake should be restricted by prohibiting extra table salt, avoiding salty foods and reducing the amount used in cooking. Although drastic salt restriction occasionally produces dramatic results, 'salt-free' diets are so unappetising that patients will not tolerate them for more than a few weeks.

Diuretics such as frusemide (p. 96) are of great value in controlling the oedema. Because of the associated oligaemia these diuretics occasionally induce renal failure by causing further salt loss. In this event, or if the oedema is resistant, relief is obtained by giving plasma, salt-free albumin or dextran intravenously along with the diuretics. Spironolactone is indicated in patients who show marked features of secondary aldosteronism, e.g. hypokalaemia.

Corticosteroids provide the main chance of cure in the treatment of minimal lesion glomerulonephritis in which the proteinuria is selective (p. 381). In the majority of cases this treatment abolishes proteinuria. Prednisolone should be given in doses of 1 mg/kg/d for about 3 weeks and then reduced to about one-third of this dose and continued for 2–3 months. In a minority of patients with minimal lesion glomerulonephritis the condition relapses after treatment when prednisolone is stopped. Such individuals are then best treated with cyclophosphamide in daily doses of 3 mg/kg for 2 months. A weekly check of the white blood cell count should be made and the dose reduced if leucopenia develops. Other adverse effects are given on page 561.

Corticosteroids, cyclophosphamide and other immunosuppressive drugs are ineffective in membranous glomerulonephritis.

CHRONIC GLOMERULONEPHRITIS

Aetiology. Chronic glomerulonephritis develops when proliferative glomerulonephritis becomes progressive and in most cases of membranous glomerulonephritis. Frequently, no history of either disease is obtained and in these, postmortem studies of the kidney suggests that the pathological change has been developing insidiously over many years. Chronic glomerulonephritis ends in chronic renal failure.

Pathology. The kidneys are small; the capsules strip with difficulty, leaving a granular surface; the peripelvic fat is increased and there is great reduction in renal cortical tissue. The normal distinction between cortex and medulla is obscured. On microscopical examination there is fibrosis or hyalinisation of most of the glomeruli with fibrous replacement of many tubules. Remaining nephrons may show hypertrophy and arteriolosclerosis is usually present.

Clinical features of chronic glomerulonephritis are attributable to the effects of chronic renal failure combined usually with arterial hypertension. As renal failure develops, the composition of the body fluid becomes abnormal, particularly with regard to its water and salt content, its acid-base equilibrium, and the concentration of nitrogenous compounds which are normally excreted by the kidney. These alterations ultimately combine to produce the clinical picture of severe uraemia which is the terminal stage of renal failure.

A history of acute glomerulonephritis or of the

nephrotic syndrome is obtained in some cases. The earlier stages of the disease may be unattended by symptoms but may come to light only by discovery of proteinuria or hypertension during the course of a routine examination. Later, because of the widespread consequences of progressive renal failure, the symptoms and signs are referable to almost every system and patients suffering from the disease present with complaints which at first sight may not suggest their renal origin. Medical advice may be sought because of polyuria, thirst, itching, loss of energy, weakness, nausea, vomiting, or diarrhoea. Polyuria develops both because of diminished power for tubular reabsorption of water and because the elevated blood urea produces an osmotic diuresis. Anaemia is the main cause of the loss of energy and it is usually normocytic. The high blood pressure may have been detected in the course of a general examination or the patient may consult the doctor for headache, loss of vision or breathlessness or because of the occurrence of cerebrovascular insufficiency.

As the disease progresses, renal function deteriorates and uraemia increases. The blood concentration of urea and other nitrogenous compounds steadily rises. The patient looks more ill and the complexion is sallow, often accompanied by a yellow-brown discolouration attributed to the retention of urinary pigment. With the exception of those who develop cardiac failure from hypertension and those in whom the chronic stage of the disease has followed rapidly upon the initial oedematous stage, the patients are not only free from oedema but usually exhibit signs of water and salt depletion. The skin and tongue are dry and the blood pressure may fall from its previous high level. Acidosis contributes to the dyspnoea and the respirations are deep (Kussmaul's respiration).

Hiccoughs, pruritus, muscular twitchings, fits, drowsiness and coma may occur. A tendency to bleed, mainly due to platelet dysfunction, may develop in the terminal phase, as evidenced by epistaxis, bleeding gums, bruises, purpura, haematemesis and melaena. Hypertensive retinopathy of any degree may be present and visual impairment may result from numerous hard exudates arranged in star shapes around the macula

(Plate I). Peripheral neuropathy due to uraemia also occurs.

Some patients complain of vague muscle or bone pain and in a few cases this becomes severe. These features are due to *renal osteodystrophy* which consists of osteomalacia, osteitis fibrosa and areas of osteosclerosis. Osteomalacia results from failure of the kidney to convert vitamin D to the active metabolite (p. 66). In young individuals this interferes with growth causing 'renal rickets'. Osteitis fibrosa arises as a result of secondary hyperparathyroidism, the parathyroid glands being stimulated by the low concentration of plasma calcium. The cause of osteosclerosis is unknown.

Investigation. During the early stages of the disease, and before nitrogen retention in the blood is detectable, the urine is found to contain protein, usually in small amounts; red blood cells and granular and hyaline casts are present in small numbers. Later glomerular filtration may be reduced to less than 10% of normal and there is a gradual rise in the concentration of plasma urea, creatinine and phosphate. The ability of the kidneys to form concentrated or dilute urine is impaired. Ultimately this power is lost completely and the urine is of a fixed specific gravity. The plasma concentration of bicarbonate diminishes as acidosis occurs. The plasma concentration of calcium is frequently reduced due to defective vitamin D metabolism and to the elevation of plasma phosphate. Potassium occasionally accumulates in the blood and may cause death by its effect on the heart.

A plain radiograph or ultrasonic examination of the abdomen may show small, irregular kidneys; the changes of renal osteodystrophy may be seen on skeletal radiography.

Course and Prognosis. The disease progresses steadily over months or years and, in the absence of treatment by dialysis or renal transplantation, leads to a fatal termination. The course may be punctuated by exacerbations of acute glomerulonephritis which hasten the progress of the disease. When nitrogen retention and acidosis are severe, the outlook is grave and most patients die in a few months or a year. Papilloedema is a bad prognostic sign and unless treatment with antihypertensive drugs is begun before uraemia becomes severe, most patients who show it die within a few months.

The cause of death is generally uraemia, frequently complicated by infection to which such patients are susceptible; in other cases the patient dies from a cerebral haemorrhage, cardiac failure or myocardial infarction. A terminal non-bacterial pericarditis is common. Haemorrhage from any site or enterocolitis are also ominous features.

Differential Diagnosis. The distinction between chronic glomerulonephritis and other causes of chronic renal failure with hypertension is difficult and may be impossible. A similar clinical picture may arise in the following diseases.

1. Other conditions which primarily affect the glomeruli with their eventual destruction include systemic lupus erythematosus, polyarteritis nodosa, amyloid disease and diabetes mellitus. Patients with these conditions may die ultimately of renal failure and uraemia.

2. Essential hypertension may occasionally lead to nephrosclerosis and uraemia and should be suspected if there is a family history of high blood pressure. In the malignant phase of hypertension from any cause, evidence of renal disease is invariably present and renal failure is rapidly progressive.

3. Congenital polycystic disease of the kidneys may be diagnosed by the family history, by palpation of the enlarged, irregular kidneys and by ultrasound or urography. Uraemic medullary cystic disease (p. 406) is also occasionally responsible for chronic renal failure.

4. Chronic pyelonephritis is more common in women, and hypertension may be absent. There may be a history of acute pyelonephritis and organisms can sometimes be cultured from the urine. The diagnosis is often suggested by the radiological appearances seen after urography.

5. Analgesic nephropathy (p. 406) is suggested by a history of analgesic abuse.

6. Bilateral hydronephrosis may be confirmed by ultrasonography or retrograde urography.

7. Congenital renal hypoplasia with bilateral small kidneys is occasionally the cause of death from uraemia in children.

8. Urinary schistosomiasis is a common cause of chronic renal failure in endemic areas in Africa and the Middle East (pp. 782 and 717).

Treatment. The natural history of chronic glomerulonephritis, unlike that of some other causes of chronic renal insufficiency, cannot be altered and there is progressive deterioration in renal function. However, the patient's feeling of well-being may be considerably improved with suitable treatment.

DIET. Protein should not be restricted until definite symptoms of uraemia develop. At this point, if long-term dialysis is contraindicated or facilities for this treatment unavailable, the protein intake should be restricted to about 40 g/day and an adequate intake of carbohydrate (250 g) and fat (60 g) provided, giving an energy value of 1700 kcal. In the terminal stages further protein restriction to 20 g/day is indicated.

FLUID. Restriction is contraindicated since, in view of the impaired concentrating power, a large volume of urine is needed to excrete end-products of metabolism. Except in the presence of cardiac failure the daily fluid intake should be sufficient to produce at least $2\frac{1}{2}$ l of urine daily.

SALT. In the absence of oedema, cardiac failure or arterial hypertension salt restriction is contraindicated. Excessive loss of sodium in the urine occurs in some forms of chronic renal insufficiency (p. 89) but not in glomerulonephritis. These patients can, however, become depleted of sodium and water as a result of nausea and vomiting in which case fluid and electrolytes must be given intravenously to restore the extracellular fluid volume. The volume and nature of the fluid required depends upon the severity of the salt and water depletion and the degree of acidosis (p. 90). An average amount for a case of moderate severity is 4 l given in 24 hours, one part of isotonic sodium bicarbonate, one part of isotonic sodium chloride and two parts 5% glucose. The infusion should be continued until the blood hydrogen ion concentration has been reduced, if possible to within the normal range, and until the patient is adequately hydrated.

INFECTION. Obvious foci of infection, e.g. tonsils, infected sinuses or root abscesses should be treated in order to reduce the likelihood of an exacerbation of acute glomerulonephritis. Antimicrobial agents, as with some other drugs, must be used with special care in reduced dosage in the presence of chronic renal failure, notably co-trimoxazole, streptomycin, gentamicin, kanamycin, tobramycin and cephaloridine. Tetracyclines should not be used because of their tendency to raise the blood urea.

ANAEMIA. This should be treated by slow blood transfusions though it is probably not desirable to increase the concentration of haemoglobin above 8·5 g/dl as a rapid rise in haematocrit causes a fall in renal plasma flow and a temporary aggravation of the uraemia. Iron therapy is ineffective unless there is evidence of iron deficiency.

NAUSEA, HICCOUGH and VOMITING. These symptoms may be relieved by chlorpromazine given in reduced doses (e.g. 25 mg i.m.) because of the danger of accumulation.

BONE PAIN. When the dominant radiographic picture is that of osteomalacia, vitamin D should be given daily as 1–2μg of alfacalcidol (p. 67). The treatment should be controlled by chemical estimations of plasma calcium and alkaline phosphatase, for there is a significant risk of producing hypercalcaemia and calcification of the tissues. This tendency is also reduced by giving aluminium hydroxide by mouth to bind phosphate in the gut and lower its plasma concentration.

CARDIOVASCULAR COMPLICATIONS. The presence of uraemia is no contraindication to the treatment of coexisting hypertension provided that care is taken to see that antihypertensive treatment does not cause a drop in renal blood flow and a rise in the concentration of blood urea. The choice and use of drugs should be made according to the recommendations given on pages 180–183. Digoxin is normally excreted in the urine, and hence in renal failure the maintenance dose should not usually exceed 0·25 mg three times per week.

REVERSIBLE FACTORS. A search should be made in every case for reversible factors which exacerbate the biochemical disturbance and these should be corrected. Renal perfusion is diminished in the presence of sodium and water depletion, following haemorrhage and when there is untreated cardiac failure or uncontrolled hypertension. The glomerular filtration rate is also reduced when there is urinary tract obstruction. Renal function can also be depressed, reversibly, by nephrotoxic drugs such as the aminoglycosides, tetracyclines and non-steroid analgesics. Infection at any site increases protein catabolism and raises the blood urea, while infection in the urinary tract may cause a reversible reduction in renal function.

DIALYSIS AND RENAL TRANSPLANTATION. *Haemodialysis*. It is possible by repeated intermittent haemodialysis to preserve the lives of many patients with chronic renal failure who are devoid of all renal function. Haemodialysis is indicated when, in spite of adequate medical treatment, symptoms of uraemia become troublesome and preferably before the patient is obliged to give up employment. It should always be started before the serious features of uraemia, e.g. pericarditis, nausea, diarrhoea or vomiting and bleeding occur. Repeated access to blood vessels is achieved by establishing an arteriovenous anastomosis, usually in the arm. Haemodialysis using cuprophane membranes, or polyacrylonitrile fashioned as hollow fibres, is best employed for periods of 4–6 hours three times weekly. In many instances patients can be trained to carry out their treatment at home, where survival of up to 10 years or more is common and where satisfactory mental and physical rehabilitation is best achieved.

Continuous Ambulatory Peritoneal Dialysis. This simple and less expensive form of long-term dialysis involves the introduction of a permanent intraperitoneal catheter, accessible from the skin surface on the anterior wall of the abdomen. Two litres of sterile isotonic dialysate fluid are introduced into the peritoneal cavity from a plastic container bag worn around the waist and left for periods of 6 hours. It is then evacuated and fresh dialysate fluid reintroduced. This cycle is repeated 4 times in each period of 24 hours, during which time the patient carries on with normal daily tasks. This form of treatment remains at the exploratory stage; some patients respond well to it, but there is a risk of recurrent peritonitis.

Renal Transplantation. The practicability of transplantation of a normal kidney from a healthy donor or a cadaver to patients with chronic irreversible renal failure should also be considered and is especially suitable in young persons. If the patient has a healthy identical twin who is willing to act as a donor, the prospects of a successful renal transplantation are excellent. However, most kidney transplantations are carried out using either kidneys from living but less closely related siblings or from cadavers. ABO compatibility is essential and it is customary to select donor kidneys on the basis of HLA compatibility. When a living donor sibling kidney is used, the best results are obtained when the donor and recipient have 3–4 HLA antigens in common; there is less evidence that matching is important in cadaver transplants, but preliminary results of matching using HLA-DR antigens are more promising. In the early years of renal transplanation, blood transfusion was avoided because of the possibility of alerting the immune system to foreign antigens and because of the danger of transmitting hepatitus B virus. More recently, it has been shown, paradoxically, that a number of units of blood transfused 1–3 months before cadaver transplant improves graft survival by about 20%, but the mechanism remains obscure (p. 416). After three years the average survival rate in living related donor grafts is about 75%, and in the case of cadaver grafts, 65%. The postoperative course is complicated by the need to give immunosuppressive drugs such as prednisolone, azathioprine, cyclosporin or antilymphocytic serum.

Dialysis and transplantation are best used flexibly in an integrated fashion. It is wise and usually necessary to establish every patient on dialysis and carry out renal transplantation when a suitable kidney becomes available, especially in the patients under the age of 45 years.

INFECTIONS OF THE KIDNEY AND URINARY TRACT

Infection of the urinary tract is an extremely common clinical problem. The infection may involve the urethra, the bladder, the ureters and the kidneys themselves. In any individual case it is difficult on clinical grounds to be certain of the extent of the invasion of the various parts of the urinary tract. Formerly it was assumed that the kidneys and the upper urinary tract are involved in every case, even when the symptoms of the infection are those solely of cystitis or urethritis. However, the great majority of patients develop recurrent symptoms of lower urinary tract infection without apparently suffering deterioration of renal function in later life, an important exception being children with vesico-ureteric reflux.

Acute Pyelonephritis

This is characterised by an acute inflammation of the parenchyma and pelvis of the kidney. The disease may be unilateral or bilateral.

Aetiology. Acute pyelonephritis is commonly associated with some obstruction in the urinary tract. In men this is often due to prostatic enlargement, in pregnant women to obstruction by the uterus and atonia of the ureters due to the action of progesterone, and in infants and children to congenital malformation of the urinary tract or vesico-ureteric reflux. Calculi, cervical prolapse, cystocele, foreign bodies or tumours may also be responsible. Pyelonephritis may occur in infancy and in adult women, however, without evidence of an obstructive lesion. Diabetes also predisposes to infection. In most cases the infection ascends via the ureter but in some, and notably the newborn, it is blood borne. About 75% of the infections are due to *Esch. coli*, the remainder being mostly due to klebsiella, streptococci, staphylococci or the proteus group of organisms.

The prevalence of urinary infections in the adult female suggests that the anatomical relation of the short urethra to the rectum is a predisposing factor. Catheterisation of the bladder is particularly liable to introduce organisms into the urinary tract; when indicated it should be carried out with the strict aseptic precautions.

Pathology. The renal pelvis is acutely inflamed and there is often a coincident inflammation of the bladder. In severe cases small abscesses may be seen on the surface of the kidney when the capsule has been stripped. On section, small cortical abscesses and linear streaks of pus in the medulla are often evident. On histological examination focal infiltration of the renal tissue by polymorphonuclear leucocytes is evident.

Clinical Features. In many cases there is a sudden onset of pain in one or both loins, radiating to the iliac fossae and suprapubic area. There may be dysuria (difficult or painful micturition) and strangury (a painful desire to pass urine though the bladder is empty), with the frequent passage of small amounts of scalding, usually cloudy urine due to an associated cystitis. The temperature rises rapidly to 38–40°C, with the general manifestations of fever. A rigor may occur, and there may be vomiting. Tenderness and muscular guarding may be present in the renal angle and the lumbar region. There is a leucocytosis. The urine in *Esch. coli* infections is nearly always acid; in other infections it may be acid or alkaline. On microscopic examination there are numerous pus cells and organisms, some red blood cells and epithelial cells. When the organisms are motile Gram-negative bacilli and the urine is acid, the infection may be assumed to be due to *Esch. coli*.

Acute pyelonephritis in infants and children, like infections of the throat and middle ear, often presents as fever without any localising symptoms. The initial feature may be a convulsion but apathy, abdominal distension and diarrhoea may occur. In the feverish child, particular attention should be paid to these sites and the urine should be examined for pus cells and organisms.

Routine culture of a midstream specimen of urine has revealed the presence of asymptomatic bacteriuria (> 100 000 organisms/ml) in about 5% of all pregnancies during the early months. If no antibiotics are given, acute pyelonephritis occurs in about 40% of such cases whereas this is rare in those in whom the urine was sterile at the original examination. Investigation by intravenous urography after the termination of pregnancy shows a high incidence of abnormalities of the urinary tract in those women with bacteriuria. Suppressive chemotherapy at the asymptomatic stage has been found to prevent the development of acute symptoms.

Course and Prognosis. With adequate treatment the disease subsides rapidly in the great majority of cases. Fever, pain, frequency and dysuria disappear and the urine usually becomes sterile within a few days.

In some cases, although the acute symptoms subside, a low-grade infection may persist, and the disease may pass into the chronic stage. More rarely the disease may be severe and cause necrosis of the papillae (*acute necrotising papillitis*). Fragments of renal tissue are then excreted in the urine and can be identified histologically. This complication, which may lead to renal failure, is particularly liable to occur in diabetic patients and in those addicted to non-steroidal analgesics (p. 558).

In view of the frequency of acute pyelonephritis, the curable nature of the condition, and the fact that chronic pyelonephritis is a common cause of renal failure and hypertension, the importance of adequate treatment of the acute stage cannot be overstressed.

Differential Diagnosis. Acute pyelonephritis should be distinguished from acute appendicitis, salpingitis, cholecystitis and diverticulitis, especially by the absence of pus and organisms in the urine in these conditions. Less commonly nowadays it may be mimicked by *perinephric abscess* due to infection by *Staph. aureus*. The characteristic clinical features are pain and tenderness in the renal region, fever and polymorphonuclear leucocytosis. Urinary symptoms are absent and there are no pus cells or organisms in the urine. Oedema may obliterate the normal hollow in the loin, and an abscess may eventually point in the loin or groin.

Treatment depends upon the infecting organism and its sensitivity, and ideally a midstream specimen of urine should be sent to the laboratory before specific therapy is begun. This specimen should reach the laboratory within 2 hours of voiding or be refrigerated at 4°C for a period not exceeding 24 hours. Since infection is usually due to *Esch. coli* treatment with sulphadimidine, trimethoprim or co-trimoxazole can be commenced and altered later if so indicated by the results of the culture or if the response is unsatisfactory. In the very severe case, and if *Esch. coli* septicaemia occurs, gentamicin is the drug of choice. Ampicillin is of value in proteus infections.

Whatever drug is employed a second midstream specimen of urine should be sent to the laboratory from 4 to 6 weeks after the completion of the initial week's course of treatment to make sure that the infection has been eradicated. If this has not been accomplished further treatment with the appropriate antibiotic must be given, depending on the bacteriological findings.

In every case the possibility of calculus, an obstructive lesion of the urinary tract or renal tuberculosis must be kept in mind and treated if found.

Chronic Pyelonephritis

Aetiology. This disease in the adult may be caused by infection above an unrelieved obstruction to the urinary tract, e.g. calculus, stricture or prostatic disease. Other cases may follow cystitis due to stasis as a result of a cystocele or interference with the innervation of the bladder, e.g. in paraplegia or multiple sclerosis. In conditions in which the outflow tract of the bladder is deranged, reflux of urine into the ureters may occur during micturition and contribute to the persistence of infection.

In the absence of obstructive lesions, vesico-ureteric reflux is an important determinant of infection and of progressive kidney damage in infancy and childhood. Chronic pyelonephritis also occurs in conditions associated with nephrocalcinosis (p. 403). *Esch. coli* is the organism responsible for most cases. Other infecting agents include proteus, *Ps. aeruginosa* and staphylococci.

Because of difficulty in culturing organisms from the urine of many patients with clinical and radiological features of pyelonephritis, the term *chronic interstitial nephritis* is often advocated as an alternative. Its use implies that the cause of the fibrosing destructive renal disease is unknown and that factors other than previous episodes of infection may be responsible. What these factors might be is unclear but they could possibly include reactions to analgesics and other drugs (p. 406).

Pathology. The changes may be unilateral or bilateral, and of any grade of severity. The fully developed case usually shows gross scarring of the kidneys, which may be much reduced in size with narrowing of the cortex and medulla. Renal scars are juxtaposed to dilated calyces. Microscopically there is patchy fibrosis with chronic inflammatory cell infiltration, tubular atrophy, periglomerular fibrosis and eventual disappearance of nephrons. The arteries and arterioles may show sclerosis and narrowing.

Clinical Features. In many cases no symptoms arise directly from the renal lesions, and the patient may consult the doctor because of lassitude, tiredness and vague ill-health or for symptoms of uraemia or arterial hypertension. The discovery of hypertension or proteinuria on routine examination may be the first indication of the presence of the disease. Symptoms arising from the urinary tract, however, may also be present and include frequency of micturition, dysuria and aching lumbar pain. Occasionally weakness and fainting may occur if the renal disorder is accompanied by excessive salt loss in the urine. The urine may contain pus cells, a small amount of protein and many epithelial cells, though in some cases it may be normal.

In all cases investigations such as rectal or vaginal examination, cystoscopy and urography must be carried out to discover the nature of any underlying mechanical factor causing obstruction to the flow of urine and to determine the extent of renal damage. Radiographs are diagnostic and show affected kidneys to be reduced in size and localised contraction of the renal substance associated with clubbing of adjacent calyces. A micturating cystogram discloses vesico-ureteric reflux.

Course and Prognosis. The course is usually a long one and is sometimes punctuated by acute exacerbations. The infection is difficult to eradicate, even when underlying mechanical obstructions are found and relieved.

Pyonephrosis may occur, especially in the presence of renal calculi. It is characterised by persistent lumbar pain, intermittent pyrexia, often with rigors, emaciation, pyuria, and, if both kidneys are involved, uraemia; one or both kidneys may become palpable.

Some cases progress to chronic uraemia, which may be alleviated for a year or two by treatment. In elderly, diabetic or paraplegic patients a fulminating infection may be the immediate cause of death.

Treatment is similar to that described for the acute disease. The chronic infection is usually more difficult to eradicate. Attempts should be made to remove obstructive lesions or renal calculi by appropriate surgical procedures. An antibiotic to which the organism is sensitive should be given for 7 days (p. 396). If the infection is not eradicated suppressive treatment may be required for many months, the antibiotic used being given in smaller doses and as indicated by the changing pattern and sensitivity of the organisms in the urine. Ampicillin, co-trimoxazole and nalidixic acid (1 g t.i.d.) are valuable for this purpose.

When the renal infection is unilateral or if pyonephrosis has developed, nephrectomy may be indicated; rarely, high blood pressure may be cured by the removal of the diseased kidney. The role of surgery in the correction of vesico-uretic reflux is undecided, particularly because the reflux tends to disappear as the child grows older.

A moderate degree of uraemia may be present which progresses little for months or years. This is especially so when hypertension is absent or minimal. Cases with more severe renal impairment should be treated as indicated on page 393. Patients who lose excessive amounts of sodium in the urine become depleted of sodium and water and this increases the uraemia. Clinical improvement can be achieved in such cases by giving 5–10 g of salt daily by mouth. The limit to the additional salt is set by the occurrence of systemic or pulmonary oedema, or by an aggravation of hypertension. Sodium bicarbonate may be substituted in part for sodium chloride when acidosis is severe.

Cystitis, Urethritis and Prostatitis

Some infections of the urinary tract may be confined to the urethra or bladder. In these, the features of systemic illness are slight and the symptoms are those of frequency and dysuria. Scalding pain is felt in the urethra during micturition. Suprapubic pain of cystitis is felt before, during and for a few moments after voiding urine. Although the bladder is empty there may be an intense desire to pass more urine due to spasm of its inflamed wall. Tenderness is often present in the suprapubic region, and the urine may have an unpleasant odour and appear cloudy. Pus cells, red cells and organisms may be seen on microscopical examination. Sometimes the urine is grossly blood-stained. Cystitis is particularly common in women and girls, and the infection is usually due to *Esch. coli*. Urethritis may be due to gonorrhoea (p. 411) or other organisms (p. 412).

In some patients with symptoms suggestive of urethritis and cystitis, no bacteria can be cultured from the urine. The term *'urethral syndrome'* has been applied to this category of patients who are predominantly female. The cause of the symptoms is unknown although a variety of explanations, which include allergy to deodorants, etc., congestion of the urethra possibly related to sexual activity and infection of the urethral glands, have been put forward.

In acute prostatitis there may be considerable systemic disturbance and the patient may complain of perineal pain. On digital examination of the rectum the prostate gland is usually very tender.

Treatment of infections is similar to that of acute pyelonephritis (p. 396) but antibiotics are rarely needed for more than one week. In the majority of instances this is effective and there is no recurrence of the symptoms. In some patients, however, the clinical features of infection persist or recur. In patients with a normal urinary tract, particularly women with recurrent urinary infection induced by sexual intercourse, the majority can be kept free of attacks by use of long-term low dose antibacterial drugs, taken after voiding urine before going to bed. Such a regimen should be commenced after a curative course of treatment, as evidenced by bacteriological culture. Some women with recurrent infection can remain free of attacks by practising pre- and postcoital micturition, or by carefully cleansing the perineum, by applying an antiseptic cream such as 0·5% cetrimide to the periurethral area prior to sexual intercourse. It is preferable to attempt these simpler measures before embarking on a prophylactic course of treatment with an antibacterial agent.

Possible causes of failure to respond to treatment, or of relapse, include:

1. Infection with organisms e.g. trichomonas, resistant to the antimicrobial agent employed.

2. Tuberculosis.

3. Continued infection from above, e.g. pyelonephritis associated with calculi.

4. Obstruction below the base of the bladder by prostatic hyperplasia, carcinoma of the prostate, or urethral stricture.

5. Atrophy of the urethra consequent upon oestrogen lack after the menopause.

6. Involvement of the bladder by: (a) malignant tumour arising in the bladder or in adjacent organs; (b) vesical calculus; (c) a foreign body may have been inserted into the bladder; (d) inflammation from adjacent structures, e.g. diverticulitis.

7. The presence of urethral caruncle, cysto-

cele, urethrocele or cervicitis in the female or meatal fissure in the male.

8. Paraplegia, in which urinary infection is frequent, persistent and often the ultimate cause of death.

Renal Tuberculosis

Tuberculosis of the kidney is invariably secondary to tuberculosis elsewhere and occurs as a result of blood-borne infection. The initial lesion develops in the renal cortex and if untreated may ulcerate into the pelvis with consequent involvement of the bladder, epididymes, seminal vesicles and prostate. The disease tends to occur in young people and may manifest itself with recurrent haematuria and dysuria due to secondary involvement of the bladder. In addition the general features of tuberculosis, i.e. malaise, fever, lassitude and weight loss, may be present.

Culture of the urine by ordinary methods may be sterile in spite of pyuria. The extent of the infection should be ascertained by cystoscopic examination, by urography and by culture of the urine from both ureters. Chemotherapy should be given as for tuberculosis elsewhere (p. 236). Partial or total nephrectomy or epididymectomy may be necessary in those in whom the disease has advanced to the stage of producing serious destruction of tissue.

RENAL FAILURE

The term *uraemia* has been used for more than a century to describe the clinical state which arises from renal failure. The symptoms of renal failure are attributable not so much to retention of abnormal amounts of urea in the blood but to disturbances in hydrogen ion concentration, abnormalities in water and electrolyte balance and the accumulation of many other products of metabolism. In addition, renal failure is accompanied in the majority of cases by arterial hypertension, and this further complicates the clinical picture.

Classification. Renal function may be impaired by disease or drugs that affect the renal parenchyma (renal uraemia), by extrarenal disorders such as acute circulatory failure (prerenal uraemia) or as a result of conditions in which there is obstruction to the outflow of urine (postrenal uraemia). The deterioration of kidney function which ensues may be acute or chronic and of varying degrees of severity.

For descriptive purposes, renal failure is conveniently considered under the following 4 headings:

1. Renal failure due to disease of the kidneys.
2. Renal failure due to prerenal disease.
3. Renal failure due to acute tubular necrosis.
4. Renal failure due to postrenal causes.

1. Renal Failure due to Disease of the Kidneys

Renal failure due to disease of the kidneys may occur acutely or develop insidiously and become chronic or persistent.

The clinical features and treatment of renal failure occurring as a result of glomerulonephritis are described on pages 391 and 393. The manifestations of renal failure due to other kidney diseases are similar but there are also the features of the underlying process e.g. bilateral pyelonephritis, accelerated (malignant) hypertension, polyarteritis nodosa, systemic lupus erythematosus, polycystic disease, diabetic nephropathy, amyloidosis, conditions causing hypercalcaemia (p. 441) and disseminated intravascular coagulation (p. 548). Less common causes include lesions of major renal arteries and damage due to nephrotoxic drugs (p. 406). The haemolytic-uraemic syndrome which may follow viral or other infections, and in which coagulation in renal blood vessels is a prominent feature, is also an important cause of acute renal failure.

2. Renal Failure due to Prerenal Disorder

Normal renal function is dependent upon the maintenance of an adequate renal circulation. The renal share of the cardiac output is normally about 25% at rest. If the cardiac output falls, the blood flow to organs other than the heart or brain is reduced. In this event, the glomerular filtration rate is reduced acutely and oliguria results. While systemic hypotension often precedes prerenal uraemia, renal ischaemia may occur in its absence. Regional vasoconstriction is a means by which the blood pressure may be maintained in the face of oligaemia, and the success of this mechanism may deprive the kidneys of a large part of their blood supply. The urine is usually small in volume and the concentration of urea in the blood gradually rises. The more important causes of prerenal failure include:

1. *Loss of blood* from any cause including complications of pregnancy, trauma or gastrointestinal bleeding.

2. *Loss of plasma* as in burns and crushing injuries.

3. *Loss of fluid and salt.*
   (a) *from the gut* in severe vomiting, diarrhoea, acute intestinal obstruction, pancreatitis, paralytic ileus and fistulous drainage.
   (b) *in the urine* in diabetic ketoacidosis.
   (c) *from the skin* in excessive sweating and severe exfoliative dermatitis.

4. *Hypotension* due to bacteraemic or cardiogenic shock or during the course of a surgical operation may reduce renal blood flow and precipitate renal failure particularly in those whose blood volume is already reduced.

5. *Intravascular haemolysis* and *rhabdomyolysis* (breakdown of muscle cells) release products which are capable of reducing the renal circulation and when severe this may lead to acute renal failure.

All these conditions should be treated by appropriate fluids given intravenously and by specific measures as indicated in the treatment of diabetic ketoacidosis, infection, etc. Prompt and effective replacement of blood, water and salt is essential. In many cases vigorous treatment in the early stages prevents the occurrence of significant degrees of renal failure. If oliguria or anuria persists in spite of the return of the circulation to normal then the structural changes of acute tubular necrosis have occurred.

3. Renal Failure due to Acute Tubular Necrosis

This disease is due to acute ischaemia affecting both kidneys, and is characterised by oliguria or anuria with urine of low specific gravity and rapidly developing uraemia. 'Tubular necrosis' is a misleading term because it does not accurately describe the histological abnormalities in the kidneys but it is in wide general use.

Aetiology. Acute tubular necrosis occurs as a complication of various conditions which are associated with renal ischaemia, and which are listed above as causes of prerenal uraemia. In addition certain drugs are capable of producing acute renal failure due to proximal tubular necrosis e.g. paracetamol, gentamicin and cephaloridine. Poisoning by substances such as sodium chlorate may also be responsible.

Pathogenesis. Severe shock and water and salt depletion are accompanied by wide-spread vasconstriction. Blood flow is reduced by the fall in cardiac output and in the kidneys afferent arteriolar vasoconstriction further curtails glomerular filtration. The latter sometimes occurs even when the systemic blood pressure is maintained. If the ischaemia is severe and of sufficiently long duration the basement membrane of the renal tubules is ruptured and focal necrosis of the cells occurs. Stasis of the circulation within the kidney is associated with some degree of intraglomerular coagulation. In addition, casts of haemoglobin or of plasma proteins sometimes form within the tubular lumen and interfere with the passage of fluid; interstitial oedema around the tubules may also raise the intrarenal pressure and constrict nephrons externally so contributing to the renal failure.

In cases due to agents such as gentamicin or sodium chlorate, direct damage to the renal tubular cells is responsible.

Rarely, but notably in cases of retroplacental haemorrhage occurring as a complication of pregnancy, the whole or a large part of the renal cortex is involved, the glomeruli as well as the tubules becoming necrotic. This is called *renal cortical necrosis.*

Clinical Features and Course. The clinical features are those of the causal condition together with those of rapidly developing uraemia. Initially the urine volume is commonly but not invariably greatly reduced to between 50 and 500 ml/d and this stage of the illness is called the *oliguric phase*. Any urine that is formed contains protein, casts and red and white blood cells. The specific gravity is usually about 1·010 early in the course of the disease, and this persists for several days or weeks.

The patient may feel well at first but after some days the features of uraemia appear. Initially these are anorexia, nausea and vomiting; apathy is followed by mental confusion and later muscular twitching, fits, drowsiness, coma, and bleeding episodes occur. At this stage the main dangers to life are (1) pulmonary oedema due to the injudicious administration of excessive amounts of fluid, (2) potassium intoxication due to the rise in the concentration of plasma potassium which is especially likely if there is haemolysis or massive soft tissue damage, (3) the occurrence of severe systemic infection to which such patients are susceptible and (4) uraemia and metabolic acidosis.

The oliguric phase of the disease usually lasts for 1 to 3 weeks. If the patient does not succumb the daily volume of urine increases and rapidly may reach several litres. This is called the *recovery* or *diuretic* phase and coincides with healing of the renal tubules, an increase in GFR, reduction in intrarenal tension and resolution of intratubular casts and intraglomerular coagulation. During this phase there is uncontrolled water and sodium loss, and, in the absence of treatment, severe muscle weakness may occur due to loss of potassium. The concentration of blood urea ceases to rise and then gradually falls. Virtually complete recovery of renal function then takes place slowly over a period of 3 to 6 months.

Treatment. With a view to preventing or minimising the renal lesion, the underlying cause should be treated urgently. The blood volume should be quickly restored by appropriate transfusion and water and electrolyte deficits should be replenished. Plasma urea, creatinine and electrolytes should be estimated and cultures of blood, urine and wounds carried out daily. The adequacy of blood transfusion and fluid therapy is best monitored by the use of an indwelling right atrial catheter and assessed by clinical response.

Patients with severe acute renal failure are seriously ill and require skilled nursing, preferably in single rooms designed to prevent cross-infection. Great care must be exercised in the use of drugs which are normally excreted by the kidneys.

THE OLIGURIC PHASE. Clinical and pathological studies have shown that the ischaemic renal lesions are usually reversible provided the patient can be kept alive during the oliguric phase. Treatment is therefore designed to minimise the need for renal function until healing occurs and this can often be achieved by simple dietary restrictions.

Water and Electrolyte Balance. This is maintained by replacing the obligatory losses of water through the skin and lungs, by giving about 500 ml water/d, and by giving no electrolytes since none are being lost from the body. In febrile patients an extra allowance of water is required to replace the fluid lost through sweating and a further small supplement equal to the volume of urine passed each day should be added. Should abnormal losses of fluid occur, as in diarrhoea, additional fluid and electrolytes will be required in appropriate amounts.

Protein and Energy. Dietary protein is restricted to about 20–40 g/d and attempts are made to suppress endogenous protein catabolism to a minimum by giving as much energy as possible as fat and carbohydrate. For this purpose a diet restricted in its protein and electrolyte content may be supplemented by a liquid glucose preparation. In the event of vomiting, oral treatment should be avoided and carbohydrate should be given in the form of 20% glucose via an indwelling central venous catheter.

In many patients in whom the acute renal failure is mild in degree and relatively short in duration this treatment prevents the blood urea from rising more than 4 mmol/l (20 mg per 100 ml) per day, and the accumulation of potassium from protein catabolism is usually not sufficient to have serious consequences. If elevation of plasma potassium concentration should occur attempts should be made to reduce it by employing methods described on page 94; these include (1) giving an intravenous infusion of 50 g of glucose and 10 units of unmodified insulin; (2) controlling acidosis by intravenous administration of isotonic sodium bicarbonate and (3) the use of a sodium or calcium charged resin which removes potassium from the body.

Haemodialysis. In some patients, however, and especially in those suffering from severe infection or trauma or massive tissue damage, or in whom blood has become loculated in one of the tissue spaces, the rate of rise of blood urea and potassium is much more rapid and occurs in spite of the application of conservative methods; in these circumstances life may be threatened from acute renal failure within a few days. The patient should then be transferred to a centre equipped with the means for extracorporeal dialysis. Daily haemodialyses may then be required over a period of several weeks before adequate renal function returns. When such a policy is adopted it is possible to be much more liberal regarding the intake of protein, fluid and energy which can be given parentally if necessary. This is desirable from the point of view of encouraging repair of damaged or diseased tissues and is rendered possible by the daily correction of the composition of the blood and volume of body fluids achieved by the artificial kidney. Essential surgical procedures may also be carried out during this period and should not be delayed until renal function recovers.

Peritoneal dialysis can sometimes be used as an alternative to haemodialysis. While this method has a place in the treatment of small children and of patients with cardiac failure, it is a prolonged and sometimes, uncomfortable procedure subject to complications, notably peritonitis.

RECOVERY OR DIURETIC PHASE. When diuresis commences, the concentration of blood urea tends to remain constant for a few days and then begins to fall. When this occurs, a light diet, containing not more than 70–80 g protein per day and ample fruit, should be provided. Sufficient fluid must be given to replace the increased and uncontrolled loss of water in the urine. The fluid intake must be increased by the volume of the previous days urinary output. Salt supplements are usually needed during the diuretic phase to compensate for increased urinary loss. On average about 3 g of sodium chloride and 2 g of sodium bicarbonate are needed for each litre of urine passed. The fruit usually compensates for the potassium loss, though in many cases an oral supplement of potassium chloride may also be required. As renal function improves and blood urea falls, a normal diet may be taken.

Prognosis. The high mortality accompanying acute renal failure of ischaemic origin has been greatly reduced by the measures described above. Prognosis depends upon the speed and efficiency with which the therapeutic measures are put into operation, the prompt recognition and effective treatment of complicating infection, and the nature and the severity of the condition precipitating the syndrome. In cases of uncomplicated acute renal failure, such as those due to simple haemorrhage, the mortality should now be less than 5% even when haemodialysis is required. In severe renal failure complicated by serious infection or multiple injuries it is about 60%, the outcome being determined by the severity of the underlying disorders and their complications rather than by the renal failure itself.

4. Renal Failure due to Postrenal Causes

Acute or chronic renal failure may result from obstruction at any point in the urinary tract due to the causes given below. In the presence of two functioning kidneys ureteric obstruction causes uraemia only when it is bilateral.

The diagnosis may be suggested by a history of previous urinary symptoms such as pain in the loins, haematuria, renal colic, nocturia or difficulty in micturition. However, in many instances the onset is clinically silent and the cause of the obstruction discovered only after appropriate investigations. In contrast to acute renal failure associated with tubular necrosis, anuria is common and the complete absence of urine suggests the need for ultrasonography, cytoscopy or ureteral catheterisation and retrograde pyelography.

Surgical treatment is required for all cases of renal failure due to postrenal obstruction. Uraemia may be severe, yet relief of the obstruction results in recovery of adequate renal function in many patients, provided that this treatment has not been delayed too long. Indeed relief of obstruction is sometimes accompanied by a massive diuresis which necessitates a high fluid and electrolyte intake.

OBSTRUCTION OF THE URINARY TRACT

Obstruction to the flow of urine from the kidney through the pelvis, ureter, bladder and urethra is a common disorder; it causes stasis and a rise in pressure within the urinary tract which predisposes to infection, stone formation and renal failure. Obstruction may occur at any level but is most often found at the pelvi-ureteric junction, in the ureter, at the neck of the bladder or in the urethra. Obstruction at the pelviureteric junction causes hydronephrosis; obstruction of the ureter results in hydroureter and later hydronephrosis; obstruction of the bladder neck or urethra distends the bladder, causes hypertrophy of its muscle seen on cystoscopic examination as trabeculation, and hydroureter and hydronephrosis. If obstruction is unrelieved, slow progressive destruction of renal tissue occurs. Superimposed infection may cause cystitis, ureteritis or pyonephrosis in which renal damage may become more rapid.

Aetiology. Obstruction may be due to an organic lesion in the lumen or in or around the wall of the urinary tract or it may arise because of a congenital neuromuscular defect at the pelvi-ureteric junction, ureter or bladder neck preventing the contraction wave and therefore the flow of urine. Vesico-ureteric reflux is an important complication in infancy. Organic causes include stone, blood clot, tumour or fibrosis following infection. An aberrant renal artery, retroperitoneal fibrosis, inadvertent ligation of the ureter at operation, carcinoma of the cervix, prostatic enlargement or phimosis may compress the lumen from outside.

Clinical features vary with the cause and site of the lesion and in particular whether it is above or below the bladder. When the obstruction is supravesical, renal colic may occur, especially if the onset is sudden. More commonly the obstruction is gradual and an aching pain in the loins, sometimes aggravated by drinking, develops. Superimposed infection causes systemic manifestations with fever and dysuria. Haematuria is common. Transmission of the increased hydrostatic pressure to the kidney in partial obstruction interferes with the counter-current concentrating mechanism and may result paradoxically in polyuria. Occasionally a hydronephrotic kidney is palpable. Sometimes the patient presents only with anuria and acute renal failure, and the diagnosis is made only after excretion urography or

ultrasound examination reveals dilated kidneys or ureters.

When the obstruction is below the bladder, there is difficulty in micturition and the urinary stream is thin in calibre and poor in force. Complete urinary retention may occur with consequent distension of the bladder, which may be visible as a swelling of the lower abdomen and palpable; anuria or overflow incontinence may ensue. In the latter event catheterisation reveals the presence of residual urine in the bladder after the patient has voided.

Treatment. In all cases the ultimate objective is to remove the source of obstruction. This is often possible, as in the case of a stone, prostatic hypertrophy or urethral stricture. In the first instance it is necessary to relieve the obstruction in order to alleviate symptoms and preserve renal function. The action required varies with the nature of the underlying disease, but sometimes it may be dealt with temporarily by draining the kidney, i.e. nephrostomy, the ureter, i.e. ureterostomy, or the bladder, i.e. suprapubic or urethral catheterisation. Temporary drainage of the obstructed kidneys can often be achieved by inserting fine catheters into the renal pelvis under ultrasound control. Antibiotics should be given if infection is severe but it is preferable to wait until the obstruction has been removed or relieved.

When the hydronephrosis or pyonephrosis affects one kidney and this is severely damaged, nephrectomy is indicated. When obstruction affects both kidneys and is irremediable appropriate treatment for renal failure should be given.

RENAL AND VESICAL CALCULI AND NEPHROCALCINOSIS

Aetiology. Urinary calculi have long presented fascinating aetiological problems which are still largely unsolved. Two or three centuries ago vesical calculus was so common in Britain that a respectable living could be made as a lithotomist, but the incidence is much lower at the present time for reasons that are not clear. It is indeed surprising that renal and vesical calculi or nephrocalcinosis do not occur more frequently since some of the constituents of urine are present in a concentration in excess of their maximum solubility in water. It seems likely that urine contains certain substances, e.g. glycosaminoglycans, pyrophosphate, and citrate, which, by forming complexes, keep otherwise insoluble salts in solution in the urine. The concentration of urate is also important as it interferes with this function. Other authorities believe that the primary cause of urinary calculi is a pre-existing renal or vesical lesion which acts as a nidus on which urinary constituents precipitate.

The following conditions are frequently associated with stone formation:

(a) Climate or occupation which necessitates living or working under conditions where excessive loss of water from sweating occurs, thus causing constituents to be precipitated because of their high concentration in the diminished volume of urine excreted.

(b) Urinary infection, obstruction and stagnation.

(c) Conditions associated with hypercalciuria which increases the liability to the formation of stones consisting mainly of calcium phosphate and calcium oxalate. These include idiopathic hypercalciuria in which the main defect is increased intestinal absorption of calcium, excessive intake of milk or cheese, prolonged immobilisation, hyperparathyroidism, Cushings syndrome, renal tubular acidosis, sarcoidosis, multiple myeloma and vitamin D intoxication.

Increased intestinal absorption of oxalate also occurs in ileal disease and may be responsible.

(d) Certain rare inherited disorders, e.g. cystinuria and primary hyperoxaluria, which may lead to the production of cystine or oxalate stones respectively.

(e) Conditions causing increased excretion of uric acid, e.g. gout and myeloproliferative disease.

(f) The pH of the urine influences the extent to which some of these conditions lead to stone formation; thus an alkaline urine tends to increase the precipitation of calcium phosphate stones and so may be responsible for their occurrence in renal tubular acidosis from any cause. Likewise an acid urine reduces the solubility of uric acid and cystine.

Today, however, in prosperous countries the great majority of renal calculi occur in well nourished, healthy young men in whom the most careful investigations reveal no cause for stone formation.

Pathology. Urinary concretions vary greatly in size. There may be particles like sand anywhere in the urinary tract or large round stones in the bladder. Staghorn calculi fill the whole renal pelvis and branch into the calyces; they are usually associated with hydronephrosis and chronic pyelonephritis. Over 90% of renal stones contain calcium but the nature of the salt varies with their origin. Deposits of calcium may also be present throughout the renal parenchyma, giving rise to nephrocalcinosis. This is especially liable to occur in cases of chronic pyelonephritis, renal tubular acidosis, hyperparathyroidism, vitamin D intoxication, and in healed renal tuberculosis.

Clinical features vary according to the size, shape and position of the stone, and the presence and nature of the underlying condition. Renal calculi or nephrocalcinosis may be present for many years and yet themselves give rise to no symptoms. While nephrocalcinosis never gives rise to pain, the most common complaint arising from renal calculi is an intermittent dull pain in the loin or back, increased by movement or a sudden jolt. Some abnormal constituents of the urine, e.g. red cells, protein or pus cells, can be found at one time or another.

Renal Colic. When a stone is small enough to enter the ureter and large enough to obstruct it, an attack of renal colic develops. The patient is suddenly aware of pain in the loin, which soon radiates round the flank to the groin and often into the testis or labia in the sensory distribution of the first lumbar nerve. The pain steadily increases in intensity to reach a maximum in a few minutes. The patient is restless, and generally tries, unsuccessfuly, to obtain relief by assuming various positions, both lying and sitting, and by pacing about the room. There is pallor, sweating, and often vomiting, and the patient may groan in agony. Frequency and haematuria may occur.

Without treatment the intense pain usually subsides within two hours but may continue unabated for several hours or some days. In many cases the pain is constant during the attack, though slight fluctuations in severity may occur. Contrary to what is often believed, it is rare for attacks to consist of intermittent severe pains, coming and going every few minutes for some hours.

Investigation. When renal colic occurs the diagnosis is usually easily made by the history and by the finding of red cells in the urine. All patients suspected of having renal calculus, including those with renal colic, should have a radiological examination of the urinary tract, including a retrograde urogram in some instances. If there is doubt about the cause of the abdominal pain, an intravenous pyelogram during the attack may be helpful. When the pain is due to a stone in the ureter, the radiograph shows a dense renal shadow with delay in the appearance of the dye in the renal pelvis. Appropriate investigations should be undertaken to discover the presence of any underlying condition which might be responsible for the development of renal calcification or lithiasis.

Treatment and Prevention. The immediate treatment of renal pain or renal colic is rest in bed, the application of warmth to the seat of pain, and the administration of analgesic drugs, e.g. pethidine (100 mg) or morphine (15–30 mg), and antispasmodic drugs, e.g. atropine sulphate (0·8 or 1·2 mg). These should be given intramuscularly and may be repeated within 2 hours.

Attempts to dissolve calculi in the kidneys have not been successful. Stones in the renal pelvis and urinary bladder must be removed surgically. Stones in the ureter usually pass naturally if left alone and surgical removal is apt to be followed by stricture and its complications. When, however, pain persists or frequent bouts of pain become intolerable, the insertion of a ureteric catheter is often followed by the passage of the stone. Urgent surgical intervention is necessary in the event of anuria. It is also required if the stone has not moved for some weeks and hydronephrosis is developing or there is continuing infection in the urinary tract. A stone larger than 1 cm in diameter generally requires surgical removal.

Suitable medical or surgical measures should be instituted for the correction of any primary cause of renal lithiasis that may have been discovered. In idiopathic hypercalciuria a diet low in calcium, by reducing the intake of milk and cheese, is advisable. If this is not effective, ben-

drofluazide in a dose of 5 mg/d reduces urinary calcium excretion by about 30%. In recurrent oxalate stones the elimination from the diet of articles which have a very high content of oxalate, such as rhubarb and spinach, may be worthy of trial. Persons who have passed several uric acid or urate stones, as may occur in gout or in patients with leukaemia benefit from allopurinol (p. 581) which also has a place in treating calcium oxalate stone disease to which urates may contribute.

Since the distribution of phosphorus occurs so widely in foodstuffs, dietary restriction for the treatment of phosphate calculi is unlikely to be of any value. Phosphatic calculi are found only in alkaline urine, hence acidifying the urine by administering ammonium chloride daily may be effective. In contrast, cystine and urate stones may be prevented or sometimes dissolved by making the urine persistently alkaline, especially if combined with a high output of urine.

Lastly, the most important therapeutic and prophylactic measure for all forms of stones is the provision of an adequate fluid intake which assists in preventing deposition of crystalloids in the renal tissue. A daily output of urine of at least 3 l is advisable hence the intake of fluid should be approximately 4 l daily. If the climate or the patients occupation causes much sweating the fluid intake requires to be greatly increased.

CONGENITAL ABNORMALITIES OF THE KIDNEYS

Congenital anomalies of the urinary tract affect more than 10% of infants and, unless they are immediately lethal, some are prone to lead to complications in later life. About 1 in 500 infants is born with only one kidney and, although usually compatible with a normal life, it is often associated with abnormalities in other organs.

Polycystic Disease

This genetically determined abnormality of renal structure may be associated with other congenital abnormalities, e.g. cystic liver (p. 568). There are two modes of inheritance. The infantile form is very rare and is inherited as an autosomal recessive; it is usually fatal within the first year of life.

The commoner or adult type is inherited as an autosomal dominant trait. It may be found during infancy, but symptoms often do not develop until adult life. Both kidneys are affected, are several times the normal size and consist of masses of cysts, predominantly cortical, with a variable amount of renal parenchyma which often shows extensive fibrosis and arteriolosclerosis.

The clinical features include pain in the renal angles, haematuria, uraemia and usually a slowly developing arterial hypertension. Often one or both kidneys can be palpated and the surface may be nodular. In addition to polycystic disease, other diseases in which the kidneys may be palpable are hydro- or pyonephrosis, solitary cyst, renal carcinoma and other tumours. It should be remembered, however, that in some normal people all of the right kidney, and occasionally the lower pole of the left kidney may be felt on clinical examination. This is particularly true in slim women. On the other hand, pathologically enlarged kidneys are not always palpable. When a kidney can be felt, as in polycystic disease, it may be possible to appreciate departures from the normal size, smooth surface and firm consistency. Diagnosis can be confirmed by ultrasound or retrograde pyelography.

In course, prognosis and treatment, polycystic disease resembles chronic glomerulonephritis and death occurs in middle age from uraemia, cerebrovascular accident or cardiac failure.

Medullary Cystic Disease

Medullary cysts are found in two widely different conditions. In *medullary sponge kidney* the cysts are confined to the collecting ducts in the renal papillae. Affected patients are usually middle aged and present with pain, haematuria or urinary tract infection. The diagnosis is made on radiographic examination in which, following excretion urography, contrast media is seen to fill dilated or cystic tubules, which are sometimes calcified. The prognosis is generally good.

In *uraemic medullary cystic disease* small cortical cysts are also present and these lead to progressive destruction of the nephrons; this condition occurs in younger patients and there is often a family history. Sometimes affected kidneys are salt-losing; this aggravates the degree of renal failure but, even when treated appropriately, serious renal failure is usual.

DRUGS AND THE KIDNEY

Drug-induced Renal Disease

The susceptibility of the kidney to damage by drugs stems from the fact that it is the route of excretion for many water soluble compounds including drugs and their metabolites. These are delivered in large amounts to the kidney which receives 25% of the cardiac output, and they may reach high concentrations in the renal cortex as the result of proximal tubular transport mechanisms, e.g. aminoglycosides, or in the medulla because of the operation of the counter-current system, e.g. aspirin.

Damage to the kidney may arise in the course of treatment with a large number of drugs and may be sufficiently severe to result in acute renal failure. Thus, streptomycin, kanamycin, gentamicin, tobramycin, some cephalosporins and iodinated contrast media may cause proximal tubular damage and proteinuria. Acute renal failure may also result from an acute allergic interstitial nephritis induced by drugs such as penicillins and phenylbutazone. The relatively soluble sulphonamides in use to-day rarely cause urinary obstruction by precipitating in the renal tract, but occasionally induce renal lesions similar to polyarteritis.

Tetracyclines accentuate uraemia by their anti-anabolic effect on protein metabolism. Amphotericin can induce renal tubular acidosis while lithium may reduce renal concentrating power and cause polyuria.

Renal failure due to intravascular coagulation occurs, rarely, from using oral contraceptives. Drug induced glomerulonephritis may complicate treatment with penicillamine or with gold.

Analgesic Nephropathy. The occurrence of chronic renal damage as a consequence of long-continued ingestion of analgesics is an important cause of renal failure. Although phenacetin is the major culprit other analgesics, such as aspirin or non-steroid anti-inflammatory drugs alone or in combination, may be responsible.

The pathological changes predominantly affect the corticomedullary junction with diffuse interstitial fibrosis and tubular atrophy. Ultimately there is a loss of tubules in cortex and medulla and acute papillary necrosis may develop. The changes are probably the result of ischaemia due to interference with the blood flow through the postglomerular vessels of juxtamedullary glomeruli. A recognised complication is the development of carcinoma of the renal pelvis.

The majority of affected patients are women who suffer from anxiety or have personal or marital problems. They are commonly divorced, anxious, apprehensive and smoke or drink alcohol to excess. Other patients have taken analgesics over many years for headache, rheumatoid arthritis or osteoarthrosis. Symptoms include polyuria and thirst and the features of recurrent urinary tract infection. Renal colic may be caused by the passage of fragments of necrotic renal papillae which can be recognised by microscopic examination of the urine.

Apart from the history of drug ingestion, diagnosis can sometimes be made by the characteristic radiological appearances of the papillae on retrograde pyelography. The contrast medium is seen as a small tract within the papillary substance; later the papillae may separate giving a ring shadow.

Treatment consists of withdrawing the offending drug and substituting another analgesic, e.g. paracetamol, if such therapy is essential. Provided the analgesic is withdrawn sufficiently early there is a reasonable prospect of some recovery of renal function; otherwise severe renal failure develops and becomes irreversible.

Use of Drugs in Patients with Impaired Renal Function

Adverse reactions to drugs are significantly more common in patients with impaired renal function. In these circumstances urinary excretion of many drugs and their metabolites is reduced. In addition uraemia is associated with alterations in the distribution of drugs in body fluids, reduced binding of drugs by plasma albumin and changes in metabolism of drugs by the liver.

Drugs should never be given to patients with impaired renal function unless specific indications for their use exist. The least toxic alternative should be chosen and the British National Formulary or other reference (p. 822) consulted to find the recommended dose for use when renal function is impaired and also the likely adverse effects of the drug. Commonly used drugs the dose of which needs to be reduced in renal failure include cephalosporins, cimetidine, hydralazine, digoxin, co-trimoxazole, aminoglycosides, narcotic analgesics, aspirin and phenylbutazone. During therapy a careful watch must be kept for any adverse effects and the drug stopped or the dose reduced should they develop. Measurements of the concentration of the drug in plasma are sometimes helpful in monitoring drug dosage (p. 820).

TUMOURS OF THE KIDNEY AND GENITO-URINARY TRACT

Renal carcinoma is the most common tumour of the kidney and is most frequently found in adult men. It was formerly called a hypernephroma on the mistaken view that it arose from adrenal rest tissue within the kidney. Haematuria is the most frequent presenting feature and blood clots may give rise to renal colic. Sometimes the tumour causes vague pain in the abdomen or flank and it may also be responsible for long continued fever. Occasionally patients present first with symptoms arising from metastases in the lungs, liver or bones. On rare occasions polycythaemia occurs, and this is believed to be due to excessive production of erythropoietin. The tumour may be palpable and is defined by radiological investigation and ultrasonography. Early surgical treatment affords the only prospect of cure.

Nephroblastoma (Wilm's Tumour) is the second most common malignant tumour of the kidney and presents in the first decade, and often the first year of life. It most commonly presents as an abdominal mass sometimes discovered accidently by the patient. Haematuria tends to occur late in the disease. The tumour is radiosensitive and responsive to chemotherapy (p. 117). The best hope of cure is early diagnosis.

Tumours of the renal pelvis, ureter and bladder are histologically similar and are almost always transitional cell carcinomas. They tend to spread locally by direct invasion but also by implantation to other parts of the urinary tract. While some are benign, e.g. papillomas, all urinary tract tumours are liable to recur even after apparently adequate treatment. The bladder is by far the most common site and epidemiological studies have shown that it is particularly likely to develop in patients who work in industries such as dyeing and printing where there may be exposure to aniline and in areas of endemicity for urinary schistosomiasis (p. 782). Haematuria is almost always the sole presenting symptom of these tumours. Features due to obstruction to the urinary tract also occur and symptoms of urinary tract infection may be superimposed.

Diagnosis is made by cystoscopy, biopsy and radiography. Bladder tumours are treated by diathermy or radiotherapy. Cystectomy with transplantation of the ureters to the colon or skin may be necessary.

Prostatic carcinoma usually presents with symptoms of urethral obstruction similar to those of benign prostatic hypertrophy. On digital examination of the rectum the prostrate is felt to be very hard and the median furrow may be obliterated. Spread through the capsule and metastases in bone occur and are often associated with a rise in the plasma acid phosphatase.

Treatment varies with the stage of the disease and consists of prostatectomy or deprivation of the testicular androgens on which the growth depends by measures such as orchidectomy or oestrogen therapy. Painful gynaecomastia is a troublesome side-effect of the latter.

Benign enlargement of the prostate gland is of unknown cause but it may be associated with a fall in androgen secretion. It is most commonly found in men over 60 years. Histologically the inner zone of the gland undergoes hyperplasia and hypertrophy and there is an increase in the fibromuscular stroma. The enlarged prostate obstructs the outflow of urine from the bladder by compressing, displacing, distorting and elongating the prostatic urethra with the effects of bladder and renal function referred to on page 403.

The clinical features are those of progressive obstruction to urinary flow. Acute urinary retention may arise if the gland suddenly increases in size because of superimposed infection or congestion, or when cardiac failure develops in the elderly. Then the patient has a sudden desire to micturate but is unable to do so, the bladder becomes tense and is tender. More chronic retention may pass unnoticed for some time but there is a gradual increase in the volume of the urine which remains in the bladder after micturition. Haematuria and bleeding from the urethra may also occur and may be the presenting symptom. On rectal examination the prostate may feel large, elastic and is uniform in consistency; however, when the median lobe alone is affected, the prostate feels normal and the condition can be recognised only by cystoscopy.

Prostatectomy is the only effective treatment and the important decision is when to operate. Acute retention should be relieved by catheterisation and drainage; sometimes this reduces congestion and the ability to pass urine spontaneously can be regained. If this does not occur, operation should be carried out in a few days.

Testicular tumours now constitute the commonest form of malignant disease in men aged 25–34 years. A seminoma presents as a painless and often uniform, rapid enlargement of the testis. A teratoma causes more nodular changes and may secrete gonadotrophic hormones producing gynaecomastia. A testicular tumour may be overlooked if it is obscured by a hydrocele or if the examination is inadequate. Spread to the abdomen and lungs can occur and cause death but with early diagnosis testicular cancer is curable. Seminomas can be treated successfully by orchidectomy and radiotherapy. Chemotherapy is also required for other tumours in which the prognosis is poorer. Tumour markers may be helpful in assessing progress (p. 107).

Sexual Disorders of Endocrine Origin

These are discussed on pages 454 to 457.

SEXUALLY TRANSMITTED DISEASES

The Venereal Diseases Regulations of 1916 defined the venereal diseases as syphilis, gonorrhoea and chancroid. These are still the legally defined venereal diseases in Britain. The incidence of syphilis fell after World War II and remains at a low level. Gonorrhoea also decreased after this war, but started to increase again in the late 1950s. At the same time the incidence of other conditions started to rise. These included viral infections (e.g. herpes simplex and warts), chlamydial infections (e.g. non-gonococcal urethritis), parasitic conditions (e.g. scabies and pediculosis pubis), protozoal conditions such as trichomoniasis and fungal infections such as candidiasis. Recently other diseases have been recognised to be sexually transmitted, including hepatitis. The incidence of gonorrhoea has now levelled off, but these other conditions have continued to increase.

Spread and Control

The fundamental factor in spread is the acquisition of infection from one sexual partner and its transmission to another. This in turn depends on the availability of partners. The most important influence in the number of partners is population movement including the migration of people from rural to urban areas and worldwide travel. Other social factors which promote spread of disease include affluence, alcohol consumption, increased leisure, personal freedom, prostitution, and ignorance. The last leads to failure to recognise infection and the continuing change of partners despite infection. Other important factors in transmission include asymptomatic disease in women and homosexual men, antimicrobial treatment and modern contraception. Unfortunately antimicrobial resistance leads to treatment failure and the spread of resistant infection. Modern contraceptives, oral contraceptives and the intrauterine device, provide no barrier to infection.

High risk groups for sexually transmitted disease include men aged 18 to 34 years and women aged 16 to 24 years, frequent travellers, prostitutes, homosexuals, members of the armed forces, merchant navy and air crew, and entertainers of all sorts. These diseases affect all socio-economic groups; no-one is immune.

Control of sexually transmitted disease in Britain is founded primarily on good clinical medicine and most patients attend specialist clinics. The basis of clinical practice is accurate diagnosis, effective treatment and careful follow-up to confirm cure. Secondly, control depends on the identification of potentially infected contacts and ensuring they attend for examination and treatment. Education is also important in control. Serological screening of blood donors and antenatal women is undertaken, but screening is less important in Britain than in countries with less well developed clinical services.

SYPHILIS

Syphilis is a chronic infection due to *Treponema pallidum*. It is systemic from the beginning, runs a chronic course characterised by florid features at some times but by long periods of latency at other times. Syphilis is infectious during the first 2 years when it may be transferable to the fetus; it responds well to penicillin and certain other antimicrobials.

The classification is shown in Table 11.2

Table 11.2 Classification of syphilis

Acquired	Early	Primary
		Secondary
		Early latent
	Late	Late latent
		Tertiary
		(benign gummatous)
		Quarternary
		(Cardiovascular p. 198)
		(and neurosyphilis p. 639)
Congenital	Early	
	Late	
	Stigmata	
	(or scars)	

The subdivision between early and late syphilis is 2 years. The course is variable and may be latent throughout. At any time syphilis may develop clinical features so all cases must be treated.

Clinical Features. ACQUIRED SYPHILIS. *Early Stage; Primary.* After an incubation period (with extremes of 9 to 90 days but commonly 14 to 28 days) the primary lesion or chancre develops at the site of infection, usually on the genitalia or, in homosexuals, at the anus. A small pink macule appears which soon becomes papular and ulcerates. The regional lymph nodes are moderately enlarged, discrete, rubbery, painless, and not tender.

Early Stage; Secondary. The primary chancre tends to heal and 6 to 8 weeks later symptoms of generalised infection appear with malaise, headache and low fever. Four cardinal signs appear — a rash, condylomata, lymphadenopathy and mucous patches — though any of them may be absent:

1. A rash is present in 75% of patients. This starts as a faint macular eruption on the trunk and proximal limbs; it develops into a generalised papular rash which is characteristically dull red, polymorphic and symmetrical, does not itch and may become scaly.

2. Condylomata lata are large flat papules that develop in warm moist areas such as around the anus.

3. Lymphadenopathy is found in 50% of patients and may be generalised. The nodes resemble those found in primary syphilis.

4. Mucous patches are found in 30% of patients; they are superficial ulcers on the mucous membranes of the genitalia, mouth and throat. They may have a characteristic white base and narrow red margin and may coalesce to form 'snail track' ulcers. Alternatively they may be so superficial as to be scarcely visible.

In over 30% of cases changes occur in the cerebrospinal fluid indicating involvement of the nervous system; clinical features of low grade meningitis may rarely be present, sometimes with cranial nerve palsies. Rarely the eyes, bones, joints (p. 571) or abdominal viscera may be affected. After several months the secondary changes gradually disappear to be followed by a latent period.

Late Stages. Latency may persist for many years.

The *tertiary stage* takes 10 or more years to develop and mainly affects skin and subcutaneous tissues, mucous membranes and submucosa, and the long bones. Lesions run a long benign course. The characteristic pathological finding is called a gumma.

Quarternary Stage. Cardiovascular syphilis (p. 198) and neurosyphilis (p. 639) usually take longer to develop characteristic features and may lead to the patient's death.

CONGENITAL SYPHILIS. The fetus may contract syphilis from an infected mother. There is no primary stage. The disease may be so severe that the child is born dead, or vesicles and bullae may present on the skin at birth. The child may appear normal at birth but fails to thrive, and within a few months develops a rash and signs of syphilitic disease of bone, joints (p. 571), liver, kidneys and other organs. In a third group of cases the disease remains latent for years until lesions of bones, joints and teeth, iritis, keratitis, nerve deafness, juvenile tabes or general paralysis appear.

Congenital syphilis is now rare in Western countries, where screening in antenatal clinics and treatment of a syphilitic woman during pregnancy usually ensure the birth of a normal baby.

Investigation. In the primary and secondary stages *T. pallidum* may be found in the chancre, papules or mucous patches by squeezing a drop of serum from one of these lesions and examining it under a microscope fitted with a dark ground condenser.

The serological tests for syphilis give positive results from about the fourth week and are always strongly positive in the secondary stage. Nonspecific antigen is used in screening tests such as the cardiolipin Wasserman reaction (CWR) or preferably the Venereal Disease Research Laboratory (VDRL) test. Hence the specificity and sensitivity of such tests is variable. False positive results may be found in infectious mononucleosis, systemic lupus erythematosus and other generalised diseases, while negative results may be observed in older patients with late syphilis. For diagnosis additional tests are required which use specific treponemal antigen e.g. *T. pallidum* haemagglutination assay (TPHA) and the fluorescent treponemal antibody-absorbed (FTA-ABS) test. Any patient in whom latent syphilis is suspected should have all these tests repeated on two separate samples of blood, the CSF should be examined to exclude neurological disease, and chest radiographs taken to exclude calcification of the ascending aorta which indicates cardiovascular disease.

Course and Prognosis. Syphilis can run a very variable course. The primary stage may not be present or may not be noticed. The secondary stage may also be transient or absent. Many cases are found in the latent stage following serological testing. 60% of patients who reach the latent stage remain in this stage without therapy unless the immunological balance is disturbed by conditions such as systemic lupus erythematosus. Modern antimicrobial therapy gives cure rates of 95 to 99%.

Differential Diagnosis. Primary syphilis must be considered in the differential diagnosis of all genital ulcers, common causes of which include herpes simplex, erosive balanitis and trauma. Less common causes of genital ulcers include scabies and secondary syphilis.

The macular rash of secondary syphilis may resemble a drug eruption, rubella and skin conditions such as pityriasis rosea and lichen planus. The papular rash may resemble drug rashes, scabies, acne vulgaris and, when scaly, psoriasis. Condylomata lata must be distinguished from condylomata acuminata or viral warts (p. 414). Ulcers in the mouth or throat may be confused with herpes simplex, aphthous ulcers, ulcerative stomatitis or the ulceration in agranulocytosis, while ulcers on the genital mucosa may be confused with herpes simplex and erosive balanitis (p. 415). Lymphadenopathy may suggest infectious mononucleosis or a lymphoma.

Syphilis has to be distinguished on clinical grounds from yaws, endemic (non-venereal) syphilis and pinta. These granulomatous diseases, caused by spirochaetes morphologically indistinguishable from *T. pallidum,* are described on pages 763 to 765.

Treatment. *T. pallidum,* though remaining very sensitive to penicillin, needs prolonged treatment. Hence longer acting forms such as procaine penicillin are used. A patient with primary syphilis requires 600 mg of procaine penicillin daily for 10–12 consective days. For secondary, tertiary or latent syphilis the course should be continued for 14 or 15 days and for cardiovascular and neuro-syphilis (p. 641) it should be prolonged for 21 days. In large patients the dose should be increased to 900 mg or 1·2 g of procaine penicillin. Tetracycline should be given to patients allergic to penicillin; for early syphilis, latent syphilis and tertiary syphilis 500 mg of oxytetracycline four times daily for 15 days is recommended while for cardiovascular and neurosyphilis the course should be continued for 21 to 28 days. All patients must be followed up to ensure cure. Contact tracing is an important part of management.

GONORRHOEA

Gonorrhoea is due to the Gram-negative diplococcus *Neisseria gonorrhoeae* which infects mucous membranes of the genital tract, rectum, pharynx and eyes. The incubation period is usually 2 to 10 days.

Clinical Features. In the male the anterior urethra is the most common site for infection. Anterior urethritis usually causes dysuria and a purulent discharge; occasionally symptoms are mild or absent.

In females the lower cervical canal is the site most commonly infected but the urethra and rectum are also involved in about half the cases. There may be vaginal discharge and dysuria, but 50% of the women have no symptoms.

The homosexual male may have rectal infection which is often asymptomatic. He may also have asymptomatic pharyngeal infection; heterosexual men and women occasionally have pharyngeal gonorrhoea.

Investigation. Gonorrhoea may be suspected clinically but diagnosis depends on laboratory investigations. Gram-negative intracellular diplococci may be seen in stained pus from infected tracts and this allows rapid diagnosis in the outpatient clinic. This finding must be confirmed by culture of exudate on selective media in the laboratory.

Course and Prognosis. Symptoms gradually resolve without treatment but it is not known how long patients remain infectious. The longer patients remain without treatment the more likely they are to develop complications. Most patients in Western countries seek treatment early so complications are rare. Infection may spread to the posterior urethra and occasionally along one vas deferens to the epididymis causing acute epididymitis and rarely epididymo-orchitis. Infection in the cervical canal may spread to the Fallopian tubes (salpingitis) and to other pelvic structures (pelvic inflammatory disease). This is the most important complication as it may lead to sterility. Pelvic infection may be associated with perihepatitis characterised by right hypochondrial pain and tenderness.

Bacteraemia is rare causing fever, joint pains and a rash — sparse peripheral haemorrhagic pustules surrounded by erythema, though other skin lesions may occur. Acute gonococcal arthritis (p. 570) and septicaemia are now extremely rare in the Western world. Infection of the conjunctiva of infants born to infected mothers causes purulent conjunctivitis and damage to sight (ophthalmia neonatorum). This too is rare in the Western world but remains an important cause of blindness in many tropical areas.

Differential Diagnosis. Gonococcal urethritis must be differentiated from non-gonococcal urethritis (below) by a Gram stained smear and culture of the discharge. The same investigations taken from the cervix, urethra and rectum allow the differentiation of gonorrhoea in the female from other causes of dysuria such as urinary infection (p. 398) and other causes of vaginal discharge such as trichomoniasis or candidiasis (p. 802). Rectal infection rarely causes clinical proctitis and therefore a Gram stained smear and culture are essential for diagnosis. Interpretation of pharyngeal smears is complicated by saprophytic neisseria so only cultures are taken from the throat.

Treatment. A single intramuscular injection of 2·4 g of procaine penicillin plus 1 g of probenecid by mouth, or 2 g of ampicillin plus 1 g of probenecid together by mouth is usually sufficient to cure most uncomplicated infections in Britain. Co-trimoxazole, preferably 8 (480 mg) tablets in a single oral dose or 3 doses of 5 tablets at 12-hourly intervals, may be given to patients who are allergic to penicillin. If one of these treatments fails it is important to establish if the patient is infected with a gonococcus which is relatively resistant to penicillin or with one of the rare, but rapidly increasing, strains totally resistant to penicillin. Relatively resistant strains usually respond to 4·8 g of intramuscular procaine penicillin or to 3·5 g of ampicillin orally, each given with 1 g of probenecid. Totally resistant strains respond to cefuroxime, cefoxitin or cefotaxime (p. 45). Patients allergic to penicillin may be given spectinomycin (p. 47). Cases with complications need multiple dose therapy such as 2 g of ampicillin plus 1 g of probenecid followed by 500 mg of ampicillin plus 500 mg of probenecid 6 hourly for 14 days.

It is essential to establish cure of gonorrhoea, and any accompanying infection, by repeating culture of secretions from infected sites. Tracing contacts is also important in the management of gonorrhoea.

NON-GONOCOCCAL INFECTION

Non-gonococcal Urethritis

In Britain, urethritis in males is more commonly non-gonococcal than gonococcal in origin. About half the non-gonococcal cases may be due to *Chlamydia trachomatis*, a member of the genus *Chlamydia* which also cause lymphogranuloma venereum (p. 413), and other diseases (p. 737); a small proportion is due to *Ureaplasma urealyticum*. A few cases are caused by trauma or herpes simplex virus; the remainder are of undetermined origin. Non-gonococcal urethritis also occurs in Reiter's disease (p. 565). The incubation period of non-gonococcal urethritis varies from a few days to a few weeks.

Clinical features resemble those of gonorrhoea but are milder. As indicated by the name the usual investigations are to exclude gonorrhoea by Gram stain and culture of infected secretions. Where available, urethral exudate may be cultured for chlamydiae.

Untreated non-gonococcal urethritis runs a prolonged low grade course. Local complications are rare and resemble those due to gonorrhoea.

Treatment is with 250 mg of oxytetracycline 6-hourly for 14 days. Cure rates are lower than in syphilis or gonorrhoea; refractory cases may be given 250 g of erythromycin stearate 6-hourly for 14 days.

Non-gonococcal Genital Infection in Women

Chlamydia may infect the cervical canal of women. It is therefore important to examine and treat partners of infected men. Uncomplicated genital chlamydial infection in women causes no symptoms or signs. Treatment is with 250 mg of oxytetracycline or erythromycin 6 hourly for 14 days.

Chlamydiae may spread upwards and cause pelvic infection; this is a more common cause of pelvic infection than gonorrhoea. Treatment is with 500 mg of oxytetracycline or erythromycin 6 hourly for at least 14 days. A woman with cervical chlamydial infection may infect her baby at birth usually causing eye infection and occasionally pharyngeal infection and pneumonia.

LYMPHOGRANULOMA VENEREUM

Lymphogranuloma venereum is caused by *Chlamydia trachomatis*, it is sexually transmitted and is widely distributed in the tropics. The different species of *C. trachomatis* can be identified by serotyping and since this method became available cases have been recognised in temperate climates.

Clinical Features. A small transient genital ulcer appears 1 to 5 weeks after infection. The regional lymph nodes enlarge and become matted together, tender and adherent to the deep tissues and to the overlying skin which may develop a characteristic dusky pink colour. There may be fever, weight loss, and rarely a macular rash and hepatosplenomegaly.

Infection may spread to the pelvic nodes. If the condition is untreated, abscesses and sinuses may develop. Proctitis and rectal ulceration, multiple sinuses and fistulae may occur. Healing is with scarring and lymphoedema may follow.

Investigation. The diagnosis may be confirmed by isolating *C. trachomatis* and by demonstrating a rise in serum antibodies preferably by means of the microimmunofluorescent test, or by the complement fixation test. Syphilis must be excluded by dark ground examination for *T. pallidum* and by serological tests.

Treatment. Once syphilis has been excluded most cases respond well to 500 mg of oxytetracycline 6-hourly for 14 days. Severe cases may require a larger dose initially and chronic cases need more prolonged treatment. Inguinal abscesses require aspiration but incision should be avoided. When sinuses have formed excision is necessary.

CHANCROID

Chancroid is due to a small Gram negative bacillus, *Haemophilus ducreyi*, 1–2 microns in length and characteristically seen on stained smears in chains arranged like fish in shoals. The disease is sexually transmitted. It is said to be common in the tropics but most cases are diagnosed clinically and over-reporting may occur.

Clinical Features. The incubation period is usually 1 to 8 days. Genital lesions start as small painful tender papules which soon form shallow irregular tender ulcers. The inguinal lymph nodes enlarge, soften and suppurate; they may become adherent. Malaise and fever occasionally accompany the local signs.

If the condition is neglected, inguinal abscesses form and occasionally genital ulcers progress to cause tissue destruction.

The multiple, tender irregular genital ulcers with suppurating lymph nodes may suggest the diagnosis but chancroid must be differentiated from primary and secondary syphilis, lymphogranuloma venereum, granuloma inguinale and genital herpes.

Investigation. *H. ducreyi* may be recognised in Gram stained smears of exudate from the genital ulcers. The organism may also be cultured but special media are required. Skin tests are no longer available. Syphilis must be excluded because primary and secondary syphilis tend to be common where chancroid is found.

Treatment. This may be with 2 g of sulphadimidine initially followed by 1 g 6-hourly for 7 to 14 days, 2 tablets of co-trimoxazole twice daily for 7 to 10 days, 1 g of streptomycin i.m. daily for 7 to 14 days or 500 mg of oxytetracycline 6-hourly for 10 to 20 days. Bathing with saline will suffice for the genital lesions. Serological tests for syphilis should be repeated after 3 months to ensure coincidental syphilis has not been missed.

GRANULOMA INGUINALE

Granuloma inguinale is due to *Donovania granulomatis* and is characterised by bipolar Donovan's bodies 1 to 2 microns long demonstrable in mononuclear cells in scrapings from the genital lesion. The disease is sexually transmitted and occurs almost exclusively in coloured people in tropical and subtropical areas.

Clinical Features. The incubation period varies from a few days to 3 months. The genital lesion starts as a small papule which enlarges to form a granulomatous ulcer which spreads to surrounding areas such as thighs, perineum and natal cleft. Lesions have a velvety appearance, varying in colour from pale pink to deep red. Granulomas develop in the inguinal region resembling enlarged lymph nodes. If the genital lesions become secondarily infected this may lead to actual lymph node enlargement. Occasional extra-genital lesions occur.

Untreated lesions may continue for years to spread at the periphery and leave an unhealthy scar which tends to break down. Fibrosis may lead to stenosis of the urethra, anus or vagina.

Well developed granuloma inguinale may be characteristic. It is important to differentiate it from primary and secondary syphilis, and from lymphogranuloma venereum, chancroid and genital herpes simplex.

Investigation. The diagnosis may be confirmed by taking a scraping from the margin of the genital lesion, staining by Giemsa's method and then identifying Donovan's bodies microscopically. A biopsy may also be taken. Syphilis must be excluded by dark ground examinations for *T. pallidum* and by serological tests.

Treatment. This may be with 1 g of streptomycin intramuscularly twice daily for 10 to 20 days or 500 mg of oxytetracycline for 14 to 21 days. Oxytetracycline should be avoided until syphilis has been excluded and serological tests for syphilis should be repeated 3 months after treatment.

SEXUALLY TRANSMITTED VIRAL DISEASES

Anogenital Herpes Simplex

This condition is due to *Herpes simplex* virus type 2 and resembles labial herpes or cold sores. The virus is spread by contact usually during sexual intercourse.

Clinical Features. There is often a relatively severe initial or primary attack with local discomfort followed by a crop of vesicles on the external genitals. The vesicles soon rupture and are often followed by further crops. The lesions may be widespread on the genitals with regional lymph node enlargement, fever and malaise. There may be root pains in the second and third sacral dermatomes and occasionally retention of urine. In homosexual men, and rarely in heterosexuals and females, the anus may be affected.

The initial illness lasts 2 to 4 weeks and in about half the patients there are recurrent attacks. These follow the same sequence of local discomfort and then a cluster of vesicles covering an area of about one square centimetre breaking down to form erosions and then healing. Recurrences last 2 to 4 days and thereafter gradually die out.

A woman with active disease may infect her baby during delivery. There may also be a link between genital herpes and subsequent carcinoma of the cervix.

The virus may be cultured from vesicular fluid or from scrapings from fresh erosions. Syphilis must be excluded.

Treatment. Lesions always heal and local bathing with saline and treatment of secondary infection with 2 tablets of co-trimoxazole twice daily for 7 days will usually suffice. Antiviral drugs have not yet an established place in the treatment of this condition but acyclovir (p. 48) may shorten the severe initial attack.

Other Sexually Transmitted Viral Diseases

Hepatitis. HB antigen is commonly sexually transmitted between homosexual men. Hepatitis is usually transient and subclinical with only minor biochemical abnormalities. A few men develop chronic active hepatitis or cirrhosis. A vaccine has been introduced which gives a high degree of protection against the spread of hepatitis B among homosexuals (p. 353).

Hepatitis A and non-A non-B hepatitis may also spread among homosexuals.

Cytomegalovirus disease of a subclinical type is widespread among homosexuals who occasionally develop mild clinical disease. Cytomegalovirus disease may also spread heterosexually.

Warts are common on the genitals and anus and spread by sexual contact. *Molluscum contagiosum* is also found on and near the genitals and is sexually transmitted.

MISCELLANEOUS CONDITIONS

Under this heading some conditions are included which are not sexually transmitted but have to be considered in the differential diagnosis of those that are.

Balanitis. This strictly means inflammation of the glans penis; the undersurface of the prepuce is often also involved, when the correct term is balanoposthitis. It is more common in men with a long or tight prepuce who have difficulty with hygiene. *Candidia albicans, Trichomonas vaginalis, streptococci* and some anaerobic bacteria cause balanitis. The affected areas are either generally or patchily erythematous with erosions in severe cases. There may be a white or purulent exudate. Diagnosis is from the clinical appearance. If one of the causes can be recognised, appropriate therapy should be given plus local saline bathing; if no cause can be identified then saline bathing alone will suffice. Diabetes, broad spectrum antimicrobials, corticosteroids and antimitotic drugs may predispose to candidiasis.

A characteristic form called circinate balanitis occurs in Reiter's disease (p. 565) with well defined round erosions which may coalesce. Balanitis xerotica obliterans is a local form of the skin condition lichen sclerosus et atrophicus; initially there is patchy erythema but later there is atrophy leading to meatal stenosis and phimosis.

Genital Ulceration. Acute genital ulceration occurs in the Stevens Johnson syndrome (p. 42), while recurrent genital ulceration occurs in Behçet's disease (p. 568). In the latter condition healing takes place leaving characteristic irregular scars often called 'splash' scars from their appearance.

Vaginal Discharge. This is a common complaint and may be due to a variety of causes including chemicals such as antiseptics in the bath water, physical trauma, or infective agents such as *Candida albicans, Trichomonas vaginalis* or bacteria. *C. albicans* produces a thick white adherent discharge and itch. *T. vaginalis* produces a thin yellow discharge and irritation. Anaerobic bacteria and *Gardnerella vaginalis* produce a malodorous off-white discharge. The different micro-organisms can be identified by microscopy and culture; local antifungals are given for yeast infections and metronidazole for trichomoniasis and anaerobic and Gardnerella infections.

Infestations and Other Skin Conditions. *Scabies* (p. 806) is commonly sexually transmitted between young adults and it is important to remember contact tracing in its management. The lesions are modified on the genitals where the burrows are coiled to produce a dull red papule.

The crab louse, *phthirus pubis* is not confined to the pubic area but may be found in other body hair such as the eyelashes. Characteristic crablike adult lice and nits (eggs attached to hairs) are seen, better with a magnifying glass than by the naked eye. The adult causes an itch or the patient may notice the parasite. Diagnosis is made by recognising lice or nits and treatment is by local application of benzyl benzoate or gammabenzene hexachloride lotion.

Skin conditions which may affect the genitals include lichen planus, psoriasis, seborrhoeic dermatitis and tinea cruris. They can usually be recognised from their appearance, and from that of the rash elsewhere. A number of premalignant skin conditions have been recognised histologically; clinically they appear as persistent red patches. Any such lesion, with no identifiable cause, not responding to therapy, should be biopsied if it persists for more than 3 months. Squamous cell and basal cell carcinomas appear on the genitals either as persistent warty growths or ulcers.

Special Problems in Homosexuals. Homosexuals form a special high risk group. They change partners frequently and have a high prevalence of early syphilis, gonorrhoea, hepatitis B and other forms of hepatitis, and infectious mononucleosis. They may also be infested with *Entamoeba histolytica* and other intestinal organisms. An immune deficiency syndrome has also been described (p. 35).

PROSPECTS IN NEPHROLOGY

The last 25 years have seen major advances in understanding the nature of renal disease and in its therapeutic control. Since 1950, renal transplantation and haemodialysis for acute and chronic renal failure have passed through a tentative and experimental phase and become established clinical procedures. Studies of renal biopsies by light, electron and immunofluoroescence microscopy have transformed concepts of glomerular disease; knowledge of immunological mechanisms and their associated effects on complement, the mediators of inflammation and coagulation, are beginning to clarify the origin of glomerular damage, and awareness that the kidney acts as an endocrine organ has increased understanding of some forms of hypertension, of vitamin D resistance and renal osteodystrophy and of renal anaemia.

Progress in the foreseeable future is likely to consist of a steady consolidation of these foundations rather than any dramatic discovery that might otherwise transform the picture. Knowledge of renal structure will be further advanced by the use of scanning electron microscopy and the application of immunofluorescent techniques to electron microscopic preparations. Improved methods of detecting and measuring immune complexes and the identification of further unknown specific antigens, including viruses, will add to the list of agents known to be responsible for glomerulonephritis. At present immunosuppressive therapy is disappointing in controlling both the naturally occurring immunological renal disorders and the immunologically based rejection of transplanted kidneys. The non-specific nature of the action of immunosuppressive drugs gives rise to serious problems of toxicity and of opportunist infection. The ultimate goal in renal transplantation is the induction of specific tolerance by which ideally the immune response against the transplantation antigens of a grafted kidney only is suppressed and all other immunological responses remain normal. Experimental work in rats gives rise to optimism that this might be ultimately achieved. A significant improvement in cadaver graft survival resulting from the empirical use of blood transfusion given several weeks before the graft remains unexplained. A number of hypotheses have been put forward; these include the induction of tolerance in the recipient's immune system perhaps by stimulating 'blocking' antibodies or suppressor cells which protect the graft. Its mechanism is unknown, but it may act by inducing some form of non-responsiveness to non-HLA and HLA antigens.

Estimates of plasma 1,OH and 1,25 OH cholecalciferol and of parathyroid hormone and calcitonin will increase the capacity to prevent renal osteodystrophy, but the isolation, precise measurement and therapeutic availability of erythropoietin appears to be more distant.

The prevention of chronic pyelonephritis and renal failure by the eradication of urinary tract infection at an early stage appears to be a goal which recedes with the passage of time. Even if it is accepted that a significant proportion of chronic pyelonephritis arises from recurrent infections in infancy, the cost and difficulties of screening large numbers of children sufficiently often to detect them present formidable obstacles.

Finally, steady miniaturisation of artificial kidneys using improved synthetic membranes and adsorbents with the ultimate aim of producing a portable, round-the-clock working artificial kidney is likely to continue.

ANNE T. LAMBIE
J.S. ROBSON
(*Diseases of the Kidneys and Genito-urinary System*)
R.N. THIN
(*Sexually Transmitted Diseases*)

FURTHER READING:

Diseases of kidney and genito-urinary system:

Avery, G.S. (1980) *Drug Treatment*. Adis Press. For information about drugs and renal disease (ch. 21, Wright, N. & Robson, J.S.).

Black, D.A.K. & Jones, N.F. (1979) *Renal Disease*, 4th edn. Oxford: Blackwell Scientific Publications. Discusses current clinical problems.

Brenner, B.M. & Rector, F.L. (1981) *The Kidney* (Vols 1 & 2). Philadelphia: W.B. Saunders. A reference book with a physiological background.

Macleod, J. (1983) *Clinical Examination*, 6th edn. Edinburgh: Churchill Livingstone. For further information about examination of the kidneys and the urine.

Passmore, R. & Robson, J.S. (1984) *Companion to Medical Studies*, 3rd edn., Vol. 1. Oxford: Blackwell Scientific Publications. For information about anatomy and physiology of the kidney. Vol. 2 (2nd edn., 1980) for pathology and Vol. 3 (2nd edn., 1975) for medicine and surgery of the kidney.

Sexually transimitted diseases:

King, A., Nicol, C. & Rodin, P. (1982) *Venereal Diseases*, 4th edn. London: Baillière Tindall.

12. Endocrine and Metabolic Diseases

Rapid progress in our understanding of the physiology of the endocrine system has had a major impact on the investigation and treatment of many endocrine disorders. Part of this progress has stemmed from improvements in the methods used for the assay of hormones. The introduction of highly specific and sensitive radioimmunoassays has enabled the clinician to diagnose endocrine dysfunction accurately. The relative simplicity of most of these assays has meant that large numbers of samples can be processed. This has resulted in a service which has allowed physicians distant from specialist centres to practise a high standard of endocrinology. Indeed, as endocrinology permeates nearly all clinical disciplines it is becoming increasingly important for all doctors to be aware of the advances in this field. Such knowledge should lead to the earlier detection of endocrine disease and hence to a reduction of the morbidity associated with it.

Laboratory studies have shown that unicellular organisms such as coliform bacilli can produce hormones (e.g. insulin). It would seem likely that evolution has led to a change in the role of these 'hormones'. Initially they were probably part of an autocrine system where they had an effect within the unicellular organism. This led to an isocrine system where secretory products of adjacent cells had a local action on each other. With the development of specialised hormone secreting cells the paracrine system emerged. In this the specialist cell secretes a hormone which acts locally on other cells. A classic example is the pancreatic islet which contains cells secreting insulin, glucagon, pancreatic polypeptide or somatostatin. These are arranged in such a way that the secretion of one cell, such as that secreting somatostatin, can directly modulate an adjacent insulin-secreting cell. Increasing complexity and size of multicellular organisms resulted in the evolution of the endocrine system where groups of specialist cells formed glands which secreted hormones directly into an aqueous compartment such as the blood stream. These chemical messengers then had a specific effect at a distance from the site of secretion on certain responsive tissues or target organs. These effects can be mediated in one of three ways. Hormones can alter the rate of synthesis of enzymes and other proteins, can influence the catalytic function of enzymes, or can affect the permeability of cell membranes.

The practice of clinical endocrinology is changing rapidly as a result of the isolation and synthesis of hormones which has stemmed from advances in the techniques of protein chemistry and recombinant DNA technology. The last few years has seen the purification and synthesis of two new hypothalamic releasing hormones, one for ACTH and the other for growth hormone; the isolation of the insulin gene has allowed the bacterial synthesis of human insulin. Human growth hormone has also been produced by this technique. The somatostatin gene has been chemically synthesised and can be inserted into a plasmid vector (p. 18). Transformed *Escherichia coli* can thus be used to synthesise somatostatin. Clearly this will rapidly lead to the *in vitro* synthesis of all the important polypeptide hormones.

Understanding of the mechanisms of hormone action will lead to still further advances in endocrinology. For example, the pulsatile release of the gonadotrophin releasing hormone is critical in determining its effect. Long acting analogues of it not only do not stimulate but actually inhibit gonadotrophin release. They can therefore be used to treat precocious puberty, as contraceptives or in the management of hormone-dependent prostatic or breast cancer. Conversely, giving the naturally occurring releasing hormone subcutaneously in a pulsatile manner by a minipump can be used to induce puberty or to treat certain types of infertility.

For the student, clinical endocrinology is a most exciting subject in which disease processes can be readily understood by knowledge of basic physiology and anatomy. For the doctor and the patient there is the satisfaction that most endocrine diseases can be accurately diagnosed and respond to the appropriate therapy.

THE HYPOTHALAMUS AND THE PITUITARY GLAND

ANATOMY AND PHYSIOLOGY

The pituitary gland is enclosed in the sella turcica, bridged over by the diaphragma sellae, with the sphenoidal air sinuses below, and the optic chiasma in the subarachnoid space above. The gland is composed of two lobes, anterior and posterior, and is connected to the hypothalamus by the infundibular stalk carrying the portal vessels from the median eminence of the hypothalamus to the anterior lobe of the pituitary gland and nerve fibres to the posterior lobe.

The Anterior Lobe

The anterior lobe consists of three main histological types of cell as identified by conventional staining: chromphobe, eosinophil and basophil. However, the correlation between these types of staining and hormone secretion is not close. Through the action of its seven hormones, four of which act on target endocrine glands while the remainder act primarily on target tissues, the anterior pituitary affects growth, thyroid activity, sexual function, lactation, the metabolism of water, carbohydrate protein and fat, as well as skin pigmentation.

Hormones of the Anterior Lobe. Secretion of each of these hormones is influenced by a stimulus provided by the hypothalamus, either in the form of a releasing hormone or factor, or by an inhibitor which suppresses secretion or by both (Fig. 12.1).

Hypothalamic hormones
CRF: Corticotrophin releasing factor
LHRH: Luteinising hormone (follicle stimulating hormone) releasing hormone
GHRF: Growth hormone releasing factor
GHRIH: Growth hormone release inhibiting hormone (somatostatin)
TRH: Thyrotrophin releasing hormone
D: Dopamine (Prolactin release inhibiting factor)

Anterior pituitary hormones
ACTH: Adrenocorticotrophic hormone (corticotrophin)
LPH: β-lipotrophin
LH: Luteinising hormone
FSH: Follicle stimulating hormone
GH: Growth hormone
TSH: Thyroid stimulating hormone (thyrotrophin)
PRL: Prolactin

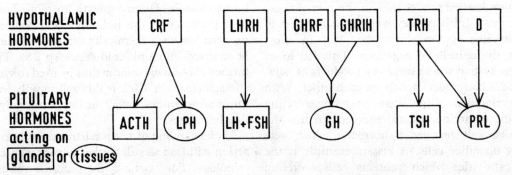

Fig. 12.1 The principal direct relationships between the hypothalamus and the anterior pituitary. Hypothalamic releasing [R] and inhibiting [I] activities are described as hormones [H] when they have been chemically identified and synthesised, and as factors [F] while their recognition still depends upon biological activity only, as determined by *in vivo* or *in vitro* bioassay studies.

The secretion of the hypothalamic factors in turn is dependent upon a wide variety of stimuli of nervous, metabolic, physical or hormonal origin, in particular from the appropriate target organs of the pituitary hormones, the thyroid gland, the adrenal cortex and the gonads.

TSH. The thyrotrophin releasing hormone (TRH) is a tripeptide formed in the hypothalamus, like the other hypothalamic releasing or inhibiting factors and passes through the portal system of vessels connecting the hypothalamus to the pituitary gland, where it promotes the secretion of the thyroid stimulating hormone (TSH).

LH AND FSH. The luteinising hormone and follicle stimulating hormone releasing hormone (designated LHRH for simplicity) is a decapeptide and acts on the pituitary to release both luteinising hormone (LH) and follicle stimulating hormone (FSH). Despite the fact that there is only one releasing hormone, LH and FSH can be secreted independently. This depends on the feedback of gonadal steroids on the pituitary which modulates the response to the releasing hormone. The latter appears to be secreted in an intermittent manner leading to pulses of gonadotrophin secretion. This pattern of secretion is critical. Continuous administration of LHRH downregulates receptors on the pituitary gonadotrophs and therefore paradoxically inhibits gonadotrophin secretion. Thus long-acting analogues of LHRH are being used for the treatment of hormone dependent prostate and breast cancer and may have a role as contraceptives. Conversely pulsatile administration of LHRH is proving to be an important new way of treating certain types of hypogonadotrophic infertility.

GH (growth hormone) is controlled by a dual system, namely growth hormone releasing factor (GHRF) and an inhibitory hormone (GHRIH). Growth hormone releasing factor has been isolated from pancreatic tumours found in patients with acromegaly, and has been shown to be similar to that present in the hypothalamus. Infusion of the pancreatic factor releases growth hormone without affecting other anterior pituitary hormones.

GHRIH is known also as *somatostatin* and has many other actions, including reduction in plasma gastrin, glucagon, insulin and in platelet stickiness. It is also produced in sites other than the hypothalamus such as the delta cells of the pancreatic islets.

PRL (prolactin) secretion differs from that of other anterior pituitary hormones in that it is under predominantly inhibitory control. The inhibitory factor is dopamine which is secreted by the hypothalamus into the portal system. Thus cutting the pituitary stalk leads to an elevation of prolactin secretion but inhibits the secretion of all the other anterior pituitary hormones. The existence of a prolactin releasing factor is controversial. Administration of TRH stimulates prolactin as well as TSH release. There is however little evidence that TRH normally controls prolactin release.

ACTH (corticotrophin). The secretion of the adrenocorticotrophic hormone (ACTH) and presumably of the hypothalamic corticotrophin releasing factor (CRF), is partly time-dependent, being most active in the morning, and least in the evening, except when this physiological diurnal (circadian) rhythm is overridden by other stimuli, particularly emotional or physical stresses.

LPH. β-melanocyte stimulating hormone (β-MSH) is now known to be an artefact created by extracting the pituitary under harsh conditions. The β-MSH amino acid sequence is contained within β-lipotrophin (LPH) which is the C-terminal part of the ACTH precursor molecule, pro-opiocortin. This core sequence is also present within ACTH (α-MSH) and in the N-terminal part of pro-opiocortin (γ-MSH) (Fig. 12.2). Thus there are several molecules derived from pro-opiocortin which function as melanocyte stimulating hormones and increase pigmentation of the skin and mucous membranes by increasing melanin synthesis in the melanocytes.

Fig. 12.2 ACTH/LPH precursor. The hatched areas represent the common core sequence contained within different molecules, each of which can stimulate melanocytes.

The C-terminal part of β-LPH (61–91) is β-endorphin, one of the endogenous substances with morphine-like actions. The first five amino-acids of β-endorphin are the same as those of the pentapeptide opioid, metenkephalin. Current evidence suggests, however, that metenkephalin is not derived from β-endorphin but from another precursor molecule.

The secretion of ACTH and β-LPH is under the control of CRF. A 41 amino acid peptide has been isolated, sequenced and synthesised which releases ACTH and hence cortisol when given to man. There is still doubt as to whether it is the only CRF. Animal studies have shown that the effect of this peptide can be markedly potentiated by vasopressin.

The Posterior Lobe

The posterior lobe (pars nervosa or neurohypophysis) contains neuroglial fibres which emanate from the supraoptic and paraventricular nuclei of the hypothalamus.

Hormones of the Posterior Lobe. The neurohypophysis secretes two hormones, arginine vasopressin (AVP) — here referred to as vasopressin — and oxytocin. The principal action of the former is to increase the reabsorption of water by the renal tubules, and because of this action vasopressin is also known as the antidiuretic hormone (ADH). The secretion of vasopressin is controlled by three main mechanisms. A rise in plasma osmolality stimulates vasopressin release which in turn results in water retention to preserve homeostasis. A fall of about 15% in plasma volume without any change in osmolality can also stimulate vasopressin secretion by activating volume receptors in the thorax. In addition the central nervous system also can play a role. Pain, for example, produces an antidiuresis.

The role of oxytocin in the male is unknown. In the female it has traditionally been thought to be important in parturition and the expression of milk from the breast. Much of the evidence has, however, been based on nonspecific assays. With more specific methods the role of the maternal hormone in human parturition has been questioned. It is possible that fetal oxytocin may be important.

DIAGNOSIS OF DISORDERED PITUITARY FUNCTION

All the protein and peptide hormones of the pituitary gland can be measured in body fluids by radioimmunoassay and access to a laboratory with a full range of these assays is critical for the proper evaluation of pituitary function. Approximate adult reference values for hormone concentrations in the plasma are given in Table 21.5 (p. 819). In addition the hypothalamic hormones, TRH and LHRH have been synthesised and can be used clinically to stimulate the release of the appropriate pituitary hormones. Furthermore, assays for the hormones produced by the target glands of the pituitary are available. Thus it is possible to assess very fully and specifically the functional activity and the secretory capacity of the pituitary gland and its target organs. Several pituitary hormones, namely TSH, ACTH, GH, and gonadotrophins are available in suitable forms for the investigation and treatment of endocrine disorders, and are useful in distinguishing between primary insufficiency of the adrenal cortex, the thyroid gland and the gonads, and secondary failure due to reduced or absent secretion of one or more pituitary trophic hormones.

One of the fundamental principles of the investigation of endocrine disorders is that if high levels of a hormone are suspected then an appropriate suppression test should be used. Conversely if there is hormone deficiency a stimulation test is normally required. Thus in assessing the increased production of growth hormone in acromegaly a glucose tolerance test is performed with measurement of growth hormone at half-hourly intervals for 2 hours along with measurement of blood glucose. Under physiological conditions growth hormone secretion is promptly suppressed by a rise in the blood glucose level, while there is either absent suppression or a paradoxical rise in patients with pituitary tumours secreting growth hormone.

Assessment of the basal function of the anterior pituitary should include measurement of serum thyroxine, an 09.00 h plasma cortisol, plasma prolactin, and plasma testosterone in the male and oestradiol in the female. When assessing the ability to secrete growth hormone in suspected hypopituitarism, insulin-induced hypoglycaemia (p. 450) is used. The test has the additional advantage that it stimulates the secretion of ACTH and hence cortisol. Prolactin is also released. Insulin-induced hypoglycaemia is also used in the assessment of growth hormone secretion in children of short stature. Alternative tests such as exercise-induced hypoglycaemia or measurement of growth hormone 2 hours after going to sleep are less reliable.

The ability of the pituitary to secrete TSH and PRL can be tested by TRH given intravenously and by measuring the serum TSH and PRL concentration before the drug and after 20 and 60 minutes. LHRH can be given intravenously at the same time and the plasma LH and FSH measured also. This test demonstrates that the gonadotrophins can be secreted in response to the releasing hormone. To test the ability of the hypothalamus to produce the releasing hormone, the anti-oestrogen clomiphene is given and the gonadotrophin response measured.

The need to measure prolactin during dynamic function tests is debatable. In prolactin deficiency it may be of value. In prolactin excess the response may indicate the cause. Thus in patients with prolactin secreting pituitary tumours the prolactin response to TRH is usually blunted (see below).

The diagnosis of disordered posterior pituitary function is considered in the section on diabetes insipidus.

Assays have now been developed for several hypothalamic hormones and factors but as yet there is no evidence that these measurements will be useful in clinical practice.

TUMOURS OF THE PITUITARY GLAND

Pathology. Pituitary tumours may be macroadenomas (associated with enlargement of the pituitary fossa or involvement of the adjacent structures) or microadenomas less than 10 mm in diameter (associated with a normal sized pituitary fossa or with minimal alteration such as a double floor). Such adenomas may be functional or nonfunctional. They may also produce hypofunction of the rest of the pituitary through pressure atrophy; such failure of function may be progres-

sive and sequential with the secretion of growth hormone and luteinising hormone declining first, followed by FSH, TSH and ACTH.

Excess production of a pituitary hormone may not necessarily be due to a tumour but to hyperplasia of the secreting cells on account of a disorder in hypothalamic control (excess production of a releasing hormone or insufficient production of an inhibiting hormone). In the case of PRL it has been claimed that the response in PRL secretion to TRH or to dopamine-receptor blockers (such as metoclopramide) is helpful in distinguishing between hyperplasia (associated with an augmented secretion) and tumour (associated with little or no response).

In the case of GH, excess production is usually due to an acidophil (or mixed acidophil and chromophobe) macroadenoma of the pituitary. On the other hand, excess secretion of ACTH (and of β-lipotrophin) is usually associated with a micro-adenoma or hyperplasia of basophil (or mixed basophil and chromophobe) cells with little or no evidence of enlargement of the pituitary fossa, except in cases of long standing or in Nelson's syndrome (p. 423).

It is important to understand that the conventional classification of pituitary tumours based on the staining characteristics of the cells may be misleading. Thus many tumours with hormone secretion have little stored hormone and hence are chromophobe. For this reason the increased sensitivity of immunohistochemistry is useful in characterising these tumours. Specific antibodies against the pituitary hormones can then be used to localise hormones.

Craniopharyngiomas are tumours or cysts developing in cell rests of Rathke's pouch, and may be located within the sella turcica, or commonly in the suprasellar space, where they frequently calcify. In either situation their clinical presentation is likely to be due to pressure on one or both lobes of the pituitary gland, on the stalk, on the hypothalamus, or on the visual pathways.

Primary carcinoma of the pituitary gland is particularly rare, but a metastatic tumour from a primary in the breast, lung, kidney or elsewhere may occur in the hypothalamus and reduce pituitary function. Other tumours, for example pinealoma, ependymoma or meningioma, may occasionally be associated with some disturbance of pituitary function. Granulomatous lesions of the pituitary or hypothalamus such as sarcoidosis or syphilis may mimic pituitary tumours.

Clinical Features. These vary, depending on the type of lesion in the pituitary gland and the effect of that lesion on surrounding structures. Enlarging tumours of the gland may present with signs attributable to increased output of hormones or to failure of secretion. Some tumours secreting hormones compress the remaining pituitary tissue, so that there may be failure of some functions of the gland in the presence of an excess of others.

Clinical features also depend upon the site and size of the tumour. Headache is the most constant but least specific symptom. Involvement of an optic nerve, the optic chiasma, or an optic tract leads to impaired visual fields. The patient occasionally notices a visual field defect, but, more commonly, examination of the visual fields by confrontation or by perimetry will be required to identify the likely point of interference within the visual pathway (Fig. 15.4 p. 602). A bitemporal field defect is the most characteristic finding associated with pressure upon the chiasma. Optic atrophy may be apparent on ophthalmoscopy. Diplopia and strabismus may follow pressure on the third, fourth or sixth cranial nerves.

Some tumours expand sufficiently to interfere with ADH secretion and so cause diabetes insipidus. Damage to the posterior pituitary *per se* will not normally produce diabetes insipidus as vasopressin secretion by the hypothalamus continues. Thus if there is diabetes insipidus it usually indicates that the tumour has a suprasellar extension. Tumours which expand upwards to impinge on the hypothalamus may cause disturbance of sleep, thirst, temperature control and appetite and also obesity.

Investigation. Enlargement of the sella turcica and erosion of the clinoid processes may be detected on radiological examination, or suprasellar calcification may be seen in a craniopharyngioma. A 'double floor' of the sella may be present if the tumour is expanding downwards with one side of the pituitary fossa being larger than the other. Computed tomography may be helpful and indeed the new generation of scanners is dis-

placing most of the invasive methods. Cysternography is another very useful investigation to determine the suprasellar anatomy. In this a water-soluble contrast medium is injected by cysternal puncture and used to outline the superior aspect of a pituitary tumour or to define an hypothalamic lesion.

Treatment. If there is evidence of pressure on the visual pathways then urgent treatment is required. In the past this was usually decompression of the tumour by a frontal craniotomy. Many tumours can, however, be decompressed by a trans-sphenoidal approach. In addition medical treatment can in some cases shrink pituitary tumours. Thus prolactinomas and growth hormone secreting tumours may sometimes be reduced in size by dopamine agonist drugs such as bromocriptine and surgery thereby avoided.

When there is hyperfunction of the pituitary, as confirmed by appropriate investigation, and this is sufficiently severe to affect the patient's welfare and prognosis, then treatment aimed at either destroying the tumour, or affecting its capacity to grow or secrete should be considered. In Cushing's disease (pituitary dependent Cushing's syndrome), prolactinomas and acromegaly it may be possible by trans-sphenoidal surgery selectively to remove an adenoma and leave sufficient normal pituitary tissue to maintain normal function. Alternatively, suppression of growth and, to a less predictable extent, of secretory capacity may be achieved by external radiotherapy usually with a linear accelerator. This treatment is nearly always given after a frontal craniotomy. Without it the recurrence rate of the tumour is about 20%.

In the case of the excess production of GH and PRL, bromocriptine (p. 423) may be used as an adjunct until such times as external radiotherapy has become effective. With microprolactinomas bromocriptine alone without any other therapy is commonly given. However, prolactinomas must be especially carefully supervised during pregnancy (fertility having been restored with bromocriptine) as they may undergo rapid expansion. The implantation of yttrium in the pituitary fossa is an alternative form of radiotherapy. It is used only in certain specialist centres. The same is true for proton beam therapy.

SYNDROMES DUE TO ANTERIOR PITUITARY HYPERSECRETION

Gigantism and Acromegaly. Hypersecretion of growth hormone by eosinophil cells may very rarely develop before the epiphyses have united and produce gigantism. Much more frequently it occurs in adult life, after union of the epiphyses, to cause acromegaly (large extremities). If hypersecretion begins in adolescence and persists into adult life, gigantism and acromegaly may be associated.

Acromegaly is characterised by an increase in the size of the bones and soft tissues of the hands, feet, supraorbital ridges, sinuses and the lower jaw. The skin becomes thick and coarse; the subcutaneous tissues increase in depth, while enlargement of the tongue, lips, nose and ears may be conspicuous. The viscera, for example the heart, thyroid and liver, enlarge. Sweating is common. Carbohydrate tolerance is reduced in about 30% of cases to the extent that diabetes mellitus develops.

As the disease progresses, the patient often develops arthritis (p. 571), kyphosis and muscular weakness. Arterial hypertension is a common complication. The disease tends to progress slowly over several years, but patients are frequently seen in whom the progress of the condition has apparently been arrested, or a phase of hyperpituitarism may pass into hypopituitarism.

Sensitive radioimmunological methods of assaying growth hormone in blood make it possible to assess with precision the activity of the condition as well as the results of treatment.

Bromocriptine is used to reduce GH levels as an adjunct to hypophysectomy or irradiation. This dopamine agonist lowers GH in about 75% of cases. The response is a paradoxical one in that dopamine elevates rather than reduces GH in normal subjects.

Cushing's Disease. Hypersecretion by basophil cells, or sometimes by chromophobe cells, leads to Cushing's disease (p. 444). This condition used to be treated by bilateral adrenalectomy. In the years thereafter some patients develop hyperpigmentation and an aggressive pituitary tumour which is usually locally invasive (Nelson's syndrome).

Hyperprolactinaemia Syndrome. This may result from a number of different causes apart from prolactinomas. Many drugs either antagonise the action of dopamine (phenothiazines, butyrophenones, metoclopramide) or deplete the hypothalamus of dopamine (methyldopa), and elevate prolactin levels (p. 419). Oestrogens also raise prolactin levels and account for the progressive hyperprolactinaemia in pregnancy. TRH stimulates prolactin secretion but it is not clear whether this is why some patients with primary hypothyroidism have hyperprolactinaemia. In renal failure prolactin levels are commonly elevated. The reason for this is obscure. Very high levels of prolactin are nearly always indicative of a pituitary tumour.

Hyperprolactinaemia may be associated with galactorrhoea and careful examination of the breasts in both sexes is important. Hippocrates was one of the first to observe that hyperprolactinaemia as evidenced by milk secretion was associated with decreased gonadal function. Thus in women amenorrhoea, oligomenorrhoea, deficient luteal phase progesterone production or menorrhagia may all be associated with hyperprolactinaemia. It is important to measure prolactin in cases of unexplained infertility.

In men hyperprolactinaemia usually presents with loss of libido or impotence. Unfortunately at this stage many have a large prolactinoma (macroadenoma) often with associated visual field defects.

Treatment with long acting dopamine agonists such as bromocriptine or newer drugs such as pergolide will lower prolactin levels and usually restore gonadal function to normal. In some patients with pituitary tumours this will not happen because of gonadotrophin insufficiency. In others there may be high levels of gonadotrophins with a premature menopause.

SYNDROMES DUE TO ANTERIOR PITUITARY HYPOSECRETION

Short Stature and Infantilism

In children hyposecretion of GH causes short stature; hyposecretion of gonadotrophins causes pituitary infantilism, implying that sexual development is subnormal for the individual's age. The term 'dwarfism' has been discarded by many endocrinologists and paediatricians because of its unpleasant connotations. Pituitary tumours are an uncommon cause of GH deficiency in children. Much more common is a genetic inability to secrete GH which is probably the result of a lack of growth hormone releasing factor. Other conditions such as craniopharyngioma are important causes of GH deficiency. In children with short stature it is essential that accurate records of height and weight are kept and entered on a percentile chart. If the child is below the 3rd percentile for height or is crossing the percentiles then further investigation is indicated.

Measurement of bone age is important. Radiographs of the non-dominant hand and wrist are taken and compared with a standard atlas to assess the progress of bone development. With GH deficiency a delayed bone age will be found. This will also be present in delayed puberty and children with constitutionally delayed puberty are often short.

Investigation of GH secretion has been outlined (p. 421). Most children will be tested with insulin-induced hypoglycaemia. In addition to GH and glucose it is important to measure plasma cortisol. Basal level of thyroxine and prolactin should be assessed. The pattern of LH and FSH response to LHRH may help in distinguishing constitutional delayed puberty from structural lesions.

Children in whom growth hormone secretion has been shown to be absent may be treated by GH; this is obtainable only from appropriate national sources because of the need to extract GH from human cadaveric pituitary glands. Intramuscular injections are given twice weekly for several years according to the response judged by serial readings recorded on standard height and weight charts.

Differential Diagnosis of Short Stature. Growth may be delayed or impaired for many reasons. Tallness and shortness of stature have genetic components. One form of impaired growth is found in Turner's syndrome (p. 9). Persistent stunting of growth is a recognised association with premature birth, anoxic forms of congenital heart disease, chronic liver or renal disease, many chronic infections, and persistent undernutrition (p. 60). Short stature of hypothalamic or pituitary origin must also be distinguished from:

1. *Cretinism and Juvenile Hypothyroidism.* If these conditions are not recognised and treated promptly, stunting of growth will occur (p. 436).

2. *Short Stature due to Malabsorption.* Coeliac disease (p. 313) may be associated with steatorrhoea and defective absorption, especially of fat, minerals and vitamins. However, in many patients there is no clinical evidence of malabsorption. Such cases can be diagnosed only by carrying out a jejunal biopsy. When the diagnosis has been confirmed treatment is with a gluten-free diet. Cystic fibrosis may simulate malabsorption due to coeliac disease. Another gastroenterological cause of short stature is Crohn's disease which may also be occult in its presentation.

3. *Achondroplasia.* This hereditary disorder of endochondral ossification is characterised by failure of the long bones of the arms and legs to grow properly, while the trunk and head develop normally. Patients with this condition are sexually and intellectually normal and frequently used to appear in circuses.

4. *Renal Disease.* Renal failure arising in early childhood is often associated with a short stature. It may be caused by neuromuscular incoordination at the outlet of the bladder, which produces back-pressure and hydronephrosis, or it may be due to polycystic disease, congenital hypoplasia of the kidneys, or most commonly, chronic nephritis. In some cases hereditary defects of renal tubular function may be responsible (p. 379). In addition to the characteristic features of renal failure, hypertension may also be present.

Hypopituitarism

Aetiology. At one time destruction of the anterior lobe of the hypophysis was commonly due to infarction and this was often a sequel to post-partum haemorrhage (*Sheehan's syndrome*). Improvements in obstetrical care have greatly reduced the incidence of this accident and hypopituitarism is now most commonly due to a chomophobe adenoma. Other causes include tumours, trauma, granulomas (syphilis, tuberculosis, sarcoidosis) and the presence of simple cysts.

Some cases are the result of failure of the hypothalamus to secrete the appropriate releasing hormones. Others may conceivably be due to an autoimmune hypophysitis.

Surgical treatment or radiotherapy of tumours of the pituitary gland is often followed by a degree of hypopituitarism calling for replacement therapy, and hypophysectomy is sometimes performed in the treatment of malignant disease elsewhere, for example carcinoma of the breast.

Clinical Features. In Sheehan's syndrome, a history is usually obtained that, several years before the onset of the presenting illness, the patient had a difficult confinement with haemorrhage and a need for blood transfusion. Lactation failed or was never established, amenorrhoea persisted indefinitely and other changes attributable to the absence of the trophic hormones gradually made their appearance. Some of the features of hypothyroidism (p. 436) may be present, but the deficiency is seldom prominent.

In all causes of hypopituitarism, LH secretion tends to be lost early in the course of the disease. In the male impotence and loss of libido are important early symptoms. Later in the established disease there may be gynaecomastia, decreased frequency of shaving and absent or scanty axillary and pubic hair.

Symptoms of adrenal insufficiency (p. 448) may be noted, but the changes in serum electrolytes found in severe adrenal insufficiency do not occur in hypopituitarism and the blood pressure is usually not so low. This is because aldosterone continues to be secreted by the glomerulosa layer of the adrenal cortex, since this function is largely independent of corticotrophin. Cortisol production, however, falls to a minimum because the essential corticotrophic stimulus from the pituitary gland is absent or inadequate.

In contrast to the pigmentation of the skin in Addison's disease, a striking degree of pallor is often one of the signs suggesting hypopituitarism. Although a mild degree of normochromic anaemia is usually present, this is insufficient to explain the pallor of the skin which is due to capillary vasoconstriction and the absence of melanin.

Coma in Hypopituitarism. Patients with hypopituitarism are liable to develop coma if inadequately treated. While the onset of coma may occur for no apparent reason, it usually follows some mild infection or injury, in the same way that an Addisonian crisis may follow some relatively trivial stress.

The coma may be due to one or more of the effects of hypopituitarism. These include adrenal insufficiency and lack of growth hormone resulting in increased sensitivity to insulin and hence hypoglycaemia. Water intoxication is another important factor, due to a disturbance of water control in patients with adrenal insufficiency. Hypothyroidism is also a component in the causation of coma; hypothermia with a rectal temperature as low as 32°C or less may develop. Failure of ventilation with anoxia and respiratory acidosis may be a lethal complication of hypopituitarism.

Differential Diagnosis. Hypopituitarism is sometimes confused with *anorexia nervosa*. The distinguishing features lie in the history and the presence of pubic, axillary and lanugo hair in anorexia nervosa. In addition, anorexia nervosa is characterised by an absent appetite and gross wasting, whereas in hypopituitarism neither is striking unless some other cause is present.

Assays of pituitary trophic hormones or the products of the target glands will help to distinguish these two disorders and others which might be confused with hypopituitarism. In anorexia nervosa the weight loss is associated with low levels of LH and FSH, and these hormones have a prepubertal circadian pattern. The response to LHRH is similar to that seen in prepubertal children (i.e. the FSH response is greater than the LH). When markedly underweight the gonadotrophin response to clomiphene is absent but returns with adequate weight gain. This suggests a functional hypothalamic abnormality.

In girls with anorexia nervosa the obvious endocrine abnormality is usually secondary amenorrhoea. There are, however, other subtle changes. The levels of triiodothyronine (T_3) are often low with the biologically inactive reverse T_3 being high. Thyroxine levels are normal. Unlike hypopituitarism the levels of GH are either normal or high; this is also true for serum cortisol levels. Prolactin secretion is normal.

Treatment. The aim should be to provide adequate substitution therapy, according to the deficiencies demonstrated, so that the patient can lead a normal life. Cortisol should be given by mouth in doses of 20 mg in the morning and 10 mg in the evening or according to the cortisol blood profile. Thyroid hormone, if required, should be given orally as thyroxine 0·15 mg daily. It is dangerous to give thyroid hormone to patients with adrenal insufficiency until they have been protected by cortisol against the possibility of an Addisonian type of crisis. Excessive doses of corticosteroids may result in the development of Cushing's syndrome. Because aldosterone secretion is maintained, mineralocorticoid replacement therapy is not required.

Sex hormone replacement therapy is important to restore normal sexual function and to prevent the development of osteoporosis. In men depot preparations of testosterone are effective either by subcutaneous implant every few months or by monthly intramuscular injections. Testosterone undecanoate can be given by mouth but produces variable blood levels and is expensive. In women cyclical oestrogen therapy is indicated in pre-menopausal patients with gonadotrophin deficiency. Ethinyloestradiol (20 μg daily) is given for 3 out of 4 weeks and a progestogen such as medroxyprogesterone acetate (5 mg daily) for the 4th week.

In patients requiring fertility, gonadotrophin therapy may be given. This can result in hyperstimulation of the ovary with multiple ovulation. Careful monitoring of the oestrogen response to the gonadotrophin will usually avoid this. Very promising results have now been reported with pulsatile LHRH therapy in many patients with hypopituitarism. This suggests that a complete absence of pituitary gonadotrophs is rare.

DIABETES INSIPIDUS

This uncommon disease is characterised by the persistent excretion of excessive quantities of urine of low specific gravity, and by constant thirst. Diabetes insipidus (DI) can be subdivided into two main types, cranial DI in which there is deficient production of the antidiuretic hormone, arginine vasopressin (AVP), and nephrogenic DI in which the renal tubules are unresponsive to vasopressin.

Aetiology. Cranial DI may rarely result from a genetic defect in vasopressin production with a dominant mode of inheritance. There is also a recessive condition in which DI may be associated with diabetes mellitus.

More commonly cranial DI develops after damage to the hypothalamus or with high stalk lesions. This may occur with tumours of the pituitary, with a craniopharyngioma, and as a sequel to basal meningitis or trauma. In panhypopituitarism, the symptoms of diabetes insipidus may not be apparent until corticosteroid therapy has been provided; an adequate level of corticosteroids is required for the condition to be expressed. In some patients no cause can be found.

Nephrogenic DI may be inherited as a sex-linked recessive condition or may be acquired. Hypokalaemia, hypercalcaemia, heavy metal poisoning and lithium therapy may all block the renal response to vasopressin.

Clinical Features. The most marked symptoms are polyuria and polydipsia. The patient may pass 5–20 or more litres of urine in 24 hours. The urine is clear and of low specific gravity and osmolality, i.e. usually less than the plasma osmolality.

The diagnosis of cranial DI depends on demonstrating that a rise of plasma osmolality induced by withholding fluids is not accompanied by a normal rise in the osmolality or specific gravity of the urine, but that when vasopressin is given, such a rise does occur. The latter test is necessary in order to show that the kidney is capable of concentrating the urine which it cannot do in nephrogenic DI.

It may be difficult to differentiate the polyuria of diabetes insipidus from that found in *psychogenic polydipsia*. This distinction can usually be made by a carefully performed water deprivation test which should be carried out during the day and should not normally last more than 8 hours. No coffee, tea or smoking is allowed before the test. The patient should be weighed at the start of the test and at intervals during it. If the weight falls by more than 3% the test should be terminated. If the weight increases this suggests the possibility of surreptitious drinking. During the procedure plasma and urine samples are taken for measurement of osmolality. At the end of test, if there has not been an antidiuresis, vasopressin is given and the urine osmolality followed over the next four hours.

In cranial DI the pre-testing plasma osmolality is usually high and with fluid deprivation often exceeds 300 mosm/kg. The urine osmolality of the DI patients is usually less than that of the plasma at the end of the test but rises when vasopressin is given whereas in normal subjects urine osmolality after 8 hours fluid deprivation is about 800 mosm/kg and does not increase when vasopressin is given.

In psychogenic polydipsia the initial plasma osmolality is usually below normal and the urine osmolality fails to rise normally with water deprivation. The renal response to exogenous vasopressin is also impaired because of the effect of long-term over-hydration on the kidney.

Other causes of polyuria are discussed on page 380.

Treatment. This is usually with the long-acting analogue of vasopressin, desmopressin (DDAVP). The amount of vasopressin required to keep the patient in water balance must be determined by measuring the fluid output. Desmopressin is given intranasally; 10–20μg once or twice daily elicits a response as effectively as vasopressin given by injection.

A variety of other drugs have been used. Chlorpropamide, the oral hypoglycaemic agent, enhances the renal responsiveness to vasopressin and can be used either in mild DI or in severe DI when large doses of DDAVP are required. As might be anticipated hypoglycaemia can be a problem. An alternative drug with a similar action is carbamazepine. Thiazide diuretics remain the only effective drug therapy for nephrogenic DI and reduce urine volume in this condition by about 50%.

Inappropriate Secretion of ADH

In a number of clinical conditions there is excess secretion of ADH leading to pathological water retention. This fails to suppress the hormone as would be expected in a normal subject. The ADH secretion is thus 'inappropriate' in that it occurs despite a low plasma osmolality. The syndrome of inappropriate secretrion of ADH is thus associated with hypo-osmolality of plasma, hyponatraemia and a urine osmolality that is often greater than that of the plasma. The symptoms relate to the degree of hyponatraemia. If the serum sodium is greater than 120 mmol/l, the patient may be asymptomatic; between 120–110 mmol/l there is usually nausea, anorexia and sometimes vomiting; below 110 mmol/l the patient becomes stuporose, may have a grand mal fit and eventually lapse into coma often with physical signs suggesting severe neurological deficit such as bilateral extensor plantar responses. These changes are all reversible if correct treatment is given.

Inappropriate secretion of ADH may be found in patients with traumatic, inflammatory or neoplastic disease of the central nervous system. It is present in about 2% of cases of small cell carcinoma of the bronchus, but can also occur with benign pulmonary disease such as pneumonia, tuberculosis or lung abscess. It is rare in malignancies other than those of the bronchus. Small cell carcinomas associated with the syndrome contain large amounts of vasopressin and can be shown to synthesise the hormone *in vitro*. In contrast, in non-malignant causes, the vasopressin is secreted by the posterior pituitary. Acute intermittent porphyria and chlorpropamide therapy are also sometimes associated with this syndrome.

The aim of treatment is to induce negative water balance by restricting fluid intake so that it is exceeded by the sum of the urinary output and the insensible fluid loss. This usually means giving 500–750 ml water per day. This is unpleasant for the patient and an alternative approach is to give drugs such as demethylchlortetracycline which produce mild nephrogenic diabetes insipidus.

THE THYROID GLAND

Anatomy and Physiology. The thyroid gland consists of an isthmus and two lateral lobes, and lies in front of and on either side of the upper part of the trachea and the laminae of the thyroid cartilage. Posteriorly it is closely related to the recurrent laryngeal nerves which lie between the trachea and the oesophagus; the gland is separated from these nerves by its fibrous sheath. The thyroid gland is provided with a rich blood supply through the superior and inferior thyroid arteries. The parathyroid glands are usually to be found lying on the posterior aspect of the thyroid, in its substance or in the sheath of the gland and in relation to the upper cornu of the thymus.

The thyroid hormones, triiodothyronine (T_3) and thyroxine (T_4), are dipeptides containing respectively 3 and 4 atoms of iodine in each molecule. Both are normally stored in the colloid vesicles as thyroglobulin (Fig. 12.3). T_3 is metabolically more active than T_4 in that it is effective in smaller doses and acts more rapidly. Only a small proportion of circulating T_3 is secreted directly by the thyroid, approximately 85% arising from extra-thyroidal monodeiodination of T_4. Alternatively T_4 may be monodeiodinated to reverse-T_3 (T_3) which is a relatively inactive isomer of T_3. More than 99% of both T_3 to T_4 in plasma are bound to plasma proteins, mainly to the specific transport protein, thyroxine binding globulin (TBG), but also to albumin and thyroxine binding prealbumin. The conversion of T_4 and T_3, possibly at the site of action, may be necessary before metabolic activity can be expressed. The action of the thyroid hormones is to increase the rate of metabolism of most tissues, especially immature ones. They also supplement the metabolic effects of catecholamines. It is only free T_4 and free T_3 that can diffuse out of the vascular spaces and be metabolically effective.

Thyroid function is controlled by thyrotrophin, the thyroid stimulating hormone (TSH) secreted by the anterior pituitary gland which in turn is controlled by thyrotrophin releasing hormone (TRH) secreted by the hypothalamus. TRH has been synthesised and is available for clinical use. There is also a negative feed-back mechanism whereby the levels of free T_3 and free T_4 influence the secretion of TSH by the anterior pituitary. The synthesis and release of thyroid hormones from the colloid into the circulation are stimulated by TSH.

Calcitonin, secreted by the parafollicular C (calcitonin) cells of the thyroid gland, is discussed on page 439.

THE INVESTIGATION OF THYROID DISORDERS

Thyroid Function

The diagnostic facilities available to determine the level of thyroid function are so precise that it should not be necessary to treat patients in the absence of a high degree of certainty concerning the diagnosis of hyper- or hypothyroidism.

Total plasma thyroxine (T_4) measured by competitive protein binding or radioimmunoassay is not influenced by exogenous iodine, but is altered by factors which affect the concentration of thyroid hormone-binding proteins (TBG). Thus, concentrations (p. 819) may be raised in people with normal thyroid function when levels of TBG are increased in pregnancy, oestrogen administration or as a congenital anomaly. Decreased levels of TBG may be due to the nephrotic syndrome, androgen therapy, liver failure or be inherited. TBG may appear to be low if binding sites are saturated with drugs such as salicylates, phenylbutazone, sulphonylureas and phenytoin. Alternatively these drugs may increase the catabolism of T_4, thus lowering the total T_4 levels.

Fig. 12.3 Synthesis of thyroxine (T_4) and of triiodothyronine (T_3). The main sites of block induced by (A) potassium perchlorate and (B) by carbimazole, methimazole and the thiouracil group of drugs are also shown.

Total plasma tri-iodothyronine (T_3) is necessary for the diagnosis of T_3 thyrotoxicosis when T_3 is elevated in the presence of a normal total plasma T_4 and other tests. It is subject to the same limitations as total plasma T_4 in relation to the level of TBG, although to a lesser extent.

T_3 Resin Uptake, Free Thyroxine Index and Effective Thyroxine Ratio. The T_3 resin uptake test is an indirect estimate of circulating thyroid hormone levels. It measures the degree of saturation of the binding sites on the thyroid hormone-binding proteins. High values are found in thyrotoxicosis but low values are recorded in euthyroid patients who are either pregnant or on oestrogen medication. The role of such a test is in the calculation of the *free thyroxine index* derived from the product of the total plasma thyroxine and the T_3 resin uptake. In euthyroid patients with abnormalities of the thyroid hormone-binding proteins and in whom the total plasma thyroxine is elevated, the T_3 resin uptake will be depressed and the free thyroxine index is more likely to lie in the normal range. Measurements of total T_4 which have been corrected for the patient's TBG are available and the result is referred to as the *effective thyroxine ratio.*

Plasma free T_3 and free T_4 levels are becoming routinely available and are likely to replace all the above methods if sufficient sensitivity and reliability can be achieved.

The Uptake of Radioactive Iodine or Technetium. The overactive gland synthesising excess T_4 has an increased uptake of iodine which can be shown by measuring the proportion of an oral tracer dose of ^{131}I taken up by the thyroid gland in a given time (e.g. 4 hours) by using an appropriate 'counter' over the neck. Alternatively, an isotope of technetium (^{99m}Tc) may be used intravenously with the thyroid uptake measured at 20 minutes, giving an even smaller dose of radiation which can be regarded as insignificant. The major fallacies in such studies are caused by iodine deficiency or enzyme deficiency beyond the stage of iodide uptake (which can give an increased uptake measurement without the presence of thyrotoxicosis) and iodine excess (which can give a low uptake measurement in spite of the presence of thyrotoxicosis). It is necessary to know how avid is the uptake of the gland before treating a thyrotoxic patient with radioactive iodine.

A radionuclide scan of the thyroid using either ^{131}I or ^{99m}Tc will indicate the distribution of functioning thyroid tissue. Scans are useful in determining the nature of a solitary thyroid nodule — whether it is functional ('hot') or non-functional ('cold'). They may also be useful in determining whether a goitre is multinodular or diffuse and whether there is a retrosternal extension of functioning tissue; the nature of a suspected maldevelopment, e.g. sublingual thyroid can also be determined. *In vivo* isotope tests should not be done in subjects who may be pregnant and in children should be done only when essential.

In the TRH test the plasm TSH level is measured before and 20 minutes after the intravenous injection of 200 μg TRH. In thyrotoxicosis the secretion of TSH by the anterior pituitary is suppressed. While this cannot be discerned within the limits of the assay of a single plasma TSH level, it can be readily detected by the failure of the plasma TSH levels to rise more than 1 mU/l in response to TRH.

Choice of test or combination of tests is made in the light of the foregoing and in relation to the individual problem and the local resources. It must be remembered that when thyrotoxicosis is due to excessive production of T_3 alone, the total serum T_4, the effective thyroxine ratio and the thyroid uptake of radioisotopes may give normal results. The measurement of the total serum T_3 concentration together with the TRH test are, therefore, the two most useful diagnostic aids in relation to thyrotoxicosis.

The Nature of a Goitre

The following tests may be helpful in elucidating the nature of a euthyroid goitre (enlargement of the thyroid gland):

Radiographs of the neck and thoracic inlet will indicate the presence of a significant goitre, whether it is compressing or displacing the trachea, and if there is a retrosternal extension. It will also show if an adenoma or the wall of a cyst is calcified. A lateral view will show if there is a retrotracheal extension of the goitre that may sometimes occur in Hashimoto thyroiditis.

Ultrasonography of the thyroid may determine whether a solitary 'cold' area on radionuclide scanning is purely cystic (and therefore almost certainly benign) or partially cystic (and therefore suspicious of being malignant).

Examination of the vocal cords will indicate whether a large or malignant goitre has damaged a recurrent laryngeal nerve.

Serum autoantibodies to thyroid cytoplasm or to thyroglobulin in high titre are indicative of Hashimoto thyroiditis in the appropriate clinical context.

Needle biopsy of the thyroid may be indicated if the nature of a goitre is still in doubt. Multiple biopsies may be taken under local anaesthetic, but the limitations of small biopsy specimens must be remembered.

HYPERTHYROIDISM

The clinical condition consequent upon overproduction of T_3 or of both T_3 and T_4 is referred to as hyperthyroidism or thyrotoxicosis. In a significant minority of patients the excess production of thyroid hormone is confined to T_3 (T_3 thyrotoxicosis) but it is likely that a greater number of cases have an initial phase of excess T_3 production followed by an overproduction of both T_3 and T_4, and it is usually at the latter stage that the diagnosis is made.

Aetiology and Pathology. The serum TSH levels in patients with thyrotoxicosis are either reduced or undetectable using current radioimmunoassay techniques. Cases of thyrotoxicosis due to excess TSH production by pituitary tumours are exceptionally rare.

In many patients with hyperthyroidism the IgG autoantibody, human specific TSH receptor antibody, can be detected in the serum and it is possible that antibodies that can stimulate the TSH receptor (thyroid stimulating immunoglobulin, TSI) may be the cause of hyperthyroidism in most instances of Graves' disease, as defined below. Other evidence of autoimmune activity directed against the thyroid gland in hyperthyroidism is the presence of lymphocytic infiltration in the gland which may be negligible, focal or extensive. There is an increased prevalence of HLA-DR3 in Graves' disease. Thus Graves' disease appears to be an autoimmune hyperthyroidism which occurs in a genetically preselected population.

In the majority of patients with hyperthyroidism the thyroid gland is either diffusely hyperactive (*Graves' disease*) or the gland consists of multiple active nodules interspersed with inactive areas. This latter state is probably the outcome of alternate stimulation and degeneration or results from the development of thyrotoxicosis upon a multinodular goitre. Toxic nodular goitres tend to occur in older patients and diffuse goitres in younger subjects. In a small percentage of patients, thyrotoxicosis is due to the presence of a hyperactive solitary nodule with suppression of the remainder of the gland through the normally functioning feed-back mechanism.

Histologically, in Graves' disease, the increased activity of the gland is manifest by reduction in the size of the thyroid vesicles which are relatively empty of colloid; the epithelium is tall and columnar in contrast to the flat cuboidal epithelium of the normal gland. The vascularity is markedly increased.

Clinical Features. Thyrotoxicosis is found much more frequently in women than in men (8:1), usually in the third to sixth decades, but it may occur at any age. There may or may not be a clinically detectable goitre. The increased blood supply to the thyroid often causes a bruit, and sometimes a thrill.

Most of the clinical features of thyrotoxicosis may be explained in terms of excess production of T_3 or of $T_3 + T_4$, although it is possible that T_4 is nothing more than a prohormone. The increased metabolism accounts for the loss in weight in spite of the increased appetite that is so often a striking feature in the clinical history. Occasionally, however, the patient overcompensates in terms of food intake and may gain weight.

Thyroid hormones potentiate the action of catecholamines, possibly by modulating amplification of the β-adrenergic signal at the level of the cell membrane. The increased cardiac output required to meet the metabolic demands, together with the effect of T_3 and T_4 on the sympathetic nervous system, tends to produce a tachycardia, or, particularly in elderly patients, arrhythmias such as atrial fibrillation or ectopic beats. The patient may complain of palpitations with or without the symptoms of cardiac failure. Sinus tachycardia, persisting during sleep, is one of the earliest and most constant signs. The pulse pressure is increased and capillary pulsation may be detectable. In the presence of coincident systolic hypertension a collapsing pulse may be noted. In the older patient cardiovascular manifestations may be the only clinical evidence of hyperthyroidism and it should be remembered that thyrotoxicosis is, along with coronary and rheumatic heart disease, one of the three commonest causes of atrial fibrillation.

There are other consequences of the effect of excess thyroid hormones on the beta-adrenergic receptors. Patients commonly complain of increased frequency of bowel motions, usually with formed stools but there may be an element of malabsorption; a lag curve in a glucose tolerance test may be demonstrable partly as a result of intestinal hurry. Retraction of the upper eyelids and a fine tremor of the fingers may occur, while the hands are often hot and sweaty because of the increased metabolic rate and the need to lose excess heat. Intolerance of warm environments is characteristic. Thyrotoxic patients, although they are hyperdynamic, have a low efficiency in terms of what they achieve. They suffer from an inability to relax both mentally and physicallly; anxiety is frequent.

Less common clinical features that cannot be so readily explained in terms of disturbed physiology include exophthalmos (p. 435), pretibial myxoedema and finger clubbing, reduced fertility and menstrual irregularities. In addition there may be thyrotoxic myopathy (p. 667), which recovers when normal thyroid function is restored.

In some cases thyrotoxicosis undergoes spontaneous remission within a period of months or years, while in other cases it follows a prolonged or intermittent course.

Thyrotoxic crises are now uncommon, as cases of hyperthyroidism are recognised and treated earlier and more effectively. They may be seen shortly after thyroidectomy in patients who have not been adequately prepared for operation or in patients who have been operated on for some other disability without hyperthyroidism having been recognised. Alternatively a crisis may be precipitated by a severe infection. The patient in crisis suffers from severe mental and physical exhaustion with delirium, delusions or mania, dehydration, ketosis, tachycardia, cardiac failure and fever.

Hyperthyroidism in the Newborn and in Children. Thyrotoxicosis may occur rarely in the newborn when it is thought to be due to the transplacental transmission of thyroid stimulating antibody. This form of hyperthyroidism is self-limiting. If thyrotoxicosis occurs before puberty there is an increase in the growth rate so that affected children are unusually tall for their age.

Investigation. The plasma total T_3, plasma total T_4 and TRH tests should be undertaken in all cases of suspected thyrotoxicosis if the facilities are available, as it is important to be certain of the diagnosis before embarking on prolonged drug therapy or using a destructive form of therapy. Reliance should not be placed on a single test which is necessarily liable to laboratory error and also subject to the artefacts mentioned on page 428. Nor should the tests be done individually in series according to the results obtained at each step as advocated by some, as this almost certainly leads to unacceptable delays in treating the patient. While a normal TRH test excludes primary thyrotoxicosis, a flat TRH test by itself does not establish the diagnosis. Insufficient experience is not yet available to rely on plasma free T_3 or plasma free T_4 measurements.

A radionuclide scan of the thyroid may be helpful in confirming the diffuse or nodular nature of the thyroid and whether or not there is a retrosternal extension of functioning thyroid tissue.

Treatment. Three effective methods of treating thyrotoxicosis are available: (1) Antithyroid drugs, such as carbimazole, initially supplemented as necessary by beta-adrenergic blocking agents, for example propranolol. (2) Surgery, after a euthyroid state has been achieved with antithyroid drugs or under propranolol and potassium iodide cover. (3) Radioactive iodine, with or without the use of propranolol or antithyroid drugs.

ANTITHYROID DRUGS. The site of action of the

different antithyroid drugs is indicated in Figure 12.3. Most commonly used are those that act by blocking the organic binding of iodine to tyrosine, carbimazole in Europe and its active metabolite, methimazole, in North America. Other drugs which act in this way are propyl and methyl thiouracil, which may occasionally be useful in the event of hypersensitivity to the drug of first choice.

Carbimazole is given initially in full suppressive doses of 15–20 mg at 8-hourly intervals for 3 to 4 weeks, according to the severity of the condition and the size of the goitre. Thereafter the dose can gradually be reduced, and, as the patient's clinical state responds, the aim should be to maintain a euthyroid state with as little of the antithyroid drugs as necessary; this ranges between 5–30 mg daily. Overtreatment with antithyroid drugs will result in TSH production by the anterior pituitary with a risk of increase in size of the thyroid. In patients in whom the natural history of the underlying process is one of exacerbation and remission, stable control may be achieved with drugs only when an excessive dose of carbimazole (but not greater than 45–60 mg/day) is combined with continuous thyroxine administration in a dose of 0·15 mg/day. The patient's response should be monitored by measuring the plasma/serum levels of T_4, T_3 and TSH.

Carbimazole or methimazole may be selected as the definitive therapy or may be used to prepare the patient for surgery. If antithyroid drugs are being used as definitive therapy they should be continued for at least 1 year and restricted to patients who do not have a large goitre. By selecting cases in this way rather less than 50% of thyrotoxic patients will go into lasting remission and will not require further therapy. The probability of remission or relapse after 6–12 months treatment with antithyroid drugs can be assessed by determining whether the patient is HLA-DR3 or not and whether TSH receptor antibodies are present in the serum.

Carbimazole, methimazole and the thiouracil group of drugs as well as potassium perchlorate, may produce toxic effects, of which the commonest is a rash and the most serious are the blood dyscrasias, agranulocytosis being most frequent.

Routine white cell counts are of little value in its early detection as it occurs with dramatic suddenness, usually but not necessarily, in the first few weeks of treatment. Patients taking these drugs must be told to report a sore throat and to stop the drug immediately until it is clear whether agranulocytosis has occurred or not. By stopping the drug promptly and by using antibiotics prophylactically serious consequences will be avoided and the leucocyte count will return to normal within 1 to 2 weeks.

Potassium perchlorate induces blood dyscrasias more commonly than other antithyroid drugs, including red cell aplasia which is usually lethal. For this reason, potassium perchlorate should be used only as a temporary expedient if hypersensitivity to other drugs has occurred and if radioactive iodine therapy or surgery under propranolol cover are not acceptable alternatives. It should never be used in a dose greater than 1 g/day.

There is no place for the use of potassium iodide as an antithyroid drug except in preparation for subtotal thyroidectomy (in combination with propranolol or when the patient has already been made euthyroid with carbimazole or methimazole), or in the management of thyrotoxic crisis.

BETA-ADRENOCEPTOR ANTAGONIST DRUGS are very useful as they can produce much symptomatic improvement by countering the effect of T_3 and T_4 on catecholamine action. Thus anxiety, palpitations, increased bowel activity, lid retraction and finger tremor may be alleviated with propranolol, 40–80 mg 6 hourly. It can therefore be useful during the interval of several weeks which is required for antithyroid drugs or radioactive iodine to be fully effective provided there are no contraindications to its use such as cardiac failure, asthma, or insulin dependent diabetes. Much higher doses (up to 1 g/day or more) may be required in severe thyrotoxicosis but must be used with care.

SURGICAL TREATMENT. This is the treatment of choice if the patient is considered too young for radioactive iodine therapy (i.e. during the reproductive years), if antithyroid drug therapy has failed or is likely to fail to produce a lasting remission, or there have been sensitivity reactions to antithyroid drugs. Thus a thyrotoxic patient younger than 40 years with a large goitre should be treated by surgery rather than by a prolonged course of antithyroid drugs in the somewhat vain hope that the condition will remit in the interval and not recur when antithyroid drugs are withdrawn.

For a woman a thin thyroidectomy scar may be more acceptable cosmetically than a goitre. Men are thought to relapse more frequently after prolonged antithyroid drug therapy than are women and some authorities advocate surgery as the treatment of choice in men under the age of 40, irrespective of the size of the goitre. The patient may state a preference once the possibilities have been explained.

Preparation for thyroidectomy is either by propranolol in increasing dosage until beta-blockade has been achieved, or by carbimazole until euthyroid. In either event potassium iodide is given for 10–14 days before surgery in a dose of 60 mg twice daily. It makes the gland firmer and less vascular and the operation easier. The effects of potassium iodide are transitory so that it is important to reserve the drug for use in the circumstances described. Potassium iodide by itself should not be used to try and achieve a euthyroid state except in thyrotoxicosis crisis.

If propranolol is used substantially as preoperative preparation it is essential that tachycardia is controlled (by increasing the dose above 80 mg 4 times per day if necessary), that the dose on the morning of operation is not omitted and that propranolol is continued for 7 days after operation. Before surgery, evidence for adequate beta-blockade should be demonstrated on exercise tolerance. Some thyrotoxic patients are very resistant to beta-blockade by propranolol; the high doses of the drug in these subjects should be reduced immediately after surgery when the serum levels of T_4 and T_3 will drop rapidly. The advantages of propranolol preparation are greater flexibility in the timing of surgery, less blood loss and quicker permanent control of the thyrotoxicosis.

Some 80% of thyrotoxic patients treated by subtotoal thyroidectomy should have no complications at least within 3 to 5 years. In some 15% there will be either recurrence of the thyrotoxicosis or post-operative hypothyroidism requiring continuous thyroxine replacement therapy. The relative proportion of each depends on the amount of thyroid tissue left at operation. Thyrotoxic patients with high titres of thyroid complement fixing antibody in the serum before operation tend to have an appreciable degree of lymphocytic infiltration in the gland and tend to develop hypothyroidism post-operatively. While the majority of patients who become hypothyroid after surgery do so within the first 6 months or a year, there is a low but steady further incidence with each year after surgery making annual review of the patient desirable. Transient hypothyroidism may occur in the first few months following surgery, presumably due to the suppression of the hypothalamo-pituitary axis following a prolonged period of elevated serum T_4 and T_3 levels.

Damage to a recurrent laryngeal nerve occurs in a small percentage of patients and will produce temporary hoarseness with subsequent appreciable recovery as the other vocal cord compensates. The normal function of both vocal cords should be confirmed before surgery and checked after surgery.

The parathyroid glands may be rendered temporarily ischaemic by interruption of their blood supply or they may be inadvertently removed, producing transient or permanent hypoparathyroidism respectively. The late onset of hypoparathyroidism is a complication of partial thyroidectomy which should be looked for in the follow up of surgical patients, as cataract and mental disturbance may develop insidiously in the presence of persistent mild hypocalcaemia. On account of the high incidence of recurrent laryngeal nerve damage and of hypoparathyroidism following second operations, thyrotoxic patients who relapse after surgery should be treated with radioactive iodine.

RADIOACTIVE IODINE is the treatment of choice for thyrotoxic patients over the age of 40 years and also for younger patients who for some other reason appear to have a short life expectancy or who have been sterilised. It has no established complications other than hypothyroidism in the years following therapy. The incidence of thyroid cancer or leukaemia following ^{131}I therapy has been shown not to be increased. Although an effect on the spontaneous mutation of the gametes in the ovary or testis has not been proved it is difficult to disprove and therefore the administration of radioactive iodine to persons of reproductive age who have not been sterilised should be discouraged unless there is no suitable alternative.

The assessment of the appropriate therapeutic dose of [131]I (half-life 8 days) presents some difficulties for the following reasons. The amount of functional thyroid tissue is not easy to assess with accuracy, the amount of radiation to the gland following a given dose can be assessed only by time-consuming dynamic studies, and even if a predicted amount of radiation per gram of thyroid tissue could be given, there remains the variation in radiosensitivity among thyroid glands of different patients. For these reasons the empirical assessment of dosage using clinical criteria gives results as good as those dependent on sophisticated physical methods, provided that an avid uptake of the isotope by the gland has been established.

Using a dose as small as 5 mCi ^{131}I with a diffuse uptake of the isotope as shown on a scan in a small thyroid or as high as 15–30 mCi for a large multinodular gland, the patient's thyrotoxicosis will be controlled in some 70% of cases following a single oral administration. It may take 2 months or longer for the dose to be effective. If the thyrotoxicosis is severe, more rapid relief may be obtained by the addition of propranolol. Carbimazole should preferably not be given prior to the administration of ^{131}I as there is some evidence that it reduces the effective radiation dose by virtue of the enzyme block which it induces. When given after ^{131}I, carbimazole masks the effectiveness of the ^{131}I and makes the assessment of the need for a further dose of ^{131}I more difficult. The use of carbimazole in conjunction with ^{131}I should therefore be reserved for patients with cardiac failure or asthma, in whom propranolol is contraindicated.

After 2 months a further dose of ^{131}I should be given in the 30% who have not responded adequately to the first dose, using a 50 to 100% higher dose in order to avoid the undesirable occurrence in a few patients of the need for repeated doses of the isotope. Large doses of ^{131}I should be given to thyrotoxic patients in cardiac failure or atrial fibrillation to ensure prompt control of thyroid function with a single dose, even though this will produce a high incidence of hypothyroidism. The patient's thyroid state can then be stabilised by replacement doses of thyroxine.

Thyrotoxicosis associated with a solitary 'hot' nodule should be treated with a large dose of [131]I (if the patient is over 40 y.) or by excision of the nodule.

The continuing incidence of new cases of hypothyroidism for many years following radioactive iodine therapy makes regular review essential until such time as the patient has become hypothyroid and is on a suitable life-long replacement dose of thyroxine. The overall incidence of hypothyroidism may be of the order of 50% at seven years depending on the dosage of ^{131}I given. Transient hypothyroidism with low plasma TSH levels may occur in the first six months after ^{131}I therapy due to the suppression of TRH and TSH secretion consequent upon sustained elevated T_4 and/or T_3 levels before therapy. Subsequent to that a rise in the plasma TSH level is an early warning that hypothyroidism may develop with low serum T_4 levels.

THYROTOXIC CRISIS. The treatment of thyrotoxic crisis consists of intravenous fluid and glucose replacement; parenteral hydrocortisone on account of possible adrenocortical exhaustion; sedation and suppression of hyperpyrexia with chlorpromazine; digoxin for cardiac failure; propranolol if cardiac failure is not pronounced; intravenous potassium iodide 60 mg twice daily as the most rapidly acting antithyroid drug; and reduction of body temperature by tepid sponging. Antithyroid drugs such as carbimazole are administered as soon as the patient is capable of taking medicines orally. Precipitating causes must be dealt with, e.g. acute infection. Prevention and early recognition are essential if deaths are to be avoided.

HYPERTHYROIDISM IN CHILDREN AND IN PREGNANCY. As the results of thyroidectomy in children and young teenagers may be less satisfactory than in adults and as radioactive iodine therapy is contra-indicated in this age group, treatment should be with carbimazole or methimazole for as many years as is necessary.

In pregnancy hyperthyroidism may be treated with antithyroid drugs or by surgery provided the operation can be carried out in the middle trimester after appropriate preparation with antithyroid drugs and preoperative potassium iodide. If antithyroid drugs are used throughout it is important to give the smallest dose that will control the thyrotoxicosis and to use an index of thyroid function that is not altered by pregnancy (p. 429). Towards term, the dose of antithyroid drugs should be further reduced in the hope of withdrawing them for the last 3 weeks of pregnancy. In this way the uncommon complication of the fetus being born with a goitre may be avoided. If antithyroid drugs are to be continued after pregnancy the baby must not be breast fed. Radioactive iodine treatment should never be used for therapy in pregnancy. The baby should be checked for neo-natal thyrotoxicosis (p. 431).

Exophthalmos

Autoimmune mechanisms involving the extra-ocular muscles, the retro-orbital fat and connective tissue are thought to be important in the pathogenesis of endocrine exophthalmos (*Graves' ophthalmopathy*). Defined as the protrusion of one or both eyeballs, exophthalmos may be detected clinically in the majority of cases by observing the white sclera both above and below the iris. In other cases periorbital oedema, which is frequently also present, may obscure this sign. The degree of protrusion and especially any progression or regression of exophthalmos should be recorded by use of an exophthalmometer.

Exposure of the cornea as a consequence of the eyelids failing to close properly will result in keratitis producing a feeling of grit in the eye and excessive watering. The conjunctiva may become injected and oedematous (chemosis). Weakness of the extra-ocular muscles may give rise to an ophthalmoplegia with double vision, which is often first detected when the patient is asked to look upwards and outwards.

In some patients exophthalmos may precede the development of frank thyrotoxicosis and present a problem in differential diagnosis, especially if the exophthalmos is unilateral when orbital or retro-orbital tumours and infections may require consideration. CT scanning is particularly helpful in this context. Support for an endocrine aetiology may be obtained by eliciting a family history of thyroid disease or by demonstrating an abnormal TRH stimulation test or thyroid or gastric antibodies in the serum.

Treatment. In a small minority of cases the exophthalmos takes a relentlessly progressive course so that the increased intra-orbital pressure causes a severe aching in the eyes and reduction in visual acuity with papilloedema. Pressure within the orbit must be relieved urgently if permanent deterioration in vision is to be avoided. Decompression of the orbital cavity by surgical means may be required, but large doses of oral prednisolone together with cyclophosphamide and plasma exchange may obviate the need for surgery. Fortunately, in most cases exophthalmos is less severe; its progression ceases and there is a prolonged phase of gradual improvement although the eyes seldom return to the normal state.

In mild cases, chloromycetin eye drops and the wearing of slightly tinted spectacles with protective side pieces to the frames will prevent the irritation of glare, dust and wind. In more severe cases lateral tarsorrhaphy, stitching together the outer margins of the eyelids, may be all that is required, thereby improving their appearance and preventing exposure keratitis.

In relation to the treatment of thyrotoxicosis it is particularly important that hypothyroidism is avoided as this does seem to aggravate any associated exophthalmos.

HYPOTHYROIDISM

Hypothyroidism may be primary due to causes within the thyroid gland itself or, less commonly secondary, due to failure of TSH production following pituitary or hypothalamic disease. Hypothyroidism, especially when it is due to primary thyroid failure, is often, but not necessarily, associated with myxoedema, a thickening of the skin or other tissues by deposition of mucopolysaccharide giving the patient a characteristic appearance.

Incidence and Aetiology. Hypothyroidism commonly occurs as a sequel to ^{131}I therapy for thyrotoxicosis. Spontaneous primary hypothyroidism is much less common than thyrotoxicosis and principally affects middle-aged females, although it can occur in either sex at any age.

Spontaneous primary hypothyroidism may be associated with a goitre or with thyroid atrophy. The commonest cause of spontaneous goitrous hypothyroidism in an adult female is Hashimoto's thyroiditis. It is believed that Graves' disease, Hashimoto's thyroiditis and primary atrophic hypothyroidism belong to a continuous spectrum of disease. This is characterised by a common familial trait towards organ specific autoimmune disease and by the frequent occurrence in the serum of thyroid and gastric parietal cell antibodies. The natural history of Graves' disease in the absence of destructive forms of therapy is the incipient development of hypothyroidism over a period of one or several decades, a further indication that both belong to the same spectrum of autoimmune thyroid disease.

Less commonly hypothyroidism may be associated with other types of goitre, for example in dyshormonogenesis (p. 438). When hypothyroidism is secondary to pituitary insufficiency, myxoedema is unusual.

Clinical Features of Primary Hypothyroidism.

ADULTS. In contrast to thyrotoxicosis the symptoms are the result of decreased metabolism, with slowing of mental and physical activity. The onset is gradual and often mistaken for ageing alone. Often the patient is the last to complain and has to be persuaded by relatives or friends to seek medical help. Frequently, the general practitioner will recognise the condition on meeting the patient for some other reason, especially after a long interval.

On questioning, the patient may admit to sensitivity to cold, dryness of the skin, coarse and dry hair, constipation, gain in weight, tiredness, vague generalised pains, deafness, forgetfulness and disordered menstrual function. The patient may also complain of tingling in the fingers from compression of the median nerve in the carpal tunnel, although it is to be remembered that patients with primary spontaneous hypothyroidism are also predisposed to Addisonian pernicious anaemia which may give rise to similar symptoms from polyneuropathy. Anaemia may also be a direct result of thyroxine deficiency.

In an advanced case the face appears swollen with puffy eyelids, thick lips and an enlarged tongue. There is often a malar flush but elsewhere the skin is pale as a consequence of thickening with myxoedema. Sweating is conspicuously absent and the skin is dry and readily flakes on rubbing. The hair tends to be more sparse than normal and lustreless. Speech is slow, monotonous and husky or, in advanced instances, deep and croaky.

Characteristically the pulse rate is slow, but if the condition has progressed to cardiac failure, tachycardia may be found. The blood pressure in uncomplicated hypothyroidism is usually normal. However, since degenerative vascular disease is frequent in hypothyroidism, the patient may have systolic hypertension. Commonly there is evidence of coronary artery disease with angina pectoris or ECG changes of myocardial ischaemia. On radiological examination the heart is frequently seen to be enlarged; in some cases there may be a pericardial effusion which is usually reversible with treatment.

Marked slowing of the recovery phase of the ankle jerk due to delayed relaxation of the calf muscles is a useful clinical sign. Patients with severe hypothyroidism may show frank psychosis with hallucinations and delusions ('myxoedema madness') or pass into a state of coma. In a severe case, failure to control body temperature is one of the most lethal complications; mortality rises markedly as the body temperature (measured by a low reading rectal thermometer) falls below 32°C.

CHILDREN. While it is easy to detect the disease in its advanced state a high index of suspicion is required to avoid missing the early case and to prevent many years of unnecessary ill health. Hypothyroidism presents as a deterioration in performance at school, lack of interest in games and an arrest or slowing of growth. These features will precede the development of clinically obvious myxoedema. As in adults there may or may not be a goitre.

INFANTS. Failure of thyroid development is responsible for the condition of *cretinism*. The defects leading to failure of thyroid development may be genetic and may be inherited as autosomal recessives: in the heterozygous state the child may be goitrous only, but in the homozygous state both goitrous and a cretin. Cretinism also occurs in areas of endemic goitre.

It is important to diagnose the state and initiate thyroxine replacement therapy as early as possible. The development of the brain is dependent on the thyroid hormones so that delay in starting treatment will inevitably lead to permanent mental impairment which will be the more severe the longer the delay. The diagnostic features are failure to achieve the normal milestones of development, constipation, poor feeding and a characteristic cry. Only in advanced cases will the child develop the obvious features of cretinism, which include a coarse facies with a broad flat nose, thick lips and a large tongue protruding from the mouth, and a pot belly with umbilical hernia.

Investigation. The measurement of total serum T_4 should be combined with a plasma TSH measurement. If abnormalities of thyroxine binding proteins are suspected, a form of free thyroxine index should be used. The measurement of serum T_3 is not helpful in suspected hypothyroidism.

All patients with primary hypothyroidism have an elevated plasma TSH level but not all patients with an elevated plasma TSH necessarily have a significant degree of hypothyroidism. While a normal or low TSH level may be associated with secondary hypothyroidism due to pituitary or hypothalamic disease, a normal serum TSH level would exclude primary hypothyroidism. No purpose is achieved by doing TRH tests when an elevated plasma TSH has already been demonstrated but a TRH test may be helpful in deciding whether secondary hypothyroidism is due to pituitary or hypothalamic disease. Screening of neonates for elevated serum TSH levels facilitates the early diagnosis of cretinism.

Radiographs of the epiphyses in children, or of ossification centres in the wrist or heel in infants, will indicate whether the bone age is delayed relative to the chronolical age. Hypothyroidism in young people is invariably associated with impaired bone development; fragmentation of the epiphysis at the head of the femur is a striking radiological sign.

Treatment. In uncomplicated adult cases treatment with thyroxine should start with 0·05 mg/day increasing to 0·1 mg/day after 3 weeks provided cardiac failure or angina have not arisen. After a further 3–6 weeks the dose may be increased to 0·15–0·2 mg/day. This is the normal full replacement dose, but a few patients may require up to 0·3 mg thyroxine/day. Patients must understand that their well-being depends on continued treatment and must not stop thyroxine when they feel better. There is no advantage in divided doses or taking tablets that consist of a mixture of T_3 and T_4.

In a patient known to have ischaemic heart disease it will usually be desirable to keep the dose of thyroxine between 0·05 and 0·1 mg/day and to use a beta-adrenergic blocking agent such as propranolol. In patients with secondary hypothyroidism it is essential to treat any adrenocortical insufficiency before starting thyroxine.

Myxoedema Coma with Hypothermia. Small doses (10–20 μg) of triiodothyronine may be given intravenously 8 hourly together with hydrocortisone and glucose. The body temperature should be restored very slowly to a level of 32°C; above this level active warming should be abandoned in favour of heat conservation.

GOITRE

This term is applied to any enlargement of the thyroid gland and on clinical examination its size, shape, consistency, symmetry, irregularity of surface, mobility and the presence of a bruit should be established. The level of thyroid activity should be determined in the manner already described. Goitre associated with thyrotoxicosis will not be discussed further. The common diagnosis of simple goitre is arrived at by the exclusion of other causes, such as Hashimoto's thyroiditis, subacute thyroiditis, dyshormonogenesis, or carcinoma of the thyroid gland.

Hashimoto's thyroiditis is characteristically a firm diffuse enlargement of the thyroid gland with or without hypothyroidism. It may give rise to an aching discomfort in the neck and to mild dysphagia. It occurs must commonly in middle-aged women. Almost all cases have antibodies in the serum to thyroglobulin or to the microsomal fraction of thyroid cytoplasm, frequently in high titre. The ESR is often elevated. Histologically the gland consists of rather small thyroid vesicles with columnar epithelium showing a varying degree of eosinophilic granularity, infiltration by lymphocytes and plasma cells, sometimes with germinal centre formation and an increase in the fibrous tissue stroma.

In most instances there will be a satisfactory regression in the size of the goitre in response to thyroxine 0·2 mg/day, which can be hastened by giving 20 mg prednisolone 8-hourly for 10 days only. Adults with Hashimoto's thyroiditis should remain on life-long thyroxine therapy irrespective of whether or not they were initially hypothyroid. In adolescence, Hashimoto's thyroiditis may be transitory. In cases of diagnostic doubt a needle biopsy of the gland under local anaesthesia may be helpful. Partial thyroidectomy in such patients rapidly produces hypothyroidism if it did not already exist and is usually unnecessary.

Subacute (de Quervain's) thyroiditis is a painful condition generally associated with some thyroid enlargement. It is thought to be due to a viral infection of the thyroid (e.g. coxsackie B) and viral antibody studies are sometimes helpful diagnostically. Thyroid function is suppressed as indicated by a very low uptake of radioactive iodine or technetium by the gland and histologically the characteristic feature is the presence of giant cells. The ESR may be markedly elevated and thyroid antibody tests are generally negative. The condition tends to regress spontaneously but may be persistent.

Thyroxine 0·2–0·3 mg/day should be given to suppress TSH secretion and, in some cases, it may be necessary to give a course of oral corticosteroids. Surgery is seldom indicated even in the protracted case.

Dyshormonogenesis. The patient who has a partial enzyme defect related to one of the steps in the synthesis of thyroid hormones (Fig. 12.3) is likely to develop a goitre in response to continued TSH secretion induced by the low serum thyroxine. While all these defects are rare, the commonest and the easiest to detect is a genetically determined defect in the binding of iodine to tyrosine which, when associated with nerve deafness, is known as *Pendred's syndrome.*

Tumours of the Thyroid Gland. CARCINOMA is uncommon, forming about 1% of all cases of cancer in Britain. The tumours may be well differentiated papillary or follicular carcinomas (or a mixture of the two) or be anaplastic. Advanced cancers are obvious by their hardness, irregularity, adhesion to surrounding tissues and associated lymphadenopathy. Early carcinoma of the thyroid gland presents as a single nodule which almost invariably has poorer function than the surrounding normal thyroid tissue. If the nodule is sufficiently large it will be detectable as a 'cold' area on radioisotope scanning. It is not possible to distinguish clinically between a single nodule that is malignant and one that is benign; all single (solitary) nodules should therefore be removed for histological examination.

Well differentiated thyroid tumours should be treated by total thyroidectomy followed by life-long oral thyroxine 0·2–0·3 mg/day according to the patient's age. Rarely metastases from a well differentiated tumour may take up sufficient radioactive iodine, after all normally functioning thyroid tissue has been ablated by surgery and ^{131}I, to allow effective therapy with a further large dose of ^{131}I. Non-functioning secondaries can be treated by local radiotherapy. Anaplastic tumours may show a good initial response to radiotherapy, but invariably recur.

Medullary carcinoma of the thyroid arises from the parafollicular C-cells; although rare, it is of particular interest as it is associated with high levels of plasma calcitonin, prostaglandins or 5-hydroxytryptamine, causing symptoms such as flushing, borborygmi and diarrhoea. Patients with this form of thyroid cancer may have neuromas on the tongue, lips or eyelids, Marfanoid skeletal proportions (p. 198), and, occasionally, phaeochromocytomas.

Total thyroidectomy and removal of affected lymph nodes are required. The tumour is not very radiosensitive. It does not take up ^{131}I. Relapse can be detected by calcitonin assay.

BENIGN TUMOURS. Solitary 'cold' lesions in the thyroid may consist of adenomas or cysts; they can be differentiated by isotope scanning and ultrasonography. Calcification in cysts is common. Cysts without an admixture of solid constituents may be aspirated and the fluid sent for cytology. Haemorrhage occasionally occurs into adenomas and for this reason, in addition to the risk of malignancy, their removal is justified.

Simple goitre may occur sporadically, but in certain parts of the world it is found more frequently and is then referred to as endemic goitre (p. 62).

The aetiology is believed to be closely related to iodine deficiency, mainly in the diet. Less commonly factors in the diet or water such as excess calcium may interfere with iodine absorption; goitrogens in the diet may prevent concentration of iodine by the thyroid. Apart from the antithyroid drugs, prolonged treatment with lithium or sulphonamides may produce a goitre. Iodides taken persistently in large doses in the form of cough mixtures or 'asthma cures' may likewise cause a goitre. In each of these examples the secretion or release of thyroid hormones is suppressed and presumably the goitre results from continuing increased secretion of TSH. An intermittent shortage in supply of iodine to the gland over prolonged periods is thought to result in the multinodular character of long-standing goitres.

A small, soft diffuse, simple goitre may occur at puberty or during pregnancy and may regress spontaneously thereafter, but in other cases it persists. If already present, it may enlarge further at these times. A simple goitre of long standing may achieve considerable size, become grossly nodular and gives rise to obstructive symptoms, particularly if there is a retrosternal extension. Deviation of the trachea may be noted clinically or radiologically and obstruction in the thoracic inlet may lead to venous engorgement of the head and neck. Bruits and thrills do not occur in simple goitres. Cretinism (p. 436) is associated with endemic goitre in areas where iodine deficiency is severe.

The treatment of sporadic simple diffuse goitre at puberty should be with thyroxine for 1 to 2 years and not potassium iodide. An adequate dietary intake of iodine should be ensured. Multinodular simple goitres are unlikely to respond to thyroxine and may require partial thyroidectomy for cosmetic reasons, or if obstructive symptoms are present or likely to occur. Postoperative lifelong treatment with thyroxine may prevent a recurrence, although hypothyroidism after partial thyroidectomy for simple goitre is uncommon.

An adequate intake of iodine, particularly in the early years of life, is the only really satisfactory way of preventing sporadic simple goitre. The incidence of endemic goitre can be greatly reduced by correcting iodine deficiency, for example, by legislation that ensures that table salt contains traces of iodine (p. 62).

Calcitonin

The parafollicular cells (C-cells) of the thyroid gland secrete a polypeptide hormone, calcitonin, apparently unrelated to the other functions of this gland. When administered by injection, the hormone lowers the serum calcium concentration. Its main effect on bone is to inhibit resorption, so that in these two important respects it could be regarded as a physiological antagonist of parathyroid hormone. It is secreted in very large quantities by medullary carcinomas of the thyroid gland, without however producing significant hypocalcaemia, and after complete removal of the source of the hormone, namely the thyroid gland, hypercalcaemia is not a feature.

Therapeutically, the hormone has been used to reduce hypercalcaemia, but corticosteroids may be more effective in doing so in sarcoidosis, vitamin D intoxication and in metastatic malignant disease in bone. In Paget's disease calcitonin relieves pain in the minority of patients in whom pain is a dominant feature (p. 587).

THE PARATHYROID GLANDS

Anatomy and Physiology. These glands, usually four in number, each measure about 5 mm in diameter. Their relation to the thyroid gland is described on page 428. The parathyroid glands control the concentration of calcium and inorganic phosphorus in the blood, both by enhancing the removal of mineral from the skeleton, and by promoting the excretion of phosphorus by the kidney.

Calcium occurs in plasma in two forms, 'diffusible' and 'non-diffusible'. The former consists of ionised calcium, and a small amount of non-ionised calcium salts of organic acids. From the point of view of neuromuscular function and the occurrence of tetany, as well as the secretion of parathyroid hormone, it is the ionised plasma calcium concentration which is important. The non-diffusible fraction is that portion which is bound to the plasma albumin; if the latter is very low, the total plasma calcium might be 2·0 mmol/l (8 mg/100 ml) or less and yet the ionised calcium could be normal. Conversely when the plasma albumin concentration is high, the plasma calcium might be 3·0 mmol/l or even more but the ionised calcium remains in the normal range.

In addition to parathyroid hormone, calcitonin and vitamin D metabolites also affect the metabolism of calcium and phosphorus, and must be considered in disorders of these elements. Assays of parathyroid hormone (PTH) are becoming more widely available but many still have considerable overlap between the normal range and hyperparathyroidism. In such cases a 'normal' PTH value is often said to be abnormal or inappropriate for the high plasma calcium. Controversy continues regarding the reliability and relevance of calcitonin assays, except in the diagnosis of medullary carcinoma of the thyroid gland.

HYPERPARATHYROIDISM

Primary hyperparathyroidism is usually due to a single parathyroid adenoma. Very occasionally it may be caused by simple hyperplasia or multiple adenomas: a functioning parathyroid carcinoma can also occur.

Secondary hyperparathyroidism is due to hypertrophy of the glands and is found in chronic renal failure which causes hypocalcaemia followed by an increase in parathyroid activity. Secondary hyperparathyroidism also occurs as a sequel to osteomalacia, malabsorption or rickets.

Tertiary hyperparathyroidism is used to describe the cases of the secondary variety of long standing in which a continuing stimulus is responsible for parathyroid hyperplasia being replaced by autonomous function in one or more parathyroid adenomas.

Osteitis fibrosa or *von Recklinghausen's disease of bone* occurs in the rare event of hyperparathyroidism involving the bones to such an extent that cyst formation occurs. Such patients usually have vitamin D deficiency and the bone lesions can be healed by vitamin D therapy.

Clinical Features. Mild, asymptomatic hyperparathyroidism is not uncommon, particularly after middle age. Patients with more severe hypercalcaemia frequently complain of weakness, loss of appetite, nausea, vomiting, drowsiness or confusion. Some of these patients also have a peptic ulcer, the symptoms from which may obscure those of hyperparathyroidism. Acute pancreatitis is sometimes a presenting feature. When bone involvement is marked, backache is a common complaint. Pseudo-gout (p. 581) may occur as can hypertension. Constipation can also be a prominent feature.

Renal calculi frequently form in association with the increased excretion of calcium in the urine. While many patients with hyperparathyroidism develop symptoms due to renal calculi, relatively few presenting with renal calculi owe their disorder to increased parathyroid activity. In other cases of hyperparathyroidism deposits of calcium form in and around the renal tubular epithelium (nephrocalcinosis p. 403). Tubular reabsorption of water may be impaired as a consequence or from the direct effects of parathyroid hormone. Polyuria and thirst may be sufficiently severe to suggest diabetes insipidus. In cases of long standing, and in those with associated pyelonephritis, the renal disease may progress to uraemia in spite of the relief of the hyperparathyroidism.

Physical examination is usually unhelpful. Occasionally a parathyroid adenoma is sufficiently large and suitably placed to be palpable or even visible as a swelling in the region of the thyroid gland. Calcification may be present at the corneoscleral junction or in the conjunctiva, seen more readily with a slit-lamp.

A parathyroid adenoma may coexist with secreting adenomas or hyperplasia in the pituitary, pancreas or adrenals. This type of association is known as *multiple endocrine adenomatosis* (or neoplasia) and may cause unusual manifestations.

Investigation. *Hypercalcaemia and Related Findings.* Hypercalcaemia is the most significant chemical finding. The fasting plasma calcium may be considerably increased above the upper limit of normal (2·62 mmol/l). It may be necessary to carry out estimations at intervals in doubtful cases, since hypercalcaemia may be episodic. A tourniquet should not be used in obtaining samples since this may be responsible for raising the plasma calcium. If the plasma albumin is low the value for the plasma calcium should be adjusted upwards.

Causes of hypercalcaemia other than hyperparathyroidism include metastatic malignant disease of bone and cancer, without bone secondaries, producing a PTH-like polypeptide. Less common causes are sarcoidosis, myelomatosis, overdosage with vitamin D, hyperthyroidism, and immobilisation especially in patients with increased bone turnover as in Paget's disease.

The plasma inorganic phosphate is usually lowered in hyperparathyroidism. The plasma alkaline phosphatase, an index of osteoblastic activity, may be raised (p. 817) depending on the degree of involvement of bone.

Radiological Examination. In the early stages there may be demineralisation or subperiosteal erosions may be noted in the phalanges. These are most marked on the radial side of the middle phalanx. There may also be absorption of the terminal phalanges. A 'pepper-pot' appearance may be seen in lateral radiographs of the skull. Cystic changes are rare. In nephrocalcinosis scattered opacities may be visible within the renal outline. There may be soft tissue calcification elsewhere. Ultrasonography and occasionally arteriography can be helpful in locating the site of an adenoma.

Parathyroid Hormone Radioimmunoassay. As discussed, an inappropriately high plasma PTH, even within the normal range, in the presence of hypercalcaemia, is indicative of hyperparathyroidism. Such assays may also be helpful in localising small tumours by identifying high concentrations of parathyroid hormone in specific veins in the root of the neck or mediastinum.

Treatment. Removal of a solitary adenoma is usually sufficient to produce clinical cure, provided advanced renal disease is not already present. Patients with multiple adenomas or generalised hyperplasia of all the parathyroids may be difficult to manage, especially when the glands lie in unusual situations such as the superior mediastinum, but surgical treatment offers the only prospect of cure.

The current management of hyperplasia is to remove all four glands and to transplant some of this tissue to the forearm. If hypercalcaemia returns then part of the transplant can be excised under local anaesthetic. Patients with bone involvement may, following removal of the tumour, show the 'hungry bones' syndrome characterised by tetany and magnesium depletion. It is not certain whether people, especially the elderly, with mild symptomless hypercalcaemia come to any harm from the continued presence of a parathyroid tumour.

Some patients with severe primary hyperparathyroidism may present as a medical emergency with hypercalcaemia. Adequate rehydration is an essential first step in management. Such patients often have a fluid deficit of several litres and when this has been replaced plasma calcium will usually fall to a level where surgery can be considered. Saline administration produces a calcium diuresis but care must be taken not to overload the circulation. Intravenous phosphate used to be given to lower calcium but has the danger of producing ectopic calcification. Oral phosphate is safer. Calcitonin is of little value in the treatment of hyperparathyroidism.

HYPOPARATHYROIDISM

This unusual condition may arise from a variety of causes, but with each the clinical feature in common is tetany. Biochemically, a depressed concentration of calcium and a raised concentration of phosphate in plasma are characteristic.

Postoperative Hypoparathyroidism. A transitory form of the disorder is common after a partial thyroidectomy, presumably due to interference with the blood supply of the parathyroid glands. After a complete thyroidectomy permanent hypoparathyroidism may occur. Hypoparathyroidism may be transient following removal of a hyperfunctioning parathyroid adenoma, the other three parathyroid glands having been suppressed by the high calcium levels.

Infantile hypoparathyroidism may be transient and associated with maternal hyperparathyroidism or calcium deficiency, or it may be associated with thymic aplasia (Di George syndrome, p. 34).

Idiopathic hypoparathyroidism may develop at any age, and is sometimes associated with autoimmune disease of the adrenal, thyroid or ovary especially in young people. In addition to tetany other features include psychoses, cataracts, aberrant calcification and moniliasis, particularly of the finger nails.

Pseudohypoparathyroidism is the term applied to a congenital variety, which may be familial. There appear to be two main types of this condition. In one PTH fails to produce an increase in urinary cyclic AMP. In the other there is a cyclic AMP rise but this does not exert its usual phosphaturic effect.

Pseudohypoparathyroidism presents with the biochemical features of hypoparathyroidism, and in addition aberrant calcification, cataracts, mental retardation and skeletal abnormalities, for example small, stocky stature and short 4th and 5th metacarpals. These patients are resistant to the action of administered parathyroid hormone; their own parathyroid glands appear to be normal histologically, plasma parathyroid hormone levels are raised, and high concentrations of calcitonin have been found in their circulation and in their thyroid glands.

Treatment. Commercial preparations of parathyroid hormone available for the treatment of parathyroid insufficiency are unsatisfactory because they have to be given by frequent injections, and soon become ineffective because of antibody formation. In the acute phase, calcium is given intravenously as for tetany; substitution therapy for persistent hypoparathyroidism and for pseudoparathyroidism is provided by calciferol. In some patients it is difficult to control the serum calcium. These can usually be successfully treated with $1,25\text{-}(OH)_2D_3$ in doses ranging from 0.25-1 μg/day or with 1-2 μg/day of 1α OH-D_3 (p. 67).

Tetany

Aetiology. There is an increased excitability of peripheral nerves due either to a low plasma calcium concentration or to alkalosis in which the proportion of the plasma calcium in the ionised form is decreased, although the total calcium concentration remains unaltered. Magnesium depletion should also be considered as a possible contributing factor, particularly in the malabsorption syndrome.

CAUSES OF DEPLETION OF PLASMA CALCIUM. (1) *Inadequate Intake or Absorption of Calcium.* This occurs in rickets, osteomalacia and the malabsorption syndrome. (2) *Hypoparathyroidism.* (3) *Chronic renal failure* where, although the plasma calcium is often low, coincident acidosis usually prevents tetany. (4) *Pancreatitis* may also be associated with hypocalcaemia.

CAUSES OF ALKALOSIS. (1) *Repeated vomiting* of acid gastric juice, as in gastric outlet obstruction from peptic ulceration. (2) *Excessive quantities of absorbable alkalis* given by mouth especially when associated with repeated vomiting. (3) *Hyperventilation*, commonly due to hysteria, lowers the arterial Pco_2. (4) *Primary aldosteronism* (p. 446).

Clinical Features. In *children* a characteristic triad of carpopedal spasm, stridor (laryngismus stridulus) and convulsions may occur, though one or more of these may be found independently of the others. The hands in carpal spasm adopt a characteristic position. The metacarpophalangeal joints are flexed, the interphalangeal joints of the fingers and thumb are extended and there is opposition of the thumb (*main d'accoucheur*). Pedal spasm is much less frequent. Stridor is caused by spasm of the glottis.

Adults complain of tingling in the hands, feet and around the mouth. Less often there is painful carpopedal spasm while stridor and fits are rare.

Latent tetany may be present when signs of overt tetany are lacking. It is best recognised by eliciting *Trousseau's sign*. Inflation of the sphygmomanometer cuff on the upper arm to more than the systolic blood pressure is followed by characteristic spasm in the forearm muscles within 4 minutes. A less specific sign of hypocalcaemia is that described by *Chvostek* in which tapping over the branches of the facial nerve as they emerge from the parotid gland produces twitching of the facial muscles.

Treatment. *Control of Tetany.* Injection of 20 ml of a 10% solution of calcium gluconate slowly into a vein will raise the plasma calcium concentration immediately. An intramuscular injection of 10 ml may also be given to obtain a more prolonged effect. In severe cases of alkalotic tetany, intravenous calcium gluconate often relieves the spasm, while more radical treatment of the alkalosis, which will vary with the cause, is being applied. If tetany is not relieved by giving calcium the administration of magnesium may be required.

Correction of Alkalosis. 1. In persistent vomiting, intravenous isotonic saline is the most effective treatment.

2. When alkalis have been given to excess their withdrawal may suffice to stop the tetany, but if not, ammonium chloride 2 g should be given 4-hourly by mouth until relief has been obtained.

3. The inhalation of 5% carbon dioxide in oxygen may be prescribed for the correction of the alkalosis of hyperventilation, or more simply, the patient should be made to rebreathe expired air from a suitable bag. The hysterical patient should also be treated by appropriate psychotherapy (p. 689).

Treatment of the Underlying Condition. When tetany follows removal of a parathyroid gland and if there is any residual parathyroid tissue, this usually undergoes compensatory hypertrophy. In the interval intravenous calcium gluconate may be required to control the tetany. If all the parathyroid tissue has been removed, prolonged replacement therapy with calciferol is commonly used to maintain a normal plasma calcium concentration. One tablet (1·25 mg) daily is usually adequate, but less, or more, may be required. The maintenance dose is determined by careful monitoring of the plasma calcium at intervals, as persistent hypercalcaemia which might follow prolonged high doses of vitamin D would lead to widespread metastatic calcification and rapidly progressive renal failure.

In chronic renal failure with hypocalcaemia the logical treatment is with either $1,25\text{-}(OH)_2D_3$ or $1\alpha\text{-}OH\text{-}D_3$ (p. 394).

Treatment may also be required for rickets (p. 68), osteomalacia (p. 70) or malabsorption (p. 313).

THE ADRENAL GLANDS

Anatomy and Physiology. The adrenal glands lie in relation to the upper poles of the kidneys. Each consists of an inner medulla which secretes adrenaline and noradrenaline and an outer cortex of three layers. These, from without inwards, are the zona glomerulosa, zona fasciculata and zona reticularis. Although over 40 steroid compounds have been extracted from the adrenal cortex, the principal hormones are cortisol, (glucocorticoid), aldosterone (mineralocorticoid) and androstenedione, androsterone and dehydroepiandrosterone (androgens).

Adrenocorticotrophic hormone (ACTH) is the only substance so far recognised that will alter the rate of biosynthesis and secretion of the glucocorticoid cortisol from the zona fasciculata and reticularis. ACTH also increases the secretion of the adrenal androgens. Aldosterone secretion by the zona glomerulosa is primarily controlled by the renin-angiotensin mechanisms (p. 379) and is not markedly affected by physiological alterations in ACTH levels.

Three major mechanisms appear to control ACTH release and thus cortisol secretion, namely, negative feedback, diurnal (circadian) rhythm and stress.

The negative feedback mechanism is thought to operate via the hypothalamus rather then directly on the pituitary but there is still uncertainty about this. Reduction in the level of plasma cortisol leads to an increased secretion of ACTH from the basophil cells of the anterior pituitary, probably effected by increased release of CRF from the hypothalamus. Conversely, a rise in plasma cortisol produces a rapid suppression of the secretion of ACTH. Cortisol secretion is thus presumably determined at the hypothalamic level, controlled by an inherent diurnal rhythmicity of CRF secretion and consequently of ACTH release. The normal range of plasma cortisol levels in an unstressed subject would be 220–720 nmol/l (8–26 μg/100 ml) at 0800 to 1000 h and less than 275 nmol/l (10 μg/100 ml) at 2200 to 2400 h.

Stress such as trauma, pain, apprehension, nausea, fever and hypoglycaemia can override the negative feedback mechanism and the diurnal rhythm.

It is from an understanding of the normal physiological mechanisms involved in adrenocortical hormone secretion that procedures have been developed to test various components of the hypothalamo-pituitary-adrenal axis and so determine the site of the lesion in cases of adreno-cortical over- or underactivity.

The glucocorticoids have effects which are antagonistic to insulin, tending to raise the blood sugar by converting amino acids derived from protein breakdown into glucose (gluconeogenesis). Glucocorticoids such as cortisol have other important actions including the suppression of inflammatory reactions which may occur in response to injury, infection or immunological mechanisms. Glucocorticoids are also lipogenic and have some mineralocorticoid effects especially when used in pharmacological doses.

Aldosterone produces retention of sodium and increased excretion of potassium and if given in pharmacological doses over a prolonged period also causes hypertension. Weight for weight, aldosterone has far greater mineralocorticoid activity than the glucocorticoids.

In addition to androgens, the adrenal cortex also synthesises oestrogen and progesterone in small quantities in both sexes. The nitrogen-retaining (anabolic) activity of the androgenic hormones is antagonistic to the catabolic effect of the glucocorticoids.

HYPERFUNCTION OF THE ADRENAL GLAND

Cushing's Syndrome. This can be defined as the symptoms and signs associated with prolonged exposure to inappropriately elevated plasma corticosteroid levels. The patients may be divided into two main groups depending on whether or not the condition derives from exposure to excessive ACTH.

1   ACTH dependent causes of Cushing's syndrome:

(i) Iatrogenic — administration of excessive quantities of ACTH or its synthetic analogues.

(ii) Pituitary-dependent bilateral adrenocortical hyperplasia, conventionally called *Cushing's disease*.

(iii) The ectopic ACTH syndrome — secretion of ACTH by malignant or benign tumours of non-endocrine origin.

2   Non-ACTH dependent causes of Cushing's syndrome:

(i) Iatrogenic — administration of supra-physiological doses of corticosteroids.

(ii) Adenomas or carcinomas of the adrenal cortex.

Cushing's syndrome associated with pituitary-dependent adrenocortical hyperplasia and adrenal tumours is four times more common in women than in men with a peak age incidence between 35 and 50 years. This contrasts with the male predominance and later age incidence found in Cushing's syndrome secondary to the ectopic production of ACTH by non-endocrine tumours, commonly carcinoma of the bronchus.

Clinical Features of Cushing's Disease. These can be interpreted largely in terms of the action of the glucocorticoids. Thus the gluconeogenic effect is seen as an elevation of the blood glucose level and glycosuria; a proportion of patients develop diabetes. The effect on the blood sugar is however not invariable because of other mechanisms that counteract any disturbance in carbohydrate metabolism, such as insulin secretion. The breakdown of protein to form glucose is reflected in the reduction of muscle, bone and connective tissue, leading to weakness, proximal myopathy, osteoporosis, easy bruising and purple striae of the skin over the abdomen, buttocks and thighs. Osteoporosis may be sufficiently severe to produce backache; radiological changes in the vertebral bodies may progress to collapse, kyphosis and shortening of stature.

The most striking features of Cushing's disease are the rounded plethoric appearance (moon face), central obesity and 'buffalo hump' (accumulation of fat at the lower part of the back of the neck) due to redistribution of body fat. There is also arterial hypertension caused by sodium retention. The loss of potassium may contribute to muscular weakness. The overproduction of adrenal androgens may lead to the development of hirsutism and acne in some patients with perhaps temporal recession of hair in females. Amenorrhoea or other disorders of menstrual function are common. Mental symptoms, in particular depression, may be prominent.

The pituitary gland in Cushing's disease is seldom grossly enlarged either in the presence of hyperplasia or of an adenoma of the basophil or chomophobe cells. Although some enlargement may be detectable on a radiograph of the pituitary fossa, usually no abnormality can be seen. Expansion of the pituitary fossa and pressure on the optic chiasma may occur due to an adenoma in Nelson's syndrome (p. 423).

In the case of an adrenocortical tumour affecting the zona fasciculata/reticularis, the clinical features will depend on the type of steroid that the tumour is synthesising. If the tumour is making glucocorticoids almost exclusively the clinical features will be indistinguishable from Cushing's disease, whereas if the tumour is making androgens predominantly the female patient will be virilised, with pronounced hirsutism, deepening of the voice, recession of the hair on the forehead, acne and clitoral enlargement, possibly with increased libido.

In males an adrenal tumour may induce feminisation, e.g. gynaecomastia, if the tumour is mainly making oestrogens.

Although many adrenocortical adenomas are benign, functional carcinomas also occur with metastases to other organs.

When Cushing's syndrome is due to the production of ectopic ACTH the striking features are the rapid development of brown pigmentation due to the very high plasma levels of ACTH and LPH (p. 419). Frequently such patients show a marked alkalosis and potassium depletion. Characteristically they do not appear Cushingoid (moon face and central obesity) presumably because of the short survival time of the underlying malignant process.

Differential Diagnosis. The main differential diagnosis of Cushing's disease or syndrome is simple obesity and simple hirsutism, especially when either is associated with mild hypertension and menstrual irregularity or when both coexist. Functional ovarian tumours may give a similar clinical picture. It can sometimes be difficult to decide when to investigate and when to exclude the possibility of Cushing's disease or syndrome on clinical grounds alone. Overactivity of the adrenal cortex is comparatively rare while simple obesity, hirsutism, menstrual irregularities and hypertension are common.

Investigation of Suspected Overactivity of the Zona Fasciculata/Reticularis. Specific radioimmunoassay (RIA) techniques for measuring serum cortisol have replaced the relatively non-specific fluorimetric method. Disordered function of the zona fasciculata/reticularis is almost invariably reflected in an alteration of the normal diurnal rhythm of cortisol secretion with high levels of serum cortisol in the evening. However, the demonstration of such an abnormality does not establish the diagnosis since stress, obesity, depression or hypertension may produce similar findings.

In subjects with normal adrenocortical function the secretion of cortisol should be readily suppressible with biologically active analogues of cortisol such as dexamethasone. These substances do not contribute to the measurement of endogenous serum cortisol by RIA. Normal subjects and patients suffering from simple obesity or from hypertension due to causes other than Cushing's syndrome will show suppression of cortisol secretion following 0·5 mg oral dexamethasone 6-hourly for 48 hours. The majority of patients with Cushing's disease will show significant suppression following 2·0 mg dexamethasone 6-hourly for 48 hours, while most patients with adrenal tumours and the ectopic ACTH syndrome will fail to do so at this dosage. A useful screening test that can be done as an outpatient by taking 2·0 mg dexamethasone orally at 2300 h and reporting to the clinic at 0900 h on the following morning when the serum cortisol is measured. In normal individuals and in simple obesity the normal morning rise in serum cortisol is suppressed, i.e. serum cortisol less than 170 nmol/*l*.

The estimation of urinary free cortisol either in a 24 hour urine sample or the measurement of the free cortisol:creatinine ratio in a single early-morning sample of urine may be useful in distinguishing between Cushing's syndrome and simple obesity.

The response in the serum cortisol levels following insulin hypoglycaemia is helpful in distinguishing between patients with true Cushing's syndrome (they show no response) and those who are stressed or severely depressed and who might show loss of diurnal rhythm and resistance to dexamethasone suppression (they show a normal response).

When abnormal production of adrenal androgens is suspected, specific steroid measurements by RIA are to be preferred to the measurement of urinary 17-oxosteroids. Examples are the measurement of dehydroepiandrosterone in suspected adrenocortical carcinoma, or measurement of cortisol, ACTH and 17 α-hydroxyprogesterone in congenital adrenal hyperplasia due to C21-hydroxylase deficiency (p. 449).

Once a diagnosis of excess activity of the zona fasciculata/reticularis has been made, some indication of the cause may be obtained by radio-immunoassay of the plasma ACTH concentration. Moderately elevated levels are seen in Cushing's disease, low or undetectable levels occur in adrenal adenoma and strikingly high levels are found in the ectopic ACTH syndrome. Computed tomography of the abdomen and chest is the technique of choice to show the adrenal anatomy and to locate a suspected ectopic ACTH secreting tumour in patients with proven Cushing's syndrome, especially small (< 1.5 cm) lung carcinoma. Adrenal tumours may also be localised by venography, which should be combined with adrenal vein sampling for estimation of the serum cortisol. Both glands should be studied as 10% of adenomas are bilateral.

Treatment of Overactivity of the Zona Fasciculata/Reticularis. This clearly depends on establishing the cause. The adrenal which is the site of an adenoma or carcinoma should be excised. In the case of the ectopic ACTH syndrome the primary tumour should be removed but unfortunately this is rarely possible. Transitory improvement may be achieved by using metyrapone (which inhibits the enzyme 11-beta-hydroxylase that is involved in the final step in the synthesis of cortisol), aminoglutethimide or trilostane to block cortisol synthesis together with appropriate electrolyte replacement with particular reference to potassium.

In relation to the more common Cushing's disease opinions vary as to the best management. Until recently the most usual form of treatment was bilateral adrenalectomy preceded by the control of adrenocortical function with metyrapone and followed by replacement steroid therapy.

Nelson's syndrome (p. 423) may be a later postoperative complication; this can be prevented either by giving external irradiation to the pituitary at the time of bilateral adrenalectomy or should there be evidence of rising plasma ACTH levels in excess of 1000 pg/ml after the operation.

External irradiation to the pituitary as the sole form of treatment is another possibility but, as in the case of excess GH and PRL secretion, its effect is slow and somewhat unpredictable in the individual patient. In experienced hands transsphenoidal microsurgery may achieve the selective removal of the pituitary microadenoma present in the majority of patients with Cushing's disease (p. 421) without significantly compromising the remaining normal pituitary tissue.

Hyperaldosteronism (Overactivity of the Zona Glomerulosa)

Hypersecretion of aldosterone may be primary in origin or secondary to some other pathological process.

In *primary hyperaldosteronism*, usually associated with an adenoma and known as *Conn's syndrome*, the most consistent symptom is weakness, often episodic, and attributable to potassium deficiency. Polyuria and polydipsia, also due to the effects of potassium depletion and impaired renal tubular reabsorption of water, commonly occur. Tetany may be an occasional presenting symptom precipitated by the metabolic alkalosis associated with potassium depletion. The blood pressure is usually raised and the condition may be mistaken for essential hypertension, or for myasthenia gravis because of the weakness. Oedema is most unusual although its presence might be anticipated from the sodium retaining effect of aldosterone. Primary aldosteronism should be treated by removal of the affected gland or if this is not possible, spironolactone should be given.

Secondary hyperaldosteronism occurs in cirrhosis of the liver with ascites, in the nephrotic syndrome and less consistently in severe cardiac failure (p. 151). Potassium depletion may not be detected in the plasma and hypertension is less likely to occur; oedema is usual from hypoalbuminaemia or heart failure. The use of spironolactone in the management of these conditions is discussed on page 97. Secondary aldosteronism may also occur in patients with unilateral renal ischaemia due to renal artery stenosis, a form which can occasionally be cured by surgery.

Plasma renin and plasma and urinary aldosterone assays are used in assessing overactivity of the zona glomerulosa.

INSUFFICIENCY OF THE ADRENAL CORTEX

Inadequate secretion of the adrenocortical hormones may be primary from acquired disease of the adrenals (Addison's disease) or because of congenital deficiency of the enzymes required for the synthesis of adrenocortical hormones (congenital adrenal hyperplasia). It may be secondary to failure of ACTH secretion due to pituitary or hypothalamic disorders (Fig. 12.4).

Addison's Disease

Autoimmune adrenal failure and, much less commonly, tuberculous destruction of the adrenals are the main causes of Addison's disease in the developed countries, while other causes such as those listed in Figure 12.4 are rare.

Autoimmune adrenal failure (previously referred to as 'idiopathic' or 'simple' atrophy)

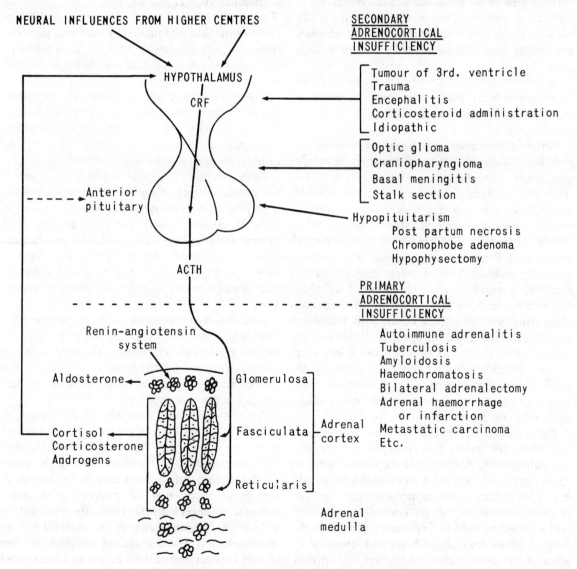

Fig. 12.4 Causes of primary and secondary adrenocortical insufficiency.

affects females twice as frequently as males and may occur at any age. It is characterised by adrenocortical antibodies in the serum, by cell mediated hypersensitivity to adrenocortical antigens, the presence of HLA-B8 and HLA-DR3 and by a high incidence of other organ-specific autoimmune diseases such as thyrotoxicosis, Hashimoto's thyroiditis, primary atrophic hypothyroidism, pernicious anaemia, premature ovarian failure, idiopathic hypoparathyroidism and also insulin dependent (Type I) diabetes. Histologically both adrenals show atrophy of the cortical cells in all three zones with lymphocytic infiltration and increase in fibrous tissue. The medulla is not significantly affected. The adrenals are usually smaller than normal and appear atrophic.

In tuberculous destruction of the adrenal there is caseation with giant cells, and calcification which may be detected radiologically in long-standing cases.

Clinical Features. The onset of adrenal insufficiency may be acute or chronic, or more commonly acute following upon chronic. The main clinical features or chronic primary adrenal insufficiency are weakness, weight loss, hyperpigmentation or vitiligo, hypotension and gastrointestinal disorders. The invariable symptoms of tiredness and malaise, both physical and mental, gradually increase. Loss of weight does not occur until the adrenal failure is well advanced and then it is invariable. Anorexia, nausea and constipation alternating with diarrhoea occur with increased frequency as the disease progresses. Eventually in adrenal crisis the gastrointestinal complaints may be the outstanding feature and an erroneous diagnosis of severe gastroenteritis may be made; pain may simulate an acute abdomen. A wrong diagnosis may cost the patient his or her life.

Pigmentation of the skin is often the clinical sign that first raises the suspicion of primary hypoadrenalism. A history of its recent onset is more significant than pigmentation of long standing. This feature is due to increased melanin and is most obvious in regions normally pigmented and exposed to light or pressure, e.g. face, neck, back of hands, knuckles, elbows and knees, or in areas of the body subject to friction and in skin creases, particularly in the palms. The mucous membranes of the mouth, the conjuctivae and the vagina may also become pigmented. Scars that have been present before the onset of primary adrenal failure remain unpigmented in contrast to those that are acquired after the onset of adrenal failure. Pigmentation may precede the other features of hypoadrenalism by many years. It often manifests itself initially by the patient acquiring a much better suntan than usual and the tan taking longer to disappear. The progressive pigmentation is due to increased secretion of LPH (p. 419) by the pituitary which occurs simultaneously with augmented ACTH release and to ACTH itself (Fig. 12.2). Vitiligo, patchy areas of depigmentation of the skin surrounded by increased pigmentation, occurs in 10 to 20% of patients with Addison's disease, particularly in dark-skinned races.

The patient may give a history of very slow recovery from an illness or operation, having escaped an acute crisis at such a time. Likewise, there may be a history of extreme sensitivity to drugs such as morphine or pethidine.

Hypotension is almost invariable whether the patient is erect or supine. It is uncommon for a patient with primary adrenocortical failure to have a systolic blood pressure greater than 110 mmHg before appropriate replacement therapy is started. Normal reflex maintenance of the blood pressure is impaired and dizziness and syncope may result from postural hypotension.

Reactive hypoglycaemia after a carbohydrate meal may occur, cortisol being one of the physiological antagonists of insulin. Hypoglycaemia is usually manifest by tiredness and lethargy, the patient having more than usual difficulty in getting up in the morning.

Loss of body hair, especially in the female, is occasionally found but is generally not so marked as in hypopituitarism. Menstrual disorders, usually amenorrhoea, are common during the onset of the disease before treatment is instituted. A significant proportion of patients with autoimmune Addison's disease suffer from premature failure of ovarian function on account of an immunological reaction against antigens that are shared between the adrenal cortex and the steroid producing cells of the ovary.

Secondary Adrenal Insuffciency

The secretion of ACTH and TSH is more resistant to pituitary damage than is the secretion of the gonadotrophins or growth hormone, so that patients with adrenal insufficiency secondary to organic pituitary disease generally show clinical features of impaired gonadotrophin secretion or of growth hormone secretion if the patient is of appropriate age for such manifestations. There is usually marked loss of axillary and pubic hair and the skin is fine provided hypothyroidism is not pronounced. A patient with secondary adrenal insufficiency will differ from one with Addison's disease by showing pallor instead of increased pigmentation of the skin. Because the secretion of aldosterone is largely independent of the pituitary, the blood pressure is better maintained than in primary adrenal insufficiency and the threat to life is less marked. Otherwise the symptoms are similar to those of primary adrenal insufficiency. In the absence of ACTH secretion the zona fasciculata/reticularis undergoes disuse atrophy.

Adrenal insufficiency induced by the prolonged use of therapeutic doses of corticosteroids is discussed on page 453.

Congenital Adrenal Hyperplasia with Insufficiency

The synthesis of aldosterone and of the glucocorticoids involve a series of enzymatic steps involving hydroxylases. Congenital adrenal hyperplasia with insufficiency may present at birth, in infancy, or in childhood, depending on the precise type and severity of the hydroxylase deficiency. In the attempt to overcome the enzyme block, negative feedback control results in increased secretion of ACTH with overproduction of the compounds synthesised before the enzyme block is encountered. This usually means the production of large quantities of androgenic steroids.

The metabolic consequences of deficiency of enzymes at the different stages of synthesis of cortisol and aldosterone are illustrated in Figure 12.5. Thus at birth, female infants may show signs of virilisation with clitoral hypertrophy and variable degrees of fusion of the labia. Male infants particularly may die from adrenocortical

Fig. 12.5 The enzymatic steps involved in the synthesis of cortisol and aldosterone in the adrenal cortex and the urinary metabolites (underlined in italics) that are likely to be increased should there be an enzyme block (e.g. in congenital adrenal hyperplasia) at the next enzymatic step. The fall in the secretion of cortisol will activate the anterior pituitary to secrete ACTH with increased stimulation of the enzymatic steps preceding the block.

insufficiency, because the genital stigmata to be seen in female infants are not present to provide an appropriate warning of adrenal disease. If the enzyme defect is less severe the patient may survive infancy and present in childhood with evidence of precocious puberty. Growth may be abnormally advanced at first but is restricted later by early fusion of the epiphyses. Thus patients with mild examples of the enzyme defects usually come under supervision when excessive tallness, premature appearance of secondary sexual characteristics or libidinous tendencies arouse parental anxieties.

Investigation of Adrenal Insufficiency

The symptoms and signs of adrenal insufficiency are so non-specific that confirmation of the diagnosis must be sought whenever suspicion arises. Tests of adrenocortical function are based on:
(1) The metabolic effects of corticosteroids.
(2) The measurement of serum cortisol levels in the resting state and following stimulation.
(3) Measurement of ACTH levels in the plasma.

1. **Metabolic Effects.** Patients with Addison's disease, in contrast to those with secondary adrenal insufficiency, may show alteration in their serum electrolytes with depressed sodium and

elevated potassium levels; this is by no means invariable even in advanced cases and must not be depended upon for diagnosis. Some degree of hypoglycaemia may occur but this also is of little diagnostic value.

2. **Cortisol Levels.** Provided the patient is not in crisis or approaching crisis, time may be taken to determine the presence or absence of a diurnal rhythm in plasma cortisol levels by taking blood at 0900 hours and 2300 hours for 2 or 3 consecutive days for determination of serum cortisol levels before treatment is started. Low levels and the absence of a diurnal rhythm could be due to a lesion at any point in the hypothalamic-pituitary-adrenal axis. Normal levels and a normal rhythm would suggest that the whole axis is normal, but the possibility exists that, while overall function is maintained, there has been a significant reduction in reserve function which could be of paramount importance in times of stress. For this reason, if either primary or secondary adrenal insufficiency is suspected clinically, the diurnal rhythm studies should be supplemented by stimulation tests.

ACTH Test. The stimulation tests should be done in a logical sequence, starting with the administration of ACTH or a potent analogue. The preparation of choice is tetracosactrin which consists of the biologically active first 24 amino acids of human ACTH and has an action of about 30 minutes when given in a dosage of 250 μg intramuscularly. Oestrogen-containing oral contraceptives, spironolactone or glucocorticoids taken within the previous 12 hours may invalidate the test. In normal subjects the serum cortisol level at 30 minutes reaches at least 550 nmol/l with an increment above basal which exceeds 200 nmol/l. A normal response excludes primary adrenocortical insufficiency, but an impaired or absent response requires further investigation using tetracosactrin depot, (lmg. i.m. every 24 hrs for 3 days). Special care should be taken in patients with a history of allergic disease in view of occasional hypersensitivity reactions to tetracosactrin depot.

In secondary adrenal insufficiency there is a characteristic stepwise increase in serum cortisol levels on each day of tetracosactrin depot administration, while in primary adrenal insufficiency (Addison's disease) there is little or no response.

For practical purposes the criteria for primary adrenal insufficiency would be failure of the serum cortisol levels to rise above 700 nmol/l by 5–12 hours after the third intramuscular injection of 1·0 mg tetracosactrin depot given on three consecutive mornings.

Since highly biologically active analogues of cortisol, such as betamethasone or prednisolone, do not cross react in the radioimmunoassay for cortisol, tetracosactrin stimulation tests can be effectively carried out even though the patient may have recently started replacement therapy using these analogues. As different steroid analogues may interfere with the assessment of serum cortisol according to the precise method used, it is important to check with the laboratory beforehand.

Insulin-Induced Hypoglycaemia. In a patient in whom secondary adrenocortical insufficiency is suspected, the next procedure should be insulin induced hypoglycaemia. Unless radioimmunoassay of ACTH is readily available, a normal adrenal response to ACTH stimulation should have been demonstrated before giving insulin because a cortisol rise in response to hypoglycaemia depends upon ACTH secretion and the patient is thus being used for bioassay.

Insulin-induced hypoglycaemia is a safe procedure provided certain precautions are taken. A history of epilepsy or myocardial ischaemia is a contraindication. Patients with hypopituitarism are very sensitive to small doses of insulin and the dose should not exceed 0·1 unit soluble insulin/kg body weight. This is given in the form of a single intravenous injection, an in-dwelling cannula with a slow infusion of saline having previously been established. The patient must be observed throughout the test with the physician checking the condition of the patient repeatedly. A good index of adequate hypoglycaemia is the presence of sweating. Should hypoglycaemia become profound and the clinical features indicate that the test should be abandoned, the situation can be readily corrected by giving glucose and hydrocortisone if necessary via the intravenous cannula. In addition to the clinical criteria of sweating, the blood sugar should fall to less than 2·2 mol/l or to less than 50% of the basal level at 30 minutes, whichever is the lower. Blood glucose and serum cortisol levels should be estimated half-hourly for 120 min. Normal peak values of the latter show a mean of 785 nmol/l with a range of 560–1060 nmol/l, the increment being a mean of 420 with a range of 200–670 nmol/l.

Useful information of growth hormone secretion and prolactin can be obtained from the samples. The serum cortisol response to insulin-induced hypoglycaemia is probably the most sensitive of the tests currently available for assessing hypothalamic-pituitary-adrenal function.

3. **Measurement of ACTH Levels in Plasma.** In the presence of low levels of serum cortisol, if the plasma ACTH level is high, one would have strong evidence of primary adrenocortical insufficiency. The measurement of plasma ACTH levels greatly facilitates the study of hypopituitarism as it is no longer necessary to use the patient's potentially normal adrenals in an *in vivo* bioassay.

Treatment of Adrenocortical Insufficiency

All patients with adrenocortical insufficiency will require replacement therapy with a glucocorticoid, while the majority of patients with Addison's disease will also need a mineralocorticoid. In congenital adrenal hyperplasia, full replacement doses of glucocorticoid will suppress ACTH secretion and prevent excessive formation of metabolites with consequent regression of the clinical features. If the nature of the enzymic block demands it, a mineralocorticoid should be added.

Cortisol (hydrocortisone) is the drug of choice for routine glucocorticoid replacement therapy. Cortisone acetate, although widely used, has the disadvantage that it has to be metabolised by the liver to cortisol before having any physiological action. Abnormal liver function results in reduced conversion of cortisone acetate to cortisol and the possibility of impaired liver function is particularly relevant in cases of secondary adrenal insufficiency taking oral androgens for concomitant hypogonadism.

Other synthetic glucocorticoids, e.g. prednisone, prednisolone, dexamethasone and betamethasone, are useful in keeping a patient in good health while adrenal function tests are being done, but have the disadvantage in long-term therapy that they do not react in the fluorogenic corticosteroid assay so that their blood levels cannot be monitored by this method.

Cortisol, cortisone acetate and the synthetic glucocorticoids have a biological action of some 6 to 8 hours.

For maintenance treatment it is best to give the glucocorticoid medication in a regime which mimics the normal diurnal variation of cortisol output. For most patients this would be 20 mg cortisol at breakfast time and 10 mg at about 1800 hours. The equivalent doses of cortisone acetate would be 25 mg and 12·5 mg respectively. While it is not possible to be dogmatic about how much glucocorticoid any individual may require as absorption and metabolism may vary, the regime described will meet the needs of most patients. To assess the requirements of those whose response appears to be unsatisfactory a *cortisol profile* should be carried out. Serum cortisol levels should be estimated before and half an hour, 1 hour and then at 2-hourly intervals after an oral dose of 20 mg of cortisol, or whatever dose seems to be clinically indicated. The plasma level usually reaches a peak after 30–60 minutes and the amount of cortisol should be adjusted to give a peak of 700–830 nmol/l and a level of about 165 nmol/l before the evening dose.

Fludrocortisone is the most useful mineralocorticoid for maintenance therapy, and the dose should be adjusted according to the serum electrolytes, the state of hydration of the patient and the blood pressure. Most patients require 0·05–0·15 mg in a single morning dose. The signs of overdosage of mineralocorticoid are those of sodium retention, i.e. hypertension, oedema, headaches and arthralgia, and also potassium depletion, hypokalaemic alkalosis and muscular weakness. The occasional patient is unable to tolerate fludrocortisone and in these cases a long-acting preparation may be given intramuscularly in a single dose of 50–100 mg every 2 to 4 weeks, e.g. deoxycortone pivalate.

The regime to be followed in secondary adrenocortical insufficiency is the same as in Addison's disease except that a mineralocorticoid is not required as aldosterone production is little affected. Any associated condition due to lack of other trophic hormones will require therapy along the usual lines.

During periods of stress, e.g. trauma, infection or operations, it is necessary for the dose of gluco-corticoid to be increased to mimic what would happen in an individual with normal function of the hypothalamic-pituitary-adrenal axis. Thus if a patient develops severe coryza or influenza the dose of oral steroids should be increased to twice their normal maintenance level for 2 to 3 days. Should gastroenteritis with or without vomiting occur the oral glucocorticoid should be changed to intramuscular hydrocortisone at an increased dose level. Consequently, it is essential that patients with impaired adrenal function, either primary or secondary, should have available ampoules of hydrocortisone hemisuccinate for injection which are not outdated and which they know how to use.

Every patient on oral steroids of whatever form should have a steroid card or preferably a bracelet giving details of the diagnosis, steroid dosage and the medical attendant's address. Should the patient be involved in an accident and be taken unconscious to a casualty department a disastrous outcome may be avoided if information that the patient is taking steroids is available. Even the most minor operation is a potential hazard to a patient with adrenocortical insufficiency. On no account should such a patient be given morphine or pethidine. For dental extraction the patient should be admitted to hospital for the day. It is usually only necessary to give twice the normal dose of glucocorticoid on the day of the extraction and possibly the following morning. Normal replacement dosage may then be resumed provided there are no complications. Larger doses of steroids and more careful monitoring of cortisol levels are required before and after more major surgery.

ACUTE ADRENAL CRISIS. This is a medical emergency. If promptly treated with intravenous hydrocortisone (as sodium succinate or sodium phosphate) and intravenous fluids there is in most cases a dramatic improvement over 12 to 24 hours in a previously moribund patient. Occasional cases will need more protracted treatment depending upon how quickly the precipitating cause, e.g. infection, is brought under control. In incipient crises, intravenous fluids may not be necessary, but in frank crises with acute circulatory failure the patient may succumb in spite of massive doses of intravenous hydrocortisone.

The intravenous fluids should consist of 5% of glucose in isotonic saline to correct hypoglycaemia and sodium loss. Hydrocortisone is best given parenterally over the first 24–48 hours until gastrointestinal symptoms settle completely and one can be sure that oral medication will be retained. The initial dose should be 100 mg intravenously 6 hourly for the first 24 hours and then 50 mg 6 hourly for the next 24 hours. If progress is satisfactory, oral cortisol (hydrocortisone) can be given thereafter in a dose of 20 mg 8 hourly. The dose or oral cortisol can then be further reduced in a stepwise fashion by 10 mg daily until normal maintenance levels are reached. Below 40 mg of oral cortisol per day a mineralocorticoid is best added to the therapeutic regime, initially in a single morning dose of 0·1 mg fludrocortisone.

Prognosis in Adrenal Insufficiency

With modern therapy the life expectancy of patients with adrenal insufficiency should be normal, within the limits imposed by any associated disease such as pituitary tumour, or other clinical disorders such as insulin dependent diabetes mellitus which may co-exist with autoimmune adrenal insufficiency. Otherwise the main risk to life is the avoidable occurrence of acute adrenal crisis and delay in its prompt management.

CORTICOSTEROIDS AND ACTH IN THE TREATMENT OF DISEASE

Extensive use is made of the anti-inflammatory actions of corticosteroids and their synthetic analogues. Alternatively, ACTH may be administered parenterally to augment the endogenous production of cortisol. The doses of steroid analogues therapeutically equivalent to 20 mg cortisol for an anti-inflammatory effect are cortisone (25 mg), prednisolone (5 mg), betamethasone (0·75 mg) and dexamethasone (0·75 mg). Of these prednisolone is the most commonly used for purposes other than replacement therapy. It is widely prescribed in the treatment of connective tissue diseases, of autoimmune disorders and conditions involving other forms of immune reaction. Corticosteroids may be used to suppress inflammation, for example in conjunction with chemotherapy in acute tuberculosis (p. 236). The use of corticosteroids in pharmacological doses is discussed under the heading of the various diseases for which they may be employed.

The Dangers of Corticosteroid Therapy

The use of corticosteroids in doses exceeding those required for replacement therapy carries certain risks which must be balanced against the possible therapeutic advantages. These risks can be subdivided into two types: (1) the undesirable metabolic consequences that cannot be separated from the anti-inflammatory effect of the steroid and (2) the suppression of the hypothalamic-pituitary-adrenal (HPA) axis that may follow the use of pharmacological doses over a prolonged period.

1. *The metabolic consequences* are those that are encountered in Cushing's syndrome and are more pronounced the higher the dose and the longer the treatment. Thus, although certain corticosteroid analogues may have slightly less mineralocorticoid activity than cortisol, fluid retention, moon face, hypertension, central obesity and striae may all be induced. The glucocorticoid action not infrequently precipitates diabetes mellitus. Osteoporosis is an insidious but frequent complication of long term therapy as a result of a decrease in bone formation and an increase in bone resorption especially in the spine and ribs. As in Cushing's syndrome, mental symptoms may be troublesome, ranging from euphoria to depression which may be so severe as to lead to suicide.

Corticosteroids may modify the normal response to a major illness so that pain, tenderness, fever or a raised ESR may be abolished, while the response to inflammation and therefore the defences against infection may be poor and healing impaired. In this way treatment with these drugs may be responsible for masking the more typical and sometimes dangerous consequences of a variety of illnesses. For example, oral corticosteroids may induce peptic ulceration with perforation without pain, and the physical signs indicative of inflammation in the peritoneal cavity may not be present.

2. *The suppression of the HPA axis* following prolonged corticosteroid therapy in doses greater than 7·5 mg prednisolone per day or its equivalent may be long standing, especially with regard to the hypothalamic-pituitary portion of the axis. This may make it difficult to withdraw steroid, the patient being as vulnerable as someone with secondary adrenocortical insufficiency due to organic pituitary disease. Stimulation of the adrenal cortex in such cases is usually possible with adequate ACTH dosage, but there is no known way of producing a comparably strong and prolonged stimulus to the hypothalamic-pituitary axis without risking adrenocortical failure.

When trying to wean a patient off corticosteroid therapy, one should first ensure that the adrenal cortex is functional by giving tetracosactrin depot (1·0 mg i.m. on 3 consecutive mornings) and measuring the plasma cortisol response at 30 minutes, 1 hour and 5 hours (p. 819). Then, after gradually reducing the dosage of oral steroid, a maintenance dose of 20 mg cortisol should be given at 0800–0900 hours and no cortisol in the evenings; the hypothalamo-pituitary axis will then have no exogenous steroid to suppress the secretion of CRF or ACTH in the early hours of the morning. In this way a normal diurnal rhythm may be restored and the HPA axis should thereafter respond normally to stress. This may take many months to achieve, while in other cases, normal function may be restored shortly after steroid therapy has been withdrawn.

Because it can be such a difficult task to withdraw corticosteroid therapy when it has been used in pharmacological dosage for a prolonged period, attempts have been made to use synthetic ACTH preparations such as tetracosactrin depot in place of oral corticosteroids. When used in appropriate doses, there is evidence that therapeutically useful elevation in the plasma cortisol level may be achieved in some patients without suppression of the HPA axis. However, this may be only a reflection of the amount of corticosteroid secreted in response to this stimulus. In children ACTH therapy has the distinct advantage over treatment with oral steroids in that it causes less inhibition of growth.

The incidence of mooning of the face and obesity is similar with oral corticosteroids and ACTH. Peptic ulceration and bruising are commoner with corticosteroids, and hypertension, pigmentation and acne with ACTH. In view of the serious risks involved very careful consideration must be given before either is employed and the practitioner must be convinced that the therapeutic benefits outweigh the disadvantages. It should also be realised that when large amounts of steroid are applied to the skin a significant proportion is absorbed.

PHAEOCHROMOCYTOMA

Phaeochromocytomas are tumours of chromaffin tissue which secrete catecholamines, predominantly noradrenaline but also adrenaline. The tumours, most of which are benign, may occur at any site along the sympathic chain, but 90% are found in the adrenal glands. Rarely the lesions may be multiple. Phaeochromocytoma is an uncommon tumour but of considerable interest because of its pharmacological effects. The clinical presentation depends upon the relative amounts of noradrenaline and adrenaline secreted. The most common sign is hypertension which may be sustained or, characteristically, paroxysmal with associated episodes of extreme skin pallor, sweating, palpitations, headache, epigastric pain and chest discomfort. Apprehension is common during a paroxysm.

Confirmation of the diagnosis of phaeochromocytoma depends on the demonstration of increased levels of catecholamines or their metabolites in the urine or plasma, e.g. metanephrine and normetanephrine. The location of the tumour can be shown by CT scanning or by angiography.

The treatment of phaeochromocytoma is by excision of the tumour if it can be identified or, failing this, alpha and beta receptor blockade may be used. In order to avoid hypertension and arrhythmias during induction of anaesthesia and handling of the tumour at operation, the preoperative preparation of the patient with α and β adrenergic blocking agents (phenoxybenzamine and propranolol) is essential. Emergencies associated with hypertensive crises should be dealt with by the intravenous administration of phentolamine in doses of 5 mg. Careful preparation before and during operation should prevent any severe fall in blood pressure resulting from hypovolaemia. If hypotension persists noradrenaline should be given intravenously in saline.

SEXUAL DISORDERS IN THE MALE

These may present in many forms. Some are due to faults arising in the mechanism of sex determination as early as conception, others to errors later in sexual differentiation of the embryo and fetus, and after birth, in sexual development. Abnormalities of the sex chromosomes may be associated with failure of sexual development so that the individual may show some of the characteristics of both sexes (intersex). The term hermaphroditism is reserved for patients in whom male and female gonadal tissue is found to coexist; it occurs much less commonly than the intersexes.

The anatomical characteristics of the male are influenced by essential hormonal factors, particularly androgen secretion. The personality and behaviour of the male are further attributes which must be considered in assessing the individual patient's needs. A few only of the more common sexual disorders occurring in the male will be discussed here. Sexually transmitted diseases are described on pages 408 to 415, and psychosexual disorders on page 697.

Hypogonadism

This term is used to include failure of one or both of the main functions of the testis, namely the production of spermatozoa and the secretion of androgens. The defect may involve only impaired spermatogenesis in the seminiferous tubules of the testis, or the interstitial (Leydig) cells of the testis may also be affected so that the secretion of testosterone by these cells is reduced or abolished. If the function of the interstitial cells is defective, then tubular dysfunction is inevitable as testosterone production is required for normal spermatogenesis.

Aetiology. Hypogonadism may arise from hypothalamic or pituitary disease (hypogonadotrophic hypogonadism) or from primary testicular disease (hypergonadotrophic hypogonadism).

Hypogonadism may be part of the syndrome of hypopituitarism. Hypogonadotrophic hypogonadism with an apparently normal pituitary gland appears to be due to failure of the hypothalamus to secrete the appropriate gonadotrophin releasing hormone.

Primary testicular failure may be due to trauma, tuberculosis, gonococcal infections, syphilis, malignant disease or orchitis as in mumps. Maldescent or failure of descent will also lead to failure of the tubular epithelium to develop. Haemochromatosis, cirrhosis of the liver and oestrogen administration may all be associated with testicular insufficiency. The disorder may also be due to abnormalities of the sex chromosomes (p. 9). Many cases remain, however, for which an aetiological diagnosis is still not possible, and these form the majority of patients who present with infertility as their only complaint (idiopathic oligospermia).

Clinical Features. The results of failure of function of the interstitial cells depend upon the age of the patient at the time of the onset of the disease. When this occurs *before puberty* the external genitalia and the secondary sex characteristics fail to develop. In these circumstances the epiphyses of the long bones do not close at the usual age and in consequence the patient may grow to an excessive height. The typical pre-pubertal eunuch develops into a tall man with a hairless face, a high-pitched voice, small genitalia and an immature personality. Some pubic hair is present and is the result of adrenal androgen production — the adrenarche.

When the onset of the disease is *postpubertal* the changes are less striking. Growth is not affected and there is regression rather than disappearance of the secondary sex characteristics. The external genitalia undergo partial atrophy. Fatigue, loss of initiative and libido and impotence are the usual complaints. In some patients, particularly when the deprivation is sudden as after surgical castration, there may be 'menopausal symptoms' such as hot flushes and profuse sweating, unless replacement therapy is provided.

Treatment. Hypogonadism due to deficiency of androgens may be corrected by replacement therapy with testosterone. A satisfactory and most economical form of therapy is the implantation of 200–600 mg of testosterone, in pellets, into the anterior abdominal wall. Renewal may be required after six to eight months. Alternatively depot intramuscular injections of testosterone can be given. An oral preparation, testosterone undecanoate, is available but is expensive. In some cases of deficiency of the germinal epithelium, especially when this is due to lack of FSH, increased spermatogenesis may be achieved by treatment with human chorionic gonadotrophin and purified LH and FSH which have been obtained from menopausal urine.

Cryptorchidism

Cryptorchidism (undescended testis) usually occurs in otherwise normal boys but may be the presenting feature of hypogonadotrophic hypogonadism. Highly retractile testes, particularly in an obese boy, may be mistaken for cryptorchidism. If the glands remain in the inguinal canal they are more liable to trauma than if situated in the scrotum. The seminiferous tubules will fail to develop in an undescended gland, and if the condition is bilateral, sterility will follow. Even in testes which remain undescended into adult life the interstitial cells function normally, so that the secondary sex characters develop in the usual way. A course of chorionic gonadotrophin should be given at about 6 years of age. If this is unsuccessful the testis or testes should be placed in the scrotum surgically.

In maldescent the testis takes an abnormal route and is liable to develop malignancy. Such testes should either be brought down into the scrotum or, if discovered in the adult, removed.

Impotence

Erectile dysfunction or failure (impotence) is thought to be due to psychological causes in the majority of cases. The incidence of this condition increases with age; vascular disease involving the internal pudendal artery or its branches is common in these patients. Whether this alone is the cause of the impotence or is the trigger for psychological dysfunction is unclear. Impotence may also be an important early symptom in organic disease such as diabetes mellitus, multiple sclerosis and tabes dorsalis. Endocrine causes of impotence are uncommon and there is usually an associated loss of libido.

Full investigation is necessary to determine whether there is primary or secondary testicular dysfunction. If there is secondary hypogonadism then hypothalamic-pituitary function apart from that relating to the gonads must be assessed. Androgen therapy will usually restore potency and libido. In some patients hyperprolactinaemia without gonadotrophin deficiency will be present; this condition responds to bromocriptine therapy. If infertility is a problem in secondary hypogonadism then gonadotrophin therapy will usually be required.

Infertility in the Male

Sterility in the husband is believed to be responsible for the infertility of approximately one half of all childless marriages. The cause is usually defective development of the germinal epithelium in the seminiferous tubules, with oligospermia or azoospermia, but may follow hypogonadism due to any of the causes described earlier. Antibodies to sperm (p. 29) may explain a small number of cases.

Klinefelter's syndrome (p. 9) is almost invariably associated with azoospermia. The additional X chromosomes may be recognised by examination of a buccal smear for Barr bodies, but usually confirmation requires a full karyotype analysis (p. 9).

In most azoospermic patients where there is defective spermatogenesis due to primary testicular dysfunction FSH levels will be high. If normal FSH levels are found in such cases this suggests that possibility of obstruction as the cause of azoospermia. Testicular biopsy may show normal spermatogenesis and analysis of the seminal fluid may be helpful. If semen has a reduced fructose concentration this suggests that there is obstruction to fluid coming from the seminal vesicles. This and other types of obstruction may be amenable to surgery as in the case of a varicocele; this condition may be overlooked if the patient is not examined standing.

In most cases of male infertility the cause of azoospermia or oligospermia is unknown. Results of treatment with gonadotrophins, clomiphene or androgens have been disappointing. Artificial insemination using sperm from the oligospermic husband (AIH) is nearly always unsuccessful and patients may opt for artificial insemination by a donor (AID). The most exciting advance for the severely oligospermic male is *in vitro* fertilisation. Specimens from men with very low sperm counts have resulted in successful fertilisation and normal pregnancies.

SEXUAL DISORDERS IN THE FEMALE

Many conditions regarded as primarily gynaecological in nature may have much wider implications. *Primary amenorrhoea*, for example, may provide an important indication of systemic disorder; it may be due to a chromosomal anomaly such as Turner's syndrome or it may be due to an autoimmune reaction against antigens shared between the steroid producing cells in the ovary and in the adrenal cortex. Hermaphroditism may present with amenorrhoea. Congenital adrenal hyperplasia, if unrecognised and untreated in childhood, pituitary tumours and developmental disorders in the genital tract may all require full gynaecological and endocrine assessment for precise diagnosis.

Secondary amenorrhoea also requires further investigation, but it is so common a feature of a wide range of conditions that by itself it has little diagnostic value. Hyperprolactinaemia (p. 423) must be considered as should amenorrhoea associated with weight loss as in anorexia nervosa.

Risks of Oral Contraception. A low level of mortality is associated with all major reversible methods of fertility control, including oral contraception (OC), compared with the risk of death from pregnancy and delivery in women using no such methods. The use of OC may be associated with coronary artery disease, hypertension, cerebrovascular accident, deep vein thrombosis, pulmonary embolism, neoplasia of the cervix of the uterus and carcinoma of the breast. These risks vary with the individual and with the duration of use and the composition of the OC.

Immediate undesirable effects which may influence the woman's acceptance of OC include weight gain, jaundice (p. 348), bleeding occurring during courses of treatment (breakthrough bleeding) and failure to bleed between courses. These complaints may subside after the first few months. Other troublesome effects include depression, hirsutism and decreased libido. The incidence of these has diminished as the dose of oestrogen in the commonly used oral contraceptives has been reduced.

Sexually transmitted diseases are described on page 408 and *psychosexual disorders* on page 697.

Disorders of the Menopause

The cessation of the menstrual cycle occurs in most women in the Western world between the ages of 45 and 50; it is the result of the gradual failure of the ovaries to produce oestrogens and progesterone. As a consequence the pituitary gland becomes more active and produces FSH and LH in greater quantity. Assays for these hormones are of value in distinguishing amenorrhoea due primarily to failure of the ovaries from amenorrhoea due to failure of the pituitary to secrete gonadotrophins.

Clinical Features. The ease with which a woman adapts herself to the change of circumstances associated with the menopause varies widely. In some the loss of reproductive capacity is associated with psychological symptoms; in others adjustment is readily achieved and may be unattended by any emotional reaction. In the group of patients who are troubled by symptoms, anxiety, emotional instability, irritability, insomnia, and particularly hot flushes and cold sweats are common complaints. Depression is frequent and occasionally may be severe with suicidal tendencies.

Obesity may first appear, or, if previously present, may increase. Hirsutism, especially the appearance of hair on the upper lip and chin, is not uncommon. Osteoporosis may present for the first time in the early years after the menopause usually with back pain. This condition occurs more commonly in women who have had a premature menopause and have not been given oestrogen. Pruritus vulvae is a complication which is frequently associated with changes in the mucous membrances of the genital tract. Leukoplakia vulvae may develop, and if untreated may prog-

ress to carcinoma. Senile vaginitis may cause considerable distress from dyspareunia, dysuria and vaginal discharge, especially if complicated by secondary infection.

Treatment. The essential treatment is explanation of the nature of the condition, coupled with specific treatment for the complications. Features attributable to oestrogen deficiency call for replacement therapy with a synthetic oestrogen such as ethinyloestradiol. The daily dose required to suppress menopausal symptoms in different individuals varies from 10 to 50 μg daily, but 20 μg is often adequate; this should be given in courses lasting for 21 days, repeated if necessary after an interval of 7 days. The patient must be warned that this treatment may be followed by vaginal bleeding as in a normal menstrual period. Other appropriate measures, such as treatment of obesity may also be required. Depression complicating the menopause responds well to psychiatric treatment.

DIABETES MELLITUS

Diabetes mellitus is a clinical syndrome characterised by hyperglycaemia, due to deficiency or diminished effectiveness of insulin. This can arise in many different ways and the diagnostic label 'diabetes mellitus' includes numerous different disorders. Lack of insulin, whether absolute or relative, affects the metabolism of carbohydrate, protein, fat, water and electrolytes, sometimes with grave consequences. The long-standing metabolic derangement is frequently associated with permanent and irreversible functional and structural changes in the cells of the body, those of the vascular system being particularly susceptible. The changes lead in turn to the development of well-defined clinical entities, the so-called 'complications' of diabetes, which most characteristically affect the eye, the kidney and the nervous system.

Diabetes mellitus is the most common of the endocrine disorders. The prevalence in Britain is over 1%, although about half of those affected remain undetected.

Aetiology. On the basis of aetiology two main categories of diabetes are recognised, namely primary and secondary diabetes.

PRIMARY DIABETES. The great majority of cases seen belong to this group, which consists of two main clinical types: *insulin-dependent diabetes mellitus* — IDDM (Type I) most frequent in those less than 50 years old and rapidly fatal without treatment with insulin and *non insulin dependent diabetes mellitus* — NIDDM (Type II) occurring mainly in the middle-aged and elderly and compatible with long survival without treatment. Although the precise aetiology is still uncertain, in both types it is the susceptibility to diabetes, rather than diabetes *per se*, which is inherited and heredity and environment interact to determine which of those with a genetic predisposition actually develop the clinical syndrome and the timing of its onset. However, both the pattern of inheritance and environmental factors differ in IDDM and NIDDM as is discussed in detail below and on page 459.

SECONDARY DIABETES. A minority of cases of diabetes occur as a result of a recognisable pathological process or secondary to the treatment of some other condition.

1. *Pancreatic Diabetes.* Diseases such as pancreatitis, haemochromatosis and carcinoma cause destruction of the pancreas and lead to impaired secretion and release of insulin. Diabetes will also follow pancreatectomy.

2. *Insulin Antagonists.* Diabetes may occur in conditions where there are abnormal concentrations of hormones antagonistic to the action of insulin in the circulation.

(a) *Growth hormone* can produce permanent diabetes in experimental animals and about 30% of patients with acromegaly are diabetic.

(b) *Adrenocortical hormones*, such as cortisol, raise the concentration of glucose in the blood by increasing gluconeogenesis and by inhibiting utilisation of glucose by the peripheral tissues. Thus, many patients with Cushing's syndrome show impaired carbohydrate tolerance; diabetes may be precipitated by ACTH or corticosteroid therapy and the stress of physical injury may operate in this way. Conversely increased sensitivity to insulin is an important feature of Addison's disease and of hypopituitarism, and this can be corrected by the administration of corticosteroids.

(c) *Adrenaline* raises the blood glucose concentration by increasing the breakdown of liver glycogen and by suppressing the secretion of insulin. Patients with phaeochromocytoma frequently show a diabetic blood glucose curve on glucose tolerance testing and the incidence of these uncommon tumours is relatively high among diabetic patients.

(d) *Thyroid hormone* in excess will aggravate the diabetic state and some patients with hyperthyroidism show impaired glucose tolerance.

(e) *Gestational diabetes* refers to the hyperglycaemia which can occur temporarily during pregnancy in individuals who have an inherited liability to develop the disorder. During normal pregnancy there is an increased production of hormonal antagonists to insulin, which in turn demands an increased rate of secretion and release of insulin. A failing pancreas may be unable to meet this demand.

3. *Iatrogenic diabetes*, in those genetically susceptible, may be precipitated by various forms of therapy, notably with corticosteroids, and thiazide diuretics.

4. *Liver disease*, particularly cirrhosis and hepatitis, may be associated with impaired glucose tolerance.

Aetiology of IDDM. The increased risk of developing IDDM is HLA linked and is primarily associated with the D locus (p. 31). Associations with alleles at the A, C, B, Bf, C_2 and the two C_4 loci occur because of linkage disequilibrium, i.e. the tendency for alleles at different loci to occur together more often in the same haplotype than is expected by chance. Two established axes, one of increased and one of reduced susceptibility have been identified. The relative risk of developing IDDM associated with DW3, DR3 is 7·3, with DW4, DR4 9·23, with DR3, DR4 14·26, and with DW2, DR2 0·12. The HLA DR determinants are probably in linkage disequilibrium with immune response (Ir) genes which are thought to exist on chromosome 6 within the HLA region. Since there is at present no way of defining Ir genes in man, the HLA antigens serve as 'markers' for genes which confer increased and reduced susceptibility to IDDM. Affected siblings of diabetics usually have one, and in many cases both haplotypes in common, irrespective of the HLA determinants that make up the haplotype.

It is postulated that the Ir genes control the immune response to environmental factors capable of damaging the β cells of the pancreatic islet. Susceptible individuals react abnormally to assault by viruses or other cytotoxic agents which leads to β cell destruction either directly or by initiating an immune reaction. Islet cell antibodies (ICA) are present in the plasma of over 80% of patients with newly diagnosed IDDM, but it is uncertain whether these are responsible for, or result from β cell damage. Prospective family studies suggest that immune-mediated destruction of the pancreatic β cells involving both humoral and cell-mediated immunological processes occurs over a prolonged period, sometimes extending over several years, prior to the development of hyperglycaemia and clinical presentation.

The possibility of heterogeneity within IDDM was suggested by the demonstration of two separate HLA DR linked axes of susceptibility. Two subtypes of IDDM have been identified. *Type 1a* is more common and occurs predominantly in those less than 30 years of age. The primary association is particularly with HLA DR4 and slightly more males are affected. Viruses are probably responsible for initiating β cell destruction and autoimmune phenomena such as ICA are transient and may result from, rather than cause, pancreatic damage. Treatment with conventional insulin preparations is associated with a high plasma titre of insulin-binding antibodies (IBA) in this type of diabetes.

Type 1b is less common, occurs mainly in women over the age of 30 years, and is primarily associated with HLA DR3. ICA tend to persist, other autoimmune diseases such as pernicious anaemia, hyperthyroidism, Hashimoto's thyroiditis, primary hypothyroidism and Addison's disease co-exist with this type of diabetes more often than can be accounted for by chance and in cases where these disorders are not present thyroid, gastric, intrinsic factor, and adrenal antibodies are frequently found. There is often a strong family history of autoimmune disease.

Aetiology of NIDDM. NIDDM is not HLA linked and there is no evidence that autoimmunity or viruses have anything to do with its development. Studies with twins and sibships have shown that genetic factors are more important in the development of this type of diabetes than in IDDM, but there is little information about what is inherited. Progress in this field has been hampered by serious problems in relation to definition and ascertainment of the condition, heterogeneity within NIDDM, lack of genetic markers and the association and interaction of environmental factors such as obesity, diet, inactivity, and pregnancy, which probably play a critical role in the clinical expression of NIDDM.

The insulin gene, situated on the short arm of chromosome 11, has been investigated as a possible genetic marker for NIDDM. Using restriction enzymes three alleles of the insulin gene have been demonstrated: an upper allele (UU), a lower allele (LL) and a third allele which is a mixture of the sequences forming the other two (UL). A significant increase has been demonstrated in the frequency of the UU allele in NIDDM compared with IDDM patients, and non-diabetic carriers of the UU allele show a delayed insulin response to oral glucose and reduced glucose tolerance with age. Thus the UU allele seems to affect blood glucose homeostasis and may confer susceptibility to NIDDM.

Simple deficiency of insulin cannot entirely account for the diabetic syndrome in NIDDM. Increased hepatic production of glucose and resistance to the action of insulin are characteristic of this type of diabetes. Insulin resistance is also seen in obesity and the majority of middle aged diabetic patients are obese. Most of the evidence supports the view that obesity is diabetogenic in those genetically predisposed to the disorder and that the rising incidence of diabetes in older people is largely related to the increasing prevalence of obesity in the population as a whole. However, obesity cannot account for all the insulin resistance in obese patients with NIDDM, and many non-obese, non-insulin dependent patients are also insulin resistant.

Insulin resistance may be due to any one of three general causes: an abnormal insulin molecule, an excessive amount of circulating antagonists and target tissue defects. The last is the common cause of insulin resistance in NIDDM. The specific mechanisms underlying this insulin resistant state are heterogeneous. In patients with relatively mild impairment of glucose tolerance the defect in insulin action is associated with a decreased number of cellular insulin receptors. Patients with more severe hyperglycaemia usually combine a reduced number of receptors with a post-receptor defect in the action of insulin and the latter seems to be the predominant abnormality. Increased amounts of circulating hormonal antagonists are not thought to be primarily involved in the aetiology of either IDDM or NIDDM. However, uncontrolled diabetes is associated with increased plasma concentration of antistorage hormones such as growth hormone, and glucagon, and the normal suppressive effect of oral carbohydrate on the secretion of these hormones is diminished. Treatment of the diabetes abolishes these abnormalities which are thought to be secondary to absolute or relative deficiency of insulin. Other types of insulin resistance are extremely rare. They include a syndrome in which antibodies are directed against the insulin receptor.

It should be noted that increased hepatic production of glucose and/or decreased peripheral utilisation of glucose cannot lead to sustained hyperglycaemia unless the pancreatic islets fail to adapt to the situation. Although the maximum, absolute, plasma immunoreactive insulin may be relatively normal in patients with mild NIDDM, a delay in the insulin response to glucose is commonly seen during a glucose tolerance test. This defect in insulin secretion appears to be selective for glucose since the response to other stimuli such as amino acids and sulphonylurea drugs is normal. It is not known whether the β cell abnormality is due to intrinsic structural or metabolic change within the islet or whether it is caused by some imbalance in neuro-endocrine input or by a change in the sensitivity of the β cell to glucose.

Chemical Pathology. Whatever the aetiology, in all cases of diabetes hyperglycaemia results from deficiency of insulin. This is absolute in IDDM and relative in NIDDM. Increased gluconeogenesis and lipolysis follow as compensatory reactions under the influence of such hormones as growth hormone, glucagon and adrenocortical hormones, in what is basically a situation of glucose lack. Thus the hyperglycaemia characteristic of diabetes arises from two

main sources, namely a reduced rate of removal of glucose from the blood by the peripheral tissues and an increased rate of release of glucose from the liver into the circulation.

CONSEQUENCES OF HYPERGLYCAEMIA AND GLYCO-SURIA. When the glucose concentration in the blood exceeds the capacity of the renal tubules to reabsorb it from the glomerular filtrate, glycosuria occurs. In most people the level of blood glucose at which this happens is approximately 10 mmol/l (180 mg/100 ml). Glucose increases the osmolality of the glomerular filtrate and thus prevents the reabsorption of water as the filtrate passes down the renal tubular system. In this way the volume of urine is markedly increased in diabetes and *polyuria* and *nocturia* occur. This in turn leads to loss of water and minerals which results in *thirst* and *polydipsia*. Severe depletion of water and electrolytes may ensue.

CONSEQUENCES OF POOR GLUCOSE UTILISATION. Impaired utilisation of carbohydrate results in a sense of *fatigue*, and causes two main compensatory mechanisms to operate in an attempt to provide alternative metabolic substrate. Both of these lead to loss of body tissue, that is *wasting*, which may occur in spite of normal or even an increased intake of food, and which is additional to any loss of weight resulting from loss of body fluid. The compensatory mechanisms are:

1. *Increased Glycogenolysis and Gluconeogenesis.* As glycogen and protein are catabolised, glucose, nitrogen, water and electrolytes, particularly potassium, are released from cells into the extracellular space. An increased urinary excretion of potassium, magnesium and phosphorus therefore occurs.

2. *Increased Lipolysis.* This is seen as a raised fasting plasma concentration of non-esterified fatty acid (NEFA), and a diminished fall in plasma NEFA in response to a carbohydrate load. The extent to which increased lipolysis occurs is proportional to the degree of insulin deficiency. If the latter is marked, the normal response to feeding, namely suppression of lipolysis, may be lost and the plasma concentration of NEFA may remain consistently elevated to three or four times the normal level.

Fatty acids are taken up by the liver and degraded through eight steps within the mitochondria of the liver cells. Each stage yields one molecule of acetyl coenzyme A. Normally most of these molecules enter the citric acid cycle by condensing with oxaloacetic acid, but in severe diabetes more is formed than can enter the citric acid cycle. Instead acetyl coenzyme A is converted to acetoacetic acid. Most of this is then reduced to beta-hydroxybutyric acid, while some is decarboxylated to acetone. These ketone bodies, when formed in small amounts, are usually oxidised and utilised as metabolic fuel. However the rate of utilisation of ketone bodies is limited. When the rate of production by the liver exceeds that of removal by the peripheral tissues, then the blood level rises.

Ketone bodies increase the osmolality of the plasma and so also lead to the withdrawal of water from the cell. They are strong acids which dissociate readily and release hydrogen ions into the body fluids. The fall in pH is reduced by the buffers of the blood, the most important being bicarbonate. The dissociation of carbonic acid is reduced, and the ratio of bicarbonate ions to carbonic acid falls, and measurement of plasma bicarbonate will show a lower value than normal. This state is called *ketoacidosis*. The rise in hydrogen ion concentration and increase in Pco_2 in the arterial blood stimulate pulmonary ventilation so that clinically hyperpnoea or 'air hunger' is observed.

The extent to which the clinical features of dehydration and ketoacidosis are seen in the individual will depend on such factors as the speed at which the condition develops and the extent to which the patient increases the intake of fluid, as well as on the degree of insulin deficiency present.

Pathology. In IDDM there is degeneration of pancreatic islet tissue, from which the beta cells have largely disappeared, leaving behind a variable number of alpha cells and a majority of small undifferentiated cells. The few remaining beta cells show evidence of excessive activity; the nuclei are commonly enlarged with degranulation of the cytoplasm. These appearances of the pancreas are consistent with the extremely low plasma insulin levels found in these patients.

In NIDDM the moderate reduction in the total mass of islet tissue which is commonly seen does not appear to be sufficient in itself to account for the degree of impaired carbohydrate tolerance present. On the other hand, the observation that in many cases the beta cells, despite prolonged hyperglycaemia and their reduced number, fail to develop cytological signs of hyperactivity, suggests that in these diabetics the beta cells may be relatively insensitive to the stimulus of an elevated blood glucose.

Long-standing diabetes is commonly associated with an abnormal thickening of the basement membrane of the capillaries throughout the body. This *per se* is not pathognomonic of diabetes. It occurs for example as part of the normal ageing process; however the increased permeability of the thickened basement membrane in diabetes is a unique pathological features. The main clinical and pathological impact of this micro-angiopathy is to be found in the retina, kidney and nervous system. (p. 477).

Clinical Features. Two main types of diabetes have long been recognised, and it is now clear that the level of plasma insulin correlates well with the clinical picture and the type of treatment subsequently required.

1. IDDM usually develops during the first 40 years of life in patients of normal or less than normal weight. The majority develop severe symptoms of diabetes acutely, over a period of several weeks or months and if treatment with insulin is withheld they rapidly develop fatal ketoacidosis.

2. NIDDM usually appears in middle-aged or elderly patients who are often obese and in whom hyperglycaemia can usually be controlled by dietary means alone or, if not, by an oral hypoglycaemic compound. Insulin is detectable in the plasma of nearly all patients in this category, and they are therefore less prone to develop ketosis. In this sense the disease is less severe than IDDM; however, the complications associated with long-term diabetes occur in both types. Many patients with NIDDM have a long history of mild symptoms which may come and go, and which may frequently be ignored or misdiagnosed for years before the true diagnosis is made.

Apart from patients with established clinical diabetes, two other categories are recognised.

1. *Potential diabetics* are persons with a normal

glucose tolerance test who nevertheless have an increased liability to develop diabetes for genetic reasons, e.g. the children of two diabetic parents; the children of parents where one is diabetic and the other has a first degree relative who is diabetic; the non-diabetic member of a pair of identical twins where the other is diabetic.

2. *Latent diabetics* are persons in whom the glucose tolerance test is normal, but who are known to have given an abnormal result under conditions imposing a burden on the pancreatic beta cells, e.g. during pregnancy, infection or other severe stress, mental or physical, during treatment with cortisone or other diabetogenic drugs, or when overweight.

PRESENTATION. Diabetes may be discovered in one of several ways:

1. Many patients are first noted to have glycosuria in the course of some routine examination. They may have had few or no symptoms, and no abnormal physical signs may be found.

2. Some patients present complaining of some or all of the classical symptoms of diabetes, including thirst, polydipsia, polyuria, nocturia, tiredness, loss of weight, white marks on clothing, pruritus vulvae or balanitis, impotence, a change in refraction usually in the direction of myopia and parasthesiae or pain in the limbs.

The severity of many of the classical symptoms of clinical diabetes are directly related to the severity of glycosuria. If relatively mild hyperglycaemia has developed slowly over many years the renal threshold for glucose will rise, glycosuria may be slight, and the symptoms of diabetes correspondingly trivial.

3. Diabetes may first present as a fulminating ketoacidosis associated with an acute infection or even without evidence of a precipitating cause, and in such cases epigastric pain and vomiting may be the presenting complaints. This is more likely to occur in IDDM and such cases are acute medical emergencies.

4. Patients may present with symptoms due to the complications of diabetes.

PHYSICAL SIGNS depend very much on the mode of presentation. Cases without complications will usually show no abnormal physical signs attributable to diabetes. In some cases vulvitis or balanitis may be found, since the external genitalia are especially prone to infection by fungi (Candida) which flourish on the skin and mucous membranes contaminated by glucose.

In the fulminating case the most striking features are those of dehydration. The intraocular pressure may be obviously reduced. A rapid pulse and a low blood pressure may then be anticipated. Breathing may be deep and sighing in the acidotic patient; the breath is usually fetid and the sickly sweet smell of acetone may be noticeable. Apathy and confusion may be present or there may be stupor or even coma.

Evidence of complications of diabetes may be noted. Ophthalmoscopy may show the typical appearance of diabetic retinopathy (p. 478). The most constant early signs of diabetic neuropathy are depression or loss of the ankle jerks, and impaired vibration sense in the legs (p. 663).

The presence of diabetic nephropathy may be indicated by proteinuria in addition to glycosuria; rarely the other features of the nephrotic syndrome may be apparent.

Potential and latent diabetic patients usually complain of no symptoms and show no abnormality on examination. However certain features are recognised as being characteristic of potential diabetes without necessarily implying that such individuals will progress to clinical diabetes. For example genetically constituted potential diabetics are predisposed to coronary and peripheral arterial disease. They may show abnormal lipid patterns in response to oral contraceptives. They have a high incidence of still-born or abnormally large and heavy babies and babies with congenital defects. Potential and latent diabetics may be much overweight at a time when there is no detectable abnormality in terms of carbohydrate intolerance.

Diagnosis. By definition hyperglycaemia remains the *sine qua non* of the clinical diagosis of diabetes mellitus. In the individual case when the classical symptoms are present, the diagnosis is often beyond reasonable doubt by the time the history taking and physical examination are complete, and it may then be confirmed by the finding of marked glycosuria, with or without ketonuria, and a random blood sugar greater than 14.0 mmol/l (250 mg/100 ml). However in many cases, particularly those with NIDDM who have few if any symptoms, and where glycosuria is frequently discovered by chance, the diagnosis is less obvious and a glucose tolerance test will be required.

URINE TESTING. *Glycosuria.* For individual screening purposes sensitive and glucose-specific dip-stick methods are available. Clinistix consists of a paper stick impregnated with an enzyme preparation which turns purple when dipped in urine containing glucose. No other urinary constituent gives this reaction: it therefore provides a rapid and specific qualitative test for glucose. A positive response indicates that the urinary glucose concentration exceeds 0.55–1.11 mmol/l (10–20 mg/100 ml), but does not measure the amount accurately. Semiquantitative measurement of urinary reducing activity can be obtained using copper reduction methods, most conveniently with the Clinitest tablet.

If a sample collected during the 2 hours following a meal is examined, then more of the milder cases of diabetes will be recognised than if an overnight specimen is tested. The most serious disadvantage in the use of the urine test diagnostically arises from individual variations in renal threshold, so that on the one hand some undoubtedly diabetic people have a negative urine test for glucose due to a raised renal threshold, and on the other those with a low renal threshold give a false positive test. In order to distinguish cases of this type from patients with mild diabetes, suitable tests of carbohydrate tolerance are required.

Detection of Ketone Bodies in Urine. Clinically important amounts of ketone bodies can be recognised by the nitroprusside reaction which is conveniently carried out using Acetest tablets or Ketostix test papers. Ketonuria may be found in normal people who have been fasting for long periods, who have been vomiting repeatedly or who have been eating a diet very high in fats and low in carbohydrate. Ketonuria is therefore not pathogonomic of diabetes, but if both ketonuria and glycosuria are found, the diagnosis of diabetes is practically certain.

RANDOM BLOOD SUGAR. In many cases the clinical diagnosis of diabetes can be made with the help of a single blood sugar estimation, which may be used as the final confirmatory test when the symptoms strongly suggest the diagnosis. In these circumstances a random blood sugar exceeding 14.0 mmol/l (250 mg/100 ml) is almost certain to indicate diabetes. However, a random blood sugar below this level does not exclude diabetes, and in this case some degree of standardisation of the conditions under which the blood sugar is measured is necessary. In practice, the oral glucose tolerance test is the cornerstone of the diagnosis of diabetes unless a grossly elevated single blood sugar measurement, with or without clinical symptomatology, has already made this clear.

THE ORAL GLUCOSE TOLERANCE TEST (Fig. 12.6). The patient, who should have been on an unrestricted carbohydrate intake of at least 150 g for 3 days or more, fasts overnight. Out-patients should rest for at least half an hour before starting the test, and should remain seated and refrain from smoking during the test. A sample of blood is taken to measure the fasting blood glucose level and 50–100 g glucose dissolved in 250–350 ml of water is then given by mouth. Thereafter samples of blood are collected at half-hourly intervals for at least 2 hours, and their glucose content is estimated.

The WHO Expert Committee on Diabetes (1980) recommended that a 75 g glucose load should be used and that the following concentrations of glucose in venous whole blood (estimated by a specific enzymatic assay) should be accepted as normal or diabetic respectively. Values for plasma glucose are about 15% higher than those for whole blood.

Glucose concentration mmol/l (mg/100 ml)

	Normal	Diabetic
Fasting	<5.5 (100)	>7.0 (120)
2 hours after glucose	<7.0 (120)	>10.0 (180)

Intermediate readings indicate the need for further evaluation of the patient, including the history obtained. It may be necessary to keep the patient under observation and to repeat the test at a later date. In pregnancy those with intermediate readings should be treated as diabetic since even minimal hyperglycaemia is associated with an increased fetal loss rate.

Differential Diagnosis of Glycosuria. *Renal Glycosuria.* Apart from diabetes, the common-

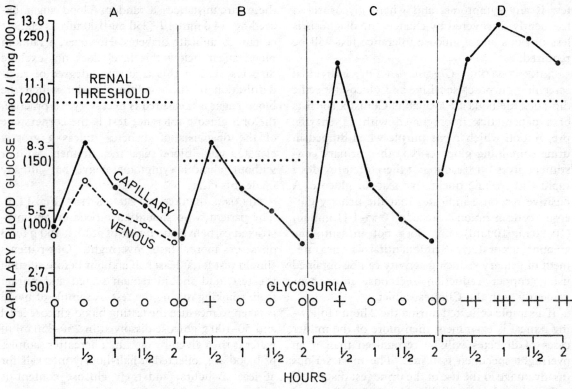

Fig. 12.6 The glucose tolerance test: blood glucose curves after 75 g glucose by mouth, showing (A) normal curve, (B) renal glycosuria, (C) alimentary (lag storage) glycosuria and (D) diabetes mellitus of moderate severity.

est cause of glycosuria is a low renal threshold for glucose, or renal glycosuria (p. 379). This is a benign condition unrelated to diabetes. Renal glycosuria also commonly occurs temporarily in pregnancy, due probably in this case to an increase in the glomerular filtration rate. Renal glycosuria is unrelated to diabetes, and is not accompanied by the symptoms associated with glycosuria in diabetes, i.e. thirst and polyuria, although pruritus vulvae and even ketonuria may occur.

Renal glycosuria is a much more frequent cause of glycosuria than diabetes in young persons, particularly in the age group 20 to 30 years, when they are commonly examined prior to entering the armed services, professions and industry. In the older age groups the reverse holds, and significant hyperglycaemia can occur without any or minimal glycosuria. For this reason if urine tests for glucose are used as a method of screening for diabetes, some cases will be missed, so that a glucose tolerance test or at least a single blood glucose estimation 2 hours after an oral dose of 75 g of glucose should be used whenever possible.

It may be important to determine the renal threshold for glucose; this can be done reliably only by testing samples of urine for glucose taken at intervals of half an hour in the course of a glucose tolerance test and relating the results to the blood glucose concentration (Fig. 12.6). This information may be important in the occasional diabetic with a low renal glucose threshold who, if attempts are made to control the diabetes on urine tests alone, may be kept in a persistent state of hypoglycaemia.

Alimentary (Lag Storage) Glycosuria. In some individuals an unusually rapid but transitory rise of blood glucose follows a meal and the concentration exceeds the normal renal threshold; during this time glucose will be present in the urine. This response to a meal or to a dose of glucose is traditionally known as 'lag storage', although alimentary glycosuria is a better term; it is not uncommon as a cause of symptomless glycosuria.

It may occur in otherwise normal people or after a partial gastrectomy, when it is due to rapid absorption, or in patients with hyperthyroidism or hepatic disease. This type of blood glucose curve is usually regarded as benign and unrelated to diabetes; although the peak blood glucose is abnormally elevated, the value 2 hours after oral glucose is normal (Fig. 12.6).

Other Metabolic Disorders. Impaired carbohydrate tolerance with associated glycosuria may occur with any of the forms of secondary diabetes (p. 458).

Carbohydrate deprivation can lead to the development of a diabetic type of blood glucose curve with associated glycosuria in normal people. It would seem, however, that the daily carbohydrate intake has to be less than about 50 g before it has a notable effect. This effect of a low carbohydrate intake may be of importance clinically in relation to the diagnosis of diabetes in a person on a weight reducing diet or if acutely ill with a low daily intake of food.

The Management of Diabetes Mellitus

Aims of Treatment. The ideal treatment for diabetes would allow the patient to lead a completely normal life, to remain not only symptom-free but in positive good health, to achieve a normal metabolic state, and to escape the complications associated with long-term diabetes. Nowadays diabetic patients rarely die in ketoacidosis in any number, but the major problem which has emerged is the chronic invalidism, due to disease of both large and small blood vessels (p. 477), of many of those whose duration of life has been extended.

Although the relationship between the degree of control and the development of serious diabetic complications is not a simple one, it would appear that the vascular abnormalities are secondary to the metabolic abnormalities occurring in diabetes, since they are found in both primary and secondary diabetes and can be produced experimentally in animals rendered diabetic by various methods. Moreover data from clinical studies strongly suggest that although genetic factors may affect the susceptibility to develop complications, the incidence of serious retinopathy is related to the degree of diabetic control achieved. It is therefore incumbent on all those who are involved in looking after diabetic patients to strive in every way to achieve as good control as is practicable in terms of blood glucose concentration.

Bearing these general principles in mind the immediate aims of treatment are therefore, first, the abolition of symptoms of diabetes while avoiding hypoglycaemia, second, the correction of hyperglycaemia and glycosuria and, third, the attainment and maintenance of an appropriate body weight.

Patients should realise as early as possible that it is upon themselves that success or failure will depend. The doctor can only advise. As adherence to a diabetic regimen demands from the patient self-discipline and a sense of purpose, every effort should be made to ensure that the object of each aspect of management is understood. Accordingly, time must be spent on the education of the patient, and the doctor must be responsible for ensuring that all diabetic patients are educated to the limit of their abilities and that as far as possible they have adjusted adequately to their condition and have sufficient knowledge to undertake the day-to-day management of their diabetes competently.

As soon as the diagnosis is certain the patient should be told and instruction and treatment begun forthwith. The average patient suffers initially from an acute anxiety reaction for which explanation is the best remedy. Moreover understanding is likely to lead to better cooperation in treatment.

Type of Treatment. There are three methods of treatment, namely diet alone, diet and oral hypoglycaemic drugs and diet and insulin. Each obliges the patient to adhere to a lifelong dietary regimen. Approximately 60% of new cases of diabetes can be controlled adequately by diet alone, about 20% will need an oral hypoglycaemic drug and another 20%, mainly younger patients, will require insulin. The principles governing the choice of therapeutic regimen when a diabetic patient is seen for the first time are discussed on page 471. A patient may pass from one group to another temporarily or permanently.

Diet. GENERAL PRINCIPLES. The treatment of all diabetic patients, especially those who require insulin, involves some dietary restrictions if control is to be satisfactory. By regulating the amount and the time of food intake, particularly of carbohydrate, and by dove-tailing the dose of insulin, or of oral hypoglycaemic agent, an attempt is made to achieve a flat profile of glycaemia throughout the day and night. It is obvious that if the intake of food varies from day to day it is impossible to work out a steady insulin or other regimen to cover it. Patients should understand that this is the main reason for dietary restriction and not the exclusion of certain 'bad' foods.

If one is to achieve a fixed daily intake and avoid the monotony of a static diet sheet, some kind of exchange system is necessary; this is the basis for the construction of nearly all diets in use today. Many doctors are intimidated by the number and variety of diet sheets published and feel that, since they are not trained dietitians, they cannot treat diabetes. A dietitian is certainly most helpful but is not indispensable; the basic principles of an exchange system of dietary treatment are simple, although the education of a patient in their use is time-consuming.

The first step in preparing any dietary regimen is to map out a time-table of the patient's day including a description of the usual meals. This is an essential step and one which is too often omitted. The total daily requirement of calories must next be decided. The diet must be nutritionally adequate for the patient's needs, and it must, therefore, be estimated for each individual patient after considering such factors as age, sex, actual weight in relation to desirable weight (Table 21.2 p. 816), activity, occupation and financial resources. An approximate range for the various groups might be (1) an obese, middle-aged or elderly patient with mild diabetes 1000–1600 kcal daily, (2) an elderly diabetic but not overweight, 1400–1800 kcal daily, (3) a young, active diabetic, 1800–3000 kcal daily. The body weight must be maintained at or slightly below the ideal for the patient's height. Thus the calorie range of group 2 may have to be extended if it is not sufficient to maintain weight, and young patients in group 3 who are overweight may have to reduce their daily intake to below 1800 kcal, perhaps temporarily.

Next the proportion of calories derived from carbohydrate, protein and fat must be allocated. The approximate ratio in the British national diet is, protein 12%, fat 42% and carbohydrate 46%. Although all sucrose should be eliminated from the diet the percentage of calories derived from carbohydrate should usually be increased slightly, those from protein increased if this is practicable, and those from fat reduced. In most diabetic diets, therefore, the percentage of calories derived from carbohydrate should be about 50%, from protein 15% and about 30–35% from fat.

The daily intake of *carbohydrate* to be prescribed ranges from the minimum sufficient to prevent ketonuria, that is, 100 g daily, to a maximum of 240–260 g. The upper limit is imposed by the fact that it is difficult to achieve satisfactory blood glucose levels throughout 24 hours with a daily carbohydrate intake greater than this. If the daily intake of carbohydrate is 240 g, aproximately 50 g carbohydrate will usually be provided by each of the three main meals, 20 g by each of three snacks and 30 g by one pint of milk (540 ml) taken in the course of the day. It is very difficult to prevent an excessive rise in the blood glucose concentration after each meal with amounts larger than this even when all the carbohydrate consumed is in the form of starch. A simple method of calculating the carbohydrate content of the diet is to allocate a figure equivalent to one-tenth of the total calories plus approximately 30–50 g to carbohydrate, that is, if a diet of 1800 kcal is prescribed it should contain about 210–230 g of carbohydrate, providing 840–920 kcal or approximately 50% of the total. All the carbohydrate eaten should be in the form of starch. Readily absorbed carbohydrates, such as glucose and sucrose, should generally be avoided because they produce a sudden rise in the blood glucose. A high intake of fibre will increase satiety and reduce constipation and may help to lower serum lipid and blood glucose.

The consumption of *protein* is largely determined by social and economic considerations and will frequently be lower than would be considered desirable. If this is the case, every effort should be made to increase the protein intake and to try to ensure that some protein is eaten at each main meal. An adequate consumption of protein is necessary in children and adolescents to ensure satisfactory growth, and since amino acids stimulate the beta cells of the pancreas to secrete insulin, in both normal subjects and those with NIDDM, a smaller rise in blood glucose occurs when carbohydrate is consumed along with protein. In both categories of diabetic patients consumption of protein will also promote satiety and so help them to keep more strictly to their carbohydrate allowance. A minimum amount of protein should therefore be specified in all diabetic diets, but in the case of those who are not obese it should be emphasised that more may be taken if desired. The daily consumption of protein will usually lie in the range of 60–110 g.

The *fat* intake should be adjusted to bring the total calories to the level desired, and will usually amount to 50–150 g daily. Because diabetic patients have an increased risk of death from ischaemic heart disease which may be related to the amount of saturated fat in the diet, the total amount of fat should be restricted even in those who are not obese. Plasma lipids, particularly cholesterol, should be checked regularly and if significantly elevated the diabetic diet may be appropriately modified (p. 486).

When the patient's requirements have been assessed the figures must be translated into practical and comprehensible instructions for the patient with the help of a diet sheet (p. 813). Each patient should be given a list of exchanges with instructions regarding the meals at which they may be taken. The diet sheet and exchanges must be discussed with the patient repeatedly and with a relative if necessary until the system is fully understood.

TYPES OF DIET. Basically there are two types of diet: (1) measured, in which the amount of food to be eaten at each time of the day is specified, and (2) unmeasured, in which the patient is supplied with a list of foods grouped in three categories: foods with a high sucrose content which are to be avoided altogether; foods containing carbohydrate in the form of starch which are to be eaten in moderation only; and non-carbohydrate foods which may be eaten as desired.

Measured Diets. In these diets the portions of food may be measured either by weighing with scales or more simply by using household measures. Measured diets are required for two groups of patients, (a) those who require insulin or an oral hypoglycaemic agent, and (b) those who are overweight and require a strict reducing regimen.

Patients in group (a) should if at all possible weigh out the portions of food initially. They should be provided with simple dietetic scales for this purpose. After a few weeks most patients are capable of assessing the weight of portions with sufficient accuracy by eye, and regular weighing becomes less necessary. However it is often valuable to check visual assessments by weighing from time to time. A method of constructing a sample diet of 1800 kcal suitable for patients in group (a) is described on page 813. It is important to realise that the exchanges or portions employed as units are arbitrary and are decided mainly in the light of the food habits of the population as a whole. The British Diabetic and Dietetic Associations have recommended that the carbohydrate unit should contain 10 g carbohydrate. In Britain the staple carbohydrate food is bread, and the basic carbohydrate exchange for the purposes of calculation is therefore taken to be $\frac{2}{3}$ oz bread which contains 10 g carbohydrate, along with 2 g protein and $\frac{2}{3}$ g fat. This is the reason why a carbohydrate exchange contains some protein and fat in addition to carbohydrate. Note also that a protein exchange contains some fat.

Diabetics who are obese should be urged to accept a reducing regime (p. 84). The method of achieving reduction in weight is the same for obese diabetic patients as for those with simple obesity. The diet on page 812 will meet the needs of many. The portions in this diet can be weighed with scales but more usually are dispensed using household measures as described in this diet. It should be explained that such a strict diet is to be followed only temporarily until the standard weight is reached; thereafter the diet may be increased, and if the patient is sufficiently intelligent, advice can then be given on how to avoid monotony by using a list of exchanges for diabetic diets (p. 813–814).

Unmeasured Diets. If insulin or oral hypoglycaemic agents are not required and marked obesity is not present it may not be necessary for the patient to follow such an accurate diet. Sometimes it may be impracticable to do so because of the patient's mental, visual or other physical incapacity or unwillingness to cooperate. Many patients develop the disease when they are already middle-aged or elderly and have a mild type of diabetes often associated with moderate obesity. For such patients an unmeasured diet of the type described on page 814 may be adequate.

Alcohol. There is no medical objection to taking alcoholic drinks in moderation provided the patient realises that account must be taken of their calorie value and sometimes of their carbohydrate content. Beer may contain 10–30 g of carbohydrate per half litre (1 pint approx.) and with the alcohol this will provide 150–400 kcal, depending on the strength of the beer. Sweet wines and cider all have a high carbohydrate content, and spirits such as whisky and gin, while free of carbohydrates, contain about 70 kcal per 30 ml.

Sweetening Agents. Advice may also be asked about sweetening agents and so-called diabetic foods and drinks. Saccharin has been employed as a sweetening agent for many years. It has no calorie value. Sorbitol, a glucose derivative, and fructose are also added to 'diabetic' foods and drinks for sweetening purposes. In moderate quantities neither will interfere with the action or requirements of insulin. If a patient is having difficulty in reducing weight or in maintaining a normal weight, then the use of substitutes for sugar should be discouraged, since they may perpetuate the patient's desire to eat sweet foods and thus make it more difficult to tolerate dietary restrictions. Diabetic chocolate has a high fat content and this must be taken into account.

Oral Hypoglycaemic Drugs. A number of compounds are effective in reducing hyperglycaemia in patients who would otherwise require insulin. The sulphonylureas, tolbutamide and chlorpropamide, and to a lesser extent the biguanide, metformin, have a place in the management of about 20% of diabetic patients. Although their mechanism of action is different, the action of both groups depends upon a supply of endogenous insulin, and it is therefore futile and dangerous to attempt to control IDDM with these compounds.

SULPHONYLUREAS. These drugs are valuable in the treatment of patients with NIDDM who fail to respond to simple dietary restriction and who are not overweight. Although their initial hypoglycaemic action is associated with an increased amount of immunoreactive insulin in peripheral plasma, their long-term hypoglycaemic effect seems to be mainly due to extrapancreatic actions. These include reduced hepatic release of glucose and improved sensitivity to insulin, possibly due to an increase in the number of peripheral insulin receptors.

Tolbutamide is the mildest, and probably also the safest, of the sulphonylureas. Since its effective action does not exceed 6 to 8 hours it should be administered two to three times a day. The dose varies between 1 and 2 g daily. It is very well tolerated and toxic reactions such as rashes occur only rarely. Tolbutamide is a useful drug in the elderly where the risk and the consequences of inducing hypoglycaemia are increased. Unfortunately, the relapse rate is relatively high.

Chlorpropamide has a biological half-life of about 36 hours, and an effective concentration can be maintained in the blood by a single dose at breakfast. The usual maintenance dose is between 100 and 375 mg daily; larger doses should not be used on a long-term basis, since above this level there is an increased risk of toxic effects, such as jaundice, rashes, and blood dyscrasia.

If alcohol is taken following chlorpropamide an unpleasant flushing of the face occurs in some patients. This is a dominantly-inherited trait associated with NIDDM. The demonstration that this reaction can be blocked with naloxone suggests that these patients may have inherited an unusual sensitivity to endorphins.

Chlorpropamide may lead to severe hypoglycaemia, which can be very refractory to treatment. Great care must be taken to avoid this, particularly in elderly patients, and once glycosuria has been abolished and symptoms relieved, the daily dose of chlorpropamide must be reduced to the minimum required to maintain control. In fact many patients who require 375–500 mg daily initially can be maintained on a long-term basis on 100 mg or less per day.

Other sulphonylureas such as acetohexamide, tolazamide, glibenclamide, glipizide and glymidine are more expensive and usually offer little advantage over chlorpropamide but may be useful in individual patients.

BIGUANIDES. The biguanides, metformin and phenformin, are less widely used in Britain than the sulphonylureas, because of the higher incidence of side-effects, particularly gastrointestinal symptoms and because there have been a significant number of deaths from lactic acidosis in patients taking these drugs, particularly phenformin. However, metformin is useful in two clinical situations. Firstly, since its administration is not associated with an increase in weight it may be preferred when it is essential to treat a patient with NIDDM who is overweight but in whom hyperglycaemia persists despite efforts to adhere to a diet and reduce weight. Secondly, as the hypoglycaemic effect of the biguanides appears to be synergistic with that of the sulphonylureas, there is a place for combining the two when the sulphonylureas alone have proved inadequate and when, as happens with 5 to 10% of patients, initial success is followed after several months, or even years, by loss of control.

Metformin is given with food in two or three daily doses of 0·5-1·0 g each. Its use is contraindicated in patients with impaired renal or hepatic function and in those who take alcohol in excess, as the risk of lactic acidosis occurring is significantly increased in such patients. Its administration should be discontinued, at least temporarily, if any other serious medical condition develops, and treatment with insulin substituted.

CLINICAL USE OF SULPHONYLUREAS AND BIGUANIDES. Patients may be started on an oral hypoglycaemic drug as soon as it is clear that dietary measures alone are inadequate. Evidence of some response is usually apparent within a week, though a full response may not occur for considerably longer. Diabetics treated successfully in this way for prolonged periods may ultimately need an alteration of dose or a change of regime temporarily or permanently; in particular they may require insulin to meet the need created by a severe infection, an operation or other stress.

There is some evidence that those taking an oral hypoglycaemic drug are at increased risk of dying from ischaemic heart disease. This may be due to a high incidence of ventricular fibrillation in diabetic patients on oral therapy who sustain a myocardial infarct. Efforts should therefore be made to control as many patients as possible by diet alone for this and other reasons (p. 471). Furthermore those taking oral hypoglycaemic drugs who develop a myocardial infarct should have these replaced by insulin during the acute illness and have a longer period of close supervision than non-diabetics, preferably in a coronary care unit.

Insulin. With one or more of the preparations of insulin available it is usually possible to keep the blood glucose within reasonable, although not physiological, limits throughout the day and night without undue risk of hypoglycaemia.

Two main therapeutic forms of insulin are available, namely (1) unmodified, rapid-onset, short-acting and (2) modified or depot, delayed-onset, long acting preparations. There are various varieties of each type some of which are shown in Table 12.1. The older insulins contain varying amounts of glucagon, pro-insulin, altered insulin and other peptides, which are largely responsible for the insulin-binding antibodies found in the plasma of all patients treated with these insulins. Highly purified, 'monocomponent' or 'single peak' insulins prepared from pig and cattle pancreases and synthetic human insulin are now available which are much less antigenic and are gradually superseding the older preparations. Care must be taken to avoid hypoglycaemia when transferring patients from the older to the newer preparations, and the higher the dose of conventional insulin, the stricter the supervision required. Insulins are available in concentrations of 20, 40, 80 and 100 International Units per ml. If required they may also be supplied in a concentration of 320 and 500 IU/ml.

UNMODIFIED INSULINS. These are clear solutions in contrast to the depot insulins which are cloudy. When injected subcutaneously, unmodified insulin is effective in 20-30 mins but the action is relatively short-lived (Table 12.1). A patient stabilised on unmodified insulin alone would therefore need at least two injections in the day.

Unmodified insulin is essential in (1) new cases with severe dehydration or ketoacidosis (2) emergencies associated with ketosis, such as acute infection, gastroenteritis and some surgical operations and (3) the treatment of nearly all young patients.

Table 12.1 Main types of preparations of insulin and duration of effect

Type	Approximate duration of effect in hours
Rapid/short — unmodified	
Soluble (regular) insulin injection (acid)	6
Neutral insulin injection	
Intermediate — modified — depot	
Insulin zinc suspension amorphous (Semilente)	12
Isophane insulin injection	12 +
Slow/long — modified — depot	
Insulin zinc suspension crystalline (Ultralente)	24
Protamine zinc insulin injection	

All these insulins are available in 'highly purified' form. This description covers several levels of purity since no precise specifications of purity are available at present. They may be prepared from beef, pork or synthetic human insulin.

MODIFIED (DEPOT) INSULINS. In some elderly patients with mild diabetes satisfactory control can be established by a single morning injection of depot insulin. Most insulin-requiring diabetics however need a depot insulin with one or two supporting doses of unmodified insulin to achieve good control throughout 24 hours. The choice of depot insulin in an individual case is determined by consideration of the patient's way of life, including the meal pattern, type of occupation, hours of work and recreation, in relation to the time of action of the various depot insulins. More insulin will be required to cover main meals and periods of inactivity, and vice versa.

Protamine Zinc Insulin (PZI). The addition of zinc and protamine to unmodified insulin delays its release from the site of injection, so that the effect of PZI is slow to start and is prolonged. Despite its prolonged action PZI alone does not usually keep the blood glucose within acceptable limits throughout the 24 hours. Glycosuria is most likely to occur before the morning injection has taken full effect, and an additional dose of unmodified insulin is generally required in the morning and sometimes in the evening, especially in young patients. Merely to increase the morning dose of PZI may result in severe hypoglycaemia later in the day or night. Indeed it is a good rule that the dose of PZI should not exceed 40 units at a single injection. When giving unmodified insulin and PZI together, the two should not be mixed in the syringe since the excess protamine in the PZI will convert some of the unmodified insulin into PZI.

Insulin Zinc Suspensions (IZS). The rate of release of these insulins from the tissues is related to the size of the insulin particles which are suspended in acetate buffer.

Three preparations are available: (1) IZS amorphous (*semilente*) insulin has a duration of action which is intermediate between that of unmodified and protamine zinc insulin. (2) IZS crystalline (*ultralente*) insulin is slower in action than IZS amorphous insulin (Table 12.1). (3) IZS (*lente*) insulin is a mixture of three parts of amorphous with seven parts crystalline.

Isophane insulin is another depot insulin similar in action to PZI, though its effect is less prolonged. Since isophane insulin contains an excess of unmodified insulin it can be mixed in the same syringe as unmodified insulin. This is convenient particularly if an automatic injector is used. Many younger patients are best treated with highly purified or synthetic isophane and soluble insulin taken twice daily.

In practice one must be prepared to try combinations of the various insulin preparations, and to vary the time at which they are administered in the light of the results of urine tests and blood glucose estimations at different times of the day until smooth control is achieved over 24 hours. It is impossible to forecast the response of a patient

PLATE I

A

A. Normal Retina. Painting of left eye showing arteries and veins, the white optic cup in the centre of a clean cut disc surrounded by a scleral ring (a normal variant). The darker red avascular area beyond the temporal side of the disc is typical of a normal macula. (Courtesy of Professor C. I. Phillips.)

B   C

B. Hypertensive Retinopathy. The upper half of this painting shows the retinal blood vessels in hypertension of moderate severity. The arteriolar blood column is narrower than normal and some sheathing of the upper temporal and nasal branches is shown. Variations in breadth of the arteriolar blood column indicates an irregular lumen. Veins at arterial-venous crossings are narrowed ('nipping'), partly because of pressure by arterioles and also because opacity of the arterial wall obscures the venous blood column. The lower half of the painting shows severe hypertensive retinopathy. Haemorrhages and soft exudates are added to the abnormalities seen in the upper half and these are more marked. (Courtesy of Professor C. I. Phillips.)

C. Severe Hypertensive Retinopathy. Retinal painting showing haemorrhages, two soft exudates, numerous hard exudates including a macular star, and irregularity of the calibre of the arterioles. (Courtesy of Professor I. C. Michaelson.)

PLATE II

A

A. Diabetic retinopathy. Retinal painting showing microaneurysms, haemorrhages, hard exudates and dilated veins. (Courtesy of Professor I. C. Michaelson.)

B. Advanced proliferative diabetic retinopathy. Retinal photograph showing heavily vascularised sheets of fibrous tissue forming in the vitreous and mainly derived from the optic disc.

C. Papilloedema. Retinal photograph showing swelling of the disc and haemorrhages on or very near the disc.

D. Thrombosis of retinal vein. Photograph showing haemorrhages and exudates in the territory of the lower temporal branch of the central retinal vein. There is also pathological cupping of the disc due to raised intra-ocular pressure which predisposes to retinal thrombosis. (Courtesy of Professor C. I. Phillips.)

to insulin, and the daily dose required to establish control varies from 10 to 100 units or more.

Choice of Therapeutic Regimen. It must be emphasised that the regimen eventually adopted in each case of diabetes is chosen by a process of trial, and that changes may be needed as more is learned about the patient. The chief indications for the main types of therapeutic regimen are:

1. Practically all young patients who develop diabetes before the age of 40 require treatment with insulin. The majority will be best controlled by taking unmodified insulin along with one of the depot insulins in the morning, and a second dose of unmodified insulin, or of unmodified and depot insulin before the evening meal. Examples of suitable commercial preparations are Velosulin and Insulatard (Nordisk Laboratories) or Actrapid MC and Semitard MC or Monotard MC (Novo Industries) or Humulin S (soluble) and Humulin I (isophane)-(Eli Lilly) taken twice daily. The first two are highly purified pig insulins, the last is human insulin synthesised by recombinant DNA technology (p. 18).

2. The majority of patients developing the disease over the age of 40 can and should be controlled by diet alone. This applies particularly to obese patients, but others who are not overweight may also do well on dietary therapy alone.

3. Those over the age of 40 who fail to achieve satisfactory control by dietary measures alone will usually respond well to a sulphonylurea if they are not obese, or to a biguanide if they are obese. If adequate control is not achieved by one drug, a combination of sulphonylurea and biguanide may be tried. If this fails insulin will be required.

4. Elderly patients who require insulin will often do well with a relatively small dose (20 units) of a depot insulin alone. A few, particularly those who would otherwise require more than 40 units a day, should be given unmodified insulin in addition and some may require insulin twice daily.

It must be stressed again that obese patients should be treated by dietary restriction and weight reduction rather than by the administration of insulin or an oral hypoglycaemic agent. The advent of the 'insulin era' has obscured the remarkable improvement in glucose tolerance which usually results from reduction in weight.

Insulin and the sulphonylureas increase the appetite, and thus may increase weight and intensify the total disability.

Initiation of Treatment. It is desirable that the patient learns to manage all aspects of the disorder as quickly as possible, and this can best be done on an outpatient basis while leading a relatively normal existence at home and at work. However, patients being stabilised on insulin have to be seen daily at first and if this is not practicable, admission to hospital will be necessary. Hospital admission will also be necessary for patients with severe ketoacidosis. The therapeutic plan must include measures directed at any of the complications to which the diabetic is prone and which may already be present at diagnosis, namely coronary artery disease and hypertension, obliterative arterial disease, nephropathy, retinopathy, cataract, neuropathy, pulmonary tuberculosis and other infections, particularly of the skin and urinary tract (p. 480).

A practical point worth mentioning, since it may give rise to distress if not anticipated, is that blurring of vision, which may occur in a severe diabetic before treatment, may become noticeably worse after starting treatment with insulin or tablets. It is due to transitory osmotic abnormalities in the eye, especially the lens, and may persist for as long as several weeks after initiating treatment.

PATIENT'S EDUCATION. Every patient who is capable of learning must be taught how to test the urine with a Clinitest set (and sometimes with Acetest tablets also), to keep a record of the results and to understand their significance.

All patients requiring insulin must learn to measure their dose of insulin accurately with an insulin syringe, to give their own injections and to adjust the dose themselves on the basis of urine and/or blood tests and other factors such as illness, unusual exercise and insulin reactions. They should be made to experience an insulin reaction (p. 473).

All patients must have a working knowledge of diabetes, i.e. they must be able to recognise the symptoms associated with marked glycosuria and to understand their significance. They must be told that many drugs have undesirable effects on the diabetic state, as may also such other factors as illness of any kind or emotional upset. They should be advised to consult their doctor or clinic at once as soon as they are aware of any deterioration in health or tests which does not respond rapidly to the simple measures that they take themselves.

All patients must know how to take care of their feet, and learn to treat any infected lesion with respect. Regular chiropody is important especially for elderly patients.

Education of the patient is time-consuming and repeated practical demonstrations may also be required. It may be supplemented by reading appropriate booklets. It is only in this way that diabetic patients can safely undertake all normal activities while maintaining good control of their disease. If the patient is a child, or is blind, mentally defective or otherwise incapable, instructions must be given to a parent or other attendant.

It is a wise precaution for diabetic patients who are taking insulin or oral hypoglycaemic drugs to carry a card with them at all times stating their name and address, the fact that they are diabetic, the nature and dose of any insulin or other drugs they may be taking, and, in addition, giving the name, address and telephone number of their family doctor and any special diabetic clinic they may be attending. Suitable cards are provided by the British Diabetic Association for the use of members.

SUPERVISION OF PATIENT. Diabetics should be seen at regular intervals for the remainder of their lives. The object is to check the degree of control and if necessary to make appropriate alterations in treatment and to watch for any complications. Records should be kept so that the doctor is immediately on the alert if changes in health occur. The frequency of visits is determined by the severity of the disability and the reliability of the patient. For the general practitioner with diabetic patients scattered widely in his practice, this supervision may be difficult. For this reason and because of the need to develop and apply new and better techniques for the control of diabetes, many hospitals arrange diabetic clinics.

ASSESSMENT OF CONTROL. At the patient's regular visit to the diabetic clinic or general practitioner, the degree of control should be assessed by considering the patient's weight in relation to standard weight, the results of urine and/or blood glucose tests, the concentration of glycosylated haemoglobin (HbA_1) and the presence or absence of symptoms of either hyper- or hypoglycaemia.

Proper assessment of control is impossible unless in the course of normal activity the patient tests samples of urine and/or blood regularly. By selecting suitable times for the tests and tabulating the results, it is easy for the doctor or the experienced patient to decide whether the dose of insulin or hypoglycaemic drug should be changed, or whether the carbohydrate content of the diet or the time when it is taken should be altered.

Urine Testing. Diabetics taking insulin should test samples of urine obtained before breakfast, before the mid-day and evening meals, and at bedtime (prior to a bedtime snack if this is taken). The patient must empty the bladder and discard the urine about 30 minutes before passing a specimen for testing. Patients treated by diet alone or with oral hypoglycaemic agents should test the first morning specimen and a sample passed about 2 hours after the main meals of the day. The majority of all the above specimens should be either free of glucose or contain $\frac{1}{4}\%$ or less.

While the patient is being stabilised, tests will have to be carried out three or four times daily; when control is established the frequency can be greatly reduced. One daily preprandial test taken serially at different times of the day is much more informative about the state of control than a single test carried out at the same time daily. Alternatively, three or four tests can be performed on a single day once or twice weekly.

Blood Glucose Estimations. It is advisable to measure the blood glucose concentration at different times of the day as an additional index of the degree of control. Some patients can be taught to take capillary blood samples and measure the blood glucose concentration in these by means of enzyme impregnated sticks (e.g. Dextrostix or BM Glycemie 20–800), if possible with a simple colorimetric meter, to improve accuracy. In assessing the result it is important to consider the interval between taking the sample and the last meal and also previous physical activity. The aim should be to keep the fasting blood glucose level less than 7·0 mmol/*l* (120 mg/100 ml) and the post-prandial peak under 10·0 mmol/*l* (180 mg/100 ml).

Glycosylated Haemoglobin (HbA₁). When haemoglobin from a normal adult is passed through a chromatographic column it separates into the major component HbA (94% of the total) and several minor, faster-moving components collectively known as HbA_1 (6% of the total). These are structurally indentical to HbA except for the addition of a glucose group to the terminal aminoacid of the β chain. This is a post-synthetic, non-enzymatic reaction and the rate of synthesis of HbA_1 is a function of the blood glucose concentration. Since the glucose linkage is relatively stable, HbA_1 accumulates throughout the life span of the erythrocyte and its concentration reflects the mean blood glucose concentration over the previous few months. Measurement of HbA_1 can therefore be used as a supplement of urine tests and blood glucose estimations to monitor the degree of diabetic control achieved.

Insulin Reactions and Hypoglycaemia. If unmodified insulin is administered to a normal person the blood glucose falls, producing symptoms that may begin to appear when the concentration is about 2·7 mmol/*l* (50 mg/100 ml) and are fully developed at about 2·2 mmol/*l*. In diabetics who are constantly hyperglycaemic, the same symptoms may develop at higher levels, e.g. 6·6 mmol/*l* or more. The symptoms may include any one or more of the following: a feeling of being weak and empty, hunger, sweating, palpitation, tremor, faintness, dizziness, headache, diplopia and mental confusion. Abnormal behaviour, leading occasionally to arrest on a charge of being drunk and disorderly, may also occur. Alternatively, and particularly in children, there may be lassitude and somnolence or muscular twitchings. Eventually coma, sometimes with convulsions, may follow.

Hypoglycaemia induces secretion of adrenaline, and this in turn causes tachycardia and tremor. Adrenaline, by mobilising liver glycogen, combats the hypoglycaemia. This homeostatic reaction partly explains why patients rarely die of hypoglycaemic coma from too much unmodified insulin. By contrast, coma is dangerous when it arises from a large dose of depot insulin or from an overdose of a sulphonylurea, particularly chlorpropamide. The latter condition, although relatively uncommon, is resistant to treatment, since the drug reduces the hepatic release of glucose, and because the half-life of the drug is so long. The brain is dependent on the blood glucose for the energy necessary for its activity. Permanent brain damage may result from prolonged hypoglycaemia which should be prevented from recurring by prompt reduction of the dose of insulin or of sulphonylurea.

Hypoglycaemia due to overdosage with unmodified insulin comes on rapidly, at the time when the insulin is having its maximum effect that is, through the morning or in the early evening, and usually elicits classical symptoms and responds rapidly to treatment. Reactions from excessive depot insulin given before breakfast usually occur in the later afternoon, at night or early next morning. These reactions may begin gradually with little adrenaline response, become persistent and profound and respond more slowly to treatment. The predominant warning symptoms are very variable and include headache, malaise, night sweats, nausea leading sometimes to troublesome vomiting, mental confusion and drowsiness, especially in the morning.

TREATMENT OF HYPOGLYCAEMIC REACTIONS. Since hypoglycaemia can easily be corrected if recognised early, diabetic patients should experience the condition under supervision. In this way they learn to recognise the early symptoms. They must be made to realise that the most frequent causes of the condition are unpunctual meals and unaccustomed exercise, and seek to avoid both or to make adjustments to meet these circumstances. They should always carry some tablets of glucose or a few lumps of sugar for use in an emergency. Unless an attack of hypoglycaemia is adequately accounted for, the patient should reduce the next and subsequent doses of insulin by 20% and seek medical advice.

If the patient is so stuporous that swallowing is impossible an intravenous injection of 25 g of glucose (50 ml of a 50% solution) should be given. This may have to be repeated. Alternatively, the insulin-dependent patient may be given a subcutaneous or intramuscular injection of 1 mg of glucagon, repeated if necessary after 10 minutes. This raises the blood glucose by mobilising liver glycogen, and has the advantage of convenience in that it can be given by anybody capable of using a syringe, but it may not be effective in severe and prolonged hypoglycaemia due to depot insulins. In addition to increasing hepatic glycogenolysis, glucagon stimulates the secretion of insulin and therefore should not be used to treat hypoglycaemia induced by an oral hypoglycaemic agent.

As soon as the patient is able to swallow, glucose should be given orally. Full recovery may not occur immediately. Further, when hypoglycaemia has occurred in a diabetic using a depot preparation of insulin or a sulphonylurea, particularly chlorpropamide, the possibility of relapse within a day or more should be anticipated.

Repeated episodes of hypoglycaemia may lead to permanent intellectual deterioration; accordingly, adjustments to prevent recurrences are essential.

THE COMPLICATIONS OF DIABETES MELLITUS

Diabetic Ketoacidosis

Prior to the discovery of insulin more than 50% of diabetic patients ultimately died of ketoacidosis. Today this complication is preventable and accounts for less than 2% of diabetic deaths. However, both the incidence and the mortality rate are still regrettably high. Failure of the patient to understand the disease, and failure to appreciate the significance of symptoms of poor control are the most common causes. Thus its prevention is largely a problem of education of patients and at times of their physicians. A clear understanding of the biochemical disorders involved (p. 460) is essential for its efficient treatment which should aim at having the patient out of danger within 24 hours.

Water and Mineral Depletion. The deficit of total body water in a severe case may be about 6 litres. About half of this is derived from the intracellular compartment and occurs comparatively early in the development of acidosis with relatively few clinical features; the remainder represents loss of extracellular fluid sustained largely in the later stages. It is at this time that marked contraction of the size of the extracellular space occurs, with haemoconcentration, a decrease in the plasma volume, and finally a fall in blood pressure with associated renal ischaemia and oliguria.

The concentration of sodium and potassium in the serum gives very little indication of total body losses, and may even be raised due to disproportionate losses of water. Sodium loss, mainly from the extracellular space, may amount to as much as 500 mmol. Potassium loss from the cells may be 400 mmol or more. The concentration of potassium in the plasma in these circumstances is dependent on the balance between catabolism of protein and glycogen and haemoconcentration on the one hand, and urinary excretion on the other. Since the former generally exceeds the latter plasma potassium is likely to be high initially, in spite of a total body deficit. However, within a few hours of beginning treatment with insulin, there is likely to be a precipitous fall in the plasma potassium. At least three mechanisms are responsible for this; dilution of extracellular potassium by the administration of potassium-free fluids, the movement of potassium into the cells as the result of insulin therapy, and the continuing renal loss of potassium.

Ketoacidosis. The mechanism of the development of this state has been described (p. 460). Apart from the clinical findings, its severity can be rapidly assessed by measuring the plasma bicarbonate, less than 12 mmol/l indicating severe acidosis. The hydrogen ion concentration in the blood is an even more valuable guide but it may not be as readily available. There are no simple and accurate quantitative methods for the determination of plasma ketones.

Clinical Features. Any form of stress, particularly an acute infection, can precipitate severe ketoacidosis in even the mildest diabetic. The most common cause is neglect of treatment due to carelessness, misunderstanding or illness, and failure to adjust the therapeutic regimen in the event of an acute infection.

The symptoms of diabetic ketoacidosis invariably include intense thirst and polyuria. Constipation, cramps and altered vision are common. Sometimes, especially in children, there is abdominal pain, with or without vomiting. Hence diabetic ketoacidosis is important in the differential diagnosis of the acute abdomen. Weakness and drowsiness are commonly present, but it should be remembered that the state of consciousness is very variable and a patient with dangerous ketosis requiring urgent treatment may walk into hospital. For this reason the term diabetic ketoacidosis is to be preferred to 'diabetic coma', which suggests that there is no urgency until unconsciousness occurs. In fact it is imperative that energetic treatment is started at the earliest possible stage.

The signs include a dry tongue and soft eyeballs due to dehydration; 'air hunger' indicated by long, deep, sighing respirations; a rapid, weak pulse, and low blood pressure; sometimes abdominal rigidity and tenderness; the smell of acetone in the breath; ultimately coma supervenes.

INVESTIGATION. This shows (1) ketonuria and severe glycosuria; (2) blood glucose usually between 22·2 and 44·4 mmol/l (400 and 800 mg/100 ml), but it may be much higher and in some cases lower; (3) low plasma bicarbonate and blood pH; (4) normal or raised serum sodium and potassium; (5) leucocytosis.

Hyperglycaemia and ketoacidosis do not always necessarily correlate well. Even at a level of blood glucose as low as 19·4 mmol/l (350 mg/100 ml), life-threatening acidosis may be present. In contrast diabetic coma can occur, usually in elderly patients, with extreme hyperglycaemia and dehydration but no ketoacidosis. This is known as *hyperosmolar diabetic coma*.

Treatment. Ketoacidosis should be treated with urgency in hospital. Intravenous therapy is required since even when the patient is able to swallow, fluids given by mouth may be poorly absorbed. Establishing an intravenous infusion can be technically difficult because of collapsed veins, but cutting down and tying in a cannula should be avoided if at all possible, because the veins may be needed again.

Treatment must be checked against the blood concentration of glucose, potassium and bicarbonate estimated at intervals at first of not longer than 2 hours. Only in this way can the metabolic disorder be corrected accurately and rapidly. The aim should be to overcome with all speed:

(1) ketosis, by means of insulin to permit glucose utilisation; (2) shock, acidosis, and water and electrolyte depletion, by means of appropriate intravenous fluids; (3) infection, if present, by means of antibiotics.

Only unmodified insulins should be used. Ketosis and dehydration render the comatose patient relatively resistant to insulin. The conventional treatment of diabetic ketoacidosis has, therefore, involved the use of large doses of unmodified insulin. It is now known that such large doses of insulin are unnecessary and that low-dose regimens are just as effective, are less complicated and may be safer.

An infusion of saline is started and 20 units of unmodified insulin given by intramuscular injection immediately and 4–6 units hourly thereafter, either by intramuscular injection or intravenous infusion, preferably using a constant-rate pump (Fig. 12.7). The blood glucose concentration should fall by 3–6 mmol/l/hour. If there is no fall in the blood glucose concentration by two hours after starting treatment, then the dose of insulin should be doubled until a satisfactory response is obtained. When the blood glucose concentration has fallen to 10·0 mmol/l (180 mg/100 ml) 5% glucose should replace or be added to the saline infusion and the dose of insulin reduced to 1–4 units i.v. hourly, or 8–16 units four hourly by subcutaneous injection.

The deficit of extracellular fluid, which is usually about 3 litres, should be made good by infusion of saline isotonic with plasma (0·9% NaCl). A suitable regimen is 1 litre in half an hour, 1 litre in one hour, and then 1 litre in two hours until there is clinical improvement (Fig. 12.7). Elderly patients or those with cardiovascular disease will require modification of this regimen and monitoring of central venous pressure may be necessary. If during the treatment the serum sodium rises above 150 mmol/l, 0·45% saline should be given.

In cases which are also severely acidotic (pH < 7·0), 500 ml of the isotonic saline may be replaced by isotonic sodium bicarbonate (1·4%) and this may be repeated if the pH remains < 7·1 mmol/l. Correction of the total deficit should not be attempted since there is some evidence that rapid correction of acidosis in

Time (hours)	Insulin (unmodified preparation)		IV Fluid	IV Potassium (rate of infusion: mmol/hour)
	Intramuscular	Intravenous (rate of infusion: units/hour)		
0	20 Units (U)		*Isotonic (0.9%)saline 1.0 litre in 30 minutes	Check urinary output Obtain results for plasma electrolytes
	6 U	6 U/hour	0.5 litre in 30 minutes	If plasma concentration (mmol/l) is:
				>6 6–4.5 4.5–3 >3
			Give	↓ ↓ ↓ ↓
	*If plasma Na+ >155 mmol/l give 0.45% saline.		mmol K+/h	0 13 26 39
1	6 U	6 U/hour	0.5 litre in 30 minutes 0.5 litre/hour	Monitor plasma concentration every 1–2 hours and change infusion rate accordingly
2	6 U If fall in blood glucose <3 mmol/l/h switch to IV	6 U/hour If fall in blood glucose <3 mmol/l/h double rate	0.5 litre/hour	
3	CONTINUE 6 U every hour UNTIL blood glucose concentration <10 mmol/l, then give 1–4 U hourly	6 U hour 1–4 U/hour	0.25 litre/hour 5% glucose: 0.25 litre /hour	

NB: Average fluid deficit = 6 litres ⟨ 3.0 litres from Extra-cellular compartment replaced by NaCl / 3.0 litres from Intra-cellular   "   "   by glucose

Procedures: Intravenous line; catheterise after 3 hours if no urine passed; nasogastric tube to keep stomach empty. Central venous pressure line if cardiovascular system compromised so that volume of IV fluid can be adjusted·

Monitor: Blood glucose and electrolytes hourly for 3 hours and then 2–4 hourly; temperature, pulse, respiration, BP hourly; urinary output; urinary ketones; ECGs, blood osmolality, arterial pH, in some cases

Fig. 12.7 Management of diabetic ketoacidosis. N.B. These guidelines for the management of a typical, 'average' case should be modified appropriately in the individual patient after considering the blood biochemistry and clinical features (p. 475).

diabetic ketoacidosis may aggravate tissue hypoxia and may also reduce the level of consciousness by causing a paradoxical acidosis of the cerebrospinal fluid. The combined administration of bicarbonate and insulin will also increase the risk of hypokalaemia and potassium should be given along with bicarbonate.

The intracellular deficit of water, usually about 2–3 litres, must be replaced by using 5% glucose and not by more saline. It is best given when the blood glucose is approaching normal. It is important to continue the intravenous glucose together with appropriate doses of insulin until the ketonuria has disappeared and the water deficit has been made good.

Acute circulatory failure should be treated as described on page 149.

Every patient in diabetic ketoacidosis is potassium depleted and nearly all will require intravenous potassium (p. 93) to prevent the development of dangerous hypokalaemia during the course of treatment. As the serum potassium is often high at presentation, potassium therapy should be started cautiously and carefully monitored by frequent estimations of plasma potassium (Fig. 12.7). ECGs are sometimes helpful, a change in the T wave indicating a falling plasma potassium. Approximately 80 mmols of potassium may safely be given by vein in the first 16 hours, but much more than this may be required and sufficient must be given to maintain a normal plasma concentration. It is customary to add 1·5 g potassium chloride (20 mmol potassium) to each 500 ml of fluid given intravenously. Once oral feeding has started potassium chloride (p. 93) should be given 4-hourly for 2 to 3 days to restore the total body deficit.

In a stuporose or comatose patient, gastric aspiration should be undertaken to avoid the risk of inhaling vomitus. The stomach will often contain a large amount of brown fluid containing altered blood.

Infections must be carefully sought and vigorously treated since it may not be possible to abolish ketosis until they are controlled.

Once ketosis has been overcome and the salt and water deficit made good (usually in about 24 hours), feeding by mouth can be started with frequent small fluid feeds each containing 25 g carbohydrate. Two examples of such feeds are:

1. 100 ml (3½ oz) fruit juice plus 15 g (½ oz) of cane sugar or glucose.

2. 200 ml (7 ozs) milk plus 10 g (⅓ oz) cereal plus 7 g (¼ oz) sugar.

Sufficient insulin should be given to prevent further ketonuria or glycosuria. Control of blood glucose can be lost very quickly and frequent blood glucose estimations are needed. Unmodified insulin should be given before each oral feed, even if the urine is free of sugar and only very small doses are required.

HYPEROSMOLAR, NON-KETOTIC DIABETIC COMA. Treatment differs from that of ketoacidotic coma in two main respects. These patients seem to be relatively sensitive to insulin and it is probably best to give approximately half the dose of insulin usually employed in diabetic ketoacidosis. Once it is known that plasma osmolality is high (calculated by the formula $2 \times$ sodium mmol/l + glucose mmol/l = 285 mosmol/l normally) 0·45% saline should be given until the osmolality approaches normal, when 0·9% should be substituted.

COMA DUE TO LACTIC ACIDOSIS. Clinically the patient is likely to be a diabetic taking a biguanide, who is very ill and overbreathing, but not so profoundly dehydrated as is usual in coma due to ketoacidosis, and whose breath does not smell of acetone. Ketonuria is no more than mild, yet plasma bicarbonate and pH are markedly re-duced. Diagnosis is confirmed by a high (usually >5·0 mmol/l) concentration of lactic acid in the blood.

Treatment is with large amounts of intravenous bicarbonate; as much as 2500 mmols may be needed. Insulin is given by continuous intravenous infusion and glucose added when the blood level falls to about 10·0 mmol/l. Dialysis may be required in very severe cases (pH <7) if sodium overload results from the administration of large quantities of sodium bicarbonate. Despite such measures the mortality in this condition is greater than 50%.

Differential Diagnosis of Coma in a Diabetic. Confusion between coma due to hypoglycaemia and that associated with ketosis should seldom arise; the distinction is clear (Table 12.2). Diabetic coma may occasionally pass undetected into hypoglycaemic coma through too enthusiastic treatment; likewise, vomiting induced by hypoglycaemia from a depot insulin may continue until diabetic coma develops.

Hyperosmolar, non-ketotic diabetic coma and coma due to lactic acidosis are distinguished by the features given above.

Vascular Disorders

Vascular disease, arterial, arteriolar and capillary, is the largest and most intractable problem in clinical diabetes. Arterial disease is easily the commonest cause of death in diabetics over the age of 50, while nephropathy accounts for more than half the deaths under 50. Strict control probably offers the best chance of delaying the onset and progress of the vascular complications of diabetes.

Atherosclerosis occurs commonly and extensively in diabetes. The pathological changes in diabetics are not specific in a qualitative sense but they occur earlier and are more widespread than in non-diabetics. Thus diabetics are more prone at an earlier age than other people to myocardial infarction and hypertension. The peripheral pulses in the legs are often diminished or impalpable, and particularly in elderly patients, intermittent claudication and ischaemic changes in the feet are frequently present. Defective circulation in the legs resulting in poorly nourished tissues

Table 12.2 Differences in coma due to hypoglycaemia and ketoacidosis in IDDM.

	Hypoglycaemic coma	*Coma with ketosis*
History:	no food; too much insulin; unaccustomed exercise	too little or no insulin; an infection; digestive disturbance
Onset:	in good previous health; related to last insulin injection	ill-health for several days
Symptoms:	of hypoglycaemia; occasional vomiting from depot insulins	of glycosuria and dehydration; abdominal pain and vomiting
Signs:	moist skin and tongue full pulse normal or raised BP shallow or normal breathing brisk reflexes	dry skin and tongue weak pulse low blood pressure air hunger diminished reflexes
Urine:	no ketonuria no glycosuria, if bladder recently emptied	ketonuria glycosuria
Blood:	hypoglycaemia normal plasma bicarbonate	hyperglycaemia reduced plasma bicarbonate

predisposes to gangrene. If a painless peripheral neuropathy is present, this may also be of aetiological importance, since the patient will tend to ignore or neglect injuries and other damage to the tissues. Diabetic gangrene usually starts in one foot, following a trivial injury, such as the cutting of a corn, or a burn from a hot water bottle. Toxic absorption from necrotic tissue and secondary infection may kill the patient unless the limb is amputated. A great deal can be done to prevent these complications by instructing diabetics with a poor circulation to wear properly fitting shoes, to use bed-socks rather than hot water bottles, never to cut their own corns and 'to keep the feet as clean as the face'. The services of a skilled chiropodist are invaluable.

Diabetic Nephropathy

Diabetic Glomerulosclerosis. A specific type of renal lesion may occur as a result of the changes in the basement membrane of the glomerular capillaries. There are two types, diffuse and nodular. The former is the more common and consists of a generalised thickening of the basement membrane. The nodular type is a development of this, in which rounded masses of hyaline material sometimes called Kimmelstiel-Wilson bodies are superimposed upon the diffuse lesion. Diabetic glomerulosclerosis can be seen by light microscopy in about 70% of diabetic patients at autopsy.

Even with well-established diabetic glomerulosclerosis the patient may exhibit only slight to moderate proteinuria. In some cases, however, marked proteinuria and the nephrotic syndrome develop with increasing renal failure and uraemia.

There is no way of preventing or modifying the progression of nephropathy once this is clinically apparent as proteinuria. In the later stages the management is the same as in other forms of chronic renal disease. Regular haemodialysis is technically possible although access to the circulation or maintenance of a shunt may be affected by diseased peripheral vessels. Results are less good than in non-diabetics and may not justify the burden placed on the patient. The place of continuous ambulatory peritoneal dialysis (p. 394) is still uncertain. Renal transplantation is more hopeful and in some centres results, in carefully selected cases, are almost as good as in non-diabetics. Unfortunately many will not qualify for active intervention because of other disabilities such as severe large blood vessel disease, neuropathy, and retinopathy.

Diabetic Retinopathy

Retinopathy is the commonest long-term complication of diabetes. In most cases it produces no symptoms but it can cause blindness and in Britain diabetic retinopathy is now the single most common cause of blindness in the middle-aged.

Clinical Features. Some aspects of these are shown in Plate II; they occur in varying combinations in different patients. Abnormalities of the capillary bed are the earliest lesions. They include capillary dilatation and closure which are not clinically visible.

In most cases *microaneurysms* are the earliest clinical abnormality detected. They appear as minute, discrete, circular, dark-red spots near to, but apparently separate from, the retinal vessels. They look like tiny haemorrhages but photography of injected preparations of retina show that they are in fact minute aneurysms arising mainly from the venous end of capillaries near areas of capillary closure.

Venous abnormalities are among the commonest manifestations of diabetic retinopathy. Dilatation, irregularity and increased tortuosity of the retinal veins are all seen.

Haemorrhages, most characteristically occurring in the deeper layers of the retina and hence round and regular in shape, are also a relatively early feature. The smaller ones may be difficult to differentiate from microaneurysms and the two are often grouped together as 'dots and blots'.

Soft exudates, similar to those seen in hypertension, occur. *Hard exudates* are more common and are specific to diabetic retinopathy. They are yellow, with irregular, sharply defined edges, varying in size from tiny specks to large confluent often circular patches. They probably result from leakage of plasma from abnormal retinal capillaries and lie over areas of neuronal degeneration.

New vessels may arise from mature vessels on the optic disc or the retina. The earliest appearance is that of fine tufts of delicate vessels forming arcades on the surface of the retina. As they grow they may extend forwards towards the vitreous. They are fragile, readily leak and at first have no visible connective tissue covering. They are liable to rupture, causing haemorrhage which may be intraretinal, preretinal (subhyaloid) or into the vitreous. Serous products leaking from these new vessel systems stimulate a connective tissue reaction *retinitis proliferans*. This first appears as a white cloudy haze among the network of new vessels. As it extends the new vessels are obliterated and the surrounding retina is covered by a dense white sheet. At this stage bleeding is less

common but retinal detachment can occur due to contraction of adhesions between the vitreous and the retina.

CLASSIFICATION. Patients with only microaneurysms, retinal haemorrhages and exudates are classified as having *simple* or *background retinopathy*, while those with preretinal haemorrhage, new vessel formation, or fibrous proliferation are classified as having *proliferative* or *malignant retinopathy*. As with nephropathy, the duration of diabetes is the most important factor influencing the occurrence of retinopathy and some abnormality, even if only a single microaneurysm, can be seen in the fundi of at least 60% of diabetics who have had the condition for 30 years.

INTERFERENCE WITH VISION. In general, prognosis for vision is good for patients with simple retinopathy and bad for those with proliferative retinopathy, of whom half are blind within 5 years. Microaneuryms, abnormalities of the veins, blot haemorrhages and exudates will not interfere seriously with vision unless they are associated with macular oedema or directly involve the macula. Unfortunately all these lesions occur most commonly in the perimacular area. New vessels may be completely symptomless until sudden visual loss occurs from a haemorrhage into the vitreous. Although these frequently clear, the risk of recurrence is high and the more frequent the haemorrhage the slower and less complete the recovery. New vessel formation is potentially reversible and therefore treatable. Fibrous tissue may obscure the retina and seriously damage sight, and retinal-vitreal adhesions may pull the retina forward and produce retinal detachment causing blindness. Retinitis proliferans is the irreversible end-stage of diabetic retinopathy which cannot be influenced by any form of treatment at present available. Early detection and treatment of new vessel formation is therefore of vital importance.

Prevention. As microangiopathy seems to be secondary to the metabolic abnormality and there is evidence to suggest that good control of the diabetes reduces the chance of its development and may delay its progression to severe diabetic retinopathy, every effort should be made to maintain a normal metabolic state in all diabetic patients. It is a common error to suppose that diabetes which is 'mild', i.e. treated by diet alone, carries little risk of complications. Whatever the type of diabetes, duration of the disorder and sustained hyperglycaemia are the main factors associated with the development of microangiopathy.

Treatment. There is no specific treatment of simple retinopathy without maculopathy which is usually not associated with significant impairment of vision. The administration of clofibrate will clear hard exudates from the retina but will not affect the underlying neuronal degeneration. It may be of value in preventing further exudation but the possible benefits must be weighed against the risks (p. 486). The diabetes and any hypertension must be well controlled.

In simple retinopathy visual loss results from macular exudates, haemorrhage or oedema. Photocoagulation can be used to destroy abnormally leaking vessels in the perimacular area and thus reduce oedema. Coagulation of the centre of rings of hard exudates may hasten absorption of the exudates. The smaller spot size and shorter duration of the argon laser enables lesions nearer the macula to be treated.

The primary aim in treating proliferative retinopathy is to destroy new vessels by photocoagulation before vitreous haemorrhage, macular damage or retinal detachment occur. Light coagulation of new vessels on the retina can be done under local anaesthesia, and in skilled, experienced hands is a simple procedure which carries little risk and can be very effective.

Because diabetic retinopathy is now a treatable condition if diagnosed early, when it is commonly symptomless, all diabetic patients must have their eyes examined regularly, every 6 to 12 months, by a competent observer. To obtain adequate visualisation of the retina the pupils must be dilated with a mydriatic. Once there is evidence of progression of simple retinopathy, and particularly whenever new vessels are seen, the patient must be referred to an ophthalmologist for further supervision and treatment.

Cataract. Very rarely a specific type of opacity of the lens (cataract) occurs in diabetic children whose disease has not been adequately controlled. Cataract also occurs in elderly diabetics, but is said to be no more common than in other people in this age group.

Infections

Poor control of diabetes is associated with a lowered resistance to infection. Alternatively latent diabetes may be unmasked by a severe infection such as a carbuncle or pneumonia. Glucose tolerance may return to normal, at least temporarily, when the infection is controlled by appropriate antimicrobial therapy. Cleanliness is a special virtue in the prevention of skin infection which is common in diabetes.

Pulmonary Tuberculosis. If a diabetic under treatment shows unexplained loss of weight, increase in insulin requirements or symptoms of pulmonary disease, clinical and radiological examination of the lungs should be undertaken. Pulmonary tuberculosis can be arrested in its early stages by prompt recognition and specific treatment.

Urinary Tract Infections. The presence of glucose in the urine provides a favourable medium for the growth of bacteria. Persistent infections of the urinary tract frequently occur, and for this reason catheterisation in particular should be avoided. Treatment consists of controlling the glycosuria and specific therapy for the urinary tract infection.

Pruritus vulvae is very commonly associated with candidiasis (p. 802) in the diabetic woman. *Candida albicans* is nearly always present. In the majority, the treatment is abolition of glycosuria which brings rapid relief. In a few cases local treatment with nystatin cream and pessaries may be required.

Diabetic Neuropathy

Mononeuropathy, generalised polyneuropathy and autonomic neuropathy are frequent complications of diabetes at any stage and may give rise to troublesome manifestations. Involvement of the autonomic nervous system may result in an impaired sympathetic response to hypoglycaemia so that the patient no longer experiences the classical warning symptoms. Motor, sensory and autonomic nerves may be involved in varying combinations (p. 663).

SPECIAL PROBLEMS IN THE MANAGEMENT OF DIABETES MELLITUS

Diabetes in Children. Fortunately diabetes is not common in childhood, but when it occurs it is relatively severe and always requires treatment with insulin. The therapeutic problem of matching the dose of insulin to the food intake raises practical difficulties but the principles of treating children with diabetes are the same as for adults who have insulin-dependent diabetes. It is important to achieve as good control of the diabetes as possible and diabetic children and their parents need to be educated in the management of their disorder to the limit of their ability.

Diet. The nutritional needs of diabetic children are essentially no different from those of other children but because of growth their caloric requirements are large in proportion to their size, by comparison with adult standards. It may be difficult to provide enough calories because children's preferences for foods are often unpredictable. On the other hand the child must not become too fat; hypoglycaemia due to too much insulin can lead to excessive appetite and hence to obesity. A dietitian can do much to help the child and the parents. Diabetic children must not have sugar or sweets, but otherwise the diet need differ little from that of their friends. It is important that everything possible should be done to avoid distinguishing them from their contemporaries. Once trained, they may take part in the same range of activities as their peers, provided that appropriate supervision is arranged. The British Diabetic Association runs special camps for diabetic children.

Insulin. Day-to-day requirements for insulin are often very variable. Children's emotions and activities fluctuate unexpectedly — sometimes wildly active and sometimes sulking. This may have an important effect on their daily needs for insulin; excessive activity may result in hypoglycaemia, whilst lethargy may lead to hyperglycaemia. The latter may also be caused by any one of the numerous infectious diseases to which all children are prone. A combination of unmodified insulin and one of the depot insulins before breakfast, repeated before the main evening meal is a suitable arrangement for most diabetic children, providing the necessary flexibility. Children and parents need to have sufficient knowledge to make daily alterations in the dose of insulin on the basis of the results of preprandial urine or blood tests and other relevant factors such as exercise and illness.

Diabetes in Pregnancy. If a diabetic woman wishes to have a child there is no reason, apart from genetic aspects (p. 484) why she should avoid pregnancy, provided that she suffers from none of the more serious complications of diabetes and provided she remains constantly under expert medical care. Nevertheless pregnancy in a diabetic woman carries certain definite risks. In the later stages of pregnancy she may develop an excessive accumulation of amniotic fluid; in addition the fetus is sometimes unusually large leading to difficulty in labour. Moreover the chances that a diabetic mother may lose her baby, either from a stillbirth or in the early neonatal period, are greater than those of a non-diabetic mother, even with the most careful supervision. Congenital malformation is more common in diabetic pregnancy and now accounts for the majority of deaths.

The proper treatment of a pregnant diabetic patient requires the close and coordinated supervision of a team consisting of physician, obstetrician, anaesthetist, nurse and dietitian. The sooner the pregnancy is diagnosed the better. Some non-pregnant diabetic women often miss one or more menstrual periods, especially if their disease is poorly controlled. For this reason a laboratory test for pregnancy is often helpful. There are grounds for suggesting that oral hypoglycaemic agents might be teratogenic, and any diabetic patient who is taking these drugs and wishes to become pregnant should change to a preparation of insulin.

Good control of the diabetes is the key to a successful pregnancy. A normal blood glucose concentration (HbA_1 8% or less) before and at the time of conception and throughout the pregnancy should be the aim. Further education of the patient may be needed in the proper management of her diet and insulin while at home. The diet, at first at least, need differ in no important respect from the diabetic diet to which she has been accustomed, but may need adjustment later, particularly with additional milk. Practical problems may be created for the physician and dietitian by bouts of vomiting that may occur in the early stages of pregnancy, and by the peculiar food fads which some pregnant women develop. The administration of highly purified unmodified and depot insulins twice daily is the best regimen for most pregnant diabetic patients.

After the diagnosis of pregnancy has been made the patient should be seen at first at fortnightly and later at weekly intervals. Continued control of the diabetes may be complicated by other factors. First, the renal threshold for glucose often falls as pregnancy advances. This is a normal phenomenon, but in the diabetic it means that the tests for glycosuria may cease to be a reliable index of diabetic control. Further, in the later stages of pregnancy, lactosuria may occasionally occur and may lead to confusion. For these reasons and because good diabetic control is mandatory, most patients will benefit from being taught to estimate their own blood glucose concentration. If excessive amounts of glucose are lost in the urine because of the lowered renal threshold, it may be necessary to give additional carbohydrate feeds between meals and sometimes at night, covered by suitable amounts of unmodified insulin to avoid ketosis. Then, too, the requirements for insulin usually increase as pregnancy advances. Frequent estimations of blood glucose are needed to ensure that an increase in insulin dosage, based on misleading urine tests, is not producing hypoglycaemia; or alternatively, that hyperglycaemia is not insidiously building up through failure to give enough insulin to meet an increase in insulin requirements.

Because of the risk in late pregnancy of sudden intrauterine death, pregnancy in a diabetic woman is seldom, if ever, allowed to proceed to term and most are delivered between the 37th and 38th week by induction of labour or if necessary by Caesarean section. Estimation of the lecithin/sphingomyelin ratio in the amniotic fluid is helpful in choosing a date for delivery. If the ratio is above 2·0 the risk of respiratory distress in the infant is low.

On the morning of delivery the usual breakfast and insulin should be replaced by an intravenous infusion of 10% glucose with 10 units of unmodified insulin added to each 500 ml. This should be given at a rate of 100 ml hourly. The blood glucose should be monitored at intervals of 1–2 hours and the rate of infusion and the dose of insulin adjusted to keep the blood glucose concentration at about 6·0 mmol/l. An alternative method is to give the insulin separately from the glucose infusion, by means of a constant-rate infusion pump at a rate of 1–2 units hourly. Whatever method is used administration of insulin should be stopped immediately on delivery and subcutaneous insulin resumed according to need as determined by urine and blood tests. Little or no insulin may be required for 12 hours after delivery. Thereafter, the pre-pregnancy dose can be gradually resumed.

A final word of warning is necessary. It has already been indicated that sugar in the urine is not unusual during normal pregnancy, either because of a fall in the renal threshold for glucose or through lactose appearing in the urine. The finding, however, of reducing substances in the urine of a pregnant woman should never be lightly dismissed as a normal phenomenon. Full clinical investigation to exclude diabetes is essential; otherwise a preventable catastrophe may follow. Since even minimal hyperglycaemia in pregnancy is associated with an increased fetal loss, the diagnostic criteria for diabetes in pregnancy are more stringent than those recommended for non-pregnant subjects (p. 463).

Diabetes and Surgery. Any surgical operation, however minor, and the accompanying anaesthetic cause metabolic stress which the diabetic is less well able to meet than the normal person. Operations under local anaesthesia do not usually require special treatment of the diabetes. For operations under general anaesthesia two points must be kept in mind: the need to provide an adequate supply of energy for the tissues, and the need to be constantly on the alert for acidosis.

In practice there are two separate problems related to elective and emergency surgery:

1. ELECTIVE SURGERY IN A STABILISED DIABETIC. All diabetics should be admitted to hospital about 3 days before even a minor operation. During this period the control of the diabetes can be checked thoroughly. Provided a diabetic goes to the

theatre in good condition, there is unlikely to be any significant change in the blood glucose plasma bicarbonate or ketone levels during the operation.

A diabetic who is not on insulin can usually be managed without special care other than careful postoperative observation of the clinical state, glycosuria, ketonuria and blood glucose concentration. However, care must be taken to avoid hypoglycaemia in those taking a sulphonylurea and conversely insulin may be required if significant loss of control occurs.

In the case of insulin treated patients it is desirable that the operation should take place as early as possible in the morning. The patient should receive no breakfast and nothing by mouth before operation and the normal dose of insulin should be omitted. Before being transferred to the theatre the fasting blood glucose level should be determined. If this lies between 7·0 and 10·0 mmol/l (120 to 180 mg/100ml) and surgery is minor, then no glucose or insulin need be given. If the level is below 5·0 mmol/l, then about 25 g of glucose should be given intravenously, preferably in hypertonic solution, in order to prevent possible hypoglycaemia (from the action of the previous day's depot insulin) during the operation. If the fasting blood sugar is over 10·0 mmol/l then some insulin will be required. About one third of the usual total daily dose is indicated, in the form of unmodified insulin, but its administration can usually be postponed until after operation. If a major surgical procedure is to be performed, intravenous 5% glucose or glucose saline should be given at a rate of 500 ml over four hours, along with unmodified insulin i.v. Either 4–20 units can be added to each 500 ml glucose or 1–3 units hourly can be given separately from the glucose infusion by a constant-rate infusion pump. The blood glucose concentration should be estimated frequently and the dose of insulin adjusted appropriately.

Recovery from the anaesthetic must be carefully supervised. The sooner the patient returns to the usual diet the better. This interval may be a few hours or several days, depending on the nature and severity of the operation. Within a few hours of recovery from the anaesthetic many patients are able to take fluid or semi-fluid feeds containing 25 g carbohydrate (p. 477) at 3- to 4-hourly intervals covered by suitable doses of unmodified insulin. After a major operation some insulin-dependent diabetics may need to have most of their energy requirements supplied as glucose, either intravenously or by mouth. If all has gone well, a single determination of the fasting blood glucose each morning will suffice. If recovery is stormy, measurements may be necessary at 4-hourly intervals or even more frequently. The determination of the plasma bicarbonate and electrolytes in the blood will also be helpful. The insulin dosage will depend on these findings, and until stability has been regained only unmodified insulin should be used.

Each specimen of urine must be tested for sugar and ketone bodies. If ketosis develops it is essential to take immediate steps to increase the metabolism of glucose by adjusting the dose of insulin.

2. DIABETES AND SURGICAL EMERGENCIES. Circumstances vary so much that it is impossible to consider them except in the most general way. The essentials are to maintain the oxidation of glucose by the tissues at a sufficient rate and to combat acidosis and electrolyte disturbances when they occur. This can be done effectively only if the state of the diabetic control is assessed continuously and accurately. A laboratory service that can provide rapid results is thus essential. As long as the surgical condition remains untreated and the 'metabolic stress' continues, the diabetic condition is likely to get worse. Once the patient's surgical condition is under control a prompt response may be expected to appropriate therapy for the diabetes.

Prevention of Diabetes Mellitus

NIDDM is a disease of the prosperous, and in wealthy countries it is one of the major health problems. The hardships of the Second World War were associated with a marked decline in the incidence of NIDDM in European countries; rationing of both food and petrol was probably responsible. The importance to health of sufficient exercise and of avoiding dietary excess has been stated repeatedly. Diabetes, like obesity and atherosclerosis, is likely to arise in genetically predisposed persons who eat too much and exercise too little. Excess of dietary carbohydrate may strain the limited capacity of the pancreas to produce insulin, especially if it is in the form of sugar or other refined carbohydrate; excess of dietary fat may accelerate the complications of diabetes; atherosclerosis is a common cause of death in diabetics. In any event the public should be warned primarily against an overall excess of calories.

Investigation of the HLA system has shown that certain individuals have an increased risk of developing IDDM and that genetic factors may also play a part in individual susceptibility to develop complications. These genetic characteristics of susceptibility and the relevant environmental factors need to be defined more precisely before appropriate preventive measures can be taken.

SCREENING. It is much easier to control the disease and to maintain the health of the patient in a state which allows a normal life to be led, if the diagnosis is made early in the course of the disease. In many patients the biochemical changes can be detected before the symptoms are sufficiently severe to make them seek medical advice. Any screening technique is expensive and should be used only if it is likely that a significant number of new diabetics will be recognised. High-risk groups, for example the first degree relatives of known diabetics, the obese and the mothers of babies weighing more than 4·5 kg at birth, will give a particularly high yield. The prevalence of diabetes in different communities varies from 0·5 to 5%. These figures vary widely according to the social and economic state of the people and the educational and medical services available.

Urine testing has been widely used as a screening procedure. As up to 3% of people may have renal glycosuria and so will have to be recalled for blood tests, and as a number of undoubted diabetics will be missed owing to their raised renal threshold for glucose, this is an unsatisfactory procedure. Whenever practicable, estimation of the blood glucose 2 hours after 75 g glucose orally is recommended as the screening procedure. Auto-analysers enable many samples to be tested daily.

Quite apart from screening high-risk groups it is not difficult to make out a case for a routine test of the urine for glucose in every full clinical examination; and all those with glycosuria (albeit of minor degree) should be considered diabetic until proved otherwise.

GENETIC COUNSELLING. Diabetic patients will often consult their doctor about the advisability of having children. They can be told that the risks of pregnancy and delivery are little greater for a diabetic mother than for a normal woman, provided she submits to the strict discipline required. The chances that she will produce a healthy baby are also good, but not quite so good as for a normal mother. The chances that her child will subsequently develop diabetes are higher than normal (Table 1.5) but most diabetics have healthy children, and how strongly a doctor should word these necessary warnings is a matter for judgement in each case. The family history, the severity of the disease in the parents and their educational and economic background, must all be considered.

Conclusion. The management of a patient with diabetes mellitus offers a special opportunity for good medical practice, there being few other chronic diseases in which efficient management makes so much difference to the patient's life. The problems presented by the aetiology of diabetes and its long-term complications continue to offer some of the most demanding and fascinating challenges in medical research today.

OTHER METABOLIC DISEASES

Metabolism is as fundamental as life itself; in medicine the term is usually restricted to disorders which can best be described in biochemical terms.

Many metabolic disorders are acquired. Others are congenital. The genetic aetiology of numerous inborn errors of metabolism has been identified with abnormalities of the structure or function of DNA and the pattern of their inheritance mapped by the study of a particular biochemical disorder. Metabolic disorders therefore may be classified in many ways, for example by the mode of inheritance or by the chemical factors involved. The specific enzyme deficiency responsible for the disorder, or the body system prinicipally affected may be named. Disorders of carbohydrate, protein or amino acid, lipid or mineral metabolism may be predominant features, and a few examples of these are given below.

The vast majority of inborn errors of metabolism are rare and it would be inappropriate to describe them here. The reader will find much further information in specialised textbooks (p. 487).

Carbohydrate. Diabetes mellitus is by far the most frequent and important disorder of carbohydrate metabolism. Rare genetic errors lead to abnormalities in the metabolism of galactose (galactosaemia), fructose (fructosuria), and glycogen (glycogen storage diseases, such as von Gierke's disease p. 579).

Amino Acids. Inborn errors account for many relatively rare diseases such as cystinuria (p. 379) and the Fanconi syndrome (p. 379). Phenylketonuria is also rare but leads to mental retardation if not detected in the neonatal period and treated with a special diet.

Purines. Gout (p. 578) is a classical example of a metabolic disorder but in practice is best considered along with other causes of arthritis.

Lipids are complex mixtures among which cholesterol and triglyceride are the most useful indices for the detection and monitoring of hyperlipidaemia. Lipids circulate as lipoproteins (chylomicrons, low and high density lipoproteins), while free fatty acids are bound to albumin (p. 336). Analysis of fasting serum lipids and particularly of lipoproteins provides a useful classification of the hyperlipidaemias as devised by WHO, and based particularly on the work of Fredrickson (Table 12.3). In this classification there are five major types (I–V) of hyperlipidaemia due either to genetic defects in lipid metabolism or to environmental factors such as diet, alcohol and drugs, including oestrogens and corticosteroids. Measurement of lipoproteins is usually not necessary for management which can generally be determined by clinical observation along with measurement of fasting serum cholesterol and triglyceride.

Hyperlipidaemias

Primary Hyperlipidaemia. Such patients can for most clinical purposes be placed in one of three groups. Two of these are metabolically heterogeneous but treatment can usually be allocated on a group basis.

Group 1 consists of those with hypercholesterolaemia and normal triglycerides (Fredrickson's Type IIa). The serum is clear, and low density (β) lipoproteins increased. Most patients have mild to moderate hypercholesterolaemia (7–10 mmol/l) and physical signs are usually absent although early arcus senilis or xanthelasma may be present. The disorder is relatively common in Britain and is a risk factor for ischaemic heart disease. It is usually weakly inherited and environmental factors, such as the dietary intake of saturated fat and cholesterol, are probably important in its aetiology.

About 5% of patients with hypercholesterolae-

Table 12.3 Classification of hyperlipidaemia. LDL = low density lipoproteins, VLDL = very low density lipoproteins, N = normal. β refers to electrophoretic mobility.

Fredrickson type	Lipoproteins elevated	Lipids		Treatment group
		Cholesterol	Triglycerides	
I	Chylomicrons	N or +	+	3
IIa	LDL	+	N	1
IIb	LDL, VLDL	+	+	2
III	abnormal VLDL (broad β pattern)	+	+	2
IV	VLDL	N or +	+	2
V	Chylomicrons VLDL	+	+	2

mia have a more sharply defined disorder transmitted as an autosomal dominant and present from birth. Serum cholesterol levels range from 8–16 mmol/l in heterozygotes and from 16–32 mmol/l in the rare homozygotes. In this disorder clinical stigmata of hyperlipidaemia are frequent. Tendon xanthomas and arthritis (p. 572) are common. Arcus senilis and xanthelasma on the eyelids are often prominent and 50% have ischaemic heart disease by the time they are 50 years old.

Group 2 comprises those with predominant hypertriglyceridaemia (Fedrickson's Types IIb, III, IV and V). The serum is cloudy, triglyceride and very low density (pre-(β) lipoproteins increased, and cholesterol may be normal or, if increased, the rise is usually less pronounced than that of triglyceride. Specific physical signs are uncommon although xanthomas can occur. Obesity, impaired carbohydrate tolerance and hyperuricaemia often coexist. There is a strong association with ischaemic heart disease and this group is also relatively common in Britain.

Group 3 is represented by Fredrickson's Type I. This is a rare disorder consisting of chylomicronaemia resulting from deficiency of extrahepatic lipoprotein lipase.

Secondary hyperlipidaemia occurs in association with diabetes mellitus, and in hypothyroidism, the nephrotic syndrome, biliary obstruction and pancreatitis.

Treatment. Control of *primary hyperlipidaemia* always requires dietary measures. Obesity must be corrected in every case. The low calorie diet on page 812 can be appropriately modified in relation to the fat content.

Groups 1 and 2 should have a fat-modified diet in which the intake of cholesterol is restricted and the total fat intake is reduced to provide about 36% of the total calories. The intake of saturated fat is reduced, while the intake of polyunsaturated fat is increased to provide a polyunsaturated: saturated fat ratio of more than 1:1. A list of foods to be avoided is given on page 814. An abnormal sensitivity to carbohydrate and/or alcohol is responsible for inducing hyperlipidaemia in some of those in Groups 2 who will require to restrict their consumption of sucrose and alcohol, even if they are not obese.

Group 3 patients improve dramatically with restriction of fat intake to about 25 g daily.

If dietary measures alone are insufficient to control the hyperlipidaemia, Group 1 patients should first be given cholestyramine. An incomplete response in these patients may be improved by the addition of nicotinic acid. Patients in Group 2 usually respond to nicotinic acid. Indications for the use of clofibrate came under scrutiny when two extensive clinical trials of this drug for the primary prevention of ischaemic heart disease revealed an increased mortality from ischaemic heart disease, cerebrovascular disorders and neoplasms, particularly of the respiratory and gastrointestinal tracts, among treated individuals. This excess mortality is unexplained but the use of clofibrate should be strictly confined to the few cases of severe hyperlipidaemia which have failed to respond to the measures outlined above and where the clinical benefit seems likely to be greater than the risk associated with medication. Those in this category are likely to include patients with the relatively uncommon Fredrickson's Type III hyperlipoproteinaemia (broad-β-band disease) which is associated with early-onset peripheral vascular disease and cardiac ischaemia and those with severe endogenous hypertriglyceridaemia (Frederickson's Type IV or V hyperlipoproteinaemia) where there is a risk of acute relapsing pancreatitis when the plasma triglyceride concentration exceeds 6–7 mmol/l.

Secondary hyperlipidaemia usually responds to treatment of the underlying condition when this is possible.

PROSPECTS IN DIABETES MELLITUS

The scale of the clinical problem presented by patients with microangiopathy, the suggestion that good control of blood glucose may prevent or retard the development of diabetic complications, the introduction of better methods of assessing diabetic control and the realisation that at present good control is achieved in only a minority of diabetic patients, has led to a search for better methods of treatment.

Improved control has been reported with battery powered portable pumps providing continuous subcutaneous or intramuscular infusion of insulin for periods of up to 4 months. In these systems insulin is delivered at fixed rates (a low basal rate and one or more higher rates before main meals) without reference to the blood glucose concentration. Their use requires a high degree of patient motivation and has the particular disadvantage that if the pump fails the onset of ketosis tends to be more rapid than with conventional treatment because there is no subcutaneous depot of insulin. These systems will not be suitable for general therapeutic use until they incorporate an automatic failure alarm and a miniaturised glucose sensor.

'Artificial pancreas' systems consist of three basic components: a glucose sensor, an insulin delivery pump, and a computer controller which regulates the administration of insulin on the basis of blood glucose concentration. Ideally such a device should be small enough for implantation and measure blood glucose without consuming blood. Existing systems use blood and are large, extracorporeal, relatively unreliable and expensive. They have few clinical applications but have some use as an investigative tool.

Pancreatic transplantation is still at an early stage of development and at present is reserved for those patients in the highest risk category whose prognisis is poor. Transplantation of isolated pancreatic islets (separated from the pancreas by digestion with collagenase and then cultured) into the splenic capsule has been very successful in small laboratory animals. Although in man there are major problems in relation to both the supply of islets and their rejection following transplantation, this may prove to be a more satisfactory approach in the long run.

From a public health standpoint the only cost effective way of dealing with diabetes is to prevent it. Some characteristics of IDDM offer hope that this might be possible. In contrast to its clinical presentation, it has been shown that the disease develops gradually and can be identified by means of complement fixing islet cell antibodies a year or more before the onset of symptoms when glucose tolerance is still normal. Even late diagnosis

might not be a bar to prevention, since one of the striking features of IDDM is a remission (or so-called 'honeymoon') period in which endogenous insulin secretion returns for weeks or months following diagnosis and treatment with insulin. This must indicate the presence of viable pancreatic beta cells and raises the possibility that they could either be protected from further damage and/or induced to regenerate.

JOYCE D. BAIRD
Diabetes Mellitus and Other Metabolic Diseases

C.R.W. EDWARDS
Diseases of the Hypothalamus, Pituitary, and Parathyroid Glands and Sexual Disorders

W.J. IRVINE
Diseases of the Thyroid and Adrenal Glands

FURTHER READING:

Endocrinology:

Hall, R., Anderson, J., Smart, G.A. & Besser, M. (1980) *Fundamentals of Clinical Endocrinology*, 3rd. edn. London: Pitman Medical.

Hall, R., Evered, D. & Greene, R. (1979) *A Colour Atlas of Endocrinology*. London: Wolfe Medical Publications.

Williams, D.H. (1981) *Textbook of Endocrinology*. Philadelphia: W.B. Saunders.

Diabetes mellitus:

Johnson, D.G. & Alberti, K.G.M.M. (1982) *New Aspects of Diabetes*. Clinics in Endocrinology and Metabolism 11, no 2.

Keen, H. & Jarrett, R.J. (1982) *Complications of Diabetes*, 3rd edn. London: Edward Arnold.

Nattrass, M. & Santiago, J.V. (1984) *Recent Advances in Diabetes*. Edinburgh: Churchill Livingstone.

Symposium on Diabetes Mellitus (1981) American Journal of Medicine 70: 101–630

Metabolic disorders:

Beaumont, J.L., Carlson, L.A., Cooper, G.R., Fejfar, Z., Fredrickson, D.S. & Stasser, T. (1970) Classification of hyperlipidaemias and hyperlipoproteinemias. *Bulletin of the World Health Organization* 43: 891. This is a definitive classification agreed by a WHO specialist committee.

Bondy, P.K. & Rosenberg, L.E. (1980) *Metabolic Control and Disease*, 8th edn. London: W.B. Saunders.

Lewis, B. (1976) *The Hyperlipidaemias. Clinical and Laboratory Practice*. Oxford: Blackwell Scientific Publications.

Stanbury, J.B., Wyngaarden, J.B. & Fredrickson, D.S. (1978) *The Metabolic Basis of Inherited Disease*, 4th edn. New York: McGraw-Hill.

13. Diseases of the Blood

BLOOD FORMATION

Up to the fifth month of fetal life blood cells are formed both in the liver and the spleen. Thereafter normal formation of the red cells, the granular series of white cells and the platelets takes place increasingly in the medullary cavity of bones and from birth onwards is restricted to these sites. Lymphocytes originate in the bone marrow. Some migrate to the thymus where they are processed to become T lymphocytes and are found in the interfollicular areas of lymph nodes, spleen and circulating in blood. Others which become B lymphocytes migrate to the follicular areas of lymph nodes and spleen.

During childhood there is a progressive diminution in the amount of red haemopoietic marrow so that in the young adult it is confined to the heads of the femur and humerus, to flat bones such as the sternum, ribs and ilia and to the vertebrae, the rest of the marrow cavity being occupied by fat. The red marrow may extend into the shafts of the long bones, replacing the fat, when there is an increased demand for blood formation.

Blood cells have a finite life span and require to be continuously replaced. Newly formed cells are provided by actively proliferating cell systems derived from mesenchymal stems cells found in the marrow, spleen and lymph nodes. The morphology of the haemopoietic stem cells is uncertain but they probably resemble lymphocytes. A stem cell has two functions. The first is to provide a continuous supply of cells committed to becoming the mature cells of the blood and the second is to replenish the stem cell compartment itself.

Stem cells probably exist at two levels, primary stem cells and secondary stem cells. Primary stem cells are pluripotential and capable of producing a series of secondary or unipotential stem cells committed to one or other of the mature cell systems. The secondary stem cells which give rise to lymphocytes probably appear at an earlier stage of differentiation of the pluripotential stem cells than those producing the erythrocytes, granulocytes and megakaryocytes. It is probable that the cells which become T lymphocytes are selected at an earlier stage of differentiation than B lymphocyte precursors.

Haemopoiesis is controlled by mechanisms that enable it to respond to fluctuation in demand. These are mainly humoral, although there may also be cell to cell interaction.

Of the three types of cell found in the blood, erythrocytes and platelets are true blood cells. They differ from most other cells in the body in that they have no nuclei. Leucocytes are cells which use the blood to migrate from the marrow or other production sites to the tissues where they function. Thus the white cells in the circulation at any one time form only a very small fraction of the total white cell mass.

The Red Blood Cells (Erythrocytes)

The earliest identifiable red cell precursor in the marrow is the pro-erythroblast, a large cell with a nucleolated nucleus and deeply basophilic cytoplasm. This cell undergoes a series of divisions rapidly so that the cells do not have time to regrow between divisions and become progressively smaller. At the same time, maturation proceeds with the formation of haemoglobin in the cytoplasm. Early, intermediate and late normoblasts can be identified (Fig. 13.1).

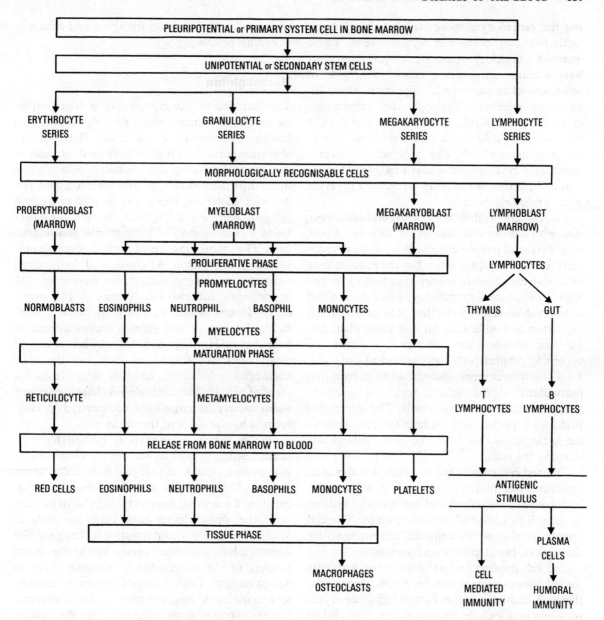

Fig. 13.1 Origin and development of blood cells.

Proliferation ceases at the intermediate nor-
moblast stage and maturation is then completed
with condensation of the nuclear chromatin and
eventual ejection of the nuclear remnant. At this
stage the cell still has the capacity to synthesise
haemoglobin, due to the presence of ribosomes in
the cytoplasm. This material (RNA) gives the cell
a faintly bluish colour with Romanowsky stains.

Supravital staining with cresyl blue causes condensation of the ribosomes to form reticular
material which makes these cells easy to identify,
and they can be counted as *reticulocytes*. The
reticulocyte matures into an adult red cell in
about 3 days and is released to the circulation
about half way through this period. Under stress,
marrow reticulocytes can be released sooner, rais-

ing the reticulocyte count without there necessarily being an increase in erythropoiesis. These 'marrow' reticulocytes can be recognised as they have a much more dense central aggregate of reticulum when stained with supravital stains. An increased number of reticulocytes reflects increased erythropoiesis. After the first few days of life there are, in health, no nucleated red cells in the peripheral blood. The presence of normoblasts indicates excessive or abnormal blood formation or irritation of the bone marrow by invasion with foreign elements.

The mature erythrocyte is a circular biconcave disc with a mean diameter of 7·2 microns. There is an excess of membrane which is partly responsible for the biconcave shape but the maintenance of this shape requires energy supplied by glycolysis. This unusual morphology gives the red cell considerable plasticity enabling it to pass through capillaries and other structures of small diameter. In some disorders the cell may lose membrane becoming progressively more spherical and rigid. As a result it is more susceptible to destruction particularly in the spleen, which is uniquely adapted to filtering out such cells. The spleen also performs a 'pitting' and 'culling' function removing inclusion bodies from red cells without destroying the cells.

The red cell membrane is a complex dynamic structure, one function of which is to maintain high levels of potassium and low levels of sodium in the cell by means of the ionic pumps. The cell membrane also carries antigenic determinants for the various blood groups on its surface.

Red cell production has specific requirements for substances such as iron for haemoglobin synthesis. A number of other factors influence erythropoiesis and include vitamin B_{12} (p. 500), folate (p. 500) thyroxine, vitamin C, androgens and possibly trace elements such as copper and manganese.

Erythropoiesis is controlled by a hormone, erythropoietin, produced mainly in the kidneys. There, cells which are probably located in the tubules, and which are responsive to tissue hypoxia, monitor the provision of oxygen to the tissues and respond to hypoxia by the production of erythropoietin. It acts mainly on the stem cell compartment stimulating increased activity. Erythropoietin also improves the speed and efficiency of erythropoiesis.

Haemoglobin

The function of the erythrocyte is based on its haemoglobin content which provides the oxygen transport mechanism of the blood. Haemoglobin also transports carbon dioxide from the tissues to the lungs buffering the carbonic acid that is formed in the red cell (p. 99). Haemoglobin is a complex molecule, being a conjugate of protein (globin) with a red pigment (haem), the latter being a combination of a porphyrin and ferrous iron. The globin fraction of normal adult haemoglobin (haemoglobin A) consists of four paired polypeptide chains, two alpha chains of 141 amino acids and two beta chains of 146 amino acids. Haemoglobin F, the fetal haemoglobin, differs by having two gamma chains instead of beta chains. Haemoglobin A2, which is found in small amounts of between 2–3% of the total haemoglobin in adults, has two delta chains instead of beta chains. Each globin chain carries one haem moiety in a specially constructed 'pocket' formed by the folds of the chain.

One molecule of oxygen is carried by each haem fraction in the haemoglobin molecule which is therefore capable of carrying four molecules of oxygen. Beta, gamma and delta chains are incapable of accepting oxygen to their haem pockets until the alpha chains have taken up oxygen. When this occurs a configurational change in the haemoglobin molecule prises open the haem pockets of the other chains, allowing them to accept oxygen. Thus the more oxygen the haemoglobin molecule has, the more easily it acquires further oxygen until saturated. In the tissues where oxygen is given up, the reverse occurs, initially easy loss becoming more difficult as the haemoglobin becomes desaturated. This function can be influenced further by a byproduct of glucose metabolism, 2–3-diphosphoglycerate (2–3-DPG). The concentration of 2–3-DPG in the red cell affects the avidity of the haemoglobin molecule for oxygen by reversible combination with deoxygenated haemoglobin. Increased levels of 2–3-DPG decrease haemoglobin's oxygen affinity and improve release to the tissues. Under hypoxic conditions, 2–3-DPG levels in the red cells increases as a compensatory mechanism. This is the first step in acclimatisation at high altitude; it occurs within 24–48 hours, long before there is any increase in red cell numbers stimulated by increased erythropoetin production.

The White Blood Cells (Leucocytes)

White blood cells are found in the blood as they migrate from bone marrow to the tissues. In any one individual the number is remarkably constant showing only minor diurnal variation. There are five morphologically distinct types of white cell. Three of these, known as granulocytes or polymorphonuclear leucocytes, are characterised by specific granules in their cytoplasm. A fourth type of cell, the monocyte, is closely related to the granulocytes. The fifth is the lymphocyte, a distinct cell, morphologically and functionally.

The Granular Series (*Polymorphonuclear Leucocytes*). These are so called because of the granules shown by Romanowsky stains in the cytoplasm of the more mature forms. Granulocytes are derived from stem cells in the bone marrow (Fig. 13.1), where their earliest recognisable precursors are myeloblasts which have large nuclei containing nucleoli and no cytoplasmic granules. Myeloblasts mature through promyelocyte, myelocyte and metamyelocyte stages with coarsening of nuclear chromatin and development of cytoplasmic granules. In later stages of maturation the nucleus becomes kidney shaped and finally segments into lobes connected by thin chromatin strands. The cells are classified as neutrophil, eosinophil or basophil according to the staining reactions of their granules.

The production of granulocytes is probably regulated by humoral factors, at least some of which are produced locally in the marrow microenvironment by mononuclear phagocytic cells and fat cells. There appears to be a close relationship between the numbers of monocytes and neutrophils.

Neutrophil granulocytes are phagocytic cells which ingest bacteria and fungi. Once mature, neutrophils may be held in the marrow for varying periods as part of a reserve pool of cells. Sooner or later the cells migrate out of the marrow and circulate in the blood for, on average, about 7 hours. They then leave the circulation by adhering to the capillary endothelium (marginating) and migrating through the vessel wall into the tissues. It is thought that this is promoted by chemotaxis. A considerable proportion of neutrophils in the blood may be marginated. Certain stress factors such as exercise and emotion may return these cells to the circulating blood causing a rise in white cell count. Their granules contain lysozyme and other substances which are discharged into the vacuole created by the ingestion of bacteria and which assist in the killing and digestion of the bacteria. The products of autodigestion from cells killed by organisms (pus cells) are potent stimulants of fresh neutrophil formation by the marrow. Pyrogens are also released. Neutrophils also ingest uric acid crystals and may disintegrate in the process, liberating tissue damaging substances and causing local inflammation.

Apart from responding to infection, neutrophils also produce a vitamin B_{12} binding protein, transcobalamin III, which explains the high levels of vitamin B_{12} in the serum in conditions in which there is a greatly increased number of neutrophils, e.g. chronic myeloid leukaemia. The degree of segmentation of neutrophils varies from unsegmented to five segments. The number of segments appears to have no functional importance. A failure to segment, with the formation of 'band' cells, occurs in toxic conditions and under such circumstances the degree of segmentation tends to diminish. This is called a 'shift to the left'. A 'shift to the right', in which there is increased segmentation, occurs in disorders such as vitamin B_{12} and folate deficiency and also in iron deficiency.

Mature neutrophil granulocytes account for more than 50% of the total leucocytes in the peripheral blood in a healthy adult; a huge reserve is held in the marrow and they are also present in large numbers in various organs and tissues.

Immature granulocytes, such as myelocytes, are found when the production of leucocytes is being stimulated by severe pyogenic infection and an increase in the cytoplasmic granulation may also be seen (toxic granulation). In adults the appearance of more primitive forms in the blood, such as myeloblasts and promyelocytes, indicates a serious disturbance of marrow function such as invasion by metastases or neoplastic change as in leukaemia.

Eosinophil granulocytes are also produced in the marrow. Factors influencing this are poorly understood but T lymphocytes appear to exert some control. Eosinophils are also phagocytic but less actively so than neutrophils. They ingest antigenantibody complexes and are concerned in processes involving foreign proteins, such as hypersensitivity reactions and in association with parasitic infections.

The *basophil granulocytes* are poorly phagocytic. The Fc portion of the IgE molecule is attached to specific binding sites on their surface. Activation of this by antigens results in degranulation of the cell with the release of histamine. Thus basophils participate in immediate hypersensitivity reactions in the same way as mast cells (tissue basophils) as described on page 24. Basophils also contain heparin which may be released to participate in lipid metabolism.

Lymphocytes originate from committed stem cells in the bone marrow. Some migrate to the thymus where they are processed to become T lymphocytes. Others become B lymphocytes and a few become cytotoxic 'killer' lymphocytes (p. 21). There are subsets of T lymphocytes called helper (or inducer) and suppressor T lymphocytes. These regulate the activity of B lymphocytes and possibly other haemopoietin cell lines. Helper T lymphocytes stimulate and suppressor T lymphocytes damp down the activity of B cells thus aiding immune function but preventing it becoming excessive.

About 75% of circulating lymphocytes are T cells. The rest are B cells and a few are 'null' cells showing neither T nor B characteristics. Both B cells and T cells respond to antigenic stimuli by transformation, in the case of B lymphocytes to plasma cells producing immunoglobulin. T lymphocytes retain their lymphoid morphology and perform their immune functions themselves (cell-mediated immunity). Other lymphocytes, K (killer) cells, undertake cell destruction.

Monocytes derive from the same precursor elements that produce the granulocyte. They partially mature into cells with an irregularly shaped nucleus in a cloudy blue cytoplasm containing numerous minute red granules. Monocytes are motile and phagocytic and migrate into the tissues where they develop further into various types of macrophages such as tissue macrophages, Kupffer cells, ostoclasts and fat cells. There they constitute the *monocyte–macrophage system*, previously known as the reticulo-endothelial system, which removes debris as well as microorganisms and collects and presents antigenic material to lymphocytes (p. 21).

The Platelets (Thrombocytes)

Platelets are derived from megakaryocytes in the bone marrow. Megakaryocytes are very large cells containing multilobulated nuclei and granular cytoplasm from which the platelets are formed by budding. Platelets are small (2–4 μm), hyaline, non-nucleated bodies with blue or purple granules. Platelet life span is estimated to be about 10 days and destruction is mostly in the spleen if the platelet is not used in haemostasis. Production appears to be regulated by thrombopoietins. The main role of platelets is in haemostasis by adhering to areas of vascular injury and promoting aggregation of more platelets. Aggregation goes through primary (reversible) and secondary (irreversible) stages with shape change and release of thromboxane A2 and other factors required in blood coagulation (p. 539).

Normal Haematological Values

These are given in Table 21.8 (p. 821).

Blood Destruction

Destruction of all formed elements of the blood occurs in cells of the monocyte-macrophage system. The survival time of the mature erythrocytes in the peripheral blood is approxiamtely 110 to 120 days. This is the period estimated by cross-transfusion experiments and represents the mean life span. A more practical technique for investigational use is one in which red cells labelled with ^{51}Cr are transfused and the time taken for half of the radioactivity to disappear is measured. By this method the half-life of the radioactivity in the red cells is 25 to 35 days and is shorter than the true half-life because of the elution of chromium from the cells. As red cells age their enzyme activity declines, the cells become defective and are removed from the blood and broken down in the monocyte–macrophage system. The degradation of haemoglobin yields iron from haem which is mostly utilised by the marrow for synthesis of fresh haemoglobin. The iron-free residual pigment, biliverdin, is converted to bilirubin and carried by the plasma to the liver for excretion. The globin is recycled.

The life span of granulocytes is probably about 3 to 4 days, of which less than 24 hours is spent in the circulation. The life span of monocytes and lymphocytes is less certain. It appears that there are short lived lymphocytes (3 days) and long lived lymphocytes (e.g. memory cells p. 21) which may re-enter the circulation at intervals for many years.

Terms Relating to Blood Disorders

Microcytosis means that the average size of the red cells is reduced. It is commonly found in iron deficiency anaemia and other disorders of haemoglobin synthesis.

Macrocytosis means that the average size of the red cells is greater than normal. It is seen, for instance, in megaloblastic anaemias but its occurrence does not necessarily mean megaloblastic change in the marrow.

Hypochromia exists when the red cells contain less than the normal amount of haemoglobin. They stain less deeply and show greater than normal central pallor. The mean corpuscular haemoglobin concentration (MCHC) is below normal. Hypochromia is commonly associated with microcytosis and is a characteristic feature of iron deficiency anaemia.

Anisocytosis means inequality in the size of the red cells. It is found in many forms of anaemia but is most prominent in megaloblastic anaemia.

Poikilocytosis means marked irregularity in the shape of the red cells. It is never present without anisocytosis and usually reflects dyserythropoiesis.

Elliptocytosis means elliptical red cells; *ovalocytosis* refers to a less marked abnormality. Such cells are found in small numbers in a variety of disorders such as megaloblastic and hypochromic anaemias. When the majority of cells are oval or elliptical it indicates a hereditary disorder of dominant type which is usually clinically benign; in less than 10% of cases, a haemolytic state exists and may cause anaemia.

Polychromasia and Reticulocytosis. Young red cells when stained by the Romanowsky method have a faint bluish colour due to residual ribosomal material. A blood film in which such cells are present in increased numbers along with those of normal pink colour is said to show polychromasia. This, like reticulocytosis (p. 489), indicates increased production of new red cells by the bone marrow.

Punctate Basophilia. Pathologically damaged young red cells may show several deep blue dots in the cytoplasm with Romanowsky staining. Such punctate basophilia may be found in any severe anaemia, but the presence of many of these cells is most commonly seen in β-thalassaemia and chronic lead poisoning where it may occur when the anaemia is slight.

Nucleated red cells are usually normoblasts and are found in the blood when erythropoiesis is very vigorous or when there is irritation of the bone marrow, as in leukaemia, or infiltration by secondary tumour.

Leucocytosis means an increase in the total number of white blood cells (over $11.0 \times 10^9/l$ in adults). This may take the form of a polymorphonuclear leucocytosis in which the increase is due to the outpouring of many young neutrophil granulocytes, as occurs in the presence of pyogenic infections such as tonsillitis or pneumonia. Alternatively it may take the form of a lymphocytosis, as is frequently found in whooping cough. Infants commonly respond to infections by producing a lymphocytosis.

Leucopenia means a decrease in the total number of white cells below $4.0 \times 10^9/l$ and usually involves a reduction only of the granulocytes (neutropenia). Leucopenia is found in tuberculosis, enteric fever, many acute viral infections, brucellosis and in hypoplastic and aplastic anaemia. Occasionally a leucopenia is found in overwhelming infections and is a bad prognostic sign. In a small number of patients it may be constitutional and represent no threat to health. In others it may be early evidence of developing acute leukaemia.

Eosinophilia is the term used when the number of eosinophil granulocytes exceeds $0.4 \times 10^9/l$. Eosinophilia is found most commonly in infections with worms, in allergic diseases, Hodgkin's lymphoma, polyarteritis nodosa and certain skin diseases. Rarely it may be familial or idiopathic.

Monocytosis refers to a monocyte count exceeding $0.8 \times 10^9/l$ and is found for example in advanced tuberculosis, malaria and in some neutropenic states.

Thrombocytopenia means a diminution in the number of blood platelets and is clinically significant only below a figure of $100 \times 10^9/l$. Capillary bleeding tends to occur when the platelet count falls below $40 \times 10^9/l$ but there is a poor correlation between the platelet count and a bleeding tendency.

Leucoerythroblastic is a term used to describe a blood picture in which primitive granulocytes and erythroblasts are simultaneously present in the peripheral blood. It is usually but not necessarily associated with anaemia and reflects bone marrow irritation as in malignant infiltration of the marrow or disordered haemopoiesis as in myelofibrosis.

Extramedullary haemopoiesis means that production of blood cells takes place outside the normal sites. It occurs not uncommonly in the first year of life when the available bone marrow space is insufficient to allow for an increased demand for blood formation.

DISEASES OF THE RED BLOOD CELLS

THE ANAEMIAS

Anaemia may be defined as a state in which the level of haemoglobin in the blood is below that which is expected, taking into account both age and sex. At birth the haemoglobin is high (20 g/dl) because the fetus has lived in a relatively hypoxic environment. After birth, oxygenation of the baby's haemoglobin in the lungs is more effective and the haemoglobin level rapidly drops, partly by removal of effete red cells and partly by reduced production, reaching about half the birth

level when the baby is 3 months of age. Thereafter the average level rises gradually until the child reaches puberty when a further rise occurs which is more marked in males than females. Adult males have haemoglobin levels on average 2 g/dl higher than adult females. This reflects the stimulus of androgens on erythropoiesis. It is thus possible for a haemoglobin level of 12 g/dl to be regarded as anaemic in an adult male, but normal in an adult female. In practice, most adults who are otherwise in reasonably good health function satisfactorily if the haemoglobin is above 10 g/dl, provided this lower level has not appeared quickly. The presence of symptoms related to anaemia depends partly on its severity but also on how rapidly the anaemia has appeared. Thus a patient who has a reduction of haemoglobin from 13 g/dl to 8 g/dl in 1 week may have severe symptoms, while another patient whose anaemia has developed slowly to a similar level over months may be asymptomatic and unaware of the anaemia.

Aetiology. A useful approach to the elucidation of the cause of an anaemia is to keep in mind that the condition results from one or more of the following three processes:

1. Loss of blood, which may be either acute or chronic (haemorrhage).

2. Inadequate production of normal red cells by the bone marrow (hypoplasia; aplasia).

3. Excessive destruction of red blood cells (haemolysis).

Most anaemias are multifactorial in their aetiology and many causes are relatively rare. The vast majority of anaemias are due to the failure of haemoglobin synthesis as a result of iron deficiency, the commonest reason for which is blood loss. This simple classification of the anaemias helps to guide the clinician in planning investigation as it reflects what is happening. Alternatively, anaemias can be classified on the basis of the morphology of the red cell as (1) normocytic (2) microcytic and (3) macrocytic. This however does not provide for dynamic concepts but is useful in providing an alternative approach.

Clinical features of anaemia are the direct consequences on the tissues of the diminished oxygen carrying power of the blood. Their occurrence and severity depend on the degree of anaemia and especially on the rapidity of its development, but are independent of its type.

The symptoms of anaemia are fatigue, lassitude, breathlessness on exertion, palpitations, audible pulse in the ears particularly in bed, anorexia, dyspepsia, dizziness, dimness of vision, headache, insomnia and paraesthesie in the fingers and toes. Myocardial anoxia causes angina pectoris, especially in older patients with coronary artery disease. Signs include pallor of the skin and, much more significantly, of mucous membranes, tachycardia, cardiac dilatation, systolic murmurs and, in severe cases, oedema of the ankles.

ANAEMIAS DUE TO BLOOD LOSS

Classification:
(i) Acute (large volume over short period).
(ii) Chronic (small volumes over long period).

Acute Blood Loss. A healthy adult can lose about half a litre of blood without ill effect. This makes it possible to provide a blood transfusion service using donors. When more than half a litre of blood is lost, compensatory mechanisms come into play which reduce the blood flow to peripheral structures such as skin and muscle, and conserve the supply for central organs. The pulse rate rises and the blood pressure is maintained. The patient is pale, cold and sweating and usually has to lie flat in order to maintain the cerebral circulation; hypovolaemic shock may ensue. At this stage the haemoglobin level of the blood is unchanged and in some cases it may even be higher than it was before the acute blood loss. If no further bleeding occurs, plasma production replenishes the volume, diluting the remaining red cells, and anaemia appears in about 24–36 hours. If blood loss is very severe, compensatory mechanisms fail and irreversible hypovolaemic shock supervenes, progressing to death. Anaemia may not have had time to appear.

In acute blood loss the primary problem is lack of blood volume which must be replaced by transfusion of whole blood, red cell concentrate, plasma or plasma substitutes. The anaemia which appears later, if transfusion is not given or if plasma or plasma substitutes are used, will be self correcting over the ensuing few weeks by in-creased red cell production unless the body iron stores are depleted. When acute blood loss is associated with other diseases, which themselves impair erythropoiesis, recovery of haemoglobin may be slow and the anaemia may become chronic. Immediately after acute blood loss there may be a transient leuco-erythroblastic blood picture. A few days later a reticulocytosis of 5–10% develops, subsiding gradually as the haemoglobin level recovers. A rise in platelet count may also be observed and is usually transient unless the blood loss becomes chronic.

Chronic blood loss in contrast to the acute process, does not give rise to reduction in blood volume or to anaemia since the body has time to compensate by increased plasma and red cell production. Eventually, however, the continued loss of red cells causes depletion of iron stores, red cell production is impaired, and anaemia appears.

ANAEMIAS DUE TO INADEQUATE PRODUCTION OF RED CELLS

Classification: Inadequate production of red blood cells may be caused by:

1. Deficiency of essential factors: iron, vitamin B_{12}, folate.

2. Toxic factors: inflammatory disease (infective and non-infective), hepatic and renal failure, drugs.

3. Endocrine abnormalities: hypothyroidism, hypoadrenalism, hypopituitarism, hypogonadism.

4. Invasion of bone marrow: leukaemia, secondary carcinoma, fibrosis.

5. Disorders of developing red cells: sideroblastic anaemia, other idiopathic refractory anaemias, hereditary disorders of haemoglobin synthesis (thalassaemia).

6. Failure of stem cell compartment: aplastic anaemia, frequently drug induced.

Iron Deficiency Anaemia

Iron deficiency is by far the commonest cause of anaemia in most parts of the world.

Iron Metabolism. Iron is essential for the synthesis of the haem fraction of haemoglobin. It is also present in myoglobin and other enzymes such as the cytochromes. Iron in food is absorbed from the upper small intestine, mainly in the ferrous form, but can also be absorbed as haem from red meat. Much of the iron in food is unabsorbable because it is irreversibly bound to other substances, for instance phytates and phosphates. Also, iron readily takes the ferric form in which it cannot be absorbed. The low pH of the stomach contents helps to preserve the iron in the ferrous form and that process is assisted by binding of iron to sugars and amino acids which protect it from conversion to the ferric form. Haem absorption is uninfluenced by these factors and it is thus a very important source of dietary iron. Some foods, for example rice and bread, are rich in phytates and other substances which prevent iron absorption. Other foods, for example spinach, have a high iron content but almost none is absorbable.

All cells obtain iron from the iron transport system (*transferrin*) in the blood by transfer across their membrane. The intestinal mucosal cell is no exception but it also receives iron by absorption from the gut lumen. When body stores of iron are adequate the intestinal mucosal cell is well supplied with iron from the blood, and absorption from the gut is discouraged although not completely prevented. When demands for iron increase, or the body stores are low, the mucosal cell becomes iron depleted and therefore avid for iron and absorption from the gut increases.

Iron adsorbed by the intestinal mucosal cell goes into a labile pool within the cell from which it may be complexed with apoferritin to form a ferritin store (see below). It may also go to mitochondria in the cell or pass to the blood transport system with which the labile pool in the cell is in dynamic equilibrium. Iron for erythropoiesis comes mainly from the iron transport system and almost all iron absorbed from the gut goes preferentially to the bone marrow and is used by the developing red cells. Increased erythropoiesis associated with a variety of disorders may increase iron absorption even when iron stores are increased. Thus some forms of prolonged anaemia, not due to blood loss or iron deficiency, can be associated with excessive iron stores.

Haem absorbed by the mucosal cell is split in the cell and iron liberated. The iron is then treated in the same way as iron absorbed by other means. Iron obtained from the catabolism of haemoglobin from destroyed red cells is recycled either to the bone marrow, or if there is excess, to the iron stores. Iron is stored in cells in two forms, (i) *ferritin* from which iron is fairly readily available, and (ii) *haemosiderin* which is a more stable form and constitutes the bulk of the iron stores. Haemosiderin is probably formed by the degradation of ferritin and can be stained by the Prussian blue reaction. This is used to provide a crude measurement of iron stores in the body.

Iron is lost from the body as the intestinal mucosal cells are sloughed off into the gut. A small amount is also excreted in sweat and urine. The total daily loss amounts to about 1 mg.

Aetiology. Deficiency of iron may be caused in a number of ways. The diet may not provide enough or it may be in an unabsorbable form. Disease of the gastrointestinal tract may give rise to malabsorption. Most commonly iron is lost from the body in greater amounts than can be balanced by absorption. This is usually by blood loss but occasionally iron may be excreted in the urine in the form of haemosiderinuria.

There are periods in life when iron deficiency may be regarded as almost physiological. At birth the normal infant has a store in the form of a very high haemoglobin level and in addition some iron is available in the liver. This is adequate for erythropoietic requirements in the first few months of life. Thereafter a mild degree of deficiency appears since milk is a very poor source of iron. If weaning is delayed to as late as one to 2 years, as is the custom in certain parts of the world, deficiency may become marked. If the child is weaned to a good diet, the deficiency is fairly quickly corrected. When prematurity and haemorrhage from the cord at birth deprive the infant of the normal store of iron, deficiency may appear sooner and be more severe.

In adolescents, in whom a marked growth spurt occurs, iron requirements may outstrip absorption. Food fads are not uncommon at this age and may contribute.

In females menstruation causes an average loss of 30 mg of iron each month requiring approximately 1 mg a day absorption in addition to the normal needs. Although this loss disappears during pregnancy, the mother must find iron for the fetus, the placenta, her own increased red cell mass and blood loss at parturition. The daily requirements will be about 2·5 mg plus her own basic requirement of 1 mg a day giving a total of 3·5 mg. In practice, the demand for iron rises as pregnancy progresses and is therefore greatest in the second half of pregnancy. Because of these factors iron deficiency is much more common in females than males during the reproductive years.

Apart from the above, iron deficiency usually indicates either an inadequate diet, some cause for malabsorption or loss of iron. The best source of iron is red meat because haem can be absorbed as such. Vegetables have variable amount of adsorbable iron; soya bean is a rich source. Foods, (e.g. bread,) may be fortified with iron to improve their quality. This improves the iron nutrition of lower economic groups whose diet is generally poor in quality and lacks regular meat because it is too expensive. Old people living alone, particularly men, are prone to allow their dietary habits to deteriorate with a low or absent meat content. Among these iron deficiency is not uncommon.

Reduction in gastric acid output, either by gastritis or resection raises the pH and reduces absorption of iron. Disorders of the small bowel mucosa, affecting mainly duodenum and upper jejunum, may cause severe malabsorption of iron as in coeliac disease.

In post menopausal women and adult men the commonest cause of iron deficiency is gastrointestinal bleeding. Erosions, ulcers, neoplasia, infective and non-infective inflammatory disease, parasitic infections and varices, whether oesophageal or haemorrhoidal, may be the site of blood loss. Hookworm infection is very common indeed and is the main cause of iron deficiency in many parts of the world.

Clinical Features. In many cases there are no symptoms and the deficiency may be discovered incidentally. In others vague symptoms of tiredness are insufficient to make the patient seek medical help. The symptomatology of severe iron deficiency is mainly that of anaemia (p. 494). However, there are some characteristic features. Cracking of the corners of the mouth (angular stomatitis), sore tongue (glossitis) and brittle finger nails are relatively common. Flattening or concavity of the nails, (koilonychia), is sometimes seen in addition to the evidence of nail cracking. Dysphagia is rare but when present should raise the possibility of a post cricoid web (Plummer Vinson syndrome). Pica, the eating of strange things, such as coal, earth, or foods in great excess such as tomatoes or greens, is more common than generally realised and may be uncovered only if the patient is specifically asked. Splenomegaly is not common unless the anaemia is severe but may reflect other disease such as portal hypertension, of which the iron deficiency is also symptomatic.

Investigation.

BLOOD COUNTS AND INDICES. The diagnosis of iron deficiency anaemia is made mainly on laboratory findings. The first abnormality to appear is microcytosis. Later, hypochromia occurs due to a reduced saturation of haemoglobin in the red cells. As the deficiency becomes more severe, other evidence of red cell dysplasia in the form of misshapen red cells and poikilocytes is seen, although the finding of oval and elliptical forms occurs quite early. Some target cells may be found but often indicate other problems, such as β-thalassaemia minor, a hereditary defect of haemoglobin synthesis.

The blood count findings are, therefore, a reduced haemoglobin level with normal or slightly reduced red cell count, a low mean cell volume (MCV) of less than 76 fl., a low mean cell haemoglobin (MCH) of less than 27 pg., a reduced mean corpuscular haemoglobin concentration (MCHC) and the blood film appearances mentioned above. The white cell and differential counts are usually normal, although hypersegmentation of the neutrophils commonly occurs. The ESR is usually lower than would be expected for the degree of anaemia or associated disease. A raised platelet count suggests that bleeding may be the cause of the deficiency.

Blood count indices vary according to whether they are produced by electronic counters such as the Coultercounter model S or by manual means. In the latter case, the MCV will not be satisfactory in many instances, as it depends on accurate red cell counting and the MCHC is then the index to use. Since the MCH, which is also dependent on an accurate red cell count, reflects both cell size and haemoglobin saturation, it is a less useful index.

The iron binding capacity of the blood reflects the level of the iron transport protein, transferrin, which is normally about one third saturated with iron. Saturation below 15% indicates iron deficiency and above 50%, iron overload, or failure to utilise available iron as in pernicious anaemia. Serum ferritin is present in minute quantities and is measurable only by radio-immunometric means. The range is wide in both sexes, mean values being higher in males. The levels, which correlate well with body iron stores, are very low in iron deficiency and raised in iron overload.

Bone marrow iron stores are found to be empty when stained by the Prussian blue technique.

DIAGNOSIS OF THE CAUSE OF IRON DEFICIENCY. Once it has been established that an anaemia is of an iron deficiency type, a cause should be sought. The direction of the investigations will obviously be influenced by the age and sex of the patient, the history and the findings on examination. Dietary histories from patients are notoriously unreliable but evidence from relatives and friends may be helpful. In the absence of any clear lead it is reasonable to start by looking for evidence of gastrointestinal blood loss with faecal occult blood tests, barium meal and enema and endoscopy. Negative barium studies should not be accepted as evidence of the absence of lesions. In tropical countries hookworm infection and schistosomiasis must be considered as likely causes but additional factors will require to be sought. In patients in whom there is a known cause of intravascular red cell destruction, such as a prosthetic heart valve, the urine should be tested for haemosiderin. Where malabsorption is suspected, investigation should follow appropriate lines (p. 310). In women during the child bearing years menstrual loss, if excessive, is a common cause as is repeated pregnancy.

Treatment. It is self evident that the patient who is iron deficient requires iron. Almost all patients can be treated by the oral route and the cheapest preparation is dried ferrous sulphate given as a tablet containing 200 mg of the salt (60 mg elemental iron) three times a day. A small proportion of patients develop 'indigestion', constipation or diarrhoea and then more expensive proprietary preparations may be tried. There are many of these and there is probably little to chose between them except that preparations employing a delayed release effect are to be avoided. They may give rise to less side effects but this reflects the fact that they do not release the elemental iron at the best absorption site. For the patient who cannot swallow tablets, proprietary liquid preparations may be used and are generally palatable.

Evidence of a response to oral medication usually appears in under 2 weeks. When there is concomitant inflammatory or neoplastic disease, response may be slower and oral therapy should not be discarded until 2 to 3 months have passed. If no response is seen, it may be that the patient is not taking the tablets for a variety of reasons. A check may be made by examining the stool which should be grey or black if the patient is taking the iron.

The rise in reticulocyte count associated with response to iron therapy is usually modest and seldom above 10%. After the haemoglobin level has returned to normal, iron should be continued for at least 6 months and in some cases a year in order to replenish iron stores. In cases of malabsorption, almost continuous therapy may be required or the parenteral route utilised.

PARENTERAL IRON THERAPY. This should be used only after iron deficiency has been clearly demonstrated. Commercial preparations of iron for injection should not be used except when one or other of the oral preparations cannot be tolerated or is found to be ineffective. The parenteral route of administration is suitable for the few patients who are genuinely unable to take iron by mouth because of pain, vomiting or diarrhoea, or who are unable to absorb iron because of some disorder of the gastrointestinal tract. It may also be used for patients who are shown or suspected to be unreliable in taking oral preparations. Iron given by injection has also been used for the treatment of the anaemia of rheumatoid arthritis, for the correction of severe anaemia in the late stages of pregnancy and following major operation.

The recommended single dose of iron-sorbitol is 1·5 mg of iron per kg of body weight given daily. It is assumed that about 250 mg of iron are required to increase the haemoglobin level by 1 g/dl of blood but the total dosage of iron should not exceed 2·5 g. Iron-sorbitol should be given by intramuscular injection and never intravenously.

Iron-dextran is seldom given intramuscularly because of local irritation and since it has been shown to cause sarcomatous change in certain animals. It can be given intravenously by what is known as the 'total dose infusion method' in a suitable diluent. Alarming systemic anaphylactic reactions can occur (p. 24).

Hypochromic Anaemia of Chronic Disease

Not all patients presenting with the haematological findings of iron deficiency are iron deficient. Such a state is usually associated with chronic inflammatory or neoplastic disease in which there is an inhibition of mobilisation of iron from the body stores. The iron storage sites in the marrow show abundant iron which is unavailable for haemoglobinisation of the developing red cells. The microcytic, hypochromic blood picture is associated with a low serum iron (p. 817) but also a normal or low iron binding capacity; the saturation of the iron binding capacity is usually less reduced than is found in iron deficiency anaemia with a similar level of serum iron. Saturation of the iron binding capacity below 15% almost always means iron deficiency. Although iron can be observed in the storage cells in the marrow virtually no sideroblasts are seen. Serum ferritin levels are normal reflecting the true state of the body iron stores.

Sideroblastic Anaemias

These are rare conditions in which red cell production is impaired by disordered iron metabolism.

The term sideroblast refers to a developing erythroblast which can be shown to have one or two iron granules in the cytoplasm. A siderocyte is a red cell containing iron granules. The iron granules are free in the cytoplasm and not associated with organelles. Both are normal findings. In certain pathological states iron accumulates in the mitochondria and appears as a ring of granules round the nucleus. These are called ring sideroblasts and are the characteristic cells of the sideroblastic anaemias. Pathological non-ring sideroblasts are cells in which there are excessive numbers of free iron granules in the cell cytoplasm. They occur in a number of conditions in which there is disordered erythropoiesis, for instance, untreated megaloblastic anaemia.

Aetiology. Sideroblastic anaemias occur in two forms:

1. A hereditary condition which usually shows a sex-linked mode of inheritance, produces a microcytic, hypochromic blood picture very similar to that of iron deficiency, is unresponsive to iron therapy and is a benign disorder.

2. An acquired group of anaemias seen mainly in the elderly, many of which are idiopathic. Others are associated with a variety of disorders, including inflammatory disease, (e.g. rheumatoid arthritis), malignant disease, pernicious anaemia, myxoedema, ingestion of drugs such as isoniazid, and rarely pyridoxine deficiency. The blood picture in these cases does not resemble iron deficiency, the mean cell volume is usually slightly raised and hypochromic red cells are seen among mainly normochromic cells.

Clinical features are those of anaemia. Often an unsuccessful attempt has been made to treat the patient with iron, particularly in the hereditary form which mimics iron deficiency.

The diagnostic feature of all these conditions is the finding of ring sideroblasts within the bone marrow when stained by the Prussian blue reaction. In addition the marrow may be hypercellular and in the acquired group there may be dyplastic changes resembling a megaloblastic disorder. Iron overload is often present. The serum iron is raised but saturation of the iron binding capacity is usually less than in haemochromatosis. With satisfactory management patients with the idiopathic acquired type can survive for a number of years. Some progress to develop frank acute myeloblastic leukaemia indicating that the sideroblastic anaemia was a pre-leukaemia condition.

Treatment includes the withdrawal of iron therapy. In some patients venesection may result in an improvement if iron overload is present. Any folate deficiency should be corrected. Rarely the disorder is caused by pyridoxine deficiency and then response will be observed to doses as small as 1 mg daily. Other cases respond to massive doses of pyridoxine up to 600 mg daily; improvement may be slow and treatment should not be abandoned in less than 3 months. When these measures are unsuccessful, transfusions with red cell concentrate may be required for the rest of the patient's life. In cases where the disorder is secondary to remediable disease, specific treatment usually corrects the sideroblastic disorder.

THE MEGALOBLASTIC ANAEMIAS

Haemopoietic tissue is one of a number of rapidly proliferating tissues in which DNA synthesis is intense. Both vitamin B_{12} and folate are essential for DNA synthesis and deficiency of one or both causes disordered cell proliferation. Haemopoiesis is particularly susceptible and division of cells is delayed and eventually halted. Morphological changes appear in the marrow cells. In the red cell series these changes are described as megaloblastic because the cells appear abnormally large. Changes also occur in the granulocyte precursors and megakaryocytes and indeed are not unique to haemopoietic tissue. Disordered morphology can be seen in other rapidly dividing cells such as those of the gastrointestinal tract. Similar morphological changes occur in other rare anaemias in which the aetiology is obscure and commonly in patients who are receiving chemotherapy for neoplastic disease especially if the treatment schedule includes drugs which interfere with DNA synthesis (antimetabolites, p. 113).

Normally in red cell production, cell division occurs rapidly. Between divisions the cells do not have time to regrow to their full size and a progressive reduction in cell size occurs. When DNA synthesis is reduced, the time between divisions is increased, more cell growth occurs and the cells become larger. In red cell precursors, haemoglobin production appears to be one of the factors limiting proliferation. Once a certain haemoglobin level has been reached, division stops. Thus in megaloblastic disorders not only do the red cell precursors have time to grow to a larger size, but they also undergo less divisions because there is no inhibition of haemoglobin formation. The end products are abnormally large and misshapen red cells which are well haemoglobinised.

As megaloblastic change becomes worse, increasing numbers of erythroblasts fail to mature and are destroyed in the marrow (ineffective erythropoiesis). Even in normal marrow a small proportion of developing cells suffer this fate but in advanced megaloblastic change the majority of the cells never mature to red cells. This massive destruction of cells in the marrow liberates large amounts of enzyme material and lactate dehydrogenase in the blood rises to very high levels. Eventually, in the absence of treatment, cell production fails. Excessive doses of antimetabolites have similar effects and may induce severe aplasia.

Vitamin B_{12} is a cobalt-containing porphyrin known as a cobalamin of which there are several. In man the assimilation of vitamin B_{12} from the lower ileum is facilitated by gastric intrinsic factor, a glycoprotein synthesised by gastric parietal cells, which complexes with vitamin B_{12}. Absorption is at specific receptor sites in the ileum. Intrinsic factor is not absorbed. Vitamin B_{12} after absorption is bound to a carrier protein, transcobalamin II, which carries it to the tissues where it is taken up by cells by pinocytosis and the vitamin B_{12} released by degradation of the complex. Transcobalamin I binds most of the measurable vitamin B_{12} in the plasma but is not a carrier protein. It may function as a circulating store. Transcobalamin III binds little vitamin B_{12}. Both transcobalamin I and III probably derive from granulocytes and their precursors.

Folates and Interaction with Vitamin B_{12}. Folic acid (pteroylglutamic acid) and related compounds are known as folates. Folic acid as such is available as a medicinal compound but the body obtains folates by the breakdown of polyglutamates in food to monoglutamates by folate conjugase in the small intestine or mucosal cell. Folate appears as methyl tetrahydrofolate in the plasma. This is changed to tetrahydrofolate (THF) by the homocysteine-methionine pathway for which vitamin B_{12} is essential. Without this, active folate coenzymes are poorly formed. 5,10 methylene THF is the form essential for the synthesis of thymidine required in DNA production. Dihydrofolate from this step is reconverted to THF by dihydrofolate reductase, an enzyme inhibited by the folate antagonist, methotrexate. Formyl THF (folinic acid) will bypass both the metabolic blocks created by vitamin B_{12} deficiency or methotrexate and acts as an antidote to this drug. Folinic acid or folic acid must not be used in treating vitamin B_{12} deficiency as they will accelerate neurological damage although they may correct the anaemia.

Deficiency of Vitamin B_{12}. This vitamin is obtained mainly from animal foodstuffs. Vegetables alone are an inadequate source. Requirements of vitamin B_{12} in the normal person amount to 1–2 μg daily. Deficiency takes at least 3 years to appear as there are large stores in the liver. It occurs because:

1. The diet may be inadequate (true vegans).

2. There may be intrinsic factor deficiency due to gastric atrophy as in pernicious anaemia, gastrectomy or, rarely, to congenital deficiency without gastric atrophy.

3. There may be disease of the terminal ileum reducing or eliminating the absorption site, e.g. Crohn's disease.

4. Vitamin B_{12} may be removed from the gut either by bacterial proliferation in blind loops or fistulae, or by parasites such as the fish tapeworm (p. 790).

Addisonian Pernicious Anaemia

The term Addisonian pernicious anaemia should be limited to megaloblastic anaemia due to a failure of secretion of intrinsic factor by the stomach other than from surgery. This disease is rare before the age of 30, occurs mainly between 45–65 years and affects females more than males.

Pathology. The marrow morphology reflects the failure of DNA synthesis with extensive maturation arrest of the red cell precursors and disparity in the maturation of nucleus and cytoplasm. Granulocyte precursors are often diminished in number and giant metamyelocytes are seen. Megakaryocytes may also be reduced in number and show dysplastic changes. There is evidence of increased blood destruction — including unconjugated hyperbilirubinaemia and increased deposition of iron (haemosiderin) in the liver, spleen, kidneys and bone marrow. The gastric mucosa is thin and atrophic. In untreated or inadequately treated cases degenerative changes in the posterior and lateral tracts of the spinal cord may be found (subacute combined degeneration).

Clinical Features. The onset is insidious and the degree of anaemia is often great before the patient consults the doctor. In addition to the symptoms of anaemia (p. 495) there may be intermittent soreness of the tongue and occasionally periodic diarrhoea.

The patient generally appears well nourished despite the fact that weight loss is a common feature. The skin and mucous membranes are pale and in severely anaemic cases the skin may show a lemon yellow tint. The surface of the tongue is usually smooth and atrophic, but sometimes it is red and inflamed. The spleen is sometimes palpable. In many cases paraesthesiae occur in the fingers and toes and occasionally there are signs of subacute combined degeneration (p. 656), which can appear before the anaemia. Dementia may also occur. In females there may be infertility. The urine contains excess of urobilinogen.

Investigation. Examination of the stained blood film shows a macrocytic blood picture. There is marked anisocytosis and poikilocytosis and in more advanced cases, fragmented red cells. Nucleated red cells sometimes show the features of megaloblastic change and can be found in the blood film, particularly if a 'buffy coat' preparation is made. This latter technique is useful if it is not possible to examine the bone marrow.

The reticulocyte count is usually low in absolute terms. Results expressed as a percentage must be assessed in relation to the reduced number of red cells. The absolute count is usually less than $100 \times 10^9/l$. Leucopenia is frequently present and is due to neutropenia. Hypersegmentation of the neutrophils is common. The platelet count is often within normal limits but may be reduced and occasionally severe thrombocytopenia is seen.

With modern counting equipment and the widespread availability of blood counts, this disorder is often diagnosed before anaemia appears as the result of finding a raised MCV. Consequently more florid, advanced cases are now seen less often.

Diagnosis is achieved in the first place by

demonstrating that the patient has a megaloblastic anaemia, based on the finding of a macrocytic blood picture with the features mentioned above, a megaloblastic marrow and a low serum vitamin B_{12} level. Serum folate levels may be raised. Thereafter a *Schilling test* will demonstrate that there is a failure of vitamin B_{12} absorption due to a lack of gastric intrinsic factor. The fasting patient is given 1 μCi of cobalt labelled vitamin B_{12} orally and at the same time 1000 μg of vitamin B_{12} is administered intramuscularly. The injected material saturates the binding proteins in the patient's blood so that vitamin B_{12} absorbed from the gut is lost in the urine. Urine is collected for 24 hours (48 hours if the patient has renal disease) and the radioactivity in the urine measured and related to the dose given orally. Normal subjects excrete more than 15% of the administered radioactivity in the 24 hour urine specimen. Patients with pernicious anaemia usually excrete less than 8% and very often less than 1% of the administered dose. The test is then repeated adding intrinsic factor to the oral dose of labelled vitamin B_{12}. If the defect in absorption is corrected, it is reasonable to assume that the patient has a failure of intrinsic factor production. Uncommonly the correction is poor due to high levels of anti-intrinsic factor antibodies in the stomach contents and higher doses of intrinsic factor may be required. Alternatively poor correction may indicate disease in the ileum.

It is possible to conduct the Schilling test using both isotopes of cobalt, one labelling free vitamin B_{12} and the other the vitamin B_{12} bound to intrinsic factor. These are given simultaneously and the urine collected. The results are assessed on the ratio of the two isotopes appearing in the urine. The Schilling test can be used for diagnostic purposes, even after the patient has been treated and is in remission.

Other tests which contribute to making a diagnosis of pernicious anaemia are the finding of *intrinsic factor antibodies* (p. 25) in the plasma in 50% of cases and the demonstration of *pentagastrin fast achlohydria*, although often this unpleasant test is omitted if the results of the Schilling test are clear. *Parietal cell antibodies* are found in 80% of patients with pernicious anaemia but are diagnostically unhelpful as they are also found in many patients who do not have pernicious anaemia.

Treatment. GENERAL. The decision to give a blood transfusion is based on general principles concerning the clinical state of the patient. When the haemoglobin level is so low as to endanger life, e.g. under 4 g/dl, it should be seriously considered. In all types of chronic anaemia of sufficient severity to require transfusion the blood should be given very slowly, preferably as red cell concentrate, because of the danger of producing cardiac failure. A diuretic should be given simultaneously with the red cell concentrate.

SPECIFIC. Hydroxocobalamin should be given in a dosage of 1000 μg twice during the first week, then 1000 μg weekly until the blood count is normal.

Within 48 hours of the first injection of hydroxocobalamin the bone marrow shows a striking change from a megaloblastic to a normoblastic state. Within 2 to 3 days the reticulocyte count begins to rise, reaching a maximum between the fifth and tenth days. If there is coexisting inflammatory disease the response may be delayed. There is a brief peak of red cell output due to the maturation of the large number of cells held in maturation arrest by the vitamin B_{12} deficiency. Reticulocyte counts may exceed 50%, the level depending on the initial erythrocyte count, but soon drop to below 10% as more normal production is resumed.

In some cases the rapid regeneration of the blood depletes the iron reserves of the body and recovery is halted. To prevent this occurring, ferrous sulphate (200 mg t.i.d.) should be given soon after the commencement of treatment. A combined deficiency of vitamin B_{12} and iron is recognised by the presence of macrocytosis and hypochromia. It is sometimes referred to as a dimorphic blood picture.

If a patient diagnosed as having pernicious anaemia fails to respond to the parenteral administration of adequate doses of hydroxocobalamin, it suggests that the diagnosis is wrong or the preparation used is not potent. The patient may be suffering from one of the other types of megaloblastic anaemia which may be partially or completely refractory to hydroxocobalamin. Such cases may respond to folic acid.

MAINTENANCE TREATMENT. The patient suffering from pernicious anaemia must be given regular doses of hydroxocobalamin indefinitely ($1000\mu g$ i.m. every 3 months). Theoretically the interval between doses may be longer but there is no merit in seeking the minimum effective dose. Blood counts should be done once a year and the assessment should never be made solely on clinical impression or on the haemoglobin level alone. With the maintenance of a normal blood count by adequate specific treatment the patient has a normal expectancy of life. There is, however, a statistically significant increase in deaths from gastric carcinoma in patients with pernicious anaemia. Patients with subacute combined degeneration of the cord should be given monthly hydroxocobalamin (p. 656).

Other Causes of Megaloblastic Anaemia due to Vitamin B$_{12}$ Deficiency

Dietary insufficiency is rare except in countries where meat and other animal food stuffs are not eaten for religious or other reasons. The deficiency is readily corrected by the parenteral administration of vitamin B$_{12}$. Thereafter the vitamin may be given by mouth.

Gastrectomy. Total resection of the stomach results in a complete loss of intrinsic factor production and therefore failure to absorb vitamin B$_{12}$. The patient will require life-long vitamin B$_{12}$ injections. Partial gastrectomy reduces vitamin B$_{12}$ absorption, in some cases to the point that deficiency occurs. Gastritis may, in part, be responsible. The Schilling test often demonstrates reduced absorption. One annual injection of $1000 \mu g$ of hydroxocobalamin is adequate prophylaxis for a patient who has had a partial gastrectomy.

Disease of the terminal ileum should be suspected if the Schilling test is not corrected by the addition of adequate amounts of intrinsic factor.

Bacterial colonisation of the small intestine (p. 311) results in an abnormal Schilling test, both without and with intrinsic factor; this is corrected by the administration of tetracycline.

Megaloblastic Anaemias due to Folate Deficiency

Folate (p. 500) occurs mainly in the form of polyglutamates in both vegetable (foliage) and animal foodstuffs. Much is destroyed by cooking and body stores are relatively small, lasting only a few weeks. It is absorbed mainly in the jejunum.

Deficiency of folate arises from:

1. Inadequate intake. Diets which totally lack fresh vegetables and meat or which consists of overcooked food, may not provide enough folate.

2. Disease of the upper small bowel, where folate is mainly absorbed. This may occur in coeliac disease or tropical sprue; very rarely extensive resection of the small bowel has a similar effect.

3. The body's demands exceeding intake.

(i) When there is very active cell proliferation, e.g. haemoloytic anaemia, leukaemias and other neoplastic disease, and during periods of acute or chronic infection.

(ii) Pregnancy, when the demands of the fetus and placental growth require large amounts of folate. In this situation folate is taken by the fetus in amounts adequate for its needs, even when the mother is folate deficient. There is no evidence that the fetus is ever affected by folate deficiency in the mother. However, a female, deficient in folate, may be infertile.

4. Interference with the dihydrofolate reductase system (p. 500). This enzyme system may be blocked by certain drugs, particularly methotrexate and pyrimethamine. In theory trimethoprim may also do this but a real danger appears to exist only in patients deficient in folate from another cause.

5. An unexplained mechanism. The antiepilepsy drugs phenytoin and primidone may cause folate depletion by an unknown mechanism not related to (4).

Approximately 60% of all cases of megaloblastic anaemia in Britain are due to folate deficiency. The majority of those suffering from vitamin B$_{12}$ deficiency have pernicious anaemia. In tropical countries most megaloblastic disease is due to folate deficiency associated with malnutrition, pregnancy and infection. Addisonian pernicious anaemia appears to be relatively uncommon in the tropics and in some areas is quite rare.

Clinical features are those of anaemia and of the underlying cause. Glossitis is less common than in vitamin B_{12} deficiency. Neurological problems are very rare.

Investigation. The blood and bone marrow findings in megaloblastic anaemia due to folate deficiency are indistinguishable from those in vitamin B_{12} deficiency as described for pernicious anaemia but serum and red cell folate levels are low. However, when the onset of folate deficiency has been recent and acute, the red cell folate, which reflects the patient's folate status over the previous 3 months, may still be within normal limits. Likewise, patients who have received folate therapy for a day or two will have a high serum folate level but may still show evidence of their past deficiency in the red cell folate. Serum folate should always be measured on a fasting specimen. The vitamin B_{12} level in the serum may also be marginally reduced for reasons that are not clear. The Schilling test, however, is normal and the vitamin B_{12} level returns to normal with folate therapy provided there is not a true vitamin B_{12} deficiency from another cause. Once folate deficiency has been established an explanation must be sought by exploring the causes of deficiency already mentioned.

Treatment. A daily dose of 5 mg of folic acid by mouth is sufficient; for maintenance therapy 5 mg once a week is almost always adequate. Folic acid must never be given, other than with vitamin B_{12}, in Addisonian pernicious anaemia or other vitamin B_{12} deficiency anaemias, because of the risk of aggravating or precipitating neurological features of vitamin B_{12} depletion. In pregnancy, megaloblastic change due to vitamin B_{12} deficiency is very rare indeed. It is therefore reasonable to give folate supplements to pregnant women. When a drug such as methotrexate inhibits dihydrofolate reductase, it is possible to employ folinic acid to overcome the metabolic block.

PRIMARY IDIOPATHIC APLASTIC ANAEMIA

This is a rare but grave disease of the stem cells which fail to a varying degree, producing serious hypoplasia of the marrow elements. An immunological mechanism may be responsible.

Clinical Features. Men are affected more often than women. The disorder may occur at any age, the peak incidence being around 30 years. The onset is insidious and the clinical problems are due to the reduction or virtual absence of production of red cells, granulocytes and platelets. Infections and haemorrhage are the most troublesome complications and may prove lethal. Bleeding occurs in the skin and mucous membranes. Haematuria and epistaxis are common. Intracranial bleeding is always a risk. Necrotic mouth and throat ulcers and monilial infections reflect the neutropenia.

Investigation. Known causes of hypoplastic and aplastic anaemia must first be excluded. A careful inquiry into exposure to drugs, chemicals and radiation should be made. A history of viral illness, particularly hepatitis, may be important. A full blood count demonstrates a pancytopenia. Neutropenia is the most marked aspect of the leucopenia, although leucopenia may not be the first to develop. The anaemia is normocytic, normochromic and often marked. Platelet production is often the most severely affected and the last to recover. The bone marrow should be examined by aspiration and trephine. The latter provides a better assessment of cellularity; aspirate may be difficult to obtain (dry tap). Sometimes an acute leukaemia is found. Studies with ^{59}Fe show poor clearance of the isotope from the blood, poor uptake and utilisation by the marrow and no extramedullary haemopoiesis.

Treatment. There are two aspects to management. The first is supporting the patient by replacement therapy. This consists of maintaining a reasonable haemoglobin level and is the least of the problems because transfusion of red cell concentrate can be given regularly. Vigorous antimicrobial therapy for infection and platelet transfusions for bleeding are required as outlined in the management of acute myeloblastic leukaemia (p. 523). Corticosteroids may be used to reduce bleeding but carry the risk of promoting infection.

The second aspect is an attempt to stimulate haemopoiesis and promote recovery. Androgenic steroids with low virilising activity are employed; these include oxymetholone by mouth or nandrolone deconate intramuscularly. High doses of methyl prednisolone may also be used. Red cell production and to a lesser extent granulocyte production benefit most from these drugs which unfortunately have undesirable and troublesome side effects when used over long periods. This is particularly so in children in whom secondary sexual characteristics may be stimulated and premature fusion of epiphyses may occur if the treatment is not suitably curtailed. Androgens may also cause cholestasis; fluid retention and prostatic enlargement may occur.

Bone marrow transplantation (p. 525) is now being advocated for this disorder in children and young adults and, in some centres, carries a better prognosis than when the disease is treated in a more conservative manner. In a few patients leukaemia supervenes and it is probable that these have been cases of leukaemia presenting in an aplastic or hypoplastic phase.

Prognosis. The course tends to be prolonged. Spontaneous improvement and recovery may occur and is one reason why treatment should be vigorous and prolonged. Androgens may be ineffective in the early phase of the disease but become effective later and should not be abandoned because of initial failure. The prognosis is undoubtedly poor and more than 50% of the patients die usually within the first year after diagnosis. Patients who survive longer than 1 year have a better chance of remission. In some instances there may be an autoimmune defect and, in the future, treatment directed towards this may prove to be of value.

Secondary Pancytopenia

This condition may be due to:

1. Idiosyncrasy to certain drugs such as chloramphenicol, phenylbutazone, oxyphenbutazone, indomethacin, sulphamethoxypyridazine, tolbutamine and troxidone or to certain industrial chemicals and insecticides chiefly benzene and its derivatives such as trinitrophenol, trinitrotuluene and gamma-benzene hexachloride.

2. The majority of drugs used in the chemotherapy of malignant disease.

3. X-rays and radio-activity.

4. Replacement of the bone marrow by abnormal cells such as tumour or by fibrous tissue.

5. Viral infections, particularly hepatitis.

6. Deficiency states such as severe lack of vitamin B_{12} or folate.

The clinical features and methods of diagnosis are the same as for primary idiopathic aplastic anaemia. The noxious agent if identified should be removed. Treatment is as for the idiopathic form. Bone marrow transplantation may be required in young patients who have HLA matched sibling donors.

ANAEMIAS DUE TO EXCESSIVE RED CELL DESTRUCTION

Haemolytic Anaemias

Red cell turnover is a normal physiological process, red cells having an average survival of 120 days. This means that all the red cells are replaced every 4 months. Various abnormalities either in the red cell or its environment may shorten its life-span and require more rapid replacement. Anaemia develops when marrow output no longer compensates. The increased output of new red cells is reflected in a raised reticulocyte count which gives an indication of the severity of the process. Under more extreme stress, nucleated red cells may be released.

The catabolic pathways for haemoglobin degradation are unimpaired but overloaded. There is an increase in unconjugated bilirubin in the blood and increased reabsorption of urobilinogen from the gut, which is then excreted in the urine in increased amounts. Bile does not appear in the urine. The level of bilirubinaemia is not greatly increased and jaundice is mild (p. 345).

Intravascular and Extravascular Haemolysis. *Intravascular haemolysis* liberates haemoglobin into the plasma where it is bound mainly by the α-2 globulin, haptoglobin, to form a complex too large to be lost in the urine. It is taken up by the liver and degraded there. Some haemoglobin is partially degraded and bound to albumin to form methaemalbumin. This is the basis for the *Schumm's test* for haemoglobin in the plasma.

If all the haptoglobin has been consumed, free haemoglobin may be lost in the urine. In small amounts this is reabsorbed by the renal tubules where the haemoglobin is degraded and the iron stored as haemosiderin. Sloughing of the renal tubular cells gives rise to haemosiderinuria which always indicates intravascular haemolysis. When greater amounts of haemoglobin are lost through the kidneys haemoglobinuria occurs, giving the urine a black appearance.

Extravascular haemolysis occurs in the phagocytic cells of the spleen, liver, bone marrow and other organs. It may not result in much depletion of haptoglobin. Furthermore inflammatory disease increases haptoglobin levels as does steroid therapy. Ahaptoglobinaemia may occur as an inherited disorder. For these reasons estimation of the haptoglobin level in the blood is not always easily interpreted. Nevertheless absence of haptoglobin is a strong indicator of haemolytic disease.

Blood and Marrow Findings. The peripheral blood shows a moderate macrocytosis and polychromasia due to the reticulocytosis. Specific red cell abnormalities may give a clue to the type of haemolytic disease. There may be a polymorphonuclear leucocytosis. The marrow shows erythroid hyperplasia. Megaloblastic change may occur and usually reflects depletion of folate reserves.

Increased erythropoietic turnover in the marrow is associated with increased levels of lactic dehydrogenase in the blood, which, in the absence of any dyserythropoietic state such as megaloblastic change, closely follows the severity of the haemolytic disorder.

If necessary red cell survival can be measured crudely using radioactive chromium (^{51}Cr). Surface counting done at the same time over liver and spleen may give an indication of where haemolysis is taking place. If transfusion has been given the patient's blood contains a mixed cell population which is not suitable for ^{51}Cr studies. In these circumstances cross-matched donor cells should be used for labelling.

Classification. Haemolytic anaemia may be caused by:

1. *Intra-erythrocytic defects:*
   (i) Hereditary: spherocytosis, haemoglobinopathies (abnormal haemoglobins and thalassaemias), disorders of glycolysis.

(ii) Acquired: red cells produced by dyserythropoietic states, e.g. vitamin B_{12} and folate deficiency.

2. *Extra-erythrocytic abnormalities:*
   (i) Antibodies (autoimmune and isoimmune).
   (ii) Physical trauma (prosthetic heart valve).
   (iii) Chemical trauma (drugs).
   (iv) Infections (malaria).
   (v) Toxic factors associated with inflammatory or neoplastic disease and metabolic failure.

HAEMOLYTIC ANAEMIA DUE TO HEREDITARY ABNORMALITIES OF THE ERYTHROCYTE

The principal disorders are hereditary spherocytosis, G6PD deficiency, haemoglobinopathies, (e.g. sickle-cell disease) and thalassaemia. G6PD deficiency and haemoglobinopathies are most common in African blacks and thalassaemia in the Mediterranean area. There has been a rise in the incidence of these disorders in other countries including Britain because of immigration.

Hereditary Spherocytosis

The exact abnormality is unknown but there are metabolic defects in the red cell membrane with increased leak of sodium ions into the cell, giving the sodium pump excessive work. Membrane loss occurs and this gradually compels the cell to lose its biconcave shape and become spherical. Spherocytes are destroyed by the spleen. The red cell life span is thus reduced giving rise to varying degrees of haemolytic disorder, often enough to cause anaemia. The haemolysis is extravascular.

Clinical Features. Symptoms vary from none to those of fairly severe anaemia. Episodic jaundice may be noted. The spleen is often but not always palpably enlarged. The severity of the disorder tends to vary in any one patient with crises of haemolysis at times. The transient hypoplasia of red cell production, which can occur in normal persons in association with viral infections, presents as *aplastic crises* in these patients because of the greatly increased red cell turnover which has become their normal state. There is an increased risk of pigment stone formation and cholecystitis may be the presenting event. Leg ulcers sometimes occur.

Investigation. The diagnosis is made by demonstrating a haemolytic state together with spherocytes in the blood film, increased osmotic fragility due to the spherocytes and the demonstration of the same disorder in other members of the family. The Coomb's test (p. 25) is negative. There is an excessive loss of urobilinogen in the urine. Red cell survival studies with ^{51}Cr show destruction of red cells almost exclusively in the spleen. The differential diagnosis is from other causes of spherocytosis, particularly the various forms of immune haemolysis (p. 512). Loss of membrane due to trauma to red cells in the circulation usually gives rise to many more schistocytes than are seen in hereditary spherocytosis.

Treatment. Splenectomy results in striking and usually permanent improvement both in the symptoms and in the anaemia. All authorities are agreed that operation should be advised when the anaemia causes persistent impairment of health, when severe haemolytic crises have occurred, when other members of the family have died from the disease, or where evidence of cholecystitis and cholelithiasis is present. Opinion differs as to the desirability of operation in mild cases with no resulting disability. The operation should be carried out during a period of remission, and in young children should be deferred until school age or older if possible. Severe haemolytic crises require treatment by blood transfusion. Blood must be matched very carefully and administered by very slow drip, as gross haemolytic transfusion reactions are common in this disease.

Folic acid, 5 mg daily, may be prescribed to support the increased erythropoiesis. Iron is of no value unless a genuine deficiency is demonstrated. In this type of haemolytic anaemia treatment with corticosteroids is not indicated.

Following splenectomy, resistance to some infections may be impaired.

Glucose 6-Phosphate Dehydrogenase Deficiency

Glucose-6-phosphate dehyrogenase (G6PD) is the first enzyme in the hexose monophosphate shunt of the Embden Myerhof glycolytic pathway from which red cells derive most of their metabolic energy. The function of the hexose monophosphate shunt is to service the enzymes glutathione reductase and glutathione peroxidase which protect the red cells against damage due to oxidation. In the absence of G6PD this protective mechanism is crippled and certain drugs in sufficient concentration can seriously injure the red cell.

It is now known that the deficiency is inherited as a X-linked recessive disorder and has a high frequency among African Blacks. In West and East Africa about 20% of males (hemizygotes) and about 4% of females (homozygous for the abnormal gene) are affected. A small number of heterozygous females are also deficient in G6PD. A similar deficiency occurs in Caucasian and Mongoloid races where it is usually more severe. Favism (haemolytic anaemia from ingestion of the broad bean, Vicia faba) is due to deficiency of G6PD of the severe Caucasian variety. In Blacks the activity of the enzyme is about 15% of normal, whereas in the others it is often less than 1% with consequently greater clinical effects. Some cases of haemolytic disease of the newborn in Caucasians have been found to be due to the same defect. This problem is rare in the type found in Blacks. Yet other types of G6PD biochemically different from the above may be associated with congenital nonspherocytic haemolytic disease and have been found in persons of pure British ancestry. In these cases splenectomy is valueless.

Many drugs in common clinical use, e.g. some antimalarials and sulphonamides, are capable of precipitating haemolysis in individuals with this defect. Infections may also potentiate the haemolytic action of drugs such as aspirin, chloramphenicol, chloroquine, and phenacetin.

Clinical Features. Persons with G6PD deficiency normally enjoy good health but are liable to haemolysis if any of the incriminated drugs or foods are ingested. However the haemolytic effect is related to the dose and will not be clinically detectable if the amount does not exceed a critical level. It is often possible to employ doses which are not toxic. The anaemia, when it occurs, may be rapid in onset, becoming obvious between 2 and 10 days after exposure to the precipitating agent and may be sufficiently severe to cause haemoglobinuria as well as the other classical signs of haemolysis. In the type of deficiency prevalent in Blacks only older cells are involved so that the haemolysis is to some extent self-limiting even when the offending agent is continued. Young red cells do have some G6PD activity and remain viable until their enzyme complement decays. Since in the Caucasian variety the enzyme deficiency is much more severe, destruction tends to be more disastrous. Anuria is an infrequent but serious complication.

Investigation. Diagnosis can be confirmed by estimating the G6PD activity of the red cell but this may not be entirely accurate if there is a considerable reticulocytosis. A number of screening tests are also available e.g. (1) the ascorbate cyanide test of Jacob and Jandl which monitors the whole glutathione regulating system of which G6PD is a fundamental part; (2) spot tests employing either the reduction of soluble tetrazolium compounds to insoluble purple formazan or the fluorescence of NADPH which is a bioproduct of G6PD activity. This last test can be performed on aged blood or blood collected on filter paper and dried. The Jacob and Jandl test has the advantage of being cheap. These tests should always be performed alongside normal controls.

Treatment is by removal of the toxic agent. Recovery is usually rapid but if the anaemia is severe, transfusion of red cells with a normal enzyme complement may be required. Thereafter the patient should be advised to avoid drugs which may precipitate the disorder.

The Haemoglobinopathies

The haemoglobinopathies can be classified into three subgroups. In the first there is an alteration in the amino acid structure of the polypeptide chains of the globin fraction of haemoglobin, commonly called the abnormal haemoglobins. The best known example is sickle-cell anaemia. Some 'abnormal' haemoglobins function as normal variants. In the second subgroup the amino acid sequence is normal but polypeptide chain production is impaired or absent for a variety of reasons; these are the thalassaemias. In the third subgroup there is the persistence of haemoglobin normally found in early life, namely haemoglobin F, into adult life. The hereditary persistence of high fetal haemoglobin is a benign condition and can be advantageous to persons carrying the haemoglobin S gene with which it is allelomorphic.

Sickle-Cell Anaemia

Abnormal haemoglobins are caused by amino acid substitutions in their polypeptide chains. These in turn reflect mutations in the structural genes controlling the production of these chains. There are four loci for these structural genes, all on autosomal chromosomes, active in postnatal life. They are designated alpha, gamma, beta and delta and are responsible for the production of the three main haemoglobins seen after birth, namely haemoglobins F, A and A2. Each of these haemoglobins contains, in common, two alpha chains and their differences reflect the possession of two gamma chains in the case of haemoglobin F, two beta chains in the case of haemoglobin A, and two delta chains in the case of haemoglobin A2. Thus the globin fraction of these three types of haemoglobin may be written $\alpha 2\gamma 2$ $\alpha 2\beta 2$ and $\alpha 2\delta 2$, respectively. Each chain in the globin fraction carries one haem moiety in its folds. It is convenient and practical to represent normal adult haemoglobins by the capital letter A and the abnormal haemoglobins by S, C and E and so on. As there are now several hundred haemoglobin variants known, the letters of the alphabet do not suffice and for some years new variants have been given names, often of the towns or districts in which they were discovered. Sickle-cell haemoglobin is the most important but haemoglobin C, D and E are also significant in some parts of the world, particularly when inherited along with haemoglobin S or with β-thalassaemia (p. 511).

Modern nomenclature includes a statement of the site of the amino acid substitution. Thus sickle haemoglobin may be defined as:

Hb S $\beta^{6GLU-VAL}$ or   Hb S $\beta^{A3GLU-VAL}$

The second method is more accurate since it defines the helix or bend in which the substitution occurs.

Control of haemoglobin synthesis is inherited

from both parents. Thus a normal adult can be depicted as having the haemoglobin genotype AA, sickle-cell trait by AS and sickle-cell anaemia or homozygous S disease by SS. The inheritance when both parents have sickle-cell trait can be shown thus:

AS ——————————— AS

AA   AS   AS   SS
Normal   Sickle-cell trait   Sickle-cell anaemia

The patient with sickle-cell trait is relatively resistant to the lethal effects of falciparum malaria in early childhood. The high incidence of this deleterious gene in equatorial Africa is thus explained by the selective advantage for survival it confers in an environment of endemic falciparum malaria. Surprisingly, patients with sickle-cell anaemia do not have correspondingly greater resistance to falciparum malaria.

Sickle-cell anaemia has been recognised among Blacks and to a lesser extent in other races since the beginning of the century. It is caused by the presence of the abnormal haemoglobin, haemoglobin S.

Pathogenesis. When haemoglobin S is deoxygenated, the molecules of haemoglobin polymerise to form pseudo-crystalline structures known as 'tactoids'. These distort the red cell membrane and produce characteristic sickle-shaped cells. The polymerisation is reversible when reoxygenation occurs. The distortion of the red cell membrane, however, may become permanent and the red cell 'irreversibly sickled'. The greater the concentration of sickle-cell haemoglobin in the individual cell, the more easily tactoids are formed, but this process may be enhanced or retarded by the presence of other haemoglobins. Thus haemoglobin C participates in the polymerisation more readily than haemoglobin A, whereas haemoglobin F strongly inhibits polymerisation. In sickle-cell anaemia most of the red cells contain haemoglobin S and little else and are very prone to sickle even *in vivo* under normal conditions. This happens particularly in those parts of the microvasculature which are sinusoidal and where the flow is sluggish. Sickle cells increase blood viscosity, traverse capillaries poorly and tend to obstruct flow, thereby increasing the sickling of other cells and eventually stopping the flow altogether. Thrombosis may follow and an area of tissue infarction results causing severe pain, swelling and tenderness (pain crises). In addition these cells are phagocytosed in large numbers by the mononuclear phagocyte system, thus reducing their life span considerably and giving rise to haemoloysis.

Clinical Features. The two major problems are chronic anaemia due to reduced red cell survival and episodes of tissue infarction.

Anaemia. Problems do not arise until about the fourth month of life when haemoglobin F containing cells have given way to haemoglobin S containing cells. The anaemia is haemolytic in type, severe, the haemoglobin seldom rising above 10 g/dl and averaging approximately 8 g/dl. Secondary folate deficiency is common and exacerbates the anaemia. When persistent, growth retardation and delayed puberty may be found. Episodes of increased sequestration and destruction of red cells occur, sometimes for no apparent reason and may lead to a swift fall in haemoglobin with rapidly enlarging spleen and liver. Aplastic crises (p. 506) occur in association with viral infections. The chronic anaemia is responsible for fatigue, reduced exercise tolerance, increased susceptibility to infection, cardiomegaly, leg ulcers and cholelithiasis. Hyperplasia of the marrow in the first year of life expands the marrow cavity producing bossing of the skull, prominent malar bones and protuberant teeth.

Infarction crises are characterised by episodes of severe pain and these punctuate the patients' lives. Commonly they occur in bones and spleen but no tissue is exempt. In the infant they classically affect the fingers and toes, producing large fusiform swellings (dactylitis). Metacarpal and tarsal bones may be affected and residual stigmata of shortening of digits due to epiphyseal involvement may occur. At any age mesenteric infarction may produce an acute abdominal emergency. The renal papilla is another site of trouble and infarction may give rise to painless haematuria. In adults aseptic necrosis of the head of the femur is a disabling complication.

Precipitationg factors include dehydration, chilling and infection, but sometimes the attacks occur spontaneously. The onset is usually rapid and the pain excruciatingly severe in the first 24 hours, thereafter abating over the next few days. Fever, increasing jaundice and malaise are common findings and, if persistent, may suggest the establishment of infection in the infarcted site. Salmonella osteomyelitis is common.

Pregnancy is hazardous unless careful antenatal care is provided and towards the end of pregnancy, infarction crises in the bones may liberate large amounts of fat and bone marrow emboli which cause diffuse microembolism of the lungs with pulmonary infarction, cor pulmonale and even death. These complications may also be seen in the less severe haemoglobin SC disease.

Sickle-cell anaemia should always be suspected in a patient who has had symptoms of anaemia since infancy and who belongs to a race which is often affected. In areas where sickle-cell anaemia is common, it should be considered in the differential diagnosis of many disorders. Patients must be adequately screened before major surgery and bloodless field surgery should never be employed, because infarction of the entire limb below the tourniquet may occur.

Investigation. Microscopic examination of the stained blood film will show some sickle-shaped red cells in patients with sickle-cell anaemia but these are not seen in patients with sickle-cell trait. The presence of haemoglobin S can be confirmed by the demonstration that the red cells will sickle within 20 minutes when mixed on a glass slide with a freshly prepared 2% solution of sodium metabisulphate under a cover slip. Positive and negative controls should be set up at the same time. Alternatively solubility tests may be employed. If neither of these is available, a small drop of blood diluted in saline may be incubated under a sealed cover slip overnight when sickling will occur. A positive result indicates the presence of haemoglobin S but does not distinguish between sickle-cell trait, sickle-cell anaemia, haemoglobin SC disease, sickle-cell thalassaemia, etc.

When suspected, the diagnosis should be confirmed by electrophoretic analysis of the haemoglobin and, if necessary, by a family study to demonstrate the inheritance. In this way true sickle-cell anaemia can be differentiated from other diseases in which haemoglobin S is combined with thalassaemia or some other abnormal haemoglobin such as C or D.

Antenatal diagnosis is discussed on page 18.

Treatment and Prevention. There is as yet no reliable method of changing the genetic constitution of an individual and therefore no means of curing this disease. Management is therefore aimed at alleviation of the symptomatology and the promotion of a lifestyle that will minimise the ill effects of the disorder. Basically this consists of the elimination of infections such as malaria and, if appropriate, life-long antimalarials should be taken. The patient should avoid becoming chilled or dehydrated. Regular folic acid supplements (5 mg daily) should be prescribed to support the greatly increased erythropoietic activity. Improvement of socio-economic circumstances is of considerable importance to the underprivileged and will go a long way to alleviating the serious results of this disease. However, acute episodes will occur whatever is done and require careful management.

Exacerbation of the chronic haemolytic anaemia is commonly associated with infections and these should be avoided or actively treated. The patient should be adequately hydrated but transfusion with red cell concentrate used only in exceptional circumstances. Most patients are habituated to a haemoglobin level of about 8 g/dl and should be transfused only when the haemoglobin drops below 5 g/dl. Clearly the circumstances in individual cases will vary so that transfusion may be needed at higher levels. Diuretics should be avoided unless cardiac failure supervenes when they should be used with caution.

The pain caused by tissue infarction crises can be extremely severe and the clinician is strongly tempted to use powerful analgesics. However, as the episodes will be recurrent, this should be avoided if at all possible and simple non-addictive analgesics such as aspirin, paracetamol and codeine used. Water and electrolyte depletion should be corrected as quickly as possible. Antibiotics will be necessary if there are infective complications such as osteomyelitis.

Many lines of prophylactic therapy of *in vivo* sickling have been tried but even those with a theoretical hope of success have proved disappointing. Sodium bicarbonate orally in large doses may help in altering blood pH but cannot be given for lengthy periods.

Prognosis. It is probable that in Africa, without medical attention, few children with sickle-cell anaemia survive to adult life. With full medical facilities and improved social and economic circumstances many patients survive and, although subject to recurrent ill health, lead a fairly normal life but are unlikely to reach old age.

Other Sickle-Cell Diseases

Sickle-Cell Trait. Most patients who are carriers of the sickle gene lead healthy lives. However, under certain circumstances they may be liable to sickling. These include bloodless field surgery and flying at altitudes over 15 000 feet (4575 m) if pressurisation is inadequate. In addition these patients are liable to attacks of painless haematuria due to infarction of the renal papillae.

Haemoglobin SC Disease. This disorder behaves like a mild variety of sickle-cell anaemia. Episodes of infarction crises are less frequent and anaemia is either absent or less severe. Aseptic necrosis of the femoral head, retinal vein thrombosis and painless haematuria are not uncommon complications.

Pregnancy is the main hazard as the same complications already mentioned under sickle-cell anaemia occur. Treatment of these should be by heparinisation and if necessary by premature induction of labour or delivery by caesarean section. Another risk is that the symptomatology may mimic closely other problems in pregnancy characterised by hypertension and proteinuria, but the treatment for these may be lethal. Sedatives should be avoided. Careful antenatal and postnatal care are required and folic acid supplements will be needed and also iron if there is a deficiency.

Haemoglobin C Disease. This is a benign haemoglobinopathy which, in its homozygous form, is not associated with much morbitiy but may cause megaloblastic anaemia in pregnancy and considerable splenomegaly in adult life. It requires no specific treatment other than folic acid supplements in pregnancy.

The Thalassaemias

Thalassaemia is an inherited impairment of haemoglobin synthesis, in which there is partial or complete failure to synthesise a specific type of globin chain. The exact nature of the defect varies and it is probable that a number of different faults occur along the pathway which translates the genetic information into a polypeptide chain. The gene itself may be deleted. β-chain synthesis is most commonly affected. When the abnormality is heterozygous, synthesis of haemoglobin is only mildly affected and little disability occurs. When the patient is homozygous, synthesis is grossly impaired and severe anaemia results.

β-Thalassaemia

Failure to synthesise beta chains (β-thalassaemia) is the commonest type and is seen in highest frequency in the Mediterranean area. Heterozygotes have thalassaemia minor, a condition in which there is usually mild anaemia and little or no clinical disability. Homozygotes (thalassaemia major) are either unable to synthetise haemoglobin A or at best produce very little and, after the neonatal period, have a profound hypochromic anaemia associated with much evidence of red cell dysplasia and increased red cell destruction. Haemoglobin F ($\alpha^2\gamma^2$) production normally ceases in the neonatal period, but because of the severe anaemia some production persists and provides much of the circulating haemoglobin. Thus these patients attempt to supply their requirements with haemoglobins that normally comprise only 3% of the total. At best they usually manage little more than 30 to 50% of the normal adult complement of haemoglobin.

Clinical Features. The anaemia is crippling and the possibility of survival for more than a few years without transfusion is poor. Bone marrow hyperplasia early in life may produce head bossing, prominent malar eminences and other changes giving a Mongoloid appearance. The skull radiograph shows a 'hair on end' appearance and general widening of the medullary spaces which may interfere with the development of the paranasal sinuses. Development and growth are retarded and folate deficiency may occur.

Splenomegaly is an early and prominent feature. Hepatomegaly is slower to develop but may become massive especially if splenectomy is undertaken. Transfusion therapy inevitably gives rise to haemosiderosis. Cardiac enlargement is common and cardiac failure, in which haemosiderosis may play a part, is a frequent terminal event.

There are several types of β-thalassaemia and a great variety of clinical manifestations which present a broad spectrum of disease. For further study the reader is referred to publications dealing with this subject in greater detail (p. 550).

Diagnosis. Thalassaemia minor is often detected only when iron therapy for a mild hypochromic anaemia fails. The demonstration of microcytes, increased resistance of red cells to osmotic lysis and a raised haemoglobin A2 fraction, together with evidence of the same abnormalities in other members of the family, establishes the diagnosis. In contrast haemoglobin A2 levels are diminished in iron deficiency states.

The diagnosis of thalassaemia major is made by the finding of profound hypochromic anaemia associated with evidence of severe red cell dysplasia, erythroblastosis, and the absence or gross reduction of the amount of haemoglobin A, raised levels of haemoglobin F and evidence that both parents have thalassaemia minor.

Treatment. Transfusion is the mainstay in the management of homozygous β-thalassaemia and if possible the haemoglobin levels should be maintained between 10 and 12 g/dl. The intraperitoneal route may be used in young children to conserve veins. Iron therapy is strongly contraindicated but folic acid supplements should be given. Attempts to remove iron by the administration of chelating agents such as desferrioxamine should be employed but fail to keep pace with the iron deposition from transfusion therapy until the patient has been transfused with over 100 units of red cells when the level of iron overload become considerable and chelating agents more effective. Splenectomy may be required for mechanical reasons or for hypersplenism. The later this can be done the better. Intercurrent infection must be treated vigorously with appropriate antibiotics.

α-Thalassaemia

The reduction or absence of alpha chain synthesis is found mainly in Southeast Asia. There are probably at least two inherited abnormalities, one associated with severe, and the other with mild inhibition of alpha chain production. Heterozygotes of either abnormality are at little disadvantage since alpha chain production is adequate. A slight excess of gamma chain production at birth may form gamma-tetramers (haemoglobin Bart's) and this can be demonstrated by electrophoretic techniques. The combination in the patient of a mild and a severe α-thalassaemia disorder results in a deficiency of alpha chain production which is less than absolute, so that some normal haemoglobin is formed. There is an excess of beta chains and these form beta-tetramers (haemoglobin H) and this may explain the syndrome of haemoglobin H disease. The inheritance of the severe α-thalassaemia abnormality from both parents is incompatible with life and such offspring are stillborn (hydrops fetalis).

AUTOIMMUNE HAEMOLYTIC DISEASE

In this disorder antibodies are formed against red cell antigens and cause inappropriate destruction of the cells (p. 25). There are two main types categorised on the basis of their thermal characteristics of the antibody. 'Warm' antibodies have a thermal optimum of 37 degrees C, this being characteristic of most antibodies. The majority are IgG. Warm type autoimmune haemolytic anaemia has antibodies of this type and these can almost always be shown to have Rhesus specificity. In some cases IgA and IgM antibodies are found, and complement binding may also be demonstrated in some cases, either with or without evidence of specific antibodies. 'Cold' antibodies have a thermal optimum of 4°C., but sometimes a thermal range of up to 37°C. Naturally occuring antibodies tend to be of this type and most are IgM.

Warm Type Autoimmune Haemolytic Anaemia

Many cases are idiopathic but some occur in association with chronic lymphatic leukaemia, lymphoma and systemic lupus erythematosus. Methyldopa may cause a warm type of haemolytic disorder; this is the commonest form of drug-induced haemolytic anaemia in Britain.

Clinical Features. Patients of all ages are affected with a slight preponderance of females. Symptoms vary with the severity of the disease and its cause and are mainly those of anaemia. In addition, in severe cases there may be fever, vomiting and prostration. Splenomegaly and sometimes hepatomegaly is present.

Investigation. The diagnosis is established by demonstrating evidence of antibody attack on the red cells by the direct antiglobulin test (Coomb's test p. 25). Antibody in the plasma may be shown by the indirect antiglobulin test. Elution of antibody from the red cells allows investigation of specificity against a panel of cells. The majority of these antibodies can be shown to have anti-Rhesus specificity (p. 514). Of these, anti-e is the commonest. Identification of specificity is useful in obtaining blood for transfusion as blood which does not carry the specific antigen can be chosen. The blood film almost always shows polychromasia and spherocytosis.

Treatment should be with prednisolone, 60 mg daily for 3 to 4 weeks, the dose thereafter being slowly reduced. Response to treatment can be monitored with reticulocyte counts and haemoglobin estimation. If relapse occurs, the dosage should be raised and maintained for a further three weeks, when reduction may be tried again. If treatment fails from the beginning or, if after 6 months of steroid therapy the patient still has active haemolytic disease, splenectomy should be considered. If splenectomy fails, immune suppression with drugs such as azathioprine may be tried. However, disease which behaves in this way usually turns out to be chronic. Blood transfusion should be avoided unless an antibody has clearly been identified and antigen-free blood is available. In life threatening situations, blood together with high doses of prednisolone may be given even though there are problems about complete compatibility.

Cold Agglutinin Disease

Idiopathic cold agglutinin disease occurs mainly in the elderly and the symptoms reflect a tendency of the red cells to agglutinate and sludge in the microvasculature of the extremities where the blood is cooled. Raynaud's phenomenon is usually present and also acrocyanosis. A low grade chronic haemolytic anaemia occurs. All these problems are worse in cold weather. Investigations demonstrate an increased red cell turnover and a 'cold' antibody in enormously high titres. The antiglobulin test is almost always positive.

Treatment consists of keeping the extremities warm. Transfusion should be avoided if possible. Steroids and splenectomy are of little value but immunosuppressive therapy may decrease antibody levels in severe cases.

Cold Agglutinin Disease Secondary to Other Disorders. Paroxysmal cold haemoglobinuria may be associated with syphilis or be idiopathic and have the Donath Landsteiner IgG antibody. Cold antibody-type disease may also occur in association with *Mycoplasma pneumoniae* infection and infectious mononucleosis when the haemolysis is usually self limiting. If found in lymphoma the haemolysis is usually more chronic.

ISOIMMUNE HAEMOLYTIC DISEASE

The term isoimmune is used to indicate that the antigen and the antibody come from different persons, although of the same species. This distinguishes it from autoimmune disease in which the antigen and the antibody are from the same individual.

Haemolytic Disease of the Newborn

This disease, previously called *erythroblastosis fetalis*, occurs in either sex at birth or within 2 to 3 days thereafter. The first-born in the family is usually healthy, but in successive children the severity of the disease increases and later children may be born dead. *Hydrops fetalis* is the most severe form, death occurring in utero; *icterus gravis neonatorum* is a dangerous illness but compatible with survival; haemolytic disease of the newborn is the mildest form.

It appears that in most cases the Rhesus (Rh) factor is the sensitising antigen. The majority (85%) of people, men and women, have red cells which contain the Rh antigen D. These people are said to be Rh-positive. Some of the children of an Rh-positive father and an Rh-negative mother are Rh-positive, since the factor is inherited as an autosomal dominant. The Rh-negative mother becomes sensitised by the Rh-positive substance contained in the fetal red cells. The resultant maternal agglutinins (antibodies to Rh-positive factor), penetrate the placental barrier and cause haemolysis of the fetal erythrocytes. In about one pregnancy in ten the mother is Rh-negative and the fetus Rh-positive. However haemolytic disease of the fetus is very rare in first pregnancies (provided the mother has not previously been sensitised by transfusion) and, fortunately, sensitisation does not occur as often as might be anticipated even in subsequent pregnancies. Indeed the risk of an Rh-negative woman having a baby with haemolytic disease of the newborn in any pregnancy other than the first is about 1 in 22.

If a mother is Rh-negative and the father Rh-positive, the maternal serum must be tested for antibodies between the 32nd and 36th week of each pregnancy. If found, delivery should be carried out in hospital. If no antibodies are detected the infant will probably escape the disease, but nevertheless the cord blood should be tested for antibodies. If present, preventive treatment can be instituted.

Very occasionally an antigen other than D is responsible for the development of haemolytic disease of the newborn.

A Rh-negative mother who has had an Rh-positive fetus may be sensitised to Rh-positive blood. If she receives a transfusion of Rh-positive blood a haemolytic reaction may occur. Consequently all women of child-bearing age or under and all pregnant women who may require transfusion must have their blood carefully typed for Rh factors as well as for the main blood groups.

Clinical features of haemolytic anaemia of the newborn are those of severe haemolytic anaemia with oedema and enlargement of the liver and spleen. Clinical jaundice is usually absent for 24 hours after birth. Thereafter deep jaundice leading to kernicterus (p. 651) may occur. The severity of the jaundice is largely due to the immaturity of the fetal liver which is unable to conjugate the large amounts of bilirubin with which it has to deal. The blood picture is very striking. The haemoglobin level, which should normally be about 18 g per 100 ml at birth, falls rapidly. Enormous numbers of nucleated red cells and a reticulocytosis of 10 to 50% are found in the peripheral blood.

In severe cases the mortality rate is 70 to 80% without treatment, death occurring within 2 weeks, but with exchange transfusion the mortality is low. Spontaneous recovery occurs in mild cases.

Treatment. Exchange transfusion should be given to all severely affected infants, as this is the only method of treatment that will overcome heart failure in the very anaemic infant and prevent deep jaundice and kernicterus in others. Delay of even a day may prove fatal and hence early diagnosis is essential. Antenatal prediction from tests for antibodies in the maternal serum gives the infant the best chance. In mild cases simple transfusion will be sufficient, and in some instances no treatment is required.

It is now believed that the most common cause of primary Rh immunisation may be transplacental haemorrhage during the third stage of labour. The likelihood of an Rh-negative woman developing anti-Rh antibodies is related to the number of Rh-positive red cells present in her circulation immediately after delivery. If this has happened the mother should receive an injection of gamma globulin containing a high titre of anti-D immunoglobulin within 72 hours of delivery. This will destroy the infant cells that have leaked into the mother's circulation and will prevent the development of antibodies in the mother and haemolytic disease in later babies.

HAEMOLYTIC ANAEMIA DUE TO OTHER ABNORMALITIES

Physical Trauma to Red Cells. Prosthetic heart valves, bacteria and intravascular fibrin formation associated with disseminated intravascular coagulation may all traumatise the red cells reducing their life span. Fragmented cells may be seen in the blood film.

Drugs, e.g. sulphasalazine or dapsone, may stress the metabolic processes of the red cells to the point of destruction even though the red cell is not enzyme deficient. Antigen-antibody reactions due to drugs acting as haptens may damage red cells directly or indirectly.

Haemolytic Anaemia due to Malaria. Haemolysis always accompanies malaria (p. 768) and in severe or prolonged attacks very considerable anaemia may ensue. Generally the degree of anaemia is related to the severity of the parasitaemia but the destruction of red cells is always in excess of that due to parasitised cells and sometimes considerably so. During an acute attack of malaria the reticulocyte count may be low but, as the patient recovers, a brisk outpouring of young red cells occurs. Recuperation may be interrupted by deficiency states, especially of folate and iron, or by other infection. Where these occur anaemia will be more severe and prolonged.

Immunity to malaria is greatest where the infection rate is highest and lowest where there is a low rate of infection or the patient is non-immune. Furthermore acquired immunity may be prejudiced by pregnancy, prolonged antimalarial therapy, splenectomy, lymphoma and allied disorders. Splenomegaly and anaemia diminish with increasing immunity but are universally found in young children. Splenectomy in patients exposed to malarial infection should be done with caution and only if lifelong prophylaxis against malaria can be ensured, otherwise disastrous levels of parasitaemia can develop and the patient die of cerebral malaria.

Inflammatory and neoplastic disease shortens the life span of the red cell. The mechanisms are complex and not completely understood. Excessive erythrophagocytosis by macrophages occurs. Red cells are damaged as they pass through affected tissue and drugs used in treatment may also harm them.

Paroxysmal nocturnal haemoglobinuria is a very rare disease in which red cell membranes acquire a susceptibility to antibodies normally present in the blood. Other blood cells may also be affected and thus thrombocytopenia is common. The disease is usually chronic but may be fatal.

TRANSFUSION WITH INCOMPATIBLE BLOOD

Transfusion with incompatible blood may arise: (1) with clerical errors leading to the wrong blood being given; (2) when the infused red cells are of the wrong main blood group due to careless typing of the bloods; (3) when the blood or recipient and donor of compatible main groups but incompatible subgroups. Direct crossmatching of recipient's serum against donor's cells greatly reduces this risk; (4) from the transfusion of Rh-positive blood to a sensitised Rh-negative recipient.

Symptoms usually begin after only a few millilitres of blood have been given, and if the transfusion is immediately stopped there may be no serious consequences. In severe reactions the patient complains of shivering and restlessness, nausea and vomiting, precordial and lumbar pain. There is a cold, clammy skin with cyanosis. The pulse and respiration rates increase and the temperature rises to 39–40°C. The blood pressure falls and the patient passes into a state of shock.

There is haemoglobinaemia, and possibly even haemoglobinuria; oliguria may occur with renal failure due to acute tubular necrosis. Jaundice appears after a few hours. In severe cases the anuria persists and uraemia develops, from which the patient may die. In others diuresis occurs even after several days and the patient recovers. In the majority the acute features subside in 24 to 48 hours.

Prophylaxis involves great care in the typing of blood and direct cross-matching before administration. The first 50–100 ml of any transfusion should be given very slowly and the transfusion stopped at once if any untoward symptoms develop. The patient should be under continuous observation during transfusion especially if unconscious.

Treatment of the established reaction involves giving hydrocortisone (100 mg i.v.), inducing a diuresis with mannitol and dealing with shock. If acute tubular necrosis occurs the measures recommended on page 401 must be instituted at once.

ERYTHROCYTOSIS AND POLYCYTHAEMIA

A raised haemoglobin level usually, but not always, indicates an absolute increase in the number of circulating red cells. In some patients it may be a spurious finding, the apparently high haemoglobin level being due to a reduction in plasma volume. This may occur because of dehydration or because of unknown mechanisms associated with stress (Fig. 13.2). A genuine increase in red cell numbers (erythrocytosis) occurs for a number of reasons which fall into three main groups:

1. When there is a physiological stimulus, as in hypoxia (p. 490) in which the production of erythropoietin is increased. Hypoxia may be due to altitude, pulmonary disease or congenital heart disease with cyanosis or where there are abnormal haemoglobins with a high oxygen affinity. The white cells and platelets are unaffected and there is no splenomegaly.

2. When there is a physiological response to a pathological stimulus. In this group the red cells are increased secondary to the production of abnormal amounts of substances with erythropoietin activity; this is occasionally found with certain benign and malignant tumours, e.g. of the kidney, liver, bronchus, uterus and cerebellum (haemangioblastoma) and with renal cysts. As in the first group the white cells and platelets are usually normal and there is no splenomegaly. However, the blood counts may be affected by the underlying disease.

3. When there is a pathological proliferation of red cells without erythropoietin stimulus. This is true or primary polycythaemia (polycythaemia vera, Fig. 13.2).

Stress or Spurious Polycythaemia. Some patients with a high haemoglobin are found to have a red cell mass which is normal or even subnormal. The cause is a reduced plasma volume. This latter disorder tends to occur in middle aged males who carry heavy responsibility or who are under stress for other reasons. It is often associated with hypertension and vascular disease. A change in lifestyle or the use of tranquillisers sometimes has a beneficial effect with recovery of normal blood values.

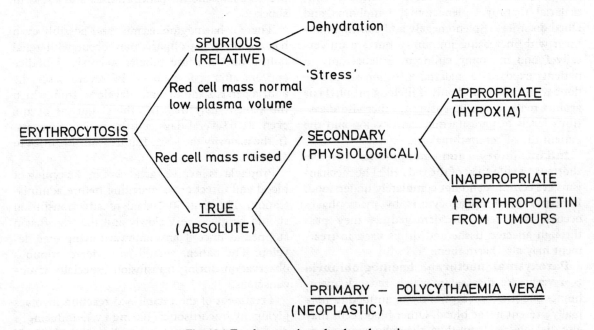

Fig. 13.2 Erythrocytosis and polycythaemia.

Polycythaemia Vera

Polycythaemia vera is one of a group of disorders of the pluripotential stem cells known as the myeloproliferative disorders (see below). These are overlapping conditions with features in common and they may progress from one form to another (Fig. 13.3).

Clinical Features. Polycythaemia vera occurs mainly in patients over the age of 40 and is more common in males than females. There may be no symptoms and the patient is diagnosed incidentally. A number, mainly males, present with peripheral vascular disease. Common symptoms among the majority of patients are lassitude, loss of concentration, headaches, dizziness, blackouts, pruritus, epistaxis and 'indigestion'. The patients often have a high colour, suffused conjunctivae, deep red palate and dusky red hands; retinal vein engorgement may be found. The spleen is palpable in 75% of cases at diagnosis. Thrombotic complications may occur and peptic ulceration is common, sometimes complicated by bleeding.

Investigation. The diagnosis is made by accumulation of evidence. The haemoglobin level is usually greater than 18 g/dl in males and 16 g/dl in females. An associated elevation of white cell and platelet count occurs in many but not all cases. The bone marrow is hypercellular with erythroid hyperplasia, very active granulopoiesis and increased numbers of megakaryocytes. Iron depletion of the marrow is usual. The red cell mass is greatly increased and the plasma volume is often normal. The neutrophil alkaline phosphatase score (p. 525) is normal or elevated and urate levels are often high. Whole blood viscosity is increased. In some patients the above results may be marginal and the diagnosis uncertain.

Treatment. Venesection is the simplest therapeutic measure and the best to use if the diagnosis is in doubt; 500 ml of blood (less if the patient is elderly) may be removed and this venesection repeated within a day or two if necessary. Venesection should continue until the haematocrit reading is reduced to 45%. Clinical improvement occurs rapidly with the reduction of blood viscosity. Iron deficiency appears, if not already present, but generally iron is not prescribed as its deficiency curbs erythropoiesis. It may be given with other methods of treatment. Venesection should be used with caution when the platelet count is very high because of the risk of thrombosis.

Radioactive phosphorus may be used when the diagnosis is certain and is an excellent form of treatment (5 mCi of ^{32}P i.v.). The full effect will not appear for three months but the white cell count and platelets respond more quickly. Further doses may be required.

Chemotherapy with busulphan (2–4 mg/day), or melphalan (2–4 mg/day) until the disease is brought under control is equally effective but requires more supervision and more frequent blood counts than radioactive phosphorus. It carries a slightly greater risk of severe marrow depression. Pyrimethamine (p. 772) may be used if no other treatment is available but can be associated with drug-induced ill health. Chlorambucil should not be used as it is associated with an increased incidence of acute leukaemia.

Prognosis. The average life span after diagnosis in treated cases exceeds 10 years. Some survive more than 20 years. Progress to a refractory state with anaemia, myelofibrosis or acute leukaemia eventually occurs if the patient does not succumb to intercurrent disease.

Other Myeloproliferative Disorders

In addition to polycythaemia vera there are a number of other myeloproliferative disorders which are closely related and are either malignant or pre-malignant. These include myelofibrosis, essential thrombocythaemia, chronic myeloid leukaemia (p. 524), chronic monocytic leukaemia (p. 527) and the myelodysplastic syndrome. There is a tendency for these disorders to terminate in an acute leukaemia phase (Fig. 13.3).

Myeloid Metaplasia and Myelofibrosis

Myeloid metaplasia is the appearance of precursors of red cells, granulocytes and platelets in abnormal sites such as the liver and spleen, and is usually associated with a leucoerthroblastic blood picture. This is not a phenomenon compensating for loss of marrow activity but is evidence of disordered behaviour by the precursor cell lines.

Fig. 13.3 Myeloproliferative disorders. Relationships with each other and with acute myeloid leukaemia [Ph′ = Philadelphia chromosome].

Myeloid metaplasia is seen in myelofibrosis. Early in myelofibrosis the marrow may have little or no fibrous tissue but as the disease progresses this increases and may eventually fill most of the marrow space.

Clinical features are very variable. Most patients with myelofibrosis suffer lassitude, weight loss, night sweats and some intolerance of heat. The spleen may be greatly enlarged in myelofibrosis and splenic infarcts may occur. Rarely splenomegaly is absent. Peptic ulceration is common and there is an increased incidence of gastrointestinal bleeding.

Investigation. Anaemia, sometimes macrocytic, is common. The white cell count varies with a diminution or increase of granulocytes and usually a leucoerythroblastic blood picture. The red blood cells show very characteristic tear drop poikilocytes. The platelet count may be very high, normal or low and giant forms are seen in the blood film. The neutrophil alkaline phosphatase score is frequently raised as are urate levels. The marrow is often difficult to aspirate and a trephine biopsy shows an excess of megakaryocytes and increased reticulin and fibrous tissue replacement. Folate deficiency is very common.

Treatment is largely supportive with blood transfusion, folic acid, and non-virilising androgen therapy. Corticosteroids may be helpful in some patients. Cytotoxic therapy should be used very cautiously. Splenectomy may be required if the grossly enlarged spleen is causing distress or because transfusion requirements are excessive but the outcome is unpredictable. Prognosis is generally rather poor. The disease is progressive with steady deterioration. Bone marrow transplantation should be considered for young patients.

Essential thrombocythaemia is a rare disorder of the elderly associated with a tendency both to bleed and to have thrombotic episodes. The platelet count is usually in excess of $1000 \times 10^9/l$ with an excessive number of megakaryocytes in the marrow. It responds well to radioactive phosphorus. Aspirin in small doses may help to counteract the thrombotic tendency. However, while it may alleviate vascular insufficiency by discouraging platelet aggregation there is the danger that excess aspirin may interfere with production of the natural anticoagulant prostacyclin (p. 547).

Myelodysplastic Syndrome. This rare disorder is found mainly in elderly patients. There is a relative failure of red cell, granulocyte and platelet production associated with an inappropriately hypercellular marrow. Often supportive management is all that is required for years. The disorder usually terminates in an acute leukaemic phase which is difficult to treat.

DISEASES OF THE WHITE BLOOD CELLS AND THE MONOCYTE-MACROPHAGE SYSTEM

The term 'monocyte-macrophage' system is now replacing the widely used 'reticulo-endothelial system' as the latter has little meaning and is inaccurate in the light of current knowledge.

NEUTROPENIA AND AGRANULOCYTOSIS

A reduction in the number of circulating neutrophil leucocytes (neutropenia) or their absence (agranulocytosis) is a potentially serious disorder.

Aetiology. In some cases the cause is an idiosyncrasy or sensitisation to, or poisoning by, a variety of drugs, notably aminopyrine, chlorothiazide, phenothiazines such as chlorpromazine, chlorpropamide, phenindione, phenylbutazone, oxyphenbutazone, troxidone, penicillin, various sulphonamides and the thiouracil derivatives. Exposure to insecticides should also be considered. Women are more commonly affected than men.

Neutropenia or agranulocytosis may follow excessive irradiation or the use of cytotoxic drugs or antimetabolites and is also found as an integral part of pancytopenia, leukaemia and some cases of hypersplenism.

In a few cases there is no discoverable cause — idiopathic agranulocytosis. Rarely the disorder is inherited.

Pathology. In many cases the bone marrow shows a virtual disappearance of the granular cells and their precursors. In some the marrow contains early myelocytes, with few mature forms — an arrest of maturation, but such appearances may indicate early recovery. In others the appearances are those of the underlying blood disease.

Clinical Features. There may be a history of exposure to one of the agents mentioned above. The onset may be either sudden or gradual. In acute and severe cases the condition begins with sore throat, fever and often rigors which may be followed by great prostration. There is rapidly advancing necrotic ulceration in the throat and mouth, with little evidence of pus formation. In fulminating cases the patient dies in a few days from toxaemia and septicaemia. In less acute cases there may be a preliminary period of malaise and weakness.

A chronic type has been described in which there is a persistence of recurring leucopenia with granulopenia. Rarely the neutropenia occurs in cycles of 3 to 4 weeks (*cyclic neutropenia*). In such cases the symptoms are chiefly recurrent malaise, low grade fever and sore throat often without ulceration.

Investigation. The outstanding and sometimes only abnormality on examining the blood is the reduction in absolute numbers of neutrophils which may be absent in the most severe cases. Where the lack of neutrophils is caused by another disorder such as leukaemia, evidence of this may be found and a reduction in the haemoglobin and platelet count observed.

Prevention and Treatment. All the drugs mentioned at the beginning of this section should be regarded as potentially dangerous and must be employed carefully. Patients taking them should be warned to report unusual symptoms, fever or a sore throat.

The most important measure in treatment is removal of the offending agent if it can be identified. The patient is at risk from septicaemia. Blood cultures should be done and the patient managed in the same way as those with the neutropenia and agranulocytosis that follows ablative chemotherapy used for acute myeloblastic leukaemia (p. 522). If the patient survives the acute phase, the outlook is fairly good, with recovery in many cases.

In more chronic cases and where there is only neutropenia, infections should be dealt with as they arise. Patients with only moderate neutropenia often have no clinical problem.

INFECTIOUS MONONUCLEOSIS (GLANDULAR FEVER)

This is a benign, acute infective disease due to the Epstein Barr (EB) virus, a herpesvirus which also causes Burkitt's lymphoma and nasopharyngeal carcinoma. Infectious mononucleosis occurs chiefly in adolescents and young adults of either sex, sporadically or in epidemics. It is mildly infectious and often spread by direct oral contact — the 'kissing disease'. The incubation period is usually about a week to 10 days but may be longer.

Clinical Features. The most common presenting features are tiredness, malaise, headache, anorexia, fever and enlargement of superficial lymph nodes, particularly the posterior cervical. Petechial haemorrhages at the junction of the hard and soft palate may occur early and be followed by sore throat with or without exudate.

A maculopapular rash often appears during the first 10 days in adults. Patients who have been given ampicillin for the sore throat develop a skin eruption due to the drug in over 90% cases. Epigastric and right subcostal tenderness is common and reflects hepatitis. The spleen is often palpable. It is usually soft and not tender. Pain in the right iliac fossa may result from mesenteric adenitis. Rarely there may be signs of meningitis or encephalitis.

Investigation. There is usually no anaemia and in the early stages the white cell count may be normal or low. A mild neutrophil leucocytosis is often present in the first few days, thereafter being replaced by an increase in the characteristic atypical mononuclear cells. These are activated T lymphocytes. EB virus selectively infects B lymphocytes and may remain latent with reactivation especially in immunocompromised persons. The proportion of the atypical cells varies greatly from case to case. The total white cell count is commonly raised to between 10 and $20 \times 10^9/l$. Another herpesvirus infection, that due to cytomegalovirus (p. 730) and also toxoplasmosis (p. 781) may cause lymphadenopathy and changes in the blood similar to infectious mononucleosis.

Heterophil antibodies develop in the serum of patients with infectious mononucleosis. After the first week the Paul-Bunnell reaction becomes positive in titres of 1:200 or more in over 80% of cases and may remain positive for weeks. The 'Monospot test' is widely used as a screening procedure. It is a simple slide test which is quick and more sensitive than the Paul-Bunnell. The Wasserman reaction may be falsely positive. IgM directed against the viral capsid antigen and a positive heterophil antibody test are considered sufficient for a diagnosis of primary EB infection.

Treatment is symptomatic. The patient should be rested during the acute phase. Metronidazole may be useful in treating the oral lesions. Although recovery is invariable some patients suffer prolonged illness, debility, with intermittent fever, sweating, inability to concentrate and depression. These symptoms may respond dramatically to corticosteroid therapy. Rarely thrombocytopenia or autoimmune haemolytic anaemia may occur; in most cases these also respond to corticosteroids.

THE LEUKAEMIAS

Leukaemias are a group of malignant disorders of the white blood cells characteristically associated with increased numbers of white cells in the blood. Leukaemias are progressive and fatal conditions most often resulting in death from anaemia, haemorrhage or intermittent infection. The course may vary from a few weeks to several years depending on the type.

Aetiology. In the majority of cases the cause of the leukaemia is unknown. Several factors, however, now appear to be associated with the development of leukaemia. These are:
1. *Ionising radiation.* There was an undoubted increase in leukaemia following the atomic bombing of Japanese cities. A striking increase in leukaemia was also observed after the use of radiotheraphy to control ankylosing spondylitis.
2. *Cytotoxic drugs.* These, particularly alkylating agents used in the treatment of cancer (p. 113), may induce leukaemia in some patients, usually after a latent period of several years.
3. *Exposure to benzene* in industrial situations.
4. *Retrovirus.* One rare form of T cell lymphocytic leukaemia appears to be associated with a retrovirus (p. 727) similar to the viruses causing leukaemia in cats and cattle.

Clinical and Haematological Features. The terms acute and chronic, when applied to leukaemias, refer to the clinical behaviour of the two main types of the disease. In acute leukaemia the history is usually brief and life expectancy, without treatment, short. In chronic leukaemias the patient may have been unwell for years and survival is measured in years. These differences are mirrored in the haematological findings. The general rule holds true that in malignant disease the more acute the clinical course, the more primitive or undifferentiated is the cell type. Thus in acute leukaemia the most primitive blast cells are characteristic whereas in the chronic forms differentiation to mature types of cell is seen.

Not all leukaemias are associated with an increased white cell count or even the appearance of abnormal cells in the blood. The term *subleukaemic* is used when the white cell count is within or below normal limits but abnormal cells are seen in the blood. *Aleukaemic* is used when there are no abnormal cells to be seen. In these cases the white cell count is usually subnormal. Almost all cases which present as subleukaemic or aleukaemic forms are acute leukaemias. The diagnosis is made from the marrow. Occasionally the acute leukaemia presents as an aplastic anaemia and declares itself later. Some of these cases also have paroxysmal nocturnal haemoglobinuria.

Classification of Leukaemia:

Acute	Chronic
1. Lymphoblastic:	1. Lymphocytic
(i) T cell type	2. Non-lymphocytic
(ii) B cell type	(myeloid)
(iii) Receptor-silent type	
(iv) Undifferentiated type	

2. Non-lymphoblastic (myeloid)

   Six varieties depending on involvement of granulocytes, monocytes, megakaryocytes and erythroid cells — FAB(French–American–British) classification.

The leukaemic process affects either the precursors of the lymphocytes or the granulocyte-monocyte series. Thus acute leukaemias may be classified as lymphoblastic and non-lymphoblastic (myeloid, myelomonocytic or monocytic). Each of these can be subclassified.

Acute lymphoblastic leukaemia can be divided into types in which the T and B receptors can be recognised by specialised techniques and a third, the most common, in which the cells are receptor-'silent' (null cells) but can be recognised by antisera raised against acute lymphoblastic leukaemia cells. A small fourth group exists in which the cells are completely undifferentiated.

The development of monoclonal antibodies has further advanced the identification and classification of these leukaemias and has superseded the antisera raised against these cells. This subclassification is of major clinical significance since it is the common receptor-silent type, which constitutes 70% of all cases, that responds well to treatment and carries a very real chance of long-term remission. When immunological techniques are not available, acute lymphoblastic leukaemia may be recognised with some certainty on the basis of Romanowsky stains, together with special staining techniques such as the PAS reaction and staining with Sudan black.

Acute non-lymphoblastic or myeloid leukaemia may also be subclassified into at least six varieties. These cannot all be detailed here but the subclassification reflects the variable degree of maturation of the granulocyte series, the common involvement of the monocyte series with the granulocytic series and also the involvement of the erythroid and megakaryocyte elements. In some, a degree of differentiation to the promyelocyte and even to the myelocyte stage can be seen and the latter may be associated with a more chronic course. In these cases the term 'subacute' is sometimes used. It is also true that not all cases pursue an acute course even though the morphology of the disease would appear to indicate that they should. They may 'smoulder'. One relatively chronic form is known as 'refractory anaemia with an excess of blasts' and this in turn merges with the myelodysplastic syndrome which includes some cases of sideroblastic anaemia.

Chronic leukaemias are similarly divided into lymphocytic and non-lymphocytic (granulocytic or myeloid). There may be a chronic monocytic leukaemia but this is probably related to the myeloid type, since it usually terminates as acute myeloblastic leukaemia.

ACUTE LEUKAEMIAS

Acute leukaemias are disorders in which there is a failure of maturation. Proliferation of cells which do not mature leads to an ever increasing accumulation of useless cells which take up more and more marrow space. Eventually, this proliferation spills into the blood. The cells in acute leukaemia proliferate more slowly than normal haemopoietic tissue, a fact that is useful in treating these patients.

Acute myeloblastic leukaemia is the most common type of acute leukaemia, except in young children in whom the lymphoblastic variety is more frequently found. In adults the incidence of acute leukaemia rises with age.

Clinical Features. The disease may begin insidiously but the clinical onset is often abrupt with 'flu' like symptoms and fatigue. There may be fever, malaise and a rapidly advancing anaemia. Epistaxis, spongy bleeding gums or other haemorrhagic manifestations including purpura are common and are due largely to thrombocytopenia. Sore throat and ulcers in the mouth or pharynx are frequent, due to reduction in normal polymorphonuclear leucocytes and anorexia with weight loss is common. Hypertrophy of the gums is often noted in monoblastic leukaemias. Muscle and joint pains may occur. The spleen and often the liver are enlarged in the later stages. There may be cervical lymphadenopathy secondary to pharyngeal sepsis but in the lymphoblastic form increase in the size of these and other lymph nodes is a common early feature.

Investigation. Blood examination usually shows a profound and increasing anaemia of normochromic type. The MCV is often raised. The white cell count may vary from a very low count of less than $1 \times 10^9/l$ to as high as $500 \times 10^9/l$ or more, but in the majority the count is less than $100 \times 10^9/l$. The blood film appearances are usually diagnostic of acute leukaemia since blast cells and other primitive cells are found. Sometimes marrow examination is required in aleukaemic forms before the nature of the disease is determined. Severe thrombocytopenia is usual but not invariable.

The marrow is involved in all cases and is the most important investigation. It is usually hypercellular with replacement of the normal marrow elements by leukaemic blast cells in varying degrees. However, it is impossible to obtain marrow by aspiration in some cases. Trephine biopsy should then be undertaken. Special staining techniques and immunological tests are used to subclassify these diseases. The presence of Auer rods in the cytoplasm of the blast cells indicates a non-lymphoblastic type of leukaemia.

Treatment. Accurate sub-classification of acute leukaemias is of great importance as treatment of the lymphoblastic and non-lymphoblastic varieties is very different. Chemotherapy (p. 113) is the major element in both, with radiotherapy (p. 111) being used in a minor role.

The first decision must be whether or not to give specific treatment. In the very elderly it may be unreasonable to subject the patient to unpleasant therapy which stands only a small chance of success for a brief period. In such cases support-ive treatment should be given and this often alleviates distress. However, with the considerable improvement in the results of treatment, the view is taken that an attempt to achieve remission should be made in most patients.

SPECIFIC THERAPY is designed to eliminate the leukaemic tissue and allow the recovery of the normal haemopoietic cells. In *acute lymphoblastic leukaemia* it is fortunate that this can be achieved in the majority of patients using a regime based on vincristine and prednisolone, with other drugs sometimes added, a regime relatively non-toxic to normal cell lines. Regrowth of the normal cells occurs as the leukaemic tissue regresses and the patient comes rapidly into remission. This phase of treatment is known as *induction*. A phase of *consolidation* follows in which other drugs are used including daunorubicin, mercaptopurine, cytarabine and methotrexate. Using the last two drugs intrathecal therapy is also given together with irradiation of the cranium to eradicate disease in the central nervous system which may have survived the initial chemotherapy. Finally a *maintenance* phase of treatment is given in which the patient receives a repeating cycle of the above drugs until 2 or 3 years have been completed in remission. Active treatment is then withdrawn because the patient probably stands more chance of death as the result of treatment than from the disease itself. Unfortunately, patients with the T cell types of acute lymphoblastic leukaemia tend to respond but relapse more frequently and the few with B cell type respond poorly. If relapse occurs in any patient the chances of achieving long-term remission are remote.

Acute non-lymphoblastic (myeloblastic) leukaemia must be managed rather differently. The three most useful drugs are daunorubicin, cytarabine, and thioguanine. All these are very toxic to normal as well as leukaemic cells. In addition daunorubicin is cardiotoxic. In order to eliminate the leukaemic tissue, a phase when the normal tissues are severely depressed must be accepted. During this phase of 'ablation' the patient may be gravely at risk from infection and bleeding as there will be severe neutropenia and thrombocytopenia. Young patients tolerate this aggressive management better than old. Treatment is generally given in '*pulses*'. A pulse of chemotherapy is a brief period of treatment between which there is an interval when no treatment is given. A number of pulses make up a course of therapy. Assessment of progress is made on blood and bone marrow findings. Once the marrow has been cleared of blast cells the normal haemopoietic tissue may be allowed to repopulate the marrow. The advantage of the more rapid proliferation of normal haemopoietic tissue is seen at this stage. As neutrophil production resumes, the patient rapidly feels better. Infections come under more effective control. Bleeding problems disappear as the platelet count rises.

At best only 50–60% of patients treated for acute nonlymphoblastic leukaemia achieve a remission. In the others the disease is to a greater or lesser extent refractory to specific therapy. When it is evident that this is the case, there is no point in giving further treatment as this merely makes the patient more ill. If chemotherapy is stopped, the patient may have a few weeks of quite good life, with suitable support.

When remission is achieved and the bone marrow recovers the patient should receive maintenance therapy. There are many regimens but most employ the same drugs as are used for induction, except that daunorubacin must be used very frugally or not at all as its cardiotoxic effects are cumulative.

Bone marrow transplantation is dealt with on page 525.

SUPPORTIVE THERAPY. The specific treatment of acute leukaemia, particularly the acute non-lymphoblastic form, would be difficult, if not impossible, without intensive supportive therapy. The easiest problem to deal with is the *anaemia* and transfusions of red cell concentrate are given to maintain an adequate haemoglobin level, preferably above 10 g/dl. Bleeding is due mainly to thrombocytopenia and is exacerbated by infection. Platelet transfusions are required. Platelets are harvested from six freshly collected blood packs and pooled to provide one donation for the patient. Two or more such donations may be required in a 24 hour period to control bleeding. Platelets may also be used for prophylaxis if bleeding is anticipated.

Infection, particularly septicaemia, is a serious and frequent problem. An infection can arise very rapidly within hours and it is necessary to act quickly when it occurs. Unexplained fever over 38°C., lasting more than 6 hours, should be regarded as septicaemia until proven otherwise, if the patient is severely neutropenic (absolute neutrophil count less than $0.2 \times 10^9/l$). Parenteral antibiotic therapy using an aminoglycoside together with mezlocillin (p. 44) and corticosteroid supplements should be administered. If a staphylococcal lesion is suspected, flucloxacillin may replace the mezlocillin. Where anaerobic infection is suspected metronidazole should be given.

In over 50% of patients blood culture is sterile and the cause of the pyrexia remains unknown. When antimicrobial therapy fails to control fever and there is severe neutropenia, white cell transfusion may be given. The preparation is usually obtained from a compatible adult relative donor, whose white cells are harvested for 4 to 5 hours, (*leucapheresis*) irradiated to kill any cells which might transplant to the recipient, and then administered. The effect can be dramatic with rapid resolution of the fever. Patients with chronic granulocytic leukaemia and a high white count make excellent donors for these problems. The leucapheresis is also of benefit to such donors by reducing the unnecessarily high white count.

Management of infection other than septicaemia should be along standard lines, always keeping in mind, however, that any infection may give rise to septicaemia. Candidiasis in the mouth, gastrointestinal tract and elsewhere tends to be intractable during periods of severe neutropenia, or if the patient is on steroid therapy; it requires treatment with antifungal agents such as nystatin or amphotericin. Topical gentian violet, although messy, often succeeds when all else fails.

A reduction in the risk of infection may be achieved in several ways. The patient may be regularly bathed in antiseptic baths (providone-iodine) and may be nursed in a protected environment, of which there are many kinds. The gut, which is a major source of infection, may be 'sterilised' using mainly unabsorbable antibiotics, and procedures such as brushing teeth or rectal examinations should be avoided.

Psychological support of the patient is of great importance. Most patients will rapidly discover their diagnosis if not told. It is usually better therefore to give the patients the opportunity to find out what they want to know and avoid telling them any untruths. In this way the patients' trust and confidence are retained and they understand why they must co-operate in an extremely stressful period of treatment. This is a delicate area of doctor-patient relationship and requires tact, sensitivity, and an understanding of the psychology of the individual. The quality of the nursing service is also very important and a team of nurses familiar with the specialised management of leukaemia is required if the best results are to be obtained.

Isolation, which may be necessary because of the risk of infection, can be psychologically very disturbing to some patients. Others prefer it. Patients are at less risk of infection with resistant organisms at home than in hospital and should be discharged whenever possible if the home circumstances permit and they are sufficiently well. Often treatment can be given on an out-patient basis. Cranial irradiation causes almost total epilation. The prospect can be devastating, especially for women. Restyling of the hair, the choice of a good wig and the firm promise that the hair will grow in again go a long way to alleviate the patient's distress.

Prognosis. At the time of diagnosis it is difficult to give a prognosis other than to say that without treatment it is very poor. It is wise to explain that a clearer view of the outlook can be given after the effects of induction therapy have been observed. The prognosis for most cases of acute non-lymphoblastic (myeloid) leukaemia is poor, the majority dying within a year. Patients with acute lymphoblastic leukaemia of the common 'null' cell variety, can be encouraged to hope that they may have the prospect of long-term remission. For those who usually do not have a particularly good outlook, hope should always be maintained, as even in some of these cases the outcome of treatment may occasionally be better than anticipated.

CHRONIC LEUKAEMIAS

Chronic Myeloid Leukaemia

The disease occurs chiefly between the ages of 35 and 60 years and is marginally more common in males.

Pathology. There is an extension of the mar-
row through the long bones. The marrow is grey and gelatinous and is crowded with myelocytes and young polymorphonuclear leucocytes. Leukaemic infiltrations occur in the liver, spleen and lymph nodes and in most other organs.

Clinical Features. The onset is insidious and the manifestations varied. Fatigue and lassitude are common. There may be slowly advancing anaemia with loss of weight, prominence of the abdomen and dragging discomfort in the left upper quadrant due to massive splenomegaly. Attacks of acute left upper abdominal pain may develop when infarction occurs in the spleen. Sternal tenderness and aching bones and arthralgia are common symptoms. Epistaxis or other haemorrhages may occur in the later stages. A hypermetabolic state may result in sweating, intolerance of heat and weight loss. Priapism is sometimes the presenting symptom. Secondary gout may also occur. However, sometimes at diagnosis the patient is asymptomatic.

The spleen is usually considerably enlarged and in occasional patients may reach the symphysis pubis. It is firm, smooth and painless but if infarction has occurred, it may be exquisitely tender and a friction rub may be heard over it. The liver may also be enlarged but lymph nodes are not usually involved.

Investigation. Examination of the blood shows an anaemia, usually normochromic, normocytic in type which increases as the disease progresses. The white cell count is usually considerably increased to between 50 and $500 \times 10^9/l$. A blood film demonstrates the full spectrum of granulocyte precursors from myeloblasts to mature neutrophils, the more mature forms being the most numerous. Myeloblasts usually number less than 10% of the total. There is also an increase in eosinophils and basophils. In the later stages, the appearance of an increasing number of myeloblasts may indicate the approach of a terminal acute phase and confirmation of this may be obtained from the bone marrow. The relative number of basophils also increases as the disease progresses. The platelet count is often high initially but with treatment usually comes down to normal levels; very high counts are sometimes found and may herald the approach of transformation to an acute phase.

The peripheral blood is more useful diagnostically than the bone marrow but the latter should be examined in order to obtain material for chromosome analysis and to exclude other conditions causing a leucoerythroblastic blood picture. The neutrophils of chronic myeloid leukaemia are usually deficient in alkaline phosphatase. Normal neutrophils stained for this enzyme can be crudely scored and usually give a result of between 20 and 100. In chronic myeloid leukaemia, the score is usually less than 5. However, a result within the normal range does not exclude the diagnosis. If initially low, the score often rises to normal with treatment.

In about 90% of cases chromosome analysis demonstrates the presence of the Philadelphia chromosome (p. 8).

Treatment. CHEMOTHERAPY. Effective palliative treatment can restore most patients to a period of symptom-free life. The method of choice is by chemotherapy using the alkylating agent busulphan (p. 113). It is given orally in a commencing dose of 4 mg daily and can bring about a temporary but satisfactory clinical and haematological remission in a high proportion of cases, with marked reduction in splenomegaly. Generally no response is seen in the first 2 weeks. Thereafter the count falls and the results plotted on semi-logarithmic paper against time give a straight line allowing prediction of the point at which the dose of busulphan may require reduction or withdrawal. On average, between 12 and 18 weeks are required to achieve a normal count, but rarely the count falls more rapidly and, unless dosage is stopped, severe and even lethal aplasia of the marrow may result. For this reason it is customary to stop the busulphan when the white cell count is between 10 and $20 \times 10^9/l$ and wait until it shows signs of rising before reintroducing the drug. Maintenance dosage of busulphan is generally 1–2 mg daily, but variation of the dose should be tailored to suit the individual patient, based on the regular blood counts which are of the utmost importance at this stage.

Alternatively a combination chemotherapy regimen employing a small dose of busulphan, 2 mg daily and either mercaptopurine 50 mg daily or thioguanine 80 mg daily may be used. Allopurinol influences the effective dose of mercaptopurine but not of thioguanine. If allopurinol is not being given the dose of mercaptopurine should be 100 mg daily. This regimen is given 5 days per week and results in a very much more rapid reduction in white cell count, taking on average 4–6 weeks, with correspondingly quicker induction of remission. Despite this, the regimen does not carry so great a risk of inducing severe aplasia as the count tends to plateau in the normal range of white cell counts. Dosage can be modified by varying the number of days per week on which the standard dose is given. The dose should be reduced when the count reaches normal levels.

Another and satisfactory way of using busulphan is to give the drug in single doses at 2 to 3 weekly intervals. Remission is induced more quickly than by the single agent daily dose method and appears to be safe. Busulphan produces minor degrees of pulmonary fibrosis in most patients. In a few, however, this may assume serious proportions and is known as 'busulphan lung'. The main symptom is severe breathlessness. If this occurs the drug should be stopped and never used again. Alternative drugs which are satisfactory include hydroxyurea, melphalan, chlorambucil and dibromomanitol. Mercaptopurine and thioguanine are effective but when used alone are rather difficult to control. Radiotherapy to the spleen can also be given and is effective in inducing control of the disease. However, it has been shown to be inferior to busulphan therapy.

SPLENECTOMY. This has been shown to be of little value; it does not appear to delay transformation to an acute phase. However, patients who present with massive splenomegaly and who run the risk of even more disabling splenomegaly in the terminal phase of the disease, may benefit from splenectomy, carried out when a good remission has been achieved.

Very high platelet counts, especially after splenectomy, appear to carry less danger of thrombotic complications than in other myeloproliferative disorders and may be well tolerated. The platelets are ineffective and may not be haemostatically adequate for major surgery, when platelet concentrates should be given postoperatively. If this is not done, there is a risk of intractable bleeding.

BONE MARROW TRANSPLANTATION. Pleuripotential stem cells from a normal marrow can be given intravenously to a patient who has been specially prepared. These cells will 'home' to the marrow and will produce enough erythrocytes, granulocytes and platelets to restore haematological normality in about 3 weeks. It takes longer, months or even years, to attain immunological stability.

Bone marrow transplantation thus offers the possibility of replacing diseased with healthy haemopoietic tissue. It provides the only long term cure for a number of serious haemopoietic disorders. There are however major problems. At present the patient should be less than 40 years old, should preferably have a suitable HLA/MLC (mixed lymphocyte culture) matched donor, a sibling if possible, and must be sufficiently stable psychologically to contend with a period of aggressive therapy during the transplantation process. The patient should be free of other disorders which might seriously limit life span.

Bone marrow transplantation is not a particularly difficult or complicated procedure but it requires highly specialised supervision and supportive facilities and a fully trained staff. It is best done in units established for the care of acute leukaemias under the primary care of haematologists, with the cooperation of immunologists, microbiologists, radiotherapists and a full laboratory service.

GVH Disease. If the graft is successful, problems of graft-versus-host (GVH) disease and interstitial pneumonitis may cause serious morbidity and death. Even low grade GVH disease, which is probably advantageous in terms of survival, can reduce the quality of life.

GVH disease is due to the cytotoxic activity of donor lymphocytes, probably T cells, which become sensitised to their new host which they regard as foreign. This may produce either an acute or chronic form of GVH disease. The acute form usually appears 14 to 21 days after the graft, although it may appear earlier or up to 70 days later. It is associated with mucositis, diarrhoea, hepatitis, cholestasis and exfoliative dermatitis. All these features may vary from being mild to lethally severe. The occurrence appears to be associated with infection, although the relationship is not fully understood. Methotrexate, cy-closporin, antithymocyte globulin and high dose corticosteroids have all been used to treat the disorder. The more severe forms prove very difficult to control.

Chronic GVH disease may follow acute GVH disease or arise independently; it occurs later than acute GVH disease. It often resembles a connective tissue disorder, although in mild cases a rash may be the only manifestation. Chronic GVH disease is usually treated with azathioprine and corticosteroids.

Indications for Marrow Transplantation. Transplantation may be syngeneic (identical twin donor) or allogeneic (non-identical donor). Autografting in which the patients own marrow is harvested to be given back again after intensive therapy may be used for disorders which do not primarily involve the haemopoietic tissues or in patients in whom very good remissions have been achieved.

Disorders for which allogeneic transplantation is currently offered include: severe aplastic anaemia, severe immunodeficiency syndromes, acute myeloblastic leukaemia in first remission, acute myelofibrosis, T and B cell lymphoblastic leukaemia in first remission and chronic myeloid leukaemia in chronic phase. Transplantation is also a possibility for acute lymphoblastic leukaemia (common type) in second remission, resistant acute leukaemia and selected patients with lymphoma.

For chronic myeloid leukaemia, autografting with the patients own chronic phase cells harvested and stored at the time of presentation has been used to treat the disease when it enters the acute phase.

Prognosis. On average patients with Philadelphia chromosome positive disease survive $3\frac{1}{2}$ years from the time of diagnosis. Philadelphia chromosome negative varieties, which are rare, carry a much poorer prognosis, the majority dying within one year. Long survival of up to 10 years or more occurs in a small proportion of patients.

In the majority the disease transforms sooner or later, either to an acute leukaemic phase, which may be either myeloblastic or lymphoblastic, or to the chronic refractory phase, with marrow fibrosis and an excess of basophils and blast cells. Unless the transformation is to acute lymphoblastic leukaemia, the outlook is extremely poor as this phase is very unresponsive to therapy. Sometimes the patient is diagnosed at the stage of transformation and this may account for some cases of acute leukaemia with the Philadelphia chromosome.

Eosinophil leukaemia is a rare variant of chronic myeloid leukaemia and shows features of the hypereosinophilic syndrome in which cardiomyopathies and endomyocardial fibrosis occur, leading to severe cardiac failure. Treatment is difficult.

Chronic monocytic leukaemia is a rare variant of chronic myeloid leukaemia. There is a monocytosis, a hypercellular marrow and variable anaemia. Management is similar to that for the myelodysplastic syndrome to which it is related.

Chronic Lymphatic Leukaemia

This is the commonest variety of leukaemia. It occurs more frequently in males than in females and the majority of patients are over the age of 45. The disease is very rare in the Chinese and other mongoloid races.

Pathology. There is moderate enlargement of lymph nodes and other lymphoid tissues throughout the body, the normal structure being replaced by a mass of lymphocytes. The histology is that of diffuse well-differentiated lymphocytic disease, nodular histology being rare. The spleen and liver are moderately enlarged and show lymphocytic infiltration. The bone marrow becomes progressively infiltrated with lymphocytes which eventually replace the erythropoietic and myeloid tissue.

In this disease lymphocytes which would normally respond to antigens by transformation and antibody formation, fail to do so. An ever increasing mass of immuno-incompetent cells accumulate to the detriment of immune function and bone marrow proliferation. The receptor profile of the lymphocytes almost always demonstrates a B cell type of disease. T cell disease occurs rarely. The light chains of immunoglobulins produced by these B cells tend to be either kappa or lambda in type (p. 22) indicating in the majority of cases, a monoclonal expansion of cells. The disease is closely related to and indeed overlaps with well-differentiated lymphocytic lymphoma (p. 533).

Clinical Features. The onset is very insidious. Tiredness and vague ill health are common although some patients are symptom free and the disorder is found incidentally. In contrast to chronic myeloid leukaemia the development of anaemia tends to be slower and the presenting feature is usually the finding of firm rubbery, discrete and painless lymph nodes in the cervical, axillary and inguinal regions. The spleen is usually palpable but smaller than in chronic myeloid leukaemia. The liver may also be enlarged. As a result of immunosuppression there is an increasing tendency to recurrent infections.

Investigation. Peripheral blood examination usually shows a mild but gradually increasing anaemia. Haemolytic anaemia may occur and is usually autoimmune in type. The white cell count may be greatly increased up to $1000 \times 10^9/l$ but in the majority of cases it is between $50-200 \times 10^9/l$. Of these cells about 95% or more are lymphocytes which are predominantly of the small variety. Lymphoblasts are rare but undifferentiated lymphocytes may increase in number in the terminal stages. The platelet count is either low normal or only mildly reduced.

Examination both by aspiration and trephine is required to assess the degree of marrow involvement. Dysplastic changes in the erythroblasts suggestive of folate deficiency may be noted and folate levels should be measured. Estimations of total proteins and immunoglobulin levels should be undertaken to establish the degree of immunosuppression which is common and progressive. In some patients immunoglobulin levels may be raised and there may be a monoclonal band. Urate levels are seldom raised because cell turnover is low.

STAGING. The disease may be staged according to the following criteria:

Stage 0:	Lymphocytes, $15 \times 10^9/l$ or more in the blood, 40% or more of cells in the marrow. No enlarged lymph nodes, spleen or liver. Hb equal to or greater than 11 g/dl, platelets equal to or greater than $100 \times 10^9/l$.
Stage I:	As in stage 0 but with enlarged lymph nodes.
Stage II:	As in stage 0 but with enlarged spleen, liver or both. Lymph nodes need not be enlarged.
Stage III:	As in the above stages, but with a haemoglobin less than 11 g/dl.
Stage IV:	As in all the above stages, but platelet count less than $100 \times 10^9/l$.

Treatment. Specific treatment is usually not required until stage III or IV of the disease is reached. The patient should be told that although the disorder is incurable it should be possible to live with it and that it may give little trouble for months or even years. Eventually specific treatment may be required and regular supervision by a haematologist becomes necessary. Patients with stage III and IV disease will require specific and supportive therapy. Folate deficiency should be corrected. Anaemia may require transfusion with red cell concentrates. If the bone marrow is severely infiltrated, initial treatment with prednisolone 40 mg daily and oxymetholone 25–50 mg daily, for several weeks before starting cytotoxic drugs, may rescue the haemopoietic elements and allow more vigorous treatment.

There is disagreement about whether treatment should be by gentle single agent therapy employing chlorambucil, either continuously in doses between 2 and 5 mg daily, or intermittently at higher doses, or by more vigorous combination chemotherapy. The latter induces more convincing remissions judged by investigational findings, but has yet to be shown to improve the well-being or the survival of the patient in the long-term; the former method of treatment is therefore recommended. Combination therapy usually includes cyclophosphamide, doxorubicin, vincristine and prednisolone. Some believe doxorubicin is the most important of these drugs, but like daunorubicin it is cardiotoxic. Both are cytotoxic anthracycline antibiotics.

Alternatively radiotherapy may be used. Total body irradiation with a very small total dose spread over 5 weeks in ten treatments can be very effective and may induce satisfactory remission with a minimum of upset to the patient. Whichever treatment is used, dosage should be controlled by accurate blood counts, the absolute neutrophil count and the platelet count being the most important.

Infections must be treated with antibiotics. If there is severe depression of immunoglobulins, gammaglobulin intramuscularly may reduce the frequency and severity of infections. When the platelet count is low, the use of intramuscular immunoglobulin may not be possible and can be replaced by fresh frozen plasma given intravenously weekly. Gammaglobulin concentrate should not be given intravenously, as it may induce severe reactions. Splenectomy may be required for autoimmune haemolytic anaemia which has proved unresponsive to corticosteroid therapy.

Hairy cell leukaemia is a variant of chronic lymphatic leukaemia now recognised to be more common than was previously thought. It is a disease of adult life affecting males four times more frequently than females. The mean age is 50 years. Patients usually present with general ill health and troublesome infections especially in the skin and are found to have considerable splenomegaly, severe neutropenia, monocytopenia and the characteristic hairy cells in the blood and bone marrow. These cells appear to be a cross between a B lymphocyte and a monocyte. The diagnostic test is to show that the acid phosphatase staining reaction in the cells is resistant to the action of tartrate. The neutrophil alkaline phosphatase score is usually high. Splenectomy is the best treatment.

Corticosteroids may help but cytotoxic chemotherapy is seldom successful and is generally to be avoided. The prognosis varies between very poor and very good.

Prolymphocytic leukaemia is another variant of chronic lymphatic leukaemia found mainly in males over the age of 60; 25% are of the T cell variety. There is massive splenomegaly with little lymphadenopathy and a very high white cell count, often in excess of $400 \times 10^9/l$. The characteristic cell is a large lymphocyte with a prominent nucleolus. Treatment is generally unsuccessful and the prognosis very poor.

Exposure to Ionising Radiation

The use of nuclear radiation both for energy production and weapons raises the risk of a nuclear accident, either in peace or in war. There is much uninformed speculation about the effects of accidental exposure, some of it grossly exaggerated. No accident, however, can be treated lightly and the facts presented here, derived from the therapeutic use of ionising radiation and the effects of the atomic bombs dropped on Japanese cities, may provide some simple basic guidelines in the event of an accident.

Relatively high doses of radiation are tolerated when only part of the body is exposed but when the whole body is involved, tolerance is greatly reduced. Given time, the body is capable of repairing some of the damage done by radiation, provided it is not too severe. This forms the basis of the calculation of maximum permissible doses for workers employed in industrial projects in which radiation in one form or another is used. The therapeutic application of ionising radiation takes these factors carefully into account and also recognises the risk of inducing secondary malignancy. Since the majority of patients treated already has malignant disease, this risk is not generally regarded as a contra-indication.

When an industrial nuclear accident occurs it is vital that all personnel leave the scene of radio-activity quickly to minimise exposure. If accidental exposure occurs, it is essential to obtain as accurate as possible an estimate of the radiation dose received and this will usually require the expertise of medical physicists. Workers, who are likely to be exposed to radiation, generally carry monitoring badges from which the doses can be calculated. If the accidental dose is relatively small, all that may be required is to remove the person from risk of further exposure. When the dose received approaches the limits of what the body can tolerate, the immediate risks are to the haemopoietic and gastrointestinal systems and can be monitored by general medical review and blood counts. Nausea and vomiting occurring under two hours from the time of exposure carry a very grave prognosis and treatment is generally useless. In patients whose symptoms develop at a later stage, support may be given in a similar way as for acute myeloid leukaemia receiving ablative therapy. Bone marrow transplantation from a sibling should be considered if facilities are available. The patient should have tissue typing performed at the earliest opportunity before his or her cells disappear.

The effects of a major atomic explosion, as from an atomic bomb, depend on where the human being is in relation to the explosion. Many are killed outright. Immediate survivors may die sooner or later from burns, both from flash exposure or the fire storm that follows, from blast and crush injuries or from radiation sickness. Radiation damage is due firstly to the intense burst of neutrons emitted at the time of the explosion and thereafter to radioactive fallout, although this is small in bombs in which the fireball does not hit the ground. Within seven hours of such an explosion the radiation from the fallout drops to 10% of what it was one hour after the explosion and after two days the radioactivity has reduced to 1%.

Survival from the effects of the Hiroshima bomb was 95% of those more than 2000 metres from the explosion, despite exposure to immediate radiation. There was virtually no fallout as the fireball did not reach the ground. There was a small but definite increase in both acute and chronic myeloid leukaemia in survivors; about 0·16% more of the population died than would have been expected. Fetuses and young children exposed at the time of the bomb showed abnormalities in some cases but subsequent survivors had normal healthy children with no increase in deformity. The incidence of other tumours in the exposed population has increased after a latent period of ten to fifteen years. These have occurred particularly in the thyroid, breast, lung, urinary tract and the haemopoietic systems. When last calculated in 1974, among a population of 54 000 exposed within 25 000 metres of the bomb, there was a total excess of death from malignant disease of 185 persons, or 0·4% of the population. Clearly the long-term effects of radiation are difficult to predict once exposure has occurred and the evidence from Hiroshima and Nagasaki is that the effect on survivors is less than was originally predicted, although the full score has yet to be counted.

The bombs used on the Japanese cities were small by modern standards. The scale of effects of the largest megaton bombs is not known but extrapolation from available evidence suggests that the population may be at risk up to 100 miles from the centre of the explosion in flat terrain. Hills and mountains may provide a degree of protection. Survivors who may benefit from medical treatment are likely to be so numerous as to overwhelm the medical and other services.

The need for prevention is obviously crucial and this responsibility involves every one of us.

THE LYMPHOMAS

This group of disorders is divided into two main types: Hodgkin's lymphoma and non-Hodgkin lymphoma.

Hodgkin's Lymphoma

This disease is characterised by progressive painless enlargement of lymphoid tissues throughout the body. It occurs in both sexes, often in adolescence and early adult life, but it may be found also in older people. The pathogenesis is unknown and the condition is usually regarded as a form of malignant disease related to other neoplastic processes of haemopoietic tissue. It is distinguished from non-Hodgkin lymphoma by the presence of Reed-Sternberg cells, now thought to be the malignant cells.

Pathology. Microscopic examination of involved tissue, usually lymph nodes, shows variable obliteration of the normal architecture, with proliferation of lymphoid cells. Reed-Sternberg cells are giant cells with paired mirror imaged nuclei and prominent nucleoli; unless they are found it may be difficult to make a histological diagnosis. In addition there may be an increase in eosinophils, neutrophils, plasma cells and histiocytes in the tissue. The numbers of well-differentiated lymphocytes vary from many to few and the degree of lymphocyte depletion forms the basis for the main pathological classification of the disease. In some cases the fibrous stroma is increased. Caseation and necrosis are most unusual. Infiltration with greyish areas of Hodgkin's tissue causes enlargement of the spleen and liver. The bone marrow, lungs, kidneys and alimentary tract may also be involved but deposits in the nervous system are rare.

The disease can be divided pathologically into sclerosing and non sclerosing types. In the latter the degree of lymphocyte depletion correlates quite well with the aggressiveness of the disease and three types are seen, (1) lymphocyte predominant, (2) mixed cellularity in which neutrophils, eosinophils and plasma cells are common and (3) lymphocyte depleted, the most aggressive variety. In sclerosing disease, called nodular sclerosing, the cellular areas may also show variable lymphocyte depletion giving some clue about the aggressiveness of the disease. The nodular sclerosing variety is the most commonly encountered with the mixed cellularity type coming second, lymphocyte predominant third and lymphocyte depleted the least often seen.

Clinical Features. The onset is insidious, usually with enlargement of one group of superficial nodes which may fluctuate in size. While the cervical nodes are often the first to be involved, the disease may also appear to start in the mediastinal and axillary nodes and more rarely in abdominal, pelvic and inguinal areas. Involved lymph nodes are usually painless, discrete and rubbery, though tenderness does occur in some cases, particularly when the nodes have enlarged rapidly. The overlying skin is freely mobile. Extension of the disease from the lymph nodes to adjacent tissues may occur, and is found particularly in the mediastinum. Pressure by node masses on neighbouring structures may cause a variety of problems, such as dysphagia, dyspnoea, venous obstruction, jaundice and paraplegia. Splenomegaly is uncommon at the onset and even when present does not always signify involvement. Absence of splenomegaly does not exclude involvement of this organ. Rarely the disease may be limited to the spleen.

General features may include progressive weakness, loss of weight and drenching night sweats. Fever may be present and in some instances is of a low grade irregular type while in others there are bouts of pyrexia with the temperature rising to 39°C and above for several days, alternating with apyrexial periods (Pel-Ebstein fever). In many cases, however, fever does not occur until the terminal stages. Pruritus is a troublesome symptom in about 10% of cases. Some patients experience discomfort at the site of a lesion shortly after an alcoholic drink.

Investigation. Anaemia is fairly common and progressive. It is usually normochromic and normocytic but occasionally there may be a haemolytic component. There is no diagnostic change in the white cells although a modest eosinophilia occurs in about 10–15% of cases. The total white cell count may be normal but is sometimes considerably raised and there is a neutrophil leucocytosis. Lymphopenia, when it occurs, is a bad sign and an indicator of lymphocyte depletion. In the terminal phase there may be leucopenia and thrombocytopenia which may be as much a reflection of treatment as of the disease. Bone marrow involvement is very uncommon at the outset but may be found later in the disease. The diagnosis can be established with certainty only by tissue biopsy, usually of a lymph node. Liver biopsy may provide the diagnosis in cases with hepatic enlargement.

STAGING. Hodgkin's disease is thought to arise in one area and spread from there to others. It is, therefore, important to establish the extent of the disease at the time of diagnosis because staging largely determines the therapeutic approach. To this end the patient requires intensive investigation including chest radiographs, bipedal lymphangiography, marrow trephine and aspirate. In some instances it is necesary to undertake laparotomy with splenectomy and biopsy of liver and various abdominal lymph nodes since lymphangiography does not demonstrate the nodes around the coeliac axis, porta hepatis and mesenteric vessels. The use of ultrasound, gallium scanning and computed tomography can add to the delineation of the extent of the disease and may be important in a patient in whom a laparotomy would be inadvisable. In time these non-invasive procedures may replace the need for laparotomy.

There are four clinical stages based primarily on the extent of the disease (Ann Arbor classification):

Stage I: Involvement of a single lymph node region (I) or extralymphatic site (IE).
Stage II: Involvement of two or more lymph nodes regions (II) or an extra-lymphatic site and lymph node regions on the same side (above and below) the diaphragm (IIE).
Stage III: Involvement of lymph nodes regions on both sides of the diaphragm with (IIIE) or without (III) extra-lymphatic involvement or involvement of the spleen (IIIS) or both (IIISE).
Stage IV: Diffuse involvement of one or more extra-lymphatic tissues, e.g. liver or bone marrow. The lymphatic structures are defined as the lymph nodes, spleen, thymus, Waldeyer's ring, appendix and Peyer's patches.

Each stage is sub-divided into 'A' or 'B' categories, according to whether they have systemic symptoms or not. The symptoms that place a patient in the 'B' category are: (1) unexplained weight loss of more than 10% of the body weight in the previous six months, (2) unexplained fever above 38°C. and (3) night sweats.

Differential diagnosis is from other conditions producing enlargement of lymph nodes and of the spleen namely (1) tuberculous lymphadenitis, which is usually confined to the neck, in which the nodes may become matted together and may show caseation and sinus formation, and there is no splenomegaly; (2) chronic pyogenic lymphadenitis (chiefly also of the neck) in which the nodes are small and tender, a source of infection can be found and there is no splenomegaly; (3) lymphatic leukaemia in which the examination of the blood and bone marrow reveal the characteristic changes; (4) infectious mononucleosis in which the lymph nodes and the splenic enlargement is transient and the blood examination and a positive Paul Bunnell or monospot test are diagnostic; (5) other types of lymphoma which can be distinguished only by microscopic examination of an excised node; (6) secondary syphilis with lymph node enlargement in which the swelling is transient, a rash is common and serological reactions are positive; (7) sarcoidosis in which the histology should differentiate.

Treatment. There are two main methods of treatment, radiotherapy and chemotherapy (p. 111). Megavoltage radiotherapy can eliminate the disease in a high proportion of patients provided the disease is localised. For this reason radiotherapy is chosen for most cases of stage I and II disease. Exceptions are when structures such as the lung are involved when chemotherapy may be used to shrink the lesion to dimensions suitable for radiotherapy. Moreover radiotherapy should not be used in stage II if three or more areas are involved, particularly if the patient has 'B' symptoms because such patients tend to relapse after this form of treatment; chemotherapy should be employed instead. As a generalisation patients with stage III or IV types of disease are treated with chemotherapy. However, stage III A patients in whom only nodes in the upper abdomen are involved do well with radiotherapy.

RADIOTHERAPY consists of treatment of the node areas. For disease above the diaphragm a 'mantle' treatment is used and includes nodes in the neck, axillae and mediastinum. In some cases, if the mediastinum is involved this field is later extended downwards to include the para-aortic region. Disease below the diaphragm is given an 'inverted Y' distribution of irradiation which includes the coeliac, para-aortic, iliac and groin nodes and follows roughly the bifurcation of the aorta. If splenectomy has not been performed the spleen should also be irradiated. In female patients the 'inverted Y' irradiation causes severe damage to the ovaries and if a staging laparotomy has been done the opportunity is usually taken to place the ovaries behind the uterus where they may be more protected.

COMBINATION CHEMOTHERAPY (p. 115) has revolutionised the treatment of advanced Hodgkin's disease. The classical combination is nitrogen mustard, a vinca alkaloid such as vincristine or vinblastine, together with procarbazine and prednisolone, given in 2-week pulses (p. 522) at 2 to 4 weekly intervals. Five pulses are given after all objective evidence of disease has gone. The minimum number of pulses is six and it is seldom necessary to give more than 12. If the patient relapses during treatment, usually about the time of the third pulse, the disease is resistant to these drugs and treatment should be changed to an alternative combination.

Nitrogen mustard (p. 113) is very unpleasant for patients and must be given intravenously. In most patients nausea and vomiting occur and can be severe, usually starting 2 to 4 hours after the injection and lasting from 12 to 24 hours in some cases. Antiemetics such as chlorpromazine or metoclopramide or both, given if necessarily parenterally in liberal doses, are helpful.

Cyclophosphamide, which is a phosphorylated nitrogen mustard, may replace nitrogen mustard in the regimen. Little advantage is gained as regards adverse effects as it is a potent epilator and also may cause haemorrhagic cystitis, etc. (p. 56).

Chlorambucil, also a nitrogen mustard analogue, has been used successfully in this regimen in place of nitrogen mustard and has the advantage that it can be given by mouth and is well tolerated. Patients can be managed easily on an out-patient basis. Nitrogen mustard and its analogues are all severely myelotoxic.

The vinca alkaloids (p. 113), vincristine, vinblastine and vindesine are relatively less toxic to the bone marrow. In particular vincristine has this advantage but is more neurotoxic than vinde-sine which in turn is more neurotoxic than vinblastine. Numbness and paraesthesiae in the fingers and toes is very common and can usually be tolerated. Paralysis of muscle groups or burning pains may force the discontinuation of the drug. Patients complain of severe constipation. This may be avoided by the use of high roughage diet and gentle aperients, if necessary. Most of these symptoms improve with time although full recovery may not occur.

Procarbazine is a myelotoxic drug which is under suspicion as possibly the most oncogenic of the drugs in this combination.

Prednisolone is almost useless in this disease on its own but has been shown to play an essential role in combination with other agents. Antituberculosis chemotherapy should be used if there is evidence of old untreated disease. Exacerbation of peptic ulceration can be controlled by cimetidine or ranitidine. Prednisolone should be withdrawn gradually over 3 days at the end of each pulse. In many instances prednisolone is a euphoriant and helps the patient to tolerate the side effects of the other drugs.

Other combination chemotherapy regimes exist but none has been shown to be as effective as the one outlined above. However, they do provide alternative chemotherapy when there is resistance to the classical combination.

Chemotherapy carries a fairly high risk of inducing sterility in males (p. 117) and this may be permanent although recovery can occur with time. To a lesser extent it is a risk in females, in whom evidence of premature menopause may also appear. Since many of these patients are young, the males in particular may require counselling about the effect of chemotherapy and be offered the possibility of sperm storage.

Prognosis. If the patient is not treated the disease is fatal. With stage IA disease, the 5-year survival rate in patients treated with radiotherapy exceeds 90%, and in stage IIA disease is greater than 70%. In more advanced disease the results of chemotherapy are very satisfactory and more than 50% of patients remain disease free after 5 years. Just how effective combination chemotherapy is, remains to be seen since many patients who were treated in this way are still alive. The prognosis so far as histological type is concerned seems to matter less when chemotherapy is used. The prognosis is relatively poor when evidence of resistance to treatment appears and very few of such patients survive thereafter for 5 years.

Non-Hodgkin Lymphoma

In this group of disorders there is a malignant monoclonal proliferation of lymphoid cells, usually identifiable as B cells. Occasionally T cells are affected. Non-Hodgkin lymphomas merge with the lymphoblastic and lymphocytic leukaemias with which they have many features in common.

Pathology and Classification. This group of lymphomas has always proved difficult to classify. At present the most widely used classification is that of Rappaport (Table 13.1). This system has major defects but it is easily understood and used and it has not been superseded, internationally, by any one classification developed since.

The first and most important division is between lymphomas in which a nodular (follicular) structure can still be seen and those in which this structure has been replaced by a diffuse sheet of cells. These two groups are known as *nodular* (follicular) and *diffuse* respectively. In both, the lymphoid cells may be either well-differentiated, poorly differentiated, mixed lymphocytic-histiocytic or histiocytic. In general, nodular lymphomas carry a considerably better prognosis than diffuse.

Table 13.1 Non-Hodgkin lymphoma
Rappaport classification

1. Nodular (follicular)	2. Diffuse
(i) Well differentiated	
(ii) Poorly differentiated	
(iii) Mixed lymphocytic-histiocytic	
(iv) Histiocytic	

One defect of this classification is that it uses the term 'histiocytic'. It is now known that true histiocytic lymphomas are very rare and the majority called histiocytic are large B cell lymphomas, consisting of primitive blast cells. Another defect is the inability to place certain lymphomas, such as Burkitt's lymphoma in the classification.

Unlike Hodgkin's lymphoma the disease in non-Hodgkin lymphoma is frequently widespread at the time of diagnosis, often involving not only lymph nodes, but also bone marrow, spleen and other tissues. Early involvement of bone marrow is typical of nodular lymphoma. Extra-lymphatic tissue involvement at the time of presentation is more common and almost every organ or tissue may be the site of initial disease. In gastrointestinal lymphomas the stomach is most frequently and the rectum least frequently involved. Thyroid lymphomas tend to be associated with gastrointestinal involvement. Some skin lymphomas are T cell in type, e.g. mycosis fungoides. Most lymphomas involving extra-lymphatic tissues are of the diffuse variety and therefore have a rather poor prognosis unless well localised.

Clinical Features. These lymphomas occur at all ages, are rare under two years and become more frequent with increasing age. Males are more often affected than females. Nodular lymphomas occur mainly in adults between the ages of 30 and 60.

Lymph node enlargement is the most common presenting finding, and is usually painless unless it has developed very quickly. The nodes are discrete and firm. The patient usually complains of tiredness, lassitude, loss of weight and occasionally fever and sweating. However, the patient may be symptom free. When the presentation is extra-lymphatic the symptoms will reflect the tissues involved. Quite often the diagnosis of lymphoma comes unexpectedly at laparotomy or during other investigative procedures. Weakness of the legs progressing to paraplegia may be due to an extradural lymphoma compressing the cord. Pressure effects in other areas may cause dysphagia, breathlessness, vomiting, intestinal obstruction or ascites and limb oedema. Pain is the main symptom of bone involvement which may present with a pathological fracture.

Physical examination often reveals more widespread node involvement than the patient has noticed. Unexplained lymphadenopathy which fails to resolve spontaneously within a few weeks should always be suspect. Moreover lymphomatous nodes may wax and wane in size and the shrinkage of nodes does not exclude a diagnosis of lymphoma. Splenomegaly usually indicates that the spleen is involved in the neoplastic process.

Investigation. Diagnosis is based primarily on histological findings from biopsy of a lymph node or other involved tissue. In some cases reactive hyperplasia is seen in the biopsy and a clinical suspicion of lymphoma is not confirmed initially. Further biopsies may eventually reveal a lymphoma.

The staging process is similar to that adopted for Hodgkin's disease except that laparotomy is seldom necessary although it may be required for diagnostic purposes when only retroperitoneal nodes are involved. Bone marrow aspiration and trephine biopsy should be done early in the investigation since marrow involvement is common and indicates stage IV disease. Blood counts usually show normal values unless there is splenomegaly with hypersplenism or a complicating autoimmune haemolytic anaemia when a reduced haemoglobin level, reticulocytosis and positive direct antiglobulin test (Coombs' test) will be found. In some cases a slight excess of lymphocytes may be present. Thrombocytopenia is uncommon. Moderate degrees of anaemia may be also present if there is considerable bone marrow involvement.

An evaluation of the cell membrane receptor characteristics of the peripheral blood and lymph node lymphocytes is helpful, particularly in cases in which the diagnosis is in doubt, but this has to be done in specialised laboratories. The demonstration of a monoclonal expansion of the B lymphocyte population is characteristic and other features may give a measure of the degree of differentiation of the cells. These techniques also assist in the identification of the rare cases of T cell lymphoma. For this a second biopsy of lymph nodes may be required. Patients accept this readily if they understand why it is being done. An assessment of immune competence is also important and immunoglobulin levels should be measured. In some cases a monoclonal band may be found.

Treatment. In the case of the more benign non-Hodgkin lymphomas, such as the nodular lymphocytic and even diffuse well-differentiated lymphocytic varieties, no specific therapy may be necessary if the disease is not advanced. Some patients can be observed for years before active measures are indicated.

RADIOTHERAPY. When treatment is required localised disease is best managed, as in Hodgkin's disease, with radiotherapy and this may be curative. However, non-Hodgkin lymphoma is often at stage III or IV when diagnosed and in these cases chemotherapy is generally the treatment of choice. Where there are pressure problems the local disease may be treated with radiotherapy in combination with chemotherapy (combined modality treatment). The more benign types of disease may also respond very well to total body irradiation, a form of radiotherapy that employs very small doses of only 150 centigrays over a period of 5 weeks in ten divided doses of 15 centigrays. This is very suitable for elderly patients as it is relatively free of side-effects.

CHEMOTHERAPY. Most cases of nodular lymphoma, with the exception of the histiocytic variety, respond very well to gentle, single agent chemotherapy and chlorambucil is the drug usually chosen. More dramatic results in terms of induction of remission may be achieved with combination chemotherapy but there is as yet no evidence that this is of long-term benefit to the patient and it may cause considerably greater morbidity. Chlorambucil may be given as continuous therapy at a dose of 5 mg daily initially, reducing to 2 mg daily as indicated by blood count. This may be given over many months in order to control the disease. Alternatively the drug may be given intermittently in higher doses. Combination with prednisolone may be useful, especially at the start of treatment when the bone marrow may be heavily involved with lymphoma. The steroid therapy may be started before as described for chronic lymphatic leukaemia (p. 527). Oxymetholone therapy may also help to rescue the bone marrow. Long-term steroid therapy should be avoided.

Combination chemotherapy is indicated for the more aggressive diffuse lymphomas of poorly differentiated lymphocytic, mixed cell or histiocytic variety. The diffuse histiocytic type should always receive the most aggressive chemotherapy as a number of cases apparently can be rendered disease free for long periods with this treatment. Radiotherapy does not appear to be able to achieve as good results. If these patients survive a year after cessation of treatment without relapse they have a chance of long-term remission. There are a number of regimes but most physicians employ a combination of cyclophosphamide, doxorubacin, vincristine, bleomycin and prednisolone. Alternatively the combination chemotherapy regime described for Hodgkin's disease may be given.

Rather less aggressive management has been used for the diffuse poorly differentiated lymphocytic variety and accordingly cyclophosphamide, vincristine and prednisolone with or without doxorubicin is generally prescribed. All these combination regimens are given as pulses (p. 522) with variable periods of rest for bone marrow recovery between each pulse. The number of pulses is usually between six and 12 in any one course. Once the disease has become resistant to the standard drugs, second line chemotherapy usually produces only brief benefit and the value of achieving this at the expense of the patient's well-being has to be evaluated in each case. It may be better to deal with troublesome disease as it arises with short courses of radiotherapy. This palliative approach can be quite successful.

As a generalisation, patients over 70 years do not tolerate aggressive chemotherapy well. Adolescents who present with an undifferentiated lymphoma, which is often initially in the mediastinum, should be managed in the same way as patients with acute lymphoblastic leukaemia. Some patients with well-differentiated lymphocytic lymphoma progress to chronic lymphatic leukaemia and should be managed accordingly.

The treatment of these disorders consists of balancing the prospects of killing off the disease with those of destroying the patient. The effect on the patient's normal tissues is usually monitored by watching the blood count. In this respect the white cell count, the absolute neutrophil count and the platelet count are the most useful. As the absolute neutrophil count drops below $0.5 \times 10^9/l$, infection with bacteria or fungi becomes an increasing risk. Similarly, bleeding is increasingly likely to occur as the platelet count drops below $50 \times 10^9/l$ although many patients tolerate very low levels for longer periods without serious bleeding. Dosage of myelotoxic drugs must be reduced once these figures are approached and some physicians would reduce the dose at higher levels. The effect of drugs may continue after they have been withdrawn and this should be kept in mind. Regular blood counts are absolutely essential for the satisfactory management of these patients.

SURGERY. In lymphomas of extra-lymphatic tissue, surgical excision may be employed and is usually supplemented with radiotherapy, with or without chemotherapy thereafter.

SUPPORTIVE THERAPY. General supportive measures such as blood transfusion with red cell concentrate should be used for anaemia when necessary. Infections should be treated promptly with antibiotics or other agents. A watch should be kept for the development of monilia infection in the mouth of patients who have developed neutropenia or are on steroids. Severe heartburn may indicate oesophageal thrush.

Prognosis. The mean survival of patients with diffuse lymphomas is in the region of 2 years and those with the histiocytic variety who do not respond well to treatment often survive less than 1 year. Patients with nodular lymphomas of lymphocytic or mixed cell type have a mean survival of 7 to 8 years and in the nodular histiocytic variety of about 3 years.

Burkitt's Lymphoma

This form of lymphoblastic B cell non-Hodgkin lymphoma occurs predominantly in tropical Africa and New Guinea, although it also occurs less frequently in other parts of the world. There is strong evidence that the Epstein-Barr (EB) virus plays an important aetiological role in its development. The majority of cases occur in children with a peak incidence between the ages of 4 and 8 years, although cases found outside the tropics show an older age distribution and a lower incidence of EB virus infection.

The disorder effects predominantly extranodal tissues with a marked predilection for the mandible and the maxillary bones. This may cause marked bony deformity, loosening of the teeth and, if the orbit is involved, extrusion of the eye with loss of sight. In the abdomen, involvement, often bilaterally, of the kidneys, adrenals, ovaries or lymph nodes may give rise to an abdominal tumour. Extradural lesions of the spinal cord may cause sudden onset of paraplegia. Other sites which may be involved include long bones, the salivary glands, the thyroid, testes and the heart. Bilateral tumours of the breast may be seen in young adult women. Lymph nodes and marrow are more frequently involved in cases outside the tropics and abdominal tumours are the most common finding.

The cytological appearance of Burkitt lymphoma is characteristic with lymphoblast-type cells showing vaculation in the cytoplasm and nucleus. Histologically the 'starry sky' appearance created by histiocytes scattered amongst sheets of primitive lymphoid cells is typical. Chromosome analysis shows an 8/14 translocation in a high proportion of cases and less often an 8/2 or 8/22 translocation. Antibody to EB virus, capsid antigen, is found in most patients with the African variety.

Response to chemotherapy, particularly if the disease is localised, is very good. Cyclophosphamide is given intramuscularly, 60 mg/kg every 2 weeks for up to six doses. Since meningeal involvement often occurs later in the disease, prophylactic intrathecal methotrexate may also be given. The response to treatment is often dramatic with resolution of the disease following the first dose of cyclophosphamide. The prognosis is good especially for patients with localised disease.

MULTIPLE MYELOMA (MYELOMATOSIS)

This is a malignant disorder of plasma cells.

Immunopathology. Normal plasma cells are derived from B lymphocytes by transformation after exposure to antigenic stimuli; individual plasma cells manufacture only one type of immunoglobulin. The finding that in myeloma, and in other related malignant disorders of B lymphocytes, all the malignant cells produce the same immunoglobulin indicates that the tumour is derived originally from one cell by cloning; the disease is therefore monoclonal. The immunoglobulin is called a *paraprotein* and appears on electrophoretic strips as a clear-cut band. Each of the five normal types of immunoglobulin (IgG, IgA, IgM, IgD, and IgE) has light chains of either lambda or kappa varieties (Fig. 2.3). In myeloma the paraprotein produced belongs to one of these immunoglobulin types and has one or other of the two light chains. In some cases only part of the immunoglobulin molecule is produced by the tumour cells, most commonly the light chains. These appear in the urine as *Bence Jones proteinuria* and if myeloma is associated only with light chains it is known as Bence Jones myeloma.

In just over half of the patients with myeloma an IgG paraprotein is produced. About 20% are IgA producing and a similar percentage are of the Bence Jones variety. IgD, IgM and IgE myelomas are rare and together amount to only 2% of cases. Patients with IgG and IgA myelomas may, in due course, develop light chain proteinuria, so called 'Bence Jones escape'. This usually indicates an accelerated phase of the disease.

In the majority of patients the bone marrow is heavily infiltrated with atypical plasma cells which are usually larger and paler staining than normal plasma cells and contain nucleoli. Some cells may be multinucleated. Progressive replacement of the marrow occurs with eventual reduction of the normal cell lines, inducing anaemia, leucopenia and thrombocytopenia. Osteoclasts are stimulated and absorption of bone occurs, producing diffuse osteoporosis. Local tumour formation by the myeloma causes punched out translucencies in the bone radiograph. Rarely the disease may present as a solitary plasmacytoma either in bone or soft tissue.

Excessive production of the myeloma paraprotein is associated with progressive reduction in normal immunoglobulin levels and impairment of immune function.

Clinical Features. The disease is very uncommon under the age of 30. It becomes increasingly frequent thereafter, having its peak incidence between 60 and 70 years. Males are affected rather more frequently than females and Black people of Central African origin two to three times more often than Caucasians. There is a long preclinical phase, in some instances up to 25 years. The disorder may be disovered incidentally by laboratory tests during this phase and the patient may thereafter be observed for years before symptoms appear.

Symptoms usually reflect bone involvement, impairment of immune function, renal damage, anaemia or hyperviscosity. The diffuse osteoporosis and local erosion of bone by myeloma result in stress pain and eventual pathological fracture. The stress pain is often wandering, difficult to locate and described as 'rheumatics'. On the other hand the first intimation of trouble may be the sudden onset of acute localised pain due to pathological fracture. These symptoms arise mainly in weight bearing bones, the vertebrae, pelvis and femur being particularly susceptible. Collapse of vertebrae is common and produces nerve root pressure symptoms and shortening of stature. Patients are often severely crippled. Weight lifting may also cause pain in the arms whereas lesions in the skull seldom give rise to pain.

The progressive impairment of immune function due to the deficiencies of normal immunoglobulins and the excess of abnormal immunoglobulins renders these patients susceptibile to infections, particularly of the respiratory tract. Pneumonia is quite frequently the presenting illness and infection very often the cause of death.

The excessive production of light chains which are lost in the urine as Bence Jones protein, may damage tubular cells and block the tubular lumen. Renal failure may supervene. Light chains deposited elsewhere may result in amyloidosis (p. 390). Mobilisation of calcium from the skeleton may be excessive and cause hypercalcaemia, which may result in nephrocalcinosis. High calcium levels may also cause lethargy and drowsiness progressing to coma if untreated.

Patients often complain of tiredness which may be due to anaemia. Bleeding and bruising problems are seldom presenting features but they may be troublesome terminally and are due both to thrombocytopenia and hyperglobulinaemia.

Hyperviscosity is a problem in some patients with very high levels of paraprotein. It may impair the circulation, notably in the central nervous system, causing headaches, vertigo, dizziness, somnolence and stupor progressing to coma.

Clinical examination may reveal tender areas in the bones, kyphoscoliosis, muscle spasm and impaired mobility, particularly with vertebral involvement. Retinal haemorrhages, exudates and gross dilation of the retinal veins, with periodic constrictions giving a 'string of sausages' appearance, suggest hyperviscosity.

Investigation. Assessment of myeloma is very dependent on laboratory findings. The degree of bone marrow involvement is reflected in the haemoglobin level, the white cell count and the platelet count and can be assessed directly with bone marrow examination. A high ESR is very characteristic but is not always present. Rarely myeloma cells appear in the blood as a plasma cell leukaemia.

The level of paraprotein production is evaluated using electrophoresis and measurement of the monoclonal band, the level being expressed in grams per litre. This measurement should be used to follow progress. Immune impairment can be assessed from the electrophoretic strip and the immunoglobulin levels. The raised level of the specific immunoglobulin involved is not a good monitor of the paraprotein level. Renal function should be assessed by blood urea and by creatinine clearance. Plasma calcium should always be determined. Plasma alkaline phosphatase is usually within normal limits despite the bone involvement unless there has been a fracture when a transient rise may occur. Plasma urate levels should also be measured.

Diagnosis depends on finding at least two of the characteristic features of the disease. The bone marrow may be pathognomonic but is not always so. A firm diagnosis may depend on the demonstration of a monoclonal paraproteinaemia and punched-out lytic areas in bone radiographs together with osteoporosis. Reactive plasmacytosis in the marrow can mimic myeloma but the increased immunoglobulins are polyclonal. Paraprotein bands may be found in lymphomas, macroglobulinaemia and so called 'benign monoclonal hypergammaglobulinaemia'; they may also be associated with a wide range of inflammatory, neoplastic and autoimmune disease. In such cases the level of paraprotein does not significantly increase with time and is usually less than $10 \text{ g}/l$.

Treatment. Local skeletal problems should be treated with radiotherapy and the general disease with chemotherapy. Melphalan is the drug of choice, although cyclophosphamide is probably as effective.

Patients in the pre-clinical phase generally do not require treatment. In the clinical phase melphalan may be given either alone as low dose continuous therapy, 2 mg daily or as high dose intermittent therapy (0·25 mg/kg/day for 4 days) in combination with prednisolone (2·0 mg/kg/day for 4 days), weaning off over the following 3 days. Such treatment should be administered in pulses every 4 to 6 weeks. The dosage of melphalan should be adjusted according to the white cell, absolute neutrophil and platelet counts. In most patients the disease is slowly brought under control. Progress should be evaluated by measuring the levels of paraprotein in the blood. When this has reached a plateau, chemotherapy may be stopped. A small proportion of patients are resistant to treatment and the disease is progressive.

In patients with the more rapidly advancing forms of myeloma more aggressive therapy may be required, using combination chemotherapy. Those who present with anaemia, hypercalacaemia and evidence of renal damage and in whom there is Bence Jones proteinuria require urgent management with high fluid intake and alkalinisation of the urine with oral bicarbonate. Corticosteroids and possibly mithramycin are given to reduce calcium levels. Careful transfusion with red cell concentrate is also required unless the haemoglobin is above 10 g/dl. Specific treatment under such circumstances should be with combination chemotherapy, bearing in mind that dose reductions may be required because of renal failure, the management of which is described on page 393. In this situation cyclophosphamide is contraindicated. Vincristine, doxorubicin and prednisolone form a useful combination.

Despite good control of the general disease, further episodes of bone pain and fracture may occur and require radiotherapy. Prophylactic irradiation of eroded vertebrae may be warranted before crush fracture has occurred. Fractures of femur and humerus require orthopaedic surgery with pinning of the bone, followed by radiotherapy. Bed rest should be minimised to avoid further loss of calcium from the skeleton. Hyperviscosity problems may require plasmapheresis (p. 33). The use of anabolic steroids can be helpful in arresting further deterioration in the skeleton.

Maintaining the morale of the patients in the face of crippling and painful disease may be difficult but they should be encouraged to look forward to gradual improvement. Given time and good management many can return from a bedridden stage to active lives.

Prognosis. Without treatment the disease progresses relentlessly to death. With treatment the outlook for the majority of patients is considerably improved and a few may survive for many years. Bad signs at the time of diagnosis are a haemoglobin level of less than 7 g/dl, severe hypoalbuminaemia and renal failure. The presence of Bence Jones proteinuria is also indicative of more serious disease. Prognosis should be guarded in any individual until the response to treatment has been assessed; this may take 6 months or more.

Waldenstrom's macroglobulinaemia is a rare disease of the elderly, more common in males than females. There is a monoclonal IgM paraproteinaemia and a tendency to develop a hyperviscosity syndrome. The marrow is infiltrated with neoplastic lymphocytes.

Untreated, the progress is often slow with eventual immune deficiency and susceptibility to infection. Chlorambucil on a long term low dose basis, such as 2 mg daily, may control the lymphocyte proliferation and the advance of the disease. Some patients are unresponsive. Plasmapheresis may be required. The majority of patients survive 2 to 5 years and some live considerably longer.

Hypersplenism

This term is used to describe the depression of leucocyte and platelet counts in the peripheral blood which is often encountered in a wide variety of conditions in which splenomegaly is a prominent feature, such as portal hypertension. The cause of the leucopenia and the thrombocytopenia is not fully understood but may in part be due to excessive sequestration of leucocytes and platelets in the enlarged spleen.

Another important effect of splenomegaly is, for reasons unknown, an increase in total plasma volume. This dilutes the red cell mass which remains normal in total amount but the dilution gives a low haemoglobin reading, down to 8 g/dl in some patients. The spurious anaemia can be identified by measurement of the red cell mass and plasma volume and is corrected only by splenectomy which may also improve leucopenia and thrombocytopenia.

HAEMORRHAGIC DISEASES

This group of disorders is composed of conditions characterised by an abnormal tendency to bleed.

Pathophysiology

The mechanism concerned in the arrest of haemorrhage can be divided into three stages. The first is spasm of damaged small blood vessels. The second is formation of platelet plugs on the damaged areas of vascular endothelium by aggregation of platelets. The third is the coagulation of blood which is the end product of a chain reaction involving many coagulation factors.

1. **The Vascular Reaction.** Spasm of small arterioles and capillary sphincters in response to injury constitutes an essential feature of natural haemostasis. It is the first reaction, slowing the blood loss and allowing other factors to operate. Eventually the spasm relaxes and if the platelets and coagulation factors have not carried out their functions, secondary bleeding develops.

2. **The Platelet.** Normal platelets do not adhere to the vascular endothelium when it is intact. The natural anticoagulant, prostacyclin, (p. 547) produced by the vascular endothelial cells from arachidonic acid, possibly helps to prevent platelet adhesion and aggregation. Platelets adhere readily to collagen under the vascular endothelium when it is exposed by injury. They also adhere to each other under the influence of adenosine diphosphate (ADP) released in damaged tissue. A platelet aggregate forms — primary aggregation. At this stage it is possible for the platelets to break off into the circulation as small emboli which usually disintegrate rapidly. Primary aggregation probably happens inside blood vessels when injury is minimal. When the injury is such that the full effect of the haemostatic mechanism is required, primary aggregation is followed by a change in the shape of the platelets. An irreversible phase of aggregation is reached, promoted by thromboxane A2 which is formed in platelets from arachidonic acid through endo-

peroxide intermediates PGG2 and PGH2 (Fig. 13.4). Another factor involved in the irreversible phase of aggregation is ADP. Platelet granules release numerous substances including fibrinogen, platelet factors 3 and 4, prostaglandins and thromboxane A2. These participate in the formation of fibrin and in the establishment of a stable haemostatic plug which differs in structure from a thrombus.

Capillary bleeding can be stopped by platelet plug formation and does not require the coagulation mechanism. This is why the bleeding time is usually normal in haemophilia and why a lack of platelets gives rise to capillary bleeding (purpura). The platelet plug is inadequate for blood vessels larger than capillaries, because the blood pressure in them is too great and without the support of fibrin formation the platelet plug is expelled when the vessel spasm relaxes. However, when the injury is slight the full train of the haemostatic mechanism will not proceed as it will be inhibited by antithrombin III and other anticoagulant factors in the blood. In this way blood flow can be maintained in blood vessels where the injury is not sufficient to require the cessation of flow.

3. **Coagulation of the Blood.** The end point of the clotting mechanism is the formation of fibrin from fibrinogen. Haemostasis, initiated by vascular spasm and platelet plug formation, is strengthened by the laying down of a fibrin mesh. The fibrin then contracts and consolidates the initial repair by binding the tissues together.

This mechanism can be activated in two ways: (1) by an intrinsic system in the blood vessels which is activated by contact with collagen exposed when the vascular endothelium is injured and (2) by an extrinsic system activated by tissue fluid. The intrinsic system is more potent but there appears to be interaction between the two. It is possible that the extrinsic system activates factor X which in turn generates the production of thrombin from prothrombin. Thrombin at this stage then acts as an enhancer of the intrinsic system.

Thirteen main coagulation factors have been named. It is now recognised that factor III (thromboplastin) and factor IV do not exist as distinct biochemical entities. Thromboplastin

Fig. 13.4 Interaction of blood coagulation, fibrinolytic, kallikrein and platelet systems. ADP = adenosine diphosphate. FDP = fibrin degradation products. a = activated.

probably represents the co-operative activity of several factors. The term, factor VI, is no longer used.

The coagulation mechanism is a biological amplifier, a cascade of activated proenzymes assisted by co-enzymes. Precursor substances or factors circulating in the blood are activated and in turn activate other factors and so on. Ionised calcium is absolutely essential at several points in the mechanism. Anticoagulation in vitro can be achieved by chelation of the ionised calcium as by using acid citrate dextrose (ACD) or citrate phosphate dextrose (CPD) to prevent the coagulation of blood for transfusion purposes.

In the intrinsic system the trigger that initiates the cascade is contact with water-wettable surfaces such as collagen. This activates factor XII which activates factor XI which in turn activates factor IX (Fig. 13.4). Activated factor IX (IXa) in the presence of co-factor VIII, platelet factor 3 (phospholipid) and calcium ions activates factor X. The precise role of the other platelet factors is uncertain.

The extrinsic system of activation is initiated by tissue damage and tissue factors activate factor X in the presence of factor VII. Factor X is the point at which the intrinsic and extrinsic systems meet and is the start of the final common pathway.

Activated factor X together with factor V, platelet factor 3 and calcium ions activates prothrombin to thrombin and this digests the fibrinogen molecule to fibrin. The effect of the amplification of the biochemical reaction is so powerful that conversion of fibrinogen to fibrin is almost instantaneous. Thus fibrin is formed sufficiently quickly to prevent it being flushed away by further bleeding.

Thrombin also activates factor XIII (fibrin stabilising factor) which stabilises the chemical structure of the polymerised fibrin. Subsequent contraction of the fibrin is dependent on adequate numbers of platelets being involved in the clotting process. When there is thrombocytopenia, retraction of the clot is poor.

Factor VIII (antihaemophilic globulin) is deficient in haemophilia. It is a molecule formed by the combination of two fractions, (1) a coagulant factor which is genetically sex linked and (2) a fraction which can be recognised antigenically and is produced by an autosomal gene (factor VIII related antigen or VIII Rag). The coagulant fraction is measured by assay of its activity in the coagulation mechanism and the factor VIII related antigen by the use of heterologous antiserum.

Factor XII is the only coagulation factor, a deficiency of which is not associated with a tendency to bleed. Deficiency of this factor is more likely to be associated with a liability to thrombosis due to failure of activation of the fibrinolytic mechanism through the kallikrein system (Fig. 13.4).

The Fibrinolytic System. This functions in much the same way as the coagulation mechanism. Plasminogen, an inert precursor, can be activated to form plasmin which digests fibrin to give soluble degradation products. In excess, it will also digest fibrinogen and other coagulation factors. This system comes into play when there is a threat of widespread intravascular coagulation and prevents or removes the deposition of fibrin in the blood vessels. This is associated with an increase in fibrin degradation products. Plasminogen is closely bound to fibrinogen and fibrin and is slowly activated after normal clotting to digest the fibrin clot. This process can be accelerated artificially with streptokinase which can be used sometimes in the lysis of thrombi.

Coagulation Inhibitors. The tendency of the coagulation mechanism to be activated is counterbalanced by inhibitory factors in the blood. These substances neutralise the activated factors rapidly. In blood vessels activation of the coagulation mechanism is minimal and these inhibitors are effective. At the point of an injury, however, the activation of the coagulation mechanism is so powerful that the inhibitors are overwhelmed. One important inhibitor is antithrombin III which inactivates thrombin (factor II) and activated factors IX, X, XI, and XII. It is required for the action of heparin. Without it heparin is useless. Patients who are deficient of antithrombin III are very liable to thrombosis.

Investigation of Bleeding Disorders

If there is suspicion that a patient has a bleeding disorder a basic screen of haemostatic function should be performed. Blood should be taken for a blood count, including platelet count and blood film and for basic coagulation investigations. A bleeding time should be done by the Ivy method. It is an excellent test of capillary and platelet function but does not uncover coagulation defects.

Coagulation investigations should include a prothrombin time to evaluate the activity of factors II, VII and X and their function in the final common pathway and the extrinsic system. A partial thromboplastin time with kaolin (the latter being used to activate the contact factors) will detect problems of significance in the intrinsic pathway or the presence of inhibitors to this pathway. A thrombin time may be done to monitor heparin-like activity such as may be produced by the presence of excessive levels of fibrin degradation products. The fibrinogen level should be measured, particularly when depletion is anticipated. If an abnormality is detected by the above tests more detailed investigation follows with factor assays, platelet function tests and tests of fibrinolysis.

The results of such investigations do not explain all the phenomena observed in patients who are bleeding. For example a prolonged bleeding time due to thrombocytopenia is not associated with insuperable haemostatic problems at a major surgical procedure such as splenectomy although haemostasis is abnormal. Equally, although the bleeding time is normal in haemophilia, major surgery would be haemostatically impossible if special measures were not undertaken (p. 544). An intact extrinsic clotting system does not compensate for a defective intrinsic system as seen in haemophilia. It would seem that the platelets are essential for controlling bleeding due to minor trauma and the coagulation mechanism for bleeding due to major trauma. Thus when platelets are deficient, capillary bleeding predominates and when the coagulation mechanism is faulty more serious deep seated bleeding occurs. These observations may partly explain anomalies in the clinical findings associated with various defects in the haemostatic mechanism.

Classification of Haemorrhagic Disorders

1. **Due to Defect of the Blood Vessels.**
(a) The vascular purpuras.
  (i) Infections, e.g. typhus, typhoid, meningococcal meningitis, measles, infective endocarditis, septicaemia.

(ii) Chemical agents, e.g. aspirin, ergot, frusemide, indomethacin, iodides, phenobarbitone, phenylbutazone, phenytoin, quinine and snake venom.

(iii) Anaphylactoid purpura (purpura simplex and Henoch-Schönlein purpura p. 569).

(iv) Metabolic purpura (uraemia, p. 392 hepatic failure p. 353).

(v) Scurvy (p. 72).

(b) Hereditary haemorrhagic telangiectasia.

2. Due to Disorders of Blood Platelets

(a) Reduced numbers of platelets: idiopathic and secondary (symptomatic) thrombocytopenic purpura.

(b) Increased numbers of platelets: thrombocythaemia.

(c) Defective platelets: hereditary and acquired thrombasthaemia.

3. Due to Defects of the Clotting Mechanism

(a) *Hereditary*:

(i) Haemophilia (factor VIII deficiency) or haemophilia A.

(ii) Christmas disease (factor IX deficiency) or haemophilia B.

(iii) von Willebrand's disease (also shows abnormalities of capillary and platelet function).

(iv) Deficiency of clotting factors other than factor XII or those listed at (i) and (ii) (all rare).

(b) *Acquired*:

(i) Deficiency of certain coagulation factors due to vitamin K deficiency.

(ii) Oral anticoagulant therapy.

(iii) Advanced liver disease.

HAEMORRHAGIC DISORDERS DUE TO DEFECT OF THE BLOOD VESSELS

Most of these disorders are discussed with the primary cause noted above.

Hereditary Haemorrhagic Telangiectasia

This rare disease is transmitted as an autosomal dominant. It is characterised by bleeding from multiple telangiectasis which consist of localised collections of non-contractile capillaries. The first and frequently the only symptom may be epistaxis but haematemesis, haemoptysis or bleeding elsewhere may occur. Telangiectases are not usually prominent till after the age of 20 and may be found on the face and hands, or in the mucous membrane of the nose, mouth and gastrointestinal tract.

Treatment of bleeding areas is sometimes difficult, but cauterisation of the lesions in the nose may be helpful. Continuous oral iron therapy is usually required, sometimes with parenteral supplements. Oestrogens may reduce bleeding from mucous membranes in some patients.

HAEMORRHAGIC DISORDERS DUE TO ABNORMALITIES OF BLOOD PLATELETS

Thrombocytopenia occurs either because (1) platelets are consumed or destroyed almost as soon as they are made (consumption thrombocytopenia), or (2) because they are not being produced (production thrombocytopenia). In the first, megakaryocytes are found in normal or increased numbers in the marrow. In the second megakaryocytes are absent from the marrow or, if present, are incapable of platelet production because they are functionally abnormal, in which case they are usually part of a neoplastic process and are morphologically abnormal. In some diseases there is both a production and a consumption problem and it may prove difficult to know which is the greater.

Idiopathic Thrombocytopenic Purpura

This is a disease characterised by a severe reduction in the number of circulating platelets. In most cases it is thought to be due to an immunological attack on the platelets, the antibody being of IgG type. However the demonstration of such an antibody is not always easy. Idiopathic thrombocytopenic purpura is seen in an acute and chronic form. The former is found mostly in young children equally in both sexes and is usually self limiting. The latter occurs at all ages and is more common in females. In the acute form a history of a recent acute respiratory tract illness is common.

Clinical Features. There may be purpura and bleeding from mucous membranes, haematuria and gastrointestinal bleeding. Intracranial haemorrhage is the greatest risk but is uncommon, particularly in children; headache, dizziness and confusion are symptoms that should warn of the risk of intracranial bleeding. In the chronic phase the severity is usually variable with remissions and relapses. Physical examination reveals varying amounts of purpura in skin and mucous membrane. The spleen is usually not palpable.

Diagnosis is established by finding severe thrombocytopenia with normal and increased numbers of megakaryocytes in the bone marrow in the absence of any overt cause. It is therefore mainly a consumption thrombocytopenia although production may be inhibited by antibody attack on the megakaryocytes. Demonstration of anti-platelet and anti-megakaryocyte antibodies is possible in some patients. There may be an associated iron deficiency anaemia.

Treatment. In young children acute idiopathic thrombocytopenic purpura following viral infection seldom requires treatment unless there is evidence suggestive of intracranial bleeding.

In adults, prednisolone (60 mg/day) should be given until the platelet count rises to normal levels when the dose should be cautiously reduced until the drug is withdrawn. Relapse may require reintroduction of a higher dose for a longer period but if this fails or if there has been no response to prednisolone in 3 to 4 weeks, splenectomy should be considered. The spleen should be removed under corticosteroid cover and platelet concentrates given, if required, only after the splenic artery has been clamped. Splenectomy is successful in about 50% of patients, giving lasting remission. In the others a chronic phase of the disorder occurs with remissions and exacerbations that may require periodic corticosteroid therapy. Elderly patients generally respond poorly to corticosteroids. Surprisingly, some patients survive chronic thrombocytopenia for years with remarkably little disability.

Secondary or symptomatic thrombocytopenic purpura occurs in association with pancytopenia, leucopenia, hypersplenism, multiple neoplastic deposits in the bone marrow, from excessive exposure to X-rays or radioactive substances, and occasionally in very severe fevers. It may be found in megaloblastic anaemia and in systemic lupus erythematosus and can follow massive blood transfusion.

Thrombocytopenia may be part of a general pancytopenia or occur alone because of sensitivity to drugs, such as chlordiazepoxide, chlorothiazide, chlorpropamide, frusemide, indomethacin, phenylbutazone, oxyphenbutazone, certain sulphonamides and tolbutamide. Here the prognosis is much better, provided the drug is withdrawn and transfusion given as required. Platelet concentrates are available in some centres.

The name '*onyalai*' has been given to a form of thrombocytopenic purpura of unknown origin which occurs sporadically in Africa. Large haemorrhagic bullae on the tongue and buccal mucosa are conspicuous features.

Thrombocythaemia and Thrombasthenia

In *thrombocythaemia* a pathologically raised number of platelets in the blood, usually in excess of $1000 \times 10^9/l$, occurs which may result in a bleeding diathesis as well as a tendency to thrombosis. This is rectified by reduction of the platelet count to normal levels (p. 518).

Thrombasthenia is a state in which the platelets, although normal in number, are defective in function. A group of very rare hereditary defects of platelets occur and are known as primary thrombasthenias. Acquired thrombasthenia is much more common and is seen in severe uraemia and after exposure to certain drugs, notably aspirin. The platelets in chronic myeloid leukaemia are ineffective and may not be adequate for major surgery (p. 525).

HAEMORRHAGIC DISORDERS DUE TO DEFECTS IN THE CLOTTING MECHANISM

Haemophilia (Haemophilia A)

Of the various factors in normal plasma concerned with the clotting mechanism the most important from a clinical point of view is the antihaemophilic factor (factor VIII, AHF or AHG), a deficiency of which leads to haemophilia. This factor is normally present in the globulin fraction of plasma.

Haemophilia is a hereditary disorder of blood coagulation, characterised by a life long tendency to excessive haemorrhage and a greatly prolonged coagulation time. The haemophilia gene is transmitted as an X-linked recessive character (p. 12). It follows that the sons of a haemophilic man do not suffer from haemophilia and do not transmit the trait to their descendants. The daughters of a haemophilic man all carry the trait. There is a 50% chance that sons of female carriers will suffer from haemophilia and a 50% chance that daughters will be carriers. In many instances no family history can be obtained and this may reflect the fact that the disorder has been handed down on the female side for several generations. Alternatively there may have been a genetic mutation.

Clinical Features. The most common manifestation is haemorrhage into joints and in severe haemophiliacs these haemarthroses may occur frequently. They usually develop spontaneously and cause pain, which may be severe, with swelling, warmth and muscle spasm. With appropriate treatment the lesion settles in a few days as the blood is reabsorbed. Repeated episodes cause damage to the joint with wasting of the related muscles, leading to deformity and crippling. These effects can be minimised by proper management. The knee joints are most frequently affected but ankles, hips, shoulder, elbows and wrists are also involved. Haemorrhage into the musculature and soft tissues is a frequent and potentially disabling complication. Intra-abdominal bleeding may present diagnostic problems and haemorrhage from the gastrointestinal tract is relatively common and can be serious.

Superficial trauma gives rise to uncontrolled bleeding which will continue unless adequately treated. Intracranial haemorrhage may occur but is relatively uncommon unless related to trauma. Surgical procedures are not possible without replacement therapy. Tooth extraction will also promote prolonged bleeding.

The severity of haemophilia varies. In the worst cases the factor VIII coagulant activity is usually less than 2% of normal. Cases with activity of between 2–5% are usually only moderately affected while those with levels about 5% have problems only with major trauma. The higher the factor VIII coagulant activity the less the clinical problem. A small number of haemophiliacs, varying between 5–15% of all cases, have factor VIII inhibitors in the serum. This greatly complicates their management.

Investigation. Diagnosis is based on the sex of the patient who is almost certain to be a male, a family history if present, the clinical picture and the demonstration of deficiency of factor VIII coagulant activity in the absence of any other haemostatic defect. Female haemophiliacs are extremely rare, requiring the marriage of a haemophiliac to a carrier female. Haemophilia must be distinguished from Christmas disease (p. 545) and von Willebrand's disease (p. 545).

Efforts have been made to detect carriers by demonstrating a disparity between the levels of factor VIII coagulant activity and factor VIII related antigen (VIII Rag). The factor VIII Rag level is higher than would be expected from the coagulant activity. However, it is hoped that immunoradiometric assay used to determine the antigenic determinant of the coagulant fraction of factor VIII will prove to be a more useful test for the carrier state. It is low in haemophilia and has been shown to be low in the haemophiliac fetus in utero.

Treatment is based on adequate replacement of the deficient factor. Factor VIII concentrate and cryoprecipitate (which contains factor VIII and is more easily prepared) are the main sources of material, both being obtained from freshly donated blood. Factor VIII concentrate may also be prepared from animal material but is strongly antigenic. Newer preparations appear to be less so. Unfortunately factor VIII has a short biological half-life of 8 hours so that repeated administration is necessary. The aim should be to maintain factor VIII activity above a level which is necessary to achieve haemostasis and the initiation of healing. For a haemarthrosis or for muscle and soft tissue bleeding a level of factor VIII above 30% of normal is usually adequate. Haematuria and retroperitoneal haemorrhage require levels above 50%, while tooth extraction and major surgery require levels approaching 100%.

In practice six or twelve packs of cryoprecipitate are usually given to the patient, with further administrations as required. Cryoprecipitate should always be of the correct blood group unless the patient is group O when cryoprecipitate from any donor can be given. The material should be prepared from donors known to be hepatitis B negative. Nevertheless, most patients receiving these preparations sooner or later develop hepatitis. In addition the frequent administration of foreign antigenic material appears to result in deterioration of immune function with altered T lymphocyte subset ratios. Possibly, as a result, they may be more susceptible to the development of the acquired immunodeficiency syndrome (AIDS) p. 35).

Teeth can be extracted under the cover of aminocaproic acid or tranexamic acid, both of which inhibit fibrinolysis, and this may greatly reduce the need for factor VIII. In mild haemophiliacs with factor VIII levels above 7% the administration of the vasopressin analogue desmopressin (DDAVP) will cause a three to four fold rise in factor VIII coagulant activity and may obviate the need to use cyroprecipitate or factor VIII concentrate. The dose of desmopressin is $0.3\ \mu g/kg$ body weight by infusion over 15 minutes and may be repeated once 6 to 8 hours later. Fluid intake should be restricted for 24 hours because of the antidiuretic effect of desmopressin. Dental extractions should always be done in hospital.

When inhibitors are present very large amounts of factor VIII may be required to overwhelm the inhibitor. Unfortunately this causes a very rapid rise in inhibitor levels and is likely to be useful for only a few days. Blood transfusion may be given when there has been much blood loss. For open wounds, topical application of a thrombogenic agent, such as thrombin, is generally helpful but does not provide a satisfactory substitute for lack of factor VIII.

Haemarthroses and muscle bleeds require initial rest for the first 24–36 hours with splinting, followed by early mobilisation to minimise the risk of contractures, muscle wasting and deformity. Analgesics should be given when pain is severe but aspirin should be avoided as it may cause gastric bleeding. Addictive analgesics should not be used if possible. If aspiration is required for an extremely tense joint the procedure should be done before replacement therapy is started. Because haemophiliacs are repeatedly exposed to blood products, the incidence of hepatitis B and liver disease is relatively high. The patients are also at risk of developing drug addiction as they require analgesics frequently.

Prevention. Severely affected patients should avoid trauma while at the same time leading as normal a life as possible. Home therapy, where patients have a supply of factor VIII and can inject themselves immediately bleeding occurs, has considerably improved the outlook for some patients. Regular administration to prevent bleeding in very severe haemophiliacs, although expensive as regards materials, may be worthwhile. All haemophiliacs should be referred to a haemophilia centre for supervision and advice, not only in relation to their treatment, but also for help with the social and educational implications of their disorder.

Christmas Disease (Haemophilia B)

This is due to deficiency of factor IX and, like haemophilia A, is X-linked. The latter is ten times more common than Christmas disease. All that has been said about haemophilia applies to Christmas disease, except that replacement therapy is with factor IX concentrate. This has a longer half-life and requires to be given less frequently.

Von Willebrand's Disease

This is a rare disorder which is usually inherited as an autosomal dominant and is seen in both sexes equally. It is not dissimilar to haemophilia with which it may be confused and probably explains at least some of the cases of haemophilia reported in females. It is due to a variable reduction of the fraction of factor VIII under autosomal genetic control: factor VIII related antigen (Rag). Normally factor VIII Rag polymerises and attaches to platelets. Without it platelets do not adhere well to collagen. This appears to explain the platelet and capillary defect which was attributed to a lack of a von Willebrand's factor. It is now known that this factor is polymerised factor VIII Rag. The lack of adequate factor VIII Rag also results in inadequate coagulant activity since factor VIII requires factor VIII Rag to function.

Clinical Features. There is excessive bleeding from cuts or other injuries. Patients who have very low factor VIII levels may develop bleeding episodes similar to those described for haemophilia although bruising and mucous membrane bleeding is commoner.

Investigation. The diagnosis is established by family studies, the finding of a prolonged bleeding time, a normal platelet count, failure of aggregation of platelets by ristocetin, impaired adherence of platelets to glass beads, a depressed factor VIII level which can be shown to be due to a deficiency of factor VIII Rag. Finally infusion of plasma or cryoprecipitate causes a prolonged rise in factor VIII levels in excess of that due to infused factor VIII, a phenomenon never seen in haemophilia and thought to be due to an increase in the polymerised factor VIII. This also corrects the platelet defects.

Treatment. Fresh frozen plasma or cryoprecipitate should be given for troublesome bleeding or surgical procedures. Superficial bleeding will usually respond to simple pressure. Desmopressin may be used for patients with factor VIII levels above 7%.

Deficiency of the Vitamin K Dependent Factors

Factor II (prothrombin) and factors VII, IX and X are synthesised by the liver. Vitamin K (p. 71) is required for this function. Deficient production occurs if the absorption of the vitamin is impaired or there is severe liver disease. When anticoagulation is required, drugs, particularly warfarin, are used to alter the synthesis of factors II, VII, IX and X; proteins are produced which are antigenically similar to these factors but do not have their procoagulant properties.

Clinical Features. Patients with simple vitamin K deficiency or overdosage with oral anticoagulants are liable to excessive bruising, gastrointestinal haemorrhage, haematuria, epistaxis and excessive menstrual loss. When deficiency is associated with severe liver disease the clinical and haemostatic problems are more complex because of the addition of other factor deficiencies, thrombocytopenia and toxic damage to the vasculature.

Haemorrhagic disease of the newborn is due to an exaggeration of the normal hypoprothrombinaemia which occurs 24–72 hours after birth when there is no bacterial formation of vitamin K in the gut.

Treatment. In simple vitamin K deficiency, whatever the cause, parenteral administration of phytomenadione (vitamin K1) corrects the factor deficiency within 24 hours. Treatment of anticoagulant overdosage is given on page 548.

The management of the bleeding problems in severe liver disease is complex and will depend on the identification of the coagulation factors involved, the platelet count and the degree to which fibrinolysis has been stimulated. Vitamin K is seldom deficient although it may be administered in the hope of producing some improvement. Fresh frozen plasma, platelets and blood transfusion may all be given. It is risky to use concentrates of factors II, VII, IX and X as these tend to induce disseminated intravascular coagulation (p. 548) unless the concentrates contain heparin. Generally, replacement therapy is best reserved for acute haemorrhage as its effects are short lived.

THROMBOSIS

In health, blood is kept in a fluid state by various mechanisms (p. 541) which may be upset in favour of thrombus formation in certain circumstances. A thrombus may be defined as an abnormal mass formed inside a blood vessel and consisting of various components of blood which have reacted together in ways similar to, but not identical to, the normal process of haemostasis.

There are two types of thrombus: (1) the white thrombus which occurs in arteries. It is formed by platelet adhesion and aggregation, with fibrin deposition in layers and may in time occlude the artery; (2) the red thrombus which consists of large amounts of fibrin and red cells and relatively few platelets. It forms mainly in veins or behind a white thrombus and is similar to the clot formed by blood in a tube. A red thrombus is soft and friable and in veins may easily be detached to cause pulmonary embolism.

Aetiology. The factors which predispose to the formation of thrombi in blood vessels fall into three main groups:

1. ABNORMALITIES OF BLOOD VESSEL WALLS due to:

(a) atherosclerosis;

(b) trauma (e.g. needles, cannulas, irritant infusions and endothelial damage over a myocardial infarction)

(c) loss of venous tone, e.g. varicosities; and

(d) infiltration of the vessel wall by neoplastic disease.

2. ABNORMALITIES OF BLOOD FLOW due to:

(a) stasis occurring mainly in veins although it may develop in the auricles of the atria in atrial fibrillation. Stasis may also be due to lack of muscular activity as in general anaesthesia, to external pressure on veins (e.g. in pregnancy or neoplasia) or to venous pooling as occurs in cardiac failure;

(b) hyperviscosity either (i) because of an increase in the cellular components of blood as in polycythaemia vera or leukaemia or (ii) because of an increase in the protein levels as in myeloma or Waldenstrom's macroglobulinaemia;

(c) turbulence, caused for instance, by kinking of arteries forcing platelets on to the vessel walls.

3. ABNORMALITIES OF THE BLOOD due to:

(a) thrombocytosis occurring in disorders such as polycythaemia vera;

(b) hypercoagulable states from an increased activation of clotting factors during and after surgery, from decrease in the activity of the fibrinolytic mechanism as in factor XII deficiency and when there is a decrease in coagulation inhibitors in the blood, for instance antithrombin III deficiency.

(c) lack of prostacyclin.

Prostacyclin. The vascular endothelium synthesises a substance, prostacyclin (epoprostenol), from prostaglandin endoperoxides produced from arachadonic acid by the enzyme cyclo-oxygenase. Prostacyclin is an unstable compound with a half life of 2 to 3 minutes; it inhibits platelet aggregation, promotes platelet disaggregation and causes vasodilation. These effects are the opposite of those caused by thromboxane A2 produced from the same precursors in platelets. It is thought that prostacyclin production is of major importance in inhibiting thrombus formation in blood vessels. Prostacyclin can also be produced in the lungs from which it perfuses the circulation. Levels of thromboxane A2 are low in people eating a seafood diet, e.g. Eskimos who are observed to have low incidence of thrombosis. This may be because the diet reduces the thrombogenic side of the mechanism by giving rise to an alternative form of thromboxane (thromboxane A3).

Aspirin inhibits cyclo-oxygenase and hence reduces the production of thromboxane A2 in platelets. However, by the same action, but in larger doses, it also probably reduces the production of prostacyclin by the cells of the vessel walls. This may explain why aspirin has been less effective in the prevention of thrombosis than was expected but the optimum dose of aspirin for this purpose has not yet been settled.

Clinical Features. Thrombosis in both arteries and veins is a major cause of morbidity and mortality. In arteries the occlusion is often crippling, if not lethal, depending on the tissue affected and whether there is a good anastamotic circulation e.g. in coronary (p. 167), cerebral (p. 628) and mesenteric thrombosis (p. 330). On the venous side the local effects are usually less damaging to health but deep venous thrombosis producing pulmonary emboli can be lethal (p. 184). This disability is likely to be severe in thrombosis of the cavernous and other venous sinuses, (p. 636) or of the renal veins, (p. 390).

Treatment. The indications for the use of anticoagulant and other forms of therapy are discussed with the individual lesions.

HEPARIN THERAPY. Heparin is a highly acidic mucopolysaccharide and is a natural, biologically produced anticoagulant. It acts by accelerating the activity of antithrombin III (p. 541). The effect is virtually instantaneous. Heparin has a half life of 60–90 minutes and disappears rapidly from the circulation. It is administered either by intermittent intravenous injection every six hours, by continuous intravenous infusion in a small volume or by intermittent (usually b.d.) subcutaenous injection. When given by continuous intravenous infusion the level of anti-coagulation may be monitored by thrombin times or partial thromboplastin times with kaolin or, if necessary, by the whole blood clotting time. Heparin is seldom used for more than 2 weeks. Prolonged treatment can cause osteoporosis. It is often combined with oral anticoagulants, the heparin being used to initiate anticoagulation until the oral anticoagulants can exert their function; heparin is then withdrawn. Overdosage may be treated either by stopping administration or, when there is haemorrhage, by giving protamine sulphate in a dose based on laboratory tests.

Heparin can be used either as an anticoagulant or as a prophylaxis against thrombosis. The doses required for the latter are much smaller (low dose heparin) and do not alter coagulation tests. At this low dose intravascular thromboses is discouraged but haemostasis is adequate for surgery.

ORAL ANTICOAGULATION. Warfarin is the drug of choice. Indanedione derivatives such as phenindione are much more likely to produce hypersensitivity reactions. Anticoagulation should be initiated carefully as some patients require lower doses than others, and indeed the dose of 20 mg of warfarin on the first day and 10 mg on the following day, which is routinely given in many centres, will be excessive in a significant number of patients. It is better to give 10 mg of warfarin on the first day and then increase the dose in those who can tolerate the drug. The maintenance dose varies widely from 2–20 mg daily. Rarely, enormous doses are required in patients who metabolise the drug in an abnormal manner.

Therapy is usually monitored by the *prothrombin time*, preferably corrected to a standard ratio to make results comparable between centres. The therapeutic range is between ratios of 1:2 and 1:4. This test does not reflect factor IX deficiency. The *thrombotest* does and is regarded by some as preferable. Also the thrombotest can be done on finger prick blood.

Since many drugs interfere with the binding of warfarin to albumin or induce enzyme activity in the liver, thereby increasing warfarin metabolism, introduction or withdrawal of other drugs should be under medical supervision and the patient advised that such changes may have serious effects unless monitored. Transient illness also affects liver function and may require dosage alteration.

Patients should carry a card indicating that they are receiving warfarin. They should be advised specifically not to take aspirin or proprietary preparations containing aspirin, but to use paracetamol for headaches and other minor discomforts.

In the treatment of overdosage, withdrawal of the anticoagulant may be sufficent. If reversal of anticoagulation is required phytomenadione (vitamin K_1) should be used. The disadvantage is that unless dosage is small it will be difficult to re-establish oral anticoagulation for some time. Alternatively fresh frozen plasma or blood may be administered if there is a need to correct the defect quickly. Concentrates of factor II, VII, IX and X may also be used in urgent situations and will correct the defect almost immediately. Such preparations usually contain a small dose of heparin to prevent the induction of disseminated intravascular coagulation. The heparin will not be enough to cause serious anticoagulation in the patient.

FIBRINOLYTIC THERAPY. Lysis of thrombi by means of streptokinase or urokinase has been used but is very expensive and potentially dangerous, especially postoperatively. Streptokinase is antigenic so that it can be given only for a limited period. This type of treatment is rarely used for longer than two days and is followed by anticoagulation.

Prevention. Low molecular weight dextrans have been used widely in surgical practice. Attempts to counteract the adhesive and aggregating properties of platelets with a variety of drugs such as aspirin and dipyridamole are being evaluated. Efforts are being made to produce a stable analogue of prostacyclin in the hope that it will prove to be a useful agent in the prevention of thrombosis.

Disseminated Intravascular Coagulation

This is a deranged state in which coagulation and lysis of fibrin produced by coagulation proceed simultaneously in the blood. It is a reflection of other problems, not a disease in itself.

Aetiology. The trigger is usually something that initiates intravascular coagulation. This may be transient or ongoing. Transient liberation of thrombogenic substances into the blood is seen classically in association with the end of pregnancy and parturition. Amniotic fluid embolism is potently thromboplastic and similar effects are seen in abruptio placentae, eclampsia and when there is a dead fetus in utero. Other triggers include malignancies, hepatic disease, severe trauma, anaphylaxis, hypoxia, venoms and sepsis. Bacterial endotoxins act indirectly through mediators such as granulocytes, platelets and damaged vascular endothelium.

Whatever the trigger, the effect is a threat to the circulation and the fibrinolytic mechanism responds, sometimes dramatically, to lyse fibrin as it is formed. This compensatory response may overshoot, and excess plasmin produced by the fibrinolytic system digests fibrinogen and other factors as well as the fibrin, causing a severe haemorrhagic state. This occurs in addition to depletion of coagulation of factors and platelets by the coagulation process which initiated the problem. The result is a severe failure of the haemostatic mechanism (Fig. 13.5). The fibrin degradation products themselves have a 'heparin like' effect which may exacerbate bleeding.

Clinical Features. Specific clinical findings are present only in severe cases. Bleeding occurs at all venepuncture sites, from mouth, nose, ears and other orifices. This is due to lysis of fibrin clots wherever they have been laid down. There is massive purpura with ecchymoses. The patient is usually gravely ill. Sometimes excessive fibrinolysis may occur locally at the site of severe trauma, such as brain operations and prostatectomy. No evidence of this phenomenon is then seen systemically but local bleeding may be prolonged.

Diagnosis of disseminated intravascular coagulation is by laboratory investigation. It is necessary to show depletion of coagulation factors and platelets and evidence of an increase in the products of fibrinolytic activity (fibrin degradation products). A full coagulation investigation with platelet counts and measurement of FDPs is required.

Treatment. When disseminated intravascular coagulation is severe, replacement of coagulation factors may be necessary. Heparin may be used when there is an ongoing stimulus to coagulation as in malignant disease. Antifibrinolytic drugs such as aminocaproic acid are given when fibrinolysis alone appears to be the major problem, usually for local haemostatic abnormalities.

In practice very severe disseminated intravascular coagulation is rare and in most cases the process is contained and excessive depletion of coagulation factors does not occur. In such cases the treatment is that of the underlying disorder.

PROSPECTS IN HAEMATOLOGY

For many years haematology has had a firm base in blood film and marrow morphology. This has determined the classification of many of the blood diseases. Electron microscopy has extended this base by demonstrating the ultrastructure of the cells. More recently immunological techniques have brought a new dimension to the subject. Dynamic concepts have appeared and resulted in new ideas about classification particularly in the field of lymphomas and leukaemias. Cells are now recognised to have characteristics not evident from light or electron microscopy. Antigens originally thought to be tumour related are now

Fig. 13.5 Disseminated intravascular coagulation.

known to be characteristic of certain stages in the differentiation of cells. This is a rapidly expanding field of knowledge and further contributions to our understanding of the nature of these diseases will undoubtedly come.

The chemotherapy of acute lymphoblastic leukaemias of the common type has proved highly successful in obtaining long remissions, even in adults. The same degree of success has not been obtained in the myeloblastic leukaemias or in the lymphoblastic leukaemia of T and B cell type. Here there is room for improvement as new drugs become available. The use of bone marrow transplantation in the treatment of acute leukaemia holds out hope for younger patients who have disease that is unlikely to be eliminated by chemotherapy. Improvements in the management of the chronic leukaemias have been awaited for a long time and while no easy answers to the problems of these diseases can be foreseen it is now clear that bone marrow transplantation may have something to offer young adults and children.

One of the most important advances of recent times has been the development of monoclonal antibodies. These are produced from 'immortal' lines of mouse myeloma cells hybridised with human cells producing normal antibody. As each antibody producing cell forms only one type of antibody the hybridised cells likewise continue to produce one type of antibody indefinitely. The antibodies produced are extremely specific, reacting with only one antigen.

Monoclonal antibodies are now used extensively for serological investigations for which previously only polyclonal antibody mixtures were available. The result has been a much sharper ability to identify specific subsets of cells and stages of cell differentiation. In addition the use of monoclonal antibodies for therapeutic purposes is being explored, both to replace old fashioned polyclonal preparations and as vehicles to carry drugs and other therapeutic weapons to specific cells. In this respect there is the possibility that human myeloma cells may be used instead of mouse myeloma cells to produce monoclonal antibodies, thus avoiding interspecies differences.

In the field of coagulation problems the understanding of the role of the prostaglandins in platelet and vascular endothelial function opens up the prospect of new therapeutic techniques to deal with the problems of intravascular thrombosis. The development of antisera to the coagulant fraction of factor VIII will hopefully improve the measurement of that factor, assist in the identification of female carriers and enable the investigator to discover at the fetal stage whether a male offspring has the disease. Perhaps similar development will also occur in relation to factor IX deficiency.

N.C. ALLAN

FURTHER READING:

Biggs, R. (1978) *The Treatment of Haemophilia A and B and von Willebrand's Disease.* London: Blackwell Scientific Publications. For detailed information on the management of these coagulation disorders.

Dacie, J.V. & Lewis, S.M. (1984) *Practical Haematology,* 6th edn. Edinburgh: Churchill Livingstone. For information regarding investigative procedures.

De Gruchy, G.C. (1978) *Clinical Haematology in Medical Practice,* 4th edn. London: Blackwell Scientific Publications. An excellent reference volume with a clinical bias.

Girdwood, R.H. (1984) *Clinical Pharmacology,* 25th edn. London: Baillière Tindall. For information about haematinics, anticoagulants and drugs used in malignant disease.

Hardisty, R.M. & Weatherall, D.J. (1982) *Blood and its Disorders,* 2nd edn. London: Blackwell Scientific Publications. A reference volume particularly useful for its section on haemoglobinopathies and thalassaemias.

Hirsh, J. & Brain, E. (1979) *Hemostasis and Thrombosis: A Conceptual Approach.* Edinburgh: Churchill Livingstone. An excellent and clearly understood introduction to coagulation.

Wintrobe, M.M. (1981) *Clinical Haematology,* 8th edn. London: Kimpton. Probably one of the best comprehensive reference volumes.

14. Diseases of Connective Tissues, Joints and Bones

Rheumatology deals with a heterogeneous group of disorders of connective tissues, joints and bones. The 'rheumatic diseases' are conditions in which pain and stiffness of some part of the musculoskeletal system are prominent. It is convenient, if rather arbitrary, to group these disorders according to whether the basis for the connective tissue pathology is primarily inflammatory, metabolic or degenerative.

Inflammatory diseases of connective tissue include rheumatoid arthritis and other types of inflammatory and infective arthritis, the spondyloarthritides and the diffuse connective tissue diseases. Metabolic disorders include the crystal deposition diseases, gout and chondrocalcinosis, while the predominantly degenerative disorders are osteoarthrosis, spondylosis and a number of painful syndromes of the soft connective tissues. Until recently these conditions have not received the attention of clinicians, medical teachers and researchers commensurate with their frequency and morbidity.

Prevalence. Rheumatic diseases affect people of all sexes, ethnic groups and ages. Their frequency increases with age so that as many as 40% of persons over the age of 65 years have some rheumatic complaint. In Britain 20 million people experience a rheumatic disorder each year. Five million suffer from osteoarthrosis, 500 000 have rheumatoid arthritis and there are 12 000 children with chronic juvenile arthritis. Eight million people consult their general practitioner annually with rheumatic complaints, amounting to 18% of all consultations in general practice. Rheumatic diseases are the most important cause of physical impairment in the community. The lives of more than one million persons are so impaired and one-fifth of these are severely disabled. In 1971 rheumatic disorders were responsible for the loss of 44 million working days and for almost £500 000 000 in lost productivity.

DISEASES OF CONNECTIVE TISSUES AND JOINTS

INFLAMMATORY DISEASES

Rheumatoid arthritis; Spondarthritis; Juvenile chronic arthritis; Infective and miscellaneous arthritis; Systemic lupus erythematosus; Progressive systemic sclerosis; Polymyositis and Dermatomyositis; Arteritis.

RHEUMATOID ARTHRITIS

In its typical and complete form rheumatoid arthritis is a chronic inflammatory, destructive and deforming polyarthritis associated with systemic disturbance, a variety of extra-articular lesions and the presence of circulating antiglobulin antibodies (rheumatoid factors). While the pattern of joint involvement is characteristically symmetrical and peripheral and its course typically prolonged, with exacerbations and remissions, atypical, asymmetrical and incomplete forms are not uncommon and give rise to difficulties in diagnosis.

Epidemiology. Rheumatoid arthritis occurs throughout the world in all climates and all ethnic groups. The overall prevalence in developed countries is about 3% with a female to male ratio of 3:1. There is an annual incidence of 0·3% so that over the age of 65 years 16% of the female population and 5% of males are affected.

The disease commences most commonly in the 3rd and 4th decades but the age of onset follows a normal distribution curve and no age group is exempted.

Incidence is higher than expected in twins and 1st degree relatives but not in spouses suggesting a fairly weak genetic predisposition. This has been confirmed by a modest but significant increase in HLA-D4 and HLA-DR4 in patients and their families. Higher incidence in urban than in rural Africans of the same ethnic origin suggests that environmental factors are important.

The disease appears to be more severe though not more frequent where the climate is cold and damp.

Aetiology and Pathogenesis. The cause of rheumatoid arthritis remains obscure. It is widely believed that an infection is the initiating factor although no causative organism has been identified. Nevertheless current concepts suggest that the disease results from altered immune reactivity and persistent antigenic stimulation in genetically predisposed persons. There is a much evidence for persistent immune overactivity, autoimmunity and the presence of immune complexes at sites of articular and extra-articular lesions, namely:

1. The presence of circulating IgM, IgG and IgA serum antiglobulins (rheumatoid factors) as well as anticollagen and antinuclear antibodies.
2. The presence of self associating IgG and IgG-IgM immune complexes within the phagocytic cells of synovial effusions.
3. Depression of synovial fluid complement components in inflamed joints associated with activation of both the classical and alternative pathways.
4. Increased numbers of plasma cells, lymphocytes and monocytes in the synovial membrane associated with local production of rheumatoid factors and lymphokines.
5. The presence of serum factors which inhibit suppressor T lymphocyte activity.
6. Amyloidosis complicating some cases of rheumatoid arthritis of long duration.

The importance of lymphocytes and cellular immunity in the pathogenesis of the disease is confirmed by the striking remission of activity which follows lymphocyte depletion by thoracic duct drainage, lymphocytapheresis or cytotoxic drug therapy.

Thus rheumatoid arthritis is considered to be both an extravascular immune complex disease and a disorder of cell-mediated immunity in which the following sequence of events leads to inflammation, granuloma formation and joint destruction:

1. Localisation of unidentified antigen in joints and processing by antigen presenting cells.
2. Release of immunopotentiating factors such as interleukin I.
3. Local synthesis of antiglobulin antibodies.
4. Formation of immune complexes and activation of the complement pathway.
5. Stimulation of neutrophil chemotaxis, cytolysis, lymphokine production and macrophage neutral protease secretion by biologically active complement components (p. 27).
6. Neutrophil and macrophage phagocytosis of immune complexes following IgG and C3 receptor recognition.
7. Release of mediators of acute inflammation — vaso-active amines, proteases, polypeptides, prostaglandins and leukotrienes.
8. T lymphocyte infiltration and production of lymphokines.
9. Macrophage and chondrocyte activation, pannus formation and enzymatic destruction of articular cartilage and bone by collagenase and neutral proteinases.

The severity of erosive damage is related to joint movement and physical stress showing that mechanical factors are also important in pathogenesis.

Pathology. The earliest change is swelling and congestion of the synovial membrane and the underlying connective tissue, which become infiltrated with lymphocytes, (especially helper T cells), plasma cells and macrophages. Effusion of synovial fluid into the joint space takes place during the active phase of the disease. Subsequently, hypertrophy of the synovial membrane occurs with the formation of lymphoid follicles resembling an immunologically active lymph node. Inflammatory granulation tissue (pannus) is formed, spreading over and under the articular cartilage which is progressively eroded and destroyed. Later, fibrous adhesions may form between the layers of pannus across the joint space and fibrous or bony ankylosis may occur. Muscles adjacent to inflamed joints atrophy and there may be focal infiltration with lymphocytes.

Subcutaneous nodules have a characteristic histological appearance. There is a central area of fibrinoid material consisting of swollen and fragmented collagen fibres, fibrinous exudate and cellular debris, surrounded by a palisade of radially arranged proliferating mononuclear cells. The nodule is surrounded by a loose capsule of fibrous tissue. Similar granulomatous lesions may occur in the pleura, lung, pericardium and sclera. Lymph nodes are often hyperplastic showing many lymphoid follicles with large germinal centres and numerous plasma cells in the sinuses and medullary cords. Immunofluorescence shows that the plasma cells in the synovium and lymph nodes synthesise rheumatoid factors.

Clinical Features. ONSET. In the majority of patients the onset is insidious with joint pain, stiffness and symmetrical swelling of a number of peripheral joints. Initially pain may be experienced only on movement of joints, but rest pain and especially early morning stiffness are characteristic features of all kinds of active inflammatory arthritis.

In the typical case the small joints of the fingers and toes are the first to be affected. Swelling of the proximal, but not the distal, interphalangeal joints gives the fingers a 'spindled' appearance and swelling of the metatarsophalangeal joints results in 'broadening' of the forefoot. As the disease progresses, with or without intervening remissions, there is a tendency for it to spread to involve the wrists, elbows and shoulders in the upper limbs, and the knees, ankles, subtalar and midtarsal joints in the feet. The hip joints are affected only in the more severe cases but neck pain and stiffness from cervical spin involvement is common. The mandibular, acromioclavicular and sternoclavicular joints are sometimes affected as indeed is every synovial joint.

In some patients the onset is 'palindromic' with recurrent acute episodes of joint pain and stiffness in individual joints lasting only a few hours or days. In about a third of such cases the disease sooner or later evolves into a more typical polyarthritis.

In 10% of patients the disease starts as an acute polyarthritis with severe systemic symptoms, including fever, weight loss, profound fatigue and malaise.

PROGRESSION. As the disease advances, pain, muscle spasm and progressive joint destruction result in limitation of joint motion, joint instability, subluxation and deformities. At first deformities are correctable, but later permanent contractures develop and the joints may become completely disorganised.

Characteristic deformities include flexion contractures of the small joints of the hands and feet, the knees, hips and elbows. Anterior subluxation of the metacarpophalangeal joints is common with ulnar deviation of the fingers. Other finger deformities lead to more loss of function. These include the 'swan neck' deformity (hyperextension at the proximal interphalangeal joints and fixed flexion at the distal interphalangeal joints), the Boutonnière or 'button-hole' deformity (fixed flexion of the proximal interphalangeal joint and extension of the terminal interphalangeal joint) and a Z deformity of the thumb. Dorsal subluxation of the ulnar styloid at the wrist is common and may contribute to rupture of the fourth and fifth extensor tendons when these are already the site of tenosynovitis.

In the forefoot, subluxation of the metatarsophalangeal joints is followed by clawing of the toes, callosities over the exposed metatarsal heads and a painful sensation of 'walking on pebbles'. In the hind foot calcaneal erosions may develop at the insertions of the Achilles tendon or plantar fascia and eversion deformities at the subtalar joint are common.

EXTRA-ARTICULAR FEATURES. Rheumatoid arthritis is a systemic disease. Anorexia, weight loss, lethargy and myalgia occur commonly throughout its course and may precede the onset of articular symptoms by weeks or months.

Raynaud's phenomenon (p. 199) is common in the prodromal period and throughout the course of the disease.

Lymphadenopathy is a frequent finding. Although it is particularly a feature of nodes draining actively inflamed joints, more generalised lymphadenopathy is not uncommon and can give rise to diagnostic confusion when arthritis is minimal or quiescent. The nodes are discrete and not tender. Histology shows a reactive hyperplasia which can occasionally be confused with giant follicular lymphoma.

Osteoporosis, muscle weakness and wasting also occur adjacent to inflamed joints and more diffusely as part of the systemic disturbance. They are seen early in the course of the disease and often progress to become prominent features in very active or advanced cases.

Tenosynovitis and bursitis are frequent accompaniments of active arthritis as tendon sheaths and bursae are also lined with synovium. 'Triggering' of the fingers may be associated with nodules in the flexor tendon sheaths which can progress to permanent flexion contractures or tendon rupture if left untreated.

Popliteal cysts (Baker's cysts) communicate with the knee, but fluid is prevented from returning to the joint by a valve-like mechanism. The high pressure generated by flexion of the knee, especially when effusions are present, can result in gradual extension or sudden rupture of the cyst into the calf. Rupture is accompanied by calf pain, swelling, tenderness, pitting oedema and a positive Homan's sign. Diagnostic confusion with deep vein thrombosis can usually be avoided by careful consideration of the history but a venogram, joint scan or arthrogram are occasionally required to establish the correct diagnosis.

Subcutaneous nodules appear at some time in the course of the disease in about 20% of patients. They are usually seen at the sites of pressure or friction such as the extensor surfaces of the forearms below the elbow, the scalp, sacrum, scapula and Achilles tendon as well as on the fingers and toes. Ulceration and secondary infection are not uncommon. Their presence is almost invariably associated with positive tests for rheumatoid factor. Rarely they are found in visceral organs.

OCULAR MANIFESTATIONS. *Episcleritis* is a fairly common and benign feature in patients with nodular seropositive disease. The intermittent inflammation of the superficial sclera is usually painless. It is not associated with visual disturbance and requires no specific therapy.

Scleritis is a rarer but more serious condition. The eye is red and painful with inflammatory changes throughout the sclera and uveal tract. The pupil may be irregular from adhesions (synechiae) which can cause secondary glaucoma and visual impairment. Scleritis often requires systemic corticosteroid therapy as well as local measures.

Scleromalacia or thinning of the sclera may follow episodes of scleritis and is seen as a blue discolouration of the white of the eye. Progression to perforation very rarely occurs. *Scleromalacia perforans* follows necrosis of a scleral rheumatoid nodule and may require grafting or enucleation of the eye.

Keratoconjunctivitis sicca occurs in 10% of patients. Lack of lacrimal secretion results in symptoms of grittiness, dryness, burning or itching associated with sticky mucous threads. The diagnosis can be confirmed by the Schirmer tear test and slit lamp examination following Rose Bengal staining.

Sjögren's syndrome is the association of xerostomia (dryness of the mouth) and keratoconjunctivitis sicca with a connective tissue disorder. In the majority of cases this is rheumatoid arthritis but the syndrome may be associated with systemic lupus erythematosis, mixed connective tissue disease, polymyositis, myasthenia gravis, progressive systemic sclerosis, autoimmune liver disease and thyroiditis.

Keratoconjunctivitis sicca and xerostomia can occur in the absence of identifiable associated connective tissue disorder when the term *sicca syndrome* is applied. It is usually associated with HLA-DR3 rather than HLA-DR4 and patients with the sicca syndrome are more likely to have widespread and serious manifestations than those with rheumatoid arthritis and Sjögren's syndrome. These include: salivary gland enlargement and malignancy; dysphagia and dyspareunia; severe dental caries; Raynaud's phenomenon and vasculitis; lymphadenopathy, leucopenia and hepatosplenomegaly; hyperglobulinaemic purpura; macroglobulinaemia; renal tubular acidosis or glomerulonephritis; pneumonia and diffuse interstitial pulmonary fibrosis.

Patients with Sjögren's syndrome may have a wide range of organ-specific and non-organ-specific autoantibodies including salivary duct and thyroid antibodies, antimitochondrial and smooth muscle antibodies, rheumatoid factors and antinuclear factors. An antibody to an extractable nuclear antigen, SS-B is characteristic of the sicca syndrome. The pathological feature which can be detected in the minor salivary glands on a simple lip biopsy is intense infiltration with lymphocytes and plasma cells. A fall in IgM levels may herald the development of malignancy.

Treatment is usually limited to scrupulous oral and ocular hygiene and the instillation of artificial tears (hypromellose eye drops). Drug hypersensitivity is sometimes a problem.

CARDIOVASCULAR MANIFESTATIONS. Asymptomatic pericarditis is a common and benign feature of seropositive rheumatoid arthritis while pericardial effusions and constrictive pericarditis occur infrequently. Rarely the formation of granulomatous lesions leads to heart block, cardiomyopathy, coronary artery occlusion or aortic regurgitation.

Vasculitis. Diffuse necrotising vasculitis is relatively common in patients with nodules and positive tests for rheumatoid factor. Clinical manifestations vary with the size and site of the vessel involved. Small vessel disease of the terminal digital arterioles or capillaries is often associated with no more than nail fold infarcts, leg ulcers or purpura.

Large areas of skin necrosis or digital gangrene have more sinister prognostic significance and may herald the onset of *'malignant' rheumatoid disease*. These patients are often febrile with severe systemic disturbance. They have multiple extra-articular manifestations of rheumatoid disease such as anaemia, scleritis, pleurisy and pericarditis. Mononeuritis multiplex (p. 662) follows occlusion of vasa nervorum. A larger vessel arteritis, histologically resembling polyarteritis nodosa, may result in catastrophic mesenteric, renal, cerebrovascular or coronary artery occlusion. Such patients frequently have evidence of circulating immune complexes, cryoglobulins and hypocomplementaemia.

PULMONARY MANIFESTATIONS. *Pleurisy or pleural effusions* occur in about 25% of men with rheumatoid arthritis. Diagnostic aspiration should be undertaken to exclude other causes. Characteristically the fluid has a high protein content, high cell count (mononuclear or polymorphonuclear) and low glucose. Pleural biopsy may show evidence of granuloma formation. Pleural or pulmonary nodules may require excision to exclude other causes.

Caplan's syndrome (p. 267) and *chronic interstitial pulmonary fibrosis* are rare manifestations of rheumatoid arthritis. The latter differs in no way from idiopathic fibrosing alveolitis which is associated with positive tests for rheumatoid factor in 30% of cases. *Obliterative bronchiolitis* is also a rare complication. Dyspnoea, from non-inflammatory small airways obstruction, begins suddenly and progresses rapidly to respiratory failure.

NEUROLOGICAL MANIFESTATIONS. *Entrapment neuropathies* result from compression of peripheral nerves by hypertrophied synovium. Median nerve compression in the carpal tunnel is the most common and may be an early clinical manifestation of the disease. Others include ulnar nerve compression at the elbow, peroneal nerve palsy at the knee and posterior tibial nerve entrapment in the flexor retinaculum at the ankle (tarsal tunnel syndrome).

Peripheral neuropathy is usually symmetrical and limited to symptoms and signs of mild 'glove and stocking' sensory loss. In patients with vasculitis sudden palsies of major peripheral nerves may be manifestations of mononeuritis multiplex but physical entrapment must be carefully excluded.

Cervical cord compression may result from subluxation of the cervical spine at the atlanto-axial joint or at a subaxial level. Atlanto-axial subluxation is a common finding in long-standing rheumatoid arthritis which can easily be diagnosed from lateral radiographs of the cervical spine taken in full flexion when the distance between the odontoid and the anterior arch of the atlas is greater than 4 mm. Although usually associated with no more than neck pain radiating to the occiput and requiring no specific treatment, it can result in cord transection and sudden death if the neck is manipulated inadvertently under an anaesthetic. Less dramatic cases of progressive cervical myelopathy may present with limb weakness, difficulty in holding up the head and tetraparesis. These lesions occur more often at the subaxial level and frequently require operative decompression and fixation. Severe disease of the cervical spine may also give rise to nerve root compression, vertebro-basilar insufficiency and spinal artery occlusion.

HAEMATOLOGICAL MANIFESTATIONS are very common in active rheumatoid disease. A normochronic normocytic anaemia of chronic disease (p. 499), characterised by a low serum iron and iron binding capacity which does not respond to oral iron, can often be complicated by true iron deficiency secondary to gastrointestinal blood loss from treatment with analgesic anti-inflammatory drugs. Much less frequently there may be a macrocytic anaemia associated with folate deficiency. Thrombocytosis is a feature of active disease.

Felty's syndrome is the association of splenomegaly and neutropenia with rheumatoid arthritis; it tends to occur in patients with seropositive, longstanding, advanced but inactive arthritis. Other clinical features include anaemia, thrombocytopenia, lymphadenopathy, weight loss, skin pigmentation and vasculitic leg ulcers. Susceptibility to recurrent bacterial infections occurs in about half of those affected but does not appear to be directly related to the neutrophil count. The mechanism for the neutropenia remains uncertain but a wide range of immunological abnormalities include granulocyte specific antinuclear antibodies, antibodies directed against leucocyte surface antigens and polymorph phagocytosis of immune complexes.

Treatment with corticosteroids is usually unsatisfactory. Splenectomy is reserved for patients with serious or life threatening recurrent infections and is followed by prolonged remission in about 60% of cases.

Complications. *Septic arthritis* (p. 570) may complicate rheumatoid arthritis in the absence of Felty's syndrome. Patients usually have longstanding nodular seropositive disease. In debilitated patients, fever and leucocytosis may be absent and signs limited to malaise and slight exacerbation of inflammation in one or more joints. *Staphylococcus aureus* is commonly implicated secondary to invasion from an ulcerated nodule or infected skin lesion.

Amyloidosis (p. 390) may be a true complication of prolonged active disease. Evidence of amyloid is found in 25–50% of cases at autopsy making rheumatoid arthritis a leading cause of secondary amyloidosis. Clinical manifestations are however usually limited to mild proteinuria with only very few patients going on to the nephrotic syndrome or renal failure.

Investigation. Active disease is associated with a raised ESR and C-reactive protein. The plasma protein profile shows increased globulin and fibrinogen and decreased albumin.

IMMUNOLOGICAL TESTS. IgM rheumatoid factors are detected by testing the ability of serum to agglutinate carrier particles coated with IgG. Polystyrene particles coated with human IgG are used in the latex slide test. Sheep or human erythrocytes coated with rabbit anti-erythrocyte antibody are used in the Rose Waaler sheep cell agglutination test (SCAT), the human erythrocyte agglutination test (HEAT) and the differential agglutination test (DAT). The latex fixation test is simple and sensitive but less specific so that it is frequently used as a screening test. The erythrocyte tests are less sensitive and more specific. Significant titres which exclude 95% of the normal population are: SCAT 1:32; DAT 1:16; latex 1:20.

The Rose Waaler test is positive in 70% of patients with rheumatoid arthritis but may not become so for a year or two. Positive tests are also found in: Sjögren's syndrome (100%); systemic lupus erythematosus (30%); mixed connective tissue disease (30%); scleroderma (30%); chronic juvenile arthritis (15%); chronic liver disease: sarcoidosis; multiple myeloma and other paraproteinaemias and in chronic infections (infective endocarditis, tuberculosis, syphilis, malaria and leprosy).

Up to 30% of patients with rheumatoid arthritis have positive tests for antinuclear factor.

RADIOLOGICAL EXAMINATION. In the early stages of the disease radiographs are normal or show no more than soft tissue swelling and periarticular osteoporosis. Progression to cartilage and bone destruction is seen as narrowing of the joint spaces and the development of marginal erosions. The earliest erosions are often seen in the metatarsophalangeal joints. Very severe destructive changes ('arthritis mutilans') are associated with gross deformities and massive bone resorption.

Marginal sclerosis and osteophyte formation are indications of secondary osteoarthrosis.

EXAMINATION OF SYNOVIAL FLUID can be of great value when the diagnosis is in doubt. Infection is excluded by microscopic examination of a Gram stained smear, culture and gas liquid chromatography for bacterial products. In inflammatory joint disease the synovial fluid is of low viscosity, turbid, clots on standing and contains many cells. By contrast fluid from joints affected by traumatic or degenerative joint diseases is clear, viscid, does not clot and contain few cells. Examination of the spun sediment by polarising light microscopy will reveal crystals of monosodium urate or calcium pyrophosphate dihydrate in patients with acute gout or pseudogout. Measurement of synovial fluid total haemolytic complement (CH50) activity can help to distinguish rheumatoid arthritis from other forms of inflammatory arthritis. Local depression of CH50 in synovial fluid is seldom seen except in seropositive rheumatoid arthritis.

ARTHROSCOPY AND SYNOVIAL BIOPSY are occasionally required to exclude diseases such as tuberculosis and synovial tumours.

Treatment. Since the aetiology of rheumatoid arthritis is unknown treatment is empirically directed towards the relief of symptoms, the suppression of active and progressive disease and the conservation and restoration of function in affected joints. To a greater or lesser extent these aims can be achieved by combining treatment of the patient — by the judicious use of drugs, rest, physiotherapy and surgery — with the modification of the environment — by paying critical attention to housing, occupation, transport, the provision of aids and appliances, and statutory social benefits.

In a chronic and progressive disease which may have exacerbations and remissions over many years as well as systemic, psychiatric and social complications, both the general practitioner and rheumatologist have a special responsibility: (1) to educate the patient to understand the nature of the disease and to develop a positive but realistic approach; (2) to develop a relationship of continuing trust and support without creating a situation of undue dependence; (3) to co-ordinate a team of orthopaedic surgeons, occupational therapists, physiotherapists, nurses, social workers, and other allied health professionals in an integrated rehabilitation programme and (4) to improve the patient's general health.

In a disorder which is as complex and changeable as rheumatoid arthritis there is a need for repeated medical, functional and social reassessment if patients are to maintain their maximum physical, psychological, social and vocational potential.

GENERAL TREATMENT IN THE ACTIVE PHASE. Physical rest, anti-inflammatory drug therapy and maintenance physiotherapy are the cornerstones of treatment for exacerbations of rheumatoid disease. Admission to hospital may become necessary when widespread active polyarthritis is associated with signs of constitutional disturbance and there has been no response to rest at home and optimum doses of non-steroidal, analgesic, anti-inflammatory drugs (NSAID).

In most patients the rest from physical and emotional stress provided by 2 to 3 weeks in hospital is sufficient to induce a marked remission of symptoms without recourse to strict bedrest. The time in hospital allows for detailed assessments by all members of the arthritis team. It ensures that the programme of medical and physical treatment best suited to the individual's needs can be started under supervision and it provides an opportunity to plan the solution of outstanding functional and social problems with appropriate aids and social services.

In a few patients a period of complete bedrest may be required to induce a remission. In these circumstances it is essential to prevent the development of 'bed deformities'. The mattress should be firm or fracture boards inserted beneath it. A back rest with the minimum number of pillows should be in position during the day and only one firm pillow used at night. Pillows behind the knees must be avoided and a bed cage with padded footrest provided. The patient should be persuaded to spend an hour each day lying flat with a small pillow under the lumbar spine and two periods of 3 minutes lying prone will go a long way to prevent the development of flexion contractures of the hips. Foot and quadriceps exercises should be performed daily by all patients confined to bed along with maintenance exercises for muscle groups in unaffected limbs and in the thoracic, gluteal and abdominal regions.

Therapy with oral iron is indicated when true iron deficiency complicates the anaemia of chronic disease (p. 499). The normochromic normocytic anaemia is resistant to oral iron and responds best to induction of disease remission. Rarely folic acid is required for a macrocytic anaemia.

LOCAL MEASURES IN THE ACTIVE PHASE. *Corticosteroids.* Where one or more joints continue to be extremely painful and inflamed, intra-articular injection of a suspension of hydrocortisone acetate, methylprednisolone acetate or triamcinalone hexacetonide will often bring symptomatic relief lasting weeks or months. The dose should be 50–100 mg of hydrocortisone for large joints such as the ankle or knee and 5–10 mg for small joints, or the equivalent doses of the longer acting synthetic steroids. Repeated injections at short intervals should be avoided, particularly in the case of weight-bearing joints. Local injection of hydrocortisone is also the treatment of choice for alleviating symptoms of median nerve compression in the carpal tunnel when this occurs during the course of an exacerbation of rheumatoid arthritis.

Rest splints can be very useful for stabilising a particularly painful joint, such as the knee or wrists, but are usually indicated only if general rest, non-steroidal anti-inflammatory drugs and intra-articular steroid injections fail to bring a symptomatic relief. Splints are also used to prevent or correct flexion deformity especially at the knee.

ANALGESIC AND ANTI-INFLAMMATORY DRUGS are the mainstay of therapy for active inflammatory arthritis. They can be very effective in relieving pain and stiffness in optimal anti-inflammatory doses but they do not alter the course of the disease and the margin between effective and toxic doses is often small.

Aspirin is widely regarded as the drug of first choice but only 50% of patients are able to tolerate adequate doses over prolonged periods. For anti-inflammatory, as opposed to simple analgesic, effect it needs to be given in doses of 4–6 g daily. It should be prescribed as soluble aspirin (the cheapest) or as enteric coated tablets when dyspepsia or occult gastrointestinal blood loss is a problem.

Alternative NSAID are listed in Table 14.1, with standard doses and leading side effects. Aspirin and indomethacin are more effective but more toxic than the newer carboxylic acid derivatives. Phenylbutazone should not be used because of the very serious risk of agranulocytosis and aplastic anaemia.

None of the newer NSAID are more effective than aspirin although many are better tolerated. In the last three years emphasis has been placed on the convenience of NSAID with longer duration of action. Cases of fatal hepatotoxicity following treatment with benoxaprofen have however emphasised the potential danger of drugs with long half lives in elderly patients with impaired renal function as well as re-emphasising the need for caution in prescribing any new NSAID preparation.

For initial treatment it is advisable to use one of the established, less expensive NSAID, with a low incidence of side effects, in adequate dosage, for a trial period of about 3 weeks. If the response is not satisfactory, another NSAID with which the clinician is familiar, can be used. The author's preference is to begin with a propionic acid derivative if aspirin is not tolerated.

Inhibition of prostaglandin synthesis appears to be a major pharmacological action of all these agents. Simultaneous inhibition of the cytoprotective effect of prostacyclin on gastric mucosa may however also be the basis for the common propensity of these drugs to cause gastrointestinal irritation. There is little to suggest that combinations are more effective or less toxic than optimal doses of single drugs.

Additional simple analgesics such as paracetamol can be given when pain relief is inadequate. Paracetamol dextropropoxyphene combinations are very widely used for this purpose. Although safe in moderate doses propoxyphene does have narcotic properties. In general, centrally acting narcotic analgesics have no place in the management of rheumatic diseases. A number of combinations of aspirin and paracetamol are marketed.

SLOW ACTING ANTIRHEUMATIC DRUGS. The use of a 'second line' or 'disease-modifying' drug should be considered in all patients where symp-

Table 14.1 Non-steroidal analgesic anti-inflammatory drugs (NSAID).

Drug	Usual dose	Side effects
CARBOXYLIC ACIDS		
Salicylic acids		
aspirin	600–900 mg × 6/day	Tinnitus, deafness, nausea, dyspepsia, GI haemorrhage
aloxiprin	1200 mg qds	
benorylate	10 ml bd	
diflunisal	500 mg bd	As above but better tolerated
salsalate	1–1·5 g bd	
trilisate	1–1·5 g bd	
Anthranilic acids		
flufenamic acid	200 mg qds	Diarrhoea, dyspepsia, headache, dizziness, renal insufficiency (rare)
mefenamic	500 mg qds	
Propionic acids		
fenbufen	300 mg mane 600 mg nocte	Occasional dyspepsia and GI haemorrhage, high incidence of rashes
fenoprofen	600 mg qds	Occasional dyspepsia and GI haemorrhage
flurbiprofen	100 mg tds	Occasional dyspepsia and GI haemorrhage
ibuprofen	4–800 mg qds	Occasional dyspepsia and GI haemorrhage
ketoprofen	100 mg tds	Occasional dyspepsia and GI haemorrhage
naproxen	500 mg bd	Occasional dyspepsia and GI haemorrhage
tiaprofenic acid	200 mg tds	Occasional dyspepsia and GI haemorrhage
Acetic acids		
diclofenac	50 mg tds	Occasional dyspepsia and GI haemorrhage
fenclofenac	600 mg bd	Occasional dyspepsia and GI haemorrhage; high incidence of rashes
Heterocyclic acetic acids		
tolmetin	400 mg qds	Occasional dyspepsia and GI haemorrhage
Indole acetic acids		
indomethacin	25–50 mg tds	Dyspepsia; GI haemorrhage, headaches, dizziness
sulindac	200 mg bd	Minimal dyspepsia; GI haemorrhage
ENOLIC ACIDS		
Pyrazolones		
azapropazone	600 mg bd	Occasional dyspepsia and GI haemorrhage; fluid retention
phenylbutazone (severe, active ankylosing spondylitis only)	100 mg tds	Dyspepsia; GI haemorrhage; fluid retention; agranulocytosis; aplastic anaemia; thrombocytopenia; acute renal failure
Oxicams		
piroxicam	20 mg daily	Occasional dyspepsia and GI haemorrhage

toms and signs of active inflammatory arthritis have persisted for 6 months despite adequate general measures and optimal doses of NSAID.

The antimalarials chloroquine phosphate (250 mg daily) or hydroxychloroquine sulphate (200 mg b.d.) may be used as an adjunct to basic therapy in such circumstances. Clinical benefit is noted in about half the patients in 4–12 weeks and the drug should be discontinued if there is no effect by 6 months. Occasional side-effects include nausea, diarrhoea, rashes, haemolytic anaemia, ototoxicity and neuromyopathy as well as a small risk of ocular toxicity after more than a year of therapy. Deposits of the drug in the cornea may produce disturbances of vision which tend to disappear when the drug is withdrawn. More rarely retinopathy can result in permanent visual impairment. If the drug is effective it is advisable to have a thorough ophthalmological assessment after 1 year and at 6-monthly intervals thereafter. In order to reduce the risks of ocular toxicity it is conventional to give the drug for only 10 months in each year. In some the dose can be halved without exacerbation of symptoms. Antimalarials do not retard the progression of radiological changes.

Penicillamine and gold are slow acting suppressive antirheumatic drugs which have been shown to decrease the progression of erosive changes as well as reduce the activity of the disease in 50–60% of patients. Because of a high incidence of toxic effects, treatment with these agents should be considered only in the following circumstances as an adjunct to basic therapy: (1) patients with active progressive disease developing erosions and/or deformities; (2) patients with nodules and/or high titres of rheumatoid factor who have persistently active disease after 6 months treatment with optimal doses of anti-inflammatory drugs; (3) patients with troublesome extra-articular features; (4) patients who have failed to respond to antimalarial drugs; (5) patients whose symptoms are controllable only with unacceptably high doses of corticosteroids; (6) patients with palindromic rheumatoid arthritis who are having frequent attacks or developing persistent inflammatory arthritis.

Penicillamine is marginally preferable to gold unless there is a previous history of severe dyspepsia because it can be given orally and because the side-effects, though numerous and potentially serious, are usually more predictable and manageable.

Treatment is commenced with a single evening dose of 125 or 250 mg and dosage is increased by no more than 250 mg monthly to a maximum of 1 g/day. Clinical benefit is noted several weeks after an effective dose has been achieved and reaches a maximum only after 4–6 months.

Early adverse effects include rashes, loss of taste, nausea, vomiting and a serious febrile reaction. Later side-effects include mouth ulcers, proteinuria and the nephrotic syndrome and more rarely diseases resembling systemic lupus erythematosus, myasthenia gravis, pemphigus and Goodpasture's syndrome. Thrombocytopenia and pancytopenia may occur at any time and are potentially the most serious toxic effects.

Patients must be monitored, initially at weekly intervals, by urinalysis and full blood counts including platelets. Proteinuria and mild thrombocytopenia are indications for cessation of therapy followed by reintroduction of the drug at lower dosage if the abnormalities disappear. It is advisable to withdraw penicillamine altogether if the side-effects recur. Febrile reactions and pancytopenia are absolute indications for drug withdrawal.

Chrysotherapy. After a test dose of 10 mg, weekly intramuscular injections of 50 mg sodium aurothiomalate are given until a response is obtained, usually at about 2–3 months. The intervals between injections are progressively increased provided the remission is maintained and the drug is continued indefinitely. The gold injections should be stopped if there has been no clinical benefit after 6 months.

Adverse effects include pruritic rashes, exfoliative dermatitis, mouth ulcers, enterocolitis, proteinuria and the nephrotic syndrome, thrombocytopaenia, agranulocytosis and aplastic anaemia, all of which are potentially serious and preclude further therapy. Patients who are HLA-DR3 positive are particularly at risk of developing a gold induced immune complex glomerulonephritis. Monitoring should include a routine urinalysis and full blood counts, with platelets initially, prior to each injection.

Pruritus may respond to antihistamines and exfoliative dermatitis, thrombocytopenia, agranulocytosis and nephropathy to corticosteroids. Patients with agranulocytosis almost invariably recover if they can be protected from serious infection; those with aplastic anaemia have a more serious prognosis. Dimercaprol (BAL) combines with heavy metals to form a stable compound which is rapidly excreted in the urine; 3 mg/kg body weight should be administered intramuscularly 6 hourly for 3–4 days in patients with aplastic anaemia who have not responded to withdrawal of gold injections after 4–5 days. An oral gold compound is available which is less toxic but less effective than injected gold.

Other Slow Acting Antirheumatic Drugs. Dapsone, sulphasalazine and the NSAID fenclofenac have been shown to have a slow acting suppressive antirheumatic action but further trials are required to establish their role in the management of the disease.

CORTICOSTEROIDS AND CORTICOTROPHIN have a very potent anti-inflammatory activity but do not possess the 'disease modifying' properties of the slow acting antirheumatic agents. Doses required to maintain adequate symptomatic relief on a long term basis are accompanied by an unacceptable level of side effects so their use is justified only in exceptional circumstances when other therapy is ineffective.

The main indications for the use of corticosteroids are: (1) in exceptionally severe exacerbations which are not remitting with rest, intra-articular injections of corticosteroids and non-steroidal anti-inflammatory drugs; (2) when all other measures fail to control persistently disabling symptoms in breadwinners or young mothers who have to return to work; (3) in some elderly patients when acute disease is threatening to render them bedbound; (4) life or sight threatening visceral disease such as severe pericarditis, polyarteritis or scleritis.

In each of these circumstances a slow acting antirheumatic agent is commenced simultaneously with a view to a gradual withdrawal of corticosteroid therapy when a remission has been obtained.

Prednisolone is the corticosteroid of choice. It should ideally be administered as a single morning dose of no more than 7·5 mg/day to minimise suppression of the hypothalamo-pituitary-adrenal axis. In practice an evening dose of 5 mg is sometimes more useful in overcoming intractable early morning stiffness. Enteric coated tablets or small doses of corticotrophin may be preferred in patients with severe dyspepsia or a previous history of peptic ulceration. In other circumstances any possible advantages of corticotrophin seem to be outweighed by the disadvantages, namely the need for injections, the difficulty in knowing the dose of steroid being effectively administered and the high prevalence of mineralocorticoid side-effects.

IMMUNOMODULATION. Since rheumatoid arthritis is associated with evidence of both overactivity of humoral immunity and suppression of some facets of cell mediated immunity both 'immunosuppressive' and 'immunostimulant' drugs have been considered for management of the disease. Increasing understanding of the complexity of regulation of the immune system and the 'immuno pharmacology' of cytotoxic and immunostimulant drugs makes it clear that these agents may have variable and even opposing effects on the expression of immune responses depending on the dosage, the timing of administration and the subpopulation of cells predominantly affected. For example, immune stimulation may result from treatment with a drug which predominantly inhibits a suppressor cell population while functional immunosuppression can follow use of an immunostimulant which selectively activates these cells.

In practice a number of cytotoxic and immunostimulant agents have been found to have both symptomatic and slow acting 'disease modifying' activity in rheumatoid arthritis. The effects, which are empirical, may be mediated as much by 'anti-inflammatory' as by the 'immunoregulatory' activity and their usefulness is very strictly limited by immediate and potential long term toxicity.

The indications for the use of these agents are limited at the present time to: (1) treatment of life threatening extra-articular manifestations which have failed to respond to corticosteroids or second line agents; (2) treatment of patients with severely active symptomatic and progressive joint disease who have failed to respond to all other forms of therapy; (3) treatment of patients receiving unacceptably high doses of corticosteroids in whom dose reduction has not been possible.

Azathioprine is a purine analogue and antimetabolite. Both high dosage (2·5 mg/kg) and low dosage (1·25 mg/kg) have been shown to be effective. The dose must be reduced to 25% in patients receiving allopurinol since azathioprine metabolism is via xanthine oxidase. Adverse effects include nausea, vomiting, stomatitis, diarrhoea, hepatitis and particularly bone marrow suppression and susceptibility to infection. Monitoring is with fortnightly or monthly full blood counts.

Cyclophosphamide is an alkylating agent with a

narrow therapeutic range (p. 115) which is effective in daily doses of 1–2 mg/kg. Adverse effects include alopecia, azoospermia, anovulation, cystitis, nausea and vomiting, susceptibility to infection, bone marrow suppression and teratogenesis. Monitoring is with fortnightly or monthly full blood counts and routine urinalysis.

Both agents are believed to carry a significant risk of carcinogenesis.

Levamisole is an antihelminthic which has been shown to augment T lymphocyte responses as well as polymorph and macrophage chemotaxis and phagocytosis in certain circumstances. It can be effective in patients with rheumatoid arthritis in doses of 150 mg once weekly. Adverse effects include febrile reactions, nausea, vomiting, urticarial and vasculitic rashes. A high risk of agranulocytosis even with weekly monitoring of blood counts precludes its use routinely.

Thoracic duct drainage, lymphocytapheresis and *total lymphoid irradiation* have been shown to be effective in inducing remissions of disease but have no place in its practical management.

MEDICAL SYNOVECTOMY. Synovial obliteration can be achieved with osmic acid or a variety of β-emitter radiocolloids if pain, effusion and synovitis persist despite local corticosteroid injections, systemic drug therapy and physical measures. Yttrium-90 silicate is used for large joints such as the knee and Erbium-159 acetate for the small joints of the hands. Joints are immobilised for 72 hours to reduce spread to regional lymph nodes. Patients under the age of 45 should be excluded.

SURGICAL TREATMENT AND REHABILITATION. In the overall management of patients with severe and progressive rheumatoid arthritis there are many circumstances when orthopaedic surgical procedures are required to relieve pain and conserve or restore locomotor function. Cosmetic operations are seldom if ever indicated.

Surgical decompression and synovectomy of the wrist and tendon sheaths of the hands are often needed when non-steroidal anti-inflammatory drugs, local injections of corticosteroids and simple physical measures have failed to relieve a carpal tunnel syndrome or flexion contractures of the fingers resulting from fibrosis and nodule formation. Flexor and extensor tendon synovectomy, the latter often accompanied by resection of a subluxated ulnar styloid, can be important measures in preventing tendon ruptures. Synovectomy of joints will not prevent disease progression but may be indicated for pain relief when drug therapy, local rest, intra-articular injections and radiocolloids have failed to provide symptomatic relief.

At a later stage, when tendons, cartilage and bone have been eroded and the mechanics of joints disturbed, reconstructive tendon surgery, osteotomy, arthrodesis and a variety of arthroplasties with or without prostheses play a major part in the rehabilitation of the patient. Forefoot pain resulting from subluxation of the metatarsophalangeal joints and clawing of the toes can be effectively relieved by excision of the heads and necks of the metatarsals if insoles and moulded shoes have failed to provide symptomatic relief. Hip arthroplasty can be remarkably effective in relieving incapacitating pain and restoring ambulation in patients with severely damaged joints. Total hip replacement is now the most frequent major elective operation undertaken in Britain where over 30 000 are performed annually. Resurfacing and total condylar arthroplasties of the knee are less consistently successful but nevertheless performed in preference to osteotomy and arthrodesis in rheumatoid patients with intractable pain and disability. Arthrodesis is however still the best solution when severe hind foot pain is associated with destruction and subluxation of the ankle and subtalar joints.

A number of 'salvage' and reconstructive operations are also available for relieving pain and restoring function in the upper limbs. Stabilisation or wrist arthrodesis, excision arthroplasty of the metacarpo-phalangeal joints with insertion of silastic spacers and arthrodesis of the PIP joints of the fingers are all procedures in appropriate circumstances to relieve pain and improve power grip. Pinch grip may be restored by arthrodesis of the interphalangeal joint of the thumb in patients with Z deformities. Radial head excision is a simple but effective procedure which will relieve the severe pain experienced on supination and pronation when the superior radio-ulnar joint is the major site of destructive change. Relief of pain and restoration of function to patients with advanced shoulder and elbow destruction is however still a major problem. Suitable prosthetic surgery for these joints is still very much in the developmental phase.

If surgical treatment is to be successful it is very important that the aims and consequences of each operation are carefully considered as part of an integrated programme of management and rehabilitation. This is often best achieved where physicians and surgeons with special experience work together in a combined rheumatology/orthopaedic clinic with other allied health professionals. Assessment of motivation, social support and environment are no less important than careful consideration of the patient's general health and detailed assessment of the extent of disease in other joints, the integrity of the cervical spine, the presence or absence of infection, arteritis or osteoporosis. In particular it must be appreciated that whereas many patients with slowly progressive disease can be maintained mobile and functionally independent by a series of major joint replacements carried out over a number of years, it is seldom possible to mobilise a patient, who has been chair or bed-bound for a long period, by multiple joint replacement during a single lengthy hospital admission. In these and other circumstances pain relief and functional independence are better served by provision of a suitable wheelchair, home adjustments, physical aids and social services.

When a patient cannot return to a former occupation it may be necessary to suggest a change of employment where less strain will be thrown on the damaged joints. Although disablement resettlement officers, industrial rehabilitation units and government retraining centres are sometimes helpful in such cases, it should be emphasised that patients have the best chance of returning to active work with their former employers. It cannot be stressed too strongly that adequate treatment in the early stages and throughout the course of the disease enables most patients to return to some form of wage earning activity. Disabilities of all kinds can be reduced even in the 25% of patients running a severe progressive course.

Prognosis. The course and prognosis in rheumatoid arthritis is very variable. In those patients with disease of such severity as to require admis-sion to hospital, review after 10 years shows that: 25% will have a complete remission of symptoms and remain fit for all normal activities; 40% will have only moderate impairment of function despite exacerbations and remissions of disease; 25% will be more severly disabled; 10% will be severely crippled. If the many patients in the community are considered whose symptoms are never of such severity as to require admission to hospital the overall prognosis is much better.

A poor prognosis may be associated with: (1) high titres of rheumatoid factor; (2) insidious onset of disease; (3) more than a year of active disease without remission; (4) early development of nodules and erosions and (5) extra-articular manifestations.

SPONDARTHRITIS

This is a group of diseases in which an inflammatory arthritis, characterised by persistently negative tests for IgM rheumatoid factor, is variably associated with a number of other common articular, extra-articular and genetic features. These spondarthritides are: ankylosing spondylitis; Reiter's disease and reactive arthritis; psoriatic arthritis; enteropathic arthritis associated with ulcerative colitis and Crohn's disease; Behçet's syndrome; Whipple's disease and juvenile chronic arthritis.

The features held in common by the seronegative spondarthritides are: (1) an asymmetrical, inflammatory seronegative oligoarthritis; (2) sacroiliitis and/or spondylitis in some cases; (3) a tendency to develop inflammatory lesions of tendinous attachments to bone (enthesopathy); (4) anterior uveitis; (5) familial association and (6) a higher prevalence of the histocompatibility antigen HLA-B27.

Current concepts of the aetiology of these disorders suggests that they may arise as an abnormal response to infection in genetically determined persons carrying the HLA-B27 antigen. In some, an inciting organism has been identified as in Reiter's disease which can follow bacterial dysentery or chlamydial urethritis, or in the reactive arthritis following infection with *Yersinia enterocolitica*. In the others the infectious agent remains obscure. It is uncertain whether possession of HLA-B27 predisposes towards disease because: (1) it is merely a marker for an immune response gene; (2) susceptibility to infection is increased as a result of cross reactivity between an HLA-B27 determined host gene product and an antigen carried by the invading organism (molecular mimicry) or (3) the inciting organism modifies HLA-B27 positive cellular receptors in such a way as to initiate an autoimmune reaction or render the cells more susceptible to cytotoxic lymphocytes.

Ankylosing Spondylitis

In its typical form this is a chronic inflammatory arthritis with a predilection for the sacroiliac joints and spine characterised by progressive stiffening and fusion of the axial skeleton.

Epidemiology. Typically ankylosing spondylitis is a disease of young men with a peak onset in the second and third decades and a male to female ratio of 9:1. About one in 250 adult Caucasian males are affected but incomplete forms may be more common and the overall sex ratio is more equal. It occurs much more frequently in the Haida Indians of British Columbia and rarely in Blacks and Orientals. There is a greatly increased incidence in the 1st degree relatives of patients with psoriatic arthritis, inflammatory bowel disease and Reiter's syndrome as well as in those with the disease itself. More than 90% of affected persons carry the histocompatability antigen HLA-B27. Chronic prostatitis is more common than would be anticipated but it has not been possible to isolate organisms from prostatic fluid. Faecal carriage of some Klebsiella species is increased in ankylosing spondylitis and this may be related to exacerbations of the disease.

Pathology. Biopsy material from peripheral joints shows changes similar to those found in rheumatoid arthritis. Bony ankylosis, however, occurs more frequently. The characteristic *enthesopathy* comprises multiple foci of inflammation with lymphocytes and plasma cells at ligamentous attachments with adjacent erosion of bone. Healing of similar lesions at the junction of the vertebral bodies and annulus fibrosus of the intervertebral discs leads to the new bone formation (syndesmophytes) which is the hallmark of the disease.

Clinical Features. The onset is usually insidious with recurring episodes of low back pain and stiffness sometime radiating to the buttocks or thighs. Characteristically the symptoms are worse in the early morning and following inactivity. Occasionally the onset may be acute, resembling a lumbar disc protrusion but on examination all movements of the lumbar spine are restricted, there is pain on sacroiliac compression and there are no associated symptoms or signs of nerve root compression. A few patients present with symptoms referable to the dorsal or cervical spine but such cases usually reveal evidence of previous sacroiliitis and lumbar spine involvement.

Chest pain aggravated by breathing results from involvement of the costovertebral joints. Plantar fasciitis, Achilles tendinitis and tenderness over bony prominences such as the iliac crest, ischial tuberosity and greater trochanter are typical. 25% of patients have an attack of acute anterior uveitis during the course of the disease and this may be the presenting feature in a few cases. In 10% a peripheral joint is first affected and in a further 10% symptoms begin in childhood as one variety of pauciarticular juvenile chronic arthritis (p. 569).

Early signs include failure to obliterate the lumbar lordosis on forward flexion, pain on sacroiliac compression, and restriction of movements of the lumbar spine in all directions. As the disease progresses stiffness increases throughout the spine, and chest expansion frequently becomes restricted. Severe spinal fusion and rigidity occurs in only a minority and in most of these is not associated with much deformity. A few develop kyphosis of the dorsal and cervical spine which can be incapacitating especially when associated with hip involvement.

Extra-articular features of ankylosing spondylitis include non-granulomatous anterior uveitis; aortic regurgitation and conduction defects; apical pulmonary fibrosis; amyloidosis; osteoporosis and myelopathy associated with atlanto-axial subluxation.

Investigation. The ESR is usually raised but may be normal. Tests for rheumatoid factor and antinuclear factor are negative and synovial fluid complement levels are not depressed.

Radiographs in the early stages may be normal. Radiological signs of sacroiliitis begin in the lower parts of the joints with irregularity and marginal sclerosis eventually progressing to fusion. In the lumbar spine there may be 'squaring' of the vertebrae owing to ossification of the anterior longitudinal ligament, syndesmophyte formation, erosion and sclerosis at the anterior corners of the vertebrae and facetal joint changes. Progressive ossification results in the typical 'bamboo spine'. Erosive changes may be seen in the symphysis pubis, the ischial tuberosities and peripheral joints. Osteoporosis and atlanto-axial dislocation can occur.

Radionuclide bone scanning may reveal evidence of sacroiliitis or spinal involvement when radiographs are negative but the increased uptake of the bone-seeking isotope is non-specific and reflects bone blood flow and turnover.

Differential diagnosis is usually from prolapsed lumbar intervertebral discs and other traumatic lesions leading to low back pain or from other types of spondarthritis.

Degenerative joint disease occurs in an older age group and is not accompanied by systemic symptoms. The radiological appearances are usually distinct although diffuse idiopathic skeletal hyperostosis can cause confusion when new bone formation is extensive and uniform. In osteoarthrosis the osteophytes extend horizontally from the edges of the vertebral bodies, there is frequently associated narrowing of the disc spaces and the sacroiliac joints are usually intact.

When ankylosing spondylitis commences in a peripheral joint all other causes of seronegative inflammatory arthritis must be considered. Involvement of the MTP joint of the great toe can occasionally be mistaken for gout, pseudogout or an infective arthritis.

Treatment. The principles are to relieve pain and stiffness, maintain a maximal range of skeletal mobility and avoid the development of deformities. Early in the disease patients should be trained to do regular exercising at home and encouraged to take up active non-contact sports like swimming. Poor bed and chair postures must be avoided.

NSAID (p. 558) are used to relieve symptoms but do not themselves alter the course of the disease. Although aspirin, propionic acids, the enolic derivatives and indomethacin should be tried first, a few patients with spondylitis find phenylbutazone the most effective drug. It can usually be given safely even over prolonged periods provided a daily dose of 300 mg is not exceeded.

Radiotherapy is occasionally indicated if the response to drug therapy is unsatisfactory. It does not affect the course of the disease and earlier regimes of treatment, when excessive radiation was employed, were associated with a tenfold increase in the risk of developing leukaemia.

Local corticosteroid injections can be helpful for plantar fasciitis and the management of other manifestations of enthesopathy. Systemic steroids are sometimes required for treatment of acute iritis.

Hip disease may require surgery and total hip arthroplasty has largely obviated the need for difficult spinal surgery in those with advanced deformity.

75% or more of patients with ankylosing spondylitis are able to remain in employment without significant loss of time from work. Restriction of chest movements does not predispose to pulmonary infection but systemic complications and especially hip involvement carry a worse prognosis.

Reiter's Disease

Classically this is the triad of non-specific urethritis, conjunctivitis and arthritis that follows bacterial dysentery or sexual exposure. Incomplete forms are frequent and include the commonest variety of inflammatory arthritis seen in young men. When arthritis alone follows sexual exposure or enteric infection with salmonella, shigella, yersinia or campylobacter the term *'reactive arthritis'* is frequently used.

Epidemiology. 1–2% of patients with non-specific urethritis seen at clinics for sexually transmitted diseases have Reiter's disease and there is a similar incidence following outbreaks of shigellosis. A male with HLA-B27 runs a 20% risk of getting the disease following an attack of shigella dysentery. Although predominantly a disease of young men, the apparent 50:1 male to female ratio is spuriously high as urethritis is frequently ignored in women and children.

Clinical Features. The onset is typically acute with the simultaneous development of urethritis, conjuctivitis (in about 50%) and an inflammatory oligoarthritis affecting the weight bearing joints of the lower limbs, 1–3 weeks following sexual exposure or an attack of dysentery. There may be considerable associated systemic disturbance with fever, weight loss and vasomotor changes in the feet.

Often the onset is more insidious and many patients present with no more than monoarthritis of a knee or an asymmetrical inflammatory arthritis of some interphalangeal joints. Symptoms and signs of urethritis or conjunctivitis may have been minimal or forgotten. In such cases, heel pain, Achilles tendinitis or plantar fasciitis are valuable clues while the presence of circinate balanitis or the rash of keratoderma blenorrhagica can clinch the diagnosis even in the absence of the classical triad and without an overt history of sexual promiscuity or dysentery. The skin lesions can vary from mild macules, vesicles and pustules on the hands and feet to marked hyperkeratosis with plaque-like lesions spreading to the scalp and trunk. These may be associated with severe nail dystrophy and massive subungual hyperkeratosis.

Ocular involvement is normally limited to mild bilateral conjunctivitis which subsides spontaneously within a month. In 10% of patients acute anterior uveitis occurs at the outset. It is distinguished from simple conjunctivitis by injection of the ciliary vessels around the cornea, by a constricted irregular or unreactive pupil and by cells in the anterior chamber on slit lamp examination. Unlike the conjunctivitis it requires urgent treatment. Chronic iridocyclitis may lead to glaucoma and blindness.

The urethritis is usually associated with minor dysuria and a clear sterile discharge. Sometimes it is asymptomatic and detected only by finding mucoid threads in the first voided specimen of early morning urine. Unusually there may be severe dysuria, haematuria and suprapubic discomfort from an associated acute haemorrhagic cystitis and prostatitis.

Initially the arthritis appears to be self limiting with spontaneous remission of symptoms within 2–3 months of onset. There is however a recurrence rate of about 15% per annum not necessarily related to further overt exposure to infection. Uveitis occurs in 30% of patients with recurring arthritis. Low back pain and stiffness from sacroiliitis are common and 15–20% of patients develop spondylitis. Other rare extra-articular features include neurological and cardiological complications, e.g. meningo-encephalitis, peripheral neuropathy, pericarditis and pleurisy.

Investigation. The ESR is often greatly raised during the acute phase and may remain so for long after joint symptoms have settled. Polymorphonuclear leucocytosis and an anaemia of chronic disease (p. 499) are further indications of active systemic disturbance. The synovial fluid has the characteristics of a low viscosity inflammatory effusion with leucocyte counts as high as 50 000/ml but it is sterile on culture. Giant synovial macrophages can be seen but synovial fluid complement levels are not depressed as they are in seropositive rheumatoid arthritis. Serum tests for rheumatoid factor and antinuclear factor are negative. Tissue typing reveals HLA-B27 in more than 70% of cases.

Radiological Examination. Periarticular osteoporosis, reduction of joint space and erosive changes can be seen when there is prolonged or recurrent inflammatory arthritis. The changes reflect the asymmetry of joint involvement and are often accompanied by marked periostitis especially in the metatarsal and phalangeal bones. Periosteal reaction around the pelvis gives a characteristic appearance of 'whiskering' and there may be large and 'fluffy' calcaneal spurs. Sacroiliitis is indistinguishable from that seen in ankylosing spondylitis but the spinal changes include early isolated bony spurs and paravertebral ossification also found in psoriasis but not in ankylosing spondylitis.

Treatment is mainly symptomatic and supportive. Rest and NSAID (p. 558) are required during the acute phases together with judicious aspiration of joints and intra-articular or other local steroid injections. Systemic corticosteroids are very occasionally required. Anterior uveitis may be a medical emergency requiring topical, subconjunctival or systemic corticosteroids.

Severe progressive arthritis and intractable keratoderma blenorrhagica very occasionally warrant cytotoxic drug therapy. The non-specific urethritis is usually treated with a short course of tetracycline but there is little evidence that it alters the course of the arthritis.

10% of patients have evidence of active disease 20 years after the onset. Spondylitis, chronic erosive arthritis, recurrent acute arthritis and uveitis are the major causes of long-term morbidity.

Psoriatic Arthritis

This is a seronegative inflammatory arthritis found in patients with psoriasis, a past or family history of psoriasis or with characteristic changes in the nails.

Epidemiology. Psoriatic arthritis occurs in about 1 out of 1000 of the general population and in 7% of patients with psoriasis. 20% of all patients with seronegative polyarthritis have psoriasis while the prevalence of psoriasis in seropositive rheumatoid arthritis is no higher than that in the general population, suggesting that the association of the skin disease with seronegative arthritis does not arise by chance alone. The onset is usually between the ages of 25–40 years and the sex incidence is equal except in those with spinal involvement where males are found to predominate.

Clinical Features. Five distinct clinical patterns of psoriatic arthritis are recognised:

1. An inflammatory arthritis involving the distal interphalangeal joints not usually affected in rheumatoid arthritis is seen in 15% of patients who almost invariably have associated nail changes (below).

2. An asymmetrical inflammatory oligo-arthritis affecting the small joints of the hand and feet is the most common clinical pattern and accounts for 70% of all cases.

3. A symmetrical but persistently seronegative inflammatory polyarthritis clinically indistinguishable from 'seronegative rheumatoid arthritis' accounts for 15% of cases.

4. Arthritis mutilans with extensive bone resorption and telescoping digits occurs in less than 5% of cases.

5. Sacroiliitis and spondylitis indistinguishable from classical ankylosing spondylitis can occur alone or in association with any of the clinical patterns of peripheral arthritis.

Extra-articular features are limited to (1) skin lesions which may be widespread scaling lesions typically over extensor surfaces or insignificant and confined to such areas as the scalp, natal cleft and umbilicus where they are easily overlooked. (2) nail changes including pitting, onycholysis, subungual hyperkeratosis and horizontal ridging and (3) anterior uveitis.

Investigation. The ESR is usually only moderately raised and there may be a mild normochromic normocytic anaemia in active cases. Tests for rheumatoid factor and antinuclear factor are negative. Radiographs showing asymmetrical disease, terminal I.P. joint involvement and relatively little peri-articular osteoporosis may help to distinguish psoriatic arthritis from rheumatoid arthritis. The changes in the axial skeleton resemble those in ankylosing spondylitis.

Treatment. NSAID are usually all that are required to control symptoms. Gold therapy can be used in persistently symptomatic progressive cases without exacerbation of the psoriasis but the antimalarials, chloroquine and hydroxychloroquine must be avoided. Immunosuppressive drugs are given very occasionally to try and control progressive arthritis mutilans or extensive incapacitating skin disease. Splints and prolonged rest are best avoided because of the increased tendency to fibrous and bony ankylosis but intra-articular steroid injections can be used with good effect in persistently active and symptomatic joints.

Prognosis is better than for rheumatoid arthritis with the exception of those rare cases with arthritis mutilans.

Other Seronegative Spondarthritides

Enteropathic Arthritis. Two patterns of seronegative inflammatory arthritis are associated with ulcerative colitis and Crohn's disease.

Enteropathic Synovitis. An acute, often migratory, non-erosive oligo-arthritis occurs in the course of the disorder in 12% of patients with ulcerative colitis and 20% of those with Crohn's disease. The knees, ankles and other weight-bearing joints are most commonly affected but the wrists and small joints of the fingers and toes can also be involved. The arthritis, which tends to follow exacerbations of the underlying bowel disease, sometimes in association with aphthous mouth ulcers, uveitis and erythema nodosum, ceases to be a problem following total colectomy in cases of ulcerative colitis. The higher prevalence in Crohn's disease may reflect the greater difficulty in eradicating the bowel problem.

Sacroiliitis (16%) and *ankylosing spondylitis* (6%) are also seen in the course of these disorders, but they pursue an independent course and often precede the bowel disease. Spinal changes which are indistinguishable from ankylosing spondylitis are associated with a high prevalence of HLA-B27 while the enteropathic synovitis is not.

In enteropathic synovitis treatment is directed at the bowel problem. The response to corticosteroids and colectomy is remarkable in such cases although the arthritis is never of such severity as to be itself an indication for these measures.

Behçet's syndrome is rare in Western Europe but more common in Japan and Eastern Mediterranean countries; there is an association with HLA-B5.

Major criteria are recurrent aphthous stomatitis, skin lesions, iridocyclitis and genital ulceration. Minor criteria are inflammatory arthritis of large joints, intestinal ulceration, epididymitis, thrombophlebitis and neuropsychiatric problems. In the presence of all four major criteria the syndrome is said to be 'complete'; in the presence of three, 'incomplete'. The arthritis is mono-articular or oligo-articular and non-erosive. It most frequently involves the knees, ankles, wrists and elbows. Occasionally the sacroiliac joints are affected.

Treatment is symptomatic with NSAID; corticosteroids and immunosuppressive therapy are reserved for the more serious systemic manifestations.

Whipple's disease is a rare disorder characterised by diarrhoea, abdominal pain, weight loss, pyrexia, skin pigmentation, malabsorption and arthritis. The pattern of the non-erosive arthritis can resemble the migratory oligo-articular enteropathic arthritis but sometimes it is symmetrical and polyarticular. Joint symptoms, most commonly affecting the knee or ankle, may precede other clinical manifestations by months or years and sacroiliitis and ankylosing spondylitis may occur.

The diagnosis is confirmed by demonstrating the presence of PAS positive macrophages in a small intestinal biopsy. Electron microscopy has demonstrated unidentified rod shaped organisms in the lamina propria and synovial membrane.

Treatment is with prolonged antibiotic therapy, usually tetracycline 1 g daily for one year. Arthralgias and arthritis settle within a month of starting treatment.

JUVENILE CHRONIC ARTHRITIS

A number of patterns of chronic arthritis commence in childhood before the age of 16 years.

Systemic Onset Juvenile Chronic Arthritis (Still's disease). In 10% of children with juvenile chronic arthritis the disease begins with a profound systemic disturbance. Lymphadenopathy, hepatosplenomegaly, pleurisy, pericarditis and a high intermittent fever are associated with myalgias, arthralgias and eventually polyarthritis. Weight loss and retardation of growth may be striking and there is often a characteristic but non-specific evanescent macular rash which tends to appear at times when the temperature is raised. This pattern of disease can occur in children of any age but is most common between the ages of 1 and 5 years.

In addition to a raised ESR and an anaemia of chronic disease, there may be a polymorphonuclear leucocytosis. Tests for rheumatoid factor and antinuclear factor are negative. Remission of systemic symptoms usually occurs within 6 months of onset but half the children have recurrent systemic attacks and one quarter go on to develop a severe chronic polyarthritis.

Polyarticular juvenile chronic arthritis can occur at any age and accounts for 20% of all cases. It is commoner in girls and four or more joints are affected. The inflammatory arthritis may begin acutely or insidiously and large joints are most commonly first affected; in some there is more widespread polyarthritis. Inflammatory arthritis in the proximity of growing epiphyses may result in growth acceleration or arrest. Early fusion and growth arrest in the cervical spine, and mandible give rise to the short stiff neck and receding chin very characteristic of adults who have had juvenile chronic arthritis. Systemic features are usually mild.

Tests for rheumatoid factor are negative but the antinuclear factor is positive in 25% of cases. The overall prognosis is good and only 10–15% have severe destructive arthritis.

Seropositive polyarticular disease occurs in 10% of children with juvenile chronic arthritis. Girls are more frequently affected than boys and the onset is usually after the age of 8 years. The disease resembles severe adult onset rheumatoid arthritis with progressive erosive joint changes in more than half of those affected. Extra-articular features include nodules and vasculitis as well as low grade fever and an anaemia of chronic disease, but these children do not get iridocyclitis. Antinuclear factor tests are positive in 75%.

Pauci-articular Juvenile Chronic Arthritis. Four or less joints are involved in half or more of all children affected and at least two distinct subsets can be identified:

1. *Young girls* with mono- or pauci-articular arthritis affecting knees, ankles, elbows or occasionally a small joint of the hand or foot. There are seldom any constitutional symptoms and the ESR is frequently normal. HLA-DR5 and positive tests for antinuclear factor appear to be a marker for chronic iridocyclitis which can occur in up to half of this group of children. Regular three monthly slit lamp examinations are required if this complication is to be detected and treated early enough to preserve normal vision.

2. *Older boys* with mono- or pauci-articular arthritis affecting hips, knees or ankles. Sacroiliitis is common and there is frequently a family history of uveitis, ankylosing spondylitis or another spondyloarthritis. 75% of these boys are HLA-B27 positive and in some the disease gradually evolves into ankylosing spondylitis in early adult life.

Differential diagnosis of acute arthritis in childhood includes bacterial, viral and reactive arthritis as it does in adults and also rheumatic fever (p. 156) and osteomyelitis (p. 586).

Henoch Schönlein (anaphylactoid) purpura is associated with abdominal pain and an acute arthritis affecting one or more joints for a few days at a time. There may be an erythematous or urticarial rash as well as non-thrombocytopenic purpura which may be seen only in areas of pressure such as over the buttocks. The disease frequently follows an upper respiratory infection in the early spring. It is a self limiting form of arthritis which usually lasts for less than 3 months.

Intussusception, rectal bleeding and haematuria are features of more severe cases and a few children have a more chronic or relapsing course with evidence of an immune complex glomerulonephritis. Serum IgA levels are raised in half the cases.

Treatment. The principles of management in juvenile chronic arthritis do not differ from those in adult rheumatoid arthritis but special consideration has to be given to maintaining the child's education and helping parents to develop a sensible, vigilant but not overprotective approach to the child's disease. Bed rest may be essential during acute phases but care must be taken to avoid development of flexion deformities of the hips and knees by regular prone lying and appropriate lightweight splints. Whenever possible the child should be kept mobile and ambulant and daily physiotherapy is given throughout to maintain a good range of joint movements and muscle strength. Hydrotherapy in a warm pool is particularly useful.

Aspirin is the drug of choice in children who tolerate salicylates better than adults. Naproxen (5 mg/kg) is safe and effective in children. Chloroquine, hydroxychloroquine, gold salts and penicillamine can be used provided the same precautions are taken as in the treatment of adult rheumatoid arthritis.

Corticosteroids are reserved for children with severe systemic disease, those with chronic iridocyclitis not responding to local therapy and a few cases where very active joint disease does not respond to other measures. The use of corticotrophin or alternate day corticosteroids should always be considered because daily doses of prednisolone as low as 3 mg/day can inhibit growth in children under age of 5 years. Older children can be taught to give their own injections of cortico-trophin if this has to be continued for any length of time. Corticosteroids do not arrest the progression of disease. Immunosuppressive drugs are used only in children with amyloidosis and persistently active disease.

Surgery is usually limited to the rehabilitation of children with deformities. Soft tissue release operations may be helpful in eliminating difficult flexion contractures and osteotomies may be required when joints have been allowed to fuse in poor positions. Total hip arthroplasty can be considered for severely destroyed joints as soon as growth has ceased.

INFECTIVE ARTHRITIS

Septic arthritis can accompany septicaemia at any age. *H. influenzae* is the common causative organism in infancy; staphylococcal and streptococcal infections are usually responsible in older children and adults. Other organisms which may be implicated are gonococci, pneumococci, meningococci, *Esch. coli, Pseudomonas* and *Proteus*. Important predisposing factors include debilitating illnesses, diabetes mellitus, immunodeficiency disorders and immunosuppression. Joint trauma, surgery, penetrating injury and intra-articular injections may lead to bacterial joint infections and may complicate rheumatoid arthritis and other established arthritides.

Clinical Features. Characteristically septic arthritis has an abrupt onset with severe pain and swelling of a single joint associated with a swinging fever, severe malaise and a polymorphonuclear leucocytosis. Large joints are most frequently affected and the joint is hot, tender and swollen with an effusion; there is marked limitation of movement. The diagnosis may be missed when more than one joint is involved, in patients with rheumatoid arthritis or when the presentation is less acute in patients receiving corticosteroids or immunosuppressive drugs.

It is essential to try to establish the diagnosis early by joint aspiration and blood culture. The synovial fluid is typically turbid with a high polymorphonuclear cell count. Organisms may be easily and immediately identified on Gram stain of a film but special culture techniques may be required especially for gonococci and anaerobic organisms.

Radiographs show no more than soft tissue swelling initially. Later there may be periarticular osteoporosis, joint space narrowing, periostitis and articular erosions. In more long-standing infections the joint margins have a peculiar 'rubbed out' appearance.

Treatment. In all cases where bacterial infection is suspected treatment should be commenced with high parenteral doses of broad spectrum antibiotics as soon as joint aspiration and blood cultures have been completed and until the responsible organism and its sensitivity have been established. Appropriate antibiotics must then be administered for several weeks. Antibiotics readily cross the inflamed synovial membrane so that there is no need to inject them intra-articularly.

The joint should be rested and immobilised with a splint and daily joint aspiration undertaken until no more fluid reaccumulates. If the fluid becomes loculated or too thick for aspiration, surgical drainage is required.

The prognosis for recovery without joint damage should be excellent and is directly related to the speed with which antibiotic therapy is instituted.

Gonococcal arthritis is more common in females than males and not infrequently commences at the time of a menstrual period within 2–3 weeks of genital infection. Joint involvement is usually asymmetrical and polyarticular with an acute or subacute, migratory polyarthralgia or polyarthritis. Tenosynovitis, an 'additive' as opposed to 'flitting' pattern of joint involvement and a macular, vesicular or pustular rash are important diagnostic clues even in the absence of overt genital gonorrhoea. The diagnosis can be established by cultures of synovial fluid, blood, skin lesions or from the genital tract but organisms are identified in joints in only 20% of cases. There is a dramatic response to penicillin, 1 mega unit daily for 3–4 days, but treatment should be continued for two weeks.

Meningococcal infection can be associated with (1) an acute transient polyarthritis that is seen simultaneously with the characteristic petechial rash, (2) a purulent monoarthritis which usually occurs after 5 days or (3) a flitting polyarthralgia in patients with chronic meningo-coccaemia. Penicillin is the treatment of choice.

Brucellosis (p. 748) is characteristically associated with polyarthralgia or transient polyarthritis. Much more rarely there may be a destructive, septic arthritis of a large joint or a characteristic spondylitis. Destructive lesions in one or more contiguous vertebrae lead to severe back pain, disc narrowing, marginal proliferation of osteophytes with early bony fusion of vertebrae. Chronic bursitis and osteomyelitis may also occur.

The diagnosis is established by blood and synovial fluid cultures coupled with rising serological titres of antibodies. Treatment is given on page 749.

Tuberculosis of joints is usually secondary to an established focus in the lungs or kidneys. Since the eradication of bovine tuberculosis in Britain, articular infection is seen mainly in debilitated, malnourished, socially deprived, elderly or immigrant groups. 50% have evidence of an established pulmonary focus. The organism is carried to the synovium or subchondral bone by blood or lymphatic spread. In more than three-quarters of all cases a single large joint is affected. Joint pain, stiffness, swelling and restriction of movements are associated with anorexia, weight loss, night sweats and malaise.

The ESR is usually only moderately raised. In the early stages radiographs show only periarticular osteoporosis and soft tissue swelling. Later there is narrowing of the joint space, bony erosion and collapse of subchondral bone with little associated periosteal reaction. The tuberculin skin test is strongly positive and diagnosis can sometimes be made by direct bacteriological examination and culture of synovial fluid. In other cases synovial biopsy is required. After antibiotic control has been established (p. 236), synovectomy is often undertaken in those with extensive disease.

Bovine infection is still common in many developing countries. In immigrant communities in Britain extra-articular tuberculosis is sometimes associated with a non-destructive allergic polyarthritis of large and small joints.

Syphilitic arthritis is now very uncommon. *Congenital* syphilis may be associated with painful para-articular swelling due to epiphyseal involvement soon after birth or painless effusions of the knees (Clutton's joints) in adolescents.

Acquired secondary syphilis may be associated with a migrating polyarthralgia resembling rheumatic fever and neuropathic arthropathy (Charcot joints) are a feature of tabes dorsalis.

Lyme arthritis is an intermittant pauciarticular inflammatory arthritis which is associated with a characteristic rash (erythema chronicum migrans). Originally limited to a small area in Connecticut it has now been shown to be a tick borne spirochaetal disease that can occur in other localities and which may respond to penicillin.

Fungal infections are rare. Blastomycosis, histoplasmosis and sporotrichosis can be associated with destructive lesions of bones and joints. Histoplasmosis and coccidiomycosis may also be associated with erythema nodosum and a benign polyarthritis.

Viral infections are commonly associated with arthralgia and transient polyarthritis, as in some cases of hepatitis B, mumps, chickenpox, infectious mononucleosis, adenoviral, enteroviral, parvoviral and arboviral infections.

Rubella. Arthritis follows 1–7 days after the rash or 2–6 weeks after vaccination in 30–40% of adults. A symmetrical inflammatory polyarthritis may be associated with symptoms of carpal tunnel compression or tenosynovitis. Joint pain, stiffness and swelling, which may be severe, usually settle in 1–4 weeks but the condition may persist with intermittent arthralgia for some months. Posterior cervical lymphadenopathy and a high lymphocyte count in the synovial fluid may be helpful in diagnosis. The latex test for rheumatoid factor and the ESR are often transiently raised.

MISCELLANEOUS DISORDERS OF SYNOVIAL JOINTS

Acromegaly is associated with a symmetrical arthropathy in 50% of cases. The small joints of the hands, wrists and knees are particularly affected as is the spine. Hypertrophy of synovium and articular cartilage are characteristically associated with periosteal new bone formation, osteophytosis, 'tufting' of the terminal phalanges and premature osteoarthrosis and hypertrophic spondylosis.

Table 14.2 SLE. Immunological abnormalities detectable in the blood

Anti-nuclear antibodies
  Anti-DNA-histone (and LE cells)
  Anti-DNA (single strand)
  Anti-DNA (double strand)
  Anti-RNA
  Anti-Sm (named after a patient)
  Anti-RNP
Anticytoplasmic antibodies (Ro and La)
Lymphocytotoxins
Depression of CH_{50} and C3 and C4
	Antibodies against erythrocytes, leucocytes and
	  platelets
	Biological false positive tests for syphilis
	Circulating anticoagulants (anticardiolipin
	  antibodies)
	Anti-thyroid (and other organ specific
	  autoantibodies)
	Rheumatoid factors
	Cryoglobulins
	Circulating immune complexes

Amyloidosis (p. 390) can be associated with carpal tunnel compression and a polyarthritis superficially resembling rheumatoid arthritis. The synovium is infiltrated with amyloid protein and the diagnosis can be made by finding fragments of amyloid tissue in the synovial fluid.

Hyperlipidaemia (p. 485). Type II can be associated with a migratory polyarthritis, and widespread xanthomas with tendon deposits. Type IV can be associated with arthralgia and morning stiffness and also hyperuricaemia and gout.

Sarcoidosis. Two distinct patterns of inflammatory arthritis may be seen. Erythema nodosum and hilar lymphadenopathy are frequently associated with a symmetrical non-destructive inflammatory arthritis especially affecting the knees, ankles and wrists. A more specific asymmetrical destructive arthritis affects similar joints especially in black people. Biopsy of the synovium in such cases shows evidence of noncaseating granulomata. Radiologically there may be 'punched out' cystic bone lesions and also 'cortical erosions' and joint destruction.

SYSTEMIC LUPUS ERYTHEMATOSUS (SLE)

This is a multisystem connective tissue disorder characterised by the presence of numerous autoantibodies, circulating immune complexes and widespread immunologically determined tissue damage.

Epidemiology. SLE affects individuals throughout the world but occurs more frequently in the United States and the Far East. American Blacks are particularly susceptible, with a prevalence as high as 1 in 250 among females. The increasing use of sensitive tests for antinuclear antibodies suggest that mild and incomplete cases are much more frequent than previously thought. The onset is most commonly in the 2nd and 3rd decades, with a female/male ratio of 9:1. In children and the elderly the sex incidence is more equal.

Aetiology and Pathogenesis. Although the cause of SLE remains obscure, current concepts suggest that this is a multifactorial disorder in which there is profound *disturbance of immune regulation*. A defect of suppressor T lymphocytes is associated with polyclonal B lymphocyte activation and the uncontrolled production of a variety of autoantibodies and immune complexes (Table 14.2).

Evidence for *genetic factors* in the aetiology of the disease includes: (1) its occurrence in monozygotic twin pairs; (2) a higher than expected prevalence of SLE, other connective tissue diseases, antinuclear antibodies and immune complexes in related family members; (3) inherited deficiency of isolated complement components, notably C2 in some patients; (4) increased prevalence of the histocompatibility antigens HLA-B8 and DR3.

Evidence for the influence of *environmental factors* includes: (1) the provocative effect of sunlight in many cases; (2) the induction of lupus erythematosus by many drugs; (3) the importance of oestrogens as determinants of disease expression. Exacerbations commonly occur in pregnancy and the puerperium and prevalence is increased in fertile women, those using oral contraceptives and men with Klinefelter's syndrome.

Clear evidence of *viral infection* exists in animal models of SLE but in humans the findings are inconclusive.

Immunologically mediated tissue damage results from at least two different mechanisms in SLE:

1. Direct antibody mediated cytotoxicity (Type II reactions). Brain damage and abortion may be a consequence of cytotoxicity by cold reactive antibodies which cross react with neural and trophoblast tissues.

2. Immune complex (and complement) mediated (Type III reactions). The renal and vascular lesions of SLE appear to be a consequence of deposition of circulating DNA — Anti DNA and other complexes in tissues.

Clinical Features. *Arthritis*, arthralgia and fever are the commonest presenting features, frequently accompanied by tiredness, anaemia, and malaise. There may be a previous history of migraine, depression or other pyschiatric disturbance. Unlike other types of inflammatory arthritis, symptoms may begin during pregnancy and there may be a past history of spontaneous abortions. The arthritis can be transient and migratory or a more persistant seronegative polyarthritis. Chronic inflammatory arthritis and tenosynovitis may lead to deformities and contractures but erosive changes are very uncommon.

Skin lesions are seen in more than two-thirds of patients. In addition to the classical, photosensitive erythematous 'butterfly' rash across the face, there may be lesions of discoid lupus, a less specific maculopapular eruption or a vasculitic rash. The last may present as purpura or periungual erythema with 'chilblain-like' lesions or digital infarcts. Livedo reticularis and Raynaud's phenomenon are common while bullous eruptions and panniculitis ('lupus profundus') occur more rarely. Alopecia can be a useful diagnostic pointer and is seen in more than 50% of patients. Painful oral or nasopharyngeal ulcers are rather less common.

Cardiopulmonary features include pericarditis, myocarditis and endocarditis, pleurisy, fibrosing alveolitis and acute lupus pneumonitis as well as a 'shrinking lung syndrome' with progressive elevation of the diaphragms and linear scars from recurrent pulmonary infarction. Lung function tests reveal impairment of ventilation and diffusion in these and many patients without overt clinical or radiological evidence of pulmonary involvement. Verrucous (Libman-Sachs) endo-carditis may be demonstrated by echocardiography.

Renal involvement occurs in half the patients and carries the worst prognosis. It may result in the nephrotic syndrome and acute or chronic renal failure. It may be limited to insignificant proteinuria or the presence of red cells or casts.

Renal biopsy is a guide to therapy and prognosis. Subendothelial dense deposits on electron microscopy and 'lumpy-bumpy' basement membrane deposits of C3 and IgG on immunofluorescence are early signs of significant immune complex disease. A diffuse proliferative glomerulonephritis on light microscopy is often associated with a bad prognosis and is an indication for vigorous treatment with corticosteroids and/or immunosuppressive drugs. Membranous glomerulonephritis may be associated with a prolonged nephrotic syndrome but the eventual outlook is usually good. Focal proliferative changes and mesangial or 'minimal change' glomerulonephritis are seldom associated with progressive renal disease.

Central nervous system involvement is seen in up to half the patients. In the majority this is limited to mild psychiatric disturbance or epilepsy but in a few there may be severe depression, dementia, organic psychosis, cranial nerve lesions, hemiplegia, transverse myelitis, chorea, cerebellar ataxia or peripheral neuropathy. The more severe manifestations are associated with a poor prognosis.

Other Manifestations. Gastrointestinal symptoms are frequent but non-specific. Abdominal pain can be due to peritonitis, perisplenitis, pancreatitis or vasculitis. Gastric or duodenal perforation may be complications of corticosteroid therapy; colonic or gall bladder perforations are more likely to be a consequence of necrotising arteritis. Lymphadenopathy is found in half the patients and a moderately enlarged spleen in 20–30%. Ocular findings include kerato-conjunctivitis sicca, episcleritis and retinal vasculitis and soft exudates.

Investigation. The ESR is usually raised in active disease but the C reactive protein rarely so in the absence of infection. Haematological findings may include a normocytic normochromic anaemia of chronic disease, a Coombs' positive haemolytic anaemia, leucopenia, thrombocytopenia or a circulating anticoagulant (Table 14.2).

IMMUNOLOGICAL FINDINGS. *Antinuclear antibodies* can be detected in the serum of more than 90% of patients but positive tests for ANF are often found in rheumatoid arthritis, juvenile chronic arthritis, Sjögren's syndrome, fibrosing alveolitis, progressive systemic sclerosis and other connective tissue diseases. Chronic liver disease, thyroiditis, Addison's disease, myasthenia gravis and leukaemia can all be associated with a positive ANF as can therapy with a variety of drugs. Positive tests in low titre have no clinical significance and are frequently found in normal elderly people. *The LE cell test* is less sensitive, very time consuming and hardly more specific.

Anti-DNA Antibodies and Immune Complexes. Antibodies to undenatured double stranded DNA have much greater specificity but are present in the serum in significant amounts in only about half the patients at any one time. High levels of anti-DNA antibodies coupled with depressed total haemolytic complement (CH_{50}) activity and low C3 and C4 complement components suggest that there is activation of the classical complement pathway by active immune complex disease (Fig. 2.6 p. 27). Further evidence for circulating immune complexes may be obtained by finding a cryoprecipitate or by using one of a number of tests for CIq binding. Tissue evidence for immune complex deposition comes from detection of complement components and immunoglobulins by immunofluorescence at the dermoepidermal junction of normal skin or in organ biopsies.

Treatment. Acute and life threatening manifestations of SLE require systemic corticosteroid therapy, often initially in doses of 40–80 mg prednisolone or equivalent daily. 'Pulse' therapy with methylprednisolone, (1g i.v. on 3 successive days) is occasionally required in patients with proliferative glomerulonephritis and rapidly deteriorating renal function. With remission of disease careful attempts are made to withdraw steroids or maintain patients on very low doses or alternate day regimes of steroid therapy. Articular symptoms and less severe inflammatory manifestations should be managed with NSAID therapy wherever possible. Anti-malarials are particularly useful in the management of patients with troublesome

skin and joint lesions and they can reduce the frequency of severe exacerbations of disease.

Immunosuppressive drugs are reserved for patients with severe diffuse proliferative glomerulonephritis who are not responding adequately to corticosteroids and for those requiring maintenance steroid doses so high as to cause severe side-effects. The combination of plasma exchange and immunosuppressive drug therapy may be useful in some patients with serious steroid resistant exacerbations.

Prognosis for life appears to have improved dramatically in SLE over the last 30 years so that overall 5 year survival should now be better than 90% with careful monitoring and the judicious use of corticosteroid and immunosuppressive drugs. Much of this apparent improvement in prognosis is, however, attributable to the detection of milder cases as a result of heightened clinical awareness and the availability of the sensitive ANF test for diagnostic purposes. Patients with severe renal, neurological and pulmonary involvement remain those at greatest risk but infection is an important cause of morbidity and mortality particularly in patients receiving high doses of corticosteroids and immunosuppressives. Pregnancy is not contraindicated provided the disease is in reasonable remission and renal, cardiac and cerebral functions are intact.

Chronic discoid lupus erythematosus is probably more common than SLE. The skin lesions are characterised by photosensitivity, erythema, scaling, follicular plugging and telangiectasia. In the majority of patients the disease is limited to the skin. ANF tests are positive but anti-DNA antibodies are not usually found and complement levels are normal. SLE may occasionally supervene.

Drug Induced Lupus. Positive tests for antinuclear factor are frequently encountered in patients receiving procainamide, hydralazine, anticonvulsants, oral contraceptives and phenothiazines. Much more rarely a syndrome resembling SLE develops. Fever, polyarthritis, skin lesions, lymphadenopathy, serositis and pulmonary infiltrates are frequent, but renal disease and neurological manifestations are rare. Complement levels are usually normal and antibodies to double stranded DNA absent. Slow acetylators of hydra lazine and those with the HLA-DR4 histocompatibility antigen appear to be particularly at risk. Remission usually follows drug withdrawal. Occasionally a short course of corticosteroids is required.

Mixed connective tissue disease is characterised by clinical features resembling systemic lupus erythematosus, progressive systemic sclerosis (see below) and polymyositis (p. 576) in association with very high titres of a circulating antinuclear antibody with specificity for a ribonuclease sensitive extractable nuclear antigen (ENA) identified as a nuclear ribonucleoprotein (nRNP).

Women are affected four times more commonly than men. The onset is usually in the 3rd or 4th decade but may be at any age. Raynaud's phenomenon with 'sausage' swelling of the fingers, skin changes resembling dermatomyositis or scleroderma and a mild inflammatory polyarthritis are typically associated with proximal muscle weakness and tenderness, abnormal oesophageal motility and minor systemic disturbance. Diffuse interstitial pulmonary fibrosis is not uncommon but cardiac, renal and central nervous system involvement are very rare. There may be a mild anaemia of chronic disease, leucopenia or thrombocytopenia. The ESR and muscle enzymes are usually moderately raised. The condition is further characterised by an excellent prognosis and a good response to low dosage steroid therapy.

PROGRESSIVE SYSTEMIC SCLEROSIS

This is a generalised disorder of connective tissue characterised by fibrosis and degenerative changes in the skin and many internal organs. Although its aetiology is unknown, it is believed to be at one end of the spectrum of diffuse connective tissue diseases where immunologically determined inflammation is followed by intimal thickening of small blood vessels and excessive production and cross-linking of collagen. Persons with the HLA haplotype A1 B8 DR3 appear to be genetically predisposed, and there is evidence of vascular hypersensitivity to cold and serotonin. A serum factor toxic to cultured endothelial cells has been described which may also select for rapidly growing clones of fibroblasts. It is less common than SLE but is seen throughout the world. Its incidence appears to be increased among miners and others, occupationally exposed to silica dust, but in general women are affected four times more frequently than men.

Clinical Features. The onset is most frequently in the 30–50 year age group although persons of all ages may be affected. Severe Raynaud's phenomenon is usually the presenting complaint and may precede other features by months or years.

Skin Changes. Initially there is often well demarcated non-pitting oedema and induration associated with 'sausage' swelling and restriction of movement of the fingers. Later the skin becomes shiny with loss of cutaneous appendages, atrophy and ulceration of the finger tips with or without associated calcinosis. The skin of the face, limbs and trunk is variably affected and there may be striking pigmentation and telangiectasia. As the disease advances, the face may become taut and 'mask-like' with 'beaking' of the nose and difficulty in opening the mouth. Tightening of skin over bony prominences results in flexion contractures and liability to trauma.

Musculo-skeletal manifestations include early arthralgia and a mild non-erosive inflammatory arthritis often characterised by 'leathery' crepitus in affected tendon sheaths or joints. Muscle weakness and wasting result from both disuse atrophy and low grade myositis.

The gastrointestinal tract is involved in the majority of cases. Reflux oesophagitis associated with a sliding hiatus hernia is a common problem and loss of oesophageal peristalsis on recumbent barium swallow examination is often detected even in the absence of dysphagia. Dilatation of segments of large and small bowel occur less frequently, causing intermittent abdominal pain, constipation, distension and obstruction; there may be diarrhoea and malabsorption secondary to bacterial overgrowth. Scleroderma may be associated with primary biliary cirrhosis and with Sjögren's syndrome.

Pulmonary fibrosis occurs in the majority of patients. In many it is limited to a symptomless defect in gaseous diffusion. In others progressive fibrosis is accompanied by increasing dyspnoea on exertion, a restrictive pattern of impaired lung function and reticulation and 'honeycomb' changes in the lower zones on a chest radiograph. Pulmonary involvement can be complicated by pulmonary hypertension and right ventricular failure, or by alveolar cell or bronchiolar carcinoma. Aspiration pneumonia may be a consequence of oesophageal involvement.

Other Manifestations. Cardiac involvement is usually secondary to systemic rather than pulmonary hypertension but pericarditis, cardiomyopathy, heart block and aortic valve lesions can also occur. Renal involvement may develop at any stage of the disease and is an important cause of morbidity and mortality. Cranial or peripheral nerve lesions occur rarely.

Investigation. In the early stages there may be a mild normochromic, normocytic anaemia and moderately raised ESR. The ANF is positive in about 50% of patients with a nucleolar or speckled staining pattern. Antibodies to single stranded RNA and to an extractable nuclear antigen are characteristic. Anti-DNA antibodies are not detected and complement levels are normal. Tests for rheumatoid factor and anti-nRNP antibodies may be positive but usually in low titre.

Differential Diagnosis and Related Syndromes. *The CRST or CREST syndrome* comprises a subset of patients whose disease is limited to calcinosis, Raynaud's phenomenon, oesophageal (esophageal) involvement, sclerodactyly and telangiectasia. An antinuclear antibody with specificity for a component of the chromosomal centromere is present in the serum.

Morphoea and linear scleroderma are localised forms of disease limited to characteristic, well demarcated, lesions of the skin and subcutaneous connective tissues. Serological findings are similar to those of systemic sclerosis and very occasionally systemic features do occur.

Eosinophilic fasciitis is a scleroderma-like condition characterised by pain, swelling and tenderness of the hands, forearms and feet where induration of the skin and subcutaneous tissues is not associated with Raynaud's phenomenon or systemic sclerosis. Carpal tunnel compression may be an early feature and the onset frequently follows abnormal exercise. Eosinophilia and hyperglobulinaemia are characteristic and the diagnosis is confirmed by finding an inflammatory cell infiltrate with prominent eosinophils in association with marked fibrosis of the subcutaneous fascia. Eosinophilic fasciitis responds to corticosteroids but is usually self-limiting.

Pseudo-scleroderma. Other conditions which may give rise to induration or brawny oedema of the skin that must be considered in the differential diagnosis of scleroderma include scleredema, scleromyxoedema, amyloidosis and acromegaly.

Treatment. No form of drug therapy has been proved to be effective in arresting the course of systemic sclerosis. Corticosteroids may produce some symptomatic benefit in early cases where inflammatory oedema or associated myositis and/or arthritis are prominent features but great care must be taken not to aggravate or precipitate hypertension. Penicillamine and colchicine have been shown to inhibit collagen cross-linking and procollagen to collagen conversion respectively, but are disappointingly ineffective in the management of the disease.

Attention should be paid to protecting the limbs from cold, the urgent treatment of chest infections and hypertension and therapy for dysphagia, cardiac, respiratory and renal failure. Articular symptoms should be managed with NSAID. Episodes of steatorrhoea often respond to a short course of a broad spectrum antibiotic.

The outlook appears to be worse in those with late onset disease, widespread skin involvement of the trunk and early renal, cardiac or respiratory system disease. The overall 5 year survival is about 70%.

POLYMYOSITIS AND DERMATOMYOSITIS

These are diffuse connective tissue disorders in which muscle weakness and inflammatory changes in muscle and skin are the predominant features. They are relatively rare but occur throughout the world in all races and at all ages. The aetiology is obscure but persons with HLA-B8/DR3 appear to be genetically predisposed.

Viral infection (overt or latent) may be one of the factors which may stimulate or precipitate the autoimmune process responsible for the disease. Skeletal muscle cells appear to be destroyed by sensitised lymphocytes.

Clinical Features. It is possible to define the following 4 rather arbitrary subsets:

1. *Adult polymyositis* occurs three times more frequently in women than men. The onset is usually insidious in the 3rd to 5th decade. The patient may experience difficulty in climbing stairs or rising from a low chair and on examination there is weakness of the pelvic and shoulder girdle muscles. Sometimes the onset is more abrupt with rapid progression of muscular weakness. Involvement of pharyngeal, laryngeal and respiratory muscles can lead to dysphagia, dysphonia and respiratory failure within a few days. In the majority of cases progression is less rapid and profound. Spontaneous remissions are followed by some return of muscle strength but there may be atrophy, calcinosis and fibrosis in damaged muscles leading to flexion contractures. Muscle pain and tenderness are unusual except in very acute cases. Mild arthralgia or inflammatory arthritis, Raynaud's phenomenon and erythematous rashes on the elbows and knuckles are frequent associated features.

2. *Adult dermatomyositis* is also more common in women. Acute or subacute muscle weakness is accompanied by periorbital oedema and a characteristic purple 'heliotrope' rash on the upper eyelids. In addition, there may be a photosensitive, erythematous, scaling rash on the face, shoulders, upper arms and chest with red patches over knuckles, elbows and knees. Muscle pain, tenderness, weight loss and malaise are common as are arthralgia and mild inflammatory polyarthritis.

3. *Inflammatory myositis associated with malignancy* is less common than was previously thought. It is seen only after the age of 40 and occurs more frequently in men than women. The onset of symptoms is usually insidious and the clinical picture does not differ from that of typical polymyositis or dermatomyositis. The associated carcinoma may not become apparent for 2-3 years. Its resection is sometimes associated with remission of the myositis.

4. *Childhood dermatomyositis* most commonly affects children between the ages of 4 and 10. Muscle weakness is usually accompanied by the typical rash of dermatomyositis. Muscle atrophy, contractures and subcutaneous calcification may be widespread and severe. Recurrent abdominal pain due to vasculitis is also a feature.

Investigation. Active disease is often associated with a normochromic normocytic anaemia, a polymorphonuclear leucocytosis and a raised ESR. Serum aminotransferases, aldolase and creatine phosphokinase are usually raised and can be useful guides to the activity of the disease. Tests for rheumatoid factor and ANF are often positive and there may be antibodies to an extractable nuclear antigen (PM-I). Electromyography may show characteristic changes which can be very helpful in distinguishing polymyositis from peripheral neuropathy. Muscle biopsy shows necrosis and regeneration in association with an inflammatory cell infiltrate.

Treatment. Prednisolone in doses of 40–60 mg daily is used initially to induce a remission. Muscle enzyme levels may fall before clinical improvement is noted. The steroid dose is then gradually reduced whilst continuing to monitor muscle strength and serum enzyme levels. Doses of 10–15 mg prednisolone daily are often needed to maintain the remission. Immunosuppressive therapy is occasionally used when there is no response to corticosteroids. The use of splints and physiotherapy to prevent contractures should not be neglected.

Prognosis is closely related to the age of onset and the presence or absence of associated malignancy. The four year survival is 80% when the disease begins before the age of 20; 60% for those under the age of 40 and 33% for older patients.

ARTERITIS

Vasculitis which occurs as part of rheumatoid arthritis, systemic lupus erythematosus, progressive systemic sclerosis and childhood dermatomyositis has been described in the relevant sections.

Polyarteritis nodosa (p. 198), Takayasu's arteritis (p. 199) and cranial arteritis (p. 199) are diffuse connective tissue disorders in which immunologically determined vasculitis is the cause of the pathological changes. Polymyalgia rheumatica is related to cranial arteritis.

Polymyalgia Rheumatica

This is a relatively common condition in elderly Caucasians, especially women. Pain and stiffness in the shoulder and pelvic girdles of at least one month's duration, are characteristically associated with a raised ESR and a dramatic response to low dosage corticosteroids.

Clinical Features. The onset is often abrupt with severe pain and stiffness in the neck, back, shoulders, upper arms and thighs, often worse in the morning. There may also be fever, weight loss, malaise and depression. Physical signs are usually limited to slight tenderness of the acromio-clavicular or sterno-clavicular joints. Occasionally there may be evidence of a mild inflammatory arthritis in a more peripheral joint. The muscles themselves usually show no evidence of tenderness or atrophy and examination of the peripheral arteries is usually normal. However, up to one-third of patients at some time develop symptoms of cranial arteritis (p. 199) and are at risk of blindness from arteritic involvement of a branch of the ophthalmic artery.

The ESR is markedly raised in the majority of cases and there may be a mild normochromic normocytic anaemia of chronic disease. Temporal artery biopsy shows evidence of giant cell arteritis in about 40% of cases but the true frequency of arteritis is probably much higher.

Treatment. The response to low dosage corticosteroid therapy is dramatic. The diagnosis must be reviewed if there is no striking remission of symptoms within 4–5 days of starting prednisolone 15 mg once daily. The ESR frequently takes longer to fall. Two to three weeks after starting therapy the dose of prednisolone is gradually reduced over several weeks. Most patients can be maintained in remission with 5–7.5 mg prednisolone daily. High dosage corticosteroids are given initially to patients with cranial arteritis (p. 199).

The natural history is for remission to occur in 6 months to 2 years although relapses are not uncommon and occasional patients have a more prolonged chronic disease. The need for maintenance corticosteroids should be reviewed by an attempt at gradual steroid withdrawal every six months.

METABOLIC AND DEGENERATIVE DISEASES OF CONNECTIVE TISSUES AND JOINTS

CRYSTAL DEPOSITION DISEASES

Gout

Gout is not a single disease. The term is used to describe a number of disorders in which crystals of monosodium urate monohydrate derived from hyperuricaemic body fluids give rise to inflammatory arthritis, tenosynovitis, bursitis or cellulitis, tophaceous deposits, urolithiasis and renal disease.

Hyperuricaemia is a necessary but not a sufficient prerequisite for clinical manifestations of gout.

Epidemiology. Gouty arthritis is predominantly a problem of post pubertal males and is seldom seen in women before the menopause. Its overall prevalence in Britain is about 0·6%. Asymptomatic hyperuricaemia is ten times more common. Serum uric acid concentrations are distributed in the community as a continuous variable and are determined by a number of demographic factors of which age, sex, body bulk and genetic constitution are the most important. Serum uric acid levels are higher in urban than in rural communities and are positively correlated with intelligence, social class, weight, haemoglobin, serum proteins and a high protein diet.

Hyperuricaemia is arbitrarily defined as a serum uric acid level greater than two standard deviations from the mean i.e. above 0·42 mmol/l in adult males and 0·36 mmol/l in adult females (p. 821).

Aetiology of Gout and Hyperuricaemia. A number of genetic and environmental factors lead to hyperuricaemia and gout by decreasing the excretion of uric acid, increasing its production or by a combination of both mechanisms (Table 14.3).

IMPAIRED EXCRETION OF URIC ACID is the problem in more than 75% of patients with gout. In most of these there appears to be an as yet undefined genetically determined defect in fractional urate excretion.

Table 14.3 Factors predisposing to hyperuricaemia and gout.

Diminished renal excretion of uric acid		Increased production of uric acid
Renal failure	Lactic Acidosis:	*Increased turnover of purines:*
	Alcohol	Myeloproliferative disorders
Drugs	Excercise	e.g. polycythaemia vera
Diuretics	Starvation	
Pyrazinamide	Vomiting	Lymphoproliferative disorders
Low doses aspirin	Toxaemia of pregnancy	e.g. chronic lymphatic
	Type 1 Glycogen Storage	leukaemia
Lead poisoning	Disease	
	Unidentified	Psoriasis — severe, exfoliative
Hypertension	inherited defect	
		Increased purine synthesis de novo:
Hyperparathyroidism		HGPRT deficiency
		PRPP synthetase overactivity
Myxoedema		Glucose-6-Phosphatase
		deficiency
Down's syndrome		Idiopathic

EXCESSIVE PRODUCTION OF URIC ACID is at least partly responsible for hyperuricaemia in 20–25% of gout patients. In the absence of significant renal impairment such patients are hyperexcretors of uric acid.

SPECIFIC ENZYME DEFECTS resulting in an increase in *de novo* purine synthesis should be suspected: (1) in the absence of disorders resulting in increased turnover of purines (Table 14.3); (2) if gout develops at an unusually early age; (3) if there is a family history of gout commencing at an early age; (4) if uric acid lithiasis is the first presenting feature.

Deficiency of Hypoxanthine-Guanine-Phosphoribosyl Transferase (HGPRT). The Lesch-Nyhan syndrome is a rare X-chromosome linked inborn error of metabolism in which gout and severe overproduction of uric acid are associated with choreoathetosis, spasticity, a variable degree of mental deficiency and compulsive self-mutilation. The enzyme defect can be detected in red cell lysates; female carriers can be identified from skin fibroblast cultures or hair root analysis and pre-natal detection can be undertaken using amniotic fluid cells. The elucidation of the mechanism whereby this deficit in a purine salvage enzyme leads to primary purine overproduction has been a key to the understanding of purine metabolism and the development of allopurinol in the prevention of gout.

Phosphoribosyl Pyrophosphate (PRPP) Sythetase Overactivity. Severe gouty arthritis and uric acid lithiasis is seen from an early age in families with inborn errors of metabolism resulting in increased activity in this enzyme. The defect can be detected in red cell lysates.

Glucose-6-Phosphatase Deficiency. Children with glycogen storage disease type 1 (von Gierke's disease) who survive to adult life develop severe gout and hyperuricaemia as a consequence of impaired uric acid excretion secondary to lactic acidosis and increased purine synthesis *de novo*. The enzyme defect can be detected only in the liver, kidney or intestine.

Idiopathic. The enzyme defect(s) responsible for most cases of gout with increased synthesis of purine *de novo* remain to be discovered.

Clinical Features. *Acute Gout.* The metatarsophalangeal joint of a great toe is the site of the first attack of acute gouty arthritis in 70% of patients; the ankle, the knee, the small joints of the feet and hands, the wrist and elbow follow in decreasing order of frequency. The onset may be insidious or explosively sudden, often waking the patient from sleep. The affected joint is hot, red and swollen with shiny overlying skin and dilated veins; it is excruciatingly painful and tender. Very acute attacks may be accompanied by fever, leucocytosis and a raised ESR and are occasionally preceded by prodromal symptoms such as anorexia, nausea or a change in mood. If untreated, the attack lasts days or weeks but it eventually subsides spontaneously. Resolution of the acute attack may be accompanied by pruritus and local desquamation.

Some patients have only a single attack, or suffer another only after an interval of many months or years. More often there is a tendency to have recurrent attacks. These increase in frequency and duration so that eventually one attack may merge into another and the patient remains in a prolonged state of subacute gout. Acute attacks are occasionally polyarticular and tenosynovitis, bursitis or cellulitis may be the presenting feature.

Acute attacks may be precipitated by sudden rises in serum urate following dietary excess, alcohol, severe dietary restriction or diuretic drugs or by sudden falls following initiation of therapy with allopurinol or uricosuric drugs. Acute attacks may also be provoked by trauma, unusual physical exercise, surgery or severe systemic illness.

Chronic Gout. First attacks of gouty arthritis are seldom associated with residual disability but recurrent acute attacks are followed by progressive cartilage and bone erosion in association with deposition of tophi and secondary degenerative changes. Severe functional impairment and gross joint deformities may be associated with chronic tophaceous gout. Tophi are frequently found in the cartilage of the ear, bursae and tendon sheaths.

Urate urolithiasis occurs in about 10% of patients with gout attending British hospital clinics. The incidence is much higher in hot climates. The formation of urate calculi is also favoured by: (1) hyperuricosuria; (2) purine over production; (3) excessive purine ingestion; (4) uricosuric drugs and defects in tubular reabsorption of uric acid and (5) low urine pH e.g. chronic diarrhoeal diseases or following ileostomy.

Chronic urate nephropathy results from a combination of renal tubular obstruction, tophus formation, hypertension, glomerulosclerosis and secondary pyelonephritis. It is rare and hardly ever occurs in the absence of well-established chronic gouty arthritis. It may occasionally be familial (autosomal dominant) without evidence of an inborn error of metabolism.

Minimal renal insufficiency is found in up to 50% of patients with gout but is largely age related. Proteinuria is found in 25% and is mild and non-progressive. Renal failure accounts for 25% of deaths in patients with gout. Most are, however, from unrelated causes and overall life expectancy is not reduced.

Other Manifestations. Gout and hyperuricaemia are frequently associated with obesity, type IV hyperlipoproteinaemia, diabetes mellitus, hypertension and ischaemic heart disease. Hyperuricaemia itself does not, however, appear to be a risk factor for vascular disease or diabetes.

Investigation. The serum urate level is usually raised but it is important to realise that this does not prove the diagnosis as asyptomatic hyperuricaemia is very common. Whenever possible synovial fluid should be aspirated and examined under polarising light. Acute attacks of gout can occur when the serum urate level is normal. This is usually seen in patients who have received treatment with allopurinol, a uricosuric agent or NSAID with uricosuric side effects such as phenylbutazone.

Joint radiographs are seldom useful in establishing the diagnosis. Although they may show characteristic punched-out erosions associated with the translucent soft tissue swelling of urate tophi, occasionally flecked with calcium, the diagnosis will be clinically apparent in such cases and in others the erosions are indistinguishable from those seen in other forms of inflammatory arthritis.

Treatment. *Acute Attack.* NSAID are the agents of choice. It is important to start treatment as early as possible, to use adequate doses and to avoid salicylates and diuretics. Patients known to have gout should keep a supply of NSAID with which they are familiar so that an acute attack can be aborted as soon as the first symptoms are noticed. Indomethacin (50 mg), azapropazone (600 mg) 6–hourly or naproxen 250 mg t.i.d. are given until the acute attack subsides. Treatment is then continued with lower doses for 7–10 days. Colchicine is highly effective but causes vomiting and diarrhoea in many patients in the doses that need to be used (1 mg stat followed by 0·5 mg 2–hourly).

Prevention. Prolonged administration of drugs which lower the serum urate level should be considered following the resolution of the acute attack in patients with: (1) recurrent acute attacks of gouty arthritis; (2) tophi or evidence of chronic gouty arthritis; (3) associated renal disease; (4) gout and markedly raised serum urate.

Allopurinol is the drug of choice for long-term prophylaxis because of its convenience and low incidence of side-effects. It lowers the serum urate primarily by inhibiting xanthine oxidase which is responsible for the conversion of xanthine and hypoxanthine to uric acid. Treatment is commenced with 300 mg once daily together with colchicine 0·5 mg b.d. to avert the acute attacks of gouty arthritis which frequently follow initiation of hypouricaemic drug therapy. It is important not to commence treatment with allopurinol until several weeks have elapsed after the last acute attack and to continue concurrent administration of colchicine for several months. The dose of allopurinol may have to be adjusted in the range of 300–900 mg daily to bring the serum urate within the normal range. If renal function is impaired lower doses (100 mg daily) should be used.

Uricosuric agents can also be very effective in lowering the serum rate level, reducing the frequency of acute attacks of gout and decreasing the size of tophi. Probenecid 0·5–1 g b.d. or sulphinpyrazone 100 mg t.d.s. are given with colchicine 0·5 mg b.d. Salicylates must be avoided as they antagonise the uricosuric effects of these drugs. Uricosuric drug therapy is contraindicated: (1) in gout with over-production of uric acid and gross uricosuria; (2) in patients with renal failure (ineffective); (3) in patients with urate urolithiasis.

Diet. There is no need for severe dietary restrictions but grossly excessive purine intake and over-indulgence in alcohol should be avoided. Gradual weight loss is encouraged in obese patients and is associated with a fall in serum urate. Severe calorie restriction must be avoided as it causes lactic acidosis and a rise in serum urate.

Surgery is occasionally required to deal with a large or ulcerating tophus.

Asymptomatic hyperuricaemia does not require prophylactic treatment in the absence of a history, family history or clinical evidence of gout. A search should be made for causes of secondary hyperuricaemia (Table 14.3). Obese subjects should be encouraged to lose weight gradually and blood pressure and renal function should be monitored annually.

Chondrocalcinosis and Pseudo-gout

Pyrophosphate Arthropathy: Calcium Pyrophosphate Dihydrate Deposition (CPPD)

In this variety of crystal deposition disorder, calcium pyrophosphate dihydrate (CPPD) crystals are deposited in fibrous and articular cartilage where they are associated with degenerative changes. Shedding of crystals into the joint space provokes an acute attack of synovitis — 'pseudo-gout'. Autopsy and radiological surveys indicate that chondrocalcinosis is a common age related finding often unassociated with symptoms of articular disease. The menisci and articular cartilage of the knee are the commonest sites.

Aetiology. Chondrocalcinosis and pseudo-gout are clearly not a single disease. The majority of cases are sporadic and no underlying cause can be found. Genetic factors are important in some families. A variety of metabolic disorders clearly predispose to chondrocalcinosis, namely hyperparathyroidism, haemochromatosis, hypothyroidism, gout, hypomagnesaemia and hypophosphatasia. No common determinant, comparable to the hyperuricaemia of gout has been identified but pyrophosphate concentrations are increased in synovial fluids. This, coupled with the association with hypophosphatasia, has suggested that the disease may be a consequence of defective pyrophosphatase activity.

Clinical Features. Pyrophosphate arthropathy can mimic many other conditions. Six clinical patterns of disease are described.

Type A: Pseudo-gout. As with gout the affected joint becomes suddenly painful, warm, swollen and tender. The knee is the site of more than half of all attacks, the duration of which can vary from a few days to four weeks. Subacute or 'petite' attacks are not uncommon and there may be polyarticular clustering of acute attacks. Men are affected more frequently than women.

Type B: Pseudo-rheumatoid arthritis. In a few patients there is a subacute inflammatory polyarthritis which may last for several months.

Type C: Pseudo-osteoarthritis with superimposed acute attacks.

Type D: Pseudo-osteoarthritis without acute attacks. Types C and D account for nearly half the patients. Women are more frequently affected. Prominent involvement of the wrists and MCP joints clearly distinguishes pseudo osteoarthritic chondrocalcinosis from primary generalised osteoarthrosis.

Type E: Lanthanic (asymptomatic) is the most common pattern.

Type F: Pseudo-neuropathic. Severe destructive changes resembling those of Charcot joints can occur in the knee and shoulder in the absence of any neurological defect.

Investigation. Acute attacks may be accompanied by fever, mild leucocytosis and a raised ESR. Radiographs show CPPD in articular cartilage, the menisci of the knees, the labrum of the acetabulum and glenoid cavity, the triangular cartilage of the wrist and the symphysis pubis. Examination of synovial fluid under polarising light microscopy allows CPPD crystals, which are positively birefringent, to be distinguished from monosodium urate crystals. X-ray diffraction techniques are however required for its precise identification and distinction from other forms of calcium phosphate and calcium hydroxyapatite which have been described in the synovial fluids of patients with degenerative joint disease.

Treatment. Joint aspiration and intra-articular injection of corticosteroids are the most effective means for treating acute attacks of pseudogout. Colchicine and NSAID are less effective than in classical gout.

OSTEOARTHROSIS

Osteoarthrosis (OA, osteoarthritis, arthrosis or degenerative joint disease) is not a single disease. Rather it is the end result of a variety of patterns of joint failure. To a greater or lesser extent it is always characterised by both degeneration of articular cartilage and simultaneous proliferation of new bone, cartilage and connective tissue. The proliferative response results in some degree of remodelling of the joint contour. Inflammatory changes in the synovium are usually minor and secondary.

Epidemiology. Radiological and autopsy surveys show a steady rise in degenerative changes in joints from the age of 30. By the age of 65, 80% of people have radiographic evidence of osteoarthrosis although only 25% may have symptoms.

Males and females are both affected but OA is more generalised and more severe in older women. Geographical surveys show differences in both the prevalence of OA and the pattern of joint involvement. OA of the hips is much more frequent in Caucasian than in Blacks or Chinese. It is particularly common in men in the north of England. Cold, damp climates are associated with more symptoms but not with greater radiological prevalence.

Aetiology and Pathogenesis. OA is classified as primary if the aetiology is unknown and secondary when degenerative joint changes occur in response to a recognisable local or systemic factor (Table 14.4). Developmental abnormalities are currently believed to be of major importance in the aetiology of OA of the hip in the vast majority of cases. Abnormal surface contacts and weight bearing alignments are thought to arise from minor degrees of acetabular dysplasia, epiphysiolysis, altered femoral neck shaft angles etc. leading to increased local mechanical stress and wear. Post traumatic malalignment and incongruity of joints are well established as important predisposing causes of premature OA.

Table 14.4 Causes of secondary osteoarthrosis.

Developmental	Perthes' disease, slipped capital femoral epiphysis, epiphysiolysis, hip dysplasia, epiphysial dysplasias, intra-articular acetabular labrum.
Traumatic	Intra-articular fracture, menisectomy, occupational e.g. elbows of pneumatic drill workers, hypermobility e.g. Ehlers-Danlos syndrome, long leg arthropathy.
Metabolic	Alkaptonuria (ochronosis), haemochromatosis, Wilson's disease, chondrocalcinosis.
Endocrine	Acromegaly.
Inflammatory	Rheumatoid arthritis, gout, septic arthritis, haemophilia.
Aseptic necrosis	Corticosteroids, sickle cell disease, caisson disease, SLE and other collagenoses.
Neuropathic	Tabes dorsalis, syringomyelia, diabetes mellitus, peripheral nerve lesions.
Miscellaneous	Paget's disease, Gaucher's disease.

Metabolic diseases lead to cartilage degeneration by very different mechanisms. In alkaptonuria (ochronosis) the genetically determined defect of homogentisic acid oxidase results in the accumulation of a pigmented polymer that binds to cartilage collagen, rendering it brittle and prone to mechanical degradation. It has been suggested that there may be other inborn errors of metabolism where unknown colourless metabolites may induce changes in the biochemical composition of cartilage matrix in a similar way and so predispose to OA. Crystal deposition of calcium pyrophosphate dihydrate or hydroxyapatite may alter cartilage matrix properties directly and low grade crystal inflammation may play a part in pathogenesis.

It is uncertain whether the degenerative joint disease seen in acromegaly (p. 571) is a consequence of joint incongruity following cartilage overgrowth or whether the endocrine disturbance results in a mechanically defective matrix. Paget's disease, Gaucher's disease and the various diseases associated with aseptic necrosis result in subchondral bone pathology, and altered stresses on the overlying articular cartilage due to subchondral bone changes.

Current concepts of the pathogenesis of OA are based on the assumption that whatever the provoking cause, the final pathway of changes in articular cartilage will be identical. Two mechanical hypotheses merit consideration. The first suggests that the initiating event is fatigue fracture of the collagen fibre network. This is followed by increased hydration of the articular cartilage with unravelling of the proteoglycans and loss of proteoglycans into the synovial fluid. There is some tentative evidence of augmented neutral protease and collagenase activity but collagen may be lost simply as a result of mechanical attrition.

The alternative hypothesis suggests that the initial lesions are microfractures of the subchondral bone following repetitive loading. Healing of the microfracture leads to significant stiffening of the subchondral bone which in turn creates a shear stress gradient in the adjacent articular cartilage. As the process evolves, the cartilage surface becomes fibrillated and deep clefts appear with reduplication and proliferation of chondrocytes within them. Simultaneous proliferative changes commence at the joint margins with formation of osteophytes. Eventually articular cartilage is lost altogether in areas of maximum mechanical stress exposing the hardened, eburnated underlying bone. Cysts may form but bony ankylosis does not occur.

Clinical Features. The joints most frequently involved are those of the spine, hips and knees. In the majority of patients the disease is confined to one or only a few joints. The symptoms are gradual in onset. Pain is at first intermittent and aching. It is provoked by use of the joint and relieved by rest. As the disease progresses, movement in the affected joint becomes increasingly limited, initially as a result of pain and muscular spasm, but later because of capsular fibrosis, osteophyte formation and remodelling of bone. There may be repeated effusions into joints especially after minor twists or injuries. Crepitus may be felt or even heard. Associated muscle wasting is an important factor in the progress of the disease, as in the absence of normal muscular control the joint becomes more prone to injury. Pain arises from trabecular microfractures, traumatic lesions in the capsule and periarticular tissues, and a low grade synovitis. Nocturnal aching may be attributable to hyperaemia of the subchondral bone.

Nodal osteoarthrosis is a clinically distinct form of primary generalised OA which occurs predominantly in middle-aged women. Characteristically it affects the terminal IP joints of the fingers with the development of gelatinous cysts or bony outgrowths on the dorsal aspect of these joints (Heberden's nodes). The onset is sometimes acute with considerable pain, swelling and inflammation. Although these lesions may be associated with a good deal of deformity they seldom cause disability. Similar lesions may affect the proximal IP joints and the disorder also frequently involves the carpometacarpal joints of the thumbs, the spinal apophyseal joints, the hips and knees. A strong family history of Heberden's nodes is usual in such cases and though the existence of multigeneration families with the disorder appears to suggest a single autosomal dominant gene, careful family studies suggest polygenic inheritance in both nodal and non-nodal primary generalised osteoarthrosis. Patients with nodal primary generalised osteoarthrosis are probably also more susceptible to secondary OA, again emphasising the multifactorial aetiology of this disorder.

Investigation. The blood count and ESR are characteristically   normal   in   osteoarthrosis.

Synovial fluid is viscous and has a low cell count. Apatite crystals can be detected on rare occasions. Radiographs show loss of joint space and formation of marginal osteophytes. Subchondral bone sclerosis, bony remodelling and cyst formation are seen in more advanced cases.

Treatment. Although the pathological changes of osteoarthrosis are irreversible much can be done to alleviate symptoms particularly in the early stages. Periods of rest and avoidance of undue trauma and physical stress to affected joints are essential. This may involve such measures as the fitting of rubber heels to reduce jarring and minimise the risk of slipping, the provision of built-up shoes to equalise leg lengths, weight loss in obese patients with OA of the knee or hip and the provision of a suitable walking stick. Occasionally patients may have to be advised to change their occupation, transfer to lighter work or give up unduly strenuous hobbies.

NSAID can be used to relieve pain and stiffness but are often disappointingly ineffective in osteoarthrosis.

Occasional intra-articular or periarticular corticosteroid injections can be very helpful especially in the knee. Hydrotherapy may be useful for patients with OA of the hip associated with pain and muscle spasm. Hip or knee arthroplasty may be necessary in advanced cases (p. 562). Arthrodesis of a knee is occasionally considered if the knee is the only joint involved.

MISCELLANEOUS LESIONS OF CONNECTIVE TISSUE

General Aspects. Musculo-skeletal aches and pains are extremely common and become more frequent with increasing age. More than one third of all 'rheumatic' complaints cannot be attributed to defined diseases of the spine, peripheral joints or connective tissues. Many are trivial, self limiting and cause little disability. Others can be more troublesome. The neck, shoulder girdle, back and gluteal regions are the common sites for many of these complaints. Muscular spasm of reflex origin is a prominent feature and must be differentiated from limitation of movement due to structural damage. Absence of signs of systemic illness and a

normal ESR will help to distinguish them from the inflammatory connective tissue diseases.

Certain factors may be of importance in precipitating attacks in susceptible individuals. Exposure to cold and damp has always been suspected as a cause of nonarticular 'rheumatic' complaints. Unaccustomed physical effort, undue fatigue, minor injuries and poor posture have also been incriminated. Any reduction in muscular efficiency will render an individual more prone to sprains of tendons, ligaments and extra-articular soft tissue structures. Loss of resilience and elasticity of the intervertebral discs can occur long before radiological evidence of disc degeneration becomes apparent and the interfacetal joints of the spine may be more exposed to strains and sprains.

Pain arising from such deep structures is poorly located and referred diffusely to the overlying skin. Pain may be referred from the cervical intervertebral joints to the occipital region, shoulder girdle and arm. 'Lumbago' and 'sciatic pain' (p. 660) without signs of root pressure may be caused by minor disc injury. More often they appear to be associated with acute or chronic 'sprain syndromes'. Although poor posture, flabby muscles and obesity may be predisposing causes, occupational factors may be of great importance. Sickness absence attributable to 'rheumatic' complaints is much higher among miners, dockers and foundry workers than it is among clerks or employees in light industry. Up to 10% of the population may have abnormally lax joints and ligaments without the stigmata of inherited connective tissue disorders such as the Marfan or Ehlers-Danlos syndrome. Such persons are particularly prone to recurrent sprains, dislocations and arthralgia — the *hypermobility syndrome*.

Diffuse muscular pain and stiffness is common in certain infections, particularly of viral origin, such as influenza, rubella and measles. Localised pain occurs in epidemic myalgia (Bornholm disease p. 270). Many anxious and depressed people complain of aches and pains, particularly in the region of the neck, shoulders or lower back.

Specific Lesions. *Shoulder pain* is frequently a consequence of extra-articular traumatic, degenerative or inflammatory lesions of the capsule or 'rotator cuff' of tendons. *Supraspinatus ten-*

dinitis is characterised by a 'painful arc' on arm abduction which can be abolished by external rotation. There is localised tenderness over the greater tuberosity of the humerus and a radiograph may show calcification in the supraspinatus tendon. Rupture of calcific material into the subacromial bursa occasionally results in acutely painful 'gout-like' attacks of inflammatory *subacromial bursitis*. Fluid aspirated from the bursa beneath the acromion contains crystals of calcium hydroxyapatite. Local injection of hydrocortisone is used to give symptomatic relief. *Bicipital tendinitis* can be recognised by pain and tenderness over the bicipital groove aggravated by resisted shoulder flexion.

'*Frozen shoulder*' is the name given to a common and disabling condition in which severe spontaneous shoulder pain is associated initially with capsular tenderness and painful restriction of all shoulder movements and later with painless restriction of movements alone. A frozen shoulder may be a late consequence of a rotator cuff lesion and sometimes follows myocardial infarction, hemiplegia, herpes zoster, breast or thoracic surgery. Treatment is with analgesics and local corticosteroid injection in the early phase and mobilising exercises after the pain has resolved. The natural history is for slow but complete recovery, the complete cycle sometimes taking as long as two years.

In the *shoulder-hand syndrome* restricted shoulder movements are associated with a painful swollen hand. The condition is characterised by burning pain, vasomotor changes and severe limitation of movements of the hand. A radiograph of the hand shows patchy osteoporosis after some weeks or months. It may be a sequel to the same disorders that precede a frozen shoulder but epilepsy, barbiturates and antituberculous drugs can also be predisposing factors. Not infrequently these patients have an hysterical personality. Treatment is aimed at mobilising the affected limb. Analgesics, a short course of systemic corticosteroids, sympathetic nerve block and physiotherapy each have their advocates in this difficult situation. The prognosis for complete recovery is less certain than in frozen shoulder.

'*Tennis elbow*' appears to follow partial tears of the origin of the extensor muscles at the lateral epicondyle. Local tenderness and pain on active wrist extension are characteristic. '*Golfer's elbow*' results from similar lesions in the origin of the common flexor tendon at the medial epicondyle. Local corticosteroid injections relieve both conditions.

DISEASES OF BONE

PHYSIOLOGY

Bone is a specialised form of metabolically active, mineralised, connective tissue. It consists of cells of monocyte-macrophage origin (bone forming osteoblasts, bone resorbing osteoclasts, resting osteocytes) and an organic matrix of type I collagen, proteoglycan and some bone specific glycoproteins. The skeleton contains more than 99% of the body calcium in the form of a crystalline calcium phosphate complex (hydroxyapatite). The tubular mid-sections of long bones (diaphyses), which make up 80% of the skeletal mass, are composed of circumferential lamellae of compact, cortical bone consisting of longitudinally orientated osteons surrounding central Haversian canals which carry the capillaries. Extracellular fluid reaches the bone osteocytes by a radial system of canaliculi and there are lateral vascular communications with the periosteal vessels through Volkmann's canals. The distal ends of the long bones (metaphyses), the vertebrae and the flat bones are composed of more loosely packed cancellous bone. Although it accounts for only 20% of the skeletal mass, the trabecular surface area of this cancellous bone is as large as that of compact bone, rendering it relatively more susceptible to metabolic diseases. From the physiological point of view it is important to realise that bone is bounded by a number of distinct cellular surfaces — the endosteal, periosteal, Haversian and trabecular envelopes.

In the growing phase of infancy and childhood the size and shape of bones changes rapidly as part of the modelling process. The marrow cavity and outer cortex expand due to endosteal resorption and periosteal accretion of bone and bone turnover may be as high as 200% per annum. Following skeletal maturity this is reduced to less than 5% but the rate of endosteal resorption is reduced less than that of periosteal accretion. Thus while the outer diameter of normal older bones is greater than that of younger ones, the cortex is progressively thinned with advancing years. Deformities and short stature may be a consequence of diseases interfering with the modelling process during the growing period. Examples include metabolic diseases such as rickets, inflammatory diseases such as polyarticular juvenile chronic arthritis, and bone dysplasias such as osteopetrosis.

Modern methods of bone histomorphometry, in which iliac biopsies are taken following double tetracycline labelling, have revealed a second form of bone turnover or remodelling. This occurs throughout life and accounts for more than 95% of turnover in the mature skeleton. Remodelling occurs in 'programmed packages'; the sequence of cellular events is invariably one of activation followed by a period of osteoclastic resorption and then a period of osteoblastic formation along the freshly resorbed trabecular surface. The whole sequence is completed in 4–6 months in healthy adults. Trauma and hyperthyroidism are two of the numerous factors that can activate the remodelling process, while oestrogens suppress it. Fluoride uncouples the remodelling sequence and stimulates osteoblastic activity.

Increased turnover of bone, whatever the cause, is associated with a rise in the plasma alkaline phosphatase and an increase in the urinary excretion of hydroxyproline and the bone specific glycoprotein, osteocalcin.

CLASSIFICATION OF DISEASES OF BONE

1. Infections.
2. Endocrine and metabolic diseases:
   (a) Rickets and osteomalacia (p. 67),
   (b) Osteoporosis (p. 70),
      (i) Postmenopausal,
      (ii) Associated with endocrine disease, e.g. in hypogonadism, hyperthyroidism, Cushing's syndrome and hypopituitarism,
      (iii) Nutritional deficiency, e.g. of calcium or vitamin C,

   (iv) Chronic wasting diseases, e.g. rheumatoid arthritis or malignancy,
   (v) Iatrogenic, e.g. corticosteroid therapy.
   (vi) Hereditary diseases, e.g. osteogenesis imperfecta (p. 11), and Turner's syndrome (p. 9),
   (vii) Idiopathic juvenile osteoporosis.
  (c) Hyperparathyroidism (p. 440).
  (d) Paget's disease.
3. Disorders of collagen, e.g. Marfan's syndrome (p. 198).
4. Mucopolysaccharidoses, e.g. Hurler syndrome (p. 17) and Hunter's syndrome (p. 17).
5. Skeletal dysplasias.
6. Neoplastic disease
   Primary, benign or malignant.
   Secondary malignant.

Infections, Paget's disease, neoplasia and skeletal dysplasias are discussed in this chapter and other diseases of bone as indicated by the page references.

INFECTIONS

Osteomyelitis is most commonly encountered in children under the age of 12. The onset is abrupt with fever, nausea, malaise and severe pain at the site of bone infection. When this is close to a joint there may be a 'sympathetic' effusion and diagnostic confusion with septic arthritis may occur. Multifocal sites of bone infection are not uncommon. Isotope scanning and careful delineation of the site of bone tenderness can be helpful in establishing the correct diagnosis but radiographic changes do not occur for some days or weeks.

Staphyloccoci are the most frequent organisms responsible and in about half the cases evidence can be found for haematogenous spread from a boil or superficial infection. Hypogammaglobulinaemia, malnutrition or debilitating illness may all be predisposing factors. Salmonella can also cause osteomyelitis and this infection is a particularly common complication of sickle cell anaemia (p. 508).

An antibiotic e.g. sodium fusidate (p. 46) must be commenced after taking blood for culture as soon as the diagnosis is suspected, and continued in adequate doses for long enough to eliminate the infection. Delay in starting treatment or inadequate therapy may result in chronic indolent bone infection (*Brodie's abscess*) with sequestrum formation. Surgical exploration and decompression are required if there is not an immediate response to antibiotics.

Tuberculous osteomyelitis has become much less common in Britain since the elimination of bovine tuberculosis but there is some evidence of a recent increase in the elderly population and immigrant communities. 50% of cases of skeletal tuberculosis affect the spine.

Typically the infection starts at the margins of vertebral bodies and invades the disc space, narrowing of which and destruction of bone leading to vertebral collapse with kyphosis. A paraspinous 'cold' abscess may form and track to the thigh, chest wall or neck. The hip, knee, ankle or wrist joint may be affected by spread from adjacent bone. Tuberculous dactylitis and sacroiliitis are unusual but characteristic lesions. The treatment of tuberculosis is described on page 236.

PAGET'S DISEASE (OSTEITIS DEFORMANS)

This is a disease of unknown aetiology characterised by softening, enlargement and bowing of bones. It is uncommon before the age of 40 years but increasingly frequent thereafter. Histologically there is increased bone blood flow and bone resorption followed by excessive osteoblastic bone formation resulting in a high rate of bone turnover, raised levels of plasma alkaline phosphatase and increased urinary excretion of hydroxyproline. This activity is reflected in abnormal isotope bone scans and radiological evidence of localised bone enlargement, altered trabecular pattern and alternating areas of rarefaction and increased density.

Clinical Features. Men are more commonly affected and there may be a family history of the disease. Often the condition is symptomless and detected only when radiological examination is made for some other reason. In others there is pain of a deep aching character often aggravated by weight bearing. The pelvis, femur, tibia, lumbar spine and skull are common sites of bone involvement. The increased vascularity may cause warmth of the affected part on palpation; rarely widespread arteriovenous shunting causes high output cardiac failure. Enlargement and deformity of bones develops when the condition is advanced. Bowing of the femur and tibia is characteristic and Paget's disease may predispose to secondary osteoarthrosis of the hip. Fractures may occur spontaneously or after minor trauma but they usually heal normally. Skull involvement may result in headache, progressive enlargement of the cranium and deafness from compression of the auditory nerves. Paraplegia can follow vertebral involvement. Osteogenic sarcoma is an uncommon late complication. The serum calcium and phosphate are usually normal with high levels of alkaline phosphatase and increased hydroxyproline excretion during phases of active disease.

Treatment. Calcitonin (p. 439) is used for the treatment of severe bone pain not controlled by analgesics. Subcutaneous injection of 100 MRC units of salmon calcitonin three times weekly can be continued for six months and recommenced if pain recurs. Mithramycin and diphosphonates, which reduce bone turnover, are less satisfactory alternatives.

Confinement to bed may be followed by rapid mobilisation of calcium with hypercalcaemia, hypercalciuria and formation of renal calculi. Such patients must be carefully monitored, given a high fluid intake and measures must be taken to lower the serum calcium if it becomes dangerously high. Secondary degenerative joint disease is treated with NSAID. Hip arthroplasty is occasionally required. Osteogenic sarcoma is treated with early surgery but has a poor prognosis.

NEOPLASTIC DISEASE

Malignant neoplasms of bone can cause diffuse skeletal aches and pains that are not infrequently dismissed as being 'rheumatic'.

Metastases from carcinomas of the bronchus, breast or prostate, are the commonest tumours of bone. Secondary deposits from most primary tumours appear typically as osteolytic areas on radiological examination and are frequently associated with a rise in serum alkaline phosphatase. Only prostatic metastases are commonly osteosclerotic and associated with a rise in serum acid phosphatase. Metastatic deposits can often be localised by skeletal isotope scans before radiological changes are apparent and widespread bone metastases can occur even in the absence of symptoms. A number of malignancies are hormone dependent and useful remissions can sometimes be obtained following hypophysectomy or administration of androgens to patients with metastatic breast cancer, or dienoestrol to those with prostatic metastases. Local radiotherapy and cytotoxic chemotherapy can occasionally be helpful in symptomatic management.

Multiple myeloma (p. 536) may also present with skeletal aches and pains associated with 'punched-out' osteolytic lesions on radiological examination. Unlike metastatic carcinoma these deposits usually fail to take up bone seeking isotopes and the serum alkaline phosphatase is normal.

Primary bone tumours are less common. Ivory *osteomas* are benign tumours which occur most frequently in the vault of the skull and are not usually associated with symptoms. Cancellous osteomas (osteochondromas or exostoses) are slender out-growths of bone which arise from the metaphyses of long bones or from the flat bones of the pelvis and scapulae. They may give rise to pressure symptoms and most frequently present during adolescence. Diaphyseal aclasis (multiple exostosis) is a rarer inherited disorder seen in younger children.

Primary osteosarcomas occur most frequently in the lower end of the femur, the upper end of the tibia or the upper end of the humerus. These are tumours of young people rarely seen after the age of 20. Swelling with or without vague aching are the presenting symptoms and the bone may be tender and warm. Radiographs show a characteristic increase in radiolucency associated with bone expansion, triangular areas of new bone formation at the periosteal margin and a 'sun-ray' appearance due to new bone formation. Early bloodborne metastases to the lungs are common and the 5 year survival is less than 10% despite treatment with radiotherapy and amputation.

Fibrosarcomas are of two types. Endosteal fibrosarcomas arise within bones and give rise to destructive lesions as they grow out. They metastasise to both the local lymph nodes and the lungs and are associated with a poor prognosis. Despite treatment with radiotherapy or amputation the 5 year survival is only 25%. In contrast periosteal fibrosarcomas seldom invade bone or metastasise to distant sites. Treatment is with local excision and this can be repeated in the event of local recurrence.

Benign chondromas arise from cartilage within the long bones or small bones of the fingers. Multiple enchondromatosis is an unusual disorder of childhood in which multiple chondromas give rise to unsightly swellings attached to bones. Malignant change is very rare in chondromas.

Chondrosarcomas occur in the long bones, pelvis or scapulae of adults, between the ages of 20 and 50. Pain and swelling are the presenting features and bone radiographs show only loss of bone density associated with some speckled calcification. Amputation is the treatment of choice and the 5 year survival is better than 50%.

Ewing's tumour is a highly malignant bone neoplasm which affects children between the ages of 5 and 15. It probably arises from the marrow endothelium and has characteristic radiographic features. Areas of osteolytic bone destruction are surrounded by layers of periosteal new bone formation giving the leasions an 'onion skin' appearance. Pain, swelling and tenderness may be associated with fever and leucocytosis so that these tumours can easily be mistaken for osteomyelitis. The 5 year survival is virutally nil despite radiotherapy and amputation.

Giant cell tumours of bone may be benign or malignant. They usually occur in young adults between the ages of 20 and 40 and present with pain and swelling of a long bone in the neighbourhood of a joint. Radiographs show a typically eccentric tumour with a 'soap-bubble' appearance. The prognosis is relatively good even for malignant tumours. Local excision is the treatment of choice.

Osteoid osteoma is a rare cause of severe bone pain which is characteristically worse at night and relieved by NSAID. The condition occurs between the ages of 10 and 30 in any bone except the skull. There may be warmth, swelling and tenderness on palpation and radiographs show some increase in sclerosis with a characteristic area of translucency surrounding a central nidus. Excision of the nidus cures the symptoms and these lesions do not recur.

SKELETAL DYSPLASIA

The skeletal dysplasias form a large and heterogeneous group of conditions which cause bone and joint deformity. Those with predominant epiphyseal involvement such as multiple epiphyseal dysplasia may be associated with premature osteoarthrosis. Those with predominant metaphyseal involvement such as achondroplasia are associated with short-limbed dwarfism (p. 424). There are disorders such as osteogenesis imperfecta, idiopathic juvenile osteoporosis and the hereditary osteolyses in which decreased bone density, fractures and bone loss are prominent features and others, such as osteopetrosis and sclerosteosis where increased bone density occurs.

Skeletal abnormalities are prominent in a number of hereditary disorders of connective tissue such as the Marfan syndrome or neurofibromatosis as well as in inborn errors of metabolism such as the mucolipidoses, and homocystinuria. The reader is referred to Fairbank's *Atlas of General Affections of the Skeleton* and to McKusick's *Hereditable Disorders of Connective Tissue* (p. 590) for details of all these groups of conditions.

PROSPECTS IN RHEUMATOLOGY

There have been no dramatic 'breakthroughs' in the understanding or treatment of the rheumatic diseases since the 13th edition of this textbook was published in 1981.

Nevertheless, our knowledge of the genetic, cellular and biochemical basis for regulation of immune responses is progressing apace with the widespread application of molecular biological probes and monoclonal antibodies. Parallel progress has been made in understanding the biochemical basis of receptor activation, intercellular co-operation and the complex networks of inflammatory mediators, as well as the organisation and regulation of the macromolecules of bone and cartilage.

Hopes that a new 'generation' of safe and effective anti-inflammatory drugs would emerge have proved to be premature, but research on inhibitors of the leukotriene pathways and selective prostaglandin inhibitors continues. Small advances have been made in understanding the mode of action of gold salts, antimalarials, penicillamine and the immuno-modulating drugs, all of which have been shown to have significant practical value in slowing the progress of inflammatory joint diseases such as rheumatoid arthritis, but there is still a very real need for similar 'disease remitting' drugs with less formidable toxicity.

Advances in diagnostic immunological tests continue to improve the definition of subsets of patients with diffuse connective tissue disorders and we can anticipate continuing progress in the diagnosis, treatment and prognosis of these diseases.

Overall, the outlook for patients with rheumatic diseases has substantially improved over the last 30 years. In particular, the remarkable developments in prosthetic surgery have transformed the lives of patients with advanced and crippling rheumatoid arthritis and osteoarthrosis of the hip. Continuing collaboration between bioengineers and orthopaedic surgeons is gradually overcoming the technical problems involved in developing suitable prostheses for severely damaged knees, elbows, ankles, shoulders and hands, so that some practical advances can be expected. Progress along these lines is, however, likely to be progress with diminishing returns. In many ways, the anatomy of the hip joint makes it uniquely suitable for total joint replacement; a similar degree of success is unlikely in other joints. Already waiting lists for hip arthroplasty are many years in length, and it is calculated that Britain would require one new 300-bedded hospital annually just to cope with this single operation. As numbers of patients with replaced joints increases, so do the problems of loosening and infection of prostheses, particularly in those with multiple joint replacement. Future efforts must clearly be directed towards preventing and curing, or at least controlling these disorders rather than simply improving salvage surgery.

GEORGE NUKI

FURTHER READING:

Emmerson, B.T. (1983) *Hyperuricaemia and Gout in Clinical Practice*. Sydney: ADIS Press.

Hart, F.D. (1982) *Drug Treatment of the Rheumatic Diseases*, 2nd edn. Sydney: ADIS Press. Multi author monograph covering all aspects of clinical pharmacology and therapeutics.

Hughes, G.R.V. (1979) *Connective Tissue Diseases*, 2nd edn. Oxford: Blackwell Scientific Publications. Concise clinical monograph on the diffuse connective tissue diseases. Includes information on clinical applications of immunological tests.

Huskisson, E.C. & Hart, F.D. (1978) *Joint Disease: All the Arthropathies*, 3rd edn. Bristol: John Wright. Thumb-nail sketch of more than 180 conditions associated with arthritis or arthralgia.

Kelley, W.N., Harris, E.D. Jr., Ruddy, S. & Sledge, C.B. (eds.) (1981) *Textbook of Rheumatology*. Philadelphia: W.B. Saunders. Major new international textbook with comprehensive basic science and clinical coverage.

Lawrence, J.S. (1977) *Rheumatism in Populations*. London: Heinemann. Source book of information on epidemiology of rheumatic diseases.

McKusick, V.A. (1979) *Hereditable Disorders of Connective Tissue*, 5th edn. St Louis: C.V. Mosby. Classical monograph.

Nuki, G. (1980) *The Aetiopathogenesis of Osteoarthrosis*. London: Pitman Medical. Recent research reviews.

Panayi, G.S. (1982) *Scientific Basis of Rheumatology*. Edinburgh: Churchill-Livingstone. 16 comprehensive reviews covering genetics, immunology, inflammation, connective tissue degradation, mechanisms of drug action and the biomechanical basis of joint actions and replacement.

Scott, J.H.S. (1983) In Macleod, J. (ed.) *Clinical Examination*, 6th edn. Edinburgh: Churchill Livingstone. Gives an account of the examination of the locomotor system.

Scott, J.T. (1984) *Copeman's Textbook of the Rheumatic Diseases*, 6th edn. Edinburgh: Churchill Livingstone. Standard British text book. Excellent and comprehensive source of information on all aspects of clinical rheumatology.

Wynne-Davis, R. & Fairbank, T.G. (1976) *Fairbank's Atlas of General Affections of the Skeleton*, 2nd edn. Edinburgh: Churchill Livingstone. Concise and beautifully illustrated introduction to skeletal dysplasias and other general disorders of bone.

15. Diseases of the Nervous System

The approach to patients presenting neurological problems must follow a logical course starting with the history and followed by the physical examination. The latter reveals neurological signs which reflect disordered neural function. The nature and distribution of these signs depend on the anatomical localisation of lesions within the central nervous system. It is a fundamental error to relate particular signs to specific pathological processes. Paralysis of one side of the body, hemiplegia, may equally well arise from a stroke or from a cerebral tumour since both lesions may similarly interrupt motor pathways. It is the history of the neurological illness which indicates the nature of the pathological process involved. A careful chronological assessment of the way in which a neurological disability has developed is essential if a diagnosis is to be made. Attention to the symptoms and signs which indicate loss of function of particular parts of the nervous system then follows for purposes of localisation.

Lesions which suddenly affect the nervous system, cause maximal disability within a few hours and after a static period of days or weeks then show a tendency to improve are usually due to vascular disturbances and sometimes to trauma. Disabilities of insidious onset and slow but inexorable progression are often due to degenerative disorders or to tumours of the central nervous system. A remittent history, wherein episodes of disability are followed by periods of improvement, with later recurrence of symptoms elsewhere in the nervous system, is characteristic of multiple sclerosis. Inflammatory lesions such as infections often develop rapidly, but less acutely than traumatic or vascular catastrophes and the recovery phase is also usually rapid. Some conditions are characterised by paroxysmal short-lived disorders of function, followed by rapid and complete recovery. A history of this type may be due to epilepsy or migraine or to transient ischaemic attacks.

These general principles are a useful guide but atypical presentations occur. Sometimes a neoplasm may produce very rapid deterioration and occasionally repetitive, minor vascular lesions give rise to a progressive, 'step-wise' deterioration of function.

Some diseases cause systematised affection of cells or fibres of similar type; these conditions, of which motor neurone disease is a good example, usually result in bilateral and symmetrical dysfunction. Tumours produce progressive involvement of adjacent neural structures causing clinical disabilities which may later be accompanied by symptoms resulting from the occupation of space by the tumour within the confines of the skull or the spinal canal.

A neurological diagnosis is achieved by the integration of all the information gained from the patient's history, the general medical examination and the neurological examination.

ANATOMY AND PHYSIOLOGY

The Motor System

Movements, whether voluntary or involuntary, are the result of the contraction or controlled relaxation of groups of muscles and never of only a single muscle. They are effected by contraction of muscles which act as prime movers and reciprocal relaxation of their antagonists. The action of the prime movers is provided with a firm base by contraction of synergists which stabilise the joints, and by appropriate adjustments of posture. The postural adjustments are largely under the control of the extrapyramidal motor system and the vestibular and spinal reflexes.

Voluntary movements require the participation of the precentral gyrus of the cerebral cortex ('motor area') and the timing and degree of contraction or relaxation of the muscles of the synergy are coordinated by the cerebellum, especially when a movement involves more than one segment of a limb.

The activities of the upper motor neurones from the motor area of the cortex, the extrapyramidal motor system and the cerebellum influence, directly or indirectly, the cells of the anterior horn of spinal grey matter or motor cranial nuclei from each of which a lower neurone runs to a group of muscle fibres. Thus the lower motor neurone is the 'final common path' for all efferent impulses directed at the muscle and the groups of anterior horn cells may be considered to 'represent a muscle' in the same sense as the cells of the motor cortex 'represent a movement'. This distinction is vital to an understanding of the signs and disorders of the motor system.

Upper Motor Neurone. The fibres arise from the cells in the precentral gyrus ('motor area'). These initiate movements of different parts of the opposite side of the body, the parts being represented in the following order from below upwards — tongue, face, hand, forearm, arm, trunk, thigh, leg, foot and perineal areas with considerable overlap. The cortical area representing movements of each of these parts is proportional to its functional importance rather than to its anatomical size. The projections of the upper motor neurones through the corticospinal (pyramidal) tracts to the contralateral motor nuclei of the brain stem and anterior horn of the spinal cord are shown in Figure 15.1.

A destructive lesion of the lateral corticospinal tract above its decussation causes a loss of some voluntary movements of part of the opposite side of the body, according to the fibres involved, but automatic associated movements, such as the stretching of a paralysed arm when yawning, may persist and other voluntary or reflex movements using the same lower motor neurones and muscles

Fig. 15.1 The motor pathways

may be preserved. This is the essential difference between paralysis of upper motor neurone type and that due to a lower motor neurone lesion.

For the same reason stretch reflexes (p. 599) are retained but these are usually of heightened activity. This indicates that the corticospinal tract normally carries fibres which are inhibitory to the stretch reflex. The pattern of cutaneous protective reflexes also changes, causing the emergence of an extensor plantar reflex.

There are thus two types of disturbance, a negative one due to loss of a particular activity, and a positive one due to the release of lower levels from control. This is a principle of general application in the nervous system and the concept is important in understanding the signs of upper motor neurone disease. Another type of positive symptom results from irritative lesions (usually incomplete damage to a nerve cell or its fibre) which causes spontaneous activity of the affected neurones. Spontaneous activity in upper motor neurones causes involuntary movements as in focal epilepsy (p. 617).

SIGNS OF A LESION OF THE UPPER MOTOR NEU-
RONE are:

1. Weakness or paralysis of movements of part
of one side of the body.

2. Increase of tone of spastic type. This is
characterised by an increased resistance to passive
movement, which is maximal at the beginning of
movement, smoothly sustained, and suddenly
lapses as passive movement is continued ('clasp-
knife' response). It occurs predominantly in flexor
muscles in upper limbs and extensor muscles in
the lower limbs (the antigravity muscles).

3. Increase in amplitude of tendon reflexes:
clonus may be present.

4. Loss of the abdominal reflexes.

5. An extensor plantar response (Babinski
reflex).

6. No muscle atrophy apart from slight wasting
which may occur as a result of disuse.

7. Normal electrical excitability of the involved
muscles (p. 607).

These signs occur with disease involving any
part of the upper motor neurone, but the exact
level at which the lesion lies may be determined
by the upper level of increased reflexes and by
associated features.

Cortex. Localised paralyses affecting, for example, one limb only, are characteristic of lesions
at the cortical level. The upper motor neurones
are spread over a wide area in the precentral gyrus
and only very large lesions could cause a hemiplegia. There may be associated evidence of cortical
dysfunction such as dysphasia and focal epileptic
fits sometimes occur.

Internal Capsule. As the fibres here are closely
packed, a hemiplegia is likely. There may be
hemihypoaesthesia and hemianopia from damage
to adjacent sensory and visual fibres respectively.

Brain Stem. Lesions in this area are rarely
confined to the corticospinal tract. One presentation comprises affection of one or more cranial
nerves on the side of the lesion and signs of
an upper motor neurone lesion on the opposite
side.

Spinal Cord. The corticospinal tracts may be
affected bilaterally. The level of the lesion in the
cord is often delineated by accompanying lower
motor neurone signs, sensory disturbance or loss
of tendon reflexes.

Lower Motor Neurone. Axons emerge from
the nuclei of the motor cranial nerves and from
the cells of the anterior horns of the spinal cord.
They pass through the anterior nerve roots to
enter a mixed peripheral nerve in which they run
to the muscles which they supply. Each lower
motor neurone has terminal branching so that it is
distributed to the motor end-plates of a group of
muscle fibres. The anterior horn cell, the axon
and a group of muscle fibres comprise the motor-
unit and each muscle is composed of a large
number of such units.

The anterior horn cell is activated by impulses
from the corticospinal tracts, from the extrapyramidal tracts, and from some afferent fibres of
the posterior nerve root responsible for spinal
reflexes. The lower motor neurone is thus an
integral part of the spinal reflex arc and is the final
common pathway for all motor impulses, involuntary or voluntary, directed to a muscle.

Normal nutrition of a muscle appears to depend on its contact with the spinal cord through
the lower motor neurone since, if it is interrupted,
the muscle rapidly wastes.

SIGNS OF A LESION OF THE LOWER MOTOR NEU-
RONE. The following signs will be present only in
those muscles supplied by the particular neurones
affected:

1. Weakness or paralysis of muscles. This
affects all movements in which they take part
whether as prime movers or synergists, voluntary
or involuntary, or in reflex contractions.

2. Loss of tone on passive movement (flacci-
dity).

3. Wasting of the affected muscles which appears within two or three weeks of an acute lesion
(atrophy).

4. Absence of reflexes subserved by the affected
neurones. Abdominal and plantar reflexes remain
normal unless the neurones to the appropriate
muscles are damaged and then these reflexes
cannot be elicited.

5. Single muscle fibres contract spontaneously
when they are no longer influenced by their
associated lower motor neurone. This phenomenon, called fibrillation, is detectable by electromyography but is invisible through the skin.
Lower motor neurones which are damaged but
still able to conduct impulses may give rise to

spontaneous contractions of bundles of fibres in the muscles supplied. Such contractions (fasciculation) may be visible, e.g. in motor neurone disease.

6. Contractures of muscles develop due to replacement by fibrous tissue and 'trophic' changes such as dryness and cyanosis of the skin, and brittleness of the nails appear partly due to impaired circulation.

7. The electrical excitability of the peripheral nerves and muscles is altered. These tests may be combined with electromyography to confirm that a weak and wasted muscle is denervated. Lesions of peripheral nerves short of complete interruption may cause slowing of conduction.

If lower motor neurones are damaged in the cord or nerve roots the muscles and reflexes affected in the ways described above will be those supplied by one or more segments of the spinal cord. If the neurones are damaged more peripherally after they have been redistributed in the nerve plexuses, the paralysis will occur in the territory supplied by the appropriate peripheral nerve and it is probable that there will be similar damage to the sensory fibres with which the motor fibres are associated in the mixed nerve.

Extrapyramidal System. This is a complex neuronal network, extending from the cortex to the medulla, from which emerge descending spinal pathways whose influence on lower motor neurones modifies voluntary motor activity. Interspersed in this latticework of fibres are areas of grey matter. Some of these are only loose aggregations of nuclei in the reticular formation of the brain stem, but there are also several well defined nuclear masses called the basal nuclei (ganglia), which include the caudate nucleus, the lentiform nucleus (globus pallidus and putamen), the substantia nigra and the subthalamic nucleus.

There are rich interconnections between the constituents of the basal nuclei and thence via the ventrolateral nucleus of the thalamus to the extrapyramidal areas of the cortex and to the medullary reticular formation. The normal functions of the extrapyramidal system are ill-understood.

SIGNS OF AN EXTRAPYRAMIDAL LESION. *Disturbance of Voluntary Movements.* There is not true paralysis in extrapyramidal disease, but rather slowness of movement and poverty of movement in that spontaneous gestures, changes in facial expression, and associated movements for postural adjustment, such as swinging the arm when walking, are lost on the side opposite to the lesion.

Disturbance of Tone. Tone may be increased as in parkinsonism or decreased as in chorea. Increase in tone, of extrapyramidal type, has characteristic features. It is present throughout the whole range of passive movement; it affects opposing muscle groups equally; it may be smooth and plastic ('lead-pipe rigidity') or intermittent ('cog-wheel rigidity') which is more common.

Involuntary Movements. There are many varieties, notably the tremor of parkinsonism (p. 648), choreiform movements (p. 651) and athetosis (p. 652).

Cerebellum. This is the most important part of the nervous system for the coordination of movement and the muscular contractions required to maintain posture.

The cerebellum receives impulses from many sources, — principally the proprioceptive end-organs, the skin, the vestibular nuclei and the cerebral cortex. The pontine nuclei and the inferior olive relay fibres from the cerebral motor cortex and basal nuclei respectively to the cerebellar cortex of the opposite side. The cerebellar cortex integrates this information about body posture, limb position and motor intention and sends efferent fibres via the cerebellar nuclei to the reticular formation, red nucleus and vestibular nucleus of the opposite side, whence fibres descend to influence motor cells in the anterior horns of the spinal cord; as these descending fibres cross again each cerebellar hemisphere controls the ipsilateral side of the body. Efferent fibres from the cerebellum also ascend to the contralateral thalamus through which the cerebral cortex is influenced. The cerebellum is therefore a great coordinating centre controlling the synergistic action of muscles during voluntary and automatic movements as well as adjusting posture.

SIGNS OF A CEREBELLAR LESION. The effects of disease of the cerebellum are best seen in acute lesions, for in chronic conditions considerable compensation occurs so that the deficit is less than might be expected. A lesion of the cerebellar hemisphere produces all its effects on the same side of the body. The principal signs are:

Hypotonia. The muscles show diminished resistance to passive movement and, when an outstretched limb is suddenly displaced, it makes a greater excursion than usual and oscillates before resuming its posture.

Disturbance of Tendon Reflexes. The reflexes are either diminished or pendular as when the knee jerk is followed by a series of diminishing oscillations.

Disturbance of Posture and of Gait. The head may be tilted towards the side of the lesion and the patient leans or may even fall towards that side. The gait is reeling with a tendency to stagger to the side of the lesion.

Disorders of Movement. Incoordination, hypotonia and the fact that muscular contraction is unregulated by the muscle spindles cause ataxia which manifests itself in different ways:

1. Dysmetria. Movements are not accurately adjusted to their object, so that the finger may overshoot or fall short of the object it is required to touch. If a movement is attempted with the eyes closed the finger overshoots towards the side of the cerebellar lesion ('past-pointing').

2. Dyssynergia. Movements which involve more than one joint are broken up into their component parts. When severe this leads to a decomposition of movement which resembles the jerky movements of a marionette.

3. Intention tremor. A combination of dyssynergia and dysmetria causes faulty correction of the badly directed limb movement so that it approaches the target in a zig-zag manner. The coarse irregular tremor increases as the target is approached. It is not more marked when the eyes are closed. The contraction of muscles necessary to maintain a posture may be similarly affected so that tremor at rest occasionally occurs in cerebellar disorders.

4. Dysdiadochokinesis. The arrest of one movement and its immediate replacement with the opposite movement requires accurate coordination of the various muscles of the synergy. Rapidly alternating movements are therefore disturbed and carried out in a clumsy, irregular, jerky fashion.

5. Rebound phenomenon. For the same reason a strong contraction cannot be arrested when resistance is suddenly removed, whereupon the limb shoots beyond the normal range.

6. Disorders of articulation and phonation. Articulation is irregular, slurred and explosive as the volume of sound is poorly controlled. A rarer form of dysarthria is 'scanning-speech' in which the syllables tend to be separated from each other.

7. Disturbance of eye movement. Jerking nystagmus in the horizontal plane is commonly seen. It is a defect of postural fixation involving conjugate gaze (p. 610). In a unilateral cerebellar lesion the movements are greater in amplitude and slower in rate when the eyes are deviated to the side of the lesion.

The Sensory System

Superficial sensation which arises from the skin has four primary components, touch, pain, warmth and cold. *Deep sensations* arising from subcutaneous structures are deep pain, pressure and proprioception which enables the recognition of movements of joints and the position of the parts of the body relative to one another. Vibration is a sensation due to rhythmical stimulation of groups of deep and superficial touch receptors.

Some of the afferent impulses carried in 'sensory' nerve fibres do not reach consciousness but convey impulses directly or indirectly to motor neurones for reflex functions or to the cerebellum for purposes of coordination, e.g. many impulses from muscle and tendon receptors.

All sensory impulses arise in the sensory receptors or end-organs which are widely distributed throughout the body. It is probable, though debatable, that specialised receptors respond to specific types of stimuli. Stimulation of an end-organ causes impulses to pass along the first sensory neurone to the spinal cord. This neurone has its cell body in a dorsal root ganglion but does not synapse until it reaches a second order neurone in the spinal cord or brain stem.

On entering the cord by the posterior nerve root, fibres subserving proprioception, vibration and a proportion of touch sensation turn medially and ascend in the posterior column of the same side to the lower part of the medulla oblongata to synapse with cells in the gracile and cuneate

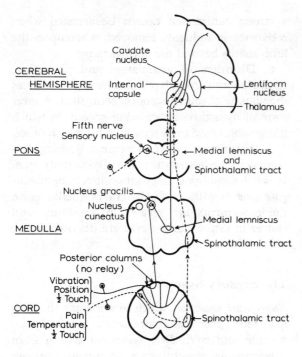

Fig. 15.2 The sensory pathways.

nuclei (Fig. 15.2). From there, the second order neurone crosses to the other side of the medulla and ascends in the medial lemniscus to the main sensory nucleus of the thalamus.

Fibres subserving pain, warmth, cold and the remainder of touch sensation synapse in the posterior horn of the spinal cord soon after entering it. Most of the second order neurones cross at the same level, or one or two segments higher, to reach the anterolateral column where they ascend to the thalamus as the spinothalamic tract. Some of these fibres do not cross but enter the ipsilateral spinothalamic tract.

As it ascends through the brain stem the tract gradually intermingles with the medial lemniscus and terminates along with it in the main sensory nucleus of the thalamus. Third order neurones, maintaining their functional specificity, are then relayed from the thalamus to the sensory area of the cortex which is situated in the postcentral gyrus.

Areas of the sensory cortex representing the different parts of the body are arranged in a similar manner to the motor cortex. Some appreciation of sensation is possible at the thalamic level but the cortical projection is necessary to allow discrimination of the intensity and pattern of stimulation. From the postcentral gyrus further connnections are made with other parts of the cortex, particularly in the parietal lobe where the information derived from superficial and deep sensation is integrated so that judgement of the size, shape, weight, texture and pattern of objects is possible. This sensory information is also integrated with information derived from the special senses to provide a mental picture of the body (body image).

This synthesis is mainly carried out in the non-dominant (right) parietal lobe. The corresponding part of the left cerebral hemisphere is important for other mental functions in which recurrent patterns of stimulation achieve the status of symbols and so are used for the receptive and interpretative aspects of speech functions. For this reason it is usually called the dominant or major hemisphere (in some left-handed people speech is mainly represented in the right hemisphere). This important part of the parietal lobe is connected with the lower part of the motor cortex of the same side so that patterns of lip, tongue, respiratory and finger movements may be used to convert ideas into motor symbols, the motor side of speech. An understanding of the link between symbol and meaning requires a knowledge of the physiological basis of the mind which we do not have at present.

Most of the afferent signals entering the central nervous system never reach consciousness. Some are used for spinal reflexes and make contact directly or through interneurones with motor neurones. Other fibres which originate in muscle receptors end at the base of the posterior horn in contact with second order neurones. These neurones turn laterally to the periphery of the cord to ascend in the anterior and posterior spinocerebellar tracts to the cerebellar cortex. Most of these ascend without crossing but some second order neurones cross to the opposite anterior spinocerebellar tract. These fibres carry some of the proprioceptive information required to enable the cerebellum to coordinate limb movements.

Still other sensory fibres, which do not carry 'sensation' in the ordinary sense, are extremely important for the maintenance of consciousness.

These are collateral branches of the main spino-thalamic pathways and of the special sensory tracts which turn medially into the upper part of the reticular formation in the midbrain. Here there is a chain of short neurones with intimate interconnections which also receives neurones from most parts of the cerebral cortex. It is therefore an important integrating centre. At its upper end it communicates with the non-specific nuclei of the thalamus which relay impulses to all areas of the cortex. Activity in this system is considered to be essential for the conscious state and may be important in some mental functions in collaboration with the cerebral cortex.

Disease of the sensory system may be accompanied by positive phenomena such as pain or paraesthesiae due to spontaneous activity or irritation of sensory neurones, or by negative phenomena in which there is loss of the ability to appreciate some modality of sensation (anaesthesia and analgesia). These symptoms occur only with disorders of the first or second order neurones, i.e. from the end-organs to the thalamus.

Suprathalamic lesions show certain differences. Paraesthesiae may occur with irritative lesions of the sensory cortex but anaesthesia does not. Instead there is a loss of sensory discrimination and of the spatial and quantitative aspects of sensation.

SIGNS OF SENSORY LESIONS. *Peripheral Nerve.* With a complete lesion all forms of sensation are lost in the area supplied by the affected nerve, but the zone of anaesthesia may be limited by the fact that neighbouring nerves overlap into its territory, the extent varying from person to person. The resistance of different types of fibres to disease need not be the same so that it is common for one type of cutaneous or deep sensation to be more affected than another and indeed some may be spared. If the afferent fibres of a reflex arc are affected, as for instance in the sciatic nerve in the ankle jerk, the reflex concerned is lost.

Some neuropathies do not affect individual nerves but rather damage fibres selectively. As a general rule the longest fibres are most susceptible and so the sensory and motor disturbance is first noticed at the tips of all the toes and fingers, irrespective of nerve supply, and spreads proximally as the advancing disease involves progres-sively shorter fibres. This produces a 'glove and stocking' distribution of sensory loss.

Posterior Root. The different forms of sensation are affected by a posterior root lesion in the same way as for a peripheral nerve but the distribution of the loss follows a dermatomal pattern. The overlap from adjacent roots may be so great that no anaesthesia can be detected. When the root is irritated, pain and paraesthesiae are experienced in the full dermatomal distribution of the root; pain may also be experienced in the deep structures such as muscles and ligaments which are supplied by the root. These structures do not necessarily underlie the dermatome. Any reflex subserved by the involved root is also lost, for example, the ankle jerk where the S1 posterior root is damaged by a prolapsed intervertebral disc.

Posterior Column. A lesion confined to the posterior column of the spinal cord will cause loss of position and vibration sense on the same side, but the sensations of pain, touch, warmth and cold will be preserved (Fig. 15.3).

The loss of the sense of position causes sensory ataxia since the patient is unable to control movements by awareness of the position achieved at each instant. Sensory ataxia differs from cerebellar ataxia in that it is more marked when the eyes are closed, because vision can compensate to a certain extent for loss of proprioceptive information. Thus there is unsteadiness in the finger-nose test which is greater when the eyes are closed but without the marked tremor of cerebellar ataxia. The gait is ataxic and the patient walks with a broad base to provide a firmer foundation and steps high to make sure that the feet clear the ground which cannot be felt with certainty. If the eyes are closed it is not possible to stand with the feet close together without swaying (Romberg's test). Vibration sense is abolished below the level of the lesion ipsilaterally.

The same symptoms will be found if the first order neurones of the proprioceptive nerve fibres are damaged peripherally but they will then be associated with other signs of peripheral nerve disease.

Spinothalamic Tract. Lesions of the anterior and lateral spinothalamic tracts in the antero-lateral columns of the cord or their continuation

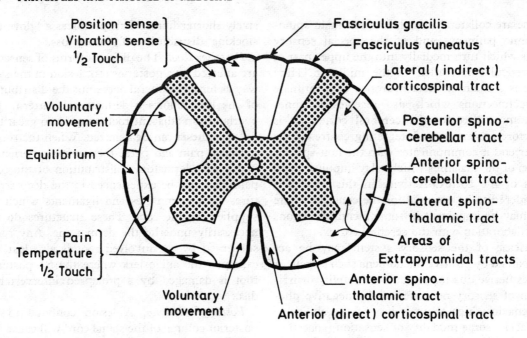

Fig. 15.3 Cross-section of spinal cord

through the brain stem cause impairment of the ability to appreciate pain, warmth and cold on the contralateral side of the body below the level of the lesion. Touch is usually modified (it feels 'different') but not abolished because of its alternative pathway in the posterior columns. This is the situation produced by the operation of anterolateral cordotomy for the relief of intractable pain.

Brain Stem. Since the spinothalamic tract and medial lemniscus run close together and eventually intermingle, lesions of the upper brain stem usually affect all forms of sensation on the contralateral side of the body. With midbrain lesions the hemihypoaesthesia will extend to the face, but with pontomedullary lesions the second order neurones from the trigeminal sensory nucleus or the nucleus and descending tract of the fifth nerve may be damaged so that sensory loss will be on the same side of the face as the lesion but on the contralateral side of the rest of the body (Fig. 15.2).

Thalamus. Lesions of the main sensory nuclei in the lateral part of the thalamus may cause spontaneous pain of most unpleasant quality in the opposite side of the body. The threshold for pain is raised on the opposite side of the body but when it is exceeded the resulting pain is exquisite

and has the same unpleasant quality which often causes considerable emotional reaction.

Loss of other modalities of sensation occurs on the opposite side of the body.

Sensory Cortex. Lesions above the thalamus do not abolish any form of sensation though the threshold may be raised. There is impairment of position sense, of two-point discrimination, of the ability to localise touch and to recognise objects in the palm of the hand (astereognosis) since shape and texture cannot be identified though the patient is able to feel the object.

Disturbance of the spatial aspects of sensation is greatest when the parietal lobe is involved, and especially in lesions of the 'minor' hemisphere this may cause disturbance of the body image and of spatial orientation. For instance the patient may be unable to recognise part of the body on the side opposite to the lesion or may feel that it is distorted. One side of external space or of the body may be ignored and this is most evident if the unaffected side of the body, or visual field, is stimulated simultaneously. When presented with this 'perceptual rivalry' the brain 'ignores' the stimulus on the side contralateral to the affected parietal lobe though a stimulus applied to that part alone would be recognised immediately.

Lesions of the dominant hemisphere in the region where parietal, temporal and occipital lobes meet (angular and supramarginal gyri) are associated with receptive dysphasia (p. 601). This is a special case of the failure to analyse the temporal and spatial aspects of sensory stimuli.

The Reflexes

Certain functions are economically catered for by the nervous system by means of reflexes, which are short chains of neurones (the reflex arc) connecting a receptor to an effector organ such as muscle or gland, so that an appropriate stimulus invariably leads to a specific response. The quantity but not the nature of the response may be modified by other stimuli or by supraspinal influences from the cortex, extrapyramidal system or the cerebellum.

There are two main categories of reflex — postural and protective. The appropriate stimuli for postural reflexes are muscle stretch and vestibular impulses. Protective reflexes are evoked by stimuli to pain receptors. They are usually superficial (cutaneous or corneal); the protective 'spasm' of muscles around a painful lesion is similar in nature.

Tendon (Stretch) Reflexes. A basic postural reflex depends on the stimulation of muscle spindles when a skeletal muscle is stretched. The afferent fibre enters the cord by a posterior nerve root and communicates directly or via a chain of interneurones with the anterior horn cells which control the stretched muscle, thus causing it to contract and so resist the displacement. A sudden tap to a tendon results in a sharp but brief contraction of the muscle. This activity may be increased by certain manoeuvres such as clenching the teeth or pulling the interlocked hands apart. This is termed *reinforcement* of the reflex and a tendon jerk should not be declared absent until reinforcement has failed to make it visible.

The stretch reflex is inhibited by receptors in the tendon if muscle tension rises too high, thus risking the integrity of its fibres. This may happen when the reflex is exaggerated by withdrawal of a normal inhibitory effect of the corticospinal tract so that the contraction is abruptly stopped. This is the mechanism of the 'clasp-knife' response.

There are also supraspinal facilitatory and inhibitory influences from the extrapyramidal system and cerebellum so lesions of these systems may abolish the reflexes.

An example of a monosynaptic stretch reflex is a knee jerk. A tap on the patellar tendon activates stretch receptors in the quadriceps muscle giving rise to impulses in first order sensory neurones which pass directly to the lower motor neurones to the quadriceps muscle making it contract. A lesion anywhere along this path will cause loss of the reflex; hence it is important in the localisation of disease to know through which spinal segment each reflex passes.

The common tendon reflexes are the brachioradialis (C 5–6), the biceps (C 5–6), the triceps (C 7), the knee (L 3–4) and the ankle (S 1).

Superficial Reflexes. These are polysynaptic reflexes originating from stimuli to superficial structures. The interneurones may connect with motor neurones at several segmental levels and so the response may be a coordinated movement, usually designed to withdraw the stimulated part from a potentially dangerous stimulus.

There are very many of these reflexes, some of which are conflicting. For example, stimulation of the sole of the foot evokes both flexion and extension reflexes. Which reflex will predominate is determined by higher influences. The nature of this influence is unknown but is believed to require the corticospinal (pyramidal) tract and damage to this tract will cause a change in the predominant reflex pattern.

PLANTAR REFLEX. When the outer border of the sole of the foot is stroked in normal people after infancy, there is plantar flexion of the great toe. In 1896 Babinski pointed out that when the upper motor neurone was damaged the same stimulus caused dorsiflexion of the toe. (Anatomically this is described as an extensor plantar response though physiologically it is part of the flexion withdrawal reflex).

When the reflex is well developed it can be elicited from the medial side of the sole of the foot or even from the lower part of the leg and the hallux response is accompanied by dorsiflexion and abduction or fanning of the other toes and even withdrawal of the limb.

The fundamental importance of the extensor

plantar or Babinski response as a sign of loss of function of the upper motor neurone is widely accepted but it may occur in transient form during temporary states such as coma or after an epileptic fit and need not indicate permanent damage. It is often extensor in normal infants during the first year of life.

ABDOMINAL REFLEXES. When the skin on one side of the abdomen is stroked with a pin, there is a reflex contraction of the underlying muscles, a reflex for protection of the viscera. This may be lost on the affected side in disease of the upper motor neurone though the sign is less reliable than the plantar reflex. For instance the abdominal reflexes may be lost early in multiple sclerosis yet retained despite severe pyramidal tract damage in motor neurone disease. The abdominal reflexes may not be obtained on either side in elderly, obese or multiparous patients and may be lost where operative incisions have severed the nerves concerned.

The abdominal reflexes are served in their peripheral course by the intercostal nerves arising from segments T 8 to 12.

CORNEAL REFLEX. A light touch on the cornea provokes a blink of the eyelids on both sides. The afferent path for this reflex is the first division of the trigeminal nerve and the efferent path is the facial nerve. Loss of both corneal reflexes is a valuable indication of a deepening level of unconsciousness from any cause but should be elicited with discretion to avoid accidental damage to the cornea.

Nervous Control of the Bladder and Rectum

Bladder. The nerve supply to the bladder is derived from three sources:

1. Sympathetic, from the first and second lumbar segments via the inferior hypogastric plexus and hypogastric nerves, which relax the bladder wall and contract the sphincters.

2. Parasympathetic, from segments S 2, 3, 4 via the pelvic nerves (nervi erigentes) which contract the bladder wall and relax the internal sphincter.

3. Somatic, from segments S 2, 3, 4 via the pudendal nerves, which contract the external sphincter of the urethra.

Afferent impulses from the bladder wall travel via the pelvic nerves and from the sphincters via the pudendal nerves. Distension of the bladder activates stretch receptors in the bladder wall and stimulates the parasympathetic fibres by means of a reflex arc through the upper sacral segments of the spinal cord; for example in the infant the bladder empties automatically when distension reaches a certain degree. Subsequently two descending pathways from higher levels assume control, one which inhibits the automatic reflex emptying, and the other which relaxes the inhibition when appropriate. The expression of urine is then promoted by contracting the abdominal and relaxing the pelvic muscles.

Interruption of the sacral reflex arc leads to retention of urine. This is accompanied by loss of bladder sensation if the lesion is on the afferent side of the arc, as in tabes dorsalis.

Damage to the anterior sacral nerve roots causes an atonic bladder without loss of sensation ('lower motor neurone paralysis'). Lesions in the spinal cord above the sacral segments may damage the inhibitory fibres, causing urgency, precipitancy or incontinence of urine, or damage to the facilitatory fibres may cause hesitancy or retention. If the higher control is completely lost there is a period of retention with overflow from a passively dilating atonic bladder until the sacral reflex begins to function as in infancy, restoring automatic bladder emptying. The bladder is hypertonic ('upper motor neurone paralysis') and may shrink if this is not prevented.

Cerebral lesions at the vertex near the motor or sensory areas may also give rise to incontinence or retention, and with frontal lobe lesions the intellectual disturbance may be associated with failure to inhibit reflex emptying.

Rectum. This has a dual nerve supply from the sympathetic (inhibitory) and the parasympathetic (facilitatory) systems. Disturbances of function similar to those in the bladder occur, but are less severe and more transient (p. 330).

Speech

Speech employs verbal symbols to communicate thoughts and information. Coherent speech requires the formulation of propositions, which are translated into conventional symbols, earlier acquired and readily accessible, which then reach external expression by means of an efficient vocalising apparatus. Disease processes may interrupt this sequence at various levels to produce different types of speech defects.

INTELLECTUAL IMPAIRMENT. Speech is deranged as a result of a generalised deficit of intellectual function which prevents the organisation of meaningful propositions. Such a disturbance reflects a diffuse impairment of cortical function which may be a temporary phenomenon in toxic confusional states (delirium) or permanent in dementia.

DYSPHASIA. This comprises disturbances of the symbolic aspects of language and these arise as a result of damage in or near the cortex of the dominant hemisphere.

The nature of the defect varies with the site of the lesion. In *expressive, motor or non-fluent dysphasia* the patient can formulate thoughts in appropriate words (i.e. internal speech is preserved) but is unable to translate them into corresponding sounds. This occurs despite an intact articulatory system and represents a specialised form of apraxia (p. 604) which results from lesions in the posterior part of the inferior (3rd) frontal convolution. Impaired comprehension of language is called *receptive, sensory or fluent dysphasia*. The patient fails to understand or carry out spoken instructions. Internal speech is disturbed and hence there is also impairment of the patient's external speech. This is an agnosic deficit (p. 604) and results from lesions of the posterior part of the upper temporal convolutions and the angular gyrus of the parietal lobe.

In clinical circumstances all the speech areas of the major hemisphere are often injured together, which results in combined receptive and expressive dysfunctions. This picture, called '*global or central dysphasia*', is usually due to occlusion of the internal carotid or middle cerebral artery which supply all the regions concerned with speech and their connections.

DYSARTHRIA. This is imperfect articulation of speech. Precise enunciation of words requires normal function and coordination of lips, tongue and palate. Any abnormality thereof results in slurring and distortion of speech. Dysarthria may be due to mechanical derangements such as cleft palate or ill-fitting false teeth. Lesions of muscles, myoneural junctions, or lower motor neurones of lips, tongue or palate will also result in dysarthria as will upper motor neurone and extrapyramidal affections of these structures.

When normal monitoring of speech is disturbed by deafness, dysarthria may ensue. This is particularly liable to occur when auditory feedback is distorted by impaired hearing in early childhood.

DYSPHONIA. Reduced volume of speech, often accompanied by hoarseness, results from dysfunction of the phonating mechanism. This may be due to weakness of respiratory movements so that air flow across the vocal cords is reduced or to malfunction of the vocal cords. The causative lesion may be in the respiratory musculature, in the peripheral nerves, or in central structures. Thus, for example, bilateral palsies of the recurrent laryngeal nerves cause aphonia. Dysphonia may be part of the picture of a bulbar palsy or it may result from extrapyramidal disease, such as parkinsonism. Complete aphonia is usually hysterical.

The Visual Pathway

The optic nerve carries second order neurones, the first order neurones being very short fibres within the retina. For much of its length the optic nerve is surrounded by a protrusion of the meningeal membranes into which cerebrospinal fluid can pass, especially if intracranial pressure is raised. For these reasons the optic nerve is liable to suffer from different pathological states than other nerves.

The visual pathway is illustrated in Figure 15.4. Sensory impulses from the retinae pass along the optic nerves to the optic chiasma where the fibres from the temporal half of the retina continue posteriorly in the lateral angle of the chiasma into the optic tract on the same side. Fibres from the nasal halves of the retinae decussate so that the optic tract carries fibres from that part of each retina which receives light from the contralateral half of the visual field of each eye (the light rays crossing in the refractory media of

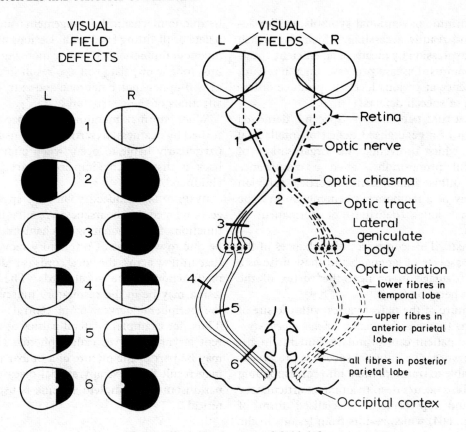

Fig. 15.4 Visual pathways and field defects

the eyes). In the same way the light rays from the upper part of the visual field stimulate the lower part of each retina and the fibres arising there remain inferior throughout their further path to the cortex.

The optic tracts continue to the lateral geniculate bodies where the fibres concerned with vision synapse and the impulses are relayed along the optic radiations to the calcarine area of the occipital cortex. The uppermost fibres which carry impulses derived from the superior quadrants of each retina (lower quadrants of visual fields) pass directly through the parietal lobe, whereas the lowermost fibres which relay impulses from the lower quadrants of the retina (upper quadrants of visual fields) sweep downwards and forwards round the temporal horn of the lateral ventricle in the temporal lobe before passing to the occipital cortex.

Throughout the whole of the visual pathway fibres from the various parts of each retina maintain approximately the same relationship with each other.

Some fibres originating in the retina and passing centrally in the optic nerve form the afferent limb of the light reflex arc of the pupils. These bypass the lateral geniculate bodies and pass medially to the superior colliculi of the midbrain where they synapse with neurones which pass to the nuclei of the third cranial nerves on each side. From these nuclei arise the efferent limbs of the light reflex (direct and consensual) to the sphincter muscles of the pupils.

No visual stimulus is required for the accommodation 'reflex' of the pupil which is more properly an associated contraction related to the movement of convergence of the eyes. This is believed to involve an unidentified cerebral path and a midbrain nucleus which controls the pupillomotor cells of both third nerve nuclei. This explains the dissociation between the light reflex and the convergence reflex which may occur in neurosyphilis and other diseases.

Clinical Manifestations of Lesions of the Visual Pathway. THE OPTIC NERVE. A complete lesion of the optic nerve produces total loss of vision in the affected eye. There is no light reflex, direct or consensual, when that eye is illuminated but both pupils contract normally when the unaffected eye is illuminated. The pupil may be slightly larger in the blind eye. If the lesion is only partial, islands of loss of vision (*scotomas*) of various shapes occur in the field of the affected eye. When the fibres originating in the macular area are damaged there is a loss of visual acuity which cannot be corrected by lenses. Direct and consensual light reflexes are depressed or absent when the abnormal eye is stimulated but the convergence pupil response is unaffected.

THE OPTIC CHIASMA. A lesion of the central portion of the chiasma involves the decussating fibres from the nasal halves of both retinae and so gives rise to bitemporal hemianopia. In practice such lesions are rarely symmetrical and hence the degree of involvement of the visual fields of each eye is often unequal. A pituitary tumour first compresses the lower fibres and so the bitemporal hemianopia begins in the superior quadrants, whereas a suprasellar cyst compresses the chiasma from above so that field loss starts in the lower quadrants.

THE OPTIC TRACTS. A lesion of an optic tract gives rise to a homonymous hemianopia, the lost half of the field of vision of each eye being on the side opposite to the lesion. The involvement of the two fields is often unequal ('incongruous'), being slightly greater in the field of the eye on the side of the lesion.

THE OPTIC RADIATION. The effects of a lesion of the optic radiation depend on its exact site. A lesion of the temporal lobe involves the lower fibres only and gives rise to a homonymous defect involving mainly the upper quadrants of the visual fields (Fig. 15.4). A lesion in the anterior part of the parietal lobe causes a homonymous hemianopia mainly affecting the lower quadrants as it affects fibres from the upper part of the retinae. A lesion at the posterior part of the parietal lobe, where both groups of fibres are

again adjacent, gives rise to a total homonymous hemianopia.

THE OCCIPITAL CORTEX. A destructive lesion of one occipital cortex gives rise to a complete (and congruous) homonymous hemianopia if it is extensive, or to a scotoma which is present in the fields of both eyes. Irritative lesions, as in the ischaemia caused by migraine, cause hallucinations of flashing lights which are referred to the contralateral field of both eyes.

The Localising Signs of Cerebral Disease

The Prefrontal Lobe. This comprises the frontal lobe anterior to the precentral gyrus. It is concerned with some aspects of psychological reactions, notably the ability to make intelligent anticipations of the future, and the emotional correlations of thought.

Disturbances of these functions cause vague psychiatric disorders which are difficult to diagnose in the early stages. The patient loses appreciation of the consequences of actions, fails to take forethought and becomes apathetic or morbidly facetious. With progressing dementia, memory and intellect become impaired and social sense is also affected. The patient becomes careless about dress and appearance and may micturate in public or become incontinent without seeming to care.

Physical signs are few but there may be generalised convulsions and a grasp reflex may be found in the contralateral hand. With this reflex, the patient involuntarily clutches at an object which is drawn lightly over the palm between the index finger and the thumb. The contralateral arm may be ataxic if the frontopontine fibres connecting with the cerebellum are interrupted. Expanding lesions of a frontal lobe may compress the underlying olfactory nerve causing unilateral loss of the sense of smell.

These signs may be missed in a routine examination. It is important, therefore, to search for them when confronted with a patient with early mental changes.

The Precentral Gyrus. Lesions in this region give rise to unequivocal signs. Jacksonian epilepsy (p. 617) occurs and monoplegia readily develops. A lesion such as a meningioma arising from the falx cerebri involving the superior ends of both 'motor areas' may give rise to signs of an upper motor neurone lesion in both lower limbs, the upper limbs being spared. When a lesion in the dominant hemisphere extends forwards from the inferior end of the precentral gyrus it gives rise to dysphasia of expressive type.

The Parietal Lobe. Lesions of this area may also present with Jacksonian epilepsy, but of sensory type, and in addition there is disturbance of the integrative and localising aspects of sensation on the opposite side of the body.

Lesions situated more posteriorly in the parietal lobe may cause:

1. Spatial disorientation — lack of the patient's ability to find the way from one place to another.

2. Apraxia — loss of the ability to perform a pattern of movements though the patient understands its purpose and has no motor or sensory deficit.

3. Agnosia — loss of the ability to recognise a previously familiar object though the patient has good vision and sensation.

4. 'Sensory inattention' or 'perceptual rivalry' — the patient tends to ignore a cutaneous or visual stimulus on the contralateral side presented simultaneously with one on the same side as the lesion, though it is perceived if presented alone. This is most prominent in disease of the non-dominant hemisphere.

5. Receptive dysphasia — lesions of the angular and marginal gyri or the posterior temporal-parietal junction cause receptive dysphasia which may be predominantly for written or spoken speech. There may be specialised types of dysfunction such as the loss of ability to count or to recognise parts of the body such as a particular finger.

6. Homonymous hemianopia — deep posterior lesions in the parietal lobe may involve the optic radiation and so cause a contralateral homonymous hemianopia (Fig. 15.4).

The Occipital Lobe. Irritative lesions cause crude visual hallucinations such as flashing lights, while destructive lesions cause a contralateral homonymous hemianopia.

The Temporal Lobe. Irritative lesions in the posterior temporal lobe may cause visual sensations which are more elaborate than with occipital lobe irritation. Patterns of moving colours or hallucinatory pictures may be experienced by the patient.

A similar lesion of the anterior part of the temporal lobe may cause auditory hallucinations (superior temporal gyrus), gustatory and olfactory hallucinations (uncus) or misinterpretations (illusions) of auditory and visual sensations. These are often associated with altered states of consciousness such as dreamy states, automatic behaviour, temporary upsets of memory (*déjà vu* p. 617) or brief amnesia.

In affections of the dominant hemisphere there may be dysphasia of receptive type.

An important sign easily overlooked is a homonymous upper quadrantanopia due to destruction of the lower fibres of the optic radiation which sweep down into the temporal lobe (Fig. 15.4).

INVESTIGATION

The selection of appropriate investigations is based on the clinical picture and should always take account of the discomforts and dangers attendant upon the techniques employed. In a few cases extreme clinical urgency will demand that the definitive test, even if invasive, be performed immediately. In most instances, however, it is wise to start with those investigations which are least disturbing and only later to proceed to uncomfortable or hazardous tests.

Radiological Examination

Plain radiographs are important preliminary investigations in many neurological problems. A chest radiograph may reveal a bronchial carcinoma and hence explain a wide variety of metastatic and non-metastatic neural complications. Plain radiographs of the skull are indicated when the clinical picture is suggestive of an intracranial lesion. They may show erosions caused by tumours; thickening of the vault of the skull may be provoked by a subjacent meningioma. Lesions such as gliomas, tuberculomas and arteriovenous malformations may be delineated by abnormal calcification.

Radiographs of the spine should be performed whenever a lesion of the cord or nerve roots is suspected. The vertebral bodies, the pedicles and the disc spaces may display abnormalities which would localise the site and suggest the cause of compression of the spinal cord.

More complex radiological investigation is discussed on pages 606–607.

The Cerebrospinal Fluid

The cerebrospinal fluid (CSF) is secreted by the choroid plexuses in the lateral, third and fourth ventricles. It leaves the ventricular system through apertures in the roof of the fourth ventricle and flows through the cerebral and spinal subarachnoid spaces. It is returned into the venous sinuses by the arachnoid villi.

An examination of the CSF used to be almost a routine procedure in the investigation of neurological disorders. It still often provides information of value, but with the development of non-invasive methods of investigation the indications for its use are fewer. A lumbar puncture is essential when acute or chronic infection of the brain or meninges is suspected, and whenever subarachnoid haemorrhage is a possibility. It should usually be performed in patients suffering from multiple sclerosis or the Guillain-Barré syndrome. It is seldom of primary importance in the diagnosis of cerebral tumours or in the investigation of epilepsy. Lumbar puncture should not be carried out if there is a suspicion of raised intracranial pressure unless there is a strong possibility of meningitis.

In health, the pressure in the lumbar subarachnoid space with the patient lying on one side is 5–15 cm of CSF. Other adult reference values are given in Table 21.4 (p. 819). Note should be made of the appearance of the fluid. Normally clear and colourless, the CSF becomes turbid if it contains many cells. If blood-stained, the fluid should be collected in three successive tubes to differentiate between a traumatic puncture in which the later collections will be less contaminated, and a subarachnoid haemorrhage in which successive tubes will be uniformly red. Blood-stained fluid should also be centrifuged to see whether the supernatant fluid has a yellow tinge (xanthochromia). The CSF may also sometimes be yellowish in deeply jaundiced patients or when its protein content is much increased.

Laboratory examination of the CSF should include a cell count, estimation of the protein and glucose content and serological examination for syphilis. In appropriate circumstances microbiological studies, bacterial or viral, should be carried out.

Cell Count. The total number of cells and the different cellular components should be counted in a fresh specimen. Normal CSF contains less than five lymphocytes per cubic millimetre. In bacterial meningitis the cell count may rise to many hundreds or several thousands per cubic millimetre with a marked predominance of polymorphs. Lymphocytosis of moderate degree is found in tuberculous meningitis and viral meningitis, though in the initial stages of these conditions there also may be an increase in polymorphs. A slight to moderate rise in the lymphocyte count may be found in viral encephalitis, in active neurosyphilis and sometimes in multiple sclerosis.

Protein. A moderate elevation of protein may be found in many intracranial diseases including acute infections, neurosyphilis, vascular lesions and many cases of cerebral tumour. Very high protein contents are found in the Guillain-Barré syndrome and when compression of the spinal cord blocks the CSF flow. A few systemic diseases, notably diabetes and hypothyroidism, may also be accompanied by a rise in CSF protein.

The total protein in most cases of multiple sclerosis is within normal limits, but the IgG level (normally 6 to 12% of the total protein) is significantly raised (greater than 20%) in approximately two-thirds of patients with multiple sclerosis whether or not the disease is active. IgG is formed by lymphocytes (oligoclonal) within the central nervous system and not by passive transfer from the blood. Oligoclonal IgG bands are present in over 90% of cases. They are not exclusive to multiple sclerosis but may be present with raised IgG (usually accompanied by a rise in total protein) in neurosyphilis, in sarcoidosis and in some disorders of connective tissue.

The *Lange colloidal gold curve* takes little time to perform and is equally informative. A first zone curve indicates a large increase in the slow γ-globulin fraction.

Glucose. The CSF glucose is related to blood glucose, being approximately 1·7 mmol per litre below the blood level. A high glucose content, therefore, may be found in diabetes. A marked reduction in CSF glucose is a feature of bacterial meningitis; in severe cases glucose may be absent. A moderate reduction in glucose is found in tuberculous and carcinomatous meningitis. The glucose content is usually normal in viral meningitis.

Serology. Tests for syphilis are described on page 410.

Microbiological Investigation. Whenever infection is suspected the CSF should be centrifuged and the deposit examined microscopically after Gram staining, and, if tuberculous meningitis is suspected, after Ziehl-Neelsen staining. Cultures should also be prepared from the CSF in cases of suspected infection and antibiotic sensitivities determined.

In certain instances viruses may be cultured from the CSF, but usually the diagnosis of viral infection depends on rising antibody titres found in paired sera rather than by isolation of the virus in the CSF.

Miscellaneous Tests. In certain situations, more specialised and refined examinations of the CSF may be carried out. For example in carcinomatous meningitis examination of a fresh CSF specimen after cyto-centrifugation may reveal malignant cells. In cases of severe meningitis antibiotic levels may be measured in the CSF as a guide to treatment.

INVESTIGATION IN RELATION TO SITE OF LESIONS

The choice of more sophisticated and specific tests is determined by the site of neurological lesions. Such investigations include clinical neurophysiology (electroencephalography, evoked potentials and electromyography), radionuclide scanning, computed tomography and other imaging techniques.

Investigation of Intracranial Disease

A wide variety of techniques is available for investigation of intracranial lesions; harmless, non-invasive tests should be employed first.

The Electroencephalogram (EEG). This records the electrical potentials of the brain after they are attenuated by passing through the skull and scalp. Potential changes are recorded simultaneously over several areas. Intracranial disease may cause normal electrical rhythms to be suppressed or, more commonly, abnormal wave forms may be engendered. Such abnormalities may be generalised or localised. The EEG is the most valuable non-invasive test to confirm encephalitis.

EEG abnormalities are more marked with acute lesions such as cerebral abscess than with slowly progressive or chronic lesions. Lesions within the substance of the brain such as gliomas produce more marked and earlier abnormalities than lesions such as meningiomas or angiomas lying outside the brain tissue. The potential changes indicate the locus of a lesion but not its pathology.

The EEG is more precise in its definition of lesions lying in the cerebral hemispheres than it is in lesions lying within the posterior fossa. It will often reveal epileptic discharges but the EEG alone cannot make a diagnosis of epilepsy. As the disorder of function is paroxysmal, a normal EEG does not exclude epilepsy.

Evoked cerebral potentials, recorded from the scalp after appropriate stimulation of the retina, auditory apparatus, peripheral nerves or skin, are used to detect conduction blocks or delayed conduction in the optic and acoustic nerves, spinal afferent roots and central tracts. Their main value is to detect subclinical lesions which may indicate that a neurological disorder is multifocal, e.g. multiple sclerosis.

Radionuclide Cerebral Scanning. This is an innocuous and useful investigation. An injected radioisotope (such as technetium) is often taken up differentially by diseased intracranial tissue compared to normal brain substance. Differing intensities of radio activities are recorded through the skull and abnormal areas mapped. In this way tumours, particularly meningiomas, can be localised and areas of infarction defined.

Computed Tomography (CT scan). This is an accurate and sensitive tool and, with contrast enhancement, will reveal the vast majority of cerebral tumours, cerebral haemorrhages, and abscesses and also cerebral atrophy. It has reduced the need for arteriography and markedly reduced the demand for pneumoencephalography. However, it is not an infallible method of investigation. Small low-density lesions such as infarcts and some gliomas may be missed. Arteriovenous malformations, small subdural haematomas and intrinsic lesions in the brain stem may also be undetected.

Emission Computed Tomography. This is a technique of imaging in which technetium-labelled radionuclides are injected intravenously and the emitted radiation from the brain is recorded by scintillation detectors. As with CT scanning, a computer is used in order to construct a two dimensional image of the brain.

The technique is highly sensitive and exposes patients to much less radiation than conventional CT scanning. It can reveal morphological abnormalities and can also define changes in function preceding structural alterations, as in vascular lesions.

The equipment is costly and is used primarily for research.

Nuclear Magnetic Resonance (NMR) Imaging. This is a procedure which utilises the magnetic properties of hydrogen nuclei within the brain. The brain is exposed to a magnetic field and the hydrogen nuclei within it are excited by radio frequency radiation and the signals thus produced are detected and computed. The brain is scanned to produce images of brain slices similar to those of conventional CT scanning.

Since grey matter contains much more water (and hydrogen nuclei) than white matter this technique vividly differentiates grey and white matter. It produces imaging of the posterior fossa which is superior to that of conventional CT scanning. As well as revealing space occupying lesions it will demonstrate small lesions within white matter such as those in multiple sclerosis. It will be particularly valuable in the diagnosis of demyelinating diseases and in those metabolic and toxic conditions where demyelination is a feature.

Cerebral Angiography. With the advent of the CT scan, angiography is rarely the primary investigation in cases of cerebral tumour. However, it still has a place in defining precise anatomy when a mass has been demonstrated on the CT scan and operation is contemplated. It is also the appropriate investigation when clinical signs point to a lesion of a blood vessel such as an aneurysm or stenosis. Carotid and vertebral arteriography are uncomfortable and potentially hazardous and should be used only if there are appropriate indications.

Pneumoencephalography. This procedure is now rarely performed. Air, introduced into the lumbar subarachnoid space, rises into the basal cisterns and into the ventricles where it can show displacement due to tumour, or dilatation due to hydrocephalus or cerebral atrophy. Pneumoencephalography should not be done if intracranial pressure is raised. It is frequently followed by severe headache for several days.

Echoencephalography. This procedure utilises the reflection of a beam of ultrasound from the mid-line structures of the brain. It is subject to many inaccuracies and with the advent of more precise imaging techniques is now rarely employed.

Investigation of the Spinal Cord

Myelography may be required for the investigation of localised damage to the spinal cord and radiculography is used to outline abnormalities of the nerve roots. The contrast media used are not harmless. These procedures should be reserved for patients in whom the radiological findings will significantly affect management.

Investigation of Muscles and Peripheral Nerves

The investigation of primary diseases of muscle may require extensive biochemical testing. Of general applicability is the estimation of serum enzymes such as aldolase, lactic dehydrogenase and, most specifically, creatine phosphokinase whose concentrations reflect the rate and extent of muscle fibre disintegration.

Peripheral nerve disorders may also require a range of biochemical investigations such as vitamin assays, blood urea, urinary porphobilinogen and glucose tolerance tests to determine the primary cause.

Electromyography (EMG). Clinical neurophysiology is, in this group of disorders, more reliable than radiology but requires informed correlation of clinical and electrophysiological signs. Needle electromyography will differentiate between neurogenic atrophy and myopathic lesions. Measurement of conduction velocity in discrete segments of peripheral nerves, roots, spinal cord and brain tracts will help to localise certain lesions of peripheral nerves and the afferent tracts. Conduction is slowed by lesions affecting the myelin but may remain normal with axonal lesions.

Judicious use of all the available techniques assists localisation of lesions and indicates the type of pathology. The physiological changes are not, however, specific for aetiology. They are redundant if there is unequivocal clinical evidence of a myopathy or neuropathy.

Combined EMG and nerve stimulation at different rates is used to detect disorders of neuromuscular transmission such as myasthenia gravis.

DISEASES OF THE CRANIAL NERVES

The cranial nerves are frequently involved in generalised disease of the nervous system. In addition, there are specific conditions affecting a single cranial nerve.

THE FIRST CRANIAL NERVE

The olfactory nerve arises from olfactory receptors in the nasal mucosa. The fine first order fibres pass through the cribriform plate in the floor of the anterior fossa of the skull. They synapse in the olfactory bulb, and second order neurones run to the olfactory area of the brain (the anteromedial part of the temporal lobe) and to higher autonomic centres via the olfactory tract which lies under the orbital surface of the frontal lobe. Thus tumours of the frontal lobe may compress this tract and cause loss of the sense of smell (anosmia) on one side of the nose.

The fragile fibres passing through the cribriform plate are readily damaged by head injuries.

THE SECOND CRANIAL NERVE

The anatomy and central connections of the optic nerve are described on page 601 and the visual field defect caused by a lesion of the nerve on page 603.

Papilloedema means swelling of the optic nerve head (optic disc). The main disorders causing papilloedema are:

1. Increased intracranial pressure due to lesions within the cranial cavity such as cerebral tumour, cerebral abscess, or meningitis. The rise in pressure of the cerebrospinal fluid causes distension of the subarachnoid space round the optic nerve and compresses the venous drainage of the retina.

2. Obstruction of the venous drainage from the orbit by thrombosis of the central vein of the retina, cavernous sinus thrombosis or, rarely, an orbital neoplasm.

3. Lesions of the optic nerve itself, some of them inflammatory, may also cause swelling of the optic disc which is usually then referred to as *papillitis*.

4. Diseases of the retinal arteries such as cranial arteritis.

5. Extracerebral conditions such as malignant hypertension and severe chronic respiratory failure.

The earliest manifestation of papilloedema is engorgement of the retinal veins, followed by an intensified pink colouration of the optic disc and blurring of its margin which usually begins on the nasal side. As swelling proceeds the physiological cup is obliterated and the whole optic disc may be elevated. If the papilloedema is severe and particularly when it is of rapid development, there may be accompanying haemorrhages abutting on to the disc (Plate II). If papilloedema is of long standing the disc becomes progressively paler as optic atrophy develops.

Often it is of clinical importance to differentiate the swelling due to raised intracranial pressure from that due to lesions of the optic nerve which present indistinguishable ophthalmoscopic appearances. The visual acuity is usually well preserved when papilloedema is due to raised intracranial pressure whilst optic neuritis usually causes marked loss of visual acuity. Papilloedema due to raised pressure gives rise to early enlargement of the blind spot. Chronic severe papilloedema may be accompanied by peripheral constriction of the visual field. Optic neuritis causes a central scotoma.

Optic neuritis encompasses inflammatory, demyelinating and some vascular diseases of the optic nerve which, in common, cause loss of vision. In many cases pain in the eye aggravated by movement, and tenderness over the eye precede or accompany the visual disturbance. There is a loss of central vision and the direct reaction to light is impaired whilst the consensual light reflex is preserved. When the lesion lies anteriorly in the nerve there may be *papillitis* (swelling of the optic disc). Where the ophthalmoscopic appearances are normal, the lesion lies posteriorly and is called a *retrobulbar neuritis*. A light flash or a moving, patterned visual stimulus evokes potentials over the occipital lobe which can be recorded using an averaging computer. These *visual evoked responses*, known also as evoked potentials (p. 606), are delayed when there is optic neuritis and the prolonged latency persists, providing evidence of an earlier optic neuritis.

Optic neuritis is most commonly due to demyelination, itself usually a manifestation of multiple sclerosis, and in this condition recovery of vision within four to six weeks is usual. Rarer causes include vitamin deficiencies, syphilis and toxins, such as methyl alcohol.

The optic neuritis associated with vitamin B_{12} deficiency and the impairment of vision accompanying excessive smoking of strong pipe tobacco (*tobacco amblyopia*) may have a common pathogenesis. Tobacco smoke contains cyanide which experimentally has been shown to cause demyelination. Hydroxocobalamin, derived from vitamin B_{12}, plays an important part in the detoxification of cyanide. If the intake of vitamin B_{12} is low and cyanide ingestion is high, demyelination of the optic nerve is liable to occur. Tobacco amblyopia may effectively be treated by large doses of hydroxocobalamin.

Nutritional amblyopia is a progressive failure of vision due to a retrobulbar neuropathy which may occur in severe malnutrition. Sometimes in West Africans and West Indians the visual failure is associated with lesions of the spinal cord (p. 656).

Optic Atrophy. Loss of fibres in the optic nerve is followed by reactive gliosis and reduced vascularisation. These pathological changes are manifest clinically by pallor of the optic disc and may result from many causes including (a) optic neuritis from the various causes listed above; (b) pressure on the optic nerve by glaucoma, tumours, aneurysms etc.; (c) long-standing papilloedema; (d) thrombosis of the central retinal artery; (e) trauma.

THE THIRD, FOURTH AND SIXTH CRANIAL NERVES

The *third nerve (oculomotor)* supplies all the external ocular muscles except the lateral rectus and the superior oblique. It also supplies the levator palpebrae superioris, the constrictor of the pupil, and the ciliary muscle. It may be involved in multiple sclerosis, meningovascular syphilis, diabetes mellitus, and cerebral aneurysms which may compress the nerve at several sites.

The manifestations of a third nerve palsy are ptosis, diplopia, external deviation of the eye (divergent strabismus, due to the action of the unopposed lateral rectus muscle) and defective ocular movement in the directions in which the muscles supplied by the third nerve move the eye. The patient complains of double vision but in a long-standing lesion one of the images is suppressed. A complete lesion of the third nerve also paralyses the constrictor of the pupil; consequently the pupil is large and fails to react to light (by the direct or consensual path) or on convergence.

The *fourth nerve (trochlear)* supplies the superior oblique muscle. A lesion of this nerve gives rise to defective movement and diplopia which is maximal when the patient attempts to look down with the eye turned inwards. The pupils are not affected. An isolated lesion of the nerve is rarely encountered, as usually there is also involvement of either the third or sixth nerve.

The *sixth nerve (abducent)* supplies the lateral rectus muscle of the eye. A lesion of this nerve causes diplopia due to inability to abduct the eye, and deviation of the eye medially (convergent strabismus) due to the unopposed action of the medial rectus muscle. The sixth nerve may be involved by pressure from an aneurysm in the cavernous sinus. Downward displacement of the brain stem due to raised intracranial pressure may stretch the nerve causing a lateral rectus palsy. The causal lesion may lie at a distance from the sixth nerve whose involvement in this manner constitutes a false localising sign.

Squint

Squint (strabismus) may be paralytic or concomitant.

Paralytic squint is due to weakness of one or more of the extraocular muscles. Defective movement of the eye can be seen when the patient uses the weak muscle to move the eye, and this usually causes diplopia. The rules for identifying the paretic muscles causing diplopia or squint are:

1. The separation of the images is greatest when the patient attempts to look in the direction to which the paretic muscle should move the eye.

2. In this position, the most peripheral image is the 'false image' from the affected eye. It is identified by covering one eye with a green glass and the other with a red one.

Concomitant squint ('lazy eye') is due to failure to maintain the correct posture of an eye which is so defective in vision that its image is suppressed by the brain. There is no muscle paresis and both eyes are capable of full movements in all directions. The most common cause is an error of refraction during childhood. If recognised and properly treated with suitable spectacles the squint can be prevented, though a 'latent squint' often remains.

Nystagmus

Nystagmus is a series of involuntary, rhythmic oscillations of one or both eyes. It may be manifest in horizontal or vertical planes or as a series of rotations of the eye about its central axis (rotatory nystagmus). The oscillations may be equal in speed and amplitude in both directions of movement (pendular nystagmus) or movement in one direction may be faster than in the other (jerking nystagmus). When there are fast and slow components, the direction of the nystagmus is arbitrarily defined by the direction of the fast component. When severe, nystagmus may be present on looking to the side opposite to the fast component — this is a measure of severity, not an indication of nystagmus to both sides. It may occur spontaneously or be induced in response to a stimulus such as rotation of the head. When testing for nystagmus it is important to keep the visual fixation point within the field of binocular vision. Some normal people show sustained fine jerking nystagmus at the extremes of lateral gaze, especially when fatigued.

Types and Causes of Nystagmus. Pathological nystagmus results from impairment of the mechanisms controlling conjugate eye movements, namely gaze, fixation, vestibular, cerebellar and peripheral mechanisms.

GAZE NYSTAGMUS. Voluntary conjugate movements of the eyes depend on pathways descending from centres in the frontal lobe to brain stem structures which then relay impulses to the nuclei of the extraocular muscles. Gaze nystagmus is usually due to lesions of the brain stem. The nystagmus is of jerking type. There is no nystagmus when the eyes are in the central position but it appears on deviation of the eyes laterally. The faster component is always in the direction of gaze.

A special form of gaze nystagmus involves only the abducting eye on conjugate lateral deviation of the eyes. This is called *ataxic nystagmus* and results from lesions of the medial longitudinal bundle in the pontine region. The ocular movements are dissociated. On looking to one side, the abducting eye shows coarse nystagmus. The other eye fails to adduct fully and if it exhibits nystagmus this is of smaller amplitude. This type of nystagmus is common in multiple sclerosis but also occurs in brain stem gliomata and Wernicke's encephalopathy.

FIXATION NYSTAGMUS. Reflex mechanisms enable the object of interest continuously to be viewed by the macular area of each eye even when the object is moving. These reflexes are mediated through pathways which run from the eye to the cortex of the occipital lobe and adjacent parietal lobe and to the superior colliculi of the brain stem. Fixation nystagmus is usually present when the eyes are in the mid position, i.e. gazing straight ahead. A common cause of fixation nystagmus (often called ocular nystagmus) is defective central vision which usually gives rise to pendular movements. Congenital visual defects produce this type of nystagmus. Rarely fixation nystagmus is associated with diffuse brain stem lesions.

VESTIBULAR NYSTAGMUS. Reflex adjustments enable the retinal images to be stabilised, even when the head is being moved in space: they are evoked by impulses arising in the semicircular canals of the labyrinth and these are relayed to the central vestibular systems via the vestibular nerve. Vestibular nystagmus may arise from lesions of the labyrinth or the vestibular nerve.

1. *Disorders of the Labyrinth.* Imbalance between labyrinthine stimuli from the two ears leads to jerking movements of both eyes. If the lesion involves the end-organs in the semicircular canals or their central connections, nystagmus is precipitated by sudden movements of the head. Lesions of the otolith organs or their central connections cause nystagmus which occurs when the head is in a particular position.

Spontaneous nystagmus is present with acute lesions of the labyrinths but tends to subside in a few days or months. This tendency to adaptation may be seen during testing, as nystagmus, brought on by movement of the head or by caloric stimulation, is not maintained. It may be difficult to elicit again if the test is repeated. It is often associated with vertigo (p. 614) and this is also brief. Cochlear function is usually affected, causing tinnitus or deafness.

Labyrinthine nystagmus may be caused by inflammatory diseases (serous or purulent labyrinthitis), degenerative middle ear disease, hypertension, atherosclerosis of the internal auditory artery, head injury and Ménière's syndrome.

2. *Lesions of the Vestibular Nerve.* Nystagmus due to lesions of the eighth nerve has the same features as labyrinthine nystagmus. It may be due to an acoustic neuroma or neuronitis. The latter is a short-lasting disease.

LESIONS OF THE CENTRAL VESTIBULAR SYSTEMS AND CEREBELLUM. Spontaneous nystagmus, or nystagmus induced by head position or head movement may be found with brain stem lesions affecting the vestibular nuclei. Spontaneous nystagmus unaffected by head position and maximal on looking to the side of the lesion is found with some cerebellar lesions. The cerebellum also participates in the coordination of eye movements, as it does in the coordination of limb movements.

Central nystagmus often occurs without vertigo, but when nystagmus is present it tends to persist and neither the nystagmus nor the vertigo shows the adaptation which is a feature of a peripheral lesion. Central nystagmus and vertigo often occur without cochlear symptoms, and may be associated with other brain stem symptoms, such as diplopia, or with asynergia of the limbs or dysarthria if the lesion involves cerebellar connections. The nature of the nystagmus may be like that of peripheral vestibular lesions, but vertical nystagmus, or nystagmus which affects each eye differently, is always central in origin.

Central nystagmus may be caused by multiple sclerosis, vascular lesions such as occlusion of the posterior inferior cerebellar artery, pontine and cerebellar tumours, encephalitis, syringobulbia, or toxic states of which alcoholism is the most common.

Postconcussional vertigo and nystagmus may be peripheral or central in type, and they are often precipitated by a particular posture of the head. Indirect disturbances of the vestibular nuclei may occur when the intracranial pressure is raised. Nystagmus is then a 'false localising sign'.

NYSTAGMUS DUE TO MUSCLE PARESIS. All the above mechanisms need an efficient effector apparatus and hence peripheral lesions of nerve or muscle may also lead to nystagmus. This common cause of nystagmus is often overlooked. If one or more of the extraocular muscles are weak, as in myasthenia gravis, then the affected eye will manifest jerking nystagmus when it is moved by the weakened muscles. Thus a partial sixth nerve palsy will result in nystagmus in the affected eye on attempted abduction.

THE FIFTH CRANIAL NERVE

The trigeminal nerve has an extensive sensory distribution through its three branches, the ophthalmic, maxillary and mandibular divisions. It supplies the skin of the face (excluding the angle of the jaw), the cornea, the sinuses, the mucous membrane of the nose, the teeth, the tympanic membrane and common sensation (but not taste) to the anterior two-thirds of the tongue. The motor division of the nerve innervates the temporal, masseter and pterygoid muscles which are responsible for the closure and opening of the jaw.

The nerve fibres and nuclei may be involved within the brain stem by conditions such as syringobulbia and thrombotic lesions, and the peripheral nerve by localised pressure such as occurs in cerebral aneurysms in the region of the cavernous sinus, and by tumours of the cerebellopontine angle. The ganglion of the nerve may also be involved by herpes zoster, giving rise to the characteristic shingles lesion over the skin of the face and causing ulceration of the cornea when the ophthalmic division is involved.

Trigeminal Neuralgia

This condition, which usually affects elderly people is of unknown aetiology and without recognised histopathology.

Clinical Features. Pain, usually paroxysmal and sharp, is the characteristic feature. It is confined to the distribution of the fifth nerve. The maxillary or mandibular divisions of the nerve are usually first involved and spread from one to the other is common but the ophthalmic division is rarely affected.

Each paroxysm lasts for only a few seconds but the stab of pain may be followed by a dull ache, or frequent attacks following one another may make the pain appear to be of longer duration. The pain is precipitated by touching localised 'trigger zones' on the affected side of the face. A cold wind blowing on the face, washing the face, chewing or even talking may be sufficient to bring on an attack.

Paroxysms may continue for days or weeks, after which a remission of equal or longer duration may follow, but remissions become shorter and less frequent as the disease progresses. The agonising pain commands the patient's full attention. It may provoke a spasm of the facial muscles. No abnormalities of fifth nerve function can be detected on examination.

When a typical history is volunteered by an elderly patient the diagnosis is obvious. If similar symptoms occur in a young person the possibility of multiple sclerosis needs to be considered. Facial pain, mimicking trigeminal neuralgia, may rarely be a manifestation of a basilar aneurysm or cerebral tumour, particularly of a neurofibroma of the fifth nerve itself. When the fifth nerve is implicated in disease processes, the pain is often continuous and there are usually signs of fifth nerve dysfunction; there may be associated disturbances of other cranial nerves or neural pathways.

Treatment. Carbamazepine (200 mg t.i.d.) is the most effective drug. Phenytoin (300 mg daily) is also useful and may with advantage be combined with carbamazepine. Either or both of these drugs will reduce the frequency and severity of the pain in the majority of patients. Clonazepam (1–2 mg t.i.d.) is a useful alternative.

Long remissions may occur. If pain persists and remissions are rare or of short duration it is necessary to interrupt the central passage of pain impulses by injection of phenol or alcohol into a branch of the nerve, if neuralgia is localised, or into the Gasserian ganglion.

Section of the sensory part of the fifth nerve or its descending root in the medulla has the disadvantage of requiring intracranial operation but permits sparing of corneal sensation which is difficult to achieve with injection of the ganglion. These procedures secure permanent relief but the face becomes anaesthetic. Loss of sensibility from the cornea demands that special care must be taken to avoid trauma with its danger of subsequent corneal ulceration.

THE SEVENTH CRANIAL NERVE

The facial nerve innervates the muscles of expression of the face and, through its chorda tympani branch, carries taste fibres from the anterior two-thirds of the tongue. Paralysis of the facial muscles may be due to: (1) lesion of the fibres of the upper motor neurones concerned with voluntary movement; (2) lesion of the fibres of the upper motor neurones concerned with emotional movement; (3) lesion of the lower motor neurones.

1. Upper motor neurone fibres originating in the lower part of the precentral gyrus are distributed to the part of the opposite facial nucleus subserving the muscles of the lower part of the face, and to the parts of the facial nuclei on both sides of the pons which supply the upper parts of the face. Accordingly, a lesion of the upper motor neurones affects more severely the

voluntary movement of the lower part of the face, contralaterally. Weakness of the upper part (the orbicularis oculi and frontalis muscles) may occur transiently but is often absent because the lower motor neurones to the upper facial muscles are supplied by upper motor neurones from both hemispheres. The patient is unable to retract the angle of the mouth on command, but in smiling and talking the mouth may move well because emotional movement is controlled by upper motor neurones which are not those concerned with voluntary movement of the face.

2. Upper motor neurones concerned with emotional movement of the face take origin further forward in the frontal lobe and so may be damaged by a lesion which spares the fibres for voluntary movement of the face. Involvement of these fibres is revealed by defective movement of the angle of the mouth when the patient smiles, with preservation of the ability to retract the angle of the mouth on command.

3. Since the lower motor neurone is the final common pathway, complete damage to the facial nucleus or nerve abolishes both voluntary and emotional movements equally in upper and lower parts of the face. Lower motor neurone paralysis restricted to part of the facial muscles can occur only when the lesion is distal to the branching of the nerve, e.g. with disease of the parotid gland, through which the nerve passes, or in leprosy.

The most common cause of damage to the nerve proximal to its branching in the parotid gland is Bell's palsy but the nerve may also be damaged by disease of the brain stem, by an acoustic neuroma, or by inflammation during its passage through the middle ear.

Bell's Palsy

This term should be restricted to cases of isolated facial paralysis of unknown cause. Bell's palsy is accompanied by oedema of the facial nerve within the facial canal. It has been suggested that the swelling may be due to a viral infection since minor epidemics of the condition occasionally occur. Swelling within the rigid facial canal results in pressure on the nerve causing paralysis of function and sometimes Wallerian degeneration.

Clinical Features. The condition occurs in both sexes at any age. The first symptom is often an ache in the region of the stylomastoid foramen which may persist for a few hours or 1 or 2 days. A unilateral facial paralysis then develops. The eye on the affected side cannot be closed and the mouth is drawn over to the opposite side so that often it may appear to the patient that there is a spasm of the normal side. Saliva and fluids may escape from the angle of the mouth. Food may collect between the teeth and the paralysed cheek when the patient is eating. The patient often complains that the affected side feels 'numb', but there is no objective impairment of sensation of the skin.

In most instances the lesion is distal to the chorda tympani and facial paralysis is the only feature. In a minority of cases when the lesion lies proximal to the chorda tympani there will be loss of taste on the anterior two-thirds of the tongue and diminished salivation. When the lesion is proximal to the nerve to the stapedius, hyperacusis on the affected side is an additional complaint.

Physical examination reveals paralysis of the upper and lower parts of the affected side of the face. The lines of expression are flattened, the patient is unable to wrinkle the brow or whistle or retract the angle of the mouth. The eye on the affected side cannot be closed, and on attempting to do so the eyeball rolls upwards.

Treatment and Prognosis. ACTH or oral corticosteroids, if started early, increase the rate of recovery, maximum benefit being obtained if they are given within 48 hours of the onset of the palsy. Dexamethasone (2 mg t.i.d.) for five days is a suitable treatment.

Recovery occurs in over 90% of patients, usually after 2 or 3 weeks and is complete after 2 to 3 months. Approximately 5% of patients have permanent loss of function and develop facial contractures and involuntary spasms of the facial muscles. Complete recovery is virtually certain if there is any return of voluntary movement within a week after the onset and is probable if recovery of function begins within a month. A guide to the prognosis is given by electrodiagnostic studies. If the voltage required to produce a contraction on the abnormal side is more than twice that on the normal side, Wallerian degeneration has probably occurred. This indicates a poor prognosis. A good response after stimulation of the facial nerve within a week of the onset indicates that there is merely a conduction block and complete recovery is likely. Recurrence of Bell's palsy is unusual.

THE EIGHTH CRANIAL NERVE

The auditory nerve has two components, the cochlear nerve which is concerned with hearing and the vestibular nerve which is concerned with the appreciation of the position of the head and its movement in space. It is impossible without special tests to differentiate lesions involving these nerves from lesions confined to their end-organs in the inner ear. Irritative lesions of the inner ear or of the cochlear nerve cause *tinnitus*, and destructive lesions *deafness*. Thus, tinnitus is often due to aural causes but it may be an early symptom of a neuroma of the eighth nerve (acoustic neuroma) which is the most important destructive lesion of the eighth nerve. It may also be damaged in meningitis, and by the toxic effects of streptomycin or kanamycin.

Irritative lesions of the vestibular part of the eighth nerve cause *vertigo* which is a subjective feeling of movement of the external environment or of the head. The movement may be rotatory or a feeling of displacement in one direction. Vertigo is accompanied by a disturbance of balance which usually causes the patient to seek support and, if sudden and severe, may throw the patient to the ground.

The most important causes of vertigo are:

1. *Cerebellar Lesions.* Vertigo may occur when the cerebello-vestibular connections are involved but this symptom is not invariable.

2. *Brain Stem Lesions.* Atherosclerosis of the basilar artery, medullary infarction or syringobulbia may cause severe vertigo when they involve the vestibular nuclei. The vertigo may be produced by particular positions of the head.

3. *Lesions of the Vestibular Nerve.* An acoustic neuroma may damage the nerve and cause vertigo. Vestibular neuronitis is a more common cause; it is a benign short-lasting condition of unknown aetiology which may occur in epidemics.

4. *Aural lesions* of many kinds, including otitis media and Ménière's syndrome, cause vertigo.

The labyrinth may be damaged in a head injury and the vertigo may then be most severe when the head is in a certain position, usually backwards and to one side. A similar type of positional vertigo may occur in brief paroxysms. It is a benign condition which may disappear after a few months. The labyrinth may be damaged by mumps and by drugs such as streptomycin, quinine and salicylates. Hearing is almost invariably affected when the lesion is labyrinthine rather than in the nerve or its central connections.

5. *Ocular Lesions.* Diplopia may be accompanied by vertigo because the false projection of one image causes confusion regarding position in space.

Ménière's Syndrome

Ménière's syndrome is characterised by recurrent paroxysms of vertigo associated with tinnitus and progressive nerve deafness. The cause is unknown but the condition is associated with dilatation of the endolymphatic system due to increase in the amount of endolymph. Many patients also give a history of migraine.

Clinical Features. The most common initial symptoms are progressive deafness and tinnitus which are frequently slight at the onset. Sooner or later vertigo occurs and is characterised by suddenness of onset and severity. It may develop so abruptly that the patient may fall, and at the height of the attack may be unable to stand. There is often accompanying nausea and vomiting, and there may be sweating, weakness and faintness. Deafness and tinnitus may be intensified during the attack, which may last for a few minutes to several hours. Examination during an attack shows rotatory nystagmus and ataxia. Between attacks there is only nerve deafness with impaired vestibular function as shown by caloric tests. The frequency of attacks tends to decrease as deafness increases but the disease may last many years.

Treatment. No treatment will abort an episode of vertigo; during severe attacks the patient should lie still and may be helped by an intramuscular injection of 50 mg of chlorpromazine. Treatment is aimed at preventing or reducing the number of attacks and includes cinnarizine (15 mg t.i.d.), prochlorperazine (5 mg t.i.d.) and betahistine (8 mg t.i.d.). All of these drugs are taken orally and are sometimes effective but none is consistently so. If attacks are frequent and disabling, destruction of the labyrinth by surgery or ultrasonics may be required.

THE NINTH, TENTH AND ELEVENTH CRANIAL NERVES

These nerves are grouped together because isolated lesions of one nerve are rarely encountered. The *glossopharyngeal nerve* (IX) transmits taste and common sensation from the posterior one-third of the tongue and motor fibres to the pharynx; the *vagus nerve* (X) is the parasympathetic nerve for the viscera of the thorax and upper part of the abdomen and also supplies somatic motor fibres to the soft palate and the larynx; the *spinal accessory nerve* (XI) supplies the trapezius and sternomastoid muscles. Unilateral lesions disturb their somatic functions but do not appreciably affect visceral function.

These nerves or their nuclei may be involved by disease of the medulla such as syringobulbia or in their course across the posterior fossa by neoplasms and basal meningitis. Lesions at the jugular foramen, such as thrombophlebitis of the internal jugular vein following suppuration in the skull or neck, may involve all three nerves as they emerge from the skull. Glossopharyngeal neuralgia is described on page 624.

THE TWELFTH CRANIAL NERVE

The hypoglossal nerve supplies motor fibres to the muscles of one side of the tongue. Upper motor neurone lesions cause spastic contraction of the muscle fibres. The tongue is small and pointed but not atrophic. Articulation is defective (spastic dysarthria) especially for the lingual sounds. There is rapid recovery of function after a unilateral lesion of upper motor neurone type, but bilateral lesions cause permanent dysarthria. This may occur in motor neurone disease or in pseudobulbar palsy (p. 630). Lower motor neurone lesions cause wasting and fasciculation of the affected part of the tongue and, when protruded, the tongue deviates to the side of the lesion.

These changes may be seen in motor neurone disease.

The lower cranial nerves may be involved by carcinoma of the nasopharynx spreading to the base of the skull so otolaryngological examination is necessary. All cranial nerves, but particularly those emerging from the base of the skull, may be affected by bone disease in that area, particularly by Paget's disease.

THE CERVICAL SYMPATHETIC NERVES

The higher centres for autonomic functions in the hypothalamus are connected with some areas of the cortex, notably the orbital surface of the frontal lobe and insula. From the hypothalamus sympathetic fibres descend through the brain stem and spinal cord to their lower neurones in the small lateral horn of the thoracic region of the spinal cord from which they pass into the anterior spinal roots from T1 to L2. Fibres destined for the head and neck emerge mainly through the first thoracic anterior root, and ascend in the cervical sympathetic chain, reaching their final destination by means of the plexuses in the walls of blood vessels.

Stimulation of the cervical sympathetic fibres causes dilatation of the pupil, protrusion of the eyeball and elevation of the upper eyelid; conversely paralysis of these fibres results in pupillary constriction, enophthalmos and ptosis (*Horner's syndrome*). In addition, sweating is impaired on that side of the face. These signs may occur in lesions of the brain stem such as syringobulbia and thrombosis of the posterior inferior cerebellar artery, in lesions of the cervical part of the spinal cord such as syringomyelia, and in lesions at the thoracic outlet such as bronchial carcinoma at the apex of the lung.

THE EPILEPSIES

Generalised Seizures (grand and petit mal); Focal or Partial Fits (temporal lobe and Jacksonian epilepsy); Status Epilepticus

An epileptic fit may be defined as a brief disorder of cerebral function, usually associated with a disturbance of consciousness, and accompanied by a sudden, excessive, electrical discharge of cerebral neurones. The electrical activity recorded by the electroencephalogram (EEG) is of high voltage relative to the background and results from an unphysiological, synchronous discharge of an aggregation of neurones.

The basic mechanism of epilepsy depends on a population of abnormal, hyperexcitable nerve cells. Such susceptible neurones are subject to excitatory and inhibitory influences from other sources. Excitatory chemical transmitters released from connecting nerve terminals tend to depolarise epileptic neuronal membranes; inhibitory transmitters lead to hyperpolarisation of membranes. The discharge of the abnormal group of cells is governed by the balance at a given time between these two opposing factors. Acetylcholine is an excitatory transmitter. Gamma-aminobutyric acid (GABA) is an inhibitory transmitter and hence has anticonvulsant properties.

Epilepsy may be generalised (grand and petit mal) or focal (partial).

In *generalised seizures* loss of consciousness is accompanied by symmetrically synchronous EEG discharges. It has been suggested that generalised fits originate in midline diencephalic areas. The site of the abnormal discharge could be in the cortex and the generalised manifestations occur because of rapid spread to brain stem structures leading to loss of consciousness and then to the secondary evocation of bilateral discharges over the hemispheres.

In *focal (partial) fits* consciousness may be retained to some extent. The discharge arises in a localised area of the cortex; it may remain circumscribed or spread to adjacent cortical regions, to the opposite hemisphere via the corpus callosum or to the brain stem. In the last case sequential activation of both hemispheres may result so that a fit, initially focal, may become generalised.

Aetiology. In many, perhaps the majority, of cases, epilepsy arises from causes which at present cannot be identified. This large category of cryptogenic or idiopathic epilepsy includes many cases in which generalised fits first occur in children whose relatives are similarly affected but also includes many other patients without a family history or with atypical fits.

Any intracranial disease may give rise to epilepsy, either as a manifestation of an active pathological process or as sequel thereof. Important causes of 'symptomatic' epilepsy include cerebral tumours, head injuries and cerebrovascular disease.

Fits may occur as a result of disease elsewhere than in the brain. Hypoglycaemia, hyperglycaemia, uraemia, heart block, ingestion or sudden withdrawal of alcohol or drugs are but a few of the conditions which may evoke seizures. About 5% of patients with epilepsy are sensitive to light, e.g. flicker, and, in many of these, attacks are induced by watching television.

Clinical Features. GRAND MAL (Tonic-clonic seizures). These fits conform to a stereotyped clinical pattern in which several stages may be recognised: (1) a *prodromal phase*, lasting hours or days, may warn the patient that an attack is impending. This is an occasional phenomenon and usually takes the form of a change of mood. (2) An *aura*, which is uncommon in grand mal fits. When it does occur, it is brief, usually being no more than an apprehension that a fit is about to happen or a 'feeling' in the epigastrium. (3) The *tonic stage*, which is an invariable part of a grand mal attack. At the onset of this stage the patient loses consciousness and, if upright, falls to the ground. A sustained, tonic spasm of all the musculature occurs and involves the respiratory muscles, so that air is forcibly expired through the partially closed glottis giving rise to a sound or 'cry'. This phase lasts 20 to 30 seconds and during this time respiratory movements are suspended so that cyanosis occurs. (4) A *clonic phase* in which the sustained tonic spasm gives place to interrupted powerful jerking movements of face, body and limbs. The movements of jaw and tongue cause saliva to froth in the mouth. This stage, also, lasts about half a minute. During the tonic and clonic stages the patient may bite and chew the tongue and may be incontinent of urine and, less often, of faeces. (5) The *stage of relaxation*: After movements cease, the patient lies in a flaccid comatose state which evolves into normal sleep. This phase often lasts only a few minutes but may be prolonged for half an hour or more. After regaining consciousness there is often a phase of variable duration wherein the patient is confused and may suffer from headache.

PETIT MAL. This term is often used imprecisely. It is best restricted to those cases showing a characteristic EEG pattern, namely bilaterally synchronous spike and slow wave complexes occurring at a frequency of three per second. This pattern occurs with three types of clinical manifestation:

1. The most common variety of attack takes the form of a transient loss of consciousness. The patient interrupts current activity and may stare blankly ahead. The whole episode usually lasts only 10 to 15 seconds, and is so brief and undramatic that it may pass unnoticed. Such 'absences' may occur very frequently in childhood. Petit mal invariably starts in childhood but may persist into adult life. Sometimes the attacks cease during adolescence or give place to grand mal fits.

2. Less commonly the brief loss of consciousness is accompanied by myoclonic jerking of the arms.

3. The least common type of attack is the akinetic seizure in which the patient falls to the ground unconscious but recovers consciousness, and is able to rise again, almost immediately.

FOCAL OR PARTIAL EPILEPSY. Since there are many neuronal regions from which epileptic discharges may originate there are many clinical variations of focal fits. Any focal discharge may spread to become generalised, and initially localised clinical disturbances may progress to mimic a grand mal fit. It is important, therefore, to establish the nature of the phenomena which occur at the onset of any form of seizure since these indicate the site of origin.

1. The *temporal lobe* is the commonest site of focal epilepsy. Most characteristic of the clinical manifestations are hallucinations of smell though these are uncommon; hallucinations of taste, hearing or sight also occur. Also indicative of temporal lobe fits are disturbances of memory including the *déjà vu* phenomenon. This refers to the patient's sensation of reliving an experience or a feeling of great familiarity with the environment. Sometimes these features are associated with intense emotional or mood changes.

In temporal lobe attacks consciousness is usually disturbed but not necessarily lost. The patient often maintains some contact with the surroundings but feels remote from them, often likening the experience to a dream-like state.

Occasionally the patient during this state will carry out well-coordinated and apparently purposeful motor acts, even of a violent or antisocial nature, without any memory of such activity thereafter (*automatism*). Temporal lobe discharges do not always give rise to such distinctive clinical features and an EEG may be required in order to reveal the temporal lobe origin of seizures.

2. *Jacksonian epilepsy* is a term best restricted to fits in which clinical disturbance of function, initially confined to a circumscribed part of the body, spreads to involve adjacent areas. There is a relatively slow 'march' of clinical events which reflects the spread of the electrical discharge to nearby cortical areas. Motor seizures usually take the form of involuntary twitching or clonic movements which begin in part of a limb, spread to involve the whole limb, then perhaps the whole of one side of the body or the involvement may even eventually become bilateral. The extent of the spread is highly variable. Consciousness may or may not be lost.

Sometimes after recovery from a Jacksonian fit, the parts affected remain paralysed. This is called a *Todd's palsy* and if prolonged for more than an hour or two suggests that there is a structural lesion in or near the cortical representation of the paralysed part.

Diagnosis. Observation of an episode by a trained person is the best and most certain method of diagnosis, but is rarely possible. A good description by, and cross-examination of, an eyewitness furnishes useful, and often conclusive evidence. The patient's own account of the attacks and the circumstances attendant upon them will sometimes give diagnostic information. The EEG is not a substitute for this type of clinical assessment nor can an EEG, recorded between attacks, alone establish or refute a diagnosis of epilepsy. The EEG may be helpful in supporting a clinical diagnosis and may be of great value in localising a cerebral cause of symptomatic epilepsy.

After the diagnosis of epilepsy has been established the next stage is to attempt to determine its cause. In practice the most important aspect of this process is to recognise patients whose epilepsy is due to a structural or progressive lesion.

Fits of recent onset, of focal nature, occurring in patients of middle age, would obviously suggest an underlying lesion, perhaps a tumour. Accompanying headache and neurological signs would strengthen such a suspicion. Fits occurring for the first time in the elderly are often due to cerebrovascular disease. They may be the result of infarction, but some are due to cerebral ischaemia secondary to cardiac arrhythmias in such conditions as the sick sinus syndrome (p. 133).

The history and examination will often furnish pointers to the aetiology of fits and hence to the need for special investigations. An EEG and skull radiographs should be obtained in all cases. Before embarking on more traumatic investigations, the need for such tests should be appraised in the light of the clinical features. In many instances observation of patients over a period is the most valuable and least distressing course of action.

Treatment. The care of the patient comprises social and psychological as well as pharmacological aspects. Patients and their relatives and too many of the general public believe that epilepsy bears a stigma. Many patients are more socially disabled by feelings of bitterness and aggression engendered by society's rejection than by their fits. Simple, rational explanations of the nature and causes of seizures should be given.

Restrictions should be kept to a necessary minimum. Children, in particular, are often in danger of being overprotected by their parents, but until fits are well controlled it is unwise for children to cycle on public roads, nor should they swim alone in the sea. An epileptic child should be educated at a normal school unless there is an intellectual deficit.

An adult should be guided into an occupation in which neither the patient nor the community is put at risk by a propensity to fits. Exposure to moving machinery and work at heights should be avoided. The legal restrictions about driving should be explained to patients. In Britain no one who has suffered from fits may drive a motor vehicle until free of attacks during waking hours for 2 years. Continued treatment with antiepileptic drugs and the occurrence of nocturnal fits do not debar the patient from driving.

Note should be made of factors which precipitate attacks. Deprivation of sleep is an important factor. Some patients have fits only during sleep, or when they are pyrexial. Others recognise that certain sensory stimuli, such as flickering light or emotional disturbances, trigger their seizures.

During a fit the patient should be protected from injury. It will rarely be possible to break the fall during a grand mal attack because the warning is too short. The patient should be moved away from fires and sharp and hard objects. A padded gag should be inserted between the teeth if this can be accomplished without force. The incident should be treated with a minimum of fuss. Embarrassment because of public attention is usually the most distressing aspect of a fit from the patient's viewpoint.

Antiepileptic drugs will usually be needed to control fits. Phenytoin, phenobarbitone, primidone and carbamazepine are all effective in grand mal and focal epilepsy. The dosage needs to be tailored to the individual needs and responses of patients. Phenytoin and phenobarbitone have half-lives which are greater than twenty-four hours and can be given once daily. Carbamazepine and primidone should be given in divided doses twice or thrice daily. An average daily dose, for an adult, of phenytoin is 200 to 400 mg, and of phenobarbitone 60 to 120 mg daily. Primidone is given in a dosage between 750 and 1500 mg daily and carbamazepine between 600 and 1800 mg daily.

Hepatic metabolism of antiepileptic drugs varies because of genetic differences, and when possible, their levels in the blood should be monitored (Table 21.7 p. 820) so that the patients can be adequately treated and toxic effects avoided. It is better to use one drug, rather than a combination; only if a single drug does not control fits should a further anticonvulsant be added. Phenytoin may be combined with phenobarbitone or carbamazepine, though, because of induced hepatic enzymes, the serum level of phenytoin may be reduced when it is given concurrently with carbamazepine. Primidone and phenobarbitone should not be given together, since primidone is partially converted into phenobarbitone.

All of these drugs may cause drowsiness; they may also cause osteomalacia (p. 67) and folate deficiency resulting in megaloblastic anaemia. Phenytoin also gives rise to gingival hyperplasia in children and coarsening of features in adults. Rarer toxic effects of phenytoin include lymphadenopathy and a syndrome mimicking systemic lupus erythematosus.

All of these drugs have some teratogenic effect which is probably most marked with phenytoin. Until more is known about the teratogenic risks of antiepileptic drugs, carbamazepine or sodium valproate are preferable to phenytoin or phenobarbitone for the treatment of epilepsy in women in the reproductive years. The risk to the fetus is less than from uncontrolled siezures, so it is advisable not to change anticonvulsants during pregnancy.

None of the above drugs is useful in the treatment of petit mal. Ethosuximide is probably the most useful drug in this condition in a dose between 750 and 1500 mg daily. Effective treatment should be guided by serum levels of the drug when possible. Ethosuximide occasionally causes nausea, drowsiness and rarely, leucopenia.

Sodium valproate differs in chemical structure from other antiepileptic drugs. It seems to act, in part, by inhibiting the enzymatic breakdown of gamma-aminobutyric acid (GABA), thought to be responsible for terminating fits. Sodium valproate does occasionally cause potentially fatal liver necrosis and commonly weight gain, but as toxic effects are comparatively rare it is a drug of first choice for petit mal and grand mal epilepsy.

Other drugs, such as diazepam, nitrazepam and clonazepam can also be used in the treatment of epilepsy.

After the patient has been free from epilepsy for at least two years, antiepileptic therapy can be gradually withdrawn in many cases.

Status Epilepticus. This refers to a continuous succession of fits occurring without any period of recovery. Status epilepticus may be fatal if not rapidly controlled. It is commoner in childhood and in patients who have intracranial lesions but it may occur in all types of epilepsy if medication is irregular or is suddenly withdrawn.

Treatment should be prompt and energetic since status epilepticus constitutes a grave emergency. Adequate respiration must be maintained and the fits suppressed. Intravenous diazepam is probably the most useful drug for the control of status epilepticus. Initially 20 mg should be injected intravenously and this should be repeated at five minute intervals until the fits are controlled; thereafter the drug is given by slow intravenous infusion (no faster than 2 mg/min), along with intravenous phenytoin (no faster than 50 mg/min) to a total of 18 mg/kg.

In those rare instances where this combination does not control status epilepticus, chlormethiazole can be given intravenously. Thiopentone and clonazepam are also used for the control of status epilepticus; the intravenous use of these antiepileptics should be restricted to situations where facilities for artificial respiration are available. If seizures continue after maximum dosage, paraldehyde or lignocaine should be given intravenously while preparing for general anaesthesia with neuromuscular blockade.

Narcolepsy

This is characterised by irresistible attacks of sleep from which, however, the patient can be aroused immediately. Several attacks may occur in a day. Narcolepsy is associated with three other phenomena; (i) *cataplexy*, in which, as a result of a sudden emotion, power is lost from the limbs, though consciousness is preserved; (ii) *sleep paralysis*, in which on waking or falling asleep the patient is unable to move though mentally wide awake; (iii) *hallucinatory states*, in which vivid and terrifying hallucinations occur, often just as the patient is falling asleep. This combination of symptoms may be associated with disease in the region of the hypothalamus. In most cases no abnormality can be demonstrated in the nervous system. There is a strong association with HLA DR2.

Amphetamine sulphate (5–10 mg b.d.) or methylphenidate hydrochloride (10 mg b.d.) reduces the frequency and intensity of narcolepsy. Cataplexy often responds dramatically to treatment with a tricyclic antidepressant such as imipramine (50 mg t.i.d.). However, tricyclics and amphetamines should not be given together. Which drug is used will depend on whether narcolepsy or cataplexy is the patient's principal disability.

CEREBRAL TUMOURS

Intracranial tumours account for 2% of deaths at all ages. Neoplasms classified histologically as malignant and benign occur but the implications of these categories differ from those in other sites. Since they grow within the rigid confines of the skull all types of neoplasm may cause disability and death by impinging on and displacing the cranial contents. The clinical features produced by an intracranial tumour depend primarily on its site of origin and its rate of growth. The histological characteristics of tumours offer a guide to rapidity of growth and to the possibility of complete removal.

Pathology. Malignant cerebral tumours rarely give rise to extracerebral metastases, but approximately a half of all brain tumours are secondary deposits from carcinoma elsewhere, particularly in bronchus and breast.

Gliomas. Of primary cerebral tumours those derived from glial cells are the commonest. These vary in cellular type, in degrees of malignancy and in rates of growth. An astrocytoma Grade 1 is a slow-growing, infiltrative tumour which may spread widely throughout the brain, sometimes for years, before causing serious disability. A Grade 4 astrocytoma (also called a glioblastoma multiforme) is a highly malignant, fast-growing tumour causing rapid clinical deterioration. Other glial tumours such as oligodendroglioma and ependymoma are graded from 1 to 4 as the degree of malignancy increases. Medulloblastoma occurs most commonly in children, arises usually in the cerebellar vermis, and is almost always highly malignant. The various types of glioma account for a quarter of all cerebral tumours. They can rarely be completely excised.

Meningiomas comprise approximately one-fifth of intracranial tumours. They are almost always benign, encapsulated, attached to the dura mater and, in the majority of instances, completely removable. Their common sites of origin are the convexities of the hemispheres, the sphenoidal ridges, the suprasellar region and the olfactory groove.

Less Common Tumours. Craniopharyngiomas (p. 421), adenomas of the pituitary gland (p. 421) and neuromas from the sheaths of the eighth and fifth cranial nerves are benign and potentially curable. Cerebral lesions resembling tumours also occur in cysticercosis, as hydatid cysts, in schistosomiasis and rarely in other helminthic infections.

Tuberculoma is still common in underdeveloped countries.

Intraventricular tumours are rare but colloid cysts of the third ventricle and papillomas of the choroid plexus can cause raised intracranial pressure and are removable.

Clinical Features. Primary brain tumours occur at all ages with a maximal incidence in the fifth decade. Medulloblastomas are commonest in children. Acoustic neuromas usually present in the third and fourth decades. Glioblastomas and meningiomas are commonest in middle life. In general brain tumours in children are situated in the posterior fossa and in those over thirty, supratentorial tumours account for 85% of cerebral neoplasms.

Cerebral tumours produce symptoms and signs by their local effects and by causing alterations in intracranial pressure and hydrodynamics.

FEATURES DUE TO LOCAL INVOLVEMENT. The local effects of a tumour on adjacent cerebral tissue may cause paralysis of function and/or excitatory effects. The neural deficits produced by a neoplasm are dependent on the site of origin of the tumour. Lesions in the various lobes of the brain can cause the types of dysfunction outlined on pages 603–604. Vascular lesions affecting these same structures cause similar disturbances but those produced by tumours are characterised by the time course of their development.

In general the focal disabilities produced by a tumour are of slow onset and are progressive. The rate of this progression is highly variable and depends on the rate of growth of the tumour and its nearness to neural structures whose interruption evokes clinical signs. Occasionally localised oedema in the brain tissue surrounding a tumour will cause a rapid progression of paralytic symptoms and the picture thus produced may mimic a cerebrovascular lesion. Sometimes, too, the initial manifestations of a metastatic tumour are of sudden onset, followed by a period of improvement. Rarely, haemorrhage into a tumour causes an acute presentation of signs and symptoms which resembles a stroke.

In addition to local paralytic effects the infiltration by tumour cells of an area of cerebral cortex often evokes excitatory responses in neighbouring cerebral neurones. Thus a discharging epileptic focus may be a manifestation of a cerebral tumour. The nature of the fit produced is variable and depends on the site of origin of the epileptic discharge and the extent of its propagation. Focal epilepsy beginning in adult life should always suggest the possibility of a tumour.

Headache is a common, but not invariable manifestation of cerebral tumour. The tumour mass tends to distort and exert traction on nearby arteries, venous sinuses or meninges which are pain sensitive structures. Headache is often localised to one area of the cranium and its site offers a rough guide to the location of the tumour. In general headache is felt on the same side as the neoplasm. Tumours which lie in the anterior and middle cranial fossae are often attended by headaches situated in front of a line joining the ears. Posterior fossa tumours usually cause headaches which are felt over the occiput or nuchal area. There are many exceptions to these generalisations. Headache commonly accompanies an increase in intracranial pressure; its features are discussed below.

FEATURES DUE TO INCREASED INTRACRANIAL PRESSURE. Since cerebral tumours occupy space within the rigid skull they may cause an increase in pressure within the cranium. The liability of tumours to do this varies and several mechanisms may be involved. The mass of the tumour itself, if large enough, will cause a rise in pressure due to relative incompressibility of the brain. Slowly growing tumours may achieve large size before there is any rise in pressure whereas a highly malignant and rapidly growing tumour, though relatively small, may cause early changes.

Raised intracranial pressure may also result from obstruction to the flow of cerebrospinal fluid. Subtentorial tumours are particularly liable to do this but even supratentorial lesions may cause obstruction to the foramen between the third and fourth ventricles. Tumours of the temporal lobe may compress the third ventricle.

Tumours lying within the ventricles themselves may cause a sudden rise in intracranial pressure in the absence of focal neurological abnormalities. Increased pressure may also occur as a result of cerebral oedema or from obstruction of the cerebral venous system by malignant tissue impairing the absorption of CSF. Whichever of these mechanisms is operative the end result is a rise in pressure within the skull causing similar clinical features.

Headache is an almost invariable accompaniment of increased intracranial pressure; the pain is felt diffusely over the head and is aggravated by manoeuvres which cause a further rise in intracranial pressure. Thus headache is intensified by bending, coughing and straining at stool. Such headaches often tend to be particularly troublesome on waking in the morning when the patient is lying flat and to be relieved to some extent when the patient stands upright and moves about, since this causes a fall in intracranial pressure.

Clouding of consciousness occurs, varying in degree from listlessness and drowsiness to deep coma, depending both on the level of the raised pressure and the rapidity of its attainment. During the early stages of this alteration in consciousness there may be behavioural and personality changes with apathy and irritability, or withdrawal and inattention, predominating.

Generalised epileptic fits are commonly produced by raised intracranial pressure from tumours at any site.

Dizziness is complained of by many patients with increased intracranial pressure. This may take the form of true rotatory vertigo or of sensations of light-headedness or unsteadiness. Such feelings of instability are often produced or aggravated by head movement.

Papilloedema (p. 608) is one of the most significant signs of raised intracranial pressure. It may be of insidious onset and slow progression but equally often a sudden rise in pressure due to cerebral oedema or obstructive hydrocephalus causes the rapid development of papilloedema attended by haemorrhages radiating out from the optic disc.

The amount of visual disturbance produced by papilloedema is variable. Often there is little change in the visual acuity but the production of transient blurring of vision when the patient stoops or bends is characteristic.

Swelling of the optic nerve head is usually bilateral but may be unilateral in the early stages. When the underlying lesion has caused optic atrophy in one eye papilloedema occurs only in the other eye. Such is the case sometimes with tumours of the inferior surface of a frontal lobe which compress the adjacent optic nerve causing optic atrophy; as the tumour grows in size raised intracranial pressure supervenes and papilloedema occurs in the other eye. This is known as the *Foster Kennedy syndrome.*

Vomiting and progressive *bradycardia* occur as the intracranial pressure continues to rise.

Brain Displacements. The rise in intracranial pressure does not necessarily occur evenly over the whole of the cerebral contents and sudden alterations in pressure relationships within the skull may lead to displacement of parts of the brain. Large supratentorial lesions may cause herniation of the hippocampal gyrus and the upper brain stem downwards through the incisura of the tentorium. This not only causes damage to the hippocampal gyrus itself but may also lead to compression of the cerebral peduncles, occlusion of the posterior cerebral artery and stretching of cranial nerves, particularly the sixth.

These developments themselves cause signs which may lead to erroneous localisation of the cerebral tumour. They are called *false localising signs.* Commonest of these is a sixth nerve palsy occurring on the side of the lesion or bilaterally. The third nerve may similarly be involved and occasionally the fourth nerve is also implicated. The cerebral peduncle on the side opposite the tumour may be compressed giving rise to upper motor neurone signs on the side of the lesion. Compression of the posterior cerebral artery may lead to a homonymous hemianopia or quadrantanopia (Fig. 15.4). Very rapid downward movement of the brain stem may lead to haemorrhage in the mid-brain with coma and death.

Another form of herniation or 'pressure cone' is the downward movement of the cerebellar tonsils so that they impact within the foramen magnum thus compressing the medulla. This may lead to further aggravation of raised intracranial pressure since the onward passage of cerebrospinal fluid into the spinal subarachnoid space is blocked. Such an event is often manifest by loss of consciousness and the rapid development of palsies of the sixth and third nerves with dilatation of the pupil on the side of the lesion being followed by dilatation on the opposite side.

Frequently when a medullary pressure cone has occurred the patient takes up a decerebrate posture, at first intermittently. These developments almost invariably lead to death.

Such brain displacements and pressure cones may occur spontaneously because of increased cerebral oedema or some other alteration in cerebral haemodynamics caused by the tumour's growth but are particularly liable to be produced if the closed CSF system is disturbed by lumbar puncture.

Investigation of cerebral tumours should, in most instances, begin with simple and non-traumatic procedures including radiography of the skull and chest followed by one of the imaging methods described on page 606. A tumour causing headache will almost invariably be demonstrable by radionuclide encephalography. CT scanning and NMR imaging may be necessary to detect small lesions presenting with focal symptoms or for precise delineation to guide a neurosurgeon. A single EEG recording may indicate a local lesion, but serial recordings may show that it is expanding. Lumbar puncture should not be used for the diagnosis of intracranial tumour.

Treatment. *Medical management* of tumours can never be anything more than temporary or palliative. Medical measures for relief of raised intracranial pressure are often demanded in circumstances when surgery is not available or when the patient's life is threatened before investigation has revealed the diagnosis. This can best be achieved by the administration of dexamethasone 4 mg four times daily, initially given by injection and later by mouth; striking improvement in a patient's conscious level is often produced and sometimes regression of focal disabilities. The use of intravenous hypertonic solutions has largely been supplanted by treatment with dexamethasone but the intravenous administration of 50% sucrose or of a 15% solution of mannitol or of a 30% solution of urea can produce marked but short lived reduction of intracranial pressure.

Cytotoxic drugs, such as cyclophosphamide, administered either systemically or through a carotid artery, offer little more than temporary palliation.

Surgery is the definitive treatment of intracranial tumours. When possible the whole of a tumour should be excised but complete removal of the tumour depends on a number of factors. The tumour may be inaccessible and thus its exposure may be attended by unacceptable brain damage. It may invade areas where excision of small amounts of tissue may cause major disability as is particularly likely to happen in the brain stem or in areas of the dominant hemisphere.

In general, benign tumours such as meningiomas and neuromas offer the best prospects for complete removal without unacceptable damage to vital structures. Meningiomas can usually be totally excised and rarely is there any recurrence. Meningiomas of the olfactory groove, those in the suprasellar area and those over the convexity of the hemispheres have a particularly favourable prognosis. Often, meningiomas of the inner part of the sphenoidal ridge and within the cerebello-pontine angles cannot be completely removed but their partial excision results in long continued improvement. Even after a successful removal of a meningioma, a number of patients may develop recurrent fits.

Craniopharyngiomas can sometimes be completely removed but often the proximity of the hypothalamus prevents total excision. Pituitary adenomas can usually be extirpated and, even when only incomplete excision is possible, further visual loss is prevented.

Colloid cysts of the third ventricle and other intraventricular neoplasms can often be removed but sometimes their complete excision is technically very difficult.

Malignant gliomas cannot be removed completely, though favourably situated tumours may benefit markedly for a time from partial removal.

Less malignant, slow growing tumours such as Grade 2 astrocytomas and oligodendrogliomas, though they can rarely be completely excised, may benefit for many years from partial removal. The prognosis for cystic astrocytoma is particularly good if the cyst is drained and as much as possible of the tumour removed. Medulloblastoma of the cerebellar vermis, found in childhood, cannot be excised completely and surgery produces little improvement.

There is a place for palliative surgery even when complete excision of a tumour cannot be attempted. Partial removal or drainage of a cyst is often of benefit. Decompression and hence relief of raised intracranial pressure may be produced by removing part of the tumour, or even by excising normal brain tissue in the frontal or temporal lobes. Removal of part of the skull vault is also effective in reducing pressure. Internal hydrocephalus may be relieved by a short-circuiting procedure in which a drain is placed in one of the lateral ventricles and led into the cisterna magna.

Prognosis. The precise surgical approach and the prognosis for a cerebral tumour can be assessed only in the light of its site, its pathological nature, its blood supply and the degree of disability it causes. Early treatment is particularly important for those tumours which are susceptible to complete removal and which menace life or sight. Early diagnosis of acoustic neuromas and pituitary tumours markedly improves the outlook for their treatment.

Death is inevitable if a malignant tumour can not be removed, though it may be postponed by palliative decompression; even so, the average expectation of life is less than six months in the case of the more malignant growths. Benign tumours can be removed completely if they grow in an accessible part of the brain, as can gliomas, or even a solitary metastatic tumour, when they are in a part of the brain such as the frontal lobe or cerebellum which can be sacrificed with relative impunity.

HYDROCEPHALUS

Hydrocephalus denotes an excessive amount of CSF within the cranial cavity. It may be a consequence of atrophy of the brain parenchyma, which results in passive dilatation of the ventricles; it is then called compensatory hydrocephalus.

Hydrocephalus may, rarely, result from oversecretion of CSF due to a papilloma of the choroid plexus.

Much more commonly hydrocephalus is caused by obstruction to the CSF circulation or to a failure of absorption. Obstruction may occur anywhere within the ventricular system due to an intraventricular tumour or from extrinsic compression due to a space-occupying lesion or oedema. The narrow channels in the third ventricle, aqueduct and fourth ventricle are particularly likely to be occluded. Inflammatory exudate may block the foramina in the fourth ventricular roof or occlude the subarachnoid space. Absorption through the arachnoid villi may be prevented by thrombosis of the sagittal sinus.

In normal pressure (normotensive or low pressure) hydrocephalus the ventricular system is dilated, initially from an obstruction to flow due to trauma, meningitis, or other cause. The initial lesion subsides. It is postulated that the force exerted outwards on the brain is proportional to the surface area of the ventricles. These having been dilated, the force exerted on the brain, by fluid at normally innocuous pressure, is increased. The brain atrophies and the conditions for progressive ventricular dilatation and cerebral atrophy are established. Dementia and ataxia result. An operation which reduces CSF pressure by a shunt from a lateral ventricle to the superior vena cava sometimes improves the patient's dementia and ataxia.

HEADACHE

Headache is a term which literally describes pain felt anywhere in the head. Custom usually restricts its usage to pains in the region of the cranial vault; facial pain and nuchal aches are excluded, but the lines of demarcation are vague and overlapping.

Headache poses certainly the commonest, probably the most ambiguous and sometimes the most difficult clinical problem in medicine. It has a multiplicity of causes but is produced by relatively few mechanisms. In the vast majority of cases the cause is trivial and reversible but in a few patients headache presages sinister intracranial disease.

The extracranial coverings and arteries are sensitive to pain. Within the cranial cavity there are few pain sensitive structures. The brain parenchyma, pia-arachnoid, ventricular linings and choroid plexuses are insensitive. Pain can be evoked from the venous sinuses, the arteries and the dura mater at the base of the brain. Displacement and distortion of these structures, particularly if rapid, cause headache. The fifth, ninth and

tenth cranial nerves contain pain fibres and direct compression of these nerves produces pain.

Clinical Features. Pain in the head may be due to lesions in nearby structures, such as the eye and ear, causing referred headache; it may be due to the cranial neuralgias, meningeal irritation, vascular disturbances, traction and distortion of intracranial structures, or to psychogenic causes.

REFERRED HEADACHES. Eye diseases such as glaucoma and iritis cause frontal headache. Ciliary spasm induced by some errors of refraction may cause pain but 'eye strain' is certainly not a common cause of headache. Nasal and sinus disease causes pain in the malar, nasal and frontal areas which responds to vasoconstriction in the form of nasal drops. Dental and aural conditions may cause pain spreading far beyond the area of primary pain. Occipital headaches occasionally result from severe cervical spondylosis. A cold stimulus on the soft palate in some people evokes a dull, frontal headache (ice-cream headache).

CRANIAL NEURALGIAS. The episodic, lancinating pain of trigeminal neuralgia (p. 612) and the continuous, burning pain of postherpetic neuralgia (p. 644), both occurring within the distribution of the fifth cranial nerve, present well-defined and usually easily-recognised entities.

Glossopharyngeal neuralgia is less common and is characterised by pain, usually of a stabbing character, felt in the pharynx and deep in the ear. The pain occurs in bouts and may be triggered by swallowing and talking. It responds to treatment similar to that given for trigeminal neuralgia.

Temporomandibular neuralgia arises as a result of derangement of the temporomandibular joint secondary to an alteration of the bite caused by loss of teeth, ill-fitting dentures or habitual overclosure of the jaws because of tension. Pain which varies from a dull ache to intense stabs may radiate from the region of the affected joint to the temporal and frontal areas, the cheek, lower jaw and occasionally to the neck. In malocclusion, a prosthetic device to prevent overclosure of the jaw is a simple and usually effective treatment.

MENINGEAL IRRITATION. Headache is an almost invariable accompaniment of encephalitis and meningitis. It is probable that meningeal inflammation lowers the pain threshold of the pain-sensitive structures at the base of the brain so that minor mechanical stimuli produce headache. The headache is usually generalised though it may be more intense in the occipital region, is of a continuous aching or boring character and is frequently associated with photophobia and drowsiness. The pain is increased by exertion and even by minor movements of the head; the accompanying pyrexia and neck stiffness usually make the diagnosis obvious.

Blood in the CSF due to subarachnoid haemorrhage produces headaches and neck rigidity similar to those of meningitis, but the pain in this condition is characteristically of abrupt and even explosive onset and may be accompanied by loss of consciousness.

VASCULAR HEADACHES. These are almost always described as throbbing in character and are aggravated by head movements. They may arise from dilatation of the intracranial or extracranial arteries after overindulgence in alcohol, in fever and in the hypercapnia of respiratory failure. Severe arterial hypertension may cause headaches in the early morning. In the elderly, localised temporal headache may be due to cranial arteritis.

Migraine (see below) is the commonest form of vascular headache. A migrainous variant, '*cluster*' *headache*, presents a distinctive picture, which is unilateral, intense and brief. Many attacks occur in quick succession during a period of a few hours or a few days, and then there is often a prolonged period of freedom, hence the name 'cluster'. The pain is usually severe and burning, primarily involves the frontal region and the eye but often spreads to the face and sometimes to the neck. It occurs most commonly in young males, characteristically wakes patients from sleep and is often accompanied by flushing of the skin, rhinorrhoea and injection of the conjunctival vessels. It is thought to be due to histamine sensitivity and attacks can sometimes be precipitated by the subcutaneous injection of 0·3 mg of histamine. Patients sometimes respond to treatment with antihistamines and to the measures used in the treatment of classical migraine.

Rare causes of vascular headaches include saccular aneurysms and arteriovenous malformations (p. 632).

HEADACHES DUE TO TRACTION ON INTRACRANIAL STRUCTURES. Headaches may occur in the pres-ence of an expanding intracranial lesion such as cerebral tumour or subdural haematoma whether or not there is a generalised rise in intracranial pressure (p. 621).

Traction headache due to reduced CSF pressure may occur after lumbar puncture; patients tend to develop their symptoms when standing or sitting and a recumbent posture produces rapid relief. Traction headaches, whether produced by raised or lowered intracranial pressure, are usually aggravated by bending, straining at stool and coughing.

Benign intracranial hypertension is a rare condition usually occurring in obese women. It causes traction headaches unassociated with any space-occupying lesion.

PSYCHOGENIC HEADACHE. Rarely headache may be a feature of psychotic illness such as schizophrenia and it may occur in conversion hysteria. Most commonly, however, psychogenic headaches are associated with anxiety and depression, and other manifestations of these affective disorders may be present concurrently. Most patients suffering from psychogenic headache describe it as of 'pressing' character. Pain tends to be localised to the front of the head or to the vertex or it may involve the whole head. It is usually not prominent on waking in the morning and in most instances tends to get worse as the day wears on. It is often described as severe, continuous and unrelieved by analgesics.

Investigation and Treatment. The extent and nature of investigations to be employed are determined by the history. Non-traumatic procedures such as radiographs of chest and skull and computed tomography should precede more traumatic investigations. A detailed history followed by a meticulous examination will help not only to clarify the diagnosis but will also be therapeutic in patients suffering from psychogenic headache. Reassurance and explanation after careful clinical assessment of these patients is often more effective than analgesics.

Migraine

Migraine is characterised by periodic headaches which are typically unilateral and are often associated with visual disturbance and vomiting.

Aetiology. The condition is believed to be due to a disturbance in the carotid or vertebrobasilar vascular tree. An initial phase of vasoconstriction causes symptoms of local cortical or brain stem ischaemia and this is followed by vasodilatation. These changes affect both intra- and extracranial arteries and it is dilatation of the extracranial vessels which causes pain by stretching the pain nerve endings in the arterial wall. Pain may be prolonged by secondary muscular contraction.

There is a genetic predisposition; approximately three-quarters of patients who suffer from migraine have close relatives similarly affected.

Migrainous attacks may be precipitated by a variety of factors such as menstruation, flashing lights, stress and anxiety. Cheese, chocolate, sherry and red wine are common precipitants and are all rich in tyramine; experimental ingestion of tyramine will often promote an attack. Reserpine, which liberates 5-hydroxytryptamine (serotonin) in the brain, can also cause migraine. It is of interest that some serotonin antagonists are helpful in treatment. The significance of these findings is not clear but it seems likely that, in some and perhaps many instances, migraine is mediated by one or more biochemical disturbances.

Clinical features. The condition usually starts after puberty and continues until late middle life. Headaches occur in paroxysms and are often related to emotional stress. Attacks occur at intervals which vary from a few days to several months.

The first symptom is due to vasospasm. This is commonly a sensation of white or coloured lights, scintillating spots, wavy lines, or defects in the visual fields. Paraesthesiae or weakness of one half of the body may be experienced or there may be numbness of both hands and around the mouth.

These symptoms may last up to half an hour, and are followed by headache which usually begins in one spot and subsequently involves the whole of one side of the head; this may be the same or the side opposite to the visual or sensory symptoms. The side affected is not constant with each attack and the headache often becomes bilateral. The pain is usually severe and throbbing and is associated with vomiting, photophobia, pallor, sweating and prostration which may necessitate the patient taking to bed in a darkened room.

The attack may last from a few hours to several days and it leaves the patient weak and exhausted. In rare cases the cerebral changes may last for several days, particularly if the motor area is involved (*hemiplegic migraine*).

Rare cases of headache resembling migraine are caused by a cerebral aneurysm or angioma ('symptomatic migraine'). In these cases the pain is unilateral and usually associated with focal signs.

Treatment. An attentive physician, a carefully recorded history and a meticulous examination followed by a full explanation of the nature and phenomena of migraine often relieves the patient's anxiety about the possibly sinister significance of the headache. These simple measures are themselves effective therapy as is the physician's continuing interest in the patient's well-being.

Neither the patient's personality nor the stresses and strains of life can be altered, but such trigger factors as flashing lights and dietary precipitants can be avoided.

If the patient suffers only occasional attacks of headache at intervals of months, it is probably unnecessary to embark on drug treatment. For those whose lives are disrupted by migraine, treatment should include prophylaxis together with appropriate treatment to abort the headaches.

There are numerous prophylactic treatments; all are inconsistently successful. Phenobarbitone, diazepam or pizotifen given thrice daily often reduces the frequency of headaches. Occasionally other drugs, such as propranolol, monoamine oxidase inhibitors and tricyclic antidepressants are helpful. Methysergide, a serotonin antagonist, is sometimes effective but is prone to produce peripheral vasoconstriction and, rarely, retroperitoneal fibrosis; it should be used only in those patients who have not responded to simpler measures and whose attacks are very frequent, severe and disabling.

Treatment of a migrainous episode is based on the use of ergotamine, which should be given as early as possible during the premonitory stages either as ergotamine tartrate (1 mg) held under the tongue or in aerosol form. Unfortunately, all the oral methods of administration of ergotamine frequently produce nausea and vomiting. In such circumstances ergotamine suppositories are sometimes helpful. Too frequent use of ergotamine may, rarely, cause peripheral vasoconstriction. It should not be given during pregnancy, nor to patients with ischaemic heart disease or hypertension. Aspirin or paracetamol with metaclopramide may suffice.

CEREBROVASCULAR DISEASES

Intracranial vascular lesions are the third commonest cause of death in Western countries. The pithy and commonly used term 'stroke' describes the sudden neurological defect that often ensues. The annual incidence of strokes of various types is more than 1% in those over 65 years old. In every 1000 of the population in any one year, two people will suffer an initial stroke and one will die from a stroke. The high morbidity caused by cerebrovascular disease in the elderly is reflected in the large number of hospital beds occupied by such patients.

Despite the prevalence of the problem and its high cost in economic terms as well as human disability, cerebrovascular disease claimed, until recently, less attention and study then some rarer conditions. Diagnoses of 'cerebrovascular accident' or 'stroke' without specification are still common. Such imprecision in assessment leads to vagueness about prognosis and apathy in treatment. Conversely, attempts rigidly to link patterns of clinical disability to blockage of individual cerebral arterial branches have been shown to be simplistic and often misleading as well as therapeutically unrewarding.

Knowledge of the natural history of intracranial vascular disease is still incomplete. Cerebrovascular disease may be due to lesions of veins and capillaries as well as arteries but the latter are much the commonest. Arterial lesions can logically be divided into two main groups: (1) Ischaemic cerebral lesions due to reduced perfusion of brain tissue by blood and often resulting in infarction. (2) haemorrhagic lesions in the brain or in the spaces between the brain and skull.

This division into ischaemic and haemorrhagic lesions is pathologically clear and although clinical differentiation is often difficult the two processes should be discussed separately.

1. ISCHAEMIC CEREBRAL LESIONS

General Considerations. Approximately a fifth of the cardiac output normally passes through the carotid and vertebral arteries to supply intracranial structures. A reduction in total cerebral blood flow to less than half of normal will impair cerebral function.

Occlusion of a cerebral artery usually, but not necessarily, leads to *infarction* in the tissue it normally supplies. A system of anastomoses and collateral channels affords a safety mechanism. The circle of Willis usually provides wide connecting channels between the two carotid arteries and the vertebrobasilar system. Perforating branches from the major cerebral arteries and from the circle of Willis pass through the brain to anastomose with capillaries derived from other branches of the anterior, middle and posterior cerebral arteries which ramify over the surface of the hemispheres and penetrate through the cortex. A similar anastomosis between centrifugal and centripetal twigs is found in the brain stem where the vertebral and basilar arteries give off penetrating and circumferential branches. At the junctions between their respective areas of supply the anterior cerebral artery anastomoses with the middle cerebral artery which in turn anastomoses with posterior cerebral branches. There are also collateral channels between the internal and external carotid circulations through their orbital branches.

These alternative routes of blood supply to the brain mean that the effects of impaired cerebral flow are determined by complex factors. Systemic hypotension tends first to produce ischaemia in the border zones between the anterior, middle and posterior cerebral arteries. Variations in this pattern occur if, in addition to generally reduced brain perfusion, there is a superimposed local blockage in one of the branches of the three major vessels.

If one internal carotid artery is occluded in the neck there is an immediate increase in flow through the other carotid artery. Young adults who sustain a blockage within one of the four major arterial trunks may manifest no ill-effects. However, the occlusion of one of these arteries in the neck in the presence of widespread arterial disease (a likely accompaniment in the elderly) may give rise to extensive infarction. The compensatory mechanisms are less effective more distally and occlusion of one of the deep penetrating branches arising from the circle of Willis often produces infarction of predictable extent.

The effects of any arterial obstruction depend, in part, upon the rate of its development. Sudden blockage is more likely to produce infarction than is the gradual reduction of an arterial lumen which allows time for the opening up of collateral channels.

Reduced blood flow is often attributed to arterial *spasm*. Cerebral vasoconstriction occurs in young people and is responsible for transient cerebral dysfunction in migraine and may, in this condition, rarely lead to infarction. Spasm also occurs if cerebral arteries are manipulated during craniotomy and as a result of irritation after a subarachnoid haemorrhage or during angiography. Ischaemia may result from vasoconstriction due to hypertensive encephalopathy or to the concurrent ingestion of tyramine and monoamine oxidase inhibitors. There is, however, no evidence that arterial spasm plays any significant part in the production of ischaemia in elderly patients suffering from cerebrovascular disease.

Atherosclerosis is by far the commonest cause of reduced blood flow and arterial occlusion. Other causes are embolism and arteritis.

Cerebral Atherosclerosis

Atheromatous changes in cerebral arteries are almost invariable findings in people over 60 years old, but even quite extensive atheroma is commonly symptomless. Atheromatous plaques may cause narrowing (stenosis) or may lead to *thrombosis* and occlusion of arteries. Fibrin, platelet and lipid emboli may arise from such plaques in the proximal vessels including the aorta and be carried distally in the cerebral circulation eventually to impact in small vessels. These mechanisms can cause localised ischaemia or infarction or a generalised, progressive loss of brain tissue.

Aetiology. There is an association between cerebrovascular disease and ischaemic heart disease. In those patients who suffer an attack of transient cerebral ischaemia more people die from myocardial infarction than from cerebral infarction. Atheroma and thrombosis are related to both conditions. Despite this association the risk factors of cerebrovascular disease are not as well understood as those in myocardial ischaemia (p. 167) and there are notable discrepancies between the two. Genetic predisposition, hyperlipidaemia and diabetes seem to be much less important factors in cerebral than in myocardial infarction. Cigarette smoking and obesity have been clearly linked to an increased incidence of coronary arterial disease but not to liability to strokes. Hypertension is a factor which seems strongly to predispose to both.

Clinical Features. Symptoms are rare before the age of 40 years, and uncommon before 50. The clinical presentations comprise (1) a 'stroke', i.e. the rapid development of focal cerebral dysfunction, due to infarction, (2) a relatively slow, or stepwise, extension of an infarct — sometimes called a stroke-in-evolution, (3) transient ischaemic attacks wherein neural disability presents suddenly and recovers completely within 1 hour, (4) progressive, diffuse loss of cerebral functions. More than one of these patterns may be manifest in a single patient. After a series of transient ischaemic attacks a patient may present with a completed stroke which may also supervene during the course of progressive, diffuse cerebral atherosclerosis.

(i) STROKE. Haemorrhage and occasionally cerebral tumour, as well as infarction, may sometimes be the cause. When due to infarction, there are often premonitory features such as headache during the few days preceding a stroke.

The onset of focal disability may occur at any time. The patient may awake with an established lesion. Very frequently the deficit evolves during a period of 1 or 2 hours. Rarely the maximal level of disability will be attained within a few minutes and occasionally impairment will progress for 1 or 2 days. Loss of consciousness at the onset occurs in a minority of cases though drowsiness is common. Severe headache is unusual. Epileptic fits, sometimes of the focal type, occasionally occur at the beginning or during the extension of a stroke.

The neurological picture presented depends on the site of infarction. The area supplied by the middle cerebral artery is most commonly involved so that a *hemiplegia* involving the face, arm and leg on the side opposite the lesion is a frequent presentation.

If the paralysis develops very rapidly it may initially be of flaccid type, but spasticity and hyperreflexia are soon manifest and usually are detected from the onset. There may be hemianopia and hemianaesthesia on the side of the hemiplegia. If the infarct lies in the dominant hemisphere dysphasia may supervene. This familiar stroke pattern reflects the frequency of infarcts in the brain territory supplied by the middle cerebral artery but it should not be assumed that the causal lesion lies within this artery. In more than half of cases presenting this picture the primary lesion lies in the internal carotid artery or in more proximal vessels.

Other clinical presentations occur. An infarct within the area normally supplied by the anterior cerebral artery often causes a hemiplegia in which the leg is weaker than the arm and which may be accompanied by disturbance of micturition, apraxia or motor dysphasia. Lesions in the posterior cerebral territory usually lead to contralateral homonymous hemianopia with macular sparing and occasionally, if the thalamus is involved, diffuse, burning pain on the opposite side of the body. This thalamic syndrome may also result from infarcts in the area served by the anterior choroidal artery.

Approximately a tenth of infarcts involve the brain stem where they are more commonly accompanied by severe headaches than are those within the hemispheres. Vertigo, ataxia and vomiting, double vision and nystagmus are common features. A crossed paralysis, with ipsilateral affection of one or more cranial nerves and contralateral long tract (usually pyramidal) signs are characteristic of brain stem infarction.

(ii) STROKE-IN-EVOLUTION. The temporal pattern of a stroke is sometimes extended. Disability may increase by step-wise progression; sudden deteriorations are interspersed with static intervals. Less commonly there is slow uninterrupted progression; the deficit spreads and intensifies. The full extent of the patient's lesion may not be exhibited for 3 or 4 days; occasionally the disability may extend for 1 to 2 weeks. This type of clinical presentation, which suggests the diagnosis of a cerebral tumour, may be associated with occlusion of an internal carotid artery.

(iii) A TRANSIENT ISCHAEMIC ATTACK is a sudden deficit followed, within the hour, by complete recovery of function. Most such episodes last only a few minutes but should be regarded as possible harbingers of a more severe stroke in the next 6 months. If symptoms persist for more than 1 hour infarction has probably occurred. Symptoms depend on the site of ischaemia. Transient loss of vision in one eye (*amaurosis fugax*) and a hemiparesis or sensory disturbance affecting the contralateral half of the body are due to ischaemia in the *carotid territory*. Ischaemia affecting the area supplied by the *vertebral and basilar arteries* may cause vertigo, diplopia, hemiparesis or loss of consciousness.

The duration and frequency of transient ischaemic attacks are variable. Some patients suffer many attacks daily for periods of a week or more; attacks then cease and may not recur for months or years. Other patients have only occasional episodes at intervals of months. The attacks in an individual patient are usually stereotyped, the pattern and duration of dysfunction being repeated.

Frequently transient ischaemic attacks are due to emboli which arise from atheromatous plaques, are carried distally, lodge in and block small arteries and then break and disperse. In other cases flow through a stenotic artery may be reduced because of hypotension and may cause transient cerebral ischaemia. Occasionally, in patients suffering from cervical spondylosis, neck rotation leads to pressure on, and reduced flow through, a vertebral artery causing ischaemia in the brain stem.

An uncommon cause of transient cerebral ischaemia is the 'subclavian steal syndrome'. This may arise if the subclavian artery is stenosed proximal to the origin of the vertebral artery. The increased blood flow needed when the arm on the affected side is exercised may be met by blood from the unaffected subclavian artery via the two vertebral arteries. Blood destined for the basilar artery from the vertebral artery on the normal side is diverted down the other vertebral artery by vasodilatation in the muscles of the arm being used. The brain stem is thus rendered ischaemic.

Such symptoms as diplopia or ataxia, produced by use of an arm, should suggest the possibility of 'subclavian steal'. A significant difference between the blood pressures measured in each arm, and a bruit audible over the supraclavicular fossa on the affected side, are signs of the syndrome.

Some episodes labelled as transient 'ischaemic' attacks may be due to small intracerebral haemorrhages.

(iv) DIFFUSE CEREBRAL ATHEROSCLEROSIS. Gradual reduction in cerebral blood flow leads to progressive brain atrophy which is reflected in a clinical picture of blunted intellectual function and multiple motor deficits. Increasing dementia (*multi-infarct dementia*) may predominate but is usually accompanied by features of bilateral lesions of the pyramidal tracts, notably supranuclear bulbar palsy (*pseudobulbar palsy*). These defects cause lability of emotional expression, dysarthria and dysphagia as well as a reduction in spontaneity, drive and movement which mimics parkinsonism. In some cases true parkinsonian features accompany bilateral pyramidal tract signs.

Sudden accelerations of disability, or transient episodes of neural deficit, usually differentiate this type of vascular disease from other causes of progressive cerebral atrophy and dementia.

Diagnosis and treatment are discussed on pages 632 and 634.

Cerebral Embolism

The role of cerebral embolism in the production of cerebral ischaemia and infarction is consistently underestimated. Post-mortem studies have shown that at least half of cerebral infarcts can be attributed to embolisation from the heart or from atheromatous plaques in the large arteries in the neck and thorax. Transient ischaemic attacks are frequently the result of emboli from these same sources.

The disability produced by the lodgement of an embolus in a cerebral artery may be of very sudden onset. However, in many instances the pictures produced by cerebral infarction due to thrombosis and those due to cerebral embolism are indistinguishable in terms of the time, course and nature of the neural findings. A firm diagnosis of embolism demands evidence of a source of emboli and the presence of multiple sites of impaction. In many cases of cerebral embolism both criteria — and particularly the latter requirement — are absent. Arrhythmia, particularly atrial fibrillation associated with rheumatic or ischaemic heart disease, may lead to the presumptive diagnosis of cerebral embolism. In contrast evidence of an embolic source within large proximal arteries is often difficult to obtain.

Direct evidence of embolisation is occasionally provided by ophthalmoscopy. Emboli, composed mainly of platelet aggregations, can sometimes be seen in the retinal vessels of the affected eye during an attack of transient monocular blindness. The likelihood of embolic infarction may be inferred if there is a history of earlier transient ischaemic attacks. The presence of an embolic site is suggested by a bruit localised to the region of the carotid bifurcation.

More cerebral emboli arise in the heart than in any other site. Thrombus following myocardial infarction is the commonest source of emboli; rheumatic valvular lesions, infective endocarditis and atrial myxoma are other potential causes of cerebral embolism. A large embolus of cardiac origin may block the internal carotid artery at its origin. Smaller emboli often lodge at the trifurcation of the middle cerebral artery. Embolism at these sites is usually followed by thrombosis and complete occlusion.

A meticulous exploration of the possibility of embolic ischaemia should be made in all cases of occlusive cerebrovascular disease since the patient's management may thus be significantly influenced (p. 634).

Arteritis

A completed stroke or multifocal, minor cerebral lesions or a toxic confusional state may be a manifestation of arteritis due to systemic lupus erythematosus or polyarteritis nodosa. Associated systemic features will usually suggest the diagnosis. Cranial arteritis (p. 199) is a frequent cause of arterial inflammation in the elderly and occasionally the disease causes cerebral infarction.

Cerebral infarction may be the presenting feature of meningovascular syphilis and the possibility should always be considered when a stroke occurs in a relatively young person. Occasionally tuberculous arteritis, associated with meningitis, may cause cerebral infarction.

2. HAEMORRHAGIC CEREBRAL LESIONS

These may be the result of (a) primary intracerebral haemorrhage associated with hypertension, (b) subarachnoid haemorrhage usually from a saccular aneurysm or (c) trauma causing extradural or subdural haematomas.

Primary Intracerebral Haemorrhage

Intracerebral haemorrhage is strongly associated with hypertension. In malignant hypertension there is fibrinoid necrosis of arterioles, and vessels so affected rupture to cause bleeding into the brain. Patients with long-standing hypertension develop hyaline changes in the muscular and elastic arterial layers which give rise to small aneurysms that are also liable to rupture. The penetrating branches of the middle cerebral artery, notably the lenticulostriate arteries, are particularly prone to develop such microaneurysms and the majority of intracerebral haemorrhages occur in the region of the internal capsule.

An intracerebral haemorrhage usually presents abruptly when the patient is awake and is prone to occur whilst he or she is engaged in physical exertion. There may be premonitory severe headache and in over a half of patients there is loss of consciousness, sometimes accompanied by an epileptic fit. Since the internal capsule is so frequently involved, a hemiplegia commonly supervenes and initially may be of the flaccid type. When the haemorrhage is massive and bleeding persists, intracranial pressure is raised; coma deepens and papilloedema develops. Haemorrhages frequently extend into the lateral or third ventricles and sometimes there is rupture through the surface of the brain into the subarachnoid space so that in many cases of initially intracerebral haemorrhage, blood is found in the cerebrospinal fluid.

A massive haemorrhage accompanied by loss of consciousness has a grave prognosis; approximately a half of patients die within a few days. Smaller haemorrhages occurring in any part of the brain may present a clinical picture indistinguishable from infarction.

Haemorrhage into the pons usually produces rapid loss of consciousness, pinpoint pupils and periodic respiration; often there is bilateral involvement of cranial nerves and pyramidal pathways. Hyperpyrexia is sometimes a feature.

Cerebellar haemorrhage is frequently of abrupt onset and is usually ushered in by occipital headache, vomiting, vertigo and ataxia. Consciousness is often lost after a few hours at which time the patient frequently develops pupillary constriction and a contralateral hemiplegia from involvement of the brain stem.

Subarachnoid Haemorrhage

Haemorrhage into the subarachnoid space is the result of rupture of an aneurysm in over 50% of cases. In about 5% the source of bleeding is an arteriovenous malformation. In older patients subarachnoid haemorrhage is usually the result of diffuse cerebrovascular disease. Other causes are trauma, extension of an intracerebral haemorrhage or a bleeding cerebral tumour.

The onset of subarachnoid haemorrhage is often marked by severe and sudden headache, which is sometimes followed by impairment or loss of consciousness. There may be focal features whose nature depends on the site of the lesion; diplopia or other cranial nerve lesions, hemiparesis and aphasia occur. Signs of meningeal irritation, i.e. neck stiffness and a positive Kernig's sign, develop. Ophthalmoscopy may reveal unilateral or bilateral haemorrhages between the retina and the hyaloid membrane. The shape of these subhyaloid haemorrhages is determined by gravity so that the upper border is horizontal if the patient is sitting upright. If the subarachnoid haemorrhage is extensive and continuous, papilloedema may occur.

The outlook for subarachnoid haemorrhage due to an extension of intracerebral bleeding is similar to that of the primary condition. If sub-arachnoid haemorrhage is due to the rupture of a saccular aneurysm bleeding is liable to recur within 6 to 8 weeks.

Saccular Aneurysm. The first manifestation of an intracranial aneurysm is often a subarachnoid haemorrhage, but sometimes aneurysms present focal features before rupture. The nature of these depends on the site of the aneurysm. An aneurysm of the internal carotid artery within the cavernous sinus usually causes pain or paraesthesiae in the distribution of the ophthalmic division of the fifth nerve, and a third nerve palsy, sometimes accompanied by palsies of the fourth and sixth nerves. Rarely, an aneurysm of the internal carotid artery will rupture into the cavernous sinus, forming a caroticocavernous fistula. This causes severe pain in and around the eye, pulsatile exophthalmos, papilloedema and complete ophthalmoplegia. A loud bruit can usually be heard over the affected eye.

Aneurysm of the supraclinoid part of the internal carotid artery may compress the optic nerve, chiasma or tract leading to impaired visual acuity and a variety of scotomata and visual field defects. These disturbances may be accompanied by paralysis of the third nerve.

Aneurysms of the middle cerebral artery tend to present with bleeding, but occasionally their presence will be heralded by focal epilepsy or by a progressive hemiparesis. Anterior communicating and anterior cerebral aneurysms may compress the optic chiasma from above, resulting in bilateral loss of the inferior part of the visual fields.

Posterior communicating aneurysms often lead to an isolated third nerve palsy. Aneurysms of the posterior cerebral artery may compress the cerebral peduncle and the adjacent third nerve causing an ipsilateral third nerve palsy and contralateral pyramidal tract signs.

Arteriovenous Malformation. A subarachnoid haemorrhage without antecedent clinical features is the commonest presentation of an arteriovenous malformation. Some present with focal epilepsy accompanied later by progressive focal signs and others cause recurrent localised headaches of throbbing character which superficially may resemble migraine. A bruit may be heard through the skull overlying a large arteriovenous malformation.

Extradural and Subdural Haematoma

Extradural haematomas are produced by skull fractures involving the branches of the middle meningeal artery. Symptoms usually develop a few hours after the injury. Coma rapidly ensues with an obvious hemiparesis. Later there are signs of tentorial herniation which often rapidly causes death so that operation should be undertaken urgently.

Subdural haematoma may occur as an acute complication of a head injury resulting from venous haemorrhage into the subdural space. The picture then resembles that of an extradural haematoma.

A *chronic subdural haematoma* may follow a minor head injury especially in an elderly person. Often the injury is so slight that it is forgotten. After an interval of weeks or months the patient may present with headache, a confusional state, or the development of focal neurological signs such as hemiparesis. Characteristically, as the subdural haematoma increases in size, there is fluctuation in the level of consciousness, and, later, signs of raised intracranial pressure may be manifest. The progressive changes may closely mimic a cerebral tumour and require investigation along similar lines. Exploratory burr holes in the skull may confirm the diagnosis and produce dramatic benefit in the case of a haematoma.

Diagnosis of Cerebrovascular Disease

Clinical Features. The diagnosis and assessment of a patient suffering from cerebrovascular disease ideally comprises four stages. Firstly, the nature of the patient's disabilities are defined and the site and extent of the lesion inferred. Secondly, other possible causes of the disturbance of function are excluded. Thirdly, the nature of the vascular pathology is determined. Fourthly, the state of the systemic circulation is investigated and associated diseases delineated.

The time course of a completed stroke will usually suggest the correct diagnosis. Occasionally patients suffering from a cerebral tumour will present with a rapidly developing disability. Multiple sclerosis and demyelinating encephalopathies present acutely but in most instances the age of onset, multiple lesions affecting the spinal cord as well as the brain and a characteristic earlier history will distinguish these conditions from cerebrovascular disease. The progression of a stroke-in-evolution may closely imitate the features of a rapidly growing cerebral tumour.

Transient ischaemic attacks may need to be distinguished from epilepsy and migraine. Consciousness is unimpaired in most transient ischaemic attacks. Migraine rarely presents after the age of 50 years whilst transient ischaemic attacks usually occur after this age. Transient ischaemic episodes are rarely accompanied or followed by headaches.

Progressive, diffuse, cerebral atherosclerosis may be difficult to distinguish from other forms of senile and presenile dementia and the diagnosis should not be made too readily. The occurrence of acute focal disabilities, interrupting otherwise steady deterioration, is in favour of diffuse cerebral atherosclerosis as is circumstantial evidence such as accompanying hypertension, peripheral vascular disease or myocardial ischaemia. In most instances the history and clinical findings will differentiate cerebrovascular disease from other intracranial lesions. In a minority of instances special investigations will be required to confirm the diagnosis.

The elucidation of the type of cerebrovascular disease is sometimes difficult. It is important rapidly to define those conditions which require life-saving, urgent or specific treatment. The history of trauma and the clinical features are distinctive in extradural and acute subdural haematoma. The diagnosis of chronic subdural haematoma can occasionally be made with confidence on clinical grounds but the possibility of this condition should be considered and investigated particularly in an elderly patient manifesting a progressive cerebral deficit accompanied by headache. Signs of meningeal irritation indicate a subarachnoid bleed which can be confirmed by CT scan or lumbar puncture. Arteritis will often be diagnosed because of accompanying systemic clinical features and by the results of simple investigations such as a raised ESR, positive ANF or positive serology for syphilis.

An attempt should be made to distinguish between patients with cerebral infarction and those who have bled into the brain. A history of transient ischaemic attacks favours a diagnosis of infarction rather than haemorrhage. The development of neural disability during sleep is likely to be due to infarction; onset during exertion suggests a haemorrhage. Blood in the CSF obviously indicates intracranial bleeding. A source of emboli is in favour of arterial occlusion rather than rupture. Hypertension is frequently associated with both infarction and haemorrhage but severe hypertension, particularly in young patients, predisposes to haemorrhage. Though these clinical hints are generally valid they do not provide firm criteria for differentiating thrombosis, embolism and haemorrhage.

The cerebral circulation cannot be considered in isolation. In any patient who suffers from cerebrovascular disease the status of heart, blood pressure, blood vessels and blood should be carefully appraised. The heart should be examined to define the presence or absence of arrhythmias, valvular or myocardial lesions and heart failure. Peripheral limb vessels and the arteries in the neck should be palpated and auscultated to detect changes in the wall and the presence of stenoses. Recordings of the blood pressure are mandatory. Abnormalities of the blood, particularly anaemia, polycythaemia and thrombocytopenia should be sought.

Investigation. The extent to which diagnostic investigations should be pursued depends on individual circumstances.

Computed tomography will not only reveal tumours but in many instances will define the nature of cerebrovascular lesions. Intracerebral bleeding gives high density abnormalities so that even very small haemorrhages are detected. Intraventricular, subarachnoid and subdural haemorrhages are readily distinguished and sequential scanning will monitor the subsequent organisation and resolution of intracerebral haematomas. Ruptured aneurysms can be differentiated from primary intracerebral haemorrhage in almost all instances and the site of the aneurysms predicted with fair accuracy.

Cerebral infarction leads to low density abnormalities which may be detectable within a few hours of onset. Some infarcts are not revealed by computed tomography but even in these cases the confident exclusion of tumours and haemorrhage enables a firm presumptive diagnosis to be made.

Other investigations are less informative. The EEG usually shows marked abnormalities after infarction or haemorrhage and serial recordings demonstrate progressive improvement. Similar EEG abnormalities due to tumour persist and become more marked. Facial thermography may indicate reduction of flow through a carotid artery. Cerebral angiography should be undertaken only if surgery is likely to be required. It should be performed if there is evidence of a tumour, vascular malformation, subdural haematoma or extracranial vascular disease in a young patient which might be amenable to surgical treatment.

Treatment of Cerebrovascular Disease

The management of patients suffering from cerebrovascular disease should be approached in a logical sequence. Initially patients may need to be protected from the dangers of unconsciousness and immobility. The causal lesion should be treated if possible and measures to improve functional recovery instituted. Patients who survive but are left with residual disability need support and rehabilitation. Finally, progression and recurrence of cerebrovascular lesions should, as far as possible, be prevented.

General Measures. An adequate airway should be established in those patients whose consciousness is impaired. The patient's fluid and nutritional intake should be maintained, employing a nasogastric tube or intravenous infusion if necessary. Pressure sores should be prevented by frequent alteration of the patient's posture, the use of pads and massage of vulnerable areas of skin. Catheterisation may be needed because of urinary incontinence. Rapid cleaning is required for the patient who is incontinent of faeces. Passive movement of limbs should be started early and the patient should be moved from bed and sat in a chair for periods during the day as soon as possible. Intercurrent urinary or respiratory infections should be treated with appropriate antimicrobial agents.

Specific Medical Treatment. A minority of patients have treatable underlying conditions. Hypertension should be controlled. Those with meningovascular syphilis should be given a course of penicillin. Those suffering from temporal arteritis or a connective tissue disease may need corticosteroids. Polycythaemia vera or anaemia should be treated appropriately.

Neurosurgery. Early referral (within 24 hours) to a neurosurgeon with a view to operation is required for patients who have bled from a ruptured aneurysm. The neck of the aneurysm should be clipped if this is technically possible. The wall of the aneurysm may be reinforced by plastic or muscle. If such a direct attack is impracticable carotid ligation may reduce the liability to further bleeding from the aneurysm. Surgical drainage of extradural and subdural haematomas usually produces dramatic and rapid improvement.

Stroke. Little can be done to reverse the effects of infarction or haemorrhage. In a very few instances blood flow has rapidly been restored through an occluded carotid artery by surgical removal of thrombus. This is effective only when the affected artery is accessible and when the operation is carried out within a few hours of the onset of the symptoms. These conditions very rarely obtain.

Treatment is aimed at minimising the extent of brain death. Around the margins of an infarct or haemorrhage there is potentially viable tissue whose function can be restored if an alternative supply of blood is available. Attempts to provoke cerebral vasodilation have not been effective and it is likely that the promotion of generalised cerebral vasodilation could be harmful by 'stealing' blood from the damaged area.

Low-molecular-weight dextran has been employed in the expectation that its effects in decreasing the aggregation of platelets and blood viscosity would improve cerebral circulation. 500 ml of a 10% solution of dextran in glucose is given intravenously as early as possible after the onset of symptoms and repeated at 12-hourly intervals for three days. There is evidence that this treatment reduces the early death rate from severe strokes but there is no long-lasting benefit.

Anticoagulants have no place in the treatment of an established stroke. Thrombolytic agents such as streptokinase are ineffective. There is thus as yet no specific medical treatment available which significantly and consistently improves the outlook for patients who have suffered a stroke.

Stroke-in-evolution. The early use of anticoagulants has been advocated to halt progression in an evolving stroke. There is some evidence that this treatment does help but there is a danger that anticoagulants may cause haemorrhage and before they are used in this situation an intracerebral haemorrhage must be excluded by investigation. There may be a place for the use of low-molecular-weight dextran in the treatment of a stroke of gradual development.

Transient Ischaemic Attacks. Anticoagulants (p. 547) seem to reduce the incidence of future strokes. Inhibitors of platelet aggregation have also been employed, namely aspirin 150 mg b.d. dipyridamole 25 mg four times daily or sulphinpyrazone 200 mg four times daily. Their efficacy has not yet been fully assessed.

Cerebral Embolism. Anticoagulants should be given, provided other conditions do not contraindicate their use.

Rehabilitation. A large number of patients are left with residual deficits as a result of cerebrovascular lesions. Much can be done to mitigate disabilities so that patients can live a largely independent life in the community. Early institution of treatment is essential. In the period immediately following a stroke, passive movements of limbs should be practised. Supervised exercises and encouragement should later aim at the development of mobility. Few patients, no matter how severe their original hemiplegia, cannot be taught to walk again. Later the patient should be guided in the performance of the activities of everyday living. Modifications of dress, housing, baths, lavatories and kitchen equipment may enable the patient to cope at home.

Throughout the period of rehabilitation communication should be encouraged, using, if appropriate, the skills of the speech therapist. The degree and extent of paralysis is less of a bar to successful rehabilitation than are disorders of perception, spatial disorientation, dysphasia and, particularly, dementia. Active cooperation between physicians, nurses, physiotherapists, occupational therapists, speech therapists and social workers improves the end result of the physical and social rehabilitation of patients who have had a stroke. The recruitment and education of relatives enables them to continue rehabilitation at home.

Prevention of Recurrence. Some of the treatments outlined above, such as anticoagulant therapy and inhibitors of platelet aggregation, are preventive measures. The most important prophylactic factor is the control of hypertension by appropriate drugs (p. 181). It has been shown conclusively that early, effective and continued reduction of high blood pressure significantly improves the outlook for both occlusive and haemorrhagic cerebrovascular disease.

The role of surgery on the carotid artery or by extracranial to intracranial arterial bypass remains uncertain because of lack of acceptable controlled trials.

Prognosis for an individual suffering from a cerebrovascular lesion depends on complex factors. There are some general guidelines. In one well-studied series of strokes the mortality within the first month after infarction was roughly 30%. From proven intracerebral haemorrhage the mortality in the same period was 80%. After a subarachnoid haemorrhage 65% died within 1 month. This investigation emphasised the poor prognosis after large haemorrhagic lesions.

Many epidemiological studies have stressed the general tendency of clinicians to overestimate the incidence of cerebral haemorrhage. Data from death certificates suggest that haemorrhage is twice as common as infarction whereas careful clinical differentiation of the two types of lesion indicates that infarction is at least five times commoner than haemorrhage and in those over 75 years of age, 20 times more frequent.

Signs of a poor outlook for a stroke, whether due to infarction or haemorrhage, are impairment of consciousness, defects in conjugate gaze and a severe hemiplegia. Of those who survive an initial stroke, life expectancy is roughly halved. Approximately 10% suffer a second stroke within 1 year of the first and 20% within 5 years. Many patients who initially present with stroke die from myocardial infarction.

The prognosis in patients who suffer transient ischaemic attacks is difficult to ascertain because of difficulties of definition. A subsequent stroke is to be expected in approximately one-third of patients who have transient ischaemic attacks and is most likely to occur within 3 years of the first attack. In 50% of patients attacks cease within 1 to 3 years of their onset. Transient ischaemic attacks are attended by a worse prognosis (in terms of survival) in people below the age of 65 than in those over that age when compared with the rest of the population.

Much further work is needed to define the factors which influence the prognosis of cerebrovascular disease.

Thrombosis of Intracranial Veins and Venous Sinuses

Intracerebral venous thrombosis may be infected or aseptic; both are relatively uncommon. Infection may spread to the veins or sinuses from the face, dental roots or middle ear; it may also follow fracture of the skull, meningitis or septicaemia. Complications such as meningitis, suppurative encephalitis or brain abscess may ensue.

Aseptic thrombosis may occur in water and salt depletion, polycythaemia, malaria and marasmus. Occasionally a cerebral venous thrombosis occurs in the puerperium or in users of oral contraceptives.

Clinical Features. *Cavernous sinus thrombosis* nearly always follows an infection such as a boil on the face. Usually the patient is gravely ill, and before antibiotics were available few patients survived. Headache and fever are marked and there is a neutrophil leucocytosis. Occlusion of the ophthalmic veins causes proptosis, chemosis and oedema of the eyelids. There are almost always complete palsies of the third, fourth and sixth nerves as well as pain in and above the eye and diminished sensation over the forehead. Papilloedema in the affected eye is common. The condition is usually initially unilateral but often becomes bilateral within 2 to 3 days.

Superior Sagittal Sinus Thrombosis. Severe headache, papilloedema, and a generalised epilep-tic seizure are followed by signs of spreading thrombophlebitis of cortical veins, including motor, sensory or visual disorders on one or both sides according to the areas of cortex infarcted.

Transverse Sinus Thrombosis. The onset is similar but extension to the superior petrosal sinus and lower cortical veins causes unilateral syndromes of local infarction. Spread to the jugular veins may cause palsies of lower cranial nerves.

Treatment. The administration of antibiotics has markedly improved the outlook for infected thromboses. Surgical drainage of an abscess may be necessary. Anticoagulants are unhelpful.

INFECTIONS OF BRAIN, MENINGES AND SPINAL CORD

SUPPURATIVE ENCEPHALITIS AND INTRACEREBRAL ABSCESS

Aetiology and Pathology. Direct infection may occur following a compound fracture of the skull or there may be local spread by suppurative thrombophlebitis from an infected ear, paranasal sinus or scalp. Metastatic infections may occur from the lungs or from infective endocarditis.

The initial infection causes a suppurative encephalitis. The pus is slowly localised by a surrounding wall of gliosis which in a chronic abscess may form a tough capsule. Multiple abscesses, communicating or discrete, occur, particularly with metastatic spread.

Clinical Features. There are three main types of presentation:

Acute Encephalitis. Soon after head injury or otitis media the patient develops headache, fever, vomiting and drowsiness progressing to coma. Focal cerebral signs may be present.

Subacute or Delayed Encephalitis. Head injury, cranial infection or infected embolism may be followed after weeks or months of apparent recovery by symptoms of encephalitis or of a chronic space-occupying lesion. During the latent interval there may be minor headache, irritability, malaise and intermittent pyrexia. These features should lead to a search for a focal cerebral lesion in patients with infections such as otitis media or bronchiectasis.

Chronic Abscess. This may follow one of the

previous types of onset or there may be nothing to suggest that the lesion is infective. The chronic abscess causes focal symptoms of a cerebral lesion (p. 603) and those of raised intracranial pressure which are indistinguishable from those of cerebral tumours. The temperature is usually normal.

Diagnosis. The possibility of an abscess should be considered if there is a progressive, focal, intracranial lesion, especially if associated with congenital heart disease. The likelihood is increased if there are signs of infection, such as pyrexia, leucocytosis or a raised ESR but these may be absent if there is a chronic abscess. The EEG may show focal abnormalities. The CSF may show a pleocytosis or a raised protein but often is normal and should not be examined if there are signs of raised intracranial pressure. CT scanning should be performed whenever the suspicion of an abscess arises. Contrast enhanced CT scanning will define the vast majority of intracranial abscesses.

Treatment. High dosage antibiotics are given as for pyogenic meningitis (p. 638). When a collection of pus has been demonstrated it should be aspirated surgically and appropriate antibiotics instilled into the cavity. This procedure may need to be repeated. After the infection has been controlled excision of the abscess may be necessary. It is important to treat the underlying cause if possible.

Spinal Epidural Abscess

This condition usually arises as a metastasis from infection elsewhere, often a boil, which may be so trivial as to be easily overlooked. Pain of root distribution is severe. It develops acutely and is followed by progressive loss of sensation and power in the lower limbs with sphincter disturbance. The signs are those of transverse myelitis (p. 657) but the local root irritation is the clue to the true cause. The temperature may be only slightly raised, but a polymorphonuclear leucocytosis is found in the blood. There may be radiological evidence of localised osteomyelitis of the spine. Paraplegia will become complete and irreversible if treatment is delayed. Large doses of antibiotics such as benzylpenicillin 600 mg 4-hourly should be given immediately and the patient transferred to the care of a neurosurgeon without delay.

MENINGITIS

Viral infection (p. 641) is now the commonest cause of meningitis. Bacterial infection has become rare since the introduction of the antibiotics, and, for similar reasons, tuberculous meningitis (p. 638) is now seldom seen in Britain. In some areas meningitis may be caused by spirochaetes (leptospirosis, p. 762; syphilis p. 409), Rickettsia (typhus fever, p. 438), protozoa (amoebiasis, p. 773) or fungi (cryptococosis, p. 805).

Inflammation of the meninges can also be due to causes other than infection, for example blood in the CSF in subarachnoid haemorrhage (p. 605). Meningeal irritation ('*meningism*') without inflammatory reaction occurs in acute specific fevers, otitis media and pneumonia in childhood. Cellular reaction (lymphocytic) may be associated with symptoms and signs of meningeal irritation in poliomyelitis (p. 643) and acute encephalomyelitis (p. 642). Malignant disease is a rare cause of meningitis.

Bacterial Meningitis

The most common organisms are *Neisseria meningitidis*, *Streptococcus pneumoniae* and *Haemophilus influenzae*.

Pathology. The pia-arachnoid is congested and infiltrated with inflammatory cells. A thin layer of pus forms and this may later organise to form adhesions. These may cause obstruction to the free flow of CSF leading to hydrocephalus, or may damage the cranial nerves at the base of the brain. The CSF pressure rises rapidly, the protein content increases and there is a cellular reaction which varies in type and severity according to the nature of the inflammation and the causative organism. The sugar content of the CSF is decreased in bacterial infections and in carcinomatosis of the meninges. If the patient is not kept in electrolyte balance the chloride content may be reduced due to loss by sweating and vomiting.

Clinical Features. Signs of meningeal irritation are present:

Neck Rigidity. The patient complains of neck stiffness and the examiner is unable to put the patient's chin on the chest by passive flexion of the neck. Spasm may be so severe, particularly in children, as to cause head retraction.

Kernig's Sign. If the patient's thigh is flexed to 90 degrees from the abdomen, it is then impossible to straighten the knee passively owing to spasm of the hamstring muscles. This manoeuvre stretches the roots of the sciatic nerve which are inflamed at their exits from the spinal theca.

Other features of meningococcal infection are described on page 747.

Investigation. Microbiological examination of the CSF (p. 606) usually determines the nature of the infection. In cases of pyogenic meningitis in which Gram stain and/or culture of CSF is negative, counter current immunoelectrophoresis of the CSF is useful for the detection of bacterial antigens.

Treatment. Meningococcal and pneumococcal meningitis should be treated initially with large doses of benzylpenicillin intravenously — 1·2–2·4 g 4-hourly for adults and 150 mg/kg/d given 4-hourly for children.

For meningitis due to *H. influenzae* chloramphenicol (p. 46) is effective given intravenously initially, and orally when the patient can swallow.

Pending the identification of the bacteria causing pyogenic meningitis, treatment of adults can be commenced with benzylpenicillin and of children with chloramphenicol. Single doses of long-acting chloramphenicol are also useful in areas where medical facilities are limited.

Tuberculous Meningitis

Aetiology and Pathology. The condition occurs most commonly shortly after a primary infection in childhood or as part of miliary tuberculosis. The usual local source of infection is a caseous focus in the meninges or brain substance adjacent to the cerebrospinal fluid pathway.

The brain is covered by a greenish, gelatinous exudate especially around the base, and numerous scattered tubercles are found on the meninges.

Clinical Features. In children the onset of tuberculous meningitis is so insidious that it may be weeks before the parents realise that the illness is serious. At first there is merely lassitude, loss of interest in toys and in play, unwillingness to talk, anorexia and constipation. Headache, at first slight, gradually becomes worse but meningeal signs may not appear for days or weeks.

In adults the malaise, headache and meningeal signs usually progress more rapidly. There may be vomiting. The temperature is intermittently raised initially but remains raised, though rarely to high levels, once meningeal signs appear. The condition then progresses more rapidly, and in untreated cases cranial nerve palsies, hemiparesis or other signs of cerebral damage, hydrocephalus with drowsiness, coma and moderate papilloedema may occur. In miliary tuberculosis choroidal tubercles may be seen.

The CSF is under increased pressure. It is usually clear but, when allowed to stand, a fine clot may form. The fluid contains up to 400 cells/mm³, predominantly lymphocytes; the count must be made on a fresh specimen before it forms a clot. There is a slight rise in protein and a marked fall in glucose. Detection of the tubercle bacillus in a smear of the centrifuged deposit from the CSF may be difficult, the clot being the most likely place to find it. Inoculation of CSF into a guinea-pig is valuable for confirming the diagnosis if this cannot be done from smears or cultures of the CSF, but as the outcome will not be known for six weeks, treatment must be started without waiting for confirmation.

Treatment and Prognosis. Chemotherapy should be started as soon as the diagnosis is made using one of the regimens described on page 236, together with pyrazinamide (p. 237). All patients should also receive prednisolone, 10 mg four times daily. If subsequent lumbar punctures suggest the development of a spinal subarachnoid block, then hydrocortisone hemisuccinate should be injected intrathecally each day in a dose of 1 mg/kg. If obstructive hydrocephalus develops in spite of treatment with corticosteroids, surgical methods for ensuring continuous ventricular drainage must be adopted. During the acute stage of the illness skilled nursing is essential and measures must be taken to maintain adequate hydration and nutrition.

The intensive regime of drug treatment should be continued for eight weeks and be followed by a continuation phase (p. 237). Prednisolone is then reduced to 20 mg daily and stopped after about three months.

Untreated tuberculous meningitis is fatal in a few weeks but complete recovery is the rule with modern treatment if it is started before the appearance of focal signs or stupor. When treatment is started at a later stage the recovery rate is 60% or less and the survivors may be mentally deficient, epileptic, deaf, blind or show some other permanent deficit.

Viral Meningitis

Acute lymphocytic choriomeningitis and other forms of viral meningitis are described on page 641.

NEUROSYPHILIS

An old and frequently reiterated neurological aphorism states that neurosyphilis may mimic any neurological disease. As a corollary it is emphasised that neurosyphilis must be included in the differential diagnosis of all neurological problems.

Neurosyphilis may present as an acute or chronic process. It may involve, singly or in combination, the meninges, blood vessels and parenchyma of brain and spinal cord and cause meningovascular syphilis, general paralysis of the insane, tabes dorsalis and combined lesions. Though the clinical manifestations produced are diverse, certain general observations are pertinent.

Pupillary abnormalities, described by Argyll Robertson, may accompany any neurosyphilitic clinical syndrome. The pupils are small, irregular and unequal. They do not react to light but respond to convergence and show an impaired response to mydriatics. The irises may be atrophied. In relatively few instances will all of these features be present. The complete picture of Argyll Robertson pupils is most frequently seen in tabes dorsalis and is distinctly uncommon in general paresis wherein some pupillary changes occur in about half of the cases. The observation of any discrepancy between the pupillary response to light and convergence, even when other manifestations are lacking, should always suggest the possibility of neurosyphilis.

Examination of the CSF reveals abnormalities in the vast majority of cases of neurosyphilis. An increase in the cell count, usually lymphocytic and of moderate degree is almost invariably present when the disease is active. A moderate rise in the protein content is usual and the gamma globulin fraction thereof is often increased. Serological tests for syphilis (p. 410) are usually positive.

Meningovascular Syphilis

The essential lesion is endarteritis obliterans which may lead to arterial thrombosis and to the formation of a granuloma or gumma. The meninges may be covered by an exudate which damages cranial nerves. Lesions may predominantly affect arteries or meninges or both structures may be involved.

Clinical Features. These usually occur within five years of the primary infection.

Intracranial Lesions. Occlusion of a cerebral artery may be due to syphilis which should be considered as a possibility in cases of stroke, particularly when cerebral infarcts occur in young people.

Basal gummatous meningitis may present with cranial nerve palsies. Meningitis over the surface of the hemispheres may give rise to headaches and fits in addition to focal signs of cortical dysfunction. Rarely, a single large gumma may present as a slowly growing cerebral tumour.

Spinal Lesions. Thrombosis of the anterior spinal artery gives rise to lower motor neurone signs at the level of the lesion. Below the affected segments, upper motor neurone disturbance is usually manifest and there may also be impairment of pain and temperature sensation.

Thickening of the dura mater in the cervical region — called *hypertrophic pachymeningitis* — gives rise to lower motor neurone lesions in the arms and upper motor neurone lesions in the legs. Meningitis accompanied by myelitis in the dorsal region causes 'girdle' pains and leads to progressive cord damage.

General Paralysis of the Insane

The principal pathological changes are seen in the cortex. There is degeneration of cortical neurones giving rise to atrophy, particularly marked over the anterior part of the hemispheres. The meninges are thickened and infiltrated with lymphocytes. General paralysis of the insane usually presents 5 to 15 years after the primary infection. Men are much more often affected than women.

Clinical Features. The initial and most characteristic feature is dementia, often of insidious onset and slow progression. Relatives or workmates usually first recognise the patient's intellectual deficit and, later, deteriorating social adaptation. Delusions of grandeur occur only in a minority of cases. Signs of upper motor neurone lesions, usually bilateral and initially mild, are usually present and tremors of the head and lips are often manifest. Less common features include epileptic fits and transient episodes of focal cerebral disturbance such as hemiplegia, hemianopia or dysphasia.

Tabes Dorsalis

The primary lesion is a degeneration of first order sensory neurones, central to the dorsal root ganglia, in the lower thoracic and lumbar nerve roots. Obvious macroscopic wasting affects the dorsal columns but all modalities of sensation may be impaired. Males are more often affected than females, usually 5 to 20 years after the primary infection.

Clinical Features. Sensory disturbances are the most common initial symptoms. 'Lightning' pains of severe, lancinating nature occur in paroxysms. They are most common in the legs. Pains radiating around the trunk in a 'girdle' distribution also occur. Paraesthesiae often affect the feet.

Other disabilities may accompany these sensory manifestations or may be presenting features. Ataxia, of sensory type, due to proprioceptive loss is often prominent. Sphincter disturbance, particularly retention of urine, may be accompanied by impotence. Failing vision or diplopia may be symptoms. Perforating, painless ulcers of the feet and swollen, unstable joints (Charcot's joints) are sometimes found. Visceral crises may cause acute symptoms and the disturbance in function may point to disease in the affected organ rather than in its innervation. Most typical are gastric crises which give rise to abdominal pain and vomiting.

Less common are laryngeal crises causing stridor, the strangury of vesical crises and tenesmus due to rectal crises.

The signs of tabes are mostly explicable on the basis of posterior root lesions. Tendon reflexes are lost, due to interruption of the reflex arcs, first at the ankles, then at the knees and later in the upper limbs. Hypotonia with resultant hyperextensibility of the joints appears. The pain fibres are affected early with delay in or impairment of the response to pin prick over a characteristic distribution. The classical areas of loss are around the nose, the trunk from the angle of the sternum to the costal margin, the inner border of the forearms and the ring and little fingers, the perineum and the distal part of the lower limbs. Deep pain appreciation is also impaired so that the tendo calcaneus, calf muscles and testes become insensitive to pressure. Vibration and position sense in the feet are also lost early, but light touch is not affected until a later stage. The combination of loss of position sense and hypotonia gives rise to severe ataxia, so that the patient walks on a wide base lifting the feet high and stamping them down in an irregular and forceful manner. Romberg's test (p. 597) is positive. The plantar responses remain flexor, but may be absent as a result of sensory loss.

Bilateral ptosis with compensatory wrinkling of the forehead and Argyll Robertson pupils constitute a typical tabetic facies. Less constant clinical manifestations also include pallor of the optic discs, defects in external ocular movement, distension of the bladder, and trophic changes such as ulcers or painless arthropathy.

Combined Neurosyphilitic Lesions

It is emphasised that the clinical syndromes outlined above represent only the commoner presentations of neurosyphilis. Combinations of pathological lesions also occur and give rise to mixed clinical pictures. Tabetic manifestations sometimes accompany those of general paralysis of the insane and the hybrid (*taboparesis*) may lead to cases of dementia accompanied by ataxia, lightning pains or areflexia; patients presenting with visceral crises may be found to have extensor plantar responses.

Treatment of Neurosyphilis. The essential part of the treatment of neurosyphilis of all types is the injection of procaine penicillin, 600 mg–1.2 g daily for three weeks (p. 411). The aim of treatment is to arrest the disease and restore the blood and CSF to normal. Further courses of penicillin must be given if symptoms are not relieved, the condition continues to advance, or the CSF continues to show signs of active disease. The first abnormality to regress is the increase in cells but these may not return to normal until three months after treatment has been completed. The elevated protein takes longer to subside and the Wassermann reaction may never revert to normal. Lumbar puncture should be repeated at 6 monthly intervals for 2 years and further courses of penicillin given so long as signs of activity remain. Evidence of clinical progression at any time is an indication for renewed treatment.

VIRAL INFECTIONS

A classification of viruses is given on page 727.

Some viruses have a propensity for invasion of nerve cells and are called 'neurotropic'. The affinity may be specially marked for one type of nerve cell; varicella-zoster virus particularly involves sensory neurones and the anterior horn cells are vulnerable to an enterovirus in poliomyelitis. Though these viruses most commonly invade their sites of predilection they may also sometimes involve the nervous system more widely; the virus of poliomyelitis often gives rise to a meningoencephalitis and the varicella-zoster virus may rarely cause motor disability.

Many viruses which usually cause diseases of other systems may sometimes implicate the nervous system. The many varieties of echo and coxsackie viruses, which are common enteric pathogens, fairly often cause neurological disease as well as more widespread manifestations in other systems. The viruses of herpes simplex and mumps, among many others, may occasionally invade the nervous system. Congenital cytomegalovirus infection can cause brain damage.

Some neurological diseases, of which encephalitis lethargica is one, are presumed to be of viral origin because of their epidemiological, clinical and pathological features though the causal agent has not been identified.

Neurological disorders are sometimes indirectly associated with viral diseases. In these instances abnormal immunological responses, evoked by the virus, cause damage to neural tissue without any viral invasion of neurones. The demyelinating encephalomyelitis (p. 647) which may follow any of the exanthemata is such an entity.

Slow viral infections may cause chronic or relapsing neurological disease. These infections exhibit a latent period of many months or years between the initial infection and the subsequent clinical illness which, once manifest, tends to run a protracted course.

Kuru is a disease which occurs only in the members of one cannibalistic New Guinea tribe. It can, however, be transmitted to chimpanzees and there is much evidence to suggest that kuru is a slow viral infection transmitted by the eating of the infected brains of dead tribal members. There is degeneration of grey matter, most marked in the cerebellum, causing a progressive ataxia.

Creutzfeldt-Jakob disease is a subacute encephalopathy characterised by presenile dementia, epilepsy, myoclonus, extrapyramidal and motor neurone signs and can also be transmitted from man to chimpanzees.

A slow viral infection has been adduced as a possible cause of a number of chronic neurological diseases, including motor neurone disease and multiple sclerosis.

Viral Meningitis

Viral infections of the central nervous system such as encephalitis and poliomyelitis may be associated with meningitis. Viral meningitis can also occur alone, without clinical manifestation of parenchymal involvement of the nervous system, in acute lymphocytic choriomeningitis and infection by echo or coxsackie viruses. Thirdly, meningitis may develop as a complication of viral infections primarily involving other organs, e.g. mumps, measles, infectious mononucleosis, herpes zoster and hepatitis.

Acute lymphocytic choriomeningitis is caused by an arenavirus, endemic in house mice.

The condition occurs mainly in children and young adults. The onset is acute and evidence of meningeal irritation develops rapidly. Focal neurological signs are usually absent. There may be a high pyrexia which gradually reverts to normal in 5 to 7 days. The CSF is under increased pressure. It is usually clear but may be turbid as there is an excess of lymphocytes which may persist long after clinical cure. There may be a slight increase in the protein but the sugar and chloride levels are normal.

Lymphocytic choriomeningitis has to be differentiated from pyogenic meningitis in which the turbid CSF contains an excess of polymorphonuclear leucocytes and the causative organism can be isolated. Tuberculous meningitis may be difficult to distinguish owing to the technical difficulties of isolating the tubercle bacillus. A normal level of sugar in the CSF is in favour of a diagnosis of acute lymphocytic choriomeningitis. If there is any serious doubt as to the diagnosis, it is better to start treatment for tuberculous meningitis while awaiting further bacteriological reports.

There is no specific treatment for lymphocytic choriomeningitis. The patient is kept at rest in bed on symptomatic measures until the temperature has returned to normal. Complete recovery is the rule.

Viral Encephalitis

All of the viruses which cause meningitis may also give rise to an encephalitis. Encephalitic features may predominate or a combined picture of meningo-encephalitis may occur. More specific types of viral encephalitis occur in epidemic forms, such as Japanese-B encephalitis (p. 737). Sporadic cases occur fairly commonly but often the causative virus is not isolated though influenza and herpes simplex viruses are fairly frequently implicated.

Pathology. The distribution and extent of lesions vary to some extent with the type of infecting virus. There is usually diffuse damage to cells in the cortex, basal ganglia and brain stem. Inclusion bodies are often present in neurones and glial cells. There is usually infiltration between neurones and in the perivascular spaces by polymorphonuclear cells initially and later by lymphocytes and monocytes. There is accompanying neuroglial proliferation. Herpes simplex encephalitis tends particularly to affect the temporal lobes and in encephalitis lethargica the substantia nigra, midbrain and basal ganglia are most prominently involved.

Clinical Features. An acute onset of headache, often accompanied by fever, is the usual clinical presentation common to all types of viral encephalitis. Disturbance of consciousness, varying from mild drowsiness to deep coma, usually supervenes early and may sometimes advance dramatically. Epilepsy of focal or generalised type is common. A variety of focal signs such as aphasia, hemiplegia or tetraplegia, cranial nerve palsies and sensory disturbances may occur but sometimes there are none. The clinical features usually do not enable a firm diagnosis of the causal agent to be made but some types of encephalitis present distinctive manifestations as follows:

Herpes Simplex Encephalitis. This is the most common type in Britain. The onset is usually acute and commonly is marked by behavioural disturbance and a confusional state resembling a psychosis. This often lasts 2 or 3 days before other features develop. Fits are very common. Papilloedema and variable focal neurological signs may be present, commonly of temporal lobe dysfunction. Progression over a few days to coma is frequent.

Brainstem encephalitis is presumed to be of viral origin but the causal agent has not been defined. There is usually an antecedent history of mild upper respiratory infection. The onset, attended by headache, is often marked by double vision and dysarthria. Later there is increasing drowsiness and progressive cranial nerve involvement.

Encephalitis lethargica occurred in epidemic form during the 1920s and sporadic cases still appear. The illness varies markedly in severity. Headache and double vision may be the only features but sleep disturbances, upper motor neurone and extrapyramidal signs may be manifest. Oculogyric crises or parkinsonism may develop during the early stages of the illness or may be a sequel.

Epidemic myalgic encephalomyelitis is a condition which is presumed, though not proven, to be of viral origin. It occurs in closed communities such as schools and hospitals. Common features are headaches, diffuse muscle pains, exhaustion, low grade pyrexia, lymphadenopathy, paraesthesiae and marked mood disturbances which may recur over long periods.

Subacute sclerosing panencephalitis is thought to be due to infection by a myxovirus which is either measles virus or a closely related agent. It occurs in children and adolescents. The onset is usually an insidious intellectual deterioration, apathy and clumsiness accompanied later by myoclonic jerks and other involuntary movements. The EEG is distinctive, showing bursts of triphasic slow waves. As the disease progresses, rigidity and dementia supervene.

Rabies presents a distinctive clinical picture described on page 731.

Progressive multifocal leucoencephalopathy is a rare condition occurring late in the course of an antecedent disease, e.g. lymphoma or carcinoma. The pathological findings comprise widely disseminated demyelinating lesions in the brain together with distinctive changes in the glial cells suggestive of invasion by one of the papova group of viruses. It is a condition of rapid and progressive nature usually leading to death within a few weeks or months of its being manifest. The clinical picture varies widely. Hemiparesis is the commonest disability but dysphasia, dysarthria and hemianopia are also frequent. Dementia may occur, as may convulsions.

Diagnosis. These various forms of viral encephalitis should first be distinguished from other intracranial diseases such as cerebral tumour or abscess, from encephalopathies, from demyelinating encephalomyelitis (p. 647) and from trypanosomiasis (p. 779). Thereafter the type of viral infection should, if possible, be determined.

The differential diagnosis depends on the nature of the clinical features and the attendant circumstances. When the predominant features are progressive focal affection of one hemisphere accompanied by headache and drowsiness, the picture may strongly suggest a space-occupying lesion and intensive investigation may be needed to exclude such conditions as cerebral abscess. When the illness is mild, neurological signs in-

definite and there are attendant general signs of viral infection the diagnosis will often be made presumptively after the patient improves.

Investigations are more helpful in excluding other lesions than in confirming the diagnosis of viral encephalitis. In a minority of instances the CSF is normal. Usually the CSF pressure and protein content are moderately raised and there is a lymphocytic pleocytosis. The sugar content is normal. The EEG is usually altered. There is a diffuse slowing of the rhythms but the findings are nonspecific except in subacute sclerosing panencephalitis.

Occasionally in herpes simplex encephalitis a radionuclide scan will show areas of increased uptake in one or both temporal lobes. This condition is potentially treatable so that it is important to establish the diagnosis when the patient's illness is severe and progressive. In such circumstances a biopsy of the temporal lobe may be justified.

Serological tests and culture may identify the infecting virus but the results of such tests are usually available too late to guide treatment.

Treatment and Prognosis. The management of most cases of viral encephalitis consists of nursing care and the prevention of intercurrent infections. When a positive diagnosis of herpes simplex encephalitis has been made, an antiviral agent such as acyclovir (p. 48) may be used.

Most patients survive and may recover completely but persisting focal defects are frequent. A significant number (perhaps 10–30%) die. The outlook is particularly poor in herpes simplex encephalitis and in subacute sclerosing panencephalitis. Brain stem encephalitis has a good prognosis; complete, if sometimes slow, recovery is almost invariable.

Poliomyelitis

Aetiology and Pathology. The disease is caused by one of three related polio viruses which comprise a subdivision of the group of enteroviruses. It is much less common following the widespread use of oral vaccines but is still a major problem in developing countries. Infection usually occurs through the nasopharynx.

The virus is liable to affect the grey matter of

spinal cord, brain stem and cortex and has a particular propensity to damage anterior horn cells especially those within the lumbar segments. There is often accompanying infiltration of the meninges with lymphocytes.

Clinical Features. The incubation period is 7–14 days. At the onset there is usually mild fever and headache which improves after a few days. Many cases do not progress beyond this stage. In other instances, after a period of well-being lasting approximately a week, there is a recurrence of pyrexia and headache accompanied by neck stiffness and signs of meningeal irritation. Paralysis may occur later. The extent is variable. Weakness of one muscle group may progress to widespread paresis. Respiratory failure may supervene if intercostal muscles are paralysed or the medullary motor nuclei are involved.

The CSF shows a lymphocytic pleocytosis, a rise in protein and a normal sugar content.

Treatment and Prognosis. In the early stages bed rest is imperative. At the onset of respiratory difficulties a tracheostomy and intermittent positive pressure respiration are required. Subsequent treatment is by physiotherapy and orthopaedic measures.

Epidemics vary widely in their incidence of abortive and nonparalytic cases and in mortality rate. Death occurs from respiratory paralysis. Paralysis is greatest at the end of the first week of the major illness. Gradual recovery may then take place for several months but any muscle showing no signs of recovery by the end of a month will not regain useful function. It is difficult to make a more definite prediction about the extent of permanent disability until three to six months after the onset. Second attacks are very rare.

Prevention is by oral vaccination (p. 41).

Herpes Zoster (Shingles)

Invasion of posterior root ganglia by the varicella-zoster virus causes pain followed by a rash over the cutaneous distribution of the affected nerve. Zoster is believed to be due to reactivation of a previous infection by the varicella-zoster virus which has lain dormant in the body. The frequency and severity of zoster increases with age and in immunocompromised patients. Chickenpox may be contracted from a patient with zoster.

Clinical Features. The first symptom is usually severe continuous pain in the distribution of the affected nerve root. After three or four days the skin in the painful area becomes reddened and vesicles appear which dry up over the course of 5 or 6 days, leaving small scars. The pain of zoster usually subsides as the eruption fades, but occasionally, especially in old people, it may be followed by a persistent and intractable neuralgia which may last for months.

Any dorsal root ganglion may be infected, most commonly those supplying the trunk where two or three adjacent dermatomes on one side only are often involved. Infection of the trigeminal ganglion usually involves the ophthalmic division; the vesicles appear on the cornea and may lead to corneal ulceration with the danger of scarring and impairment of vision (*ophthalmic herpes*).

Segmental muscle wasting may occur sometimes from involvement of the motor root. The virus occasionally invades the spinal cord or the brain, giving rise to myelitis or encephalitis.

Treatment. Idoxuridine (p. 48) may be applied to the skin in a 5% solution in the early stages of the evolution of the rash; 0·1% drops are used for corneal infections. The treatment of post-herpetic neuralgia is difficult. Analgesics should be continued, but addictive ones, such as morphine must be avoided.

DEMYELINATING DISEASES

Loss of myelin sheaths occurs with many disorders of the central and peripheral nervous systems but there is a particular category with certain clinical and pathological features in common in which loss of myelin is considered to be the primary change and the axis cylinders may be spared or, if affected, are damaged secondarily. The lesions are almost entirely confined to the white matter of the central nervous system. They are initially inflammatory in type but differ from lesions known to be caused by direct viral infection and so they are grouped separately from viral encephalitis.

MULTIPLE SCLEROSIS

Multiple sclerosis, also known as *disseminated sclerosis*, is the commonest of the demyelinating diseases. It affects about 1 in 2000 of the population in Britain.

Aetiology. The cause of the disease is unknown but there is much information about its prevalence and about the factors associated with its development. Incidence varies widely in different geographical areas. It is very low in the tropics and high in the temperate zones of both northern and southern hemispheres.

Migrants from a high to a low prevalence area have a reduced risk of developing multiple sclerosis. Those who migrate from a low to a high prevalence area are at greater risk than had they remained in their original environment. These effects apply only to those who move before the age of 15 years. Migrants at a later age bear the same liability to the disease as do the people of their country of origin.

A genetic susceptibility is suggested by an increased frequency of HLA-A3, B7 and DW2/DRW2 and particularly of the B cell alloantigen, BT101, in European patients with multiple sclerosis. There is also a greater occurrence of the disease in close relatives of sufferers than in the general population.

The part played by an autoimmune mechanism, possibly induced by a slow viral or a persistent measles infection, is also being studied but the results are inconclusive. One theory is that in genetically susceptible individuals the disease follows a dormant viral infection, either directly or via an immunological mechanism.

Pathology. The acute lesion consists of a circumscribed area in which the myelin sheaths have undergone destruction while the axis cylinders show only irregular swelling. The plaque has a swollen pinkish appearance because blood vessels are dilated, but there is little infiltration with inflammatory cells. Reactive gliosis follows, so that the chronic lesion becomes a glial scar with a shrunken greyish appearance. The lesions are widely scattered in the white matter of the brain, especially round the ventricles, in the spinal cord, and in the optic nerves.

Despite the disseminated distribution there is a tendency for spinal cord and brain stem lesions to occur in symmetrical situations.

Clinical features are diverse. It is impossible to outline a 'typical' history. Characteristic features are a relapsing and remittent course and widespread lesions which result in varied symptomatology.

The first manifestation may occur at any age but onset before puberty or after the age of 60 years is rare. Initial symptoms present between 20 and 40 years of age in the majority of cases. Women are affected about one-and-a-half times as often as men.

Weakness of one or more limbs developing acutely is probably the commonest presentation. Unilateral retrobulbar neuritis is also a frequent mode of onset as are paraesthesiae affecting a limb or felt in a girdle distribution around the trunk. Diplopia, vertigo and ataxia are also common initial features. Less frequent are epilepsy, aphasia, hemiplegia, facial palsy and bouts of facial pain resembling trigeminal neuralgia.

In most instances the symptoms and signs of the initial manifestation recover completely within 1 to 3 months of the onset. A period of well-being follows and after a very variable interval there is a recurrence. In a few instances there is no remission; the initial disability progresses and more widespread deficits develop. A minority of patients suffer three or four further exacerbations during the year following the onset. Another small group remains well for more than 10 years after the first disturbance. In many cases neural deficits recur within 2 years of the first incident.

The outlook for the second and subsequent manifestations is variable. Some patients continue to show exacerbations with virtually complete recovery for many years. In other instances successive relapses are attended by diminishing degrees of improvement. Eventually half of the sufferers enter a chronically progressive stage with persisting and increasing disability.

The signs depend on the site of the demyelinating lesion. Pallor of one or both optic nerve heads is common and is particularly prominent over the temporal halves of the discs even in patients who give no history of an earlier retrobulbar neuritis. Many patients develop diplopia from involvement of the third or sixth cranial nerves. Nystagmus is often found and is usually of cerebellar or ataxic type (p. 610).

Signs of motor dysfunction are usually found at some stage, particularly involving the upper motor neurone. The abdominal reflexes are often absent early in the course of the disease and remain so. Later upper motor neurone signs in both legs and arms become more marked. Spasticity and paraplegia in flexion and flexor spasms ensue.

In people who develop the disease in middle age the only manifestation is often a slowly progressive, moderate paraparesis without remission but without severe exacerbations. Motor deficits are often temporarily but strikingly aggravated after a hot bath.

Cerebellar signs include the staccato, interrupted rhythm of scanning speech, ataxia and intention tremor; they are usually found during the progressive stage of the disease and are especially disabling.

Sensory symptoms are almost invariable at some time during the course of the disease. Paraesthesiae of varying type and distribution occur. Objective impairment of superficial sensation is usually less prominent than would be anticipated from the intensity of symptoms. A distinctive symptom is a tingling or 'electric shock-like' sensation which radiates into the arms, down the back, or into the legs when the patient flexes the neck. This is sometimes called the 'barber's chair' sign. It is most commonly due to multiple sclerosis but is not diagnostic thereof since it may occur in other diseases of the cervical cord such as compression, syringomyelia or vitamin B_{12} deficiency.

Localised muscle wasting, parkinsonian tremor and choreoathetotic movements are rare and it is unusual for the spinothalamic tracts to be involved to such an extent as to cause painless burns and trophic lesions. As the disease progresses sphincter disturbances occur, notably frequency and urgency of micturition or hesitancy and retention.

Some patients exhibit a sustained euphoria; others are fully aware of their disabilities and may become depressed. Late in the course of the disease there is often significant intellectual impairment.

Investigation. The diagnosis of multiple sclerosis depends clinically on the demonstration of lesions occurring at different times and at different sites in the central nervous system. Sometimes the occurrence of multiple lesions may not be apparent clinically but delayed evoked cerebral potentials (p. 606) after visual, auditory or somatosensory stimulation may indicate the presence of earlier lesions. Disseminated lesions in the white matter can be detected by nuclear magnetic resonance imaging (p. 607).

There is no specific test which will confirm the diagnosis. A raised gammaglobulin in the CSF in the presence of a normal total protein is present in approximately 70% of patients suffering from multiple sclerosis. More sophisticated tests, utilising the electrophoresis of CSF protein, have shown that oligoclonal bands of IgG are present in over 90% of patients with multiple sclerosis but they are also found in other diseases (p. 605).

In some cases the diagnosis of multiple sclerosis has to be achieved by a process of exclusion. It is important in all patients to eliminate potentially curable conditions such as syphilis or vitamin B_{12} deficiency. The appropriate investigations, and the lengths to which they should be pursued, depend on the particular clinical syndrome presented. In cases of slowly progressive spastic paraparesis, as commonly occurs in late onset multiple sclerosis, a myelogram may be needed to exclude compression of the spinal cord.

Treatment. There is no curative treatment but much can be done to support the patient during the course of the illness. Corticosteroids promote more rapid and complete recovery during acute exacerbations; 2 mg of dexamethasone given orally three times daily, for five days, is an adequate course of treatment. There is no evidence that prolonged administration of corticosteroids significantly alters long-term prognosis. A variety of other treatments has been tried, including immunosuppression and transfer factor, but the results have been disappointing.

Spasticity may become severe in multiple sclerosis and baclofen in a dose of 20 to 60 mg daily is sometimes helpful. Severe, painful flexor spasms may be relieved by the intrathecal injection of phenol in glycerine. Spinal cord stimulation is an interesting but ill-understood method of treatment. Electrodes are inserted into the epidural space and the dorsal columns are repetitively stimulated. In some series more than half of the patients so treated have shown improvement, particularly in sphincter control.

Of prime importance in the management is encouragement and support of patients and their relatives. Regular medical supervision contributes to this end. Patients with motor disabilities should avoid any gain in weight. Periods of physiotherapy help the disabled patient. Assisted and passive movements and walking exercises improve gait as well as the patient's morale. In general the patient should be advised to avoid long periods in bed during intercurrent infections. Pressure sores should be prevented by advice about changes in posture and skin care; should they occur they must be treated early and vigorously in hospital.

Walking aids such as tripod supports or frames and the provision of wheel-chairs and motor vehicles together with the advice of an occupational therapist may enable the patient to function more easily at home and at work and to enjoy some form of social life. Nurses and social workers should regularly visit patients at home to assist in their care and to ensure that all the help which the community can provide is made available.

The care of the bladder is particularly important. Infections should be treated with an appropriate antibiotic. Male patients suffering from incontinence, urgency and frequency can be relieved by continuous drainage, through a tube attached to the penis, into a portable urinal strapped to the thigh. In some patients bladder neck resection is helpful. Various appliances are now available which help incontinent female patients. A permanent in-dwelling catheter, changed at intervals of a month or two, often makes life more comfortable and helps to prevent pressure sores.

Prognosis is variable. Multiple sclerosis does not inevitably lead to immobility and a chair-bound or bedridden existence. Approximately 5% of patients die within 5 years of the onset of the disease but a rather larger proportion remain well and retain unrestricted mobility for 20 years. The disease may run a progressive, disabling course, or may be relatively benign. It is not possible to predict the outlook with confidence in any individual patient though there are some useful indicators.

A favourable course often follows when retrobulbar neuritis is the initial manifestation, particularly when it occurs unaccompanied by any other neural deficit. A long gap between the presentation and the next recurrence often presages a fairly good prognosis, and particularly so if both manifestations recover completely. If motor function is only slightly impaired during the early years of the disease, crippling disability is usually long delayed. Repeated episodes of purely sensory deficit with complete recovery point to a benign course. Those whose initial manifestation is relatively late have usually a better prognosis. In those who show the so-called middle-aged spinal form the disease remains confined to a very slow progressive paraparesis.

Males generally seem to be more severely affected than females. An onset in the late teens or early twenties is often attended by a bad prognosis. Incomplete recovery from the initial attack is a sinister feature. Early recurrence, within 6 months of the initial manifestation, also suggests that relapses are likely to be frequent and disability rapidly progressive. Early manifestations of motor disability or brain stem and cerebellar dysfunction usually forecast a poor outlook. However, at any stage of the disease striking improvement may follow sudden deterioration.

Acute Demyelinating Encephalomyelitis

This is a group of related acute disorders occurring without obvious cause about a week after diseases such as measles and chickenpox or following vaccination. There are areas of perivenous demyelination widely disseminated throughout the brain and spinal cord probably due to an immunological reaction.

Headache, vomiting, pyrexia, delirium and signs of meningeal irritation are presenting features. Fits or coma may occur. Flaccid paralysis and extensor plantar responses are common but sensory loss is unusual. Cerebellar signs may be present especially when the disorder follows chickenpox. The CSF may be normal or show a small increase of mononuclear cells and protein.

Neuromyelitis optica is a restricted form of the disease characterised by massive demyelination of the spinal cord and both optic nerves.

ACTH 80–120 units by injection or prednisone 60 mg by mouth daily for several days followed by a maintenance dose for 2 to 3 weeks is beneficial. These drugs must be used with caution in chickenpox if encephalitis develops before the rash has subsided as it may become confluent and haemorrhagic. The usual care of the paralysed and incontinent patient is required.

The mortality rate is high in neuromyelitis optica and in postvaccinal encephalomyelitis but is low in the postexanthematous cases. If the patient survives, the recovery may be remarkably complete and second attacks are very rare.

DISEASES OF THE EXTRAPYRAMIDAL SYSTEM

In diseases of this system voluntary movement is disturbed, involuntary movements appear and muscle tone is altered.

PARKINSONISM

Parkinsonism is the name given to a clinical syndrome comprising impairment of voluntary movement (hypokinesis), rigidity and tremor. Its incidence is approximately 1 in every 1000 of the population rising to about 1% in those over 60 years.

Aetiology. Parkinsonism is caused by lesions in the basal nuclei and is associated particularly with damage to the interconnecting system between the substantia nigra and the corpus striatum. The nigrostriatal pathways utilise dopamine as a neurotransmitter, and parkinsonism is associated with dopamine deficiency. The precise pathophysiology and the interdependent biochemical abnormalities in parkinsonism are incompletely defined.

The commonest entity, accounting for perhaps three-quarters of cases, is *paralysis agitans* (also called idiopathic parkinsonism or Parkinson's disease) which is of unknown origin. It has been suggested that a slow viral infection might cause paralysis agitans. Parkinsonism is a recognised sequel of encephalitis lethargica and rarely results from other encephalitides caused by such viruses as coxsackie type B and Japanese B. Parkinsonism is frequently — and usually wrongly — attributed to cerebral atherosclerosis. Many patients suffering from parkinsonism also show signs of cerebral atherosclerosis, but it is probable, in most instances, that the two conditions — both common in the elderly — occur coincidentally. Discrete cerebrovascular lesions affecting the substantia nigra may, very occasionally, cause parkinsonism.

Of the known causes, drugs are the commonest, and notably those of the phenothiazine group. Parkinsonism may occasionally follow a single head injury and is often a sequel of repeated head trauma in the 'punch-drunk' syndrome. There are other infrequent causes of parkinsonism, namely cerebral tumours, notably those causing midbrain compression, parasagittal and sphenoidal ridge meningiomas, meningovascular syphilis, carbon monoxide poisoning, manganese poisoning and copper deposition in Wilson's disease.

Pathology. In parkinsonism the most consistent histological change is cellular loss and depigmentation of the substantia nigra. In paralysis agitans the characteristic pathological changes accompanying loss of cells are Lewy bodies (hyaline masses of cytoplasm and sphingomyelin) in the central areas of the substantia nigra. In postencephalitic parkinsonism the cell depletion affects the whole substantia nigra and is usually more severe than in paralysis agitans. Other changes, such as atrophy of the globus pallidus and patchy cortical atrophy, are inconstant.

Clinical Features. Two-thirds of patients first develop symptoms in the fifth or sixth decades. Initial manifestations are usually so slight and develop so insidiously that a gap of 2 or 3 years may elapse between the onset of the condition and its diagnosis. Occasionally the presentation is acute and progression is rapid; this is particularly likely in postencephalitic or drug-induced cases.

Tremor is usually the feature which causes the patient to seek advice. It first involves the fingers and spreads to proximal parts of the arms; it may later extend to the tongue and legs. The tremor is slow and in the earliest stages involves rhythmical movement of the thumb towards the fingers. The fully developed movement comprises a combination of adduction and abduction of the thumb, flexion and extension of the interphalangeal and metacarpophalangeal joints as well as pronation and supination of the wrists. Tremor is present at rest and often is lessened during purposive activity. Stress and embarrassment aggravate the tremor's amplitude. These factors are operative during clinical testing so that requested movements may be accompanied by increased, rather than reduced tremor. Head tremors are rare in parkinsonism. Tremor may never be present during the course of the condition and often diminishes as rigidity progresses.

Rigidity is usually detectable early. Resistance to passive movement is increased throughout the range of movement of a joint. Concurrent tremor may lead to the 'cog-wheel' phenomenon — a superimposed jerky sensation. Profound rigidity is accompanied by fixed abnormalities of posture. The patient is flexed at neck, hips, elbows and knees. The hands are flexed at the metacarpophalangeal joints and hyperextended at the interphalangeal joints; these deformities, accompanied by adduction of the thumb across the palm, present a characteristic picture.

Hypokinesis, comprising delay in initiation of movements together with paucity, slowness and lack of precision of movements, is the most disabling feature. Of insidious onset it may first be manifest by a gradual reduction in size and legibility of a patient's handwriting. Other fine movements, such as fastening buttons and laces, are impaired, and later feeding and even turning over in bed become difficult. There is often difficulty in rising from a chair and in starting to walk. Loss of normal arm swinging when the patient walks is a very early sign of hypokinesis.

Later the gait displays characteristic features. Steps are short and shuffling. Walking is usually slow but is sometimes accompanied by periods of uncontrolled acceleration when walking downhill. This phenomenon, called festination, causes patients to take ever more rapid, smaller and smaller steps as they chase their own centre of gravity. Falls often result.

Normally pliant emotional movements of the face are slow in starting, reduced in amplitude and prolonged in their accomplishment. Blinking is usually reduced but spontaneous blepharospasm is an occasional feature, particularly in postencephalitic parkinsonism. Blinking provoked by tapping the glabella does not show the normal habituation.

Impaired pupillary accommodation is a common finding in all types of parkinsonism. Sustained, involuntary, conjugate deviation of the eyes, usually upwards, called oculogyric crises, may last for minutes or hours; they occur in postencephalitic and drug-induced parkinsonism.

Speech is often affected. Some loss of voice volume is almost invariable. Delayed initiation and dysarthria are common. The cadence is slow; inflection is restricted so that speech becomes monotonous.

Hypokinesis may be overcome for short periods under the influence of a strong emotional drive such as fear or anger. Though the defects in voluntary movement are often striking and disabling, power is well preserved.

Signs of upper motor neurone involvement are not found in uncomplicated paralysis agitans, but they may be detected if there is accompanying cerebral atherosclerosis; they commonly occur in postencephalitic and post-traumatic parkinsonism and are found in those rare instances where parkinsonism is due to a cerebral tumour.

Differential Diagnosis. Physiological tremor often is exaggerated in the elderly and by anxiety, alcoholism and thyrotoxicosis. It is much faster than parkinsonian tremor, tends to occur only in one plane and lacks the abduction/adduction movement of the thumb.

Cerebellar atrophy is of fairly frequent occurrence in elderly patients who manifest intention tremor. Such a tremor is relieved when an affected limb is supported and relaxed and increases as the limb approaches a target.

Depressed and hypothyroid patients are often apathetic and lack normal facial expressiveness so that their appearance may suggest a diagnosis of parkinsonism.

Atherosclerotic dementia, with its attendant apathy, is often associated with increased tone due to bilateral upper motor neurone signs and may mimic parkinsonism. Other clinical features such as an exaggerated jaw jerk, increased tendon reflexes and spasticity rather than rigidity differentiate this condition from parkinsonism.

Treatment. Ideally, this should be aimed at the cause. The drug-induced condition is the only type which is both relatively common and curable if the offending drug is discontinued. In the majority of parkinsonian patients the cause is not known and treatment is designed to ameliorate disability. The most generally effective therapy for established cases is a combination of an anticholinergic preparation together with levodopa and a dopadecarboxylase inhibitor.

Anticholinergic drugs produce modest improvement in early parkinsonism. There are a number of synthetic preparations, such as benzhexol hydrochloride (2 mg or 5 mg), benztropine (2 mg) and orphenadrine (50 mg). One of these drugs is introduced in small amounts, such as one tablet twice daily, and the dose is increased until dryness of the mouth or blurring of vision supervenes. The dose is then reduced slightly to obviate these effects.

Dopamine Replacement. Levodopa has strikingly improved the treatment of parkinsonism. Given by mouth in doses varying from 2 to 8 g (average 5 g daily) levodopa reduces disability in more than two-thirds of patients and is particularly effective in relieving hypokinesis. The drug causes many side-effects, some of which develop early, e.g. nausea, vomiting, and cardiac arrhythmias; these are reduced if the drug is given together with a dopadecarboxylase inhibitor.

More than 90% of an orally ingested dose of levodopa is metabolised in extracerebral tissues and does not reach the brain. Selective inhibition of extracerebral dopadecarboxylase reduces the amount of levodopa required to produce a therapeutic effect and also diminishes the side-effects caused by peripheral breakdown of levodopa. Preparations are available which combine levodopa with extracerebral dopadecarboxylase inhibitors, e.g. 250 mg of levodopa and 25 mg of carbidopa or 50 mg of benserazide. One such tablet is equivalent in its therapeutic effect to 1 g of levodopa. This combined therapy, like levodopa itself, must be introduced in small amounts (half of a tablet twice daily) and increased gradually by a half tablet every 4 days.

The long-term and centrally determined side-effects of levodopa are not reduced by combined therapy. Induced involuntary movements and psychiatric disturbances are very troublesome and may demand reduction or temporary cessation of treatment. Particularly disabling is the so-called 'on/off' effect which develops in patients who have been treated, often with considerable success, for more than 2 years. Manifestations of this phenomenon include unsteadiness of gait, hypotonia, anxiety and, commonly, akinesis. These disabilities tend to develop and regress suddenly.

Accompanying the 'on/off' effect in some patients and persisting between the acute manifestations are unusual defects in higher cerebral function, including disinhibition, aphasia, apraxia and memory impairment. It seems likely that the frequency of occurrence of these distressing phenomena increases as treatment becomes more prolonged. Their alleviation requires withdrawal of levodopa therapy for several weeks, after which patients will often again tolerate and derive benefit from the drug.

Treatment with any antiparkinsonism drug should not be stopped abruptly. The 'on/off' effect should be distinguished from 'end of dose' deterioration requiring administration of doses at shorter intervals, perhaps every 2 hours.

Monoamine oxidase inhibitors should not be given to patients taking levodopa (p. 682).

Alternative treatment includes dopamine agonists of which the most useful is bromocriptine. An initial dose of 2·5 mg twice daily is gradually built up to 30 to 40 mg daily. The drug may be given alone or in combination with levodopa. Amantadine hydrochloride (100 mg b.d.) produces some effects both therapeutic and untoward, resembling those of levodopa but less in degree; improvement is maintained for only a few months in most cases. Other drugs, notably amphetamine and tricyclic antidepressants, have mild antiparkinsonian properties.

Stereotactic thalamotomy is now rarely employed; however, it may be helpful in occasional patients whose disability is unilateral tremor unresponsive to medical treatment.

Prognosis. There are extreme variations in

the rate of progression and the degree of disability produced. Twenty per cent of patients suffering from parkinsonism at any given time cannot cope independently with the normal activities of living. The mortality of patients suffering from parkinsonism is three times that of the general population of similar age. Levodopa, though it ameliorates disability, does not slow the progress of the basic pathology. There is increasing evidence that the rate of progression may be accelerated by premature use of levodopa.

Other Disorders of the Extrapyramidal System

Wilson's Disease (Hepatolenticular Degeneration) is described on page 366. In the cerebral type necrosis and sclerosis of the corpus striatum cause basal ganglion syndromes in adolescence. Most common is choreoathetosis, but parkinsonism may be caused according to the site mainly affected. There is usually cortical involvement leading to progressive dementia in which loss of emotional control is a feature.

Kernicterus is a disorder of the basal ganglia and auditory nuclei occurring in association with neonatal haemolysis, particularly in premature infants. It may be caused by haemolytic disease of the newborn (p. 513), but prematurity is more important than Rh incompatibility.

Premature babies have a functional immaturity of the glucuronyl transferase enzyme system of the liver, and, as a result, unconjugated bilirubin formed by haemolysis is not conjugated. Unconjugated bilirubin rapidly rises to toxic levels which depress oxidative metabolism of brain cells, and in particular those of the basal ganglia. The danger decreases rapidly about 10 days after the birth in normal full-term infants when the liver enzyme system matures, but the premature baby is in danger for a longer period.

Convulsions, coma, opisthotonos and rigidity may be early manifestations but athetoid movements or spastic paralysis, deafness of nuclear type, and mental deficiency may not appear until the baby is several months old.

Prevention depends on the early detection of haemolytic jaundice, especially in the premature child, and its prompt treatment by exchange transfusion. (p. 514). There is no treatment for established kernicterus and the future management is that of the child with cerebral palsy.

Chorea. Choreiform movements are irregular, jerking, ill-sustained and unpredictable, easily recognised when fully developed. In milder forms the condition may seem to be no more than restlessness or fidgeting. Often chorea is accompanied by athetoid movements. Chorea may be the sole neurological manifestation of systemic lupus erythematosus, idiopathic hypoparathyroidism or polycythaemia vera.

Sydenham's chorea (St. Vitus' dance) occurs in adolescents and is commoner in girls. It often follows a streptococcal throat infection. The onset may be abrupt or insidious. Choreiform movements are usually generalised and are accompanied by emotional lability so that often the condition is thought initially to be psychogenic. Pregnancy may precipitate a recurrence of chorea.

Because of the agitation, the patient, in all but the mildest cases, should be admitted to hospital and preferably nursed in isolation. Diazepam or haloperidol should be prescribed. An initial course of penicillin should be given.

Most patients recover within a month, though more prolonged illnesses occur and relapses are common. Since many patients later develop valvular heart disease their future observation and management should be as for rheumatic fever.

Huntington's chorea is of autosomal dominant inheritance and usually first presents in the thirties. Choreiform movements, often particularly prominent in the face, are accompanied by progressive dementia. The movements may be well controlled by tetrabenazine (50–200 mg/d) which is usually tolerated in this condition. The mental deterioration is untreatable and institutional care may be needed as the disease progresses.

Ballism and Athetosis. Flinging limb movements of wide amplitude are called *ballismic movements*. They resemble chorea but are much more violent. It is sometimes an arbitrary decision whether one calls movements severe chorea or ballism. Usually they suddenly affect one side of the body (hemiballism or, if less dramatic, hemichorea) as a result of a vascular lesion in elderly patients. Spontaneous improvement usually occurs over a period of weeks and during this time tetrabenazine may decrease the disability. When hemiballism persists it can be treated by stereotactic thalamotomy.

Athetoid movements are relatively slow, confluent, writhing and usually most prominent at the periphery of the limbs. They are often accompanied by choreiform movements and by forced axial rotations of the trunk and neck (torsion dystonia). Athetosis usually results from cerebral hypoxia or trauma at birth or during the neonatal period and from kernicterus. Drug treatment is usually ineffective, though tetrabenazine, haloperidol or diazepam occasionally produce improvement in mild cases. Stereotactic procedures, indicated only in severe disability, sometimes help.

DIFFERENTIAL DIAGNOSIS. The involuntary movements of chorea, athetosis and ballism must be distinguished from *tics* which in most cases are not due to organic disease. Tics are usually rapid, repetitive, co-ordinated and stereotyped movements, most of which can be mimicked. Their pattern varies widely but an individual's tic tends to be reproduced faithfully. Common mild tics, including blepharospasm, sniffing, and shrugging movements, may be irritating but rarely need treatment. When well established in an adult they are virtually irremediable. In contrast, many children develop tics, often elaborate facial movements which cause much parental concern but which almost always disappear.

In adults, tics of recent development may be induced by drugs. Amphetamine addiction leads to repeated, rapid chewing movements of the jaws. Complex tongue, mouth, and cheek movements may result from taking phenothiazines or levodopa. Withdrawal of the causal drug usually leads to rapid cessation of the movement.

Spasmodic torticollis is a form of tic which comprises involuntary turning of the head to one side and starts most commonly in the thirties. Initially rapid and correctable rotating movements may give place to long-sustained and later to fixed deviation of the neck.

DEGENERATIVE AND CONGENITAL DISEASES

In many diseases of unknown cause, there is clinical and pathological evidence of damage which is confined to a special type of neurone, e.g. motor neurone disease. Although no causative factors have been identified, it seems probable that many of the following disorders will ultimately be classified together as being due to 'biochemical lesions'. The metabolic functions of the neurone are controlled by its cell body but when any gradual failure of any of these processes occurs the effect is first seen at the end of its axon, so that there occurs a progressive 'dying back' of the neurone from its termination towards the cell body, associated with loss of nucleo-protein in the cell (chromatolysis). This is the typical feature of the pathology of the degenerative and congenital disorders.

Motor Neurone Disease

This rare disorder of unknown cause is the paradigm of a systematised neurological disease.

Loss of motor neurones and gliosis can be demonstrated in the motor cortex, in the motor nuclei of the brain stem and in anterior horn cells of the spinal cord. In the cord, there is also loss of myelinated corticospinal fibres.

Clinical Features. Motor neurone disease is characterised by the insidious onset and uninterrupted progression of combinations of lesions of upper and/or lower motor neurones. Fasciculation (p. 594) is common. Motor neurone disease is twice as frequent in males and is rare before 40 years of age. The commonest age of onset is in the sixth decade. Some patterns of evolution are frequently manifest and are usefully categorised because they offer a guide to prognosis.

PROGRESSIVE BULBAR PALSY comprises dysarthria, dysphonia and dysphagia. Impaired articulation is usually the earliest feature but difficulty in swallowing, hoarseness and loss of voice volume supervene. There are signs of true, as well as supranuclear, bulbar palsy. Wasting and fasciculation of the tongue are accompanied by spasticity thereof and a pathologically brisk jaw jerk. Features of bulbar palsy eventually develop in the later stages of the other types listed below.

AMYOTROPHIC LATERAL SCLEROSIS is probably the commonest mode of presentation and is characterised by lower motor neurone signs in the upper limbs and upper motor neurone signs in the legs.

Wasting and weakness of the small muscles of the hands, usually the earliest manifestation, are accompanied by spasticity of the legs and extensor plantar responses. Wasting and fasciculation spread to the proximal arm muscles and the leg musculature; increased tendon reflexes in the arms may later indicate involvement of the upper motor neurones.

PROGRESSIVE MUSCULAR ATROPHY implicates only lower motor neurones for long periods. It usually presents with foot drop, which is often initially unilateral but eventually becomes symmetrical. Wasting and weakness of the hands, proximal spread of lower motor neurone affection in the limbs and the addition of upper motor neurone involvement occur after an interval of years.

COURSE. These labelled entities are frequently recognised but variant patterns are common. As the disease progresses the pictures of the different categories merge so that the final picture usually includes severe bulbar palsy as well as upper and lower motor neurone signs in all four limbs.

Diagnosis. Some aspects of the clinical features of motor neurone disease, irrespective of the particular type of natural history, are useful in diagnosis. There are no sensory signs. Sensory symptoms, with the exception of pain, are rare. Aches caused by the use of weakened muscles and painful cramps in the legs are fairly common. Paraesthesiae, unless clearly attributable to a coincidental cause, are not a feature of motor neurone disease and their presence should lead to critical reappraisal of the diagnosis.

Fasciculations, though not pathognomonic of the condition, are seen almost invariably in motor neurone disease in which they are usually more obvious and more widespread than in any other disease.

Though the initial manifestations of motor neurone disease are commonly unilateral, they usually become bilateral, and indeed symmetrical, in the vast majority of instances, within a few months.

In few other conditions do severely wasted muscles subserve pathologically brisk tendon reflexes. This phenomenon, sometimes called tonic atrophy is common to all types of motor neurone disease other than progressive muscular atrophy during its early stages.

Defects in external ocular movements and sphincter disturbances are extremely rare. Full awareness and normal intellectual abilities are usually preserved intact throughout the course of the illness. The CSF is almost always normal.

Three pathological processes which are potentially treatable may closely mimic motor neurone disease and should always be excluded. (i) An occult carcinoma (particularly of the bronchus) may produce systematised motor neurone lesions. A chest radiograph should always be obtained in patients presenting the features of motor neurone disease, and if there are indicative clinical features further investigations should be performed. (ii) Diabetic amyotrophy (p. 663) may resemble motor neurone disease and accordingly diabetes mellitus must be excluded. (iii) Meningovascular syphilis can present a picture similar to that of motor neurone disease and syphilitic serology is therefore an essential investigation.

Treatment and Prognosis. No medical treatment improves the outlook in motor neurone disease. Management includes the provision of walking aids and wheel-chairs and the maintenance of morale. Physicians have a duty to support patients and their relatives and to relieve distress in the disease's terminal stages.

Motor neurone disease is inexorably progressive and invariably fatal. Death usually results from pneumonia and respiratory failure and within 2 years of the onset of bulbar palsy. Amyotrophic lateral sclerosis is compatible with 4 or 5 years of life from the initial manifestation. Progressive muscular atrophy runs the most prolonged course; death usually occurs in 8 to 10 years from the onset.

The final state, of anarthria, aphagia and widespread limb weakness, in a person fully aware of the position, is extremely distressing for the patient and the family.

Spinal Muscular Atrophies

Common disorders — often wrongly diagnosed as motor neurone disease or as myopathies (p. 666) — are neurogenic muscular atrophies caused by genetically determined abnormalities of the anterior horn cells. In the spinal form of *peroneal muscular atrophy* (Charcot-Marie-Tooth syndrome) the lower motor neurone lesion is distal, but others are commonly proximal. Various forms are classified according to the age of onset. The *Werdnig-Hoffman type*, of infantile onset, is severe and rapidly progressive, whereas the adult-onset spinal muscular atrophy often progresses slowly. The lower motor neurone palsies with fasciculation may be mistaken for the graver motor neurone disease. Specialised investigation is required for reasons of prognostication and for genetic counselling though treatment is confined to orthopaedic management.

The Hereditary Ataxias

This is a group of related hereditary or familial disorders in which the systems of neurones which 'die back' (p. 652) are mainly the spinal and brain stem tracts leading to the cerebellum, the cortico-spinal tracts, and the optic nerves. Different combinations of these elements form recognisable clinical pictures, which usually 'breed true' in a family. The group forms a link with hereditary disorders of the peripheral nerves such as peroneal muscular atrophy (p. 653) and with neurofibromatosis (p. 655) and these may occur in association with the hereditary ataxias either in one individual or in the same family. Congenital deformities, particularly pes cavus, are also commonly present.

Cerebellar degeneration commencing in later life may be due to carcinomatous neuropathy (p. 668).

Clinical Features. The onset may be any time from infancy to middle life. Symptoms are slowly progressive. Where cerebellar or spinocerebellar neurones are involved there is progressive ataxia of gait, followed by intention tremor of the arms, dysarthria of explosive type and, in some types, nystagmus. Where the main lesion is in cortico-spinal tracts there is a hereditary spastic paraplegia. Optic atrophy and loss of bladder reflexes may occur.

Friedreich's ataxia is the most common type, usually familial but occasionally sporadic. There is degeneration of the spinocerebellar and corti-cospinal tracts, and of the posterior columns. There is therefore very severe ataxia. Tendon jerks are lost at an early stage, muscle tone is decreased and the plantar reflexes are extensor. Muscle, joint and vibration senses are impaired as the posterior column degeneration progresses. Scoliosis and pes cavus are almost invariable and other congenital abnormalities such as spina bifida are common. There may be an associated hypertrophic cardiomyopathy (p. 186).

Treatment and Prognosis. There is no specific treatment. Co-ordination exercises and occupational therapy will help the patient to overcome the disability in the early stages but a wheel-chair life becomes inevitable later. Scoliosis and pes cavus may require appropriate appliances or orthopaedic surgery. All diseases of this group are progressive but compatible with a long life.

Syringomyelia

Cavities, filled with fluid and surrounded by glial tissue, lying near to the centre of the spinal cord, are the characteristic pathological lesions in syringomyelia.

Aetiology. The most important factor is failure of development of the foramina of Magendie and Luschka. Cerebrospinal fluid cannot escape into the subarachnoid space from the fourth ventricle since its roof is imperforate. Pressure rises within the closed ventricular system and is communicated to the central canal of the cord which expands along irregular paths of least resistance.

The expanding cavity usually disrupts second order spinothalamic neurones, often interrupts the lateral columns, and may extend laterally to damage anterior horn cells (Figs 15.2 and 15.3). Clinical signs predictably reflect the interruption of function of these neural structures; this is usually maximal in the lower cervical region.

Dilatation of the central canal of the cord may also result from increased pressure in the canal associated with congenital malformations of the brain in the region of the foramen magnum, e.g. herniation of parts of the cerebellum through the foramen magnum (*Arnold-Chiari syndrome*) and cysts.

Clinical Features. Symptoms are of insidious onset, and slow progression. Patients usually present in the third or fourth decade but signs may be detectable much earlier. A most characteristic sensory feature is 'dissociated' sensory loss, i.e. loss or depression of pain and temperature sensation with preservation of the modalities of touch, vibration and position. The patient often recognises this sensory loss and seeks advice because of it. Less commonly, when pain fibres are irritated, pain in the arms is a presenting feature. Loss of protective sensory functions leads to trophic lesions such as painless burns and ulcers on the hands and sometimes painless, disorganised joints (Charcot's joints) in the upper limbs.

Wasting of the small muscles of one or other hand is often manifest early. Loss of one or more reflexes in the arms is almost invariable. Characteristically there are upper motor neurone signs in the legs. Hyperreflexia in the legs and extensor plantar responses are common.

Upward extension of the cavities to involve the lower brain stem (*syringobulbia*) leads to dissociated sensory loss on the face, palatal palsy, Horner's syndrome and nystagmus. Kyphoscoliosis, pes cavus and spina bifida are often found.

Investigations should be aimed at defining potentially treatable anomalies around the foramen magnum. Radiographs of this area may show bony malformations. CT scanning or myelography demonstrates cysts or malformations of the medulla.

Treatment and Prognosis. Where causative congenital lesions are demonstrated early, surgical treatment is indicated. Decompression of the foramen magnum, opening the roof of the fourth ventricle, aspiration of the cavity in the cord and occlusion, by muscle, of the upper end of the central canal, may prevent progression of the disease. If surgical treatment is not feasible, management is directed towards preventing injury. In the rarer cases where pain is a problem, it may be relieved by radiotherapy aimed at the cavity. If untreated the condition is slowly progressive, and worsens if the brain stem is involved.

Neurofibromatosis (Von Recklinghausen's Disease)

This is an autosomal dominant disorder in which fibromas are derived from the neurilemmal sheath of the peripheral nerves, nerve roots or cranial nerves. Tumours such as gliomas, meningiomas and phaeochromocytomas may be associated with neurofibromatosis.

Clinical Features. A patient may show only one or many of a wide range of cutaneous or of peripheral or central neurological abnormalities. Some of the more common are *café-au-lait* patches of skin pigmentation, cutaneous fibromas and benign tumours of peripheral nerves which are discrete, movable lumps arranged along the course of nerves. The nerve trunks may be thickened or there may be a diffuse plexiform growth.

Solitary neurofibromas may occur on a spinal nerve root or on a cranial nerve, especially the eighth. The tumours may also occur within body cavities, in the eyes and within the bones where they cause cystic change or kyphoscoliosis. New tumours gradually appear throughout life but the progress is slow. Any tumour may become malignant (sarcoma) but the chances of it doing so are small.

Biopsy of a tumour is rarely necessary. With intracranial and intraspinal types the protein level of the CSF is very high. Radiological examination may show that an internal auditory meatus or intervertebral foramen is widened if it contains a neurofibroma.

Treatment. No treatment is required unless there is cerebral or spinal compression, or sarcomatous change, when removal of the tumour is necessary.

NUTRITIONAL NEUROLOGICAL DISEASES

Malnutrition may cause lesions in a number of sites in the nervous system. Deficiencies, particularly of the B vitamin group, are important causes but there are often multiple contributory factors and vitamin deficiencies may be combined with protein deficiency and toxins, notably alcohol. The various neurological syndromes that ensue are best considered on an anatomical basis.

Lesions of the Cerebral Cortex. Vitamin B_{12} deficiency may cause a toxic confusional state and, if the deficiency is prolonged, may result in dementia. Pellagra (p. 77) gives rise to marked impairment of higher cerebral function, delirium and dementia. An isolated deficiency of pyridoxine (p. 79) occasionally occurs in infants and causes irritability and epileptic fits.

Alcoholics may develop a slowly progressive dementia with cerebral atrophy due in part to a direct toxic effect of alcohol but associated multiple vitamin deficiencies also contribute.

Brain Stem Lesions. Rapidly developing, severe deficiency of thiamin may cause *Wernicke's encephalopathy* (p. 75). Pathologically there are petechial haemorrhages in the brain stem and widespread patchy necrosis of neurones. Clinically there are disorders of ocular movement with nystagmus often accompanied by memory defect and confabulation (*Korsakoff's psychosis* p. 75). The condition, if untreated, may be fatal but thiamin, if started early enough, produces dramatic improvement.

Central pontine myelinolysis occurs in alcoholics. There is widespread destruction of myelin in the pons involving all the long tracts. The picture usually develops suddenly with tetraparesis, dysphagia and anarthria and is often terminal.

Cerebellar Lesions. Ataxia of gait and of leg movements with little affection of the arms is due to degeneration of the anterior superior vermis of the cerebellum in alcoholics; if the patient continues to drink alcohol more widespread cerebellar dysfunction develops. The contributions of dietary deficiency and the toxic effect of alcohol are not clearly defined but withdrawal of alcohol and giving vitamins result in marked improvement.

Spinal Cord Lesions. VITAMIN B$_{12}$ DEFICIENCY: This condition is also called *subacute combined degeneration of the spinal cord* and is characterised by demyelination affecting particularly the posterior columns and corticospinal tracts of the spinal cord. There is usually involvement of the peripheral nerves.

The condition is associated with Addisonian pernicious anaemia (p. 501) and rarely follows gastrectomy. It usually develops gradually in the middle aged. The most common presenting symptoms are paraesthesiae of the toes and, later, of the fingers. Motor symptoms, notably weakness and ataxia, become progressively more severe as the spinal cord is more extensively involved.

The physical signs depend on the degrees of involvement of the peripheral nerves and of the posterior and lateral columns of the spinal cord. Glove and stocking impairment of superficial sensation is almost invariable. Calf tenderness is often increased. Position and vibration sense are usually markedly impaired in the legs. The tendon reflexes may be brisk but commonly the ankle jerks are lost. The plantar responses are usually extensor. Occasionally there may be an associated toxic confusional state. It responds to treatment, but without treatment, dementia follows.

The diagnosis should be considered whenever a patient presents with symmetrical paraesthesiae or with unexplained dementia. Associated features such as glossitis, megaloblastic anaemia and achlorhydria will strongly support the diagnosis but need not be present. Diagnosis should be confirmed by the estimation of vitamin B$_{12}$ in the serum.

The treatment of vitamin B$_{12}$ deficiency comprises large doses of hydroxocobalamin, 1000 micrograms daily for a week, weekly for three months and monthly thereafter. The response to treatment depends on the stage at which it is initiated. The signs due to a peripheral neuropathy often recover completely; ataxia may markedly improve; severe spasticity and dementia often persist.

TROPICAL SPINAL ATAXIA occurs mainly in West Africa. In most cases the picture is one of sensory spinal ataxia but sometimes there is upper motor neurone involvement and amblyopia with optic atrophy.

This type of spastic paraparesis seems in most cases to be due to chronic exposure to excess dietary cyanide in those who live largely on a diet of cassava, which is rich in cyanide. A similar type of spastic paraparesis with amblyopia occurs in West Indians, but the nature of the aetiology in these cases is ill-defined.

LATHYRISM. The consumption of peas, a common constituent of Indian diets, may produce an acute or slowly progressive spastic paraplegia if the pulses include *Lathyrus sativus* which contains a neurotoxin. A similar type of spastic paraplegia was described in European prisoners of war in the Far East. This was probably due to multiple vitamin deficiencies though the precise agent was not identified.

Peripheral Nerve Lesions. Deficiencies of one or more of the vitamins of the B complex lead to neuropathy. Thiamin, nicotinic acid and pyridoxine deficiencies may cause a symmetrical, mixed sensory-motor neuropathy (p. 663). In many instances, particularly in alcoholics, there are combined deficiencies of these vitamins. If treated early, nutritional polyneuropathy responds well to a mixed diet and generous doses of the vitamin B complex.

The *burning feet syndrome* is due to a mild but painful sensory neuropathy which occurs among the elderly who subsist on an inadequate diet. The cause is deficiency of the B group of vitamins. Patients complain of severe, lancinating or burning pains in the feet and distal parts of the legs, particularly in bed at night. Signs of polyneuropathy are sparse or absent. The response to vitamin B complex, given orally, is usually good.

DISEASES OF THE SPINAL CORD AND PERIPHERAL NERVES

COMPRESSION OF THE SPINAL CORD OR NERVE ROOTS

Aetiology and Pathology. The more important causes of spinal cord compression are:

1. *In the vertebral column:* crush fracture of a vertebral body; posterior protrusion of an intervertebral disc; secondary carcinoma (from breast, prostate, bronchus or other sites); myelomatosis and tuberculous disease of the spine.

2. *In relation to the spinal meninges:* epidural abscess; tumours (meningioma, neurofibroma; infiltration with lymphomatous and leukaemic deposits); syphilitic meningitis.

3. *In the spinal cord:* tumours (gliomas, ependymoma and metastatic deposits).

Tumours, disc protrusions and trauma account for the majority of cases of spinal cord compression. It is convenient in practice to divide the tumours into those arising outside the spinal cord (extramedullary), which constitute about 80%, and those arising within (intramedullary).

A space-occupying lesion within the spinal canal may involve nerve tissue directly by pressure, or indirectly by interfering with the blood supply. Oedema from venous obstruction impairs the function of the neurones. Ischaemia from arterial obstruction leads to necrosis of the spinal cord. The earlier stages are reversible but severely damaged neurones do not recover so it is most important to diagnose and treat spinal compression without delay.

Clinical Features. The onset of symptoms of spinal cord compression is usually slow but it may be acute with trauma or metastases, especially if there is arterial occlusion. Pain localised over the spine or in a root distribution is the most common initial symptom. It may be aggravated by spinal movement or by coughing, sneezing or straining at the toilet which cause temporary elevation of spinal fluid pressure. Paraesthesiae and numbness or cold sensations may also develop early, especially in the lower limbs. Motor symptoms, which usually appear later, consist of heaviness, stiffness or weakness of a limb. Urgency or hesitancy of micturition, leading eventually to urinary retention is usually a late manifestation.

The signs found on examination vary according to the structures involved. There may be a local kyphosis if there is vertebral disease, and local tenderness may be present with this or with extradural abscess. A bruit may be heard with a stethoscope over the site of a vascular tumour (angioma).

Involvement of the posterior roots gives rise to hyperaesthesia and later to sensory loss over the appropriate dermatome. When the anterior roots are affected there are signs of a lower motor neurone lesion at the corresponding level.

Interruption of ascending fibres in the spinal cord causes sensory loss below the level of the lesion which may be of superficial sensation or of proprioceptive sense, according to which tracts are mainly involved (Fig. 15.3). Light touch, however, is often affected early. Interruption of descending fibres gives rise to upper motor neurone signs below the level of the lesion and control of the sphincters may be lost.

If damage is confined to one side of the cord the *Brown-Séquard syndrome* results. On the side of the lesion there is a band of hyperaesthesia with below it loss of proprioceptive sense and upper motor neurone signs. On the other side there is loss of spinothalamic sensation (pain, warmth and cold) as fibres of that tract decussate soon after entering the cord.

The distribution of these signs varies with the level of the lesion. Lesions above the fifth cervical segment give signs of an upper motor neurone lesion and sensory loss in upper and lower limbs (tetraplegia). A lesion between the fifth cervical and first thoracic segments gives signs of a lower motor neurone lesion and segmental sensory loss in the upper limbs and signs of an upper motor neurone lesion in the lower limbs. A lesion in the thoracic cord causes a spastic paraplegia with sensory loss having a horizontal upper level on the trunk. A lesion in the lumbosacral cord gives signs of a lower motor neurone lesion in the appropriate segments of the lower limbs and sensory loss. Spinal lesions lower than the first lumbar vertebra cannot damage the spinal cord but may damage the roots of the cauda equina.

Examination of the CSF is of great value but withdrawal of fluid may alter the pressure balance above and below the lesion in the cord and lead to rapid exacerbation of compression. For this reason, if lumbar puncture confirms the diagnosis, the patient should be referred without any delay to a neurosurgeon and if the diagnosis is highly probable on clinical grounds the puncture should be postponed until it is convenient to operate on the patient. The cell content is normal but there is a great excess of protein and xanthochromia is present (*Froin's syndrome*). Radiological examination of the spine may reveal abnormalities at the site of the lesion but often further investigation is required.

Diagnosis. Pain, which is so often a presenting symptom of spinal cord compression, may be wrongly attributed to such conditions as pleurisy, cholecystitis or 'rheumatism', but a careful examination will reveal signs of sensory impairment.

If there is indisputable evidence of spinal cord damage it is essential to decide the site of the primary lesion. A general examination may reveal evidence of disease elsewhere making it likely that the lesion in the cord is secondary to this. A search should be made for a primary tumour in another organ, enlargement of lymph nodes, the cutaneous signs of neurofibromatosis and the presence of sepsis which could lead to extradural abscess. An abscess should always be considered if pain is severe and signs of cord disease develop rapidly as immediate treatment is imperative.

If the lesion causing compression arose initially in the spinal cord it is necessary to distinguish it from conditions such as multiple sclerosis, syringomyelia, motor neurone disease and subacute combined degeneration. Multiple sclerosis appearing for the first time in middle-aged people may present as a slowly progressive lesion of the spinal cord. The differentiation from spinal cord compression is, however, so difficult and of such importance that there should be no hesitation in seeking expert advice.

Treatment and Prognosis. Surgical relief of the compression is a matter of great urgency since recovery from severe paralysis is unlikely. A delay of even a few hours may be critical in extradural abscess. Exploration is also often required to ascertain the pathological nature of the lesion. If a benign extramedullary tumour is found, it may be removed. In malignant tumours, leukaemic infiltration, and in most intramedullary lesions decompression helps little if at all. Radiotherapy may halt the course of the disease and may be of help in the relief of pain.

Prognosis depends on the severity and duration of the compression before it is relieved. In addition, the nature of the cause must be taken into account. Thus decompression for a malignant lesion may be undertaken though it will be of only temporary benefit.

Paraplegia

Paraplegia may result from many causes, e.g. tumours, trauma and other forms of spinal compression (p. 657), multiple sclerosis, subacute combined degeneration of the cord and, in India, lathyrism.

Treatment must be directed to the cause but management of the paraplegia itself is most important if complications, which may in themselves lead to death, are to be avoided. Pressure sores, urinary infections, renal calculi, faecal impaction and contractures can all be prevented.

SKIN. The skin is liable to be damaged with the formation of pressure sores because of the loss of sensation, diminished blood supply and the immobility. The patient must be nursed on a specially made rubber mattress and every two to four hours should be turned to a position which will avoid pressure on bony prominences such as the sacrum and heels. This is most easily done by nursing the patient in a Stryker frame.

The skin must be kept dry and clean. If a pressure sore forms, the patient must not lie on the affected side and scrupulous asepsis must be observed until healing takes place. Skin grafting may be required. Nutrition must be maintained by a well-balanced diet containing adequate amounts of protein, vitamin C and iron.

BLADDER. If retention occurs, aseptic intermittent catheterisation must be carried out. An indwelling catheter may then be inserted and attached to a water-seal drainage bottle. It should be clipped and allowed to drain at regular intervals to establish reflex emptying of the bladder. As the rhythm becomes established the catheter is withdrawn and the patient trained to micturate reflexly at fixed times. Emptying of the bladder should be assisted by manual compression of the lower abdomen by patient or nurse.

It is not advisable to give antibiotics prophylactically but if infection develops, it must be treated promptly. An adequate consumption of fluid should be ensured. Frequent turning and early ambulation where possible are the best measures for reducing the dangers of urinary stagnation and calculus formation.

BOWEL. Constipation must be prevented by suitable diet and laxatives. If it occurs it must be relieved by enemas; otherwise the faeces will become hard and impacted and may require to be removed manually.

PARALYSED PARTS. Spasticity readily leads to the development of flexor spasm and contractures in the limbs. This danger can be reduced by regular passive movement of the limbs and by nursing the patient in such positions as will discourage flexion of the joints. The weight of the bedclothes should be taken from the lower limbs by a cradle to reduce reflex stimulation and prevent drop-foot deformity. If there is no hope of recovery, flexor spasms may be abolished by intrathecal injection of phenol in glycerine or by section of anterior nerve roots.

REHABILITATION. When the cause of paraplegia is not progressive, a great deal can be done by rehabilitation. Patients may learn to walk with calipers or to use a wheel-chair. They may thus be able to care for themselves and may even follow suitable occupations and take part in a variety of recreational activities.

Cervical Disc Herniation and Cervical Spondylosis

Degenerative changes occur in the cervical intervertebral discs in the same manner as in the lumbar region (p. 660) and may lead to herniation. This may affect one disc only, most commonly that between the sixth and seventh cervical vertebrae, or there may be involvement of several discs with secondary osteoarthrosis. The latter changes (cervical spondylosis) are especially liable to interfere with the blood supply to the spinal cord, and thus lead to further damage.

The clinical syndromes of acute cervical disc protrusion and chronic cervical spondylosis may occur at different times in the same patient, depending on the anatomical relation of disc protrusions and osteophytic outgrowths to the nerve roots and spinal cord, and on secondary postural or traumatic factors. Acute herniation is usually laterally situated and causes compression of a nerve root but does not involve the spinal cord. The chronic degeneration of discs is associated with midline herniation and so spinal cord compression may result.

Acute Protrusion of a Cervical Intervertebral Disc. This may occur at any age, usually without apparent trauma to the neck. The patient complains of attacks of pain in the neck. In severe attacks pain is referred to the skin segmental area of one of the lower cervical nerve roots and to the muscles, bones and joints which it supplies. Hyperaesthesia and hyperalgesia may be found in the affected segment but sensory loss sometimes occurs. Depression of tendon reflexes utilising the affected root is common and lower motor neurone paresis of root distribution is also an occasional finding. The neck is held stiffly, and pain is produced by its movement.

Cervical Spondylosis. This term is used for the disorder resulting from chronic cervical disc degeneration. The highest incidence is in the decade 60 to 70. The symptoms are of two types depending on whether the protrusion is lateral or dorsomedial.

(1) Lateral herniation of discs, with secondary calcification and osteophytes encroaching on the intervertebral foramina, causes radicular symptoms like those of the acute disc syndrome just described, but the onset may be subacute or insidious and involvement of more than one root on one or both sides is common.

(2) Dorsomedial herniation of discs which become calcified results in transverse bars which cause pressure on the spinal cord and on the anterior spinal artery which supplies the anterior two-thirds of the cord.

The onset is insidious. Upper motor neurone weakness involves one or more limbs and the legs may be spastic before the upper limbs are involved. Sensory loss is most common in the upper limbs where it has a dermatome pattern. Involvement of the spinothalamic tracts may cause disturbance of pain and temperature sensation in the lower limbs, and in some cases muscle-joint sense is also defective. Pain and limitation of movement of the neck are not marked features unless a particular posture causes nipping of a nerve root.

Investigation. Radiological examination shows narrowing of the disc spaces and osteophyte formation with loss of the normal cervical lordosis. Oblique views show encroachment by osteophytes on the intervertebral foramina. The CSF is normal unless its circulation is obstructed, when the protein may be raised. It may be necessary to confirm the diagnosis by myelography.

Treatment. The acute syndrome is treated by rest in bed or by intermittent neck traction followed by immobilisation of the neck in a light metal or plastic collar. It is important to watch for progressive cervical cord compression but decompressive surgery is rarely required.

The Lumbago-Sciatica Syndrome

Lumbago is pain in the lower part of the back; sciatica is pain in the distribution of the sciatic nerve. They are not, therefore, disease entities but symptoms and they are often associated.

Aetiology and Pathology. The most common cause is herniation of an intervertebral disc.

Other causes are much rarer but important to recognise. They include spinal tumour (neurofibroma and meningioma), ankylosing spondylitis, malignant disease in the pelvis, and tuberculosis of the vertebral bodies. Degenerative changes in the intervertebral discs may appear as early as 20 years of age, but herniation is often precipitated by trauma such as twisting the spine, lifting heavy weights while the spine is flexed or during childbirth. The nucleus pulposus may bulge or rupture the annulus fibrosus, giving rise to lumbago by pressure on nerve endings in the spinal ligaments and by producing changes in the vertebral joints, and to sciatica by causing congestion of, or pressure on, the nerve roots.

Clinical Features. The onset may be sudden or gradual, and may follow closely upon trauma to the back. Attacks of lumbago may precede sciatica by months or years.

Lumbago is characterised by sudden severe low back pain when the patient is bending, preventing straightening. The sciatic pain is felt in the buttock and radiates down the posterior aspect of the thigh and calf to the outer border of the foot. It is exacerbated by coughing or sneezing which raises the pressure in the veins and the spinal subarachnoid space. Paraesthesiae and later numbness may be felt over the distribution of the involved nerve root, most often the first sacral. In severe cases, weakness of the calf muscles or foot-drop may occur, according to which roots are involved. The signs associated with prolapse of an intervertebral disc may be divided into two groups.

Signs Due to Altered Mechanics of the Lumbar Spine. Muscle spasm causes flattening of the lumbar curve and scoliosis at the level of the prolapsed disc. Tenderness may be found when pressure is applied to the side of the vertebral spines in the region of the affected disc.

Signs Due to Pressure on the Nerve Root. Involvement of the *first sacral* root causes loss of the ankle jerk, weakness of eversion and plantar flexion of the foot, and sensory loss over the outer border of the foot. The glutei may be wasted on the affected side. Involvement of the *fifth lumbar* root causes weakness of dorsiflexion of the toes and sometimes foot-drop. Sensory loss occurs on the dorsum of the foot and the lateral aspect of the leg over the fifth lumbar dermatome. The ankle jerk is not affected. Involvement of the *fourth lumbar* root causes weakness of inversion of the foot and of the quadriceps muscle and loss of the knee jerk. Sensory loss is over the medial aspect of the leg.

A valuable sign of root pressure is limitation of flexion of the thigh on the affected side if the straight leg is raised (Lasègue's sign).

Investigation. Other causes of sciatic pain can be excluded by pelvic examination and by radiological examination of the lumbosacral spine. There may be no apparent radiological change in acute disc herniation, or there may be narrowing of the disc space with osteophyte formation at the margins of the vertebral bodies. Myelography is required only if the diagnosis is in doubt or for purposes of localisation before operation. Intraspinal neoplasm as the cause should be suspected if the CSF protein is raised.

Treatment. The initial treatment in all cases is rest in bed on a firm mattress supported by fracture boards. Rest must be absolute with prohibition of the sitting position. Compromise in this respect and permission to leave bed for toilet purposes are the usual reasons for failure of this treatment. The roots most commonly involved are the first sacral and the fifth lumbar, in which case the patient should be kept supine and no rotation of the spine permitted; but in disc protrusion involving the fourth lumbar root the lateral position with flexion of the hips is best suited to relax tension on the affected root and hence to relieve pain. Bed rest is continued for two to four weeks, after which gradual mobilisation with back-strengthening exercises is carried out over a further period of 10 to 14 days. For middle-aged or elderly patients with chronic residual backache and a tendency to acute attacks of lumbago, a spinal support may be of value. Cases which do not respond to rest, or in which there have been recurrences, may require surgery.

PERIPHERAL NEUROPATHY

The cells of origin of peripheral nerves lie in the anterior horns of the spinal cord and the dorsal root ganglia. Axons represent elongated processes of these cells. They are enveloped by a series of Schwann cells which form the fatty myelin sheath. Pathological processes which primarily affect cell bodies may first manifest themselves at the distal ends of axonal processes.

Many diseases affect peripheral nerves whose pathological reactions may be (1) parenchymal where the lesion affects (a) nerve cells and their axons, or (b) the myelin sheath; (2) interstitial where the pathological process primarily affects the connective tissue or blood vessels of nerves. Although these rather stereotyped reactions do not lead to distinctive clinical features, a knowledge of the pathological nature of a neuropathy is helpful in assessing its prognosis. The clinical classification of peripheral nerve lesions comprises (1) involvement of one or more individual peripheral nerves or (2) a generalised polyneuropathy.

Mononeuropathy

This term refers to affection of a single nerve. Trauma is a common cause. Sustained pressure or stretching of nerve occurs in a variety of situations. The radial nerve is implicated as, for instance, in the 'Saturday night' palsy which results from bizarre sleeping postures caused by drunkenness. The ulnar nerve at the elbow and common peroneal nerve at the head of the fibula may be compressed. The signs are those of lower motor neurone paresis and sensory loss in the distribution of the respective nerves. Complete recovery of function in four to six weeks is almost invariable.

Diabetes, particularly if insulin dependent, is a common cause of an acute mononeuropathy affecting a peripheral (or cranial) nerve. Recovery is usually complete in 4 to 8 weeks.

ENTRAPMENT NEUROPATHY. Nerves may be compressed whenever they pass through or near rigid anatomical structures, particularly fibro-osseous tunnels; this is one of the most frequent affections of peripheral nerves.

Compression of the median nerve in the carpal tunnel is the commonest example. It occurs most frequently in middle-aged women and is then usually unaccompanied by other disease. It may also be a complication of pregnancy, myxoedema, acromegaly or rheumatoid arthritis (p. 555). The patient complains of pain, numbness, tingling or an 'electric shock' feeling in thumb and fingers supplied by the median nerve, especially after using the hand or in bed at night when it may waken the patient from sleep. There is sometimes objective sensory loss of the radial three and a half digits and there may be weakness and wasting of abductor pollicis brevis and opponens pollicis muscles. The condition is often bilateral.

Rest and splinting at night should be tried. Local injection of hydrocortisone is sometimes effective if there is no muscular wasting. Thyroxine therapy relieves the carpal tunnel syndrome in myxoedema. The syndrome occurring in pregnancy usually disappears in the puerperium but until then may be controlled by the use of diuretics. If these measures are unsuccessful the condition can be relieved by surgical decompression of the nerve in the carpal tunnel.

The *lower trunk of the brachial plexus* may be compressed at the thoracic outlet, especially if there is a cervical rib. Nocturnal pain in the arm and sensori-motor disturbance in the C8-T1 distribution are relieved by rest and physiotherapy. Operative treatment is rarely necessary.

The *lateral cutaneous nerve of the thigh* may be entrapped at the inguinal ligament giving rise to paraesthesiae and pain over the anterolateral aspect of the thigh (meralgia paraesthetica).

Mononeuritis Multiplex

In this condition several spinal nerves are involved concurrently or serially. Clinically signs are limited to discrete neural territories. Leprosy is a common cause of this picture in some geographical areas (p. 758). Polyarteritis nodosa, rheumatoid arthritis (p. 555) and other connective tissue disorders, diabetes mellitus and sarcoidosis may also give rise to multiple peripheral nerve lesions.

Localised Radiculopathy

Neuralgic Amyotrophy. Demyelination of a localised group of nerve roots sometimes follows vaccination or inoculation; an immunological mechanism may be responsible. It may also occur after infection, injuries or operations.

The patient complains of severe pain over one shoulder girdle, sometimes spreading up the neck or down the arm. Simultaneously, or two or three days later, paralysis develops in the painful muscles. These are usually supplied by the fifth and sixth and less commonly the seventh cervical roots so that the deltoid, spinati, and serratus anterior muscles are usually involved, and frequently also the muscles of the upper arm. The tendon jerks disappear in the affected limb and wasting is rapid. Sensory loss is slight or absent. If present it is usually on the outer aspect of the upper third of the affected arm. The brachial plexus is often tender. Sometimes paralysis of single nerves of the upper limb occurs and occasionally both shoulder girdles are involved. Constitutional symptoms are mild or absent. The CSF is normal or shows only slight lymphocytosis.

Pain usually subsides in one to two weeks. Recovery from paralysis is slow. It usually takes several months, but eventual complete recovery after two or more years is usual. Recurrent attacks of neuritis in the same or the opposite shoulder rarely occur. Corticosteroids may be tried in the early stages.

Generalised Polyneuropathy

When the causal lesion lies in the nerve cell body the first manifestations are at the distal end of the longest nerves. This gives rise to the typical picture of a generalised polyneuropathy with distal paraesthesiae first affecting the feet and later the hands, and progressing proximally up the limbs. These sensory symptoms are associated with diminution of superficial sensation over 'stocking' and 'glove' areas. There is also distal weakness with diminished or absent tendon reflexes. There are variations of this stereotyped picture, e.g. the Guillain-Barré syndrome.

Aetiology. There are a large number of causes; some of the most important are listed:

GENETICALLY DETERMINED NEUROPATHIES: the peripheral type of peroneal muscular atrophy; progressive hypertrophic polyneuritis; hereditary sensory neuropathy.

DEFICIENCY NEUROPATHIES: deficiencies of vitamins B_1, B_2, B_6 and B_{12}; folate deficiency.

TOXIC NEUROPATHY: lead, arsenic, mercury, triorthocresylphosphate; a variety of organic chemicals such as carbon tetrachloride, acrylamide and aniline dyes; a large number of drugs including chloroquine, phenytoin and vinca alkaloids; solvent abuse.

NEUROPATHIES ASSOCIATED WITH INFECTIONS: leprosy is true infective neuropathy; polyneuropathy may complicate a number of infections including influenza, measles, and typhoid fever; some neuropathies are due to exotoxins notably diphtheritic polyneuropathy; the Guillain-Barré syndrome.

CONNECTIVE TISSUE DISORDERS: polyarteritis nodosa; rheumatoid arthritis, systemic lupus erythematosus and occasionally giant cell arteritis.

METABOLIC NEUROPATHIES: diabetes mellitus; renal and hepatic failure; acute intermittent porphyria.

MALIGNANT DISEASE: carcinoma of the bronchus and other malignant tumours.

Descriptions of the many neuropathies listed above would be repetitive. Diabetic neuropathies illustrate the various clinical patterns of the polyneuropathies and the Guillain-Barré syndrome is a relatively common and life threatening disease. These conditions will be discussed in more detail.

Diabetic Polyneuropathy

Peripheral neuropathies of various types are commonly associated with diabetes mellitus. Conversely diabetes is a frequent cause of peripheral neuropathy. In general, diabetic neuropathies occur more often in older patients and their incidence increases when control of diabetes is poor.

The following main categories of diabetic neuropathy are not mutually exclusive, and mixed pictures occur.

Distal, symmetrical, mixed sensory-motor polyneuropathy is a common form of diabetic neuropathy. It occurs most frequently in elderly, long-standing diabetics. Distal, symmetrical paraesthesiae is the commonest presenting feature. There is usually glove and stocking sensory loss and distal weakness with loss of ankle jerks. Exacerbations may occur when control of the diabetes is inadequate but this type of distal neuropathy also occurs in well-controlled diabetics and responds poorly to treatment.

Motor neuropathy (diabetic amyotrophy) is an asymmetrical, predominantly motor and proximal form of neuropathy. It often occurs in elderly diabetics and is sometimes the presenting feature in patients who have no other symptoms of diabetes. There is usually asymmetrical wasting of the quadriceps with diminution or loss of knee reflexes. With good control of diabetes, complete recovery is usual though resolution may take one or two years.

Sensory neuropathy is a distal, symmetrical, sensory neuropathy. Patients complain of numbness and paraesthesiae of the feet spreading up the legs and later involving the fingers. Glove and stocking sensory loss is common. As the condition progresses there is loss of position sense and vibration sense in the legs with the development of sensory ataxia. Trophic lesions such as ulcers and Charcot joints may supervene. Since many patients with diabetes have pupillary abnormalities due to recurrent attacks of uveitis this picture may resemble tabes dorsalis and indeed is sometimes called diabetic pseudotabes.

Autonomic neuropathy. Impotence is probably the most frequent symptom of autonomic diabetic neuropathy. There is sometimes also involvement of the nerve supply to the intestine causing diarrhoea which is usually nocturnal or postprandial. Impaired cardiovascular reflexes are found in 20% of diabetics but symptomatic postural hypotension is uncommon. Other manifestations are tachycardia and disturbances of sweating and micturition.

The Guillain-Barré Syndrome (Acute Post-Infection Polyneuropathy)

About two-thirds of the patients with this neuropathy have had an infection 1–4 weeks before its onset. This and other features are considered to indicate an immunological pathogenesis resulting in multifocal demyelination in spinal roots and peripheral nerves.

The presenting clinical features vary. Pain in the back is common. There may be tingling affecting the distal part of the limbs and ascending proximally. In about 50% of patients motor symptoms predominate, with weakness which may be profound and rapidly progressive and which often affects proximal more than distal limb musculature. Facial muscles are commonly involved. The most striking findings on examination are diffuse weakness and widespread loss of reflexes. The rate of spread is variable. Occasional patients will develop quadriparesis with respiratory failure within a few hours of the initial symptoms. In other cases there will be a progression for one to two weeks.

The protein content of the cerebrospinal fluid is markedly raised in most patients at some time during the illness though it may be normal during the first ten days. There is usually no rise in cells.

The most important aspect of the management of patients with the Guillain-Barré syndrome is the maintenance of respiration. During the initial stages of the illness careful monitoring of respiratory function is essential. A deterioration in respiratory function tests or subjective feelings of dyspnoea should lead to early tracheostomy and the institution of intermittent positive pressure respiration. Some patients, especially with a recurrent type of the disease, are helped by plasma exchange.

The prognosis is good providing respiration is maintained. Approximately 90% of patients will recover completely within 3 to 8 weeks; 5% will die and 5% will be left with residual paralysis.

ACUTE INTERMITTENT PORPHYRIA may cause a neuropathy similar to that of the Guillain-Barré syndrome. Acute intermittent porphyria is characterised by attacks of unexplained colicky abdominal pain, constipation and psychiatric disturbances, notably confusion and emotional lability. Tachycardia and hypertension are frequent. The condition is due to a hereditary deficiency of an enzyme in the pathway of haem biosynthesis and an attack may be precipitated by phenobarbitone, oral contraceptives, sulphonamides, pentazocine, methyldopa, chlorpropamide, alcohol and other drugs. The diagnosis is confirmed by the finding of porphobilinogen in the urine (p. 382).

Diagnosis, Prevention and Treatment of Polyneuropathy

Diagnosis. The clinical picture will usually localise the lesions to the peripheral nerves. Nerve conduction velocities will, in most cases, confirm the presence of impaired conduction in nerve trunks. This will be gross in most cases of peripheral segmental demyelination and relatively minor in lesions affecting nerve axons. Occasionally, particularly in those with interstitial neuropathies, a sural nerve biopsy will establish the cause. Sometimes the pattern of the clinical picture, as in the Guillain-Barré syndrome, will indicate the likely diagnosis. Although the presence of a polyneuropathy is easily established clinically, the definition of a cause may be difficult. The presence of associated diseases, drug ingestion or exposure to toxic chemicals should be sought in each case. The possibility of diabetes mellitus should always be excluded.

If the constellation of findings from the history, the family history or the clinical signs does not indicate a likely aetiology then it may often prove impossible to establish a cause for a peripheral neuropathy.

Prevention and Treatment. Any new drug which is liable to cause neuropathy must be used with care and industrial hazards should be avoided by protective clothing, exhaust ventilation and other techniques advised by the industrial medical officer.

When polyneuropathy has developed as a result of exposure to a toxic substance the first step is to remove the patient from further exposure. When the cause is nutritional every effort should be made to restore the original body weight; plenty of protein is desirable supplemented by generous doses of the vitamin B complex. If the cause is metabolic the appropriate treatment must be initiated without delay, e.g. for diabetes.

In severe cases bed rest is essential since the nervous control of the heart may be defective and cardiomyopathy is sometimes associated. The limbs should be supported in the optimum position, and passive movements carried out several times a day. A cage should protect the feet from the weight of the bed-clothes. Respiratory insufficiency may require tracheostomy or institution of intermittent positive pressure respiration (p. 217). When recovery begins, active movements should be carried out under the supervision of a physiotherapist.

DISEASES OF MUSCLE

Diseases of muscle are not diseases of the nervous system, but as some of their manifestations may be readily confused with neurological conditions myasthenia gravis and myopathy are described here.

MYASTHENIA GRAVIS

This condition is characterised by progressive failure to sustain a maintained or repeated contraction of striated muscles.

Aetiology and Pathology. Nicotinic receptors of acetylcholine in the post-junctional membrane of neuromuscular junctions are blocked or lysed by a complement-mediated autoimmune reaction between receptor protein and anti-acetylcholine receptor antibody. The antibody is produced by B lymphocytes defectively controlled by T lymphocytes because of a disorder of the thymus gland. About 15% of cases, mainly of late onset, have an encapsulated or locally invasive thymoma. The majority, including all young cases, have one of a number of thymic abnormalities, the most characteristic being germinal centres in the medulla of the gland. The latter group has a marked personal and familial relationship with other autoimmune diseases (p. 29), and many have inherited an immunoreactive gene which is linked to some of the HLA haplotypes; in a North European population these are HLA-B8 and DRw3. Inheritance of this gene is not obligatory for myasthenia and nothing is known about possible triggering factors for the spontaneous disease. Penicillamine may be one such breaker of immunological tolerance.

Clinical Features. The disease usually appears between the ages of 15 and 50 and females are more often affected than males. It tends to run a remitting course especially during the early years. Relapses may be precipitated by emotional disturbances, infections, pregnancy and severe muscular effort.

The cardinal symptom is abnormal fatiguability of muscles; movement, though initially strong, rapidly weakens. Intensification of symptoms towards the end of the day or following vigorous exercise is characteristic.

The first symptoms are usually intermittent ptosis or diplopia but weakness of chewing, swallowing, speaking or of moving the limbs also occurs. Any muscle of a limb may be affected, most commonly those of the shoulder girdle, so that the patient is unable to undertake work above the level of the shoulder, such as combing the hair, without frequent rests. Respiratory muscles may be involved and respiratory failure is a not uncommon cause of death. Asphyxia occurs readily as the cough may be too weak to clear foreign bodies from the airways. Muscle atrophy may occur in long-standing cases. There are no signs of involvement of the central nervous system.

An invaluable diagnostic aid is the increase in muscle strength produced by an intravenous injection of a short-acting anticholinesterase, edrophonium hydrochloride. An initial dose of 2 mg is injected and a further 8 mg given half a minute later if there are no undesirable reactions such as fasciculation, sweating and colic. Improvement in muscle power occurs within 30 seconds of the injection and usually persists for 2 or 3 minutes. Ptosis or defects in eye movements are the most convenient parameters of improvement but diminution of dysarthria or increase of power in the limbs can also demonstrate a response to edrophonium.

Treatment. The principles of treatment are: (i) to maximise the activity of acetylcholine released at the remaining receptors in the neuromuscular junctions by nerve impulses and (ii) to limit or abolish the immunological attack on motor end-plates.

The duration of action of liberated acetylcholine is greatly prolonged by inhibiting its hydrolysing enzyme, acetylcholinesterase. The most commonly used anticholinesterase drugs, pyridostigmine and neostigmine, are chosen for rapid action lasting 2–8 hours (wide individual variation). Longer acting drugs are cumulative and even moderate overdosage so prolongs acetylcholine half-life as to cause depolarisation block of motor endplates and also of muscarinic endings, leading to muscular fasciculation and paralysis, pallor, sweating, excessive salivation and persistently small pupils; the last is the most valuable sign of this *cholinergic crisis*. Smaller doses cause diarrhoea, colic and other autonomic effects. These can be controlled by propantheline (15 mg as required) or, on occasion, by atropine (0·6 mg parenterally). These anticholinergic drugs are best avoided as they dilate the pupils and so remove the best marker for impending cholinergic crisis. Pyridostigmine is the anticholinesterase of choice, 60–120 mg given orally at intervals determined by supervised trial (2–8 hours). For exceptional muscular effort, neostigmine (15–30 mg) acts more promptly but for a shorter time. It may be given intravenously in an emergency but parenteral administration requires experience and is rarely necessary.

Sudden exacerbations of myasthenic or cholinergic weakness may require intermittent positive pressure respiration to save life. Early intubation before a crisis has developed will normally remove the need for a tracheostomy.

The immunological disorder is treated by various procedures. Thymectomy should be performed as soon as feasible in any patient with myasthenia not confined to the extraocular muscles, unless the disease has been established for more than 7 years; the indication for surgery is the stage of myasthenia gravis, not the presence of a thymoma.

Plasma exchange (plasmapheresis), by removing antibody from the blood, may give marked improvement but, as this is usually brief, such therapy is normally reserved for myasthenic crisis or for pre-operative preparation. Corticosteroid treatment may cause rapid improvement but this is commonly preceded by marked exacerbation of myasthenic symptoms and should be initiated only in a hospital with ventilation equipment. Various high and low dose, daily or alternate day dosage schedules are in use with apparently similar results. As it is usually necessary to continue treatment for months or years, with the possibility of adverse effects, corticosteroids are not recommended for first line management. In an attempt to reduce these risks, trials of azathioprine and other immunosuppressant drugs or of radiation of lymphoid tissues are being made. No anti-immunological therapy has yet proved superior to thymectomy, an operation with practically no mortality when performed early.

Prognosis is variable. Remissions sometimes occur spontaneously. When myasthenic affection is confined to the eye muscles prognosis for life is normal and disability slight. Rapid progression of the disease more than 5 years after its onset is uncommon. Thymectomy, perhaps followed by high dosage steroid treatment, often leads to marked improvement so that disability is minimal and life expectancy normal. When the disease is associated with a thymoma, even though this is removed, the outlook is markedly worsened.

MYOPATHY

Myopathy is a generic term comprising all primary diseases of muscle. It may be subdivided into genetically determined, congenital, metabolic and drug induced myopathy. Inflammatory myopathy (polymyositis) is described on page 576. There are obvious exceptions, but it is a useful generalisation that myopathy affects mainly the proximal muscles of the limbs whereas neuropathic disease (polyneuropathy or motor neurone disease) affects mainly the distal muscles.

Genetically Determined Myopathy

Progressive muscular dystrophy is a group of hereditary disorders characterised by progressive degeneration of groups of muscles without involvement of the nervous system. The wasting and weakness are symmetrical, there is no fasciculation, tendon reflexes are preserved until a late stage and there is no sensory loss. Several clinical types have been described; from a prognostic viewpoint there are three major groups.

The *Duchenne type* is transmitted by an X-linked recessive gene and occurs almost exclusively in males (p. 13). The disease usually appears within the first three years of life, beginning in the pelvic girdle and lower limbs and later spreading to the shoulder girdle. About 80% of cases show an initial pseudohypertrophy involving the calf muscles, quadriceps, glutei, deltoids and infraspinati. Contractures are common. The affected muscles are larger and firmer than normal, but are nevertheless weak. The weakness gives rise to a characteristic waddling gait, and when rising from the supine position, the child rolls on to his face and then uses his arms to push himself up. Death occurs from inanition or respiratory infection by the middle of the second decade.

Limb girdle type (Juvenile scapulohumeral type of Erb). The gene carrying this disorder is inherited as an autosomal recessive, affecting both sexes. It usually appears in the second or third decade. It starts in either the shoulder or pelvic girdle and later spreads to involve both. The rate of progression is variable; it may be slow, with long periods of arrest, but severe disablement usually occurs within 20 years and the patient does not survive to middle age.

Facio-scapulo-humeral type (Landouzy-Déjerine). This type is inherited by an autosomal dominant gene so that several siblings of both sexes may be affected. It appears at any age, first in the facial muscles and then in the shoulder girdle. After many years the pelvic girdle may also be involved. The disease progresses very slowly with periods of arrest and is compatible with a long life.

The *diagnosis of muscular dystrophy* is readily confirmed by electromyography (EMG) or muscle biopsy. Aldolase, or creatine kinase and other enzymes which are usually intracellular, are increased in the serum, especially in the rapidly advancing Duchenne type. Serum enzyme changes may be found before other clinical signs, enabling early detection of the disease in siblings. Less severe changes of the same type are found in women who carry the abnormal gene of the Duchenne type.

Treatment. No effective treatment is known. Deterioration may occur with excessive confinement to bed. Physiotherapeutic and orthopaedic measures may be required to counteract deformities and contractures.

Myotonic Dystrophy. Myotonia consists of slow relaxation of muscles due to hyperexcitability of the muscle cell membrane.

Myotonia congenita (Thomsen's disease) is inherited as an autosomal dominant and appears in early childhood. The only symptom is the slow relaxation of a muscle if it is contracted voluntarily or by mechanical stimulation. The patient may be unable to relax the grasp or to open the eyes if they have been closed tightly. The muscles may be unusually powerful in early life.

Myotonia atrophica is also autosomal dominant and appears between the ages of 20 and 30 years. There is wasting of the facial and temporal muscles, sternomastoids, shoulder girdle, forearms, quadriceps and leg muscles, and all these and the tongue show myotonia after voluntary contraction or after percussion of the muscle. Ptosis is prominent. Unlike most muscular diseases, distal muscles are more severely affected than proximal. There is also cataract, frontal baldness and gonadal atrophy leading to impotence and sterility in men and amenorrhoea in women.

Treatment. There is no treatment for the muscular dystrophy, but if myotonia is troublesome it can be relieved by procainamide, 0·5–1·0 g q.i.d., quinine sulphate 300–600 mg t.i.d. or phenytoin 100 mg t.i.d.

Congenital, Metabolic and Drug Induced Myopathy

Congenital myopathies are rare and present in infancy with muscular weakness and limpness. Serum enzymes tend to be normal or slightly raised. The EMG is usually myopathic. The mode of inheritance is variable. They are named according to the type of structural abnormality found in the skeletal muscle fibres. Most cases are non-progressive or only slowly progressive.

Metabolic Myopathy. *Thyrotoxic Myopathy.* Mild weakness of the proximal muscles of the limbs is a common feature of thyrotoxicosis. In a few patients muscular wasting and weakness predominate, and the other manifestations of hyperthyroidism may not be obvious. Treatment of the hyperthyroidism results in recovery from the myopathy. Ophthalmoplegia is discussed on page 435.

Corticosteroid Myopathy. Weakness of the pelvic girdle may occur in Cushing's syndrome and as a result of treatment with corticosteroids.

Familial periodic paralysis is characterised by attacks of profound weakness, lasting for several hours and often occurring after exertion or after a heavy carbohydrate meal. In the common variety the attacks of weakness are accompanied by a fall in the serum potassium level.

Drug Induced Myopathy. A wide variety of drugs may cause disorders of muscle. Often muscle cramps and mild weakness are the first symptoms. Lithium or beta-blockers may cause mild symptoms which disappear when the drug is withdrawn. Alcohol may cause a spectrum of muscle diseases varying from a mild, proximal weakness to severe muscle necrosis with myoglobinuria.

Neurological and Myopathic Complications of Carcinoma

Cerebral invasion or spinal compression may be the presenting feature of a metastasis from an unsuspected primary neoplasm or may augment the disability already caused by tumours arising elsewhere in the body, particularly in bronchus and breast. More than half of all cerebral tumours are secondary deposits and this high incidence emphasises the need for a careful search for a primary neoplasm in those patients who present with an intracranial space-occupying lesion.

Paraneoplastic syndromes (p. 108) may arise at a distance from a primary carcinoma in the absence of metastases. The relationship between the underlying malignant process and such neurological manifestations remains obscure in most instances. Neural disturbances may occur at any stage during the development of the primary lesion and may antedate the symptoms directly attributable to the carcinoma by weeks or months. At the time of neurological presentation the primary carcinoma often cannot be defined even by radiological techniques. Nor does the course of the neurological complication consistently parallel the development of the carcinoma.

Immunological mechanisms, conditioned nutritional deficiencies and the direct effects of toxins produced by tumours have all been adduced as explanations of attendant neurological dysfunction but there is little supporting evidence for any of these hypotheses. In contrast it is likely that progressive multi-focal leucoencephalopathy (p. 643) results from viral infection when immunological responses are impaired by malignant disease.

Clinical Features. The neurological features evoked by distant carcinoma are protean; they may affect singly, or in combination, muscles and peripheral nerves as well as central neural structures and the brain. The syndromes presented are most conveniently categorised anatomically.

Myopathy, Myositis and Myasthenia. A proximal weakness of late onset, usually first affecting the legs may be due to a lesion of muscles secondary to a distant carcinoma. Histologically the muscles may show changes of a non-specific myopathy or there may be collections of inflammatory cells, characteristic of polymyositis. Sometimes the weakness is markedly exacerbated by exertion producing a myasthenic syndrome and may be improved by an intravenous injection of edrophonium hydrochloride. The electromyographic picture in these carcinomatous myasthenic syndromes differs from that produced by myasthenia gravis.

Peripheral neuropathy is probably the commonest of the distant neurological complications of carcinoma. Clinically the neuropathy is usually of mixed sensory-motor type. The cerebrospinal fluid protein content is often raised.

Spinal Cord Affection. Carcinomata may produce a picture which resembles motor neurone disease with loss of anterior horn cells, accompanied sometimes by upper motor neurone signs. Necrosis affecting the cells and the tracts of the spinal cord, maximal in the thoracic segments, is a rare complication of carcinoma.

Subacute degeneration of the cortical layers of the cerebellum is an uncommon manifestation of distant carcinoma. Ataxia, affecting upper and lower limbs, is a presenting feature.

Encephalopathy has occasionally been found in patients suffering from carcinoma. The most common presentation is an insidious and progressive dementia with memory disorder. This may be accompanied by features of brain stem involvement and upper motor neurone signs.

Treatment of the neurological complications is that of the primary lesion. Improvement, and occasionally complete remission, of a myasthenic-myopathic syndrome may occur with removal of the primary tumour but this is by no means invariable. In most instances the response of the neurological complications is unpredictable.

PROSPECTS IN NEUROLOGY

The most obvious advances in the diagnosis of neurological disorders are concerned with the imaging of intracranial contents by non-invasive techniques such as computed tomography and nuclear magnetic resonance imaging. Advances in radionuclide techniques also permit high resolution dynamic imaging of the brain, and positron-emission tomography allows study of the time varying distribution of certain metabolic reactions in the brain. Advances in clinical electrophysiology are adding precision to identification of conduction disorders of the peripheral and central nervous system.

These spectacular aids to localisation are not necessarily the most significant growth areas of the future. These are the increasing knowledge of the distribution and function of neurotransmitters and their pharmacological manipulation, the development of potent antiviral agents, and the advances in knowledge of the immunopathology of the nervous system and muscle and its treatment. Identification of the chemical abnormality of specific genes, with potential genetic engineering for inherited disorders is expected in the near future. These highly significant developments offer prospects for prevention and treatment of many chronic 'degenerative' diseases of the nervous system at present regarded as untreatable.

J.A. SIMPSON

FURTHER READING:

Brain, Lord & Walton, J.N. (1977) *Diseases of the Nervous System*, 8th edn. London: Oxford University Press. A comprehensive text written for postgraduate students, but a suitable reference work for undergraduates.

Jennett, W.B. (1977) *An Introduction to Neurosurgery*, 3rd edn. London: Heinemann. A succinct and clearly written introduction to surgical neurology.

Macleod, J. (1983) In: *Clinical Examination*, 6th edn. Edinburgh: Churchill Livingstone. Contains an account of the examination of the nervous system designed to be read in conjunction with this chapter.

Matthews, W.B. (1982) *Diseases of the Nervous System*, 4th edn. Oxford: Blackwell Scientific Publications. A concise, readable account of neurological disorders intended for undergraduates.

Weller, R.D., Swash, M., McLellan, D.L. & Scholtz, C.L. (1983) *Clinical Neuropathology*. Berlin: Springer Verlag. A valuable short account of pathological processes related to clinical neurology. It includes clear accounts of biochemical disorders of the nervous system.

16. Psychiatry

Psychiatry is the study and treatment of disorders of the mind and of behaviour. The mind, or psyche, is usually defined as the part of the person consisting of the thoughts, the feelings and the function of willing. Psychiatric disorder, therefore, can be viewed to occur whenever there is an impairment of thinking (cognition), feeling (affect) or willing (volition). In a paranoid reaction, for instance, the patient wrongly thinks he or she is being persecuted by an ill-intentioned acquaintance; in depressive psychosis the patient is incapacitated by a persistent feeling of intense gloom; and in schizophrenia some patients are inactive, ineffectual and lacking in volition.

Psychiatry is the proper concern of all doctors, not only of psychiatrists. Only a small proportion of the psychiatric illness in the community is seen and can be treated by psychiatrists. In a country with as many doctors as Britain only 1 in 20 cases of psychiatric disorder is treated by psychiatrists. The epidemiological evidence makes it clear that the great proportion of psychiatric morbidity falls in the clinical domain of non-psychiatrists — general practitioners mainly but also physicians, surgeons, obstetricians and gynaecologists. Neurologists should also be singled out, for they treat many psychiatric patients.

Patients with emotional disorders tend to consult their doctors more often than patients with physical diseases and complain of a wider variety of symptoms. As a result, they are often referred to a succession of clinics for specialist investigation and commonly undergo minor or major surgery without avail. This involves a waste of both doctors' and patients' time, which could be avoided if the psychological disorder had been recognised at an earlier stage. Another reason for requiring all doctors to be psychiatrically informed and skilled is that psychiatric disorder and physical illness frequently occur in the same patient.

It follows that the priority is to ensure that psychiatric knowledge and skills, and professional attitudes appropriate to adequate provision of psychiatric care, are part of the clinical equipment of all doctors. They must know the symptoms, signs and syndromes in psychiatry, and they should all be aware of the psychological, pharmacological and physical treatments that are effective in psychiatric illness.

The basic skills are the ability to take a psychiatric history and to examine the mental state; such technical competence enables the doctor to elicit the clinical features of psychiatric disorder presented by the patient. This constitutes the psychiatric examination which is described on page 675.

MENTAL HEALTH

As a basis for understanding the abnormal, all doctors must know what constitutes mental as well as physical health. Before defining this it is necessary to consider the development of personality and the mechanisms of psychological defence.

Personality Development. Personality is socially acquired, given its genetic basis, over the course of time. The individual arrives at an adult psychological state after passing successively through a series of maturational stages. A baby is born into a family, which provides immediate social support and responses. From the start the baby's 'personality' consists of the totality of its actions, but also of the reactions made particularly to the caring parent.

1. During the stage of *primary attachment* the baby is helpless and receptive, dependent utterly on succour; such total care occurs as a result of nurturing impulses in the mother, fostered from the first days by the relationship and the interactions which develop in the nursing couple. The baby's cries, its smiles after some weeks, its need of nourishment and the relative satisfaction or distress deriving from its alimentary experiences, its fear of strangers from 8 months, all combine to bring out the protectiveness of the parental family. During this first stage, the baby is perforce relatively passive; its needs are for care and nourishment.

2. During the *stage of initial socialisation*, from 9 months to 2 years of age, the infant comes to gain sphincter control and to become more socialised as a member of the family in other ways also, starting to learn the language and its usage, and coming to grasp the rules of the parental household.

3. The *stage of family role identification* extends from 2 to 6 years of age. One of its characteristics is that the child now has sufficient awareness of family interactions and social norms to want to become informed about such matters as the difference between the sexes, where babies come from and how they are made. Boys begin to imitate and assimilate aspects of their father's behaviour and character, while girls also become less concentrated in their attachment to the mother; they can show the most intense affection for their fathers, a passion that apparently needs recognition and an affectionate response for proper personality growth between 2 and 6 years.

During the *oedipal phase* (as this third stage is called in the psychoanalytic literature), the child is often intensely frustrated by diminutive size, puny strength and subservience to the powerful parents at a time when perception, knowledge and mastery of the environment evolve rapidly as physical and mental abilities develop.

4. *At 6 years, the child enters the social world outside the home.* The child is socially obliging, very actively adapting to school life and is becoming increasingly an independent personality, able to be away from the parents for substantial portions of the day. If the parents are not seriously deficient as culture carriers, through neurotic illness or crippling social handicaps, the child now comes closely to grips with the norms, the roles, the stereotypes and the obvious and prevailing cultural values. The child is extremely impressionable, as advertisers on television well know, eager to add to personality and experience by observing and borrowing from the behaviour and ideas of others.

5. At *puberty* the child's personality can enter a period of relative flexibility, when it may be given 'a second chance' and can set aside some trait patterns and in their place substitute new attitudes and beliefs. With the bodily and sexual changes of this period come demands for new orientations and relationships; a special requirement is for a friend. Children, just before entering their teens, either do succeed in achieving a close friendship or else they may suffer from a sense of unpopularity or loneliness.

The early teenage years are when *identity formation* either occurs or else fails to happen, when identity diffusion will result. Then the youngsters continue in a state of not knowing what they want to be or what aims their capacities and potential may permit. The boy may be timid and lacking in confidence, or compensatorily brusque and hostile; the girl may inwardly bewail her female state, be perturbed at having menstrual periods and feel uncertain and wretched in social relationships especially as these relate to the future prospect of being courted. When identity formation does occur successfully, the adolescent decides on life goals and works towards them more or less hopefully, while feeling common cause with enough age-mates to be a member of a group.

6. At about 18 years, the late adolescent becomes capable of *intimacy*, able to regard the welfare of another loved person as no less important than one's own. Then adulthood follows, with the capacity for *generativity*, with the intention and the potential to provide responsibly and reliably for others.

When the question of psychological normality of a patient is at issue, this chronological and subjective progression through biographical epochs has to be borne in mind. Psychological theory holds that each of these different stages is not obliterated by the one succeeding it but, like layers of an onion, one developmental phase superimposes the challenges (and the person's solutions to them) over and around the earlier solutions achieved. The residues of past developmental periods persist to give individuality to the person. When particularly upsetting setbacks (psychologically traumatic experiences) are encountered, a *fixation* may result, the person not negotiating developmental challenges but instead remaining unduly preoccupied with the issues of that earlier life epoch. Often the facts about the psychic trauma are not remembered, as when a small boy is parted from his parents for a surgical operation he does not comprehend.

Jean Piaget was a pioneer in discovering that intellectual development also proceeds in stages, and that in the early years of life unrealistic thinking prevails. Only in middle childhood, from 7 to 8 years onwards, does the child acquire logical thinking, and even then abstract thinking and reasoning is not possible until about 13 years of age. Thus the first four stages of emotional development described above take place in parallel with magical, prelogical modes of thought.

This information makes it clearer why there are infantile psychic remnants in the thinking of many disturbed adults. Although knowledgeable about sex, a woman can fear she is pregnant despite intercourse not having occurred; a man can be distressed that he 'caused' the death of his mother by behaving harshly to her when she was terminally ill. Thinking that departs from reality or distorts it is often related to early demands which the child found unmanageable, or to distress which was intolerable emotionally at that time of life, such as the loss of a parent through death, or the family breaking up.

Adults, when handicapped by a persistence of immaturity, need not constantly manifest distortion of thinking or feeling in their behaviour. Only when a fresh setback occurs in adult life may they decompensate in behaviour and *regress* to act in extreme variance from their everyday demeanour, for example with dependency and passivity (as when confronted by major surgery), or with obstinacy or hostility.

Mechanisms of Defence. As a consequence of excessive strains occurring early in life with which the personality was insufficiently mature to cope, the person can make use of psychological devices, 'mental tricks', to alter the inner environment or the surrounding reality and create an illusion of safety and predictability. A girl, unable to clarify sexual issues at the age of 5 years, perhaps lacking a reassuring relationship with a kindly father, may use *denial* excessively. There are women who remain unaware of their sexual impulses and behave like school-girls forever — 'pregenital' personalities, some writers name them. A person may *overcompensate* — a timid, insecure boy setting out to acquire the outward characteristics of a tough male when he reaches adulthood. A boy who copes with upsetting homosexual desires at puberty by means of *repression*, in later life can be in greater emotional difficulty should he use the mechanism of *projection*; if psychotic, such a man may have an auditory delusion that other people are alleging he is a homosexual. A sexually deprived single woman, using the same mechanisms, may be profoundly distressed, in the course of a paranoid reaction, by her erroneous beliefs that neighbours view her as sexually promiscuous; her own suppressed wishes are not admitted to her awareness but are exteriorised so that she believes others falsely suspect her of immorality.

There are other psychological mechanisms in the range of distortions and evasions to which troubled people can have recourse in extremity. By *reaction formation* we imply that individuals give forth the opposite of facts they cannot acknowledge about themselves: the son dominated by his father often becomes not a domineering man, but a timid, ingratiating, subservient adult — perhaps overwhelmed by an intimidating wife. However, such a man can change character drastically and turn on his oppressor; the bedroom is the commonest setting for matrimonial murder when the victim is the wife; the husband dies often in the kitchen.

Of course, psychological defence mechanisms rarely present so dramatically, and for clinical purposes more precise observation of smaller cues is required. We all use defence mechanisms at times of great stress: the surgeon's matter-of-fact manner is sometimes seen as necessary suppression of sympathetic emotions which could impair his competence, and his *selective inattention* to pathetic life circumstances may be altogether appropriate in an emergency. A civilian disaster is not the time for anguish over the human condition, if one is a surgeon with an operation to carry out.

The defences which a person assumes psychologically can be of much social value to others. A latently homosexual youth leader may be a boon to a neighbourhood — until his *sublimation* no longer serves, perhaps if he drinks excessively and loses his customary mental controls. School teachers and clergymen who interfere sexually with boys are in this category, and some doctors who become sexually involved with patients.

In the course of clinical work, we judge a patient to assess whether he or she is spontaneous and unconstrained, or whether in contrast the patient when troubled denies mental conflict and imaginatively but unknowingly distorts surrounding reality in order to gain psychological relief.

Psychological Normality

In common with medical practice generally, individuals are often considered psychiatrically normal if no evidence of disorder is clinically present. An epidemiologist doing a population survey may use an *empirical definition of normality* and regard as normal everybody who has not seen a psychiatrist nor consulted a general practitioner for any nervous ailment during the preceding year.

Another concept of normality at times invoked is an *ideal norm*, conveying an aspiration towards a desired state of well-being (such as is expressed in the preamble to the World Health Organization constitution), devoutly to be wished but not to be found in this world: 'Health is a state of complete physical, mental and social well-being and not merely the absence of disease or infirmity'.

Psychiatrists occasionally write about normality, or aspects of it, in such inspirational terms that only too evidently they are not describing people as they are but as they would be, if a theoretical schema or 'mental health' blueprint were to become actual.

The third concept is a *statistical norm*, implying the state of most people contained in the community of which the patient is a member. In this sense, without straining after the ideal, we can indicate features characteristic of psychiatric normality in mature adults. Each of these can be readily identified, especially when the doctor has additional background information from prior acquaintance with the patient or members of the family.

Individuals who have successfully negotiated the sequence of stages in personality development are *appropriately autonomous*; they can manage their own affairs and tasks without undue reliance on others and can be depended on to meet obligations and to discharge responsibilities appropriate to their occupation, social circumstances and interests. The statement that a mature person can work, love and play perhaps reflects this capacity for autonomy.

A second feature of normality is *accurate self-perception*, the person not overestimating nor belittling his or her abilities. A third characteristic is correct *reality-testing*, the environment being perceived in an undistorted way. A fourth feature is *adjustment*, the person taking things as they are and making the best of them. The final two qualities of maturity are *integration* (relative coherence of the parts of the personality in contrast to gross self-contradictions), and *achievement*, the person using skills and interests in such a way that efforts are productive.

DIAGNOSTIC DECISION-MAKING

The doctor's first consideration when examining a patient for psychiatric disorder, is to question whether the patient may be suffering from a psychosis, one of the serious disorders to which the term 'insanity' used to be applied. The psychoses are the serious illnesses which interfere with a patient's perceptions, thinking and feelings so profoundly that, at times, what he says to his fellow-men no longer makes sense to them and he is regarded as insane. The doctor scans the understanding obtained by means of history-taking and examination of the mental state, perhaps augmented — when the patient is uncooperative — by information from a relative or other informant. The doctor judges whether the syndrome presenting indicates an illness of psychotic quality and severity. Syndrome identification is of course possible only if the doctor has knowledge about the signs and symptoms of the two main classes of psychoses: the organic psychoses due to cerebral impairment, and the functional psychoses presumed to be related to an as yet undiscovered disturbance of cerebral biochemistry.

The Major Disorders (The Psychoses)

Organic Mental Disorders. In these organic brain syndromes the functioning of the brain is impaired either by a physical lesion (trauma, tumour or infection) or by a toxic or degenerative process. Organic brain syndromes when acute are known as *delirium*. Examples are the toxic confusional states occurring with brain trauma, cerebral anoxia, infection, or intoxication with barbiturates, amphetamines or alcohol.

The chronic organic psychoses, where there is an irreversible brain lesion, are the *dementias*. The commonest are those associated with ageing: atherosclerotic and senile dementia. Mild degrees of dementia make the patient forgetful, easily confused, irritable and emotional; more severe dementia results in disorientation, gross loss of memory and deterioration in personal habits.

Functional psychoses are the major psychiatric illnesses occurring without brain disease or impairment. It is postulated that a neurophysiological or neurochemical aetiology will be found, resulting from the operation of complex causes. The two most common forms are *major depressive illness*, in which the principal symptom is a profound disturbance of the patient's mood, and the *schizophrenias* in which patients' thoughts become bizarre and disorganised, so that they lose contact with their fellows and surroundings.

The major disorders are discussed further on pages 678 to 684.

The Minor Disorders

The second step in the decision-making process towards a psychiatric diagnosis, having excluded the presence of psychosis, is for the doctor to determine whether the patient suffers from a 'minor' psychiatric disorder. The following forms of minor disorder are differentiated:

1. The Psychoneuroses. Clinical recognition of one of the forms of psychoneurosis depends on the doctor knowing the signs and symptoms of each syndrome and of being able to elicit the relevant clinical data from the patient. The psychoneuroses are the most common forms of psychiatric illness encountered in general medical practice. They are subdivided into *anxiety, hysterical, obsessive, depressive* and *phobic psychoneurosis*.

2. Personality Disorder. This term is used to describe patients whose personalities differ markedly from the normal population.

The third diagnostic rule, after the presence of possible psychosis or of psychoneurosis has been considered, is to make an appraisal of the personality of the patient. An individual's personality is regarded as normal if his or her actions and reactions are not grossly different from customary behaviour in society. When a personality is diagnosed as disordered, the implication is that the person deviates observably in behaviour, presenting a type of abnormal personality which is well recognised clinically. The abnormal personality manifests in recurrent disturbance in relationships with other people. In addition to their social difficulties, such people can be recognised to have traits (e.g. hostility, passivity) not found to the same degree in the personalities of normal people. Patients with moderate degrees of personality disorder are distressed by their inability to get on constructively with others and often seek treatment; otherwise they do so when they are further disabled by psychoneurosis or psychosomatic illness. Those with gross degrees of disorder (sociopathy) interfere disruptively in the lives of their relatives and associates and may come into conflict with the law; they may not regard themselves as abnormal and reject any efforts to treat them.

It is by no means unusual, indeed it is usual, for psychiatric illness and personality disorder to coexist. When the associated illness is of psychotic dimensions, the symptoms may so distort behaviour that a reliable estimate of the pre-illness personality will be possible only after recovery from the insanity. When the illness is a neurotic reaction, however, the functioning personality remains sufficiently intact for a personality diagnosis to be made at the same time as the illness is appraised. A personality disorder may also be associated with sexual deviation, alcoholism, drug dependency or psychosomatic illness.

3. Psychosexual Disorders. People not conforming sexually to the prevailing norm most often consult (or are brought to) their doctor only when their abnormality has become seriously disturbing to their relatives or has put them into conflict with the law. Some, however, are themselves distressed by their deviation and may on occasion need psychiatric treatment for complicating psychiatric disorder, such as a depressive illness or paranoid reaction. Now that sexual relations between consenting adult males is no longer a crime in many countries, homosexuals are less vulnerable socially.

4. Alcoholism and Drug Dependency. An alcoholic is an excessive drinker who is unable to stop although to do so has become necessary because of health impairment, marital strife or difficulties at work. An addict is physically or psychologically dependent on a drug which is used repetitively, and suffers distressing side-effects when deprived of it.

5. Psychosomatic Illnesses. The term is applied to the extremely common physical illnesses, such as some cases of asthma, peptic ulcer, dermatitis or ulcerative colitis, which emotional factors help to precipitate or to prolong.

These 'minor' disorders are discussed further on pages 684 to 698.

Mental Handicap

The fourth and final diagnostic decision is to be clear about a patient's intellectual status. Mental subnormality is an impairment of the intellect present from birth or an early age, unlike psychiatric illnesses which supervene after a more or less normal psychological development. Two categories are distinguished:

1. *Mild mental retardation* (I.Q. 50 to 70). Although the intelligence level is below normal (I.Q. 85 to 115), the child may benefit from special teaching and social training.

2. *Severe mental retardation* (I.Q. 49 and below) refers to those so handicapped that they require very considerable attention and support and are incapable of leading an independent existence. The most common single cause of severe subnormality is Down's syndrome. A definite cause of subnormality is found only in a minority of cases, and then various clinical conditions can be responsible, e.g. phenylketonuria or hypothyroidism. Patients who are mentally subnormal may also suffer from other mental illnesses. They may, for example, become depressed or schizophrenic, but when this happens the symptoms of their mental illness will be modified by their basic handicap of mental retardation.

THE PSYCHIATRIC EXAMINATION

It must be emphasised that attention should be paid to the patient's emotional state not only when a frank psychiatric illness is suspected, but in the course of any thorough clinical examination. Psychiatric disorders can be elicited while taking the history and while examining the patient's mental state. The procedures for conducting these two aspects of the psychiatric examination are described in *Clinical Examination* (p. 700) and will be indicated only briefly here.

The Psychiatric History. Taking a psychiatric history is one of the chief clinical skills in psychiatry. The technique differs from history-taking in internal medicine, being rather less directive, the doctor to a greater extent, perhaps, allowing the patient to raise apparently unconnected subjects and expand in directions initiated by the patient rather than the clinician. In internal medicine there may be a course of enquiry which the doctor wants to pursue; this is also so with psychiatric history-taking, but inevitably the patient will have personal information to give which may be unexpected. Hence the clinician is well advised to be especially receptive and to encourage disclosures which the patient initiates. Psychiatric disorder is most commonly missed because the doctor fails to attend to and understand what the patient communicates.

The following areas need to be explored in the course of taking the history:

(i) The date of the examination and the reason why the patient is seeking help.

(ii) The presenting complaints and the patient's detailed account of the present illness.

(iii) The patient's parental family: an account of father, mother, each brother and sister (with patient's birth order in the sibship), and the home atmosphere.

(iv) The personal history, including early childhood; schooling and other education; sexual development and experience; work record; friendships; marriage.

(v) Previous illnesses, physical and psychiatric.

(vi) The personality before illness, with an account of the patient's interests, social activities, traits and such other information about subjective experiences and life events as the patient can provide.

Taking the history is also the first therapeutic step. Psychological treatment begins the moment that the patient and doctor meet. The doctor's attitude to the patient and to the illness should be powerful therapeutic factors which operate immediately. If history-taking is done patiently, thoroughly and objectively the individual feels a personal interest is being taken and that his or her problem is being understood. A spontaneous account of the illness by the patient should be encouraged. Too systematic an approach to the history often results in a mass of facts being obtained, but the real problem, from the patient's aspect, may be entirely overlooked.

Examining the Mental State. As the interview proceeds, the doctor already is observing the patient's current mental functioning. The examination of the mental state is carried out in a systematic manner, paying attention in turn to the separate aspects of observable behaviour which disclose the state of mind.

Appearance and Behaviour. The appearance of the patient may be immediately informative, a dejected posture suggesting depressive illness; if the gestures the patient makes are tense and restless, clues may be provided which guide the doctor to enquire after further evidence of anxiety.

Mood. Whether the patient feels cheerful or depressed, confident or fearful, suspicious or bewildered, will become evident when the doctor asks the appropriate questions. 'How do you feel in yourself?' may be enough, but many patients need some help before they can unburden themselves of fears, anxieties or feelings of intense unhappiness. Some patients are ashamed to mention emotional disturbances, such as a phobia, i.e. unreasonable intense anxiety experienced in certain settings, e.g.

in open or confined spaces. The patient may show a lack of emotional response; a very gross failure in rapport should alert the doctor to the possibility that the patient may have schizophrenia.

Thought Processes. The way a patient thinks is evident in the patient's talk, which may be abnormal through incoherence, changes of topic, or bewildering shifts from one topic to another; all these can be features of schizophrenia. The patient may speak very rapidly, with puns and rhymes, as occurs in mania. Talk may be laboured, slow and flat and indicate a depressive state. Repetitive thoughts characterise obsessional psychoneurosis, an important feature of which is an *obsession*, a persistent idea which the patient cannot get rid of; the repetitiveness may be extremely distressing even when the patient recognises the idea as absurd.

Perceptions of Environment. The doctor next ascertains if the patient's perceptions are accurate. A girl may be unduly sensitive to glances or chance remarks. The patient may suffer from *illusions*, misinterpretations of sensations arising from real stimuli: a patient with delirium tremens may misinterpret furniture as menacing persons. *Hallucinations* are sense perceptions, such as visions, which occur in the absence of any kind of external stimulus. *Delusions* are false beliefs, such as that one is being slowly put to death, to which the patient adheres even when demonstrably wrong; a man with a hypochondrial delusion, e.g. a depressed patient convinced he has venereal disease, persists in his morbid notion despite evidence to the contrary. A schizophrenic may be firmly of the belief that he has changed sex.

Intellectual Functions. While listening to what he tells us, we can at the same time pick up clues about the patient's intellectual level from his choice of words and from the ease or difficulty with which he expresses himself. The best clues to the basic intellectual level are given by the patient's scholastic record and by the type of job which he has been able to perform in adult life.

If there is reason to suspect that he may be intellectually impaired, one can test his general information by posing simple questions, such as asking him to name the head of state, the capitals of the larger countries in Europe, or to perform simple sums of mental arithmetic. We note whether he knows the date and time of day, and recognises where he is and to whom he is talking: this tests his orientation for time, place and person.

Impairment of mental function is commonly shown by inability to concentrate, to 'take things in', and hence to remember recent events. This may become apparent during the interview or it may be elicited by asking the patient to remember a name and address or a telephone number and then asking him to repeat it after an interval of 1 or 2 minutes. The final step in the examination of the mental state is an assessment of the patient's degree of insight into his condition; that is, does he recognise that he is ill or is he wrongly convinced that it is his environment and his fellows that are at fault?

When the history has been taken and an examination of the mental state completed, a thorough *physical examination* should be carried out and, following this, appropriate investigations when required. Such intervention needs to be handled well. Investigations which are necessary must be carefully planned, and quickly executed, and then a halt must be called. The pernicious habit of 'just having one more test' must be avoided as it undermines the confidence of the patient in the certainty of the diagnosis; the practictioner must be able to decide how much evidence is required to elucidate the nature and the cause of the disorder and, having obtained it, must act upon it.

Diagnosis and Formulation. The doctor is now in a position to make a formal *diagnosis*, deciding from which psychiatric syndrome the patient suffers, i.e. whether the patient's illness falls in the general class of organic mental illness, functional psychosis, psychoneurosis or personality disorder.

The next step is the *formulation*, a brief statement in which is summarised the doctor's understanding of the disorder and the person suffering from it, including the main setbacks or conflicts with other people, in the sequence in which they occurred.

PSYCHIATRIC INTERVIEWING

When the clinician undertakes to see the patient for a series of interviews, particularly when psychoneurosis or a personality disorder is present, a more detailed investigation of the psychological state is embarked upon. To do so, the clinician must acquire the necessary skills by receiving training in psychiatric interviewing, and must gain theoretical understanding of the common developments which occur as the therapeutic relationship is established and progressively extended. The clinician has available four well-documented theoretical approaches to interviewing on which to base his or her own style and approach; at times a combination of approaches is best suited to a particular patient.

1. The *descriptive approach* is most akin to medical history-taking and examination and leads to syndrome identification. As in other branches of medicine, it is appropriate in psychiatry to think in terms of disease entities, that is, to assume that the patient is suffering from a particular disease with its specific aetiology, pathology, signs and symptoms, which can be elicited by history-taking and examination.

2. The *analytical approach* enables the doctor to elicit any relevant complexes or pathogenic ideas of which the patient may be partially or totally unaware. The name 'dissociation' is given to the process by which distressing thoughts, memories or ideas disappear from awareness, and then reappear in disguised form e.g. as a dream or a physical symptom.

In addition to their symptoms, patients can also be found to have disturbances in their relations with people close to them. These self-defeating patterns of behaviour in personal relationships have been learned by life experience; the early life of the neurotic or psychosomatic patient has included some painful, frustrating or damaging experiences which disturbed his peace of mind and continue to interfere with his performance. Moreover, the minor psychiatric disorders differ from diseases by being biographically meaningful. We can often understand why that person became ill in that way at that particular time as we come to understand the course of his life and to comprehend his dilemma in relation to the people of importance to him. A psychoneurosis, in this sense, symbolises a personal predicament of the patient.

3. A third interview procedure is the *interpersonal approach*, the doctor now exploring a patient's significant interpersonal relationships; much psychiatric illness, as we shall see, accompanies

difficulties patients currently have in their associations with the people most important to them.

4. Finally, the *phenomenological approach* is the method whereby doctors, by an effort of imagination, use their own life experience to enable them intuitively to grasp what the patient is suffering; such empathic perception of the patient's present predicament in living calls on the clinician to attempt a feat of fellow-feeling by which understanding of the patient derived from the other three approaches can be extended.

Professional Attitudes of the Doctor

Three habits of mind are relevant to psychiatric work, in addition to those clinical attitudes which are necessary for the practice of medicine in general.

1. First, the clinician needs, for purposes of comprehensive interviewing, to surrender temporarily the relative detachment and authority appropriate to the practice of internal medicine, and instead to adopt a more receptive, less directive, clinical style. Much of the patient's experiences relevant to the psychiatric illness are locked up in the patient and get disclosed only if security, trust and some hope of being helped can be aroused in the patient. A paranoid patient who believes that there is a plot against him may conclude the doctor is part of the plot, unless by warmth and encouragement the doctor reassures the patient and brings him out of himself; a phobic patient may consider a fear of open spaces too ridiculous to disclose to the doctor, especially if already that doctor seems abrupt and critical.

Michael Balint wrote, in *The Doctor, His Patient, and the Illness* (1968), that medical training handicaps many clinicians for psychological work. He had in mind that when a person becomes a doctor that person sets aside to some extent the innate perceptiveness, readiness to be informed by the patient and to be led by him into unexpected avenues. The question-and-answer interviewing technique in medicine, and the professional status as the expert who knows what course the clinical discussion should take, often constrains the patient. The 'small but necessary personality change' the doctor has to make, for purposes of psychiatric interviewing, is to be more passive, less decided in advance about matters to be explored, and more ready to receive private disclosures from the patient. Indeed, at first patients often impart a 'cover story', a version of the illness and personal troubles which they hope will not offend the doctor; only when they confirm for themselves that the doctor is not censorious and remains open to receive further revelations will patients give utterance to more distressing facts.

2. The second professional attitude of importance in psychiatric work is related to a skill which has already been indicated. The doctor must practise minimal intervention and allow the patient to be the more active.

3. Third, the doctor doing psychiatric work requires an orientation of self-scrutiny, reflecting constantly on the impact exerted on the patient and asking oneself whether the patient is being influenced as intended. A readiness continuously to study one's own personality in clinical action and the responses made to patients enables the doctor progressively to increase knowledge about the life experiences of others, skills for alleviating personal distress, and capacity for gaining self-knowledge. The doctor's personality is the chief clinical tool. It is always to this personal attribute that the psychiatrically ill patient will respond, over and above the clinical expertise the doctor exercises when engaged on the exploration, diagnosis and management of any disorder of the patient's mind or personality.

PSYCHIATRIC DISORDERS

Classification of Psychiatric Disorders

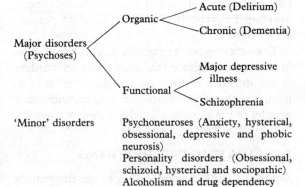

'Minor' disorders   Psychoneuroses (Anxiety, hysterical, obsessional, depressive and phobic neurosis)
Personality disorders (Obsessional, schizoid, hysterical and sociopathic)
Alcoholism and drug dependency
Psychosexual disorders
Psychosomatic disorders

Mental handicap (mental retardation)

THE ORGANIC MENTAL DISORDERS

Psychiatric symptoms may arise in the course of physical illnesses which either primarily or secondarily affect the brain. The mental symptoms of general paresis or the occurrence of delirium during the course of febrile illnesses are two well-known examples. It is important to recognise the particular mental symptoms which occur in organic mental syndromes, since their presence should lead to the search for physical factors which may not otherwise have declared themselves.

The organic mental disorders can be divided into two groups: *delirium*, which is an acute syndrome, and *dementia* which is a chronic disease. Generally speaking the acute form is potentially recoverable, being the result of temporary effects on the brain from toxic processes or disorders of metabolism, while the chronic form is the expression of more severe and progressive tissue changes in the brain and is thus not reversible. The mental symptoms of each of these organic syndromes are not specific to the causative disease and will be the same whatever may be the underlying physical disorder producing the delirium or dementia.

The terminology now used in the United States is similar, since the introduction in 1980 of the American Psychiatric Association's third edition of the *Diagnostic and Statistical Manual of Mental Disorders* (DSM III).

Delirium

This acute syndrome may be produced by such varied conditions as (i) drug intoxication (alcoholism, LSD), (ii) physical disease such as infections (encephalitis, typhoid fever); (iii) diseases of the brain, (iv) electrolyte imbalance and metabolic disorders (hepatic failure, uraemia), (v) vitamin deficiency (Wernicke's encephalopathy), and (vi) cerebral hypoxia (severe respiratory or heart failure).

In addition to the physical symptoms appropriate to the primary disorder there are often found slurred speech, tremor, nystagmus, diplopia and sluggish pupillary reactions. The characteristic mental symptoms are: insomnia and restlessness; disorientation; impairment of the sensorium (clouding of consciousness) so that alertness and attention are diminished; confusion; hallucinations, particularly in the visual sphere; ideas of persecution (paranoid ideas); and a feeling of fear or terror. All the symptoms and particularly the level of consciousness are variable. The patient may be in a state of restlessness varying from simple tossing and turning to such activities as aimlessly searching in the bedclothes or agitation. He may appear orientated for time and place and be able to recognise visitors at one moment, only to be quite confused soon after. The patient will often give the easiest answer to a question without regard to the truth and may supplement his faulty memory and perception by invention (confabulation), as when he describes in detail a large meal which he says he has just had, when in fact he has eaten nothing.

Visual hallucinations are characteristic of delirium, and are usually vivid and may be terrifying. Many are based on illusional misinterpretations of objects seen in the room; thus patterns on the wallpaper may become an advancing army of hideous and menacing reptiles. Hallucinations of other senses may occur.

Doubt and suspicion are readily induced by the impaired mentality leading to misinterpretations and may blossom for a short time into transient and rather ill-defined delusions of persecution.

An acute organic syndrome is commonly precipitated by withdrawal of alcohol, or of barbiturates, from patients who have become habituated to taking them in substantial amounts. When the syndrome is due to alcoholism it is known as delirium tremens (p. 695), but its features do not greatly differ from those of delirium from other causes.

The course and prognosis of delirium depend, of course, on the underlying physical disease, and treatment of this in most cases clears up the mental symptoms completely. Sometimes, however, delirium may be an episode in a progressive dementia.

Treatment. The use of chlorpromazine (25–50 mg t.i.d. by mouth or 100 mg i.m.) has transformed the management of acute delirium, enabling the majority of patients to be cared for in a side-room of the medical or surgical ward where their primary disease is being treated. Thioridazine in similar doses has less hypotensive effect.

In all these conditions the patient can be helped by explanations and friendly support; patients who are frightened and bewildered tend to regress to a state of childlike dependency and welcome a firm reassurance from someone whom they are willing to trust. They cannot, however, be kept calm if staff changes expose them to many strange faces or if they are bewildered by too many novel events.

Some patients have catastrophic reactions following operations on the eyes, when they must submit to being blindfolded for some time, and others have reacted adversely to the accompaniments of cardiac resuscitation or renal dialysis. These acute psychoses contain an element of panic. Nitrazepam (5–10 mg) or dichloralphenazone (1–4, 650 mg tablets) are suitable hypnotics.

Dementia

This chronic organic syndrome is very prevalent, affecting one person in 20 by the age of 70 and one person in five over the age of 80. Dementia may be caused by a wide variety of diseases of the brain. The most common of these are Alzheimer's disease (presenile and senile dementia) and cerebrovascular disease, the latter referred to also as 'multi-infarct dementia'. Other important causes include cerebral trauma, inflammations (neurosyphilis, encephalitis), multiple sclerosis, intoxications and deficiency disorders (alcoholism, pellagra, vitamin B_{12} deficiency), prolonged hypoglycaemia, carbon monoxide poisoning, cerebral neoplasm, and degenerative disorders such as Huntington's chorea.

It will be noted that some conditions (encephalitis, alcoholism, vitamin deficiencies) may also cause delirium. The cerebral changes brought about at first by these factors result in delirium and can be reversed by treatment, but if they are allowed to continue unchecked too long, permanent cerebral damage occurs, giving rise to dementia.

The clinical picture of dementia varies to some extent with the cause, the previous personality of the patient, the age of onset, and the rate of progression, but in all cases the mental symptoms are seen to involve the intellect, memory, emotions and behaviour, although the actual degree of impairment depends on the factors mentioned above. Insomnia is often an early symptom and may lead to nocturnal restlessness and confusion as the disease advances. Judgement and reasoning are involved early, and the disability caused by this will depend on the extent to which these faculties are utilised in the patient's daily life and work; it will be more noticeable in a teacher than in an unskilled labourer.

Impairment of memory is the most prominent finding, particularly in relation to recent events, and in the later stages this may combine with defective perception to produce disorientation in place and time. Impairment of higher control leads to emotional instability and outbursts of violence or sexual aberrations at variance with the patient's previous character. There may be wide fluctuations of mood with euphoria or depression but finally, as mood flattens, the patient sinks into apathy. Delusions are common, and may be either centred on the patient, when they are grandiose or self-condemnatory and hypochondriacal according to the mood, or centred on others, when they tend to be paranoid.

As the structure of the personality disintegrates, patients neglect their appearance and become lax in personal cleanliness; careless incontinence occurs. Focal neurological signs may be found, e.g. dysphagia, apraxia, agnosia, hemiplegia, and epileptic attacks, either focal or generalised.

Pneumoencephalography formerly and now computed tomography reveal the increase in the size of the ventricles and in the width of the sulci present in brain atrophy. Dementia in the elderly is usually due either to cerebral atherosclerosis or is of senile type. Table 16.1 shows the differences between the two syndromes.

Table 16.1 Dementia in the elderly

	Cerebrovascular	Senile
Age of onset	From 45 onwards	After 65
Impairment of intellect	Late in illness	Early
Deterioration of personality	Late	Early
Course	Steplike	Progressive
Brain damage	Focal	Global
Physical symptoms	Present	Absent
Physical signs	Present	Rare and late
CT scan	May show multiple infarcts	Cortical shrinkage and dilatation of ventricles

FUNCTIONAL PSYCHOSES

Major Depressive Illness

Depression is a mood which all of us experience from time to time, usually as a result of some distressing circumstance. In contrast, patients suffering from major depressive illness complain of a prolonged dejected state. They seem to have become ill for no reason they can identify, their low spirits and subjective misery causing them to feel altogether different as people. Such patients are suffering from depressive psychosis. Also known as endogenous depressive illness, in the new American classification (DSM-III) the condition is called major affective disorder.

The patient may have been subject previously to mood swings or have had an over-scrupulous rigid personality following too strict upbringing. Major depressive illness may be induced by physical illness such as influenza or by drugs, notably corticosteroids and oral contraceptives. There is a genetic predisposition, particularly in bipolar illness when both depressive and manic episodes occur. Like the less severe psychoneurotic depressive reaction (p. 690), major depressive illness may be precipitated by external events particularly those which impart a sense of loss, separation or disappointment. Much more often it arises without detectable external influences. It is commoner in patients of middle age or older, but certainly does occur in the young and also in children.

Clinical Features. In addition to a mood varying from mild depression to black despair the manifestations are: insomnia of a type characterised by early waking after 2 to 3 hours sleep; diurnal variation of mood, in which the depression often lifts considerably towards evening; slowness of thought and inability to make decisions; ideas of guilt, unworthiness and self-blame which are often delusional in intensity, i.e. they are impervious to reasoned argument or demonstration of their falsity; and various somatic manifestations such as anorexia, loss of weight, amenorrhoea, pressure headache, backache, constipation, retardation of physical activity (more rarely aimless over-activity or agitation), and hypochondriacal delusions. Such a patient may sit bowed and immobile on the edge of a chair obviously in the depths of misery, weeping silently, and answering questions in slow monosyllables; but in the earlier stages the physical appearance is much less striking and the diagnosis depends on the doctor's ability to elicit the symptoms described above.

Severe depressive psychosis, especially when associated with restlessness and agitation (p. 699), with delusions of unworthiness and preoccupation with thoughts of death, is an extremely distressing condition and fraught with risks of suicide. This is the main hazard and the risk is often greatest at the onset of major depressive illness or when treatment begins to relieve the depression and reduce the accompanying psychomotor retardation. Severe cases should be admitted to psychiatric care in hospital.

In *manic-depressive psychosis*, the bipolar form, patients can suffer from morbid elation and hyperactivity in addition to attacks of depression. They look excessively cheerful, speak rapidly, shifting from one idea to another, often joking, teasing, making puns and paying poor attention to the environment. They are overconfident, over-optimistic and overimportant. They may suffer from grandiose delusions and behave in an extravagantly spendthrift way. They usually do not realise they are ill, and may react with violence if crossed or restrained. Failure to diagnose mania can have very serious consequences for a patient, who can run up vast debts or jeopardise his social position drastically by ill-judged, embarrassing or boisterously inappropriate and undesirable behaviour.

Treatment The first task after diagnosing major depressive illness is to proceed without delay to treat the patient with one of the potent antidepressant drugs. One has to bear in mind, however, that these do not take effect until after some 6 to 14 days. There are two principal groups of antidepressant drugs:

1. Tricyclic drugs (e.g. imipramine, amitriptyline and trimipramine), the monoamine reuptake inhibiting drugs (MARI).

2. The monoamine oxidase inhibitor (MAOI) drugs (e.g. phenelzine, mebanazine and tranylcypromine).

1. *Tricyclic drugs* constitute the treatment of choice for most cases of major depressive illness. In order to be effective, they have to be given in

sufficient dosage. It is usual to prescribe 25 mg t.i.d. for one week, and 50 mg or more t.i.d. subsequently. Trimipramine may be given as a single dose (50–100 mg) at night. Amitriptyline is also available in 50 or 100 mg sustained-release tablets for use at night. A course of tricyclic drugs should be taken for 3 to 6 months; if they are stopped too soon the symptoms of depression may recur. A patient who fails to respond to one drug may benefit from another.

Tricyclic drugs give rise to some disagreeable anticholinergic effects, for example on the eyes, causing difficulty in focussing. Imipramine may make the patient feel even more on edge and restless during the first few days and it may also cause some difficulty in micturition. Amitriptyline tends to make some patients feel uncomfortably drowsy and causes dryness of the mouth. These side-effects usually recede with continued use and become quite easily tolerated once the patient begins to experience a lifting of the mood and a return of former energy.

2. *The monoamine oxidase inhibitors* (p. 681) are especially helpful in the treatment of 'atypical' depression (or prolonged phobic symptoms), occurring in patients with good previous personalities. Patients on MAOI drugs should be warned not to partake of substances rich in tyramine (such as cheese, chianti and some types of beer) because these may interact with the drug to provoke a hypertensive crisis, with splitting headaches and a risk of subarachnoid haemorrhage. The MAOI drugs also potentiate other drugs, including pethidine, opiates, barbiturates, phenothiazines, amphetamine and alcohol, all of which should be avoided while a patient is taking this form of antidepressant. Caution is needed when changing from a MAOI drug to a tricyclic or vice versa: a drug-free interval of a week is advisable.

Electroconvulsive therapy (ECT) administered under intravenous anaesthesia and modified by muscle-relaxant drugs may be indicated if the patient has not improved after antidepressant medication has been given for about 4 weeks.

Lithium carbonate is effective in controlling manic-depressive states. The patient needs to be in hospital at the start of treatment. It may also prevent the recurrence of manic attacks when used as maintenance therapy, in daily doses of 800–1600 mg, out-patients returning for weekly estimation of plasma lithium (p. 820) and a check on adverse effects which include nausea, vomiting, tremor, myopathy and cardio-respiratory symptoms.

Rehabilitation. As a general rule, it is wise to postpone any practical decisions about business, change of work or domestic matters until the patient has regained a normal mood. Once the patient has responded to drugs or ECT it is essential to review personal circumstances and to help make plans to cope with the difficulties which may have precipitated the illness. Moreover, the patient may need to know that the illness sometimes takes a recurring form and that advice must be sought if symptoms return. However, major depressive illness, once of gloomy prognosis, is now eminently treatable, and with appropriate care few such patients become chronic hospital inmates.

Schizophrenia

Schizophrenia is the illness with symptoms corresponding most closely to the popular conception of madness. The personality becomes disintegrated, and detached from the social environment. The mental life becomes split up. The cardinal features are: disorder of thinking, which becomes incoherent, disjointed and rambling; incongruity of emotion; impulsive actions and utterances; and hallucinations (most commonly, in the form of threatening or unfriendly voices). Patients express bizarre delusions with little or no appreciation of why it is that their ideas are unacceptable to those around them.

Delusions and hallucinations may also occur in other forms of mental illness, such as severe depressive illness, mania, or delirium, but certain other features are especially suggestive of schizophrenia. These include (1) *passivity feelings*, in which the patient is convinced that his (or her) actions are controlled by some alien power, (2) *thought insertion* and *thought broadcasting*, in which he feels that other people put thoughts into his mind, and are able to read his thoughts, and (3) *paranoid delusions* in which he believes that he is surrounded by hostile forces which watch him and secretly intervene to do him harm.

Patients with depressive illness may also develop paranoid ideas, but these are coloured by their all-pervading feelings of guilt. For example, a depressed patient may believe that he is being watched by secret police because they have found out that he has committed a terrible crime. The paranoid schizophrenic, on the other hand, is quite sure that it is his unseen enemies who are the hostile villains, and he their innocent victim.

Schizophrenic patients tend to have little insight into the fact that they are ill and in need of treatment. When their behaviour is becoming alarming, it may be necessary, in their own interests, to admit them compulsorily to hospital. In Britain application is made by the patient's nearest relative supported by recommendations by the patient's family doctor and a psychiatrist. The patient's case must be reviewed after 28 days. In many cases he will continue in hospital voluntarily. A mentally ill patient who is a danger to himself or others may also be admitted compulsorily as an emergency for 3 days in England and Wales and 7 days in Scotland. This certificate is signed by only one doctor and can be used when the patient is already in hospital.

The features indicated above are the more florid manifestations of schizophrenia. The patient's functioning declines, in regard to the capacity for work, social relations and self-care. Milder signs, less easy to recognise, include instances of unexpected rudeness or tactlessness, and abrupt and inexplicable behaviour with a marked withdrawal from ordinary social contacts. Such persons may be considered awkward or unsociable and it is only when they reveal quite bizarre ideas, shout back at their hallucinatory voices, or otherwise behave in a conspicuously strange manner, that one realises that they are not merely eccentric, but mentally ill.

Treatment. Phenothiazine drugs such as chlorpromazine, and the butyrophenones (e.g. haloperidol) have changed the prognosis of schizophrenia but it should be remembered that even before there was any specific drug treatment for this illness, many cases made a spontaneous recovery from the stage of the psychosis in the course of 3 to 9 months. These drugs offer symptomatic relief of the patient's delusions, hallucinations and alienation from reality, rather than a radical cure of this little-understood disease. There is abundant evidence that the way in which the patient is treated, in hospital and in the community, will influence both the degree of recovery and the probability of a subsequent relapse.

Schizophrenic patients do badly if they are allowed to withdraw too completely from social contacts and practical activities; but they also do badly if they are involved in emotionally demanding relationships, to which they are unable to respond.

Many, if not most, schizophrenics must be regarded as having particularly vulnerable personalities and many emerge from the acute stage of their illness with some residual defects ('end states'). Those left with moderate or severe deficits, perhaps as many as a third, then lead impaired lives, and require skilled rehabilitation. These patients are not necessarily intellectually impaired — they may be highly intelligent — but they are seldom able to cope with positions of responsibility, particularly when they are required to supervise, or interact with other people. Many such partially recovered patients do best in tasks in which they can work on their own, with only rather formal contacts with their fellows.

Nowadays the great majority of schizophrenic patients, after discharge from hospital, can be treated at home, taking their prescribed drugs for at least the first year or two. The doctor should be ready to enlist the help of a community nurse or of a social worker if patients appear to be having difficulties either at work or in their domestic relationships.

During the acute stage of the illness, chlorpromazine or thioridazine is effective medication, 150–1000 mg being given each day in divided doses. About 60% of patients with acute schizophrenic symptoms can be expected to improve significantly within a matter of weeks. A suitable maintenance dose for a schizophrenic patient in remission is 50 mg twice daily. Chlorpromazine is also given by intramuscular injections (50–100 mg) in order to control stages of agitation or over-excitement. Postural hypotension is an important side-effect which is more marked with elderly patients, who should be given smaller doses. Haloperidol (up to 30 mg/d orally or i.m.) may be substituted for chlorpromazine.

A long-acting phenothiazine, fluphenazine decanoate (12·25–25 mg each 2–4 weeks) can be given intramuscularly on a maintenance basis for chronic schizophrenics treated as out-patients who are unreliable with oral medication.

All the phenothiazines can have adverse extrapyramidal effects, and anti-parkinsonian drugs (p 650) may also have to be taken. Restlessness and dystonia of the jaw and neck can occur. Another drug effect is tardive dyskinesia, continuous movements of the head and tongue, which may persist for years.

When the schizophrenic psychosis is of acute onset, and the previous personality relatively sociable and well-adapted, the outcome is better. It is important for doctors to know about the condition and recognise it when it occurs, because competent and early psychiatric treatment can spare the patient and the relatives extreme harm, through social catastrophe or accident.

THE PSYCHONEUROSES

There are two conditions to be met before the doctor can regard an illness as psychoneurotic. First, one of the typical syndromes (to be described below) must be in evidence. Second, the person must have experienced a recent setback, usually a disturbance in his relationship with a person or persons important to him. Often, when the first condition applies, the doctor may need to act on the basis of a clinical diagnosis without having elicited the biographical corroboration, but it must be remembered that the omission exists and needs to be remedied, otherwise serious mistakes can be made. Symptoms resembling those of neuroses, e.g. hysterical states, can occur with cerebral trauma or disease or in a functional psychosis.

The interpersonal or social setback preceding the onset of psychoneurotic illness need not be gross. However, it will be highly charged emotionally, in the context of the patient's biography, sometimes fitting as a key does into a lock with an earlier similar setback. It then seems understandable that the recent miscarriage of a relationship (the dynamic cause) has disorganised the adaptation of a person previously sensitised by an earlier emotional trauma (the predisposing cause). A woman who becomes ill with psychoneurosis when afraid that she may be deserted on discovering that her husband has become attracted to another woman, may be found by further questioning to have lost her loved father through his death before her teens. The threat of the present loss is more understandably distressing in relation to the earlier deprivation.

Psychoneurosis, one of the 'minor' disorders, is an illness taking the form of one of the well-described syndromes in this category of disability: anxiety, hysterical, obsessional, depressive or phobic neurosis.

With all these characteristic syndromes the patient will be only partially disabled, many aspects of personality and social competence being unaffected. The man or woman can often cope with work and household responsibilities, and hence usually be treated as an out-patient. Reality testing is not impaired in any gross way, i.e. the misperceptions of the human and material environment characterising psychotic illness do not occur.

There is a great amount of psychoneurotic illness in every community, for psychoneurosis is much the most common psychiatric disorder. Many individuals will be mildly disturbed and may not need medical treatment. A man with a fear of heights is not disabled if he works on the ground in a community made up of low houses; the same man who moves for postgraduate work to New York, for example, where he may have to attend seminars in skyscrapers, can become seriously impaired. On the other hand, flying phobia developing in any member of aircraft personnel is instantly incapacitating.

Not all patients will accept with equanimity a diagnosis of psychoneurosis when their preferred concept of their illness is a physical one. This will often be evident from the initial reluctance with which some patients accept advice for psychiatric referral. A sickness of one's body is not regarded as a matter for which one is culpable. In contrast, a disturbance of one's mind could be regarded as an affliction of one's very self, and therefore a weakness in one as a person.

It has been demonstrated that the higher the social class of the patient, the more acceptable is a psychiatric diagnosis. The same correlation between socio-economic disadvantage and somatisation is evident in transcultural psychiatric studies: in the East and in Africa, patients in much greater numbers than in developed countries present psychogenic illness in the form of physical complaints. Indeed, as university health service experience with medical and other students has shown, even sophisticated patients often tend to complain first about somatic symptoms such as headache or stomach discomfort (and many doctors are more receptive about physical illnesses), and only afterwards proceed to relate a personal problem or to describe emotional distress.

The most important clinical rule is the need not only to elicit any psychoneurotic syndrome which may be present, but also to uncover the intrapersonal emotional conflict preceding the onset of the illness.

Anxiety Neurosis

Anxiety is a state of fear, manifestating with a feeling of inner tension and somatic symptoms such as sweating, tremor and tachycardia. Anxiety neurosis is the most common form of psychoneurosis. Although anxiety is a symptom of many psychological disorders, in this syndrome it dominates the clinical picture and other symptoms such as depression are but minor features of the total illness.

Aetiology. Hereditary factors play a part, although a relatively small one, in the genesis of anxiety neurosis, manifestations of anxiety being found in 15% of parents and siblings of patients, which is more than in the population as a whole (5%). Twice as many women as men are affected.

In addition to the genetic trait, even more important aetiologically are emotionally disturbing experiences during the formative years. Often it is found that the patient's early years were attended by prolonged insecurity. For example, a parent may have been so burdened by problems that the child felt unloved, if not unwanted; a brother or sister may have seemed to get preferential treatment; or a mother's own profound anxieties may have imparted an excessive timidity to her child, gravely undermining the child's self-confidence.

This emotional trauma may not be apparent for several years, particularly if the experiences of school life and early adolescence prove free from alarming or painful incidents: but a setback in early adult life may precipitate adult emotional illness. Painful events, such as a bereavement, a reverse in a love affair, disappointment in one's career, being obliged to contend with disagreeable or frankly hostile people at work, or being involved in prolonged domestic strife, may cause a vulnerable individual to succumb to feelings of anxiety which interfere materially with the ability to cope with the daily routine. The adult setback will often be found to have been similar in quality to the earlier childhood emotional trauma.

Clinical Features. The illness may take many forms. It may occur as an acute anxiety attack, often severe in intensity, referred to in the United States classification (DSM-III) as panic disorder. Another form is a chronic anxiety state, known as generalized anxiety disorder in DSM-III. It is present since adolescence in mild degree, but subject to periodic exacerbations occurring at the time of social setbacks, disappointments in close relationships, or work stresses.

The outstanding feature of all forms is anxiety, with its accompanying feeling of inner tension and unpleasant anticipation. Sometimes the anxiety is fear of a potential danger but often it is a diffuse dread. The fear and foreboding fluctuate in intensity, being sometimes a mild feeling of tension or nervousness, at other times a state of panic, in which the patient may be overwhelmed by a feeling of terror, which is no less disturbing because the reason for it is not apparent to the patient.

A *phobia* implies that anxiety is associated with a specific form of activity such as travelling in a bus or train, and so much may this be dreaded that the patient is eventually house-bound through being unable to travel at all. The state of anxiety gives rise to other symptoms. The ability to concentrate is impaired and decisions are difficult to make. There may be a continuous state of restlessness or extreme irritability. The patient may fear becoming insane or committing suicide though, in fact, both are extremely rare in anxiety neurosis. Preoccupation with bodily functions (*hypochondriasis*) and fear of serious illness (*cancerophobia*) are frequently manifested. Continued stress exhausts the patient who, lacking energy and perseverence, may be unable to continue at work.

Somatic symptoms are also prominent. There is a general tenseness of muscles, with hyperactivity, especially of the hands. A fine tremor of the fingers is often present and profuse perspiration, particularly of the palms and forehead, is common. The pulse rate is raised, the blood pressure labile and overactivity of smooth muscle commonly manifests by frequency of micturition or of defecation. Breathing is often rapid and feelings of nausea and flatulence occur; headaches of tension type, dizziness and unsteadiness are frequent. The patient sleeps badly, finding it difficult to get off to sleep and being easily disturbed. Appetite is poor, and loss of weight may be a pronounced feature. Disturbances of menstruation are common.

Not infrequently the patient omits mention of the distressing emotional state and complains to the doctor only of the somatic accompaniments of anxiety; unnecessary special investigations can be initiated or diagnostic errors made if the doctor omits to ask about the state of the patient's mood.

Treatment. PSYCHOTHERAPY. When the formulation of the case indicates that emotional factors are prominent, some form of psychotherapy is required; the patient needs an opportunity for exploration and clarification, and for gaining greater insight into the nature of his difficulties. Simply informing the patient that there is nothing wrong with him, or that he must pull himself together, is useless. Even telling the patient that his difficulties are psychological and identifying the emotional problems in his life is unlikely to be of benefit, because although he may acquiesce verbally, his emotional tension will not be thereby lessened.

A series of interviews, for which periods of at least half an hour or longer should be set aside, are needed when the patient is encouraged to talk about his difficulties. Initially, the discussions should be allowed to proceed in any direction the patient desires; subsequently, aspects of his problems which come to seem relevant may be suggested by the doctor as themes for more detailed discussion. The error that is commonly made with this form of psychotherapy is for the doctor

to talk too much and give advice. In order that the patient may achieve a better knowledge of himself, it is essential that he should do most of the talking, the doctor saying little, but maintaining an attitude of interest and expectation. If the patient's flow of talk is arrested, encouragement can often be given, without diverting him from his present theme. Thus, if he says 'I wasn't able to cope at work', and then becomes silent, after giving him ample time to resume spontaneously, the doctor may say, 'You found the job too much for you?', which starts the patient off again.

The effect of this approach is first that the patient feels better for having talked to someone about his troubles. A second effect is that frequently the patient comes to grasp more accurately the nature of his problems, and will, at that stage, often accept suggestions and interpretations which, if given earlier, would have been rejected. What emerges is that the patient is having difficulties with a person of importance: a spouse, a parent, or an employer, for example, and that there is a need for an improvement in the patient's own participation in the relationship. Thus a man may be too dependent on his wife, too docile to his parent, or too subservient to his employer — in which case his interviews should encourage greater assertiveness.

When the psychoneurotic illness takes the form of somatic symptoms and fear of bodily disease is prominent, it is not sufficient to tell the patient that there is no evidence of organic pathology. It is necessary to let him know that his distress and his symptoms are recognised as genuine and need exploration. It is often possible to use events in the patient's own experience to illustrate the influence of emotion on bodily functions. Many people can recognise what it feels like to be sick with excitement, to be aware of a pounding of the heart in moments of fear or to experience frequency of micturition when keyed up before an examination.

Patients are helped greatly when they can go one stage farther, to confront the painful situation and to master it, e.g. the patient can say to his employer that he considers he is being exploited and his abilities insufficiently recognised. When this is done, there is commonly an immediate, even if temporary, relief from the distressing symptom, together with a sense of accomplishment which encourages the patient to persevere with further efforts of self-discovery.

In the treatment of all forms of neurotic illness it is important to decide what can best be done, within the limitations of resources for treatment and in the circumstances of each individual patient.

Brief psychotherapy focuses upon recent events in the patient's personal experience and explores their emotional significance. By this method, many patients can be helped to reconstitute the way of life which, for the particular person, represents normal mental health.

Explorative psychotherapy, which calls on patients to take stock of their relationships with people close to them and to modify some of their habitual patterns of behaviour, is more time-consuming and aims to produce personality change as well as relief from the symptoms of the illness.

DRUG THERAPY. Drugs can be particularly helpful in tiding a neurotic patient with anxiety over an especially difficult period of subjective distress. They do not, however, do anything to resolve the causes of the patient's symptoms, and unless this is altered either through psychotherapy or through a significant change in personal circumstances, the symptoms will tend to recur and the patient may become dependent on the palliative drug.

The use of drugs to obtain reduction of distressing mood disturbance is often a necessary preliminary to effective psychotherapy. A very anxious patient will not be able to concentrate sufficiently to benefit more than partially from clarification of conflicts discussed during an interview. Diazepam (6–40 mg/d) and chlordiazepoxide (10–60 mg/d) are effective anxiety-reducing drugs. The phenothiazines, though widely used (up to 150 mg/d), are more likely to give rise to lethargy or drowsiness but thioridazine, in the same dosage, can be of value when the patient is both fearful and restless.

Adrenergic blocking agents, such as propranolol, are effective in selected patients. Like all medication in treatment of psychoneurotic illness, it is no more than a part of a therapeutic approach in which the doctor's ongoing participation is crucial.

Hysterical Psychoneurosis

Hysterical psychoneurosis is a protean group of disorders, commonly encountered in all branches of medicine. Essentially a hysterical neurosis consists of the production of the symptoms or signs of a 'physical' illness by a patient for some personal purpose, without being fully aware of the motive in doing so. Familiar examples are sudden 'blackouts' or 'loss of memory' by which a patient deals with a particularly painful or humiliating occurrence.

Aetiology. Heredity is even less important in the development of hysterical neurosis than it is in anxiety neurosis. Environment, by contrast, provides those situational factors which precipitate the development of hysterical symptoms. Lack of emotional security in the early years can encourage and prolong a state of child-like dependency. The lack of development of confidence to tackle practical difficulties makes a person rely on others to solve problems and such a person may later react with hysterical illness. Gross hysterical symptoms occur frequently in association with educational and intellectual disadvantage, and are a particularly common occurrence in developing countries.

Conversion Hysterical Neurosis. This type of psychoneurosis includes the illnesses in which the patient presents with a physical symptom, such as sudden blindness, or paralysis of one or more limbs, or total loss of sensation in a part of the body. Neurological examination will often reveal that the disability does not correspond to the anatomical areas served by motor or sensory nerves; instead, the lesion illustrates the patient's own idea of what it is like to lose the power of the right hand, or to be unable to walk. In many cases, the patient has acquired a concept of a particular affliction as a result of seeing someone who was similarly handicapped. The form the symptom takes may be determined by identification with another person, as when the daughter, after her mother's death, develops the symptoms of her mother's last illness.

The grosser forms of conversion symptoms are not so common today as they were a generation ago, but still occur particularly frequently as a complication of injuries where a compensation award enters the picture. A striking feature of conversion hysterical neurosis is that although the patient may be quite severely incapacitated by the symptoms, he appears remarkably unconcerned about them. This is because the disability due to the illness has in fact intervened to remove a cause of anxiety, so that the patient feels strangely relieved, although not aware of the reason for being so calm.

The list of conversion hysterical symptoms and signs is extensive, for there are few clinical features which may not be encountered in the many forms of this diverse disorder. Some features, however, occur more commonly than others and may be arbitrarily divided into two groups, sensory and motor. *Sensory symptoms* may be of the special senses, such as blindness and deafness, or in the somatic sphere, when cutaneous and deep sensibility in their various forms are lost. The sensory loss does not obey anatomical or physiological laws but follows the patient's concept of disability. Cutaneous sensory loss may have a sharp horizontal upper margin on the limb. In monocular blindness, the patient may on occasion see with the 'blind' eye and the light reflex is preserved. There may also be subjective sensory symptoms such as headache, pain, tinnitus and so on.

Motor symptoms consist of aphonia, mutism and paralysis and rigidity of movements. Positive clinical features in the motor sphere consist of tremors, tics and explosive utterances, spasm of ocular muscles, and fits. These fits may vary from simply falling to the ground to bizarre attacks with wild movements of arms and legs. Carpopedal spasm and other manifestations of tetany may result from hysterical hyperventilation. In the 1980 United States classification (DSM-III) this illness is named conversion disorder and considered a subtype of the 'somatoform disorders', which have as essential features physical symptoms suggesting physical illness for which there are no demonstrable physical findings to explain the symptoms.

Dissociative Hysterical Neurosis. The second type of hysterical psychoneurosis includes the numerous altered states of awareness, such as faints, fits, amnesias, trances, twilight states and forms of multiple personality. A fugue state is one in which the patient wanders away from home in a condition of altered awareness. Hysterical stupor, when the patient lies motionless showing no reaction to the environment, is sometimes seen; in pseudodementia (seen on occasion in a prison setting) the patient behaves as if insane. The term 'dissociative disorder' is used in DSM-III.

Anorexia Nervosa. In this condition, classified with the hysterical psychoneuroses, patients aim to become very slim and to stay so. Frequently preoccupied about food, the patient stubbornly seeks to lose weight. The determination to diet is a disorder of motivation. Exertion of the will, so that over-riding priority is given to becoming thin, is the chief feature of the illness. It often follows teasing about being plump.

Young girls are mainly affected, and boys much more rarely. If questioned suitably, the patients often reveal preoccupations (sometimes so distorted as to reach delusional proportions) relating to sex, sometimes following misinformation by parents; however, these patients also give evidence of great fear at growing up and accepting mature responsibilities. They are often in a hostile relationship with their mothers. Frequently there have been upsetting life experiences, such as separation from or death of a parent. In addition to dread of sexual development, girls with anorexia nervosa often show athletic preoccupations and are overactive physically. The usual mood state is cheerful high spirits, but depression can occur. Patients usually show unconcern about their physical deterioration and reject treatment, which often has to be very firmly advised and provided.

Gonadotrophic and other hormone disturbances occur (p. 425). Amenorrhoea at times precedes marked emaciation.

Those anorexics who in addition induce vomiting and use purgation have a worse prognosis.

Increasingly often, patients present with *bulimia*, sometimes not preceded by anorexia nervosa, characterized by orgies of overeating followed at once by self-induced vomiting.

In-patient psychiatric treatment with psychotherapy to achieve emotional maturation is usually necessary, in addition to correction of the eating disorder.

Diagnosis of Hysterical Psychoneurosis. This can be the most difficult in medicine. Three steps are required: the first is to identify the psychoneurotic syndrome on the basis of its characteristic symptomatology, as described above. The second step to be taken, should any doubt still exist, is to demonstrate that there is no organic disease which can account for the symptoms and signs. Error in diagnosing hysterical psychoneurosis would be infrequent, however, if the diagnosis were not made until the third step was also taken: this consists of discovering what disappointment or setback preceded the development of symptoms. The precipitating cause of an hysterical illness is usually an emotionally charged experience, with unpleasant consequences socially or personally to the patient who excludes it from consciousness and replaces it with symptoms.

If evidence of previous hysterical breakdowns can be uncovered, the diagnosis is more firm. It should be kept in mind, however, that the stress of organic disease may provoke a superadded hysterical reaction in a person so disposed. An axiom worth remembering is that suspected hysterical neurosis appearing for the first time in a stable person in middle life has almost always an organic basis.

Treatment may be a difficult problem. Removal of a symptom can often be achieved by a prolonged interview in which intense persuasion is used; but if the precipitating situation is unaltered, relapse is usual. The method may be justified, however, in certain circumstances as when aphonia prevents discussion, or when loss of memory in hysterical amnesia prevents the patient from communicating his identity or revealing the events which precipitated his illness.

The principles described for psychotherapy in the treatment of anxiety neurosis are also relevant in hysterical psychoneurosis. When hysterical personality disorder is also present, special aspects of management become necessary, as described on page 694.

Obsessional Psychoneurosis

An *obsession* is a constantly recurring thought which the patient recognises as his own, but of which he tries to rid his mind because it is foolish or repugnant. In spite of his efforts to dismiss the thought, it persists in returning so that in the end he becomes tormented by it. A *compulsion* is a similarly insistent urge to perform, or to repeat, some act which the patient consciously repudiates as meaningless or troublesome; he struggles against the urge, but finds himself experiencing very acute anxiety, which is allayed only by giving in and performing the compulsive act.

Obsessive-compulsive symptoms may occur as episodes of illness in otherwise normal individuals. They may become aggravated during an episode of psychiatric illness. Sometimes obsessions and/or compulsions are the outstanding, if not the only, symptoms of which a patient complains. In this condition the patient, although perfectly lucid and in contact with the environment, may be severely handicapped by the unrelenting pressure of unwelcome thoughts and impulses. The illness is also remarkable in that a person almost incapacitated by obsessional symptoms can appear normal to the external observer, until the appallingly repetitive thoughts are disclosed.

Aetiology. Obsessive-compulsive neurosis has an hereditary factor: one-third of the parents of obsessional patients and one-fifth of their siblings have obsessional traits. Many observers believe that the meticulous, rigid routine imposed by such parents is more conducive to obsessional neurosis in the child than the hereditary endowment itself. Environmental factors, other than the influence of obsessive parents during the formative years, appear to contribute less to the causation of obsessional neurosis than is the case with the other syndromes of neurosis.

Clinical Features. Obsessions may be arbitrarily divided into ideas (or images), impulses and ruminations. The *ideas* consist of thoughts, images (often obscene) and strings of words and phrases, which constantly recur to the patient despite resistance to them, and recognition that they are absurd and meaningless.

Impulses are urges to some act such as killing offspring, or jumping under a train, or to less fearsome activities like laughing at sorrow or arranging objects in a certain set manner. Fears of some act may accompany impulses. A fear of knives develops from an impulse to use them for murderous ends. Likewise, a patient may not be troubled by obscene thoughts but rather by the fear that he may have such thoughts; he fills his mind with neutral thoughts lest obscenity should intrude. The idea representing an obsessive impulse keeps on invading the patient's consciousness.

Ruminations comprise the practice of constantly turning over problems in the mind, seeking an answer to a question. Religious scruples are of this order, when the patient has repeatedly to examine and re-examine his conscience, uncertain as to whether he has offended or not.

These symptoms are often intermingled one with another, and may be of all degrees of intensity. Sometimes they are merely a nuisance, not interfering seriously with life, but preventing enjoyment and causing tension. In other cases they become so severe as to arrest all activity and make the ordinary daily round an impossible task. Thus a patient who was a house painter stood for three hours, unable to paint a crack on the wall until he had the 'right' thoughts in his mind. A housewife may spend all her time washing her hands for fear they should be contaminated, and so be unable to do her housework.

When the obsessions are severe they cause great anxiety and tension, the patients becoming increasingly agitated as they fight against the compulsion. In addition, they frequently become depressed, since life becomes so difficult and escape from the obsessions seems to be impossible. Suicide is, however, relatively uncommon except when depressive symptoms complicate the illness.

Treatment. The patient with obsessional illness does not respond well to treatment, but often the condition is self-limiting, at least in its acute phases. The patient should be encouraged by being given the assurance that his doctor knows that his irrational, obscene or murderous thoughts are not indicative of his true nature, and that they are harmless. Behaviour therapy based on learning theory is sometimes helpful. The patient should be encouraged to avoid situations which foster the development of the obsessions and should diversify interests as much as possible. The best antidote for obsessive ruminations is for the patient to keep at work, occupied with practical tasks which demand attention.

Severe obsessional symptoms may be helped by a tricyclic antidepressant drug. Clomipramine has been used, 75–450 mg daily in divided doses.

Depressive Psychoneurosis

This type of illness is at times also named *reactive depression*. Characteristically the morbidly depressed state comes on after a personal setback which often takes the form of a loss of a person important to the patient, for example through death or separation as occurs with a divorce or a broken engagement. Careful exploration will show that the recent disappointment reflects one that occurred earlier in the patient's life. A typical example is the onset of depressive neurosis after a woman is left by her husband, and further interviewing discloses that she had lost a beloved father as a child. When the illness corresponds to an abnormal grief response after the death of a significant person, the term 'bereavement reaction' is sometimes used.

Only occasionally is admission to a psychiatric hospital required, the patient often responding well to out-patient psychotherapeutic interviews.

It may be confusing but it is nevertheless of the greatest importance to emphasise that mixtures of depressive psychoneurosis and major depressive illness are extremely common. The clinical task is to scrutinise any case of depressive illness to determine the presence and amount of any component of 'endogenicity', i.e. so-called biological features including loss of energy, sleep disturbance, loss of appetite, constipation, impairment of libido, and — in severe cases — gross self-blame. In such mixed states antidepressant drugs are indicated, and good practice calls for a combined psychotherapeutic and pharmacological approach.

The 1980 United States classification omits the term depressive psychoneurosis, contending that these patients can be assigned to one or another illness entity, depending on the main clinical features. Mixtures of depressive symptoms with anxiety reaction occur frequently; some neurotically depressed patients are also hypochondriacal.

Phobic Psychoneurosis

These widely prevalent illnesses consist of unjustified fear which is firmly related to a precise stimulus, either a place or an object. The patient may be terrified at being in a supermarket, a bus, an open space (*agoraphobia*), or a closed place (*claustrophobia*). Fear of flying can be a nuisance to a housewife and may deter the family from taking overseas holidays, a major handicap to a business executive, and an occupational disaster to a pilot or other member of air crew.

The phobic place or object can be so innocuous as to seem ridiculous, and dreading ridicule the patient may not be able to summon the courage to disclose the affliction to the doctor. Direct questioning may be needed to explore cues which are offered, such as a patient never coming unaccompanied to consult the doctor.

Phobias can at times be referred to parts of the body, hence the use at times of such terms as 'cardiac neurosis' and 'cancerophobia'. Patients can be terrified that they may have an urge to urinate when a toilet may not be accessible; when afflicted with this syndrome, patients know exactly the locus of every public lavatory in their neighbourhood.

The subjective benefit to the patient of suffering from a phobic state (rather than, say, an anxiety reaction or an obsessional illness) is that life can be perfectly manageable as long as the phobic stimulus is avoided. A person with a dog phobia need only find a dogless route to work, if one exists.

Antianxiety medication, such as chlordiazepoxide or diazepam, can assist such patients greatly, in association with psychotherapeutic interviewing which encourages the patient to 'go against the phobia'. A requisite of treatment is that the doctor should comprehend the terror experienced by the patient (often related to childhood traumatic experience) and avoid a belittling response even when the patient's fear is grotesquely unjustified.

Behaviour therapy has a high rate of success. It is based on devising for the patient a hierarchy of experiences relating to the phobic object or situation, in which increasing exposure is gradually built up, always avoiding excessive anxiety. Someone with a dog phobia may look with the doctor or clinical psychologist at canine pictures, starting with a benign species and coming at length to an Alsatian; then real dogs can be introduced to the interview, first a docile, aged pet and perhaps later quite daunting beasts encountered on a walk can be approached with due circumspection.

PERSONALITY DISORDERS

In every large community there are a number of people who do not conform to the prevailing norm. Statistically speaking, a person can be outside the range of normal either by being exceptionally gifted or by being so grossly underendowed as to be an eccentric or a social misfit; but it is the latter who are more likely to come to medical attention.

The personality disorders began to gain notice only late during the development of psychiatry as a medical discipline; they have been recognised increasingly as the out-patient responsibilities of psychiatrists have extended, and as psychiatric units have developed in general hospitals. The diagnostic differentiation between psychiatric illness and personality disorder is the more necessary because very often the two coexist. Indeed, clinical convention has it that hysterical psychoneurosis commonly supervenes in individuals with hysterical personality, obsessional neurosis in those with obsessional personality disorders, etc. In addition to their presentation with psychotic illnesses and psychoneuroses, people with abnormal personalities often appear clinically with psychosomatic disorders and may be chronic hospital attenders.

Abnormal personalities may not enter the medical ambit at all, but be encountered in penal settings. Still others may continue unrecognised in the community and escape anonymity only when widespread screening of the population occurs, as in a wartime when obligatory intake to the armed forces exposes all adults to clinical scrutiny.

The central feature of abnormal personality is some degree of persistent abnormality of behaviour which is frequently, but not necessarily, antisocial in its manifestations. The abnormality varies considerably in degree, ranging in severity from schizoid and hysterical people who are often valuable if somewhat unstable members of the community, to psychopaths who are socially destructive.

In the 1980 United States classification the personality disorders are classified on a separate axis from the psychiatric illnesses, encouraging multiple diagnoses wherever possible.

Obsessional Personality Disorder

Obsessional persons give scant regard to the emotional aspects of a situation or an interaction. They are rigid rather than flexible, overattentive to details rather than to the wider scope of an event or encounter, and prefer to have everything predictable and orderly. They often appear officious, sometimes so pedantically that they can be comical, and not only control themselves excessively but also attempt to dominate others. They appear to behave in an unduly egotistical manner, and respond in an overriding way when involved in a venture calling for co-operation. They are over-careful, methodical, punctual and overorganised, to the extent of becoming uncomfortable and even upset if their routines are disturbed by an unexpected development. They have a set of fixed standards and points of view, from which they can deviate only with great difficulty. They are uninfluenced, therefore, by the wishes, needs, opinions or views of other people.

The meticulousness and preservation of sameness extends to the person's mode of dress, which can be scrupulously neat. They can be overconscientious, and often work compulsively. Such persons, in consequence, can be of particular usefulness in bureaucratic posts calling for scrupulous concern with minutiae. They may be highly obstinate when faced by any requirement that they should deviate from the straight and narrow path.

At times such persons appear to leave some loophole, so that the conformity, inhibition and rigidity is waived in some context or other. The precise, neat youngster, who must have everything in place, may for example permit himself to have his clothes cupboard in disorder, or may periodically forget thrift to overspend in a foolish self-indulgence which rationally is at odds with his habitual miserliness.

The gross form of the disorder is easy to recognise. The milder forms may be less obtru-sive, and may be particularly evident only at times of pressure, as when an examination is looming for a youngster or when a house-proud woman has relatives coming to stay in her home.

Schizoid Personality Disorder

Schizoid persons are essentially solitary. They are aloof in their loneliness, detached and distant from other people. The term 'introverted' is applied to this disorder in the 1980 United States classification (DSM-III). Such individuals have few close relationships, and may be much more preoccupied with some impersonal activity in the realms of electronics, physics, mathematics or engineering. Often the engrossing venture is a personal fad or invention, which may be of negligible application in ordinary life, but may be pursued with a single-minded devotion inappropriate to a mere hobby or interest.

Cold, quiet and shy, the person's abnormality may already have been apparent early in childhood, from an inability or disinclination to mix, and a preference for solitary pursuits. The lack of friendships may have been upsetting to the parents; as schizoid individuals grow up, they can themselves be distressed by their incapacity for any intimacy in their association with others.

The person may appear odd or eccentric and in awkward isolation may be seen as a figure of fun or seem excessively secretive. Schizoid people are often solitary workers, who cannot function satisfactorily in a team. Bookish, reserved, out of touch with others, relatively blind to social cues, their personal lives may appear barren. However, this remote exterior may belie the strong emotions which some schizoid people cannot express. Others find a vehicle for their private feelings, and may keep a diary, or indulge in daydreaming, or succeed in establishing some relationship in which the expression of emotion is allowed.

Schizoid persons are rigid and brittle. They have little empathy with other people, of whose intentions, feelings and wishes they remain unaware. When attempting to appraise others intuitively, they are often wildly wrong, thereby complicating their already attenuated relationships. They can be made profoundly uncomfortable when well-meaning but misguided mentors or doctors attempt to have them mix more, or urge them to become intimate with other persons, perhaps other isolates as lacking in interpersonal skills as themselves.

Schizoid persons are at times mistrustful, seeing slights where none is intended. Suspicion can become the prevailing response to others, in the belief that they are being exploited, misused or disparaged. Some clinicians would differentiate this development separately, diagnosing such a personality as *paranoid*.

Hysterical Personality Disorder

People of this type can be identified on the basis of a constellation of behaviours: they seek to please and influence others; they crave attention; they are insincere; and they are given to excessive displays of emotion. They were often victims of inadequate maternal care in childhood.

Hysterical individuals appear to be exploitative, with an eye always on others. They talk for effect, not to convey any honestly felt opinion. One feels their need for appreciation, and their readiness to express themselves with that aim in view. They over-react in order to evoke a response from others.

Psychiatrists probably over-diagnose this type in abnormal women, attaching the label very much less often to men. The person is showy, histrionic in manner and dress, with a quality of spuriousness and exaggeration, even theatricality, in what she does. The condition is named 'histrionic personality disorder' in DSM-III. The exhibitionism appears intended to impress others, even to shock them. Speech is superficial, with plentiful hyperbole ('heavenly', 'ghastly'), which only heightens the effect of shallowness. Women of this type suffer from sexual timidity and frigidity, the more distressing to them because their frequently seductive manner and provocative dress invites advances with which they cannot cope; hysterical men also have difficulty in establishing a close relation with one woman, and may seek intimacy in a series of attachments of short duration.

The management of an hysterical personality disorder is discussed on page 694.

Sociopathy

Sociopaths suffer from the most severe form of abnormal personality. Because of serious defects in the capacity for feeling, they are often described as 'affectionless'. Lacking in conscience they have great difficulty in realising that other people are harmed when they behave antisocially. The name for the condition in DSM-III is 'antisocial disorder'. Loveless, indifferent and destructive, they cannot form satisfactory relationships, and major failures repeatedly occur in marriage, work and social life. They come into conflict with the norms, customs and laws of the community.

Impulsiveness is usually evident, sociopaths dismaying those associated with them by uncontrolled, often destructive outbursts in the absence of sufficient provocation. Such precipitate and deplorable action has been spoken of as 'short circuit reactions', to indicate that often the person is aware of the build-up to the outburst and will often admit after the aggressive or destructive episode to feeling calmer and relieved of tension.

Sociopaths do not show ability to modify destructive behaviour reactions, or to learn from even drastic setbacks; they may be punished repeatedly for the same unacceptable behaviour, and yet continue it; the individual's antisocial patterns are often monotonously repetitive. Kleptomania, gambling or physical assaults may each be associated with excitement which the sociopath seeks and indulges repeatedly; the antisocial behaviour can be seriously destructive to others, as in cases of sadistic attacks on children or of fire-raising.

The lack of regard for the possible consequences of their actions is also impressive, sociopaths appearing not to care about the outcome, and being inconsiderate even of persons on whom their welfare depends. They disregard their obligations to others. The lack of concern amounts often to callousness. The Mental Health Acts in Britain allow for the compulsory hospitalisation of the 'seriously irresponsible' sociopath, and so does the legislation of many other countries.

Social relationships are shallow and transient. Sociopaths are not loyal to individuals or to groups. They have poor judgement of situations, and often lie their way out of complications. They are indifferent to the welfare of others. Swindling and deception are frequent features.

Two types of sociopathy are distinguished:

Aggressive Sociopath. The hostility displayed in attacks on other people, damage to property, thefts and fraud may bring the sociopath to legal attention.

Passive Sociopath. Persons of this type are seriously inadequate and cannot adapt to social requirements; they are chronically inept, passive and dependent. Many are placid and responsive; others are cold, withdrawn and apathetic. They may exist as aimless drifters, to be found in places where hobos congregate. Even if supported in a family or protective environment such as a half-way house or hostel, such people may be further incapacitated by the complications of drug addiction or alcoholism.

Management Implications of Personality Disorders

The chief medical relevance of personality disorder, in terms of the doctor-patient relationship, is that patients respond to the clinician in accordance with their particular personality deviation. For this reason, diagnosis of the personality type permits the management to be planned realistically, so that the doctor does not expect a degree of co-operativeness which the patient is not equipped to provide. In addition, the doctor will be better able to predict the patient's pattern of behaviour in the future.

For example, the long-term management of a woman with an hysterical personality disorder has much in common with that of a frightened or petulant child. It consists in convincing her that you are on her side, even while refusing to comply with some of her requests. Treating a patient with such personality disorder is often a test of nerve; in the face of dramatic protestations and apparently alarming social crises, one must quietly but firmly insist upon facing the painful realities from which the patient has taken flight. If one has succeeded in gaining her confidence, helplessness and distress will sometimes disappear with dramatic suddenness, but all too often they are replaced by subsequent turmoil. The hysterical patient finds it difficult to abandon the defences against alarming feelings which she has been using since her early adolescence. In addition these patients are especially prone to develop an emotional dependence upon their doctors, which must be recognised and brought to their attention kindly but firmly. The family doctor can give helpful advice to other people in the patient's immediate environment, warning them that hysterical acting-out behaviour only becomes aggravated if too much attention is paid, and encouraging them to avoid entering into the patient's pattern of self-deception. It is usually much easier for the onlookers than for the patient herself to see the real motivation of her symptoms, but of course, it is no use simply telling her — she has to discover for herself why she behaves in the way she does.

The achievement of a long-term cure of an hysterical personality disorder is a formidable task since it requires the patient to mature emotionally. Not surprisingly, both patients and their doctors often tacitly agree not to attempt it. Instead, the doctor may concentrate upon dealing with the most pressing difficulties of the patient's immediate predicament and may settle for her remaining a somewhat demanding and dependent patient. In that case, the goal for each consultation can be to ensure that the patient departs calmer and with more self-esteem than when she arrived. The doctor helps the patient discover some modifiable aspect in a problem which she had considered insoluble.

ALCOHOLISM AND DRUG DEPENDENCE

Addiction to alcohol or drugs represents a form of psychological dependence and indicates that the patient has been unable to attain adequate satisfaction or self-esteem in his or her personal life. Addictions to drugs and to alcohol are associated with a high risk of suicide. The underlying lack of self-confidence is often so deep-seated that prolonged treatment and rehabilitation is necessary once the drug or alcohol has been given up. In the 1980 United States classification these conditions are named 'substance use disorders'.

Alcohol. Alcoholics are often brought reluctantly to their doctors by close relatives who can see more clearly than the patients how seriously their lives are being interfered with by the addiction. These unwilling patients are particularly difficult to treat; but the prospect is very different when the patient is distressed by the dependence and is anxious for change.

Alcoholism is one of the most serious public health problems in all developed countries. Mental disorders due to alcoholism are responsible for a large proportion of admissions to Scottish mental hospitals. It is an insidious condition, because the enjoyment of alcohol is socially accepted and even encouraged. There is a relationship between alcohol consumption in a country and rates of alcoholism; alcohol consumption has been increasing steadily in countries such as Britain, the United States (32 per cent higher in 15 years), West Germany (61 per cent), the Netherlands (83 per cent) and Finland (50 per cent). The Irish have a high alcoholism rate, while Chinese and Jews are rarely alcoholic.

The process by which an occasional drinker becomes an excessive drinker, and finally dependent on drink, can be gradual; acquaintances, and even friends are reluctant to draw attention to a man's excessive drinking because the alcoholic is liable to fear being shunned and is prone to take offence. Here, however, doctors have a clear responsibility because often an intercurrent illness, chronic dyspepsia or haematemesis, or even a street accident will bring the patient to medical care, and a carefully taken history (especially if supplemented by information from others in the patient's family) will reveal the increasing dependence upon alcohol.

Sometimes an unexpected hospital admission, interrupting a sustained high intake of spirits, results in the onset of *delirium tremens* which compels attention to the seriousness of the drinking problem. This acute psychosis is characterised by gross peripheral tremors, great restlessness, confusion, misidentification of people and places and delusional ideas. These delusions may be agreeable but much more often they are threatening or even terrifying, especially when accompanied by hallucinatory visions. Because of these complications, hospital admission may be necessary when starting to treat an alcoholic.

The fully established syndrome of alcoholism is characterised by: (1) a need for alcohol as for a drug, customary activities being difficult to perform without it: (2) taking of alcohol apart from social occasions; (3) tolerance, the person being able to drink increasing amounts without becoming incapacitated; (4) the abstinence response, i.e. unpleasant symptoms occurring as the blood alcohol level falls, e.g. tremor, sweating, wakefulness and tension; (5) loss of tolerance; becoming incapacitated before imbibing the amount of alcohol needed; (6) restitution, i.e. the rapid development of the entire syndrome after drinking is resumed following a period of abstinence.

Treatment of Alcohol Addiction. This consists initially of 'drying out', which often calls for hospital admission. Withdrawal symptoms can be controlled by phenothiazines, diazepam, haloperidol or chlormethiazole. The last is an hypnotic related to thiamin. It is probably the drug of choice in severe alcohol withdrawal syndromes including delirium tremens. In these circumstances it should not be used for longer than 1 week because of the danger of dependency. Vitamins B and C intravenously may also be of value.

The next phase of treatment, once the patient is abstinent, is to explore, by means of a series of interviews, the personal and other problems which require attention. Psychiatric assistance is needed if obvious psychological disorder is apparent once the drinking has stopped. Those abstinent alcoholics who consider themselves in danger of relapse can ensure their sobriety by taking disulfiram (0·5 g/d) or citrated calcium carbimide: when on these drugs, the patient will have an unpleasant reaction after taking only a small amount of alcohol.

The main requirement of treatment is that the alcoholic should become totally abstinent. Many alcoholics are active and valuable members of society and can maintain this necessary abstinence if given appropriate medical supervision.

Alcoholic women who are pregnant require urgent and skilled care to avoid damage to the fetus. The fetal alcohol syndrome is characterised by impairment of growth, mental retardation and dysmorphic features. Women who drink alcohol only socially would be well advised not to do so during pregnancy.

Morphine. Dependence is seen in doctors,

nurses, pharmacists and dentists, and at times in patients who become addicted through therapeutic use. The desired euphoric effect can be achieved by subcutaneous injection, but as tolerance grows intravenous injections are used. Hypodermic tattooing of the skin, thrombosed veins and pinpoint pupils are indications of the condition. Treatment, such as substitution with methadone, is best done at a centre with the necessary facilities.

Heroin. Dependence is increasing rapidly in incidence, and many addicts are young people. The drug has a marked euphoriant effect; it acts quickly and its desired action also dissipates quickly. The abstinence syndrome is particularly unpleasant. Many addicts cannot be cured, and their management then is by supplies of the smallest dose of the drug preventing the withdrawal symptoms, or by substitution of methadone in place of heroin.

Cocaine. Those addicted to cocaine take the drug in the form of snuff, smoke or intravenously. It is a stimulant, like amphetamine. The most well-known toxic symptom is formication, the sensation of insects crawling under the skin. Use occurs mainly in those addicted also to heroin, the effect of cocaine alone being unsatisfactorily brief. Physical effects are anorexia, emaciation, nausea, insomnia and convulsions.

By the Drug Addiction Act of 1968 issue of heroin and cocaine is limited in Britain to named doctors, usually psychiatrists in designated treatment centres. Social complications are damaging, disorganised behaviour leading to loss of friends and inability to work, and to trouble with the law because of possession, purchase or sale of the drug.

Lysergic Acid Diethylamide (LSD) is used mainly by young people. Taken by mouth, it has dramatic effects lasting about 6 hours. Illusions occur, colour is intensified, mood changes include euphoria, awe or anxiety, a curious blurring between the individual and the environment is experienced, and phantasy thoughts, flight of ideas and delusions serve to heighten the mystical nature of the 'trip'.

Physical dependence does not occur, but some users become psychologically dependent. Proponents of the drug as a 'mind expander' sometimes overlook the serious hazards. These include psychotic reactions with paranoid delusions which can last many weeks, and non-psychotic reactions chiefly terror; both can result in self-injury or suicide. A bad LSD experience can be cut short by chlorpromazine, used intramuscularly in severe cases.

Cannabis (hashish, marihuana, 'pot') is also used very commonly by the young, sometimes only a few times; there is no evidence that occasional use is harmful. At first the user feels 'high', and then drifts into a peaceful, drowsy state heightened by unusual mental images. Skin flushing, rapid pulse and dilated pupils may convey that a person has taken cannabis, usually by smoking a 'joint'. Many addicts use more than one drug. That physical dependence can occur is doubted, but marked psychological dependence is common.

Barbiturate. Many middle-aged or elderly women come to rely upon a nightly dose of sleeping tablets and some of them find that if they take two or three during the day, this helps to relieve tension and anxiety. Gradually, they begin to show the signs of chronic barbiturate overdosage, namely, slight ataxia, absent-mindedness amounting at times to confusion as to time and place, defective judgement, loss of emotional control, slurred speech and tremor of the fingers. A sudden cessation of barbiturates can be followed by a major epileptic fit. The withdrawal syndrome can be alarming, with headaches, insomnia and vomiting, and a delirious state with delusions. Small doses of barbiturates may need to be administered. A patient cured of one addiction, e.g. alcoholism, may start using another drug, e.g. barbiturate, which is erroneously regarded as innocuous.

Another pattern of usage is in young people who obtain the drug illicitly and take it often with their associates and with other drugs.

Amphetamine formerly used in the treatment of obesity and still used for narcolepsy, soon came to be abused, particularly by teenagers, either alone or combined with barbiturate to provide a rapid lifting of the spirits and feeling of wellbeing. The use of amphetamine readily gives rise to a psychological dependency, when the daily dose taken can increase vastly, tolerance developing with continued use. The amphetamine addict has an impression of increased mental and physical drive and competence. There are also restlessness, irritability and excitability. Amphetamine can give rise also to an acute psychotic reaction with auditory and visual hallucinations and delusions of persecution. These features can be clinically indistinguishable from those of paranoid schizophrenia, but they clear up in about 3 weeks time after withdrawal of the drug. Since the Misuse of Drugs Act (1971), amphetamines are listed as controlled drugs in Britain, special regulations applying to prescribing them. The drug is justified medically only in occasional cases of narcolepsy.

Volatile substances (glue sniffing; solvent abuse) have received much publicity in recent years, because of their abuse by children and adolescents particularly in deprived communities. The most widely used is toluene, but benzene, lacquers, cigarette lighter fluids, paint thinners and xylene have been employed. The glue is sniffed from smears on rags, from plastic bags, or directly from tubes. This practice promotes stimulation ('jags'), but tolerance develops, and amounts are sniffed which lead to damage to the brain and other organs. Volatile solvents are among the most dangerous of the psychoactive substances to which users can become addicted.

Multiple drug abuse is frequent. Those who misuse alcohol also regularly make non-medical use of other drugs e.g. benzodiazepines. This occurs especially in those with access to medicines, such as doctors, nurses or pharmacists. But members of the general public, from adolescents to those in middle-age, also frequently have poly-dependency, tobacco and pharmaceutical agents complicating, say, a drinking problem.

PSYCHOSEXUAL DISORDERS

These include sexual deviation (paraphilia) and conditions such as premature ejaculation and vaginismus.

Sexual Deviation

Sexual deviants are people who are unable to obtain physical and emotional satisfaction in nor-mal sexual intercourse, but can do so only in ways which to a greater or lesser degree are socially condemned. Practices which alarm, threaten or injure other persons, such as *exhibitionism* (exposing the genitals to a stranger), *paedophilia* (having sex with immature partners of either sex) or *sadism* (deriving sexual pleasure from inflicting pain) are still regarded as antisocial and are punishable by law. On the other hand, public opinion has become somewhat more tolerant of deviant practices which do not interfere with other people. The change of opinion found expression in the Sexual Offences Act 1967, which, for the first time in English history, excluded homosexual acts, carried out in private by consenting adults, from any legal sanction.

Homosexuality. People who are responsive erotically to partners of the same sex are frequent in the population. Four percent of adult men are exclusively homosexual, and another 13 per cent are so for years of their lives. For women the rates are half as much. During the 1970s increasing numbers of homosexuals have 'come out' and publically declared their sexual orientation. After debate and public pressure the American Psychiatric Association in 1974 ruled that homosexuality as such would no longer be listed as a mental disorder, creating instead a new category of 'sexual orientation disturbance'.

Forms of deviant sexual behaviour also include *transvestism* (deriving gratification from wearing the clothing of the opposite sex) and *fetishism* (when the person becomes sexually stimulated by parts of the body not usually experienced as erotogenic — e.g. the feet — or by articles of clothing or other objects). These conditions seem to be the result of distorted experiences at the stage of development when boys and girls learn their sexual roles.

Deviant forms of sexual gratification often prove very resistant to change. If the patient suffers because of them — and many sexual deviants appear to be content with their lot — treatment often has to be limited to damping down the intensity of the sexual drive, e.g. by the administration of oestrogens to males or to helping the patient (and perhaps also the spouse) to accept the peculiarity.

Psychosomatic Disorders

These are the physical illnesses which are caused in part by psychological factors or, when present, are maintained by psychological factors. Examples of such conditions are many cases of peptic ulcer, bronchial asthma, colitis and various forms of dermatitis. The implication of the term 'psychosomatic' is that tension arising from a long-standing emotional conflict can induce changes in bodily function (e.g. excessive secretion of gastric acid; bronchospasm) which, when repeated over a period of time, can in turn lead to actual tissue damage.

For many years, attempts have been made to delineate particular personality types associated with different forms of psychosomatic illness. A review of this literature, however, fails to reveal a specific type of personality in relation to each of these disorders. Instead, psychosomatic subjects tend to be characterised by relatively constant emotional elements, the chief of which are dependency, anger or fear, which appear to be the most harmful when they are denied conscious expression. Repressed dependency needs have been particularly associated with peptic ulcer and ulcerative colitis, repressed anger with asthma and hypertension.

Individual cases, however, when studied in depth, are not easily fitted into any common mould. Modern psychosomatic theory has, therefore, retreated to the more general observation that all patients with physical illness accompanied by a conspicuous psychological component have long-standing problems in the control of their own internal emotional experiences, and in the conduct of their relationships with people who matter in their private lives. It is probable that genetic factors, which have endowed some of us with a particularly vulnerable organ or organ system, will dictate both the occurrence of a psychosomatic illness (which often indeed co-exists with neurotic symptoms) and the choice of the organ which is affected.

Treatment of the emotional disturbance and disregard of the local physical factors, or vice versa, will seldom lead to benefit for the patient, and an assessment must be made in each case of the relative importance of both factors, so that whichever appears to have the greater aetiological significance can be the main target for therapy, while the lesser factor is in no way neglected. The family doctor is often in the best position to know the unrealised ambitions, the frustrations at work or at home, or the marital unhappiness which may form the background to the patient's physical illness. A knowledge of the family history may also reveal that hereditary predisposition plays a part in determining the form of the illness, as for example in migraine.

PSYCHIATRIC DISORDERS IN RELATION TO AGE

The individual is confronted with new problems in adaptation at all the main stages of change, namely puberty, adolescence, pregnancy or following childbirth, at the menopause and on retirement. Mental disorders occur particularly at these times.

Childhood. Psychiatric disorder in children is now a major subspecialty of psychiatry. In childhood very significant phases in the development of personality are taking place; the child is at the mercy of the environment, utterly dependent on the adequacy of the parents and the provisions they make. In addition to behaviour disorders including untoward fear, aggressiveness, jealousy, stealing, school phobia and truancy, children require treatment for such distressing syndromes as enuresis, soiling (involuntary defecation), psychoneurotic illnesses, psychotic disorders including early infantile autism, and the handicaps such as stammering, dyslexia, extreme hyperactivity and organic brain damage.

The doctor responsible for the health of the child needs to collaborate closely with the child psychiatrist, with institutions which may be involved including the school, and with professional colleagues who contribute in any treatment, especially the clinical psychologist and the social worker. The parents must always be implicated clinically. The outcome of a programme of management often depends crucially on the comprehensiveness and adequacy of the co-operation between those involved.

Adolescence. Psychoses are rare until adolescence, when they increase in frequency; psychotic illnesses thereafter are increasingly common with advance of age. At adolescence, the period between puberty and young adulthood, the young person has to cope with more complex social involvement, sexual commitment and occupational challenge, while also separating from parents and detaching from their domestic arrangements. The personality changes of normal adolescence may be upsetting to some parents, teachers or other adults; a period of turmoil when the adolescent is aggressive, defiant or rebellious may precede the achievement of a stable adult personality. A previously polite child may become rude and sarcastic in the course of developing assertiveness and independence.

Often the youngster surmounts troublesome behaviour if the family, school and community are understanding, encouraging and tolerant. But certain disturbances of adolescence require clinical attention. These include delinquent behaviour, deviant sexual practices with consequences which are harmful socially or damaging to the young person, inadequate school attainment, mood disturbance such as depression sometimes with attempts at suicide, withdrawal, social isolation and apathy, and, of course, bizarre behaviour with psychotic features such as delusions or hallucinations which may signal the onset of schizophrenic illness.

Adolescents can develop any of a range of psychiatric disorders, such as the adjustment reaction of adolescence, psychoneuroses, the functional psychoses, personality disorders, acute organic psychoses, drug and alcohol misuse and psychosomatic disorders.

Adulthood. Mental disorder may be associated with pregnancy or the puerperium. Puerperal psychoses may be schizophrenic in type or, more rarely, manic-depressive. Psychoneurotic illnesses also occur in the postpartum period.

The majority of patients receiving psychiatric treatment are middle-aged. However, when the numbers of first hospital admissions are calculated in relation to the proportion of the general population in each group, the psychiatric admission rate to hospital rises steadily with increasing age, particularly after the sixth decade. In middle age, depressive psychosis is sometimes accompanied by intense anxiety, resulting in the syndrome of *agitated depressive psychosis*. The patient is characteristically restless, overwrought, hopeless, with extreme self-blame and low self-regard, and expressing nihilistic, guilty or hypochondriacal delusions. The previous personality in such patients is often characterised by over-conscientiousness or obsessionality.

Retirement from work can be a source of anxiety, especially for people who derived particular satisfaction, status, or esteem from working with others. Depressive illnesses with a sense of worthlessness or apathy can be a real burden for some at this stage of life. Women are often at risk in earlier middle life when their children leave home and make their separate existences, especially when mothering formed a predominant role in the woman's pattern of adjustment, unaccompanied by additional interests and commitments.

The Elderly. The care of the elderly plays an increasingly large part in contemporary society. Dementia has been discussed on page 680 but of great clinical importance is the fact that many elderly people with dementia can also become depressed. It is a most serious omission to fail to recognise this common illness in the elderly, who may be incapacitated by such superadded psychiatric disability, but become able to cope again when relieved of the morbid gloom and apathy by antidepressant therapy.

What is also not widely appreciated is the fact that episodes of neurotic illness, with anxiety states, phobias, hysterical symptoms or compulsions are also encountered in this age group, and are no less amenable to simple psychotherapy than at other ages. In the after-care of these older patients it is important to remember that social isolation is an important threat to their mental well-being. This becomes even more important when physical disability or deafness further restricts their opportunities of making contact with other people. Here voluntary agencies as well as local authority welfare and preventive services can do useful prophylactic work, but the family doctor is often in the best position to recognise when an ageing (and perhaps recently bereaved) patient is in special need of help.

Elderly patients easily develop delirium, and then adapt poorly to sudden changes of scene and bewildering happenings. It is helpful for them if they can be visited by only a few nurses and doctors who take pains to identify themselves; their sick-room should be well lit and they should be encouraged to keep a few familiar possessions on their bed-side table. Since patients with even very slight clouding of consciousness are prone to misunderstand what is happening round about them, any changes of routine or new procedures should be explained to them in advance, in simple terms and if necessary more than once.

Conclusion

Psychiatric disorder can present diverse problems throughout an individual's life and also clinical challenges not only to psychiatrists but to all who practise medicine.

H. J. WALTON

FURTHER READING:

Bancroft, J. (1983) *Human Sexuality and its Problems*. Edinburgh: Churchill Livingstone.

Kendell, R. E. & Zealley, A. K. (eds) (1983) *Companion to Psychiatric Studies*, 3rd edn. Edinburgh: Churchill Livingstone. A postgraduate textbook written by Edinburgh teachers.

Madden, J. S. (1979) *A Guide to Alcohol and Drug Dependence*. Bristol: John Wright.

Shepherd, M. & Zangwill, O. L. (eds) (1983) *General Psychopathology. Handbook of Psychiatry I*. Cambridge: Cambridge University Press An authoritative and comprehensive text, to appear in 5 vols.

Silverstone, T. & Turner, P. (1978) *Drug Treatment in Psychiatry*, 2nd edn. London: Routledge & Kegan Paul.

Trethowen, W. H. (1979) *Psychiatry*, 4th edn. London: Baillière Tindall. A useful text for undergraduate students.

Walton, H. J. (1979) In Macleod, J. (ed.) *Clinical Examination*, 5th edn. Edinburgh: Churchill Livingstone. For a detailed description of the psychiatric examination.

17. Acute Poisoning

Self-poisoning is a very common and urgent medical problem. The number of patients admitted to hospital because of it has increased steadily in Britain over the last 30 years, so much so that this type of behaviour has become endemic in our society. In England and Wales, there were 33 600 hospital admissions due to acute poisoning in 1962, whereas in recent years the figure has been well in excess of 100 000, representing 10 to 30% of all admissions to acute medical units in Britain with a general average of 15%. These hospital statistics are formidable, but the true incidence is probably much higher. Many symptomless children and up to 40% of adults who reach Accident and Emergency Departments may be sent home because the physical effects are mild. Many patients, estimated to be about 30%, are not even referred to hospital but are treated at home by their general practitioners. In Britain, therefore, it is more likely that the true incidence of poisonings is over 300 000 per annum.

The mortality due to acute poisoning in Britain has fallen in recent years but according to official statistics approximately 3500 deaths occur due to poisoning each year. It has been estimated, however, that about 80% of all deaths from acute poisoning occur outside hospital and so it is important that hospital statistics should not be considered alone as an index of the physical consequences of poisoning in the community. The fall in mortality has occurred, despite the increase in incidence, for two main reasons. Carbon monoxide poisoning has become rare since the relatively non-toxic natural gas replaced coal gas in domestic supplies, and prescriptions for barbiturates have been much reduced with the

substitution of safer hypnotics such as benzodiazepines. Improved methods of treatment have also played their part, and in any good district hospital the mortality resulting from acute poisoning should be less than 1%.

The major causes of death by poisoning are now dextropropoxyphene, barbiturates, tricyclic antidepressants, salicylate and paracetamol. Perhaps as a result, there are two peaks in mortality; the first occurs in the 15 to 25 age group mainly from analgesics, and the second in patients over 65 due to barbiturates with, in addition, coexisting physical disease. At all ages the number of females who die tends to be greater than males, but this is probably a reflection of the fact that acute poisoning is commoner in women than in men. Among the 25 to 30 year olds, suicides constitute one in 10 of all deaths, and in doctors, death from acute poisoning is as common as death from carcinoma of the lung.

The problem of acute poisoning is not restricted to Britain but is experienced in all the developed and many developing countries of the world. In the United States of America five million poisonings occur every year and the number is increasing. Acute poisoning is the fourth most common cause of accidental death in that country and the reported mortality is over 5000 per annum. Poisoning is the most common medical emergency in paediatric hospitals. At all ages it accounts for 10% of all emergency home visits and 5 to 10% of adult medical admissions. In most European countries a similar problem exists, but direct comparison, especially in terms of mortality statistics, is difficult due to the wide variations in which deaths from poisoning are recorded and coded. Morbidity statistics are subject to even greater discrepancy and much more standardised information is required before the true international situation can be assessed.

This chapter deals with the clinical features, diagnosis, treatment and prevention of acute poisoning. Food poisoning is discussed on pages 753–754. Brief reference is made to industrial and agricultural poisons. The effects of exposure to ionising radiation are discussed on page 528.

Classification and Causes of Acute Poisoning

Acute poisoning can be accidental or intentional.

Accidental Poisoning. Death from accidental poisoning has increased almost three-fold in the past 30 years, women being more likely than men to die in this way. In Britain the mortality from this cause is approximately 15 per million population; in other European countries there is considerable variation. In Scandinavia, for example, the rate is about 20 per million. Except in children, it is doubtful if the official statistics reflect the true incidence of accidental poisoning. For example, it is difficult to believe the official figures that more adults die each year from accidental barbiturate poisoning than from suicidal poisoning by these drugs. Certification is often purposely made inaccurate to save family feelings. Confused elderly patients may develop acute accidental poisoning because they are often given many medicines and they are prone to make mistakes in the dosage and frequency of the administration of drugs. This is particularly the case when inappropriate psychotropic therapy is prescribed.

SUBSTANCES INVOLVED IN ACCIDENTAL POISONING. Children are most frequently involved due to the careless storage of medicines and household products. Common causes include ingestion of medicine (e.g. aspirin, tricyclics, antihistamines or iron), a wide range of household substances (e.g. paraffin, detergents or bleach) weed killers (e.g. paraquat) and, rarely, poisonous berries. Inhalation of organic solvents (e.g. glues and cleaning fluids) and occasionally carbon monoxide from incomplete combustion due to faulty gas appliances or motor car exhaust pipes, also occurs.

Accidental poisoning may also be caused by arthropods (e.g. common insects, scorpions, spiders, and ticks), marine animals (e.g. poisonous and stinging fish and cone shells), snakes, fungi (mushrooms) and vegetables (pp. 706–711).

Intentional Poisoning. This is due to a wide variety of causes ranging from a minority of patients who are determined on self-destruction, i.e. *suicidal poisoning*, to a large group who indulge in *self-poisoning* which some prefer to call *parasuicide*. The term *attempted suicide* is best discarded as it implies a motive to an act of self-administered poisoning, which is frequently incorrect. The majority of people who deliberately take poison do not wish to die; in fact, they often take positive precautions to ensure that help will be available. Self-poisoning is usually a conscious, often impulsive act undertaken to manipulate a situation or a person and secure redress of circumstances which have become intolerable. Frequently relatives and society rally to help and the situation which has caused so much distress is rectified. Mistakes, however, do occur through misjudgement of dosage or a lack of available help, and an act which was committed primarily to draw attention to a particular situation may end in death. Self-poisoning often occurs in a setting of poverty or alcoholism and with a background of a broken home in childhood. The alarming increase in the incidence of acute poisoning is largely due to self-poisoning which accounts for approximately 90% of all adult poisoned patients admitted to hospital. Such behaviour now constitutes a major social problem. This is the case particularly in areas of dense conurbation and is less marked in small towns and rural communities.

Homicidal poisoning, which is another form of intentional poisoning, is rarely encountered now in hospital practice.

SUBSTANCES AND METHODS USED IN INTENTIONAL POISONING. *Self-poisoning.* Perhaps the most important cause for the increase in self-poisoning is the ready availability of drugs in the community. There is no doubt that the dramatic increase in the frequency and size of individual prescriptions over the last 30 years in Britain, in the National Health Service, has tended to encourage the mistaken belief in the community that the taking of pills is the answer for all life's ailments.

Almost any substance may be used for self-poisoning, but evidence of the importance of availability is the changing pattern of drugs taken in overdosage over the years. Ten years ago 60% of admissions were due to barbiturates and other hypnotics, notably methaqualone. As a result of campaigns and voluntary restrictions by doctors in prescribing, the incidence of these drugs in acute overdosage is now only 10%. In contrast, psychotropic drugs, especially sedatives and antidepressants, which are now commonly prescribed, are frequent causes of poisoning. Benzodiazepines account for 40% of poisonings and tricyclic antidepressants 13%. Salicylates and paracetamol amount to 10%. The incidence of acute salicylate poisoning, particularly in children, has been reduced in recent years. This is due to an increased awareness of the toxicity of salicylates in overdosage, resulting in more careful prescribing habits together with the provision of child-proof containers and individually wrapped tablets. For similar reasons acute poisoning with the analgesic combination of paracetamol and dextropropoxyphene, has become less common.

Combinations of drugs are taken in about 60% of overdoses and alcohol is involved in 70% of poisonings in men and about 50% in women. These combinations may cause problems in assessment of the severity of poisoning and in treatment; chemical analysis also may be difficult.

Suicide. The methods adopted for deliberate self-destruction vary from country to country and between sexes. In Britain women most often use drugs with drowning second choice. Self-injury, such as hanging, is most common in men with drug overdosage second. In America, shooting is the first choice in males, but takes second place to drugs in women. For reasons stated, coal gas poisoning, which was previously common, now seldom occurs.

Diagnosis of Acute Poisoning

Information Service. The impact made by poisoning on medical services has led to increasing demands for information regarding the tox-icity of substances and drugs. In the last 25 years, therefore, there has been a proliferation of poisons information and poison control centres in many countries. Information can be obtained immediately on a 24-hour basis regarding the ingredients of a substance and the approximately fatal dose of a poison. In many of these centres the best method of treatment can be discussed with a physician trained in clinical toxicology. In order to provide as comprehensive, accurate and up-to-date information as possible with ready accessibility, much of the data has been computerised, especially in the United States where, in addition to regional centres, extremely comprehensive information may be obtained at national level.

Clinical Features. For the majority of poisons the clinical features are non-specific. Fortunately, the diagnosis is usually apparent from the history obtained from the patient, relatives or friends or on circumstantial grounds such as finding tablets beside the patient. Difficulty arises when there is no such information and the physician is faced with the diagnosis of the unconscious patient. It is helpful to remember that in the age group 15–40 years acute poisoning is the commonest cause of unconsciousness in the absence of head injury.

Pin-point pupils, vomiting and depressed respiration suggest overdosage of morphine and related alkaloids or of cholinesterase inhibitors. In young people in particular, a history of marked and sometimes rapid changes in level of consciousness with associated respiratory and perhaps cardiac arrest is often associated with dextropropoxyphene poisoning, especially if taken with alcohol. Widely dilated pupils, bladder distension, absent bowel sounds, cardiac arrhythmias and upper motor neurone involvement characterise tricyclic antidepressant toxicity. Sweating, tinnitus, deafness and hyperventilation strongly suggest acute salicylate poisoning.

In general, however, it is impossible to provide clear clinical diagnostic guidelines because the range of substances available for poisoning is so great and their potential toxic effects are so variable in an individual patient. Too much importance is often placed on the state of the pupils, changes in limb reflexes and other neurological features. For example, inequality of pupil size, abnormalities of eye movements and nystagmus, which may have great significance in patients with primary neurological diseases, may all be due to drug effects. In patients with acute poisoning, therefore, assessment of the level of consciousness, which for many poisonings is the most practical means of determining the severity of toxicity, is best kept as simple as possible as in the Edinburgh method: grade 0 — fully conscious; grade 1 — drowsy but responsive to vocal command; grade 2 — unconscious but responsive to minimal painful stimuli; grade 3 — unconscious but just responsive to strong painful stimuli and grade 4 — unconscious with no response to stimuli.

Other useful clinical features are evidence of self-injury especially on the flexor aspects of the arms and wrists and on the face and hands. Also all patients suspected of self-poisoning should be examined carefully for venepuncture marks, abscesses or skin ulceration on the arms, hands and feet, which suggest recent 'mainlining' by a drug addict. Many household products, such as volatile hydrocarbons and solvents, have characteristic smells which aid diagnosis when they are ingested or inhaled. There may be buccal damage after the ingestion of strong acids or alkalis, phenols and cresols, although with some serious poisonings, such as paraquat, this may not become apparent for up to 36 hours after ingestion.

Identification of Poisons. More secure identification has now become possible by the marking of an increasing number of tablets and capsules with a code letter and number. Others can be recognised by their characteristic colour or shape. Coloured diagrams are available to aid this.

Laboratory Analysis. The only conclusive identification of acute poisoning is laboratory analysis using specimens of blood, gastric aspirate or urine as appropriate. Simple, rapid screening methods using thin layer chromatography are available for approximately 90% of common poisonings and can be of considerable help to the clinician. Confirmatory and more precise quantitative measurement is usually done by gas chromatography which is sometimes combined with mass spectrometry. Although these analyses can be carried out, the results seldom influence treatment but may be of value for medico-legal purposes. Simple clinical methods of analysis are available for salicylates and paracetamol.

General Therapeutic Measures

Treatment should not be delayed by spending excessive time in attempting to identify precisely the poison involved, since the essential immediate management of poisoning is dependent on the application of well-established basic therapeutic principles.

The major considerations are the establishment and maintenance of adequate respiration and circulation. Removal and inactivation of the poison should also be achieved where possible. The first-aid treatment is often the responsibility of the general practitioner outside hospital and if carried out effectively, contributes substantially to reducing both mortality and serious morbidity. Particular care should be taken during the transport of unconscious patients to hospital.

Maintenance of Respiration. A clear airway is essential. Dentures, vomitus, foreign bodies and excess secretions should be carefully removed from the mouth and fauces; if necessary an oropharyngeal or cuffed endotracheal tube should be inserted depending on the level of consciousness. All unconscious patients who do not have the protection of an endotracheal tube should be transported or nursed in the semi-prone position. Artificial respiration is required if respiration is depressed. Mouth to mouth respiration should be given, but, where facilities are available, more effective ventilation is achieved by administering oxygen using an Ambu bag or Water's cannister through a face mask or endotracheal tube. When significant respiratory depression persists more formal methods of mechanical ventilation become necessary (p. 217). Antibiotics should be given only if there is good evidence of aspiration or respiratory infection.

Maintenance of Circulation. Serious cardiac arrhythmias should be treated by the administration of anti-arrhythmic drugs (p. 139), particular attention being paid to the pharmacological actions of the poisoning to guard against adverse interactions with the therapy. The details of the treatment of acute circulatory failure are described on page 149. The foot of the bed should be raised, heat loss prevented and high flow oxygen given. A catheter should be inserted into the bladder of all 'shocked' patients in order to monitor urinary output with a urinometer. Otherwise catheterisation should be avoided unless bladder distension cannot be controlled by intermittent suprapubic manual compression. Cardiac resuscitation may be required on an emergency basis (p. 138).

Removal or Inactivation of the Poison. Patients with gassing must be removed to fresh air as quickly as possible. When a liquid or solid poison capable of cutaneous absorption is in contact with the patient's clothes these must be removed and any poison on the skin washed off. Care should be taken during these procedures to avoid personal contamination. When the poison has been swallowed within the previous hour, conscious patients should be given orally 50–100 g of activated charcoal.

EMESIS; GASTRIC ASPIRATION AND LAVAGE. A decision as to whether emesis or gastric aspiration and lavage should also be undertaken will depend on three factors: (i) the substance ingested, (ii) the state of consciousness of the patient, and (iii) the length of time since the poison was ingested.

(i) *Nature of Substance Ingested.* The only contraindication to inducing vomiting or passing a stomach tube is the knowledge that paraffin oil (kerosene) or other petroleum distillates have been swallowed, as the entry of even a small quantity of these substances into the lungs results in a severe pneumonia. Great care must be exercised in passing a stomach tube in corrosive poisoning, in alcoholics, in patients who have had gastric surgery and in the very young and elderly.

(ii) *Level of Consciousness.* The second factor to be considered is the state of consciousness. Fully conscious patients should be made to vomit by giving syrup of ipecacuanha (15 ml followed by 200 ml of water) which is an effective emetic. Its limitation is that there is a delay in the onset of its action. The dose may be repeated on one further occasion if vomiting does not result after 20 minutes. This is the treatment of choice in young children as, apart from the trauma involved, a sufficiently large tube cannot be passed to achieve effective removal of gastric contents.

In a semiconscious patient, emetics are to be avoided in view of the danger of aspiration pneumonia, but gastric aspiration and lavage can be employed provided the cough reflex is still present. In the deeply unconscious patient, gastric lavage is particularly important, but, as the cough reflex may be absent, it is a highly dangerous procedure unless the lungs can be first protected by the insertion of a cuffed endotracheal tube.

(iii) *Time Since Ingestion.* If 4 hours have passed since ingestion very little or no recovery of the drug will be achieved by inducing vomiting or by gastric lavage. If it is known that the poison was taken less than four hours previously, gastric aspiration and lavage is indicated provided the factors already discussed have been considered. In salicylate poisoning these procedures are of value up to 24 hours after ingestion. In the case of tricyclic drugs a worthwhile recovery may be achieved up to 12 hours after ingestion.

Technique of Gastric Aspiration and Lavage. With the foot of the trolley raised about 0·5 m and the patient lying on the left side a wide-bore Jacques stomach tube, English gauge 30, should be passed. Rubber tubes are most suitable for routine use, but if there is any suspicion that the patient may have hepatitis, not uncommon in drug addicts, disposable plastic tubes should be used and appropriate precautions taken by staff. A gag may be necessary to prevent biting on the tube. When the tube has been inserted, its position in the stomach is verified by aspiration of stomach contents or by blowing a little air through it and auscultating over the abdomen when a bubbling sound will be heard.

Aspiration is best achieved by lowering the funnel to which the stomach tube is attached, to a level well below the patient's head. Aspiration is advisable prior to lavage as initial lavage will drive some of the stomach contents into the duodenum and promote absorption. When no further material can be aspirated, repeated careful lavage with tepid water should be undertaken, using the same apparatus and no more than 300 ml for each single washout. Lavage should be continued until the returning fluid is clear. Except in the specific instances given on pages 707–711, little is achieved by employing lavage fluid other than water.

On occasions, after lavage, some further impairment of consciousness may occur. In general, therefore, the stomach should be left as empty as possible in view of the dangers of subsequent aspiration pneumonia, especially if an endotracheal tube has not been inserted.

OTHER METHODS OF ELIMINATION OF POISONS. If considerable absorption has occurred the patient may be gravely ill, hence measures to enhance elimination of the poison may be required. These can be carried out only in hospital because of the technical skill and special apparatus required; they include forced diuresis (p. 709), peritoneal dialysis, haemodialysis and exchange transfusion.

Haemoperfusion. Attempts have been made to develop safer ways of increasing removal of toxic substances from the body. The most effective of these is haemoperfusion whereby heparinised blood from the patient is passed through a column containing charcoal coated with synthetic acrylic hydrogel or alternatively ion-exchange resins. These methods may be life-saving for some severe poisonings, such as those due to medium and short-acting barbiturates, glutethimide, methaqualone, meprobamate and ethchlorvynol, for which previous techniques of elimination were inadequate. These techniques are still not free of dangers. Haemoperfusion, therefore, is indicated only in seriously ill patients in whom intensive supportive therapy fails.

ANTIDOTES. It is widely but erroneously believed that for each toxic substance there is a specific antidote. There are, in fact, no antidotes for the majority of substances producing poisoning. Certain pharmacological antagonists are, however, of value, and can be life-saving. Examples are naloxone (opiate poisoning), cobalt edetate (cyanide poisoning), desferrioxamine (iron poisoning) and n-acetylcysteine (paracetamol poisoning). Details of the use of these are given on pages 706–709.

Other Therapy. *Hypothermia.* A rectal thermometer which records low temperatures is required for the accurate assessment of hypothermia. Since it reduces the oxygen demands of the tissues, hypothermia is not a deleterious feature provided the patient is nursed in a space blanket and in a warm moist environment, unless the rectal temperature is below 35°C, when it may cause hypotension, sludging of the blood, confusion, coma and cardiac arrest.

The patient with hypothermia below 35°C should be rewarmed rapidly by external methods (e.g. a radiant heat cradle over the torso) and oxygen given. If there is hypotension or increased peripheral vascular resistance, warm fluids are administered intravenously. Metabolic acidosis is controlled by sodium bicarbonate (p. 101).

Epileptiform convulsions should be treated with diazepam (p. 619).

Fluid and electrolytes require careful monitoring and appropriate replacement therapy as necessary.

Psychiatric Assessment. As most instances of poisoning in adults are deliberate acts of self-poisoning it is very important that all patients, whether suffering from apparent accidental or intentional poisoning, should have a psychiatric assessment. Self-poisoning is often an important feature of various psychiatric disorders and of depression in particular. It is greatly to the benefit of the patient if the initial psychiatric interview takes place as soon as possible after the act before the patient and the relatives have time to discuss the event and thereafter present the same rationalised and often false picture. The incidence of repeated acts of self-poisoning has been shown clearly to be reduced by early psychiatric consultation.

Notes on Clinical Features and Treatment of Poisoning and Envenomation by Specific Agents *(Including common insect stings and poisoning by marine animals, mushrooms, scorpions, snakes, spiders, ticks and vegetables)*

The following descriptions are directed primarily towards adults. For children, appropriate adjustments in doses of drugs suggested in treatment regimens would require to be made.

Amphetamine Group. *Clinical Features.* Alertness, excitement, tremor and insomnia are common. Confusion, aggressiveness, hallucinations and even homicidal tendencies may occur. Initial excitement may give way to lethargy and depression. Brisk reflexes, tachycardia and hypertension occur and nausea, vomiting, diarrhoea and abdominal colic may be severe. In very heavy overdosage convulsions and deep unconsciousness are characteristic.

Treatment (1) General measures. (2) Droperidol (5–15 mg) or haloperidol (5–10 mg) by slow intravenous injection are the recommended treatments. Alternatively, chlorpromazine 100 mg intramuscularly. (3) In severe poisoning, forced diuresis using intravenous ammonium chloride to make the urine acid.

Barbiturates. *Clinical Features.* Absorption is unpredictable but drowsiness and coma develop rapidly. The duration of cerebral depression varies greatly with the type of barbiturate taken, the dose and the tolerance of the patient. In general a large dose of short- or medium-acting barbiturate causes more severe poisoning than long-acting phenobarbitone. Changes in the pupils and limb reflexes are very variable and are unreliable guides to the severity of the poisoning. Withdrawal features such as restlessness, insomnia, delirium and convulsions may occur. Ventilatory depression and hypotension may be severe. Hypothermia is common and if severe may be associated with renal failure. Bullous lesions occur in 6% of patients with acute barbiturate overdosage especially with short- or medium-acting drugs.

Treatment. (1) General measures with particular emphasis on respiratory and cardiovascular support. (2) When these measures fail, haemodialysis for phenobarbitone and barbitone, and charcoal haemoperfusion for short- and medium-acting barbiturates.

Benzodiazepines. *Clinical Features.* Drowsiness, ataxia, dizziness, hypotension and ventilatory depression may all occur, but the toxic effects are usually surprisingly mild.

Treatment. General supportive treatment is adequate in almost all cases.

Beta-adrenoceptor Antagonists. *Clinical Features.* Bradycardia and hypotension with low output cardiac failure. Bronchospasm. Cardio-respiratory arrest may occur. Drowsiness, delirium, fits and hallucinations. Hypoglycaemia.

Treatment. (1) Gastric aspiration and lavage if appropriate and intensive supportive measures. (2) When bradycardia is severe, atropine 0·6 to 3 mg intravenously (50 μg/kg in children), followed if necessary by isoprenaline 2 mg diluted in 500 ml normal saline or 5% dextrose at a rate of 20 to 40 drops per minute depending on the response. A cardiac pacemaker should be inserted. (3) If significant hypotension occurs, the inotropic action of glucagon is beneficial — 50 to 150 μg/kg intravenously over one minute, followed by an infusion of 1 to 5 mg/hour. In severe cases dobutamine infusion 2·5 to 20 μg/kg/min. may be effective. (4) For bronchospasm, salbutamol by nebuliser. Intravenous salbutamol or aminophylline may be required. (5) Intravenous glucose for hypoglycaemia.

Corrosives. *Clinical Features.* Stains and burns of the mouth and lips. Burns of fauces, abdominal pain and shock may result. Hepatic or renal damage occur.

Treatment. (1) General measures. (2) Gastric lavage is contraindicated in severe poisoning. (3) Neutralise acid or alkali. Milk by mouth is often the most effective available treatment. (4) Analgesics, blood transfusion and correction of acid-base balance all may be required.

Cyanides and Hydrocyanic Acid. *Clinical Features.* Odour of bitter almonds with shallow breathing; pink colour of skin and mucosae; widely dilated pupils and shock.

Treatment. This is very urgent. (1) General measures. (2) Cobalt edetate 600 mg in 20 ml intravenously over one minute. (3) If no recovery in the next minute, repeat 300 mg cobalt edetate. (4) If ingested, gastric lavage with 25% sodium thiosulphate. (5) Correct acidosis with i.v. sodium bicarbonate.

Dextropropoxyphene. See opium alkaloids.

Digoxin. (p. 142).

Dinitro-ortho-cresol Weedkillers. *Clinical Features.* These may develop very rapidly. Yellow skin and burns of the lips and mouth. Anxiety, restlessness, fatigue, convulsions and coma. Tachypnoea, pulmonary oedema, hyperpyrexia and intense sweating are common. Acute renal and liver failure may result.

Treatment. (1) Wash exposed skin. (2) Sedation with chlorpromazine 100 mg intramuscularly. (3) General measures. (4) Tepid sponging to reduce temperature.

Domestic Bleach. *Clinical Features.* Local irritation if in contact with skin. If inhaled, cough and possible pulmonary oedema. If ingested, burning sensation of mouth and fauces. Nausea and vomiting.

Treatment. (1) Gastric lavage with 2·5% sodium thiosulphate or alternatively with milk. If severely ill sodium thiosulphate (1%) 250 ml intravenously.

Insect Stings. Stings from ants, wasps, hornets and bees usually result only in local pain and swelling, unless the sting is on the mouth or tongue when local oedema may cause respiratory distress. Occasionally deaths may result from very extensive stings or more commonly due to severe anaphylaxis in individuals previously sensitised particularly to bee stings.

Clinical Features. (1) Local pain and oedema. (2) Severe cases may become shocked; local tissue necrosis, acute haemolysis and acute nephritis may occur.

Treatment. Bee stings are alkaline and wasp, hornet and ant stings are acid. Local application of an acid or alkaline solution is soothing and systemic antihistamines may be helpful. The barbed bee stings should be removed as soon as possible as the venom gland attached continues to release venom. In severe sensitivity reactions, subcutaneous adrenaline (0·5 ml) and hydrocortisone (100 mg) intravenously may be life-saving. Allergic patients should carry adrenaline for immediate self-injection. In some, desensitisation has proved helpful.

See also scorpion, spider and tick.

Ethanol. See page 695; blood levels page 817.

Fish, poisonous. See marine animals.

Iron Salts. *Clinical Features.* These are more severe in children but this poisoning is potentially dangerous at all ages. The poisoning occurs in three stages. The predominant initial features are epigastric pain, nausea and vomiting. Haematemesis is frequent and may cause shock. Respiration and pulse are rapid. These symptoms may settle after a few hours and there may then be a quiescent period lasting for up to several days, suggesting that all is well, but then frequent black and offensive stools may be passed, followed by acute encephalopathy and circulatory failure. Most deaths occur in this second stage, but even if the patient survives, acute liver and renal failure may develop later and both carry a high mortality.

Treatment. Speed is essential. (1) An intramuscular injection of 2 g desferrioxamine is given immediately (1 g in a child). (2) Gastric lavage is performed following which 100 ml 5% sodium bicarbonate is left in the stomach. (3) This is followed by an intravenous infusion of desferrioxamine in saline, dextrose or blood. The amount should not exceed 15 mg/kg body weight/hour up to a maximum of 80 mg/kg in 24 hours. (4) Full supportive treatment for convulsions, shock, acidosis, blood loss and electrolyte disturbance.

Marine Animals. Poisonous fish are numerous and widely distributed around the world. In some areas they are a common source of poisoning.

CIGUATERA POISONING. This is common, particularly in the Indo-Pacific and the Caribbean. It occurs sporadically after eating reef-dwelling fishes, which are popular items of diet. It is impossible to identify fish which are poisonous from others which are not and the toxins responsible are unaffected by all forms of preparation and cooking. Ciguatoxin is the cause of poisoning and the primary source is thought to be an alga (*Gambierdiscus toxicus*) eaten by herbivorous fish such as parrot fish and surgeon fish. Ultimately carnivorous fish such as barracuda also become poisonous. Outbreaks of this poisoning are very sporadic. Also curious variations in the clinical presentation occur between people of different races.

Clinical Features. The onset of symptoms is usually 1–6

hours after eating toxic fish, but may vary from a few minutes to 30 hours. Numbness and paraesthesiae of the lips, tongue and throat are common, followed by abdominal pain, diarrhoea, headache, arthralgia and myalgia. In 20% patients, dyspnoea, hypotension and paresis occur.

Treatment. Principally symptomatic with bed rest and analgesics. Most patients recover after about three days, but sometimes the convalescence may be prolonged with persisting arthralgia and myalgia.

SCROMBOID FISH POISONING. The flesh of scromboid fish, such as mackerel, tuna, bonito and skipjack, has a high free histidine content. Many bacteria decarboxylate histidine to histamine and, if fish become contaminated by these organisms, large amounts of histamine accumulate in the flesh.

Clinical Features. Flushing, headache, dizziness, abdominal cramps and symptoms of gastro-enteritis occur. These usually develop 30 minutes after ingestion and the upset lasts for about 4 hours.

Treatment. Symptomatic.

SHELLFISH POISONING. Paralytic shellfish poisoning results from eating filter-feeding shellfish such as mussels, clams, oysters and scallops contaminated by the toxic protozoa, *Gonyaulax catanella* and *G. tamarensis.* The neurotoxin involved is called saxitoxin. These protozoa tend to colour the sea when present in numbers and fishing communities are well aware that it is dangerous to eat molluscs when the tide is red, blue or green.

Clinical Features. Circumoral paraesthesiae, a 'floating' feeling, headache, nausea, vomiting and diarrhoea are common with, in severe cases, weakness, dysarthria and respiratory depression.

Treatment. (1) Gastric aspiration and lavage. (2) Symptomatic and supportive therapy. A less severe, but similar, poisoning results from eating shellfish contaminated by another dinoflagellate, *Gymnodinium breve.* The resultant illness is self-limiting, requiring only symptomatic treatment.

TETRODOTOXIC POISONING. This is generally known as 'puffer fish poisoning'. These and similar fish are found in all warm and tropical seas and fresh water varieties occur in South-east Asia, India, North and West Africa and the Caribbean. Although less common than ciguatera, the mortality from this poisoning is as high as 50%. The toxin responsible is tetrodotoxin, which is one of the most powerful neurotoxins known.

Clinical Features. Early symptoms are circumoral paraesthesiae, malaise, hypotension, dizziness and a feeling of 'floating in air'. In severe poisoning, ataxia, dysphagia and profound descending neuromuscular paralysis develop.

Treatment is symptomatic as there is no known antidote.

VENOMOUS MARINE ANIMALS. Serious illness from venomous marine creatures is rare in temperate waters. Poisoning by sea snakes is described under snake bites.

VENOMOUS FISH. Although many species occur, only two major groups are of real significance, the sting-rays and scorpion fishes. All sting-rays inhabit warm or tropical coastal waters with the exception of one fresh water variety in South America. These fish will sting only if stood upon by mistake. Scorpion fish include the zebra fishes, the true scorpion fishes and the stone fishes. The spines of these fish are their offensive weapons and they are all capable of aggressive stinging. The stone fishes are particularly poisonous and zebra fishes are important as they are becoming popular for domestic aquaria.

Clinical Features. Immediate intense pain and swelling at the site of the sting. Severe tissue necrosis may occur and systemic features include nausea, vomiting and diarrhoea. Cardiac arrhythmias may occur.

Treatment. (1) Analgesics as required with local anaesthetic. (2) Careful cleansing of the wound and surgical removal of the sting sheath if it has been retained. (3) The venoms are heat-labile and if possible the wound should be immersed in water as hot as can be borne for 1 hour. (4) In the case of stone fish antivenoms are available.

VENOMOUS MOLLUSCS. Only two members of this very large species are venomous to man. These are the cone shells and the octopuses. The cone shells are not uncommon causes of poisoning as the colourful shells are eagerly collected. These predatory gastropods catch their prey by shooting out a dart-like tooth attached to a muscular venom gland. The only octopuses of importance are the small blue ringed octopuses of Australia which have toxic saliva and this may flow into wounds made by the beak of the octopus.

Clinical Features. There is a local inflammatory response with generalised paraesthesiae. This is rapidly followed by muscular paresis which in severe poisoning may result in respiratory failure. Fatalities have occurred.

Treatment. Symptomatic and supportive therapy.

VENOMOUS COELENTERATA. These include the hydroids, jelly-fish, sea anemones and corals. Although many of these animals may cause painful and at times disfiguring stings, few fatalities have resulted. The most important are the Portuguese man-of-war (*Physalia physalis*), sea wasps (*Cubomedusae*) and the true jellyfishes *Chironex fleckeri* and *Chiropsalmus quadrigatus.* Some authors suggest that only *Chironex* should be considered truly lethal. The precise toxins are not yet fully identified but haemolytic, dermatonecrotic and cardiotoxic substances have all been isolated.

Clinical Features. All species cause intense pain at the site of envenomation and large wheals appear which may become necrotic, leading to extensive scar formation. Severe abdominal and generalised pains may result. In severe poisoning the patient rapidly loses consciousness with cyanosis and hypotension. Death may occur quickly or be delayed for some hours.

Treatment. (1) Analgesics and local anaesthesia if required. (2) Any tentacles must be carefully removed using adhesive tape. The tentacles should not be removed with the bare hand as they may still be capable of causing stings for many hours after removal from the water. Common vinegar can be used to inactivate adhering tentacles, but alcohol solutions should not be used as this may stimulate further stinging. (3) General supportive measures. (4) Antivenom for sea-wasp stings is available. At certain seasons 'Irukandji stings' affect bathers in the sea off N.E. Australia. They are caused by minute *Carybdeid* (simple sea-wasps). Acute poisoning develops in a few minutes characterised by violent abdominal and generalised pains, vomiting and prostration. After a few days of acute illness, full recovery always occurs.

Mushrooms. Serious poisoning is uncommon in Britain. Considering the many types of fungi, a relatively small number are poisonous. The difficulty is that identification of these harmful species is not easy and often dangerous mushrooms grow in the same places as edible varieties. The commonest types of mushroom poisoning results from eating species containing heat-labile toxins, many of which have not been identified. These cause acute and sometimes severe abdominal colic with diarrhoea, nausea and vomiting developing about two hours after ingestion. These symptoms may result in fluid and electrolyte deficits, especially in children, requiring correction and antiemetics, but are of short duration. Occasionally the features are those of muscarine toxicity with parasympathetic stimulation which can be counteracted with atropine 0·6–2·0 mg in the adult. If the patient is excited or disorientated, atropine should not be given and chlorpromazine prescribed instead. The Common Ink Cap (*Coprinus atramentarius*) contains coprine which has a disulfiram-like action and, if taken with alcohol, provokes acute vomiting.

A trend amongst adolescents has been to ingest 'Magic' mushrooms (*Psilocybe semilanceate*) and *Panaeolus foenisecii* containing psilocybin and psilocin, which are hallucinogens. The amount required to obtain a 'trip' varies greatly from individual to individual and so some develop acute toxic effects. Acute gastroenteritis may result with visual hallucinations lasting up to 6 hours. Occasionally the symptoms last for several days and acute psychiatric upset has been reported continuing for weeks.

DEATH CAP (AMANITA PHALLOIDES). This mushroom accounts for 90% of all deaths due to mushroom poisoning in Britain. It contains two types of toxin; phallotoxins, which cause severe gastroenteritis within 6–12 hours of ingestion, and amatoxins, which also may cause gastric upset, but the major effect is delayed and results in liver and renal tubular damage. These toxins are heat-stable and may survive cooking.

Clinical Features. After an initial delay of 6–12 hours and occasionally as long as 24 hours, acute and usually severe gastro-enteritis with abdominal colic. The patient may then seem to improve before the onset of liver and renal damage.

Treatment. (1) If possible the mushrooms eaten should be identified, ideally by an expert in mushrooms. It is useful to remember that the later the onset of abdominal symptoms, the more likely it is to be a serious poisoning. (2) Gastric aspiration and lavage. (3) Careful medical care for liver and renal failure if these develop. Haemodialysis and haemoperfusion are ineffective in removing the toxins but the former may be required for renal failure and the latter for liver failure.

Other species of mushroom which produce similar toxic effects to *A. phalloides* are the North American *Deadly Agaric* (*A. verna*), *A. virosa* and some types of *Galerina*.

Opium Alkaloids (Dextropropoxyphene). *Clinical Features.* Pinpoint pupils, pallor, nausea and vomiting, depressed respiration and coma are characteristic. These effects are potentiated by alcohol and when these are combined in acute overdosage sudden respiratory and cardiac arrest may occur even in previously healthy young people.

Treatment. (1) General measures. (2) If ingested gastric lavage with very dilute potassium permanganate — 1 in 10 000. (3) Naloxone 0·4 mg intravenously and 0·8 mg repeated intravenously three minutes later, if required. In heavy overdosage larger quantities may be necessary. The patient should be kept under close observation and naloxone repeated if required.

Organophosphorus Compounds. *Clinical Features.* These insecticides are very toxic. Constricted pupils; cold perspiration; salivation, nausea, vomiting and diarrhoea; twitching, which may go on to convulsions; bradycardia; bronchospasm, intense bronchorrhoea and pulmonary oedema.

Treatment. (1) Remove contaminated clothing and wash skin, but take care to wear protective gloves. (2) General measures including meticulous care of the airway. (3) Atropine 2 mg intravenously, but if cyanosis is present this must first be corrected by oxygen therapy. The atropine is repeated at 5 to 10 minute intervals to achieve full atropinisation and this is maintained for at least 2–3 days. (4) Pralidoxime should be given in addition to atropine in a dose of 30 mg/kg intravenously at a rate not exceeding 500 mg per minute and repeated every 30 minutes as necessary. More recently obi-

doxime 3 mg/kg body weight by intramuscular injection has been reported to be more effective than pralidoxime as it has a faster action and crosses the blood-brain barrier. When these cholinesterase reactivators take effect the dosage of atropine should be reduced to avoid atropine toxicity.

Paracetamol (Acetaminophen). *Clinical Features.* Nausea and vomiting initially, but at first symptoms are often nonspecific. After 36 hours in severe poisoning (plasma paracetamol levels above 200 μg/ml at four hours after ingestion) more serious toxic effects may develop including hypotension, hypothermia, metabolic acidosis, hypoglycaemia, bleeding tendency and delirium. The main danger, however, is acute liver failure which tends to occur several days after ingestion and carries a high mortality.

Treatment. (1) General measures. (2) In moderate or severe poisoning (likely over 20 × 500 mg tablets) the liver damage may be prevented provided the following treatment is given within 12 hours of the poisoning. An initial dose of n-acetylcysteine 150 mg/kg in 200 ml 5% glucose is given intravenously over 15 minutes, followed by an infusion of 50 mg/kg in 500 ml 5% dextrose in 4, 8 and 8 hours (total 300 mg/kg in 20 hours). (3) Intravenous glucose may be required to correct hypoglycaemia. (4) The best investigation to assess impending acute liver failure is the prothrombin time ratio. If this rises above 3·0 full medical prophylaxis to combat hepatic encephalopathy must be started. (5) Charcoal haemoperfusion for fulminant liver failure. (6) Haemodialysis for acute renal failure.

Paraffin and Petroleum Distillates. *Clinical Features.* Pallor; vomiting and diarrhoea; cough and dyspnoea.

Treatment. (1) Do not wash out stomach (p. 705). (2) Antibiotics if aspiration has occurred. (3) General measures.

Salicylates. *Clinical Features.* Young children are much more susceptible to the toxic effects of salicylates than adults, particularly to the complex and altering metabolic disturbances which occur. Coma is common in children, in contrast to adults in whom coma is seen only in very severe poisoning. In adults, plasma salicylate levels above 3·6 mmol/*l* (50 mg/100 ml) indicate moderate or severe poisoning. In this situation, characteristic features are tinnitus, deafness and blurring of vision. Restlessness, sweating and increased metabolic rate also occur. Hyperventilation results in respiratory alkalosis. There may be vomiting and this, together with hyperventilation and profuse sweating, often results in severe dehydration. Hypokalaemia is common. The initial respiratory alkalosis is frequently followed by a metabolic acidosis, which may be severe, especially in children. Despite these formidable fluid, electrolyte and acid-base disturbances the patients may seem less ill than they really are. Marked acidosis should be regarded as a very serious feature as it may herald sudden respiratory or cardiac arrest.

Treatment. 1. General measures, but gastric aspiration and lavage should be done in all patients when practicable. 2. In moderate or severe poisoning *forced alkaline diuresis* should be given. The following should be mixed together and given intravenously at a rate of 2 litres hourly for 3 hours:

Saline (0·9%) ....0·5 litre
Glucose (5%) .... 1 litre
Sodium bicarbonate (1·26%) ....0·5 litre
Potassium chloride ....3 g

If this regimen of diuresis cannot be given because of renal or cardiac impairment, peritoneal dialysis or haemodialysis are effective. Careful monitoring of fluid replacement, electrolyte and acid-base status must be carried out during this treatment.

Scorpion Stings. Many genera of scorpions are found in

the tropics and subtropics. Stings can cause dangerous poisoning. In Mexico, for example, 1000 deaths occur per year. Paired poison glands are situated in the terminal segment of the jointed tail.

Clinical Features. (1) Intense local pain occurs immediately around the single puncture site, followed by erythema, swelling and sometimes ecchymosis. (2) Severe systemic features may follow, especially in children, such as sweating, salivation, nausea, vomiting and respiratory depression. Disseminated intravascular coagulation may occur, and in Trinidad, acute but usually reversible pancreatitis is a feature of stings from the scorpion, *Tityus trinitatis*.

Treatment. (1) A firm pressure bandage should be applied to limit the spread of the neurotoxic venom. (2) Analgesics and general supportive therapy. (3) In children, antivenom (5 ml i.m.) should be given if available. (4) Specific treatment of disseminated intravascular coagulation, if present.

Snake Bite. In Britain there is only one indigenous poisonous snake, the adder (*Vipera berus*) which seldom causes significant poisoning. Serious snake bites may still occur as dangerous snakes are kept in zoos and by amateurs, often in less than ideal circumstances. There are three families of medically important venomous snakes. All have fangs at the front of their mouths whereby they inject venom from the parotid glands. The *Elapidae* (cobras, mambas, kraits, tiger snakes, and coral snakes) are found in all parts of the world except Europe. They have short fangs and are land snakes, the venom of which produce neurotoxic features. Local tissue necrosis may occur, a feature characteristic of venom of Asian cobras and the African spitting cobra. The *Hydrophidae* (sea snakes), which abound in the Asian-Pacific coastal waters, also have short fangs and characteristic flattened tails. The venom of these snakes is myotoxic. The *Viperidae*, which have long erectile fangs, are divided into *Viperinae* (true vipers) such as the European adder, Russell's viper and Carpet viper. These occur in all parts of the world except America and the Asian-Pacific area. The second sub-group is the *Crotalidae* (pit vipers) such as rattlesnakes, Fer-de-lance and Malayan pit viper which have a small heat-sensitive pit between eye and nostrils. The venom of the *Viperidae* is vasculo-toxic.

At least 50% of people bitten by snakes suffer few or no toxic effect as little or no venom has been injected. On the other hand, in serious poisoning the mortality is high if adequate medical care is not given. The natural mortality without effective treatment is 10% in *Elapidae* poisoning within 5 to 20 hours of the bites, 10% for sea snakes within 15 hours and 1 to 15% in *Viperidae* within 2 days. In the early stages snake bite is very unpredictable and all patients must be carefully monitored for at least 12 hours.

First Aid Measures. Arterial tourniquets are no longer indicated and incision/excision of the bite area should not be done. Firm pressure bandaging of the bite area and immobilisation of the part substantially delays spread of the venom. Patients are often very apprehensive and should be reassured and sedated if necessary.

Clinical Features. Local pain and fang marks are very variable and of no help in diagnosis.

Viperidae. Local swelling starts almost immediately. This is also a feature of poisoning in bites by Asian cobras and the African spitting cobra, but may not develop for up to 2 hours. Early signs of systemic poisoning, which may develop within 15 minutes of the bite include vomiting, hypotension and signs of abnormal bleeding from or into any site. Later signs include increase in local swelling which may become massive over 48 to 72 hours with associated bruising. Blister formation

around the site of the bite is common and spreading blisters suggest a large dose of venom and may precede necrosis. Local tissue necrosis with an offensive putrid smell is typical of cobra bites. Shock may occur and haemorrhage into a vital organ which is often fatal may occur up to a week after the bite if antivenom has not been given.

Elapidae. There is seldom any local swelling. Vomiting, hypotension and a polymorph leucocytosis suggest systemic envenomation. More specific signs of muscle weakness such as ptosis, glossopharyngeal palsy and cough indicate severe poisoning and may be delayed for 10 hours after the bite. There is a danger of respiratory paralysis and ECG changes and rises in cardiac enzymes occur.

Hydrophidae. The early features are similar to *Elapidae*. More specific signs are generalised myalgia, with the appearance of myoglobinuria 3 to 5 hours later. Paresis of the limbs may follow with respiratory paralysis within a few hours of the bite, although it may be delayed for up to 60 hours. Hyperkalaemia may result in cardiac arrest and acute renal failure may occur.

Treatment. (1) The site of the bite should be cleansed and then left strictly alone; otherwise the risk of infection is increased. Antibiotics are indicated only if there is evidence of local necrosis. If skin necrosis occurs, sloughs should be excised with skin grafts applied as appropriate. (2) General measures, including intravenous fluids, should be given to support vital functions. (3) sedatives are required if the patient is apprehensive. (4) Appropriate antitetanus prophylaxis should be given taking account of the patient's immune state. (5) Antivenoms should be given only if there is clear evidence of systemic poisoning. Some local effects, however, especially necrosis, may be avoided or minimised if antivenom is given within 4 hours of the bite. This is the case in bites by Asian cobras, African spitting cobras, puff adders and rattlesnakes. In *V. berus* bites, the only poisonous snake in Britain, adult patients may have prolonged and painful local swelling which can be effectively treated by Zagreb Antivenom if given within the first few hours. All antivenoms may cause severe allergic reactions which may be fatal. Appropriate precautions, therefore, are mandatory. The potency of the antivenom should be checked by first making sure that it is clear and has no opacities. Depending on the severity of poisoning, 20–100 ml antivenom is diluted in 2 to 3 volumes of isotonic saline. This is then given by slow intravenous infusion (15 drops per minute). Adrenaline (1:1000 solution) must always be immediately available. If a reaction occurs the drip is stopped temporarily and 0·5 ml adrenaline injected intramuscularly. Provided the adrenaline is given at the first sign of anaphylaxis, it is rapidly effective and the drip can be restarted with care. Several injections of adrenaline may be indicated. There is marked variation in the requirements of different patients for antivenom. Therefore it is important to give sufficient antivenom to counteract the toxic effects of the poisoning and children require the same doses of antivenom as adults. This is especially important in neurotoxic poisoning.

Spider Bite. Only a few genera of spiders are harmful to man. *Lactrodectus* species are found only in warm climates, including the Mediterranean area and some parts of central Europe. The Black Widow Spider (*L. mactans*) is the most dangerous and occurs only in the tropics. The Funnel Web Spider (*Atrax Robustus*) also quite often causes venomous bites. These spiders are shy, inhabiting dark corners of sheds, basements and foundations of houses and outside privies. Death may occur in up to 6% of cases, especially in young children.

Clinical Features. (1) Burning of the bite site. (2) After about 1 hour, generalised muscular pain, which may simulate an acute abdomen, nausea and vomiting. (3) Pyrexia, sweating and the patient may become shocked.

Treatment. (1) 10–20 ml calcium gluconate (10%) by slow intravenous injection. (2) Analgesics. (3) Supportive treatment. (4) If severe systemic toxicity give specific antivenom if available.

In the South States of America, Central and South America, the Brown Recluse Spider (*Loxosceles reclusa*) and related species may be found in houses and outbuildings. The spider often crawls into clothing and bed clothes. Poisoning is relatively uncommon but important as it results in necrosis at the site of the bite, which is slow to heal. Systemic features of fever, vomiting and rashes may occur and occasionally haemolysis and thrombocytopenia. Analgesics should be given as required and antihistamines and corticosteroids are considered helpful.

Tick bite. Tick paralysis is due to venom in the saliva of certain hard ticks. If such a tick remains attached to the skin for some days there is increasing and spreading paralysis with a danger of respiratory failure. If the tick is removed in time the patient recovers. Intensive supportive measures with mechanical ventilation may be required.

Tricyclic Antidepressants. *Clinical Features.* These features appear one to two hours after ingestion, but seldom last longer than 18–24 hours. Dry mouth, dilated pupils, urinary retention and absent bowel sounds are common. Varying degrees of loss of consciousness result but deep coma is not common. Hallucinations and pressure of speech occur. Cardiac arrhythmias may be severe, especially in children, and hypotension may result. Torticollis and ataxia may be pronounced in children, but at all ages brisk reflexes are common and tonic-clonic movements occur. Ventilatory depression, on occasions, is severe.

Treatment. 1. General measures. 2. Gastric lavage is effective up to 12 hours after ingestion. 3. Supportive therapy is all that is required in the great majority of patients but, if inadequate, physostigmine salicylate (1–3 mg) by slow intravenous injection will abolish the central nervous system effects and some of the cardiac complications. If necessary, the injection may be repeated after 10 minutes. 4. Cardiac arrhythmias may respond to 40 mEq sodium bicarbonate by rapid intravenous infusion over 20 minutes. If this is ineffective, appropriate antiarrhythmics should be given.

Vegetable Toxins. The harmful effects of the ingestion of aflatoxin (p. 720), unripe cassava (p. 656) and bush teas (p. 367) are mentioned elsewhere.

EPIDEMIC DROPSY (ARGEMONE POISONING). This results from ingesting mustard oil contaminated by extracts from the seeds of the poppy weed, *Argemone mexicana*, which contain the toxin, sanguinarine. This substance interferes with the oxidation of pyruvic acid, which accumulates and causes dilatation of capillaries and small arterioles. Haemangiomas may develop. This poisoning commonly occurs when curried dishes are prepared with contaminated mustard oil and is seen mainly in India and in Indian communities elsewhere.

Clinical Features. The time of onset is variable. Nausea, vomiting, diarrhoea and fever occur followed by the development of peripheral oedema and cardiac failure. There is erythematous mottling of the skin and raised haemangiomas on the skin and mucosae may appear. Severe glaucoma may result.

Treatment. All contaminatd mustard oil must be identified and further exposure avoided. Supportive therapy for cardiac failure is effective, but the response may be slow. A high protein diet is beneficial.

VOMITING SICKNESS OF JAMAICA (ACKEE POISONING). The unripe fruit of the common West Indian and South American tree, *Blighia sapida*, contains a water-soluble toxin, capable of blocking gluconeogenesis in the liver. If eaten, especially by undernourished children, severe and prolonged hypoglycaemia may result. Vomiting, loss of consciousness and convulsions are common. Continuous intravenous infusion of glucose should be started as soon as possible. Without treatment the mortality is high.

Industrial and Agricultural Poisoning

Lead, cyanide (p. 707), mercury, beryllium (p. 268) and cadmium are potential causes of industrial poisoning. In agriculture many highly toxic weedkillers, including paraquat and the dinitro-ortho-cresol group, and organo-phosphorus insecticides have been developed in recent years. They have been responsible for only a small number of cases of acute poisoning in Britain owing to effective legislation for controlling their use. In some countries, however, they have caused many deaths.

PREVENTION OF ACUTE POISONING

An indication of the size and complexity of the problem has been given in the introduction to this chapter. Thus, in Britain, acute poisoning now accounts for approximately 15% of all acute medical admissions to hospital. The scope for preventive action is clear.

About 60% of patients consult their doctors in the month prior to taking the overdosage and many do so within a week of their action. Also a considerable number poison themselves again after discharge from hospital or during active treatment for psychiatric conditions such as depression. There can be no doubt, therefore, that doctors can make a very important contribution to the prevention of poisoning by learning to recognise the danger signs of imminent overdosage and take appropriate preventive action. General practitioners are particularly well placed for this purpose as not only can they assess the personality concerned, but also the social and family circumstances which are often the main cause of the problem. For example, it has become apparent that some poisoning incidents in young children occur as an expression of abuse by their parents. Improvements are required in the social services in order that their response to such difficulties should be more immediate and effective; but even now doctors should make more use of agencies such as the Marriage Guidance Council, Alcoholics Anonymous and the Samaritans.

At all ages a major predisposing factor is the ready availability of medicaments and toxic household products. In the prevention of poisoning in children, the best method is to keep all medicines in a locked cupboard. Poisoning by household preparations is also common in children under the age of 5 years and is likely to continue as long as these articles are stored in places accessible to inquisitive toddlers. A potentially very dangerous practice is the storage of toxic chemicals such as weedkillers in old lemonade or beer bottles.

Another important factor in acute poisoning is that many tablets and capsules are supplied in a variety of attractive colours and shapes, often similar to popular sweets and therefore very attractive to children. This danger is increased by parents who, often with the best intentions, encourage their children to take medicines by suggesting that the tablets are in fact sweets. Also, many potent and dangerous drugs are dispensed as pleasant elixirs and syrups with an increased danger of overdosage in the unwitting youngster or careless adult. An effective preventive measure has been the development of drug containers which children find difficult to open, and this could with value be expanded to include a much wider range of medicines. An increasing number of drugs are also being supplied in individual wrapping, a useful deterrent for patients inclined to impulsive self-poisoning. These measures may add substantially to the price of production of drugs, but when one considers the cost of hospital and social care, the additional expense is justified.

The major cause of acute poisoning incidents is intentional self-poisoning which, as has been stated, is usually of an impulsive and conscious type. The availability of drugs is particularly relevant in this group. Patients should therefore be constantly encouraged to dispose of unused drugs from previous prescriptions and it follows that doctors should make every effort to prescribe

numbers of tablets carefully calculated for the immediate needs of the patients. Also, sedative and psychotropic drugs should be prescribed only when there is a clear and genuine medical indication. In the recent past the numbers of prescriptions in Britain for these types of drugs rose in a most dramatic way and there is no reason to suspect that serious psychiatric illness had undergone any major increase in the same time. This suggests that much prescribing of sedative and antidepressant drugs was inappropriate and was given often for psycho-social problems rather than significant psychiatric disorder. On the other hand, patients who are significantly depressed must be kept under careful observation when therapy is commenced because the antidepressant may cause partial improvement, but also make these patients capable of taking active measures towards self-destruction.

There have been various attempts in the field of health education with the aid of schools, national press and television to make the general public aware of the need for preventive measures, but these campaigns are often of limited duration and quickly lose their impact. The medical profession as a whole has not played a very direct role in these educational exercises and much more could be done in this regard. In Britain, poisons information services answer questions only from members of the medical profession, but experience in other countries suggests that the scope of these services could be widened with benefit to the community. In the United States, for example, poison control centres have provided information and advice direct to the general public and fulfilled a valuable educational role whereby, for example, parents have become more aware of the importance of keeping drugs and household products out of the reach of toddlers. As a result in many parts of the United States, the incidence of childhood poisoning has fallen substantially.

Considering the large number of people involved and the vast range of possible toxic substances used in industry, accidental industrial poisoning is uncommon in Britain. This is largely due to the vigilance and initiative of industrial medical officers and to the effectiveness of legislation which regulates the safe storage, transport and use of potentially toxic substances. Also, many essential processes in industry involving the use of dangerous poisons have been made safer by the introduction of automatic mechanical techniques which avoid exposure of workers to the risk.

Inevitably, the management of patients with acute poisoning rests with the medical profession and the social services, and it is easy to criticise their apparent inability to improve the situation. The basic problem, however, lies within the community. Until a more responsible attitude emerges with a willingness to be more supportive towards the emotional problems of individuals, there seems little doubt that acute self-poisoning will continue to be an expression of a plea for help to correct a situation which for the individual has become intolerable.

ALEXANDER A.H. LAWSON

FURTHER READING:

*Practical manuals for quick consultation
    in an emergency:*
Dreisbach, R. H. (1980) *Handbook of Poisoning*, 10th edn. Los Altos, California: Lange Medical Publications.
Matthew, H. & Lawson A. A. H. (1979) *Treatment of Common Acute Poisonings*, 4th edn. Edinburgh: Churchill Livingstone.
Vale, J. A. & Meredith, T. J. (1981) *Poisoning: Diagnosis and Treatment*. London: Update Books.

Specialised reference books:
Avery, G. S. (1980) *Drug Treatment*, 2nd edn. Sydney: ADIS Press; Edinburgh: Churchill Livingstone.
Brown, S. S., Mitchell, F. L. & Young, D. S. (Eds.) (1979) *Chemical Diagnosis of Disease*. Amsterdam: Elsevier/North Holland Biomedical Press.
Dukes, M. N. G. (Ed.) (1980) *Meyler's Side Effects of Drugs*, Vol 9. Amsterdam: Excerpta Medica.
Gilman, G. A, Goodman, L. S. & Gilman, A. (Eds.) (1980) *The Pharmacological Basis of Therapeutics*, 6th edn. New York: Macmillan.
Griffin, J. P. & D'Arcy, P. F. (1980) *Drug Induced Emergencies*. Bristol: John Wright.
Halstead, B. W. (1965–1970) *Poisonous and Venomous Marine Animals of the World* (3 vols.). Washington: Government Printing Office.
North, P. M. (1967) *Poisonous Plants and Fungi*. Poole: Blandford Press.
Polson, C. J., Green, M. A. & Lee, M. R. (1983) *Clinical Toxicology*, 3rd edn. London: Pitman Medical.
Russell, F. E. (1980) *Snake Venom Poisoning*. Philadelphia: J.B. Lippincott.
Wade, A., Reynolds, J. E. F. (Eds.) (1977) *Martindale's Extra Pharmacopoeia*, 27th edn. London: Pharmaceutical Press.

18. Tropical Diseases and Climatic Disorders

Many factors affect the patterns of disease around the world. Important among them are climate, which helps determine the range of pathogenic microbes in the environment, and wealth which provides the means to avoid and control the microbes through education, development, sanitation and health services. The majority of tropical countries are hot, humid and poor. They cannot feed themselves and have rudimentary health services that cannot educate or protect their exploding populations. Infectious diseases and malnutrition are rife, especially among children. Cosmopolitan diseases, such as measles or diarrhoea may take on special significance, while others like malaria (p. 768) or sleeping sickness (p. 779) are confined to certain areas for climatic reasons. Disease due to infection is the main determinant of childhood mortality, the strength of the working man, the health of the mother and the pattern of systemic disease including neoplasia.

This chapter considers the patterns of disease seen in tropical countries and describes some of them. Diseases due to infection, with particular reference to those encountered in the tropics, are described in Chapter 19. The rapid economic growth of the developed nations and the technological advances in air travel mean that no country of the world can be considered remote any more, nor its diseases exotic. Rich and poor countries are becoming increasingly interdependent and doctors should be aware of the health problems of countries other than their own. Worldwide travel has also led to a rapid increase in the importation of tropical diseases into temperate countries, by refugees, immigrants, tourists and businessmen. British students should be familiar with these diseases.

PATTERNS OF DISEASE IN TROPICAL AND DEVELOPING COUNTRIES

Patients in the tropics suffer from disorders of all the major systems and psyche, as they do in temperate and developed countries. In tropical countries, however, the aetiological factors may be different, especially in the case of infectious disease which still represents the greatest problem. The genetic constitution of patients in many parts of the world makes them resistant to certain conditions and predisposes them to others. The battle against acute disease is often a single episode in a long campaign against chronic infection and malnutrition. Clinical patterns of illness in the tropics, therefore, differ in many ways from those in temperate zones. Although the principles of diagnosis and treatment will be the same, multiple pathologies and diagnoses are the rule rather than the exception and treatment may need to be modified in the light of the background factors. The preponderance of children in the tropics and the high incidence of diarrhoeal and parasitic disease and malnutrition creates special problems.

THE BACKGROUND TO DISEASES IN THE TROPICS

Climate. A large number and variety of microbial agents and parasites flourish in the moist heat of the tropics and subtropics. Insects and other arthropods abound and many of them serve as vectors of infections. Numerous species of animals, especially rodents, live close to man and are reservoirs of disease. Close contact with animals exposes man to a wide range of zoonotic diseases.

714

Venomous animals are relatively common, as are toxic plants and fungi that may contaminate foodstuffs. Desert and mountain people suffer fewer infectious diseases. Heat (p. 722) and altitude (p. 725) impose special physiological demands on the body.

Genes and Race. The best example of genetically determined disease is sickle-cell anaemia in which homozygous producers of haemoglobin S become anaemic and often die in infancy. The heterozygous carrier of haemoglobin S, on the other hand, is healthy and enjoys a measure of protection against the severe complications of malaria. Other examples of racially determined responses to disease are seen in leprosy, which is worse in Caucasians and Mongolians than in Blacks, and in tuberculosis, the pattern in Indians differing from that in Europeans.

Nutrition and Agriculture. The presence or absence of malnutrition depends on the availability of food, its cost and the correctness of its use and also on infection, especially gastrointestinal. Traditional practices and taboos may limit the use of use of available food, e.g. the banning of eggs and milk in pregnancy. Malnutrition impairs both the cellular and humoral components of the immune response and predisposes children to infection which further drains the body's nutritional reserves and retards growth. Moderate degrees of undernutrition are much commoner than the gross malnutrition syndromes and may be overlooked.

Dietary toxins are found in some areas and produce conditions such as tropical spinal ataxia from cassava in Africa (p. 656), veno-occlusive liver disease from seneccio alkaloids in Jamaica and elsewhere (p. 367) and hepatoma from aflatoxin in badly stored nuts and cereals (p. 720).

Infections. Acute infectious diseases, especially respiratory infections, measles and gastroenteritis, still account for the high infant mortality in some parts of the tropics where up to 40% of children die before the age of 5 years. Acute infections may precipitate the syndromes of malnutrition, which may then be complicated by further infection, for example measles leading to kwashiorkor and cancrum oris.

Many of the decimating diseases of the past are now controlled by vaccination (yellow fever), vector control (malaria and sleeping sickness) and general improvement of living standards (plague and relapsing fever), but control is imperfect and the diseases reappear as, for example, malaria in the Indian subcontinent and relapsing fever among refugees. Other epidemic diseases such as cholera in Asia and meningococcal meningitis in Africa remain largely uncontrolled and still kill hundreds of thousands of people annually. Efficient vaccines exist for many diseases, such as yellow fever, poliomyelitis, measles and tetanus, but they have made little impact because of the cost and practical difficulty of administering them.

Chronic infections do serious damage to important organs, such as the liver or kidneys in schistosomiasis, the heart in trypanosomiasis cruzi (Chagas' disease), the lungs, bones and lymph nodes in tuberculosis, the bone marrow reserves of iron in ancylostomiasis, and of folate in malaria, the small bowel in strongyloidiasis and the muscles in leprosy. These organs may then fail prematurely if increased demand is imposed on them by work, pregnancy or additional disease. Such infections produce chronic ill health in millions of children and even more so in adults. Amyloidosis is common. Very often the degree of suffering is not sufficient to take people to hospital, even if one is available, but the ceaseless pruritus and gradually failing vision of onchocerciasis, the persistent diarrhoea of schistosomiasis mansoni and the immobilising cellulitis of the guinea worm are examples of conditions sufficiently debilitating to reduce performance, deepen poverty and lead to malnutrition. These chronic infectious diseases are enormous economic burdens on the nation as well as on the patient and the family.

Epidemiological Factors. These determine the distribution, prevalence, incidence and endemicity of a disease, especially if it is infectious, and so alter its pattern in the community. In many places, especially the urban slums, the lack of a supply of clean water and absence of any hygienic system for disposal of sewage and refuse, ensure the prevalence of infections transmitted orally from faeces. Endemic malaria, poliomyelitis and viral hepatitis affect the indigenous children, who either die or become immune so that adults suffer less from these diseases. Non-immune adults, such as tourists, invading soldiers or refugees are, however, fully susceptible unless specifically protected. Particular requirements of organisms, vectors, hosts or intermediate stages of parasites make rabies a sporadic disease, meningococcal meningitis a disease of the Sudan savanna, cholera a riverine disease, onchocerciasis a rural disease, Chagas' a poverty disease, and hookworm primarily a farmer's disease. Cooking and eating habits determine the prevalence of paragonimiasis, clonorchiasis and tapeworm infection.

Immunity and Autoimmunity. The natural immunity of animals to some human infection such as smallpox, which has only man for its host, has enabled this disease to be abolished, whereas the eradication of yellow fever is prevented by the susceptibility of monkeys to it. Natural immunity of individuals may possibly explain why some people do not suffer certain infections, but immunity acquired in childhood is a more usual explanation. Leprosy and tuberculosis, for example, commonly cause subclinical but immunising infections in children living in an endemic area, so that clinical disease is seen mainly in teenagers and young adults in whom naturally acquired immunity has failed.

Most human infections are terminated or controlled by an efficient immune response. When the response is inefficient the organism multiples unchecked, causing either death, or chronic disease as in lepromatous leprosy or onchocerciasis. Immunity is usually accompanied by hypersensitivity, which often causes more damage than the organism itself, as in tuberculoid leprosy or hepatosplenic schistosomiasis. Sometimes the immune response seems to be inappropriate, as in the tropical splenomegaly syndrome of chronic malaria, or to be grossly exaggerated, as with the hyperglobulinaemia of trypanosomiasis. In sharp contrast with their prevalence in temperate countries, autoimmune diseases are relatively uncommon in the tropics.

Poverty, Politics and Progress. The poverty of so many tropical countries is often tragically deepened by the strife that accompanies attempts to progress. Development itself may introduce new health problems. The construction of dams and irrigation canals may create breeding sites for the vectors of malaria, yellow fever, schistosomiasis or onchocerciasis. Penetration into forests uncovered Lassa and Marburg viruses (p. 732) in Africa, and has caused much mutilation from espundia (p. 778) in Brazil. New settlements in the Middle East are plagued by cutaneous leishmaniasis (p. 777).

Variations within the Tropics. As well as the gross but general differences between patterns of disease in tropical underdeveloped and temperate developed countries, there are many variations within the tropics. A certain condition may be present in only one climatic belt, continent or even community, but be very important there; examples are loiasis in the West African rain forest, Chagas' disease in South America and kuru among the Fore people of New Guinea.

GEOGRAPHICAL INFLUENCES ON DISEASES OF THE MAIN SYSTEMS

Diseases due to infection are considered in chapter 19; their distribution throughout the world is shown in Figure 18.1.

CARDIOVASCULAR DISEASE

Acclimatisation to a hot, humid environment demands a 20% increase in cardiac output and later an increase in plasma volume. A diseased heart is less able to acclimatise.

Rheumatic heart disease is worldwide, especially where there is overcrowding due to urbanisation and industrialisation. In Mexico, one tenth of all deaths is due to rheumatic heart disease. A restrictive cardiomyopathy (p. 187) due to endomyocardial fibrosis is just as important in children and young adults in parts of East and West Africa, Sri Lanka and Southern India, Brazil and Colombia. In West Africa restrictive cardiomyopathy may be a sequel to the hypereosinophilia of a filarial infection. Cardiomyopathy is due to alcohol in parts of Africa and to thiamine deficiency in parts of South-east Asia and Southern Africa. In some countries cardiomyopathy is a common cause of heart failure as is anaemia due to hookworms, sickle-cell disease or kwashiorkor.

Infective endocarditis is often secondary to skin

Fig. 18.1 Geographical distribution of disease due to infection (Based on information supplied by the Ross Institute of Tropical Hygiene, London)

	Area												
	Africa					Asia and Pacific				America			Europe
Disease	A1	A2	A3	A4	A5	B1	B2	B3	C	D	E	F	G
Malaria	††	††	*	†	*	†	††	††	†	†	*		
Schistosomiasis	†	†	*	††	*	*	1			†	*		
Trypanosomiasis 2	†	†	*	*						†			
Leishmaniasis	*	3,†	3,*	†	*	†	†	†	*	†	†	*	
Cholera 4	*	*	*	*		*	††	†		*			
Amoebiasis	†	†	†	†	†	†	††	††	†	††	†	*	*
Typhoid fever	†	†	†	†	*	††	††	††	*	†	†	*	*
Leprosy	††	††	†	††	*	*	††	††	†	†	*	5,	5,
Onchocerciasis	††	†		†		6,*				6,*			
Lymphatic filariasis	††	††	†				†	††	††	†	*		
Paragonimiasis	*						7,*	††	7,*				
Clonorchiasis								††	†				

*endemic	1 Small foci in B2, near Bombay and Madras
†highly endemic	2 Sleeping sickness in A, Chagas' disease in D
††very highly	3 Visceral in A2, both in other areas
endemic	4 Situation varies with gradual spread of seventh pandemic
	5 Only a few small residual foci in F and G
	6 Yemen only in B1, north of equator in D
	7 Nepal and Sri Lanka in B2, Korea in C

sepsis but is no more common than in temperate climates whereas pericarditis is much more frequent and is usually either pyogenic or tuberculous. Chagas' disease, which accounts for 10% of all necropsies in Brazil, is an outstanding cause of myocarditis; other causes in the tropics are African trypanosomiasis, typhoid fever, diphtheria, rickettsial infections and acute schistosomiasis.

In some rural tropical communities blood pressure does not increase with age. The 'normal' blood pressure is usually lower than in temperate communities, essential hypertension is rare and pregnancy hypertension less frequent, but in other communities, essential hypertension is becoming common. Atherosclerotic and especially coronary heart disease is virtually unknown in many rural populations, whose plasma cholesterol levels are low and fibrinolytic activity high, but is increasing in affluent groups in cities. Cor pulmonale is also rare in the tropics except where schistosomiasis is highly endemic.

Other forms of arterial disease are rare, but primary arteritis of the aorta, which can affect any of its major branches and of which the Takayasu syndrome is an example, is relatively common in Japan, South-east Asia and parts of Africa. In East and Central Africa an arteritis of unknown origin causes peripheral gangrene.

With the exception of tropical phlebitis, venous diseases such as haemorrhoids, varicose veins and deep vein thrombosis with its complication of pulmonary embolism are rare in the tropics.

TROPICAL PHLEBITIS of uncertain origin occurs in tropical Africa. Vascular granulation tissue is laid down, especially in the wall of the vein which becomes thrombosed and painful. Splenic vein thrombosis may cause necrotic infarction and liquefaction in the spleen. The patient is usually febrile. The venous lesion gradually resolves and the circulation is re-established. Treatment is symptomatic.

RESPIRATORY DISEASE

Acute respiratory infection is the commonest cause of childhood death all over the world, especially where measles is still prevalent. Most adult respiratory diseases in the tropics are also due to infection. Pneumococcal pneumonia and tuberculosis are commonest, followed by histoplasmosis in parts of South America, paragonimiasis in South-east Asia, filariasis (pulmonary eosinophilia) in India and the pulmonary complications of hepatic amoebiasis and schistosomiasis. Chronic bronchitis is rare in most rural areas, although common in North and Central India and parts of New Guinea where it is attributed to woodsmoke in huts. In countries that are starting to become industrialised, diseases such as silicosis and byssinosis are appearing.

DISEASE OF THE ALIMENTARY TRACT AND PANCREAS

Diarrhoea is the second commonest cause of death in childhood the world over and the most frequent in infancy in countries of poor hygiene if the mother is not breast feeding. In adults, infectious disease are the most important causes of alimentary disorders, especially acute gastroenteritis, giardiasis (p. 775), typhoid and other salmonelloses (p. 751), ileocaecal tuberculosis, amoebic and bacillary dysentery (p. 755), schistosomiasis mansoni (p. 784) and, in some countries, tropical sprue (p. 719).

In many developing countries the rural diet is rich in hand-milled grain fibre (bran) which is not only nutritious in vitamins, protein and iron and helps protect against deficiency diseases such as beriberi, but also makes a bulky soft stool which is passed two or three times daily. This bowel habit is associated with a virtual absence of appendicitis and diverticular disease. Other diseases which are rare in the tropics include Crohn's disease and ulcerative colitis. Cholecystitis is infrequent except as a complication from biliary flukes (p. 787). The prevalence of peptic ulcers varies greatly between different regions; when it is high, gastric outlet obstruction is common. In certain parts of the tropics calcifying pancreatitis is common in children and young adults and may be related to protein deficiency associated with a highly alkaline vegetarian diet. In others it may be associated with alcohol.

Acute Gastroenteritis

Ten million people die each year from acute gastroenteritis, especially infants and children in the tropics. Many infectious agents may be responsible, including rotavirus, coronavirus, other enteroviruses, enterotoxogenic *Escherichia coli*, *Salmonella* and *Giardia lamblia*. Attacks are often associated with bottle, as opposed to breast, feeding, and with weaning. Most attacks are self limiting within a few days, but if diarrhoea and vomiting are severe and treatment is not available, death may follow dehydration as in cholera (p. 755). Infantile diarrhoea is also the single most important cause of malnutrition in the tropics. Treatment is by rehydration. Mothers can be taught to make up glucose electrolyte solutions (p. 757) from prepared packs and give it to their children to drink, thus reducing the need for intravenous rehydration in hospital.

Tropical Sprue

Tropical sprue may be defined as malabsorption of two or more unrelated substances occurring in a patient in or from the tropics, in the absence of other intestinal disease or parasites. Its manifestations resemble those of coeliac disease (non-tropical sprue, p. 313).

Aetiology. This is unknown but the prevalence of sprue in certain well defined tropical countries and localities, and its epidemiological pattern, suggest that an infective agent may be involved initially. In established sprue the jejunal contents are grossly overpopulated with aerobic enterobacteria which seem to play a role in maintaining the disease. Sprue is not due to gluten or any other demonstrable sensitivity and there is usually no evidence of preceding malnutrition, but folate deficiency, as in pregnancy, may precipitate the disease. Not all cases necessarily have the same aetiology, which may account for occasional reports of sprue from Africa and elsewhere where the disease is not usually encountered.

Sprue occurs mainly in Asia, including Sri Lanka, Southern India, Malaysia, Indonesia, Hong Kong and China, some Caribbean Islands, Puerto Rico and parts of South America. It is a problem mainly in European residents in Asia but also does occur in the indigenous populations. It is common among travellers returning to Europe overland from India and Nepal.

Pathology. The changes closely resemble those of coeliac disease, although they tend to be less advanced. The jejunal villi are blunted or, rarely, absent and there is a subepithelial infiltration with plasma cells and lymphocytes. In severe cases the ileum is also affected. These changes are associated with malabsorption of fat, protein, carbohydrate and vitamins and the presence of diarrhoea which may lead to depletion of water, electrolytes, iron and calcium. A macrocytic anaemia is common with megaloblastic change in the bone marrow due to folate deficiency. Vitamin B_{12} deficiency takes longer to develop.

Mild changes in the jejunal mucosa are common in asymptomatic indigenous peoples, without gross malabsorption, throughout the tropics (*tropical enteropathy*).

Clinical Features. Although the onset of sprue may be acute with explosive diarrhoea and occur within a few weeks of arrival in the tropics, it is more often insidious with increasing lassitude, mental apathy and depression, loss of weight, anorexia and flatulence. Remissions and relapses are a characteristic feature. In severe cases 10 stools or more may be passed daily, especially in the morning or during the night. Defecation is urgent and often follows meals. The stool is bulky, frothy, pale and fatty, loose, foul-smelling and floats in the lavatory pan and is difficult to flush away. Vomiting may occur with nausea, abdominal distention and borborygmi. The tongue becomes sore, fiery red, fissured and painful, and there may be difficulty in swallowing. As the disease progresses much weight is lost.

Continued malabsorption leads to specific deficiencies; follicular keratosis (p. 66), angular stomatitis (vit. B), osteomalacia and tetany (vit. D), bleeding (vit. K) and hypoproteinaemic oedema, but peripheral neuropathy is rare. Loss of fluid and electrolytes causes dehydration, muscular weakness and cramps.

Diagnosis. The clinical features and the history of residence in an area noted for tropical sprue will suggest the correct diagnosis if care is taken to recognise the early and the mild cases as well as the late presentations. Evidence of malabsorption should be sought. Macrocytosis occurs early. Serum and erythrocyte levels of folate are low. Anaemia may also be hypochromic from defective absorption of iron. Jejunal biopsy shows partial villous atrophy which is not specific for tropical sprue. Jejunal mucus and fluid is examined to exclude parasites. Barium meal and follow through examinations are necessary only to exclude other disease.

Differential diagnosis is from other forms of steatorrhoea. Additional causes in the tropics are infections of the intestine with *Giardia intestinalis*, *Strongyloides stercoralis* or *Capillaria philippinensis*. Early symptoms of sprue may erroneously be attributed to amoebiasis or neurosis.

Treatment. Dehydration and potassium

deficiency must be corrected. Tetracycline, 1 g daily in divided doses for 28 days, will usually eliminate the jejunal bacterial overpopulation, reduce diarrhoea and improve absorption. In addition folic acid, 5 mg daily (10 mg intramuscularly in severe cases), is given as this seems in many patients to improve absorption as well as to relieve symptoms due to folate deficiency. The jejunal mucosa soon returns to normal. It has not yet been established whether to give a small prophylactic dose of folic acid daily to prevent a relapse in patients remaining in the tropics or to administer folic acid only if a relapse occurs.

Vitamin B_{12} deficiency requires intramuscular injections of hydroxocobalamin, 1000 μg twice in 1 week, followed by a dose of 250 μg once a fortnight for 6 weeks in addition to folic acid. Anaemia is corrected and the danger of developing subacute combined degeneration of the spinal cord is avoided. Deficiencies of other vitamins and iron should be corrected. It is often helpful to give a multivitamin preparation containing 10 mg thiamin, 5 mg riboflavin and 50 mg nicotinamide twice daily for a few weeks.

Complicated diets are no longer advised but the diet initially should be bland and appetising, limited in fat and carbohydrate and high in protein. After recovery, the diet should contain meat, liver and green vegetables which are rich in folate. Folic acid supplements should be given to women who have had sprue should they become pregnant. Often, after apparently successful treatment, mild diarrhoea and flatulence may persist. These are usually due to secondary hypolactasia and respond to a lactose-free diet.

DISEASE OF OTHER SYSTEMS

Liver Disease. This is a serious cause of disability and death throughout the tropics and subtropics. The microscopic structure of liver from a normal person in tropical Africa differs from that in a European. The hepatocytes are irregular in size and staining and frequently contain more than one nucleus. Portal tracts are infiltrated with mononuclear cells and a variable degree of fibrous tissue. Black pigment may be present in Kuppfer cells or portal tracts. These changes probably reflect the insults to which the liver is exposed in the tropics, including protein and vitamin malnutrition, alimentary infections and toxins, and systemic infections, notably malaria and schistosomiasis. The effects of protozoal and helminthic infections on the liver are discussed on page 367.

In most areas where hygiene is poor, type A viral hepatitis is endemic and especially affects children. Cirrhosis of the liver and hepatoma are common in adults and a relationship has been postulated with hepatitis B virus which is extremely common in some parts of Africa where the prevalence exceeds 10% of the population. Aflatoxins, produced by fungi from badly stored groundnuts and grains can cause hepatoma.

Renal Disease. Schistosomiasis haematobium (p. 783), which is the commonest cause of haematuria in endemic areas, may grossly damage the bladder and ureters. Skin infection with streptococci is a frequent precursor of acute glomerulonephritis. Pyelonephritis is common and in males often follows a gonococcal stricture of the urethra. *Plasmodium malariae* (p. 391) and schistosomiasis (p. 782) are important causes of the nephrotic syndrome in children. Lepromatous leprosy (p. 759) may also result in glomerulonephritis. Bancroftian filariasis (p. 795) is a frequent cause of orchitis, epididymitis and hydrocele in endemic areas.

Endocrine and Metabolic Disease. The prevalence of chronic fluoride poisoning is high in some areas (p. 63). Diabetes mellitus seems to be common throughout the tropics, but with few cardiovascular complications. The prevalence of other endocrine disorders is less certain though goitre is endemic in some localities (p. 62).

Blood Disease. In many tropical countries anaemia is common and often severe. This is largely explained by the high frequency of protozoal, helminthic and bacterial infections and the prevalence of malnutrition. The aetiology of anaemia in the tropics varies from one country to another, and from one area to another, and effective management can only follow the clear appreciation of local patterns of disease, nutrition and social custom.

Ancylostomiasis (p. 793) is a major cause of iron deficiency anaemia. Although Addisonian pernicious anaemia occurs in all races, it is relatively uncommon in tropical countries where megaloblastic anaemia is much more frequently due to nutritional deficiency.

The various types of haemolytic anaemia which occur in temperate climates are also encountered in tropical countries. Haemolytic anaemia in the tropics is frequently due to malaria. In addition two types of genetic abnormality resulting in haemolytic anaemia are also particularly common, namely deficiency of the enzyme glucose-6-phosphate dehydrogenase, and the haemoglobinopathies. Haemolysis also occurs in acute bartonellosis (p. 757) and may be caused by the venom of certain snakes (p. 710).

Connective Tissue Disease. Autoimmune disease is rare in most tropical countries. The incidence of dermatomyositis, scleroderma, lupus erythematosus and rheumatoid arthritis is low, but differs between races. In Malaysia lupus erythematosus is commoner in Chinese than in Malays. Acute tropical polyarthritis, of obscure aetiology, is a common self-limiting disorder. Reiter's disease is frequent in Africa and causes much disability.

Disease of Muscle. Painful tender muscles, but without suppuration, are a feature of several systemic infections, notably dengue fever (p. 736), trypanosomiasis (p. 779) and relapsing fever (p. 765), and are characteristic of trichinosis (p. 800) and cysticercosis (p. 788).

TROPICAL MYOSITIS. The cause of suppurative myositis in the tropics is uncertain. Abscesses explored early are sterile but, later, culture of the pus usually yields *Staph. aureus*. Pyomyositis starts with fever and painful induration of one or more of the large muscles, mostly in the lower limbs. The indurated area subsequently suppurates and a large abscess may form and be associated with a swinging temperature and leucocytosis. The affected area is swollen, hot and tender. When the pus is superficial, fluctuation can be detected.

Diagnosis of tropical myositis is usually not difficult although meningitis or peritonitis may be simulated. The differential diagnosis includes Calabar swellings (p. 795), sparganosis (p. 790), scurvy and an underlying osteomyelitis. When an abscess has formed, it should be incised, the pus evacuated and an appropriate antibiotic given.

Disease of the Nervous System. Infections still cause much of the neurological disease throughout the tropics, e.g. pyogenic and tuberculous meningitis, rabies and arthropod-borne viral encephalitis, malaria, tetanus, poliomyelitis, cysticercosis and hydatid disease. In some African countries as many as 1% of children suffer an attack of paralytic poliomyelitis. Locally important neurological diseases include trypanosomiasis in Africa, bartonellosis and Chagas' disease in South America, and eosinophilic meningitis in the Far East. Leprosy is the commonest cause of peripheral neuritis in the world and Chagas' disease of systemic autonomic neuropathy. Tuberculoma is a frequent and amoebic abscess a rare cause of an intracranial space-occupying lesion. In some tropical communities cerebrovascular accidents and trauma are becoming the chief causes of neurological disease. Certain diseases, such as tabes dorsalis, multiple sclerosis, parkinsonism and vitamin B_{12} neuropathy are rare. In countries that eat undercooked pork, cysticercosis is the commonest cause of epilepsy.

There are several syndromes, due to dietary deficiencies or toxins, which are locally important. These include beriberi in the poorer areas of South-east Asia, Wernicke's encephalopathy among the Bantu in southern Africa and pellagra among maize eaters.

Tropical spinal ataxia may be caused by cyanide in undercooked cassava (p. 656). Causes of spastic paraplegia in the tropics include lathyrism in India and the horn of Africa, Burkitt's lymphoma in African adolescents, schistosomiasis in Africa, hydatid disease in the Middle East, and, commonest of all, spinal tuberculosis.

Ophthalmic Disease. Eye disease is a major cause of suffering and poverty in the tropics; it often proceeds to blindness. The most frequent causes are keratitis, glaucoma and cataract which commonly occur as complications of neonatal ophthalmia, trachoma, onchocerciasis, malnutrition and leprosy. In Zambia, for example, 3 per 1000 of the population are blind.

Psychiatric Disease. The prevalence of psychiatric diseases in the tropics is similar to that in temperate countries, but some of the precipitating factors and symptom-complexes are different. Included among the causes of organic confusional states are alcoholism, meningitis, syphilis, malaria, trypanosomiasis and typhoid fever.

Functional psychoses present in the same ways as in temperate countries, but acute emotional disturbances, especially in Africans, often present with schizophrenic features such as hallucinations and paranoia; the prognosis is, however, good. Fear, implanted by witchcraft, may have profound effects and, in addition, the subject may have been made to swallow potent poisonous charms. Neuroses are especially common in people from underdeveloped countries who are suddenly moved to a strange environment. Symptoms are often florid and usually hysterical, the patient having little understanding of their cause.

Malignant Disease. Patterns of malignant disease vary greatly between different communities. Some tumours are rare — for example, carcinoma of the colon or lung in Africa and Asia — and some extremely common locally. Hepatoma is frequent in parts of Africa and in the Singapore Chinese. Carcinoma of the mouth is the commonest cancer in India and Sri Lanka and carcinoma of the nasopharynx associated with the Epstein-Barr virus is frequent in Kenya and among Chinese in S. E. Asia. Four of the commonest tropical neoplasms, hepatoma, nasopharyngeal carcinoma, Burkitt's lymphoma and Kaposi's sarcoma are due to viruses, probably in association with another carcinogen.

KAPOSI'S SARCOMA, or idiopathic multiple haemorrhagic sarcoma of the skin, is a multifocal malignancy composed of new blood vessels and large spindle cells. It presents as firm, bluish-brown nodules in the skin, usually on the limbs. It is common in parts of tropical Africa and occurs in Western societies in homosexual males with the syndrome of acquired immuno-deficiency (p. 35).

FURTHER READING:

Cook, G. C. (1980) *Tropical Gastroenterology*, Oxford, Oxford University Press.
Greenwood, B. M. & Whittle, H. C. (1981) *Current Topics in Immunology Series: 14: Immunology of Medicine in the Tropics*, London, Edward Arnold.

DISORDERS DUE TO CLIMATE

Acclimatisation to Heat and Heat Injury; Exposure to Strong Sunlight; Solar Keratosis; Prickly Heat; Heat Exhaustion; Tropical Anhidrotic Asthenia; Heat Hyperpyrexia; Cold Injury; High Altitude Acclimatisation and Deterioration; Mountain Sickness.

Acclimatisation to Heat and Heat Injury

In cool climates heat production in the body is balanced by loss from the surface chiefly by radiation and convection. When the atmospheric temperature is above that of the body, evaporation of sweat is all-important in the maintenance of a stable body temperature, assisted to a minor degree by insensible loss through the skin and lungs.

Acclimatisation to heat is an essential preparation for workers exposed to excessive heat in certain industries in cool climates as well as for people who go to the tropics. This can be achieved by undertaking exercise daily under artificially produced or natural hot weather conditions for 10 to 14 days. The total volume of circulating fluid increases and is accommodated in the expanded vascular bed; this is accompanied by a diminished pulse rate and an increased cardiac output. Salt excretion by the kidneys and in sweat is reduced, mainly as a result of increased production of aldosterone. The sweat glands also become more active, responding more rapidly and efficiently to increases in body temperature; consequently the rise in body temperature in response to exercise diminishes. With these adjustments the individual is better able to work and remain well under conditions of high atmospheric temperature provided an adequate intake of water and salt is maintained.

Heat syncope occurs in people dressed in unsuitable clothes in a warm atmosphere with poor air circulation, during exercise or on suddenly standing up.

Sunburn. This is caused by exposure to ultra-violet light. The skin of those with fair complexions, green eyes and red hair is especially sensitive to strong sunlight. Natural tolerance to the sun may be won by gradual exposure which enables the skin to acquire protective pigmentation.

Short periods of unaccustomed strong sunlight produce erythema and itch. Prolonged exposure causes pain, oedema and bullae, accompanied by malaise, headache and nausea. Severe cases may suffer from prostration and even acute circulatory failure. When a large area of skin has been damaged, this may interfere seriously with sweating and predispose to heat hyperpyrexia (p. 724).

No treatment is needed for mild sunburn, but for severe cases rest in bed in a cool room is required with sedatives to relieve the pain. Shock and dehydration must be corrected. Large blisters should be pricked. Calamine lotion should be applied to intact skin. Antihistamine drugs given by mouth help to relieve pruritus. Some protection is afforded by creams or lotions containing 5% para-aminobenzoic acid which absorbs ultraviolet light.

Solar Keratosis. After prolonged residence in the tropics atrophic patches are liable to develop on exposed parts of the body. The backs of the hands, the neck and the forehead are most commonly affected. These areas may later develop small patches of hyperkeratosis which occasionally progress to carcinoma. This process is most severe in albinos.

The skin should be protected as far as possible from the sunlight by clothing and creams. Hyperkeratotic areas can be removed by the application for one week of 5% fluorouracil ointment.

Prickly Heat. (*Miliaria Rubra*). Many Europeans living in the tropics, especially when humidity is high, suffer from prickly heat. This arises from blockage of sweat ducts within the prickle cell layer of the epidermis so that sweat escapes into the epidermis and causes severe irritation. The lesions consist of numerous minute papules, surrounded by erythema, which become vesicular or pustular. The pus is sterile, although scratching may lead to secondary pyogenic infection. The lesions are most numerous on covered parts of the body.

The principles of treatment are to reduce sweating to a minimum and to overcome the blockage of the sweat ducts. If the patient can be transferred to a cool environment such as an air-conditioned room, the blocked ducts may become patent within a week or two. In severe cases it may be necessary to move to a cooler climate. Calamine lotion relieves the irritation.

In prevention, excessive washing and irritation from clothing should be avoided and a bland soap containing hexochlorophane used. Clothing must be loose fitting, changed frequently and thoroughly rinsed after washing. Obese patients must lose weight. Curries, condiments and alcohol, which cause sweating, should be avoided.

Tropical Anhidrotic Asthenia. The majority of patients with this disorder have suffered from prickly heat which has left extensive areas of skin, especially on the trunk and limbs, incapable of sweating properly. The condition develops insidiously towards the end of the hot weather, with headache, giddiness, lack of energy, diminished sweating and often marked polyuria, the dilute urine containing chloride. Fever is common and hyperpyrexia may develop. The patient must live in a cool climate for several months until the skin has recovered and sweating has returned to normal.

Heat Exhaustion. This is brought on by a period of great heat or by extra effort in hot weather, when the patient has not taken enough fluid and salt to balance the increased loss by sweating. The amount of fluid lost as sweat during a working spell in a hot environment may be as much as 6 to 8 litres and even in persons fully acclimatised to heat, this may entail a loss of approximately 2 g sodium chloride per litre of sweat. Ill-health, especially gastrointestinal disturbances with vomiting and diarrhoea, will increase the risk of heat exhaustion.

Warning signs include headache, giddiness, loss of appetite, nausea, cramps and irritability. Lack of thirst may disguise the severity of dehydration until tachycardia, hypotension and a cold clammy skin develop (the 'cold moist man', c.f. the hot dry man p. 424). A cool environment and cold drinks with added sodium chloride (10 g/l) are adequate for mild cases; others require intravenous rehydration. When heat exhaustion is not recognised and treated, the patient may pass into heat hyperpyrexia.

Heat Hyperpyrexia (Heat Stroke)

This occurs in those exposed for considerable periods to unusually high environmental temperatures, independent of exposure to direct sunlight. Unacclimatised people are more liable to suffer, but a prolonged period of very high temperature may affect even those who are fully acclimatised, including local inhabitants. The disorder is always associated with cessation of sweating, and the rectal temperature may reach 42° to 43°C or even higher. Predisposing factors are those which interfere with the production and evaporation of sweat — unsuitable clothing, poor ventilation and heavy work in conditions of high temperature and humidity. Old people and those with congenital absence of sweat glands, with cystic fibrosis or skin diseases are particularly vulnerable. Hyperpyrexia may follow heat exhaustion when dehydration leads to cessation of sweating.

Pathological and Clinical Features. The most important changes are in the central nervous system. There is general congestion of the brain with increased pressure of the cerebrospinal fluid. Microscopic examination may show degeneration of nerve cells, particularly in the hypothalamic region and base of the brain.

The onset is usually dramatic with no warning in a person who appears to be neither dehydrated nor deficient in salt, but who may have noticed that perspiration has diminished. Loss of consciousness is rapid and may be preceded by prodromal signs of cerebral irritation. On examination a dry burning skin is found (the 'hot dry man'). When the temperature reaches between 41° and 42°C unconsciousness supervenes and without treatment the patient dies. Hyperpyrexia may be complicated by acute circulatory failure, hypokalaemia, acute renal or hepatic failure and haemorrhage.

Treatment. The aim is to reduce the temperature as quickly as possible in order to prevent permanent damage to vital structures. In the field, the patient is moved into the shade, the clothing removed and the skin kept wet and fanned vigorously. In hospital this is done by spraying the naked patient with water or loosely wrapping the individual in a cool wet sheet and promoting evaporation by fanning. Ideally the water should be at 15°C and the airstream at 30–35°C. The use of iced water, or immersion in cold water causes vasoconstriction and hinders heat loss. Cooling should be stopped when the rectal temperature has fallen to 39°C. The airway must be maintained and oxygen given. When return to consciousness is delayed, lumbar puncture and withdrawal of excess fluid may help.

Potassium deficiency should be corrected and severe haemorrhage controlled by blood transfusion. Acute circulatory failure (p. 149), acute renal failure (p. 401) or hepatic failure (p. 356) may require treatment. Parenteral antimalarial therapy (p. 771) should be given concurrently if malaria is a possibility. During convalescence control of body temperature will remain unstable. With energetic treatment 90% of patients recover.

Prevention of Ill-effects of Heat. Careful selection should be made of those required to work under hot atmospheric conditions. General physical fitness, youth, mental stability and acclimatisation are important. Fever, gastrointestinal disease, obesity, alcoholic excess and lack of sleep all predispose to the ill-effects of heat. It is highly important that the skin should be healthy and that sweating should be normal.

When the atmospheric temperature is very high, leading to excessive sweating, even the fully acclimatised require to take extra fluid and salt. A daily intake of up to 15 litres of cool drinking water and 30 g of sodium chloride (3 flat teaspoonfuls of salt) per person may be needed to prevent water and salt depletion. The extra salt is taken with food and in the drinking water or in enteric coated tablets.

In addition, everything possible should be done to improve working conditions by arranging for a free circulation of air and for a reduction of high temperature and excessive atmospheric humidity by air-conditioning. Clothing should be light and loose fitting. Hard or prolonged manual work should not be undertaken when atmospheric conditions are exceptionally unfavourable. Off-duty living conditions should be made as cool and comfortable as possible.

Cold Injury

Frostbite. Dry cold, below 0°C, freezes poorly insulated tissues such as fingers, especially in people exercising at altitudes where oxygen demand is high and availability low. The warning sign is intense pain in fingers or feet. Superficial frostbite causes blistering of skin, and deep frostbite necrosis of tissues leading to gangrene. Frostbite is treated by rapidly rewarming the whole patient with good insulation and hot drinks, and by warming the affected part in water at 40°C.

Accidental Hypothermia. This can be due to sudden immersion in a cold pond or sea, or to gradual but steady heat loss from exposure or from evaporation off the wet clothes of a poorly clad hill walker on a rainy day. The old and the sick become hypothermic if they are not well insulated at night. Clinical features and treatment are described on page 706.

High Altitude Acclimatisation and Deterioration

The partial pressure of atmospheric oxygen decreases with altitude (p. 491). Physiological acclimatisation starts at about 7000 ft (2100 m) and most people feel the need to acclimatise by about 12 000 ft (3650 m). Pulmonary ventilation and perfusion increase, plasma volume decreases and renal excretion of bicarbonate increases. These and other changes serve to maintain arterial oxygen tension until erythrocyte production raises the haemoglobin and haematocrit. Above 14 000 ft (4270 m) heart rate and cardiac output increase and pulmonary artery pressure rises. Physically fit young people acclimatise best and do better with each ascent. Lowlanders, however, never attain the performance of highlanders. Lack of acclimatisation is shown by increased respiration, Cheyne-Stokes respiration, mild headache and irritability, easy fatiguability and sleeplessness.

Acclimatisation continues successfully up to 17 500 ft (5330 m) above which arterial oxygen saturation falls to 70% and physical performance starts to decline. Short bursts of work can be undertaken, but at the risk of the production of an exaggerated lactic acidosis. Prolonged residence above this height causes anorexia, weight loss, decreasing mental and physical capacity and increasing susceptibility to infection. There are no permanent human habitations above 15 000 ft (4575 m).

Acute mountain sickness is experienced by people who go up too high too quickly; some suffer at 8000 ft (2440 m), others reach 19 000 ft (5795 m) without trouble. The earliest symptoms are headache, nausea and vomiting, followed by lassitude, muscle weakness, breathlessness, dizziness, rapid pulse and insomnia. Retinal haemorrhages may occur.

The symptoms are probably due to intracellular oedema and may herald the onset of two severe, possibly fatal, complications: pulmonary oedema and, less commonly, cerebral oedema. Paradoxically the robust young man is prone to pulmonary oedema, probably due to overconfidence. Cerebral oedema causes drowsiness, irritability, confusion, fits and coma. Its presence may be confirmed by the detection of papilloedema.

These complications are prevented by ascending gradually and by acetazolamide which probably acts by causing a metabolic acidosis and an increased drive to ventilation. They are treated by descending rapidly and by giving oxygen. Frusemide (40–120 mg), or morphine (15 mg) is the treatment for pulmonary oedema, and dexamethasone (p. 622) for cerebral oedema.

Venous thromboses, which may lead to pulmonary embolism, may afflict the partially acclimatised; they are due to increased viscosity of blood and are prevented by adequate hydration and exercise.

Chronic mountain sickness is due to alveolar hypoventilation and chronic hypoxia and may affect highlanders as well as acclimatised lowlanders. It causes cyanosis, cardiac failure, pulmonary hypertension and neuropsychiatric symptoms. It is treated by taking the patient down to sea level.

A.D.M. BRYCESON

FURTHER READING:

Clark, E., *et al.* (1975) *Mountain Medicine and Physiology.* London: Alpine Club.
Dickinson, J. G. (1982) *Terminology and Classification of Acute Mountain Sickness.* British Medical Journal 285: 720.
Edholm, O. G. & Bacharach, A. L. (1965) *Exploration Medicine.* Bristol: John Wright.
Ellis, F. P. (1976) *Heat Illness.* Transactions of the Royal Society of Tropical Medicine and Hygiene 70: 402–411.

19. Diseases Due to Infection

with particular reference to those encountered in the tropics

In the introductory chapter, 'Infection and Disease', general topics relating to infection and its treatment were discussed. In the preceding chapter, the importance of infection in tropical and developing countries has been stressed. In this chapter, an account is given of diseases due to infection other than those that are more appropriately described in the system mainly involved, for example infective endocarditis, pneumonia and other respiratory infections, viral hepatitis, infections of the kidney and genito-urinary tract, infectious mononucleosis and infections of the nervous system.

The sequence in this chapter is determined by the infecting agent and consists of diseases due to:

1. viruses and chlamydia (see below).
2. rickettsia (p. 738)
3. bacteria (p. 742)
4. spirochaetes (p. 762)
5. protozoa (p. 768)
6. helminths (p. 782)
7. fungi (p. 801)
8. arthropods (p. 805)

The chapter concludes with a section on advice to travellers about the prevention of disease.

DISEASES DUE TO VIRUSES AND CHLAMYDIA

No single classification of viral diseases is entirely satisfactory for the clinician, whether by viral structure and nomenclature, by method of transmission or by type of disease. Viruses are divided into two groups according to whether they contain DNA or RNA in their genome, and are subdivided further into families according to their structure (Fig. 19.1).

The important families of DNA viruses of man include the papovaviruses that cause warts, adenoviruses causing respiratory infections (p. 220), the poxviruses causing smallpox and vaccinia, and the herpes viruses causing herpes simplex infections, chickenpox and zoster, infectious mononucleosis (p. 519) and cytomegaloviral infections. Parvoviruses cause a mild exanthem in children and transient arthralgia mainly in adults.

The RNA viruses are more numerous. The reovirus family includes the rotaviruses which are important causes of infantile diarrhoea (p. 718), and the orbivirus of Colorado tick fever. The picornavirus family includes: (1) the enteroviruses of man — (a) poliomyelitis viruses (p. 643), (b) the coxsackie viruses that cause pleurisy (p. 270), myocarditis (p. 186) and pericarditis (p. 187), and (c) the echoviruses causing meningitis (p. 641); (2) hepatitis A (p. 349); and (3) the rhinovirus of the common cold (p. 219).

The paramyxoviruses cause parainfluenza (p. 220), measles, mumps and respiratory syncytial disease of infants (p. 224). The orthomyxoviruses include the agents of influenza (p. 221), and the rhabdovirus causes rabies. A retrovirus may be associated with leukaemia (p. 520) and the acquired immunodeficiency syndrome (p. 35). The other families of RNA viruses of human importance are the arenaviruses (Lassa fever, Bolivian and Argentinian haemorrhagic fevers; lymphocytic choriomeningitis p. 641), the coronaviruses (p. 220), the bunyaviruses which cause some of the arbovirus infections and, finally, the togaviruses which include most of the arboviruses and also cause rubella.

Some viruses, which include the agents of

| NON-ENVELOPED | ENVELOPED |

Fig. 19.1 Families of animal viruses. Human viruses and the diseases they cause are listed on page 726: ds — double stranded; ss — single stranded. Adapted from Matthews, R.E.F., Intervirology, 1979, *12*, 158 S. Karger AG Basel.

hepatitis B (p. 351) Marburg and Ebola virus disease, and the slow-virus encephalitides (p. 641) are not yet classified. It will also be noted that not all the viruses shown in Figure 19.1 are associated with disease in man.

Chlamydia cause psittacosis and ornithosis (p. 225), urethritis (p. 412), lymphogranuloma venereum (p. 413) and trachoma.

The diseases due to viruses and chlamydia described in this section are: *measles, rubella, mumps, herpes simplex and cytomegalovirus infections, chickenpox, smallpox, rabies, Lassa fever, Marburg and Ebola virus diseases, other haemorrhagic fevers, arbovirus infections (yellow fever, dengue, Rift Valley fever and Japanese B encephalitis) and trachoma.*

Other diseases due to viruses and chlamydia are discussed elsewhere as indicated by the cross references given above and on page 726.

MEASLES

Measles is caused by a paramyxovirus which spreads by droplet infection. One attack confers a high degree of immunity. Most people suffer from measles in childhood, and a mother who has had the disease confers passive immunity on her infant for the first 6 months of life. Measles is very severe with a high mortality in many tropical countries. The incubation period is about 10 days to the commencement of the catarrhal stage. A quarantine period is not necessary.

Clinical Features. *Catarrhal Stage.* Measles commences in much the same way as a common cold. There is an acute febrile onset, with nasal catarrh, sneezing, redness of the conjunctivae, swelling of the eyelids and watering of the eyes. In addition a cough, hoarseness of the voice due to laryngitis, and photophobia usually appear by the second day.

At this stage, a diagnosis of measles may be made from the presence of Koplik's spots on the mucous membrane of the mouth. These are small white spots surrounded by a narrow zone of inflammation. Though often numerous on the inside of the cheeks, they may be sparse and confined to the region around the opening of the parotid duct. The disease is highly infectious during the catarrhal stage and the child is miserable and irritable.

Exanthematous Stage. After 3 or 4 days of the catarrhal stage, the diagnostic Koplik's spots disappear while the dark red macular or maculopapular rash develops. The rash is first seen at the back of the ears and at the junction of the forehead and the hair. Within a few hours there is invasion of the whole skin, and there is usually some accentuation of fever. As the spots rapidly become more numerous they fuse to form the characteristic blotchy appearance of measles. The face is ordinarily the most densely covered area. When the rash is fully erupted, usually in 2 or 3 days, it tends to deepen in colour and then fade into a faint brown staining followed by a fine desquamation of the skin. The malaise and the fever subside as the rash fades.

Complications. Convulsions occur in young children and are commonest as the rash is appearing. Secondary infection by haemolytic streptococci, pneumococci or staphylococci may cause otitis media or pneumonia. Persistent conjunctivitis may be followed by corneal ulceration which, if neglected, may result in impairment of vision. Stomatitis, gastroenteritis, appendicitis and encephalitis may also occur. In the undernourished child measles may precipitate kwashiorkor.

Treatment. The patient should be isolated if possible and excluded from school for 10 days from the appearance of the rash. Most cases of measles, in spite of the high temperature, remain uncomplicated, and antibiotics should be prescribed only for unequivocal bacterial complications.

Prevention. ACTIVE IMMUNISATION. One injection of live attenuated measles virus should be given subcutaneously in children over one year old who have not had the disease. In the United States an aggressive immunisation programme has led to the virtual eradication of measles from that country.

PASSIVE IMMUNISATION. Human normal immunoglobulin, given intramuscularly, is recommended for the prevention or attenuation of measles, particularly for contacts under 18 months of age and for debilitated children. The dose is 250 mg for children under one year old and 500 mg for those over this age.

RUBELLA (GERMAN MEASLES)

Rubella is caused by a togavirus which spreads by droplet infection. One attack confers a high degree of immunity. It tends to affect older children, adolescents and young adults and spreads less readily than measles. The disease in children is trivial. In adults the illness may be more severe, but of short duration and of little importance except when it develops in a woman during the first four months of pregnancy. In such cases the child may be born with a congenital malformation such as a cardiac or mental defect, cataract or deafness. The risk of damage to the fetus by the rubella virus varies from over 70% during the first 4 weeks of pregnancy to virtually zero after the end of the fourth month. The disease is not notifiable. The incubation period is usually about 18 days. A quarantine period is not necessary.

Clinical Features. In children the constitutional symptoms are so slight that the illness is rarely suspected until the rash is seen. The spots are pink macules which appear first behind the ears and on the forehead. The rash spreads rapidly, first to the trunk and then to the limbs. A minor degree of conjunctival suffusion is common. Tender enlargement of the suboccipital lymph nodes is usual. Sometimes many groups of lymph nodes are affected and the tip of the spleen may be palpable. In adolescents and adults the onset may be acute with fever and generalised aches, but even then the illness lasts for only 2 or 3 days.

Polyarthritis, is the commonest complication. Encephalomyelitis and thrombocytopenic purpura are very rare. Complete recovery from all of them is the rule.

The diagnosis can be confirmed by isolation of the virus from the throat or by demonstration of a rising titre of antibody in the blood.

Treatment and Prevention. No treatment is available. If infection is known to have occurred during the first 16 weeks of pregnancy there is such a high chance of fetal abnormality that termination should be recommended. It is therefore advisable to immunise all girls between their 11th and 13th birthdays who have not had the disease as shown by the absence of serum antibodies to the virus. Women of child-bearing age who are found to be serologically negative should also be offered vaccine provided that they are not pregnant and are willing to avoid pregnancy for 12 weeks after vaccination.

MUMPS

Mumps is caused by a paramyxovirus which spreads by droplet infection and affects mainly children of school age and young adults. The infectivity rate is not high and there is serological evidence that 30–40% of infections are clinically inapparent. The incubation period is about 18 days. A quarantine period is not necessary.

Clinical Features. Malaise, fever, trismus and pain near the angle of the jaw is soon followed by tender swelling of one or both parotid glands. Indeed, parotid swelling alone is often the first feature. The submandibular salivary glands may also be involved. The swollen glands subside in a few days, and may be succeeded by swelling of a previously unaffected gland. Orchitis occurs in about one in four males who develop mumps after puberty; it is usually on one side only, but if it is bilateral, sterility may be a sequel. Obscure abdominal pain may be due to pancreatitis or oöphoritis. Acute lymphocytic meningitis is another mode of presentation. Encephalomyelitis is rare.

Most cases of mumps can be diagnosed on clinical grounds alone, but the diagnosis can be confirmed in doubtful cases by the demonstration of specific antibodies, or the virus may be cultured from the saliva, or from the cerebrospinal fluid in meningitis.

Treatment. Oral hygiene is important when the mouth is very dry due to lack of saliva. Apart from the relief of symptoms as they appear, no other treatment is necessary. Orchitis can be relieved by prednisolone (40 mg daily for 4 days). Cases of mumps should be isolated until the gland last affected has subsided.

HERPES SIMPLEX AND CYTOMEGALOVIRUS INFECTIONS

Herpes simplex (Herpesvirus hominis) is a common DNA virus which frequently causes nonspecific illness; hence many people have serum antibodies to the organism. It has now assumed greater importance as a cause of serious, and sometimes fatal, infections in immunocompromised patients. There are two strains of *Herpesvirus hominis*, Type I and Type II, the latter being principally responsible for sexually transmitted anogenital infections (p. 414). Infections caused by these viruses can be categorised as primary or recurrent.

Primary infections include ulcerative stomatitis (commonest in infants), keratitis (dendritic ulcer), finger infections (often in nurses), vulvo-vaginitis and encephalitis. In neonates and the immunosuppressed the infection may be disseminated, involving many organs and tissues, and can be fatal. The newborn may contract the infection from the mother's genital tract during birth and active genital *H. simplex* infection is therefore an indication for Caesarean section.

Recurrent *H. simplex* infections are commonest in the distribution of the trigeminal nerve, the lesions most frequently developing on the lips and adjoining skin (herpes labialis or 'cold sore'). The lesions start as macules, become vesicular and then pustular. Attacks of herpes labialis may be precipitated by various stimuli including sunlight, menstruation, viral and bacterial infections, or emotion. Genital lesions also commonly recur. Between attacks the virus lies dormant in the posterior root ganglion of the affected nerve.

The virus can readily be cultured from lesions and infection is confirmed by rising serum antibody titres.

The *H. simplex* virus is susceptible to idoxuridine and acyclovir although most infections resolve spontaneously. Drops containing idoxuridine or acyclovir are effective in eye infections and intravenous acyclovir is indicated for disseminated infections in immunocompromised patients. Acyclovir is also recommended for *H. simplex* encephalitis, which has a mortality of up to 80%, but its efficacy in this infection has not yet been confirmed. An oral preparation of acyclovir has recently been made available for the treatment of infections of the skin and mucous membranes. Unfortunately, there is no evidence that acyclovir will eradicate the *H. simplex* virus from posterior root ganglia and recurrent attacks cannot therefore be prevented. However, there is evidence that acyclovir will shorten the duration of the acute infection, provided that it is given early enough in the course of the illness.

Cytomegalovirus (CMV) infection is very common all over the world. The name refers to a characteristic enlargement of involved cells. Although most CMV infections are symptomless, this herpesvirus can also cause severe congenital abnormalities, a disease resembling infectious mononucleosis (p. 519) and disseminated infection in immunocompromised patients. CMV infection commonly occurs in the acquired immunodeficiency syndrome (p. 35). There is no specific therapy.

CHICKENPOX

Chickenpox (varicella) is caused by a herpesvirus (varicella-zoster virus) which spreads by droplets from the upper respiratory tract or by contamination from the discharge from ruptured lesions of the skin or through contact with herpes zoster (p. 644). Herpes zoster is due to reactivation of infection with the varicella-zoster virus and may be accompanied by a varicelliform rash.

Chickenpox is highly infectious and chiefly affects children under 10 years of age. Most children are little incommoded by this disease but, as often happens with viral infections, adults may develop a more severe illness including a prodromal rash. Second attacks are very rare. In patients on corticosteroid or immunosuppressive therapy the disease may be severe or even fatal. Most recorded fatalities have been suffering from leukaemia and it is probable that the blood disorder has been the major factor in reducing resistance to the virus. The incubation period is 14–21 days.

Clinical Features. Constitutional symptoms are usually brief and mild, and the first sign of the disease is often the appearance of the rash. Lesions are sometimes present on the palate before the characteristic rash appears on the trunk

on the second day of the illness. Then the face and finally the limbs are involved. The spots reach their maximum density upon the trunk, and are more sparse on the periphery of the limbs. Macules appear first and within a few hours the lesions become papular and then vesicular. The vesicles are unilocular, very superficial and thin-walled. The shape is elliptical rather than spherical. Within 24 hours the lesions become pustular. The vesicles and pustules are so fragile that they may be ruptured by the chafing of garments. Damage from scratching is also frequent, since itching may be troublesome. Whether or not the pustules rupture, they dry up in a few days to form scabs. The spots appear in crops, so that lesions at all stages of development are seen in any area at the same time.

The course of the disease is usually uneventful but secondary infection may occur. Serious complications, which are rare, include chickenpox pneumonia (p. 224), proliferative glomerulonephritis (p. 385), and acute demyelinating encephalomyelitis (p. 647).

Treatment. No treatment is required in the majority of cases. At the first sign of secondary infection a local antiseptic should be applied to the skin, e.g. chlorhexidine. If bacterial infection progresses, an antibiotic should be prescribed. Children who lack natural immunity owing to leukaemia, immunological deficiency, or treatment with corticosteroid or cytotoxic drugs, and who have been in contact with chickenpox or shingles should have an injection of human anti-varicella gammaglobulin (zoster immune globulin).

Spread of infection can be prevented by isolation of the patient and the sterilisation of all soiled articles, but the disease is usually so mild that in domiciliary practice these precautions are not normally required.

SMALLPOX

As a result of an intensive WHO programme of case detection and vaccination, it is confidently believed that smallpox has been eradicated. Apart from two laboratory-acquired infections in 1978, the last known case occurred in Somalia in 1977. Major smallpox produces a severe constitutional disturbance associated with a peripherally distributed rash with lesions which, in any one area, progress in unison from macules through papules to pustules. The mortality rate may be as high as 40%.

A similar virus causes *monkeypox* in primates in jungle areas of Central Africa, with lesions resembling those of smallpox. Some human cases have occurred in those in contact with infected primates but inter-human spread is exceptional.

The virus of smallpox is being maintained in a few designated laboratories, particularly in order to be able to differentiate such diseases as monkeypox from smallpox. Only staff employed in the vicinity of these designated laboratories, of which there are none in Britain, now require to be vaccinated against smallpox. Limited stocks of smallpox vaccine are available for this purpose and in case, contrary to all expectation, the disease should reappear.

RABIES

Rabies is caused by a rhabdovirus which infects central nervous tissue and salivary glands. It affects a wide range of animals and is conveyed by bites and licks on abrasions or on intact mucous membranes. Transmission by droplets in confined spaces has also been demonstrated. In Europe the maintenance host is the fox and in recent years the disease has spread from Poland westwards through Germany and has progressively penetrated through France. Man is most frequently infected from dogs but cats and other animals may be responsible. In the U.S.A. skunks are an important host and may infect man, while in Central and South America vampire bats also cause death of domestic animals and occasionally man. Insectivorous bats only rarely convey the infection. There have been several cases of rabies transmitted by corneal grafts taken from people who had died of undiagnosed rabies.

Clinical Features. The incubation period, during which the virus is spreading centripetally along axons to the brain, varies in man from a minimum of 9 days to many months but is usually between 4 and 8 weeks. Severe bites, especially if on the head or neck are associated with short incubation periods.

Although only a proportion of people bitten by a rabid animal develop the disease, once it is manifest it is almost invariably fatal. At the onset there may be insidious fever and a return of pain or paraesthesia at the site of the bite. After a prodromal period of from 1 to 10 days, during which anxiety may be increasingly evident, the characteristic fear of water, responsible for the alternative name of 'hydrophobia', becomes evident in many cases. Although the patient is thirsty, attempts at drinking provoke violent contractions of the diaphragm and other inspiratory muscles and thereafter the sight or even the sound of water may precipitate these distressing spasms and attacks of panic. Delusions and hallucinations may develop accompanied by spitting, biting and maniacal behaviour, with lucid intervals in which the patient is acutely anxious. Cranial nerve lesions develop and terminal hyperpyrexia is common. Death ensues, usually within a week from the onset of symptoms.

In a small proportion of cases there is an ascending paralysis without mental excitement and these patients survive, on average, 12 days. This type is particularly associated with bites from vampire bats.

During life the diagnosis is usually made on clinical grounds but rapid immunofluorescent techniques to detect antigen in corneal impression smears or skin biopsies have been successfully employed.

Treatment. A few patients with rabies have survived. All received some post-exposure prophylaxis. Intensive care is needed with facilities to control cardiac and respiratory failure. Usually only palliative treatment is possible once symptoms have appeared. The patient should be heavily sedated with diazepam 10 mg 4–6 hourly, supplemented by chlorpromazine 50–100 mg, if necessary. A gastrostomy is the kindest way to give fluids and food.

Prevention. *Pre-exposure prophylaxis* is required by those who handle professionally potentially infected animals, those who work with rabies virus in laboratories and those who live at special risk in rabies endemic areas. Protection is afforded by two intradermal injections of 0·1 ml human diploid cell strain vaccine given 4 weeks apart, followed by yearly boosters.

Post-exposure Prophylaxis. The wound should

be thoroughly cleansed, preferably with a quaternary ammonium detergent or soap; damaged tissues should be excised and the wound left unsutured. Rabies can usually be prevented if treatment is started within a day or two of biting. Delayed treatment may still be of value. For maximum protection hyperimmune serum and vaccine are required. The biting animal should be confined, if possible. If it is healthy after 5 days, it does not have rabies and treatment is stopped. If it dies, or is killed, the brain is examined by immunofluorescence for Negri bodies. If positive, or if the animal escapes, treatment is continued.

The safest antirabies antiserum is human rabies immune globulin. The dose is 20 i.u./kg body weight, once. Half is infiltrated around the bite and half is given intramuscularly at a different site from the vaccine. The dose of hyperimmune animal serum is 40 i.u./kg. Hypersensitivity reactions, including systemic anaphylaxis are common.

The safest vaccine, free of complications, is human diploid cell strain vaccine 1·0 ml is given intramuscularly on days 0, 3, 7, 14, 30 and 90. Of the older vaccines, the Semple-type, containing killed virus, is potent and widely available. It causes a serious neuro-paralytic accident in one in 1600 recipients. The dose is 5 ml subcutaneously into the anterior abdominal wall, daily for 14 days, with boosters 10, 20 and 90 days later. The duck embryo vaccine is safer (one accident in 30 000) but less reliably potent. Where human products are not available and when risk of rabies is slight (licks on the skin, scratches or abrasions, or minor bites of covered arms or legs) it may be justifiable to delay starting treatment up to 5 days while observing the confined animal or awaiting examination of its brain.

Control of Spread. Human rabies is an infrequent disease even in endemic areas. Its fearful manifestations, however, justify stringent attempts being made to prevent its spread. In endemic areas household dogs should have a yearly dose of a Flury canine (live) vaccine, and stray dogs killed. Importation of all animals into uninfected countries should be strictly controlled, with isolation in quarantine for a minimum of 6 months. Vigilance and appropriate measures of control over infected maintenance hosts, such as

the fox, are urgently required where areas of endemicity are extending.

LASSA FEVER

This disease, first observed in 1969, is due to an arenavirus, a group which also includes the viruses responsible for Argentine and Bolivian haemorrhagic fevers. Outbreaks have so far been limited to subsaharan West Africa where serological studies have shown that the infection is widespread. The natural reservoir is the multimammate rat and spread is probably through urine. The mode of human infection is unknown but case to case transmission in hospital occurs through direct inoculation and possibly inhalation.

Clinical Features. The disease has the general features of a viral infection, high fever, intercostal myalgia, bradycardia, a low blood pressure and leucopenia. Adherent yellow exudates on the pharynx are particularly characteristic. The fever lasts between 7 and 17 days. In severe cases liver and renal failure, electrolyte imbalance, haemorrhage and acute circulatory failure develop. Mortality rates of overt infections have been as high as 50% but mild and subclinical infections also occur.

The virus may be isolated in maximum security laboratories from serum, pharynx, pleural exudate and urine but diagnosis will usually be established from 'paired sera', the later specimens being taken 6–8 weeks after the onset of infection. The diagnosis should be considered in Britain in patients presenting with fever within 21 days of leaving West Africa.

Treatment and Prevention. Strict isolation and general supportive measures, preferably in a special unit, are required. There is no proved specific therapeutic measure. The administration of convalescent immune plasma has been followed by recovery and is therefore recommended for prophylaxis after accidental exposure to infection.

MARBURG AND EBOLA VIRUS DISEASE

In Marburg, West Germany, in 1967 a severe infectious illness broke out among laboratory workers who had handled tissues from a batch of vervet monkeys imported from Uganda. In 1976 outbreaks of the disease occurred in Sudan and Zaïre from a focus on the Ebola River. The viruses causing these two outbreaks have a unique identical structure but are antigenetically distinct. Sporadic cases have occurred elsewhere in Africa. The natural animal reservoir of these viruses is not known nor is the usual mode of spread, but man-to-man transmission can take place. In these outbreaks the mortality has varied from 25% of treated patients to over 90% in the untreated, but successive human passage seems to reduce virulence.

After an incubation period of 5 to 9 days, the illness presents suddenly with fever, severe myalgia and diarrhoea. By the fourth or fifth day the fauces become inflamed and a bright red, follicular rash appears on the extensor surfaces of the limbs; it spreads to the trunk and face, becomes maculopapular and finally confluent and livid. There may be lymphadenopathy. About the sixth day, in severe cases, bleeding associated with thrombocytopenia starts usually in the gastrointestinal tract. The virus also attacks the brain, kidneys and lungs. Fatal complications, often between the sixth and tenth days of the illness, include haemorrhage, secondary infection, encephalitis, renal failure and pneumonia.

Treatment consists of supportive measures, replacement of blood and the management of complications. Immune plasma may be beneficial if given at an early stage. No vaccine is available.

OTHER HAEMORRHAGIC FEVERS

The term haemorrhagic fevers is increasing in popularity but covers too wide a field of medicine to be of much value. Infections due to many different organisms may cause bleeding, and through several different mechanisms. Common among them are certain arbovirus infections (yellow fever, dengue, Kyasanur forest disease, Omsk haemorrhagic fever, chikungunya, Crimean haemorrhagic fever), Marburg-Ebola virus disease, Rocky Mountain spotted fever, relapsing fever, meningococcal septicaemia, plague and other gram negative septicaemias, and trypanosomiasis, all of which are described elsewhere in this book.

There still remain a number of other viral infections that are commonly associated with severe haemorrhage.

Bolivian and *Argentinian haemorrhagic fever* are caused by Machupo virus and Junin virus, respectively. Both are arenaviruses, like that of Lassa fever. Both have a reservoir in *Calomys* rodents which excrete the virus in urine. Both cause epidemics in rural workers, characterised by fever, with severe haemorrhage developing about the fifth day. Treatment with convalescent plasma greatly reduces the mortality.

Haemorrhagic fever with renal syndrome has occurred in outbreaks in Korea, Manchuria, Eastern Europe and Scandinavia. The virus (Hantaan virus) normally infects certain small rodents that pass it in their faeces. The infection causes severe capillary congestion, leakage and haemorrhage, especially in the renal medulla, so that oedema and acute renal failure develop, with oliguria and the passage of cells and protein in the urine. Untreated the mortality is about 30%, but with proper treatment for acute renal failure (p. 401) and blood transfusion if necessary, all patients should recover.

ARBOVIRUS INFECTIONS

So called because they are *ar*thropod *bo*rne, the hundred or so arboviruses are divided into groups according to their antigenic characters.

Group A are togaviruses all of which are transmitted by mosquitoes. The group includes three important causes of encephalitis in the New World, Eastern, Western and Venezuelan equine encephalitis, and several important fevers of Africa (Chikungunya, O'nyong-nyong, Sindbis and Semiliki Forest fevers), South America and Australia (Ross River fever).

Group B are also togaviruses, many of which cause encephalitis or haemorrhagic fevers. Yellow fever, dengue, Japanese B encephalitis, and West Nile, St Louis and Murray Valley fevers are transmitted by mosquitoes. Russian and European spring-summer encephalitis, Omsk haemorrhagic fever, Kyasanur forest disease of India and louping ill of Britain are transmitted by ticks.

Bunyamwera group of bunyaviruses, all of which are mosquito borne, are responsible for a large number of fevers, especially in the New World, including California encephalitis.

The remaining arboviruses, many of which are bunyaviruses, are placed in small groups or are ungrouped. Included here are the sandfly fevers, Rift Valley fever, and the haemorrhagic fevers of Crimea, Congo and Korea.

Arboviruses often cause epidemics. Clinically many infections are mild; even with the potentially serious ones, subclinical cases outnumber severe cases one hundred or one thousand times. The immunity that follows is often life-long and is an important determinant of the pattern of disease in the exposed community. Normally immunity protects and prevents further epidemics, but in the case of dengue, it may also sensitise and predispose to more severe disease if the person is infected with a different, but cross reacting type.

The incubation period is usually less than a week. The presentation is with fever which may disappear after a few days, either permanently or to return accompanied by the clinical features and complications characteristic of the particular infection. In many arbovirus infections there is a maculopapular rash, conjunctival suffusion, photophobia and orbital pain. Arthralgia and myalgia are common; pain may be severe and immobilising. Lymphadenopathy is found in a few infections.

The most serious complications of arbovirus infections are encephalitis and haemorrhage. When inoculated into mice most arboviruses cause encephalitis, but relatively few do so in man. The important ones are listed above, but their distribution is wider than their names suggest. The clinical features of encephalitis are described on page 642.

The causes of haemorrhage in arbovirus infections are not fully understood. In some, such as dengue, disseminated intravascular coagulation is important; in others, notably yellow fever, haemorrhage follows severe hepatitis when deficiency of prothrombin and other coagulation factors develops. Thrombocytopenia occurs in many arbovirus infections, and may contribute. Acute circulatory failure may follow haemorrhage, or occur on its own, possibly due to increased capillary permeability, as in dengue.

Diagnosis may be possible on clinical grounds during the course of an epidemic. For virological confirmation blood is transported on ice for inoculation into mice or tissue culture. It may be possible to isolate virus from cerebrospinal fluid if there are signs of encephalitis. Serological diagnosis depends on demonstrating rising titres of antibodies, usually by complement fixation or haemagglutination-inhibition. Such antibodies are however usually only group specific. Neutralising antibodies may be genus specific, but are more time consuming and expensive to assay.

Prevention of arbovirus diseases rests mainly on vector or reservoir control, but vaccines are available for some, including yellow fever, Kyasanur forest disease and Japanese, European Spring-Summer encephalitis and Japanese B encephalitis.

Yellow Fever

The togavirus of yellow fever is transmitted to monkeys and man by the bite of an infected *Aedes* mosquito. The virus is in man's blood for 2 days before the onset of fever, for the first 4 days of the fever and exceptionally for longer. The mosquito becomes infective for man 10 to 20 days after ingesting infected blood and remains infective for its life which may be as long as 7 months. Life-long immunity is conferred by the infection, which is often subclinical and babies born to immune mothers are protected for 2 to 4 months.

Yellow fever is normally a zoonosis of monkeys that inhabit tropical rain forests in West and Central Africa and South and Central America, among whom it may cause devastating epidemics. It is transmitted by mosquitoes living in tree tops. *Aedes africanus* is the vector in Africa and *Haemagogus* species in America. The infection is brought down to man either by infected mosquitoes when trees are felled, or by monkeys raiding human plantations. In the latter case *Aedes simpsoni*, which breeds in the axils of banana plants, may transmit the disease to man. In towns yellow fever may be transmitted between humans by *Aedes aegypti* which breeds efficiently in small collections of water. The distribution of this mosquito is far wider than that of yellow fever and poses a continual risk of spread.

Pathology. The main lesions are found in the liver and kidneys but haemorrhages may take place into many organs. If the disease has not been rapidly fatal the tissues will be jaundiced. Liver cell necrosis and fatty degeneration are widespread but maximal in the mid-zonal region. Characteristic inclusions, 'Councilman bodies' (p. 349) and 'Torres bodies', are usual. The kidney shows acute tubular necrosis and subcapsular haemorrhages.

Clinical Features. The incubation period is from 3 to 6 days. A mild attack consists of a short fever accompanied by proteinuria, with little or no jaundice. The classical attack falls into three phases: the initial fever, a period of calm and a subsequent period of reaction or intoxication. In very severe attacks there is no calm period.

The onset of the fever is sudden, sometimes with a rigor. The fever is highest on the first day and then declines. There are severe supraorbital headaches, backache and pains in bones. The face is flushed, the conjunctivae injected and the tongue is coated and its edges are red. The patient becomes prostrated; vomiting may be pronounced and the vomit may contain bile or altered blood. If vomiting persists the prognosis is grave. There is increasing epigastric pain, mental irritability and photophobia. The pulse rate falls more quickly than the temperature, and bradycardia is marked by the third day. This disproportion between pulse and temperature is very characteristic (Faget's sign). There is a persistent leucopenia. The urine contains protein in increasing quantities and, later, casts appear and the volume decreases. At the end of four days the temperature reaches normal and the second stage, the period of calm, is reached. Recovery may now take place without further fever and there is no residual damage.

In more serious cases the third stage, of intoxication, follows after a few hours, the temperature rising but the pulse still remaining slow. Jaundice becomes pronounced and the liver palpable and tender. The urine contains bilirubin and red cell casts. There is bleeding, sometimes profuse, from gums, nose, stomach, intestine and urinary tract; petechiae, conjunctival haemorrhages and ecchymoses in the skin may appear. The patient remains mentally clear and anxious until near death, which is only briefly preceded by coma. The pulse rate increases rapidly in the late stages. In fulminating infections the patient dies within a few days of the onset. Death rarely occurs in those who survive for 12 days. In some outbreaks meningo-encephalitis has been a prominent feature.

Diagnosis and Treatment. In an endemic area fever, leucopenia and proteinuria with or without jaundice should suggest the possibility of yellow fever. Virus may be isolated from the blood in the first few days. There will be a rising titre of antibodies. In fatal cases retrospective diagnosis by histological examination of the liver is important on public health grounds. The disease is notifiable under the International Health Regulations. There is no specific treatment. The patient should be nursed under a mosquito net for the first 4 days of the illness because the blood is infectious. Dehydration should be corrected by intravenous glucose saline and blood transfusions should be given if blood loss is severe. Acute renal failure is treated as described on page 401.

Prevention. A single vaccination with the 17 D nonpathogenic strain of virus, available at internationally recognised centres, gives full protection for at least 10 years, the period of validity of the vaccination certificate. Ten days after vaccination adequate antibodies are present in the blood and the certificate of vaccination becomes valid. The vaccine does not produce appreciable side-effects in adults, unless they are allergic to egg protein, when desensitisation may be necessary. Vaccination is not recommended in children under 9 months of age because of a slight risk of encephalitis. No ill-effects have as yet been observed from vaccination during pregnancy.

Only travellers possessing valid certificates of vaccination against yellow fever are allowed to proceed from an endemic area to 'receptive areas', by which is meant countries free from the disease but in which the potential vectors exist. In this way the disease has not yet entered Asia. As an additional precaution mosquito control of airports should be maintained. The urban disease can be eradicated by the abolition of the breeding places of *Aedes aegypti*, by the use of residual insecticides in houses and by mass vaccination in endemic areas. If susceptible mosquitoes are present and the virus persists in forests, humans living near are at risk.

Dengue

Six antigenic variants of dengue virus have been described. It is transmitted to man by mosquitoes, chiefly *Aedes aegypti*. Man is infective to the vector 18 hours before the temperature rises and for at least 3 days after the onset of symptoms. The mosquito can transmit the disease 8 to 12 days after feeding on a patient suffering from dengue and remains infective for life.

The disease is a risk in many tropical and subtropical countries, especially in coastal areas. It is most prevalent during the hot season when the mosquitoes are numerous. One attack usually gives immunity for about 9 months and after several attacks a considerable degree of permanent immunity is attained. Some cross-immunity exists between dengue and other members of the B group of arboviruses, including the virus of yellow fever.

Clinical Features. The incubation period is usually 5 to 6 days. The disease varies considerably in its severity. It may be a sharp illness with marked constitutional symptoms and signs lasting for 7 to 10 days or a milder disease resembling sandfly fever. Subclinical infections are common. A prodrome of malaise and headache for 2 days may precede the acute onset, characterised by fever and intense backache and generalised pains especially severe in the orbital and periarticular areas. Painful movement of the eyes, photophobia, conjunctival injection and lachrymation, nausea, vomiting, anorexia, prostration, insomnia and depression are often features of the disease. In severe cases the temperature may remain elevated for 7 to 8 days. An afebrile interval lasting 24 to 48 hours may intervene at the end of the third day when symptoms subside temporarily, to be followed with a recurrence of symptoms and a further febrile period of a day or two ('saddleback fever'). There is bradycardia, cervical lymphadenopathy and leucopenia.

A rash may appear, especially during the second febrile period. It is morbilliform but the colour resembles that of scarlet fever. It usually begins on the dorsum of the hands and feet and spreads up the arms and thighs to the trunk. After the temperature has fallen, depression and prostration often persist.

Dengue haemorrhagic fever occurs in South East Asia, rarely elsewhere. After 3 to 4 days of fever bleeding starts with petechiae, ecchymoses, epistaxis and melaena, and proceeds to acute circulatory failure. Even with treatment of these complications, 10% of patients die.

Disseminated intravascular coagulation and complement activation which leads to vascular damage are thought to be triggered by hypersensitivity to the virus.

Diagnosis is usually easy in an endemic area when a patient has the characteristic symptoms and signs. However, mild cases may resemble other viral diseases and a severe attack may be mistaken for anicteric yellow fever, but the absence of urinary changes will help to differentiate it. The virus can be recovered from the blood and antibody titres rise.

Treatment and Prevention. There is no specific treatment. The severe pains can be relieved by aspirin or paracetamol, but occasionally opiates are required. Blood transfusions and corticosteroids are indicated in the haemorrhagic varieties.

The patient is nursed under a mosquito net. Breeding places of *Aedes* mosquitoes should be abolished and the adults destroyed by insecticides.

Rift Valley Fever

This disease is caused by an arbovirus which normally infects sheep and goats in East and South Africa. It is usually conveyed by a culicine mosquito, especially *Culex pipiens*. Cattle and other domestic animals may act as amplifying hosts. Sporadic infections have followed direct contact with infected meat and from inhalation. In 1975 an outbreak occurred in South Africa with 12 cases of encephalitis, 4 fatal. Since 1977 there have been large outbreaks in Egypt with four clinical types; uncomplicated fever resembling dengue fever, or fever with retinal changes, with haemorrhages and jaundice or with meningo-encephalitis. Deaths occurred among the latter two groups. There is no specific treatment.

Japanese B Encephalitis

This arbovirus is transmitted to man by the bites of infected culicine mosquitoes which have fed on infected animals or birds, notably nestling herons. Pigs and other domestic animals are important sources of infection acting chiefly as amplifiers of the virus brought to them by mosquitoes. The virus is widespread in the Pacific Islands from Japan to Guam, in the Philippines, Taiwan, Borneo, Malaysia and Singapore and is spreading slowly west across the Indian subcontinent. Devastating epidemics, with a high mortality rate, have occurred. In endemic areas, serological surveys indicate a high incidence of subclinical infection and only sporadic cases may be encountered. Inflammatory and degenerative changes are found in the brain.

Clinical Features. Many infections are subclinical but overt disease may occur at any age, although children are particularly susceptible. With the development of encephalitis the patient experiences a very severe headache, fever, often with rigors, and vomiting. The physical signs in severe cases are neck rigidity, congestion of the optic fundi, imperfectly reacting pupils, muscular twitching and tremors; and, in severe cases, progressive coma, muscular rigidity and cranial nerve palsies. The cerebrospinal fluid is under raised pressure and an increase of cells and protein appears within several days. The acute illness may last from a few days to 2 weeks or longer. Convalescence is prolonged and tedious. Persistent neurological damage is a feature only in children or after prolonged illness in adults. The mortality rate in overt disease varies from 15 to 40%.

The virus has only rarely been recovered from the blood or cerebrospinal fluid but in fatal cases may sometimes be obtained from the brain. Increasing titres of specific antibodies in the blood is the usual basis for diagnosis.

Treatment and Prevention. There is no specific treatment and the value of corticosteroids has not yet been established. Skilled nursing and aids for the patient in coma, may be life-saving. The elimination of breeding places of the vector mosquitoes, the control of piggeries, and the use of insecticides, where practicable, should be instituted. A vaccine is available.

DISEASES DUE TO CHLAMYDIA

Chlamydia cause psittacosis and ornithosis (p. 225), urethritis (p. 412), lymphogranuloma venereum (p. 413) and trachoma.

TRACHOMA

Trachoma is a specific communicable keratoconjunctivitis caused by *Chlamydia trachomatis*. Transmission is usually by contact or from fomites in unhygienic surroundings. Some infections occur during birth from infected genital passages.

Vast numbers of people suffer from trachoma in the hot dry dusty areas of the subtropics and tropics but it is also present in Southern Europe, and among immigrants in Britain. The disease varies markedly in incidence and in severity in different geographical areas. In endemic areas the disease is commonest in children.

Pathology. The infection lasts for years, may be latent over long periods and may recrudesce. The conjunctiva of the upper lid is first affected with combined vascularisation and cellular infiltration; pannus, spreading to the cornea causes corneal opacity and impairment of vision. Cicatricial deformity of the upper tarsal plate is an early finding.

Clinical Features. The onset is usually insidious and infection may not be apparent to the patient. Early symptoms include conjunctival irritation, and blepharospasm. In underdeveloped areas, unless discovered on surveys, the condition may not be reported until vision begins to fail.

Trachoma may also present as an acute ophthalmia neonatorum.

The early follicles of trachoma are characteristic, but clinical differentiation from conjunctivitis due to other viruses may be difficult at this stage. Intracellular inclusions may be demonstrated in conjunctival scrapings by staining with iodine or immunofluorescence. Chlamydia may be isolated in chick embryo or cell culture.

Treatment and Prevention. Local ophthalmic ointment or oily drops of 1–3% tetracycline may be used twice daily for 3 months. In mass therapy in endemic areas such topical application twice daily for 3 to 6 consecutive days each month for 6 months has given good results. An oral sulphonamide daily for 3 weeks is a useful addition. Deformity and scarring of the lids, corneal opacities, ulceration and scarring require surgical treatment, after control of local infection.

Personal and family cleanliness should be improved. Proper care of the eyes of newborn and young children is essential. The finding of a case, particularly in a child, should lead to examination of the whole family. Population surveys should lead to discovery and treatment of asymptomatic infections. Trachoma clinics are required in areas of high endemicity.

DISEASES DUE TO RICKETTSIAE

Typhus Fevers; Rickettsialpox, Trench Fever; Q Fever.

Rickettsiae are natural inhabitants of the cells of the intestinal canal of arthropods. Some species may parasitise higher mammals including man. Infection is usually conveyed to man through the skin from excreta of arthropods but the saliva of some biting vectors is infected. Transovarian infection in arthropods to the next generation occurs in ticks and mites, which serve as reservoirs as well as vectors of infection.

Pathological and Clinical Features. In man rickettsiae multiply in vascular endothelial cells especially of capillaries and other small vessels, producing lesions in the skin, central nervous system, heart, lungs, kidneys and skeletal muscles. Endothelial proliferation, associated with a perivascular reaction (nodules of Fraenkel) may cause thromboses and small haemorrhages. In epidemic typhus the brain and in scrub typhus the cardiovascular system and lungs are particularly attacked.

The common clinical findings in this group of diseases are fever, severe prostration, mental disturbance and often a rash. The rash in epidemic, endemic and scrub typhus is at first central, but in tick typhus it starts peripherally. In Q fever only a sparse rash is occasionally seen.

An eschar is often found in tick and scrub typhus and in rickettsialpox, but not in epidemic and endemic typhus or in Q fever. An eschar is a necrotic sore, often scabbed, at the site of the bite and is due to vasculitis following immunological recognition of the inoculated organism. Regional lymph nodes often enlarge.

Diagnosis. The Weil-Felix reaction, which is the non-specific agglutination by the patient's serum of the strains of organisms Proteus OX 19 or OXK, helps in the differentiation of human infections (Table 19.1). A fourfold rise in titre is diagnostic.

Table 19.1 Weil-Felix reaction

Disease	Vector	Weil-Felix reaction	
		OX 19	OXK
Epidemic typhus	Louse	+ + +	negative
Endemic typhus	Flea from rat	+ + +	negative
Rocky Mountain spotted fever	Tick	+	negative
Other forms of tick typhus	Tick	+	variable
Scrub typhus	Larval mite	negative	+ + +
Q fever	None or tick	negative	negative
Rickettsialpox	Mite from mouse	negative	negative
Trench fever	Louse	negative	negative

Species specific antibodies may be detected by complement fixation, microagglutination and fluorescence in specialised laboratories. Rickettsiae may be isolated from the blood in the first week of illness by intraperitoneal inoculation into male guinea pigs, mice or voles.

TYPHUS FEVERS

There are epidemic (louse-borne), endemic (flea-borne), tick-borne and scrub (mite-borne) typhus fevers.

Epidemic Typhus Fever

Louse-borne or epidemic typhus is caused by *R. prowazeki* and is transmitted by infected faeces from the human body louse, *Pediculus humanus* usually through scratching the skin, or sometimes by inhalation. Patients suffering from epidemic typhus infect the lice which leave when the patient is febrile. In conditions of overcrowding the disease spreads rapidly. During interepidemic periods the disease may be maintained by inapparent or latent cases or perhaps by infected fleas and rats. The disease is prevalent in parts of Africa especially Ethiopia and Rwanda, the South American Andes and Afghanistan. Large epidemics have occurred in Europe, usually as a result of war.

Clinical Features. The incubation period is usually 12 to 14 days. There may be a few days of malaise but the onset is more often sudden with rigors, fever, frontal headaches, pains in the back and limbs, constipation and bronchitis. The face is flushed and cyanotic, eyes congested, and the patient soon becomes dull and confused.

The rash appears on the fourth to the sixth day and often resembles measles. In its early stages it disappears on pressure but soon becomes petechial with subcutaneous mottling. It appears first on the anterior folds of the axillae, sides of the abdomen or back of hands, then on the trunk and forearms. The neck and face are seldom affected.

During the second week symptoms increase in severity. Sores collect on the lips, and the tongue, dry and brown, becomes shrunken and tremulous. The spleen is palpable, the pulse feeble and the patient stuporous and delirious. If the patient recovers, the temperature falls rapidly at the end of the second week and convalescence ensues. In fatal cases the patient usually dies in the second week from general toxaemia, cardiac or renal failure or pneumonia.

Common complications are bronchopneumonia, parotitis, venous thrombosis and gangrene of fingers, toes, nose or genitalia. In endemic areas indigenous people may suffer relatively mildly. A mild relapse (Brill's disease) may occur after many years.

Diagnosis and Treatment. The clinical features are diagnostic when there is an epidemic of the disease but in mild cases may be much less distinctive. Laboratory aids to diagnosis are discussed on page 738 and treatment on page 740.

Endemic Typhus Fever

Flea-borne or 'endemic' typhus caused by *R. mooseri* is endemic world-wide. Man is infected when, by scratching, he introduces the faeces or contents of a crushed flea which has fed on an infected rat. The incubation period is 8 to 14 days. The symptoms resemble those of a mild louse-borne typhus. The rash may be scanty and transient. Laboratory aids to diagnosis are discussed on page 738 and treatment on page 740.

Tick-borne Typhus Fevers

1. Rocky Mountain Spotted Fever

The causal organism, *R. rickettsi* is transferred by the bite of hard (*Ixodid*) ticks which carry the infection to rodents and dogs and on occasion to man. It is widely distributed and increasing in western and south-eastern states of the U.S.A. and also in South America. The pathological changes are similar to those in epidemic typhus. Haemorrhages and gangrene of the genitalia, ears and digits are more common.

Clinical Features. The incubation period is about 7 days. There may be an eschar at the site of the bite, with enlargement of the regional lymph nodes. Symptoms closely resemble those of louse-borne typhus. The rash appears about the third or fourth day, at first like measles, but in a few hours the typical maculopapular eruption develops. Each day it becomes more distinct and papular and finally petechial. The rash first appears on the wrists, forearms and ankles, spreads in 24 to 48 hours to the back, limbs and chest and lastly to the abdomen where it is least pronounced. The fully developed rash often affects also the palms, soles and face. Petechiae may appear in crops. Cutaneous and subcutaneous haemorrhages of considerable size may appear in severe cases. The liver and spleen become palpable. Complications are as in louse-borne typhus. Untreated, the course of the disease may be mild or rapidly fatal.

Diagnosis and Treatment. There may be a history of a bite by a tick. The character of the rash, appearing first at the periphery, is helpful. Laboratory aids to diagnosis are discussed on page 738 and treatment on page 740. Detection of organisms by immunofluorescence in frozen sections of skin biopsies is quick and efficient.

2. Other forms of Tick-borne Typhus Fever

The causal agents of African tick-borne typhus are *R. conori* and a substrain *R. conori pijperi*. They cause typhus in South and East Africa, the reservoir hosts being dogs and rodents. 'Fièvre boutonneuse' of the Mediterranean is similar, as is also the infection in Queensland where *R. australis* is the causal organism. Infected hard ticks may be picked up by walking on grasslands, or dogs may bring the ticks into the house. An eschar and lymphadenitis are usual. A maculopapular rash may cover the trunk and limbs and affect the palms and soles but may be scanty. There may be delirium and meningeal signs in severe infections but recovery is the rule except in the debilitated. There are no haemorrhages into the skin.

Scrub Typhus Fever

Mite-borne or 'scrub' typhus is caused by *R. tsutsugamushi* transmitted by the bite of infective larval trombiculid mites. It occurs in the Far East, Assam, Burma, Pakistan, Bangladesh, India, Indonesia, S. Pacific Islands and Queensland.

Pathological and Clinical Features. The pathology is similar to that of louse-borne typhus, but lesions in the lungs are more prominent. In most cases one or more eschars develop, surrounded by an area of cellulitis and enlargement of regional lymph nodes. The incubation period is about 9 days.

The onset of symptoms is usually sudden with headache, often retro-orbital, fever, malaise, weakness and cough, occasionally with diarrhoea. The conjunctivae become injected. In severe cases the general symptoms increase, with apathy and prostration. An erythematous maculopapular rash often appears on about the fifth to the seventh day and spreads to the trunk, face and limbs including the palms and soles with generalised painless lymphadenopathy. The rash fades by the fourteenth day. The temperature rises rapidly and continues as a remittent fever with sweating until it falls by lysis about the twelfth to the eighteenth day. In severe cases the patient is prostrate with cough, pneumonia, confusion and deafness. Cardiac failure, renal failure and haemorrhage may develop. Convalescence is often slow and tachycardia may persist for some weeks. Mild subclinical cases are common.

Diagnosis and Treatment. In endemic areas diagnosis is often possible on the clinical findings. Laboratory aids to diagnosis are discussed on page 738 and treatment below.

OTHER RICKETTSIAL DISEASES

Rickettsialpox is due to *R. akari*, transmitted from the domestic mouse by a mite. It appears to be restricted to New York and Philadelphia where mice are now adapted to live in communal rubbish chutes of apartment houses.

The illness starts with a papule, which develops into an eschar, and is followed a week later by the sudden onset of fever, sweating, backache and a rash, maculopapular at first but which soon vesiculates and crusts, healing without scarring.

Trench fever is caused by *R. quintana* and is spread to man by louse faeces. It was prevalent in the First World War among troops in the trenches and again in the Second World War in the USSR. The disease is otherwise rare.

The incubation period is 10 to 20 days. The onset is sudden with headache, severe pains in trunk and limbs. The temperature rises sharply and remains raised for 5 to 7 days. The initial illness is like a mild case of typhus fever but febrile relapses are common, usually at intervals of 5 to 6 days and may be debilitating.

Treatment of the Rickettsial Diseases. The various fevers due to rickettsiae vary greatly in severity but respond to tetracycline and chloramphenicol. Tetracycline is given in a dose of 250 mg 4 times daily. In severe infections the dose is 500 mg 4 times daily for the first 3 days. The fever usually settles within 2 or 3 days. As there is a tendency to relapse tetracycline should be continued for 5 to 7 days after the patient is afebrile. In endemic areas good results have been obtained in louse-borne typhus and scrub typhus by a single dose of 100 mg doxycycline.

Patients suffering from louse- or flea-borne typhus are a danger to others unless they have been disinfested.

Nursing care is important, especially in epidemic typhus. Attention is paid to oral hygiene, skin and hydration. Tepid sponging is needed if the temperature rises above 40°C. Delirium may require sedation and haemorrhage may require blood transfusion. If headache is intense and fails to respond to aspirin or codeine, lumbar puncture should be performed to relieve the increased intracranial pressure and to detect any concomitant bacterial meningitis. Relapsing fever and typhoid are common intercurrent infections in epidemic typhus, and pneumonia in scrub typhus. They must be sought and treated. Convalescence is usually protracted especially in older people.

Prevention. For louse- and flea-borne typhus and in trench fever steps should be taken to get rid of all lice and fleas and their faeces. An insecticide powder can be insufflated into the undergarments of those at risk without their undressing; 5% carboryl or 0·5% malathion are replacing 2% gamma-benzene hexachloride and DDT to which lice are becoming resistant. Residual insecticide powder on floors and bedding prevents fleas hatching. To prevent flea-borne typhus, food stores and granaries should be protected from rats. Rats and their fleas must be destroyed.

Attendants on patients with louse-borne typhus should wear protective clothing smeared with an insect repellent such as dimethylphthalate (DMP). The patient should be washed, and an insecticide applied all over, especially to the hairy parts. Clothing should be disinfested with insecticide in plastic bags, or sterilised in a domestic tumble drier or autoclaved.

To guard against tick-borne typhus, dogs should be regularly disinfested of ticks with forceps and should not be allowed to sleep in bedrooms. Protection of the legs when walking through grasslands may reduce the risk of picking up infected ticks. The early removal of ticks and cleansing the site of the bite are also important. Floors of log cabins in the U.S.A. should be creosoted annually.

Mite-borne typhus is acquired when man enters scrub country in endemic areas. Protection against the larval mite can be secured by wearing suitable clothing, the inside of which has been smeared once a week with a mite-repellent such as DMP. Mites can be destroyed by aerial spraying of infected areas with Aldrin or Dieldrin, repeated every 3 months.

Active Immunisation. Those likely to be at risk can be protected by vaccines prepared from killed cultures of *R. prowazeki*, *R. mooseri* or *R. rickettsi* cultured in eggs. Three doses each of 1 ml should be given subcutaneously at intervals of 7 to 10 days and booster doses of 1 ml should be given at 6-monthly intervals or yearly. No protective vaccine is available against mite-borne typhus.

Chemoprophylaxis. It is likely that doxycycline (100 mg/weekly) would protect those at risk.

Q FEVER

Q (Query) fever is caused by *Coxiella burnetii*, a rickettsia-like organism, which is widespread in nature and is carried by many insects, ticks and animals, including cattle and sheep. The exact method of transmission of the organism to humans is unknown although air-borne spread is considered to be one important route and unpasteurised milk is another. The organisms are highly resistant to drying.

Clinical Features. The incubation period of Q fever is from 7 to 14 days. The clinical features of the illness are protean ranging from subclinical infection to fatal encephalitis or endocarditis (p. 165). Acute Q fever usually starts like influenza with pyrexia followed by myalgia, headache and sweating. Many cases resolve without specific therapy. Some patients have a cough and radiological examination may reveal an atypical pneumonia. Less common features of Q fever include myocarditis, epidydimo-orchitis, hepatitis, uveitis and osteomyelitis.

The diagnosis of Q fever should be especially considered in patients living in rural areas and those whose hobbies take them into the countryside. *C. burnetii* does not grow in the media used for routine blood cultures and it is therefore important to consider Q fever as a possible cause in patients with clinical evidence of endocarditis who have sterile blood cultures. The diagnosis of Q fever is confirmed by the detection of serum antibodies to the two polysaccharide antigens of *C. burnetii*; acute infection is confirmed by a fourfold rise in phase II antibody titres in paired specimens of blood taken at intervals of between 10 and 14 days. Phase I antibody titres rise more slowly than phase II and the persistence of both suggest chronic infection; endocarditis is confirmed by the presence of raised serum antibody titres to the phase I antigen.

Treatment. *C. burnetii* is sensitive to the

tetracyclines, clindamycin and chloramphenicol. Acute infections usually respond to one of the tetracyclines in a dose of 500 mg 4 times daily for 2–3 weeks. The treatment of chronic infections, especially if there is endocarditis, requires prolonged therapy; tetracycline plus clindamycin is recommended for Q fever endocarditis.

DISEASES DUE TO BACTERIA

Streptococcal infections; Staphylococcal infections; Diphtheria; Tetanus; Anthrax; Meningococcal infections; Gonococcal infection (p. 411); Whooping Cough; Brucellosis; Plague; Tularaemia; Melioidosis; Salmonella infections (typhoid and paratyphoid fevers, food poisoning); Bacillary dysentery; Cholera; Bartonellosis; Leprosy; Mycobacterial Ulcer.

STREPTOCOCCAL INFECTIONS

A number of different streptococci cause disease in man. These include *Streptococcus pyogenes* (scarlet fever, impetigo and erysipelas), *Strep. faecalis* (pyelonephritis and endocarditis), *Strep. viridans* (endocarditis), anaerobic streptococci (liver abscess and pulmonary infections) and Group B streptococci (neonatal infections). All can cause septicaemia which may be rapidly fatal. The present section describes infections caused by Group A haemolytic streptococci (*Strep. pyogenes*).

Haemolytic streptococcal infection results in features which vary with the invasiveness of the organism, its capacity to produce toxins, the site involved and the reaction of the host. If the resistance is low and the invasive properties of the haemolytic streptococcus are high, a rapidly spreading erysipelas, cellulitis, lymphangitis or bacteraemia, may result. The haemolytic streptococcus may produce a specific exotoxin causing a widespread punctate erythema. When the infection is associated with such a rash the syndrome is known as scarlet fever. The same type of streptococcus may produce in one person acute tonsillitis, in another scarlet fever and in a third erysipelas.

Scarlet Fever

Although scarlet fever is at present a mild disease, it may not necessarily remain so, as fluctuations in its severity have been recorded for the past 200 or 300 years. The primary site of infection in scarlet fever is usually the pharnyx or the tonsils but the disease may follow haemolytic streptococcal infection in other sites, e.g. in the genital tract after childbirth resulting in 'puerperal' scarlet fever or in wounds resulting in 'surgical' scarlet fever. It is transmitted by airborne infection, or more rarely by milk or ice-cream contaminated by streptococci. The disease is notifiable. The incubation period is about two to four days. Quarantine is not necessary.

Clinical Features. Scarlet fever occurs most commonly in children. It has a sudden onset and the more severe cases present with a sore throat, shivering, pyrexia, headache and vomiting. There is inflammation of the fauces; the tonsils are enlarged and may be covered with a follicular exudate. The exudate may be distinguished from the membrane seen in diphtheria by its yellow appearance and the ease with which it is wiped off. There is tender enlargement of the tonsillar lymph nodes. The rash, which usually appears first behind the ears on the second day, rapidly becomes a generalised punctate erythema. It is most intense in the flexures of the arms and legs. The face is not affected by the rash, though it is usually flushed due to fever, and the region round the mouth is pale. The tongue is initially furred but shows prominent red papillae, an appearance known as the 'white strawberry' tongue. In two or three days the fur peels leaving the 'red strawberry' tongue. The rash fades in about one week and is succeeded by desquamation.

A profuse growth of haemolytic streptococci can usually be obtained from a throat swab. A high antistreptolysin O titre (ASO) may be demonstrated in the serum.

The complications are less common than formerly as a result of the mild form of the disease and the introduction of effective chemotherapy. Extension of infection along the Eustachian tubes may lead to acute suppurative otitis media. Suppurative cervical adenitis and sinusitis also occur. Rheumatic fever and nephritis are rare sequelae which develop two or three weeks after the onset of any haemolytic streptococcal infection.

Treatment and Prevention. The treatment of scarlet fever is the same as for streptococcal sore throat. Most cases respond rapidly to phenoxymethylpenicillin (250 mg for children and 500 mg for adults t.i.d. for 7 days). An institutional epidemic calls for chemoprophylaxis with penicillin or erythromycin.

Erysipelas

Erysipelas is an acute haemolytic streptococcal infection of the skin. It occurs in both sexes and is much commoner in the elderly than in the young. A quarantine period is not necessary.

The onset is abrupt with heat and pain in the infected skin together with a systemic upset. There is a rapidly spreading red patch of inflamed skin with underlying oedema of the subcutaneous tissues. The edge of the patch is palpably raised and clearly defined and the lymph nodes draining the area become enlarged and tender. As the oedema subsides vesicles and bullae appear in the central part of the affected area. The face is involved in at leat 80% of all cases of erysipelas as a result of the spread of streptococci from the nose.

Erysipelas is usually brought under complete control within 48 hours of treatment with penicillin; hence the prognosis is now excellent for a disease which used to be very serious.

STAPHYLOCOCCAL INFECTIONS

Staphylococcus aureus is responsible for a wide variety of suppurative conditions such as infected lacerations, styes, boils, carbuncles, abscesses, osteomyelitis, pneumonia, endocarditis, umbilical cord sepsis, enterocolitis and bacteraemia with pyaemic abscesses. Many infections, particularly boils, carbuncles and abscesses, are due to autogenous infection as the organisms can be grown from the nasopharynx and skin of up to 30% of healthy persons. The staphylococcus is readily spread from these sites and from clothing to contaminate the dust in which it survives in the dry state for weeks or months. In hospital this organism is an important cause of wound infection, pneumonia and neonatal sepsis. Under suitable conditions it multiplies freely in food and milk to produce a heat-stable toxin which is an important cause of food poisoning (p. 753).

When the severity of the disease warrants antibiotic therapy, the choice depends on whether the infection has been acquired inside or outside hospital. In the latter case the organism may be sensitive to penicillin. If the illness is severe treatment should be commenced with the cloxacillins (p. 44), unless the patient is known to be allergic to the penicillins when erythromycin (p. 45), fusidic acid (p. 46) or clindamycin (p. 46) should be given.

The *toxic shock syndrome* is a condition caused by the toxins of certain *Staphylococcus aureus* strains and principally occurs in women using some types of tampon, the infection originating in the vagina and presenting with fever, rash and shock. The syndrome has also been described as a complication of staphylococcal infections of the skin, lungs and breasts.

DIPHTHERIA

By 1950 diphtheria, which was formerly a common and lethal disease in Britain, became so rare as a result of prophylactic inoculation that many doctors have never seen it. Yet in many parts of the world diphtheria is still an important cause of illness.

Infection with *Corynebacterium diphtheriae* occurs most commonly in the upper respiratory tract and sore throat is frequently the presenting feature. The disease is usually spread by droplet infection from cases or carriers. The organisms remain localised at the site of infection and the serious consequences result from the absorption of a soluble exotoxin which damages the heart muscle and the nervous system.

The infection may occur rarely on the conjunctiva or the genital tract, or it may complicate wounds, abrasions or diseases of the skin.

The average incubation period is two to four days. Cases are isolated until cultures from six daily nose and throat swabs are negative.

Clinical Features. The diagnostic feature is the 'wash-leather' elevated membrane of variable extent on the tonsils with a well-defined edge and surrounded by a zone of inflammation. The membrane is firm and adherent. There may be swelling of the neck and tender enlargement of the lymph nodes. In the mildest infections, especially in the presence of a high degree of immunity, a membrane may never appear and the throat is merely slightly injected.

The disease begins insidiously. The temperature is seldom much raised although tachycardia is usually marked. The infection may remain mild if the membrane is confined to the anterior nares or the larynx or the tonsils. With anterior nasal infection there is also nasal discharge often tinged with blood. In laryngeal diphtheria there is a husky voice, a high-pitched cough, and a danger of respiratory obstruction which can be fatal if tracheostomy is not carried out. Tonsillar diphtheria usually causes a sore throat. When the infection spreads towards the uvula, to the fauces and then to the nasopharynx, the patient is often gravely ill and apathetic. The complexion is pale, the pulse rapid and of poor volume and the blood pressure low. Death from acute circulatory failure may occur within the first 10 days. Those who survive the earlier toxaemia may later develop arrhythmias or cardiac failure. Electrocardiographic changes are common and are due to myocarditis. These are reversible and there is no permanent damage to the heart in those who survive.

Involvement of the nervous system sometimes occurs, and after tonsillar or pharyngeal diphtheria it usually commences with palatal palsy on about the tenth day of the illness. The voice assumes a nasal quality, while regurgitation of fluids through the nose and sluggishness of palatal movements may be observed. Paralysis of accommodation soon follows and may be inferred from the patient's complaint of difficulty in reading small print.

A week or two later, though somewhat rarely, weakness and paraesthaesia in the limbs due to polyneuritis may develop. In exceptional cases paralysis of the respiratory muscles may necessitate the use of a mechanical respirator. Recovery from such neuritis is always ultimately complete.

Treatment. Upon making a clinical diagnosis of diphtheria, the case should be notified to the community medical authorities and sent urgently to a hospital for infectious diseases. Antitoxin should be injected intramuscularly without awaiting the report on a throat swab if the clinician considers that diphtheria is likely to be the cause of the illness. Every moment of delay increases the danger to the patient, because toxin, once fixed to the tissues, can no longer be neutralised by antitoxin. However, horse serum, in which antitoxin is contained, being a foreign protein, is liable to cause undesirable reactions. Firstly, there may be an immediate anaphylactic reaction with dyspnoea, pallor and collapse or even death. Secondly, within 7 to 12 days serum sickness, with fever, urticaria and joint pains may occur. If there is a previous history of inoculation of horse serum, the symptoms commonly appear in 3 or 4 days. As anaphylaxis is potentially lethal, every patient must be asked whether they have ever had antiserum before and whether they suffer from any allergic disorder. In all cases a small test injection of serum should be given half an hour before the full dose.

When a reaction does occur after the test dose in an allergic subject, rapid desensitisation must be undertaken with extreme caution. In all cases an ampoule of 1/1000 adrenaline solution must be close at hand to deal with any immediate type of reaction (0·5–1·0 ml i.m.). An antihistamine is also given.

In a very severe case the risk of anaphylactic shock is outweighed by the mortal danger of diphtheritic toxaemia and up to 100 000 units of antitoxin should be injected intravenously if the test dose has not given rise to symptoms. For cases of moderate severity 16 000–32 000 units i.m. will suffice, and for mild cases 4000–8000 units.

Penicillin should be administered for one week to eliminate *C. diphtheriae*. Patients allergic to penicillin can be given erythromycin.

Prevention. The mortality in diphtheria, combined with the fact that the risks and cost of treatment are considerable, emphasise the necessity for active immunisation. This should be given in accordance with the instructions on page 41.

If diphtheria occurs in a closed community, a daily examination of the throat of all contacts should be made during the incubation period and swabs taken for the detection of carriers and potential cases. Those with positive throat swabs or with the slightest suspicion of clinical diphtheria should be isolated and given erythromycin which is more effective than penicillin in eradicating the organism in carriers. All contacts should also be advised to have active immunisation or a booster dose of toxoid.

Cases, convalescents and healthy carriers are isolated until six daily throat swabs are negative on culture.

TETANUS

This disease results from infection with *Clostridium tetani*, which exists as a commensal in the gut of man and domestic animals and is found in the soil. Infection enters the body through wounds, often trivial, such as those caused by a splinter, a nail in the boot or a garden fork or following septic infection such as a dirty abrasion. The disease is thus most commonly found in agricultural workers and gardeners. If childbirth takes place in an unhygienic environment *tetanus neonatorum* may result from infection of the umbilical stump or the mother may develop the disease.

In circumstances unfavourable to the growth of the organism, spores are formed and these may remain dormant for years in the soil. Spores germinate and bacilli multiply only in the anaerobic conditions which occur in areas of tissue necrosis or if the oxygen tension is low as a result of the presence of other organisms, particularly aerobic ones. The bacilli remain localised but produce an exotoxin with an affinity for motor nerve endings and motor nerve cells. Involvement of the former by direct spread causes local tetanus. The anterior horn cells are affected after the exotoxin has passed into the blood stream and their involvement results in rigidity and convulsions. Symptoms first appear from two days to several weeks after injury — the shorter the incubation period, the more severe the attacks and the outcome may well be fatal with an incubation period of only a few days.

Clinical Features. Much the most important early symptom is trismus — spasm of the masseter muscles which causes difficulty in opening the mouth and in masticating, hence the name, 'lockjaw'. This tonic rigidity spreads to involve the muscles of the face, neck and trunk. Contraction of the frontalis and the muscles at the angles of the mouth gives rise to the 'risus sardonicus'.

There is rigidity of the muscles of the neck and trunk of varying degree. The back is usually slightly arched and the board-like abdominal wall resembles that seen a few hours after the perforation of a peptic ulcer, but there is little or no tenderness.

In the more severe cases sudden violent spasms lasting for a few seconds to 3 or 4 minutes occur spontaneously or may be induced by stimuli such as moving the patient, knocking the bed or making a noise. These convulsions are painful, exhausting and of very serious significance, especially if they appear soon after the onset of symptoms. They gradually increase in frequency and severity for about one week and the patient may die from exhaustion, asphyxia or aspiration pneumonia. In less severe cases convulsions may not commence for about a week after the first sign of rigidity and in very mild infections they may never appear. Autonomic involvement may cause cardiovascular complications such as hypertension.

Rarely the only manifestation of the disease may be *local tetanus* — stiffness or spasm of the muscles near the infected wound — and the prognosis is good if treatment is commenced at this stage. If local tetanus follows wounds of the head and neck, the resulting irritation or paralysis of cranial nerves may resemble tuberculous meningitis or encephalitis and in cases of doubt the cerebrospinal fluid should be examined; in tetanus it is normal. Lumbar punctures should be avoided except in cases of real doubt.

The diagnosis is made on clinical grounds. It is rarely possible to isolate the infecting organism from the original locus of entry. Spasm of the masseters due to dental abscess, septic throat or other causes is painful, in contradistinction to tetanus. Conditions which can mimic tetanus include hysteria and phenothiazine overdosage.

Tetanus is still one of the major killers of adults, children and neonates in the tropics where the mortality rate can be nearly 100% in the newborn and around 40% in others.

Treatment. This should be begun as soon as possible. The essentials are as follows:

1. *Prevention of further Absorption of Toxin from the Wound.* A single intravenous injection of immune serum containing 1000–3000 i.u. of anti-

toxin should be given immediately the diagnosis is suspected. Whenever possible human antitetanus globulin should be used. The wound requires to be thoroughly cleaned and drained if there is evidence of necrotic tissue, foreign body or sepsis. Surgery should not be undertaken until 1 hour after the injection of antitoxin. Benzylpenicillin should be administered in doses of 300 mg 6 hourly.

2. *Control of Spasms.* The patient should lie in a quiet room with subdued lighting and with the bedclothes supported by a cradle. A notice should be put outside the door requesting silence. All necessary manipulation of the patient should be done gently and with due warning, for unexpected stimuli are particularly liable to provoke spasms. Expert nursing, preferably in an intensive care unit, is of supreme importance.

In most cases spasms may be controlled by diazepam. In more serious cases curare should be given, but only when facilities for assisted respiration are available. The aim of such measures is to control spasms which are terrifying, exhausting and occasionally fatal.

3. *General Measures.* Nutrition and fluids are of vital importance to enable the patient to survive an ordeal which may be prolonged. In milder cases it may be possible for the patient to swallow fluids or to tolerate a stomach tube left *in situ*. If oral treatment is impossible, intravenous feeding should be commenced without delay. Aspiration of bronchial secretions and antibiotic treatment of pneumonia may be necessary. It is vital that the patient should be repeatedly reassured that a complete recovery from this terrifying illness will be made.

Prevention. Active immunisation should be given (p. 41). Contaminated injuries must be treated by débridement. The immediate danger of tetanus can be greatly reduced by the injection of a dose of a long-acting preparation of penicillin followed by a 7-day course of oral penicillin. When the risk of tetanus is judged to be present, further protection may be given by a subcutaneous injection of 250 units of human tetanus antitoxin, and an intramuscular injection of toxoid which should be repeated 1 month and 6 months later. For those already protected only a booster dose of toxoid is required.

ANTHRAX

Anthrax is a disease of domestic animals which become infected by inhaling or ingesting spores of *Bacillus anthracis* passed in faeces. Grazing lands remain infective for years. In man anthrax is an occupational disease of farmers, butchers and dealers in hides, animal hair and wool and handlers of bone meal from endemic areas. Anthrax is endemic in primitive conditions, where skins are used as sleeping mats, for clothing or for carrying water, and where diseased cattle are eaten.

Pathology. The primary lesion in man may be in the skin, nares, pharynx, larynx, lung or intestinal tract, from any of which sites the infection may spread to lymph nodes and lead to a bacteraemia and infection of spleen, lungs, meninges and brain. The microscopical changes are those of haemorrhagic inflammation with areas of necrosis and interstitial oedema. There is a neutrophil leucocytosis of the blood and infiltration in the tissues without abscess formation.

Clinical Features. The incubation period is usually 1 to 3 days. When the infection is acquired from a skin or hide or from handling or slaughtering an animal, a cutaneous lesion develops on an exposed part of the body, commonly the face. It begins as an itching papule which enlarges and forms a vesicle filled with serosanguineous fluid surrounded by gross oedema — the 'malignant pustule'. The lesion is relatively painless and accompanied by slight enlargement of regional lymph nodes. The vesicle dries up to form a thick black 'eschar' surrounded by blebs. Occasionally there are multiple lesions. In endemic areas patients may exhibit only slight constitutional symptoms and little oedema but in nonimmune persons high fever, toxaemia and fatal septicaemia may develop.

When infected meat is eaten, an ulcer with much surrounding oedema may be seen in the pharynx or more commonly the infection causes a severe gastroenteritis which frequently terminates fatally. Older people may escape unscathed, presumably because of previously acquired immunity.

Those who acquire the infection by inhalation, 'wool-sorters' disease', may develop an acute laryngitis or a virulent haemorrhagic bronchopneumonia. Anthrax may also present as meningitis.

Diagnosis. The appearance of a cutaneous lesion and the environmental and occupational history should suggest the diagnosis. A stained smear of fluid taken from the edge of a malignant pustule demonstrates the organism, which may be confirmed in an atypical case by culture and pathogenicity tests in mice, rabbits or guinea-pigs. *B. anthracis* is also recoverable from laryngeal and pulmonary anthrax and from the CSF in meningitis. If a group of people who have feasted on an animal which has sickened and died are taken abruptly ill with fulminating gastroenteritis, anthrax should be suspected. *B. anthracis* may be cultured from the faeces.

Post-mortem examination is not to be lightly undertaken because of the risk of spreading the infection. Suspected animal products can be investigated by the use of anthrax immune serum.

Treatment and Prevention. Treatment is with penicillin. For mild cases 600 mg of procaine penicillin is given intramuscularly every 12 hours, but for severe cases up to 12 g of benzylpenicillin, intravenously may be necessary daily. The organism is also sensitive to sulphonamides, tetracycline, chloramphenicol and streptomycin.

The disease is controlled in cattle by slaughter and deep burial of the diseased animal and by vaccination of healthy animals at risk. Imports from endemic areas should be subject to strict control and sterilisation. Persons at risk through their occupation should be vaccinated.

MENINGOCOCCAL INFECTIONS

Infections caused by the Gram-negative diplococcus, *Neisseria meningitidis*, are serious and not infrequently fatal. In the Sudan savanna belt of Africa special climatic conditions predispose to annual outbreaks of 10 000 to 100 000 cases. Spread is by the airborne route and epidemics occur, particularly in cramped living conditions or when the climate is hot and dry. The organism invades through the nasopharynx producing bacteraemia and usually also pyogenic meningitis. The meningococcus is the commonest cause of bacterial meningitis in Britain where an increasing proportion of meningococci have become sulphonamide-resistant; fortunately, all strains remain sensitive to penicillin.

Clinical Features. The disease may present in a fulminating form with abrupt onset and prostration associated with shock and a widespread purpuric rash. The progression of the infection may be relentless even with specific therapy and the patient can die within hours of the first symptom. Disseminated intravascular coagulation (p. 548) can also occur in the course of meningococcal infections.

Meningitis (p. 637) is a much commoner presentation. Upper respiratory symptoms for 1 to 2 days are followed by fever, vomiting, headache and usually a petechial rash. This frequently starts with a few lesions on the buttocks spreading to involve limbs and trunk. The spots can remain petechial but occasionally large purpuric areas may form. The patient, often a child, is febrile and toxic, and signs of meningeal irritation are common. Convulsions may occur, especially in babies.

Chronic meningococcaemia is a rare condition in which the patient can be unwell for weeks or even months with recurrent fever, sweating, joint pains (p. 570) and transient rash.

Investigation. There is a polymorph leucocytosis. The CSF is turbid due to the presence of many neutrophils, the protein content is raised and the glucose reduced. Diagnosis is confirmed by culture of *N. meningitidis* from blood or CSF or by antigen detection (p. 638). Microscopic examination of CSF may show Gram-negative kidney-shaped diplococci in the polymorphs. However, in some cases, particularly if the patient has been treated with an antibiotic prior to admission to hospital, Gram stain and culture of CSF may be unhelpful and an early clinical diagnosis is therefore of the utmost importance in a disease which can be so rapidly fatal.

Treatment and Prevention. Benzylpenicillin, given initially by intravenous injection, is the antibiotic of choice for meningococcal infection. The dosage used in meningitis is given on page 638. Treatment may also be required for shock (p. 50) or for disseminated intravascular coagulation (p. 548).

Close contacts of patients with meningococcal infections, especially children, should be given a 5 day course of the tetracycline, minocycline, or 2 days of rifampicin. Vaccines are available for the prevention of disease caused by meningococci of Groups A and C but not Group B which is the commonest serogroup isolated in many countries including Britain.

WHOOPING COUGH

Whooping cough (pertussis) is a highly infectious disease caused by *Bordetella pertussis*. It is spread by droplet infection. Clinical diagnosis in the early and most infectious stage is virtually impossible so that epidemics occur. The incubation period is 7 to 14 days to the catarrhal stage. A quarantine period is not necessary. Whooping cough occurs at all ages but approximately 90% of cases are children under 5 years of age.

Clinical Features. The first stage of whooping cough consists of a highly infectious upper respiratory catarrh lasting about one week during which conjunctivitis, rhinitis and an unproductive cough are present. The distinctive paroxysmal stage follows and is characterised by severe bouts of coughing. The number of such paroxysms in 24 hours varies from an occasional attack to 40 or 50 and they are more severe at night. Each paroxysm consists of a succession of short sharp coughs, gathering in speed and duration and ending in a deep inspiration during which the characteristic whoop may be heard. It may be absent in older children and in adults because the air passages are so much wider. The last paroxysm of a series frequently ends with vomiting. The paroxysmal stage lasts from one to several weeks and is followed by the stage of convalescence during which the cough becomes less frequent and the sputum less tenacious. After the illness there is usually a lasting immunity.

The most important complications of whooping cough are pneumonia and segmental or lobar collapse which may be followed by bronchiectasis. Fits may be induced by cerebral anoxia. Subconjunctival or periorbital haemorrhage, ulceration of the frenum of the tongue, and prolapse of the rectum are relatively unimportant results of the stress of coughing. Neonates are highly susceptible and the mortality is greatest in the first year of life.

The diagnosis of whooping cough is very difficult in the catarrhal stage when the disease is most infectious. It can be confirmed in the laboratory by the isolation of *Bordetella pertussis* taken from the posterior wall of the nasopharynx on small swabs passed along the floor of the nose. Examination of the blood shows a lymphocytosis which, however, may not develop until the disease is well established. The diagnosis is easy in the paroxysmal stage when the whoop has developed, but by this time the danger of transmission of infection has largely disappeared.

Treatment. Erythromycin may reduce the severity of the infection if given during the catarrhal stage. Antibiotics are of no value if the spasmodic stage has been reached and they should not be used unless secondary infection occurs. The milder case need not be kept in bed, and is better out of doors. A cough suppressant such as methadone may be helpful in controlling the severity of paroxysms. When the illness is of long duration and vomiting is frequent, skilled nursing will be required to maintain nutrition, especially in infants and young children. Feeds are usually accepted and retained if they are given immediately after the vomiting which frequently follows a paroxysm of coughing.

Prevention. Active immunisation (p. 41) can occasionally cause convulsions or rarely neurological damage and adverse publicity regarding this had led to a marked decrease in the number of children who are immunised against the disease. However, the adverse effects of the vaccine have to be balanced against the risk of contracting a potentially serious disease, especially in young children. Many of the deaths from whooping cough occur in the first three months of life and hence very special care must be taken to avoid exposure of infants to the risk of contracting the disease.

BRUCELLOSIS

(Undulant Fever; Malta Fever; Abortus Fever)

Brucellosis is caused in Northern Europe by infection with *Brucella abortus* which is usually spread to man by the ingestion of raw milk from infected cattle. It is also an occupational hazard of veterinary surgeons, laboratory personnel, slaughterhouse workers and others. The infection has now been virtually eradicated from cattle in Britain. In Malta and many other countries the disease is frequently due to *Br. melitensis* and is transmitted by infected goats or sheep. In the U.S.A. and the Far East *Br. suis* acquired from pigs may be the causative organism. The incubation period is about 3 weeks.

Clinical Features. The disease commences as a blood stream infection and the clinical manifestations are gradual in onset and variable. The symptoms in order or frequency are sweating, weakness, headache, anorexia, pain in limbs and back, constipation, rigors, and joint pains. The spleen may be palpable. The temperature characteristically shows undulations, during which febrile and afebrile periods alternate over periods of a week or so. In other cases the pyrexia may be continuous and sweating profuse. Arthritis, spondylitis, bursitis and osteomyelitis may occur (p. 571). Untreated, the disease may last for a few days or continue for many months, and in the latter case the patient often becomes extremely depressed. Neutropenia and lymphocytosis usually occur in the more severe cases.

The diagnosis of brucellosis is most readily confirmed by agglutination and complement-fixation tests. Blood culture in special media should be attempted but it is frequently negative in *Br. abortus* infections in man. Other conditions causing prolonged fever must be considered in differential diagnosis (p. 39).

Treatment and Prevention. Tetracycline 500 mg 6 hourly or co-trimoxazole 2 tablets twice a day for 21 days is usually effective. The spread of brucellosis by milk is prevented by pasteurisation or boiling. Veterinary surgeons and others handling infected animals need to exercise scrupulous hygiene.

PLAGUE

Plague has been a recurrent scourge of man from ancient times and earned the name of the Black Death. Now it is limited to rodents in the wild with occasional sporadic human cases or local outbreaks. The causative organism, *Yersinia pseudotuberculosis subsp. pestis*, is a small Gram-negative bacillus. It is spread between rodents by their fleas and if domestic rats become infected then infected fleas leaving a dead rat may bite and infect man. In the late stages of human plague *Y. pestis* may be expectorated and inter-human spread by droplets, 'pneumonic plague', may result. This can also be caused by the accidental inhalation of a laboratory culture or by hunters inhaling dust containing viable organisms from infected wild rodents or fleas. Recent outbreaks have predominantly been in Vietnam and East Africa with sporadic cases in U.S.A. and elsewhere.

Pathology. Rarely a vesicle with surrounding cellulitis is evident at the site of the flea-bite. The more usual initial lesion is acute haemorrhagic inflammation in and around the lymph nodes regional to the site of entry of the organisms. Disseminated intravascular coagulation causes subpericardial and meningeal haemorrhages. There may be haemorrhagic foci of consolidation in the lungs, enlargement of lymph nodes and spleen and multiple small necrotic foci in the liver. In some severe cases there may be little or no swelling of regional lymph nodes; these are the cases clinically presenting as 'septicaemic plague'.

In deaths from 'pneumonic plague' the findings are those of acute congestion in one or more lobes of the lungs and evidence of disseminated intravascular coagulation. Patients suffering from pneumonic plague treated with antibiotics may develop pulmonary abscesses. *Y. pestis* are numerous in all affected organs. Post mortem examination is dangerous.

Clinical Features. The incubation period is short, 3 to 6 days, but less in pneumonic plague.

Bubonic Plague. The onset is usually sudden with a rigor, high fever, dry skin and severe headache. Soon aching and then also swelling at the site of the affected lymph nodes begin. The most common site of the bubo, made up of the swollen lymph nodes and surrounding tissue, is one groin. Some cases are relatively mild but in the majority signs of toxaemia rapidly increase, with a rapid pulse, dilated heart and mental confusion. The spleen is usually palpable.

Septicaemic Plague. Those not exhibiting a bubo usually deteriorate rapidly. Pneumonia and expectoration of blood-stained sputum containing *Y. pestis* may complicate bubonic or septicaemic plague.

Pneumonic Plague. The onset is very sudden

with cough and dyspnoea. The patient soon expectorates copious blood-stained frothy, highly infective sputum, becomes cyanosed and rapidly deteriorates. Radiographs of the lung show a lobar opacity.

Diagnosis. A report of deaths among rats should alert suspicion of an outbreak. Early diagnosis is urgent. An aspirate from a bubo, sputum, or the buffy coat is used to make a smear which is stained with methylene blue to show the characteristic organism. For confirmation the aspirate or blood can be cultured. A leucocytosis helps to distinguish septicaemic plague from typhoid fever. Plague is notifiable under the International Health Regulations.

Treatment. If the diagnosis is suspected on clinical and epidemiological grounds, treatment should be started as soon as, or even before, samples have been collected for laboratory diagnosis. Streptomycin should be given by intramuscular or intravenous injection every 6 or 12 hours, at a daily dose of 30 mg/kg for 7 days. Tetracycline, 10 mg/kg every 6 hours orally or intravenously, is also given for 14 days.

Treatment may also be needed for acute circulatory failure, disseminated intravascular coagulation or hypoxia.

Prevention. Prophylaxis against bubonic and septicaemic plague largely depends on preventing biting by fleas carrying plague. Rats should be controlled. Powders containing 1·5% Dieldrin or 2% Aldrin applied to floors and blown into rat holes kill all the fleas and remain active for 9 to 12 weeks.

For personal protection there are two vaccines, the killed vaccine given in two or three doses, and the attenuated requiring one dose only. Both vaccines cause fever and do not protect against pneumonic plague. Booster doses are required after 3 to 6 months. Patients are isolated and attendants must wear gowns, masks and gloves. Samples are handled carefully, wearing gloves. Contacts should be protected by tetracycline 2 g daily, or a sulphonamide such as sulphadimidine 3 to 6 g daily for a week.

TULARAEMIA

Tularaemia is an infection due to *Francisella tularensis* transmitted to mammals and birds by the bites of infected blood-sucking flies and ticks. It is often seasonal. Man may be accidentally infected in a laboratory or while skinning infected wild rabbits or hares. In Norway lemmings are another source. The micro-organisms enter through dermal abrasions, the conjunctiva or mouth. Contaminated water, infected meat and the bites of infected arthropods are less common sources of human infection.

The disease is found in the Americas, Japan, the USSR, and most European countries.

Pathological and Clinical Features. Focal areas of necrosis occur especially in lymph nodes, spleen, liver, kidneys and lungs. There may be cutaneous, oral or ophthalmic lesions when infection is by these routes. The commonest presentation is of a papule at the site of inoculation, which becomes swollen and painful and suppurates, causing an ulcer up to 2 cm in diameter. Regional lymph nodes become tender, enlarged and may suppurate. There may be a systemic illness with fever, often prolonged. Sometimes the conjunctiva is the site of entry, and is inflamed. Sometimes the presentation is only glandular.

The rarest, but most severe form of the disease is septicaemia. There is a sudden onset of high fever, with malaise, prostration, aching limbs, vomiting, diarrhoea and mental confusion. Pneumonia, pleurisy and pericarditis are common complications.

The organism may be isolated by repeated blood culture on special media or guinea-pig inoculation. An intradermal test using killed *F. tularensis* may be positive as early as the third day and positive agglutination and complement-fixation tests after 10 to 12 days.

Treatment and Prevention. Intramuscular streptomycin 1 g daily for 10–14 days is better than tetracycline 250 mg 6 hourly for 2 weeks. Masks should be worn in the laboratory and gloves should be used when skinning rabbits and hares in endemic areas. Adequate cooking renders infected meat safe for eating.

MELIOIDOSIS

Melioidosis is caused by *Pseudomonas pseudomallei*, a micro-organism closely related to *Ps. mallei*, the cause of glanders, which is a rare disease of horses and grooms. *Ps. pseudomallei* is a saphrophyte found in puddles following recent rain. Infection is through abrasions of the skin. Diabetics and patients with severe burns are particularly susceptible.

The disease is commonest in the Far East and S.E. Asia and occurs rarely in India, Africa, Australia and America.

Pathological and Clinical Features. A bacteraemia is followed by the formation of abscesses in the lungs, liver and spleen. There is high fever, prostration and signs of pneumonia, with enlargement of the liver and spleen and sometimes dysenteric symptoms. A chest radiograph resembles that of acute caseous tuberculosis. In more chronic forms multiple abscesses also recur in subcutaneous tissue and bone. Culture of blood, sputum or pus may yield *Ps. pseudomallei*. Except in fulminating infections, antibodies may be detected by indirect haemagglutination, direct agglutination, and complement-fixation tests.

Treatment. In acute cases prompt treatment, without waiting for cultural confirmation, with tetracycline 3 g daily and chloramphenicol 3 g daily, in divided doses, may be life-saving. Treatment is maintained for weeks or months until cavities have healed.

SALMONELLA INFECTIONS

There are more than 1500 Salmonella serotypes. The large majority originates in animals, especially poultry, and is transmitted to man either directly or in food. The exception is *Salmonella typhi* which invariably has a human source.

Salmonellae can cause a number of different conditions namely:

1. Typhoid and paratyphoid fevers.
2. Food poisoning producing gastroenteritis, sometimes associated with septicaemia which may lead to metastatic abscess formation or endocarditis.
3. An asymptomatic carrier state which may follow 1. or 2.

Typhoid and Paratyphoid (Enteric) Fevers

In many countries where sanitation is primitive, typhoid and paratyphoid fevers, which are transmitted by the faecal-oral route, are an important cause of illness. Elsewhere they are relatively rare. Nevertheless, outbreaks occur from time to time and the infection may be contracted by persons travelling abroad.

Aetiology. The enteric fevers are caused by infection with *S. typhi* and *paratyphi* which are specific human pathogens. Other members of the Salmonella group, many of which cause infection in animals, produce disease in man ranging from mild food poisoning to more serious infection which may simulate many of the features of paratyphoid fever including bacteraemia.

Typhoid and paratyphoid infections have a world-wide distribution and occur endemically wherever sanitation is poor and the water supply is liable to be contaminated by human excreta. In Britain spread is usually by carriers, often food handlers, through the contamination of food, milk or water; infected shell fish are occasionally responsible for an outbreak. In carriers the bacilli may live in the gallbladder for months or years after clinical recovery and pass intermittently in the stools and less commonly in the urine.

Pathogenesis. After a few days of bacteraemia, the bacilli localise mainly in the lymphoid tissue of the small intestine. The typical lesion is in the Peyer's patches and follicles. These swell at first, then ulcerate and ultimately heal, but during this sequence they may perforate or bleed.

The incubation period of typhoid fever is about 10 to 14 days; that of paratyphoid is somewhat shorter. Quarantine is not necessary, but contacts are kept under surveillance for three weeks.

Clinical Features. *Typhoid Fever.* The onset may be insidious. The temperature rises in a stepladder fashion for 4 or 5 days. There is malaise, with increasing headache, drowsiness and aching in the limbs. Cough and epistaxis are not uncommon; constipation may be present although in children diarrhoea and vomiting may be prominent early in the illness. The pulse is often slower than would be expected from the height of the temperature.

At the end of the first week the typical rash may appear on the upper abdomen and on the back as sparse slightly raised, rose-red spots which fade on pressure. It is usually not visible on non-white skin. About the seventh to tenth day of illness the spleen becomes palpable. Often about this time constipation is succeeded by diarrhoea and generalised abdominal distension with tenderness in the right iliac fossa. Bronchitis may develop and there may be delirium.

By the end of the second week the patient may be profoundly ill unless the disease is modified by antibiotic treatment. In the third week toxaemia increases and the patient may pass into coma and die. The prognosis may worsen at this stage due to haemorrhage from or perforation of the ulcerated Peyer's patches. In those who recover the temperature falls by lysis, the appetite returns, distension disappears, and strength improves. After an initial recovery recrudescence of the disease may occur.

Paratyphoid Fever. The most common variety in Britain is due to *S. paratyphi B*. The course tends to be shorter and milder than that of typhoid fever but the onset is often more abrupt with acute enteritis. The rash may be more abundant and the intestinal complications less frequent.

Complications. Haemorrhage and perforation may occur at the end of the second week or during the third week of the illness. The bleeding may be sudden and severe. The features of shock suggesting that a haemorrhage has occurred are described on page 297. Perforation usually occurs from ulcers near the ileocaecal valve. Additional complications may involve almost any viscus or system as a result of the septicaemia which is present during the first week. Pneumonia, thrombophlebitis, myocarditis, myositis, arthritis, periostitis, osteomyelitis, meningitis and cholecystitis are all recognised complications.

Investigation. In the first week of the disease the diagnosis may be difficult as in this invasive stage with bacteraemia the symptoms are those of a generalised infection without localising features. A white blood count may be helpful as there is typically a leucopenia. In a suspected case, blood culture is the most important diagnostic method, particularly during the first week of the disease. During this period the organism may not grow from the stool and urine. The faeces will contain the organism more frequently during the second and third weeks. Agglutinating antibodies to the causative organisms form after the second week of the disease. The *Widal reaction* is a serological test for the detection of these antibodies and can be useful in supporting a clinical diagnosis of enteric fever particularly when cultures are negative.

Treatment. The patient should be treated in bed and preferably in isolation. A high standard of nursing is required with special attention to the maintenance of nutrition and fluid intake, care of the mouth and the prevention of pressure sores. Scrupulous precautions must be taken against the spread of infection by the provision of special gowns and adequate washing facilities by the bedside, and sterilisation by disinfectant of excreta and of articles used by the patient.

Chloramphenicol should be given for 14 days initially in a dose of 1 g t.i.d. reducing to 500 mg 6 hourly. Co-trimoxazole (or amoxycillin) is an alternative to chloramphenicol in typhoid fever and is the drug of choice for paratyphoid fever. Pyrexia may persist for up to 5 days after the start of specific therapy. Even with effective chemotherapy there is still a danger of complications, of recrudescence of the disease and of the development of a carrier state. For the first few days a semifluid diet should be given, followed by a low roughage diet. A second course of chemotherapy must be given in the event of a relapse and this usually produces good results. The chronic carrier should be treated for several weeks with co-trimoxazole, as chloramphenicol has proved ineffective; in some cases cholecystectomy may be necessary.

The treatment of haemorrhage is described on page 298. Prior to the introduction of chloramphenicol the treatment of perforation was by immediate recourse to surgery, which carried a high mortality in the seriously ill. Such patients can be treated conservatively while chloramphenicol is continued, but advice from a surgeon should be sought as laparotomy may be indicated.

The patient should be considered as infective until six consecutive stools and urines are found to be negative on culture.

Prevention. Those who propose to travel to or live in countries where enteric infections are endemic should be inoculated with the monovalent typhoid vaccine (p. 807).

Food Poisoning

Food poisoning includes a number of disorders, presenting with diarrhoea and vomiting, due to acute gastroenteritis developing up to 48 hours after the consumption of food or drink. It is customary not to include under this term the enteric fevers, dysenteries (p. 754) and cholera (p. 755) which are also spread by infected food and drink. In contrast to enteric fever which is relatively uncommon and cholera which has been almost unknown in Britain for the past 100 years, there is an increase in the reported incidence of bacterial food poisoning.

Food poisoning may also be due to intestinal allergy, e.g. to shell fish, or to children eating unripe fruit or other unsuitable foods. Rarely a poisonous substance may be eaten, e.g. *Amanita phalloides*, in mistake for a mushroom, or a chemical poison in food may be unwittingly consumed, an extreme example being arsenic administered murderously in the tradition of the Borgias. Food which has been placed in a container previously used for holding a chemical poison may be contaminated. Placing acid fruit juices in cheap enamel or zinc vessels may result in the liberation of antimony or zinc.

Aetiology. Bacterial food poisoning is usually divided into the infective and toxic types.

INFECTIVE TYPE. The organisms mainly responsible are the Salmonella group and *Campylobacter jejuni*. Certain birds, rodents, cattle and less frequently reptiles, such as pet tortoises, are sources of Salmonellae. The domestic fowl is one of the commonest sources and modern methods of poultry husbandry involving battery-rearing and deep-freezing of carcasses encourage the spread and transmission of infection.

Salmonella typhimurium causes at least three-quarters of the cases of food poisoning of the 'infective' type in Britain. Food may be contaminated with infected excreta of mice or rats, or the bacteria may be transferred by flies or by human carriers employed in the handling of food. The size of the infecting dose of bacteria bears a close relationship to the speed of onset of symptoms and to the severity of the illness. This indicates the dangers of bacterial multiplication which may take place when food is contaminated and there-after remains warm for many hours or days. The types of food which are particularly likely to be affected are twice-cooked meat dishes, stews, soups, milk and synthetic cream. The danger of food poisoning is greatly reduced if such foods are kept in a refrigerator. Ducks tend to be carriers of salmonella organisms in the oviduct and alimentary tract, and ducks' eggs are not suitable for the preparation of lightly cooked foods. Hens' eggs are rarely affected.

Enterocolitis caused by *Campylobacter jejuni* is now recognised as a very common form of food poisoning. Sources of this infection include poultry, dogs and milk.

Food poisoning due to *Bacillus cereus* is a hazard of eating rice which has been cooked and then consumed at a later date following re-heating. Infective gastroenteritis in adults may also be caused by viruses such as the rotavirus which is more commonly responsible for infantile gastroenteritis.

TOXIN TYPE. Such poisoning is most commonly caused by the enterotoxin of *Staph. aureus*. This frequently originates from a food handler suffering from a septic lesion. Incubation at a suitable temperature leads to growth of the organism and production of toxin which is relatively heat resistant and may not be destroyed by cooking. Strains of *Clostridium welchii*, many of them relatively resistant to heat, may contaminate certain foods, particularly meat. Pre-cooking of stews and pies may not destroy all the spores and the keeping of such food will lead to the formation of heat-stable toxins which can give rise to gastroenteritis, sometimes severe.

Outbreaks of food poisoning affecting large numbers of persons occur in canteens, restaurants, hospitals and other institutions.

Clinical Features. The simultaneous occurrence of symptoms in more than one member of a household or institution often simplifies diagnosis. The incubation period is a useful pointer to the aetiology. If vomiting starts within 30 minutes of the ingestion of suspected food, it is likely to be due to a chemical poison; if it arises 12 to 48 hours later, it is probably due to a salmonella or campylobacter infection. The incubation periods of staphylococcal and clostridial food poisoning are usually intermediate between these extremes being from 1 to 12 hours.

The principal symptoms are nausea, vomiting, diarrhoea and abdominal colic. Staphylococcal food poisoning may be associated only with vomiting while diarrhoea and abdominal pain are more prominent with *Cl. welchii* toxins. In severe cases there may be prostration, collapse and dehydration. In the chemical and toxin types of food poisoning the onset tends to be sudden and severe and the patient may rapidly become shocked. Recovery however usually occurs within 24 hours. In the infective type, symptoms develop more slowly and there is usually pyrexia and toxicity. The patient may be ill for several days. The stools are watery and offensive, and may contain blood and some mucus, in contrast to bacillary dysentery where there is also pus. Salmonella septicaemia may be associated with osteomyelitis, septic arthritis, endocarditis or meningitis.

Severe abdominal pain and blood in the stool are common in campylobacter infections. Rarely, septicaemia may complicate gastroenteritis, and endocarditis has been reported. Campylobacter enteritis may be confused with ulcerative colitis and rectal biopsies can appear similar in both diseases.

Botulism is a rare form of bacterial food poisoning due to the ingestion of one of the most potent poisons known to man, namely the toxin produced by *Cl. botulinum*. Imperfectly treated tinned food or preserved fish may be contaminated with the organism and be the source of the toxin. The clinical features differ from all other types of bacterial food poisoning and consist chiefly of vomiting and pareses of skeletal, ocular, pharyngeal and respiratory muscles. The mortality rate can be high.

Investigation. A specimen of the patient's stool or vomit together with the suspected food, if available, should be sent for culture. Campylobacter and organisms of the salmonella group can usually be readily isolated. In more severe cases blood should be sent for culture. Notification of salmonella infection and other types of food poisoning is compulsory in Britain.

Treatment. Most cases are mild and can be treated at home. Solid food should be withheld and the patient instructed to take fluids only. A pinch of salt added to one pint of water flavoured with a small quantity of fruit juice provides a satisfactory oral replacement solution. Patients who are severely ill or dehydrated require intravenous fluid therapy (Table 19.2 p. 757).

Symptoms normally pass off spontaneously in a day or two. When acute symptoms cease, a semi-fluid low-roughage diet may be taken containing bread, butter, eggs, fish, soft puddings and jellies. Codeine phosphate or loperamide is useful in controlling diarrhoea.

Antibiotics should not be given for acute diarrhoea and vomiting as they are ineffective and frequently exacerbate symptoms. If salmonella bacteraemia is suspected or confirmed, ampicillin, 1 g every six hours should be given by intramuscular or intravenous injection. Co-trimoxazole is a satisfactory alternative. If there is associated septicaemia or endocarditis, gentamicin or chloramphenicol is indicated. Campylobacter enteritis is treated with erythromycin.

If the poisoning is thought to be due to a chemical or a poisonous food, the patient's stomach should be washed out with tepid water, using the technique described on page 705 and the stomach contents kept for analysis.

Prevention. In Salmonella food poisoning the carrier state persists on the average for about 14 days after infection but may be much longer. A reduction in the high incidence of food poisoning can best be achieved by improving the standards of personal hygiene, especially in those handling food, and by stressing the importance of hand-washing after using the lavatory. Increasing facilities for low temperature storage of food which has to be kept for some hours or days before being consumed is of the greatest importance. It is essential to keep frozen poultry at room temperature for at least eight hours before cooking or pathogens at the centre may survive unharmed.

DYSENTERY

Dysentery is an acute inflammation of the large intestine characterised by diarrhoea with blood and mucus in stools. Its causes are bacillary or protozoal infection. Amoebic dysentery is described on page 773.

Bacillary Dysentery

The bacilli belong to the genus *Shigella* of which there are three main pathogenic groups, *dysenteriae*, *flexneri* and *sonnei* the first two having numerous serotypes. In Britain the majority of cases of bacillary dysentery are caused by *Shigella sonnei* although in recent years there has been a significant increase in imported infections caused by *Sh. flexneri* whereas sonnei dysentery has decreased.

Epidemiology. Bacillary dysentery is endemic all over the world. It occurs in epidemic form wherever there is a crowded population with poor sanitation, and thus has been a constant accompaniment of wars and natural catastrophes. Spread may occur by contaminated food or flies but contact through unwashed hands after defecation is by far the most important factor. Hence the modern provision of plenty of handbasins, disposable towels and hot air driers goes a long way towards the prevention of the faecal-oral spread of disease. Outbreaks are not uncommon in mental hospitals, residential schools and other closed institutions. The disease is notifiable in Britain.

Pathology. There is generalised inflammation of the large bowel which may extend to involve the lower part of the small intestine. Sigmoidoscopy shows that the mucosa is red and swollen, the submucous veins are obscured and mucopus is seen on the surface. Bleeding points appear readily at the touch of the endoscope. Ulcers may form.

Clinical Features. There is great variation in severity. Sonne infections may be so mild as to escape detection and the patient remains ambulant with a few loose stools and perhaps a little colic. Flexner infections are usually more severe while those due to dysenteriae may be fulminating and cause death within 48 hours.

In a moderately severe illness, the patient complains of diarrhoea, colicky hypogastric pain and tenesmus. The stools are usually small, and after the first few evacuations, contain blood and purulent exudate with little faecal material. There is frequently fever, with dehydration and weakness if the diarrhoea persists. On physical examination there will be tenderness over the colon more easily elicited in the left iliac fossa. In sonne infection the patient may develop a febrile illness and diarrhoea may be mild or even absent; there is usually some headache and muscular aching. Arthritis or iritis may occasionally complicate bacillary dysentery as in Reiter's disease (p. 565).

Diagnosis depends on culture of faeces. Amoebic infections usually have a less acute onset than bacillary dysentery.

Treatment and Prevention. Diarrhoea may be controlled by codeine or loperamide. A fluid or semifluid low-roughage diet should be given depending on the severity of the diarrhoea but if this is severe, it will be necessary to replace the water and electrolyte loss by intravenous therapy.

Bacillary dysentery is usually a self-limiting disease and antibiotics or sulphonamides are not indicated in most cases. In severe infections, especially those caused by dysenteriae or flexner strains, ampicillin 500 mg 6 hourly or co-trimoxazole two tablets twice daily should be given. In many countries including Britain the majority of shigellae are now sulphonamide-resistant.

The prevention of faecal contamination of food and milk, the isolation of patients, and the identification of carriers, are methods which are theoretically important but may be difficult to apply except in limited outbreaks. Hand-washing is very important.

CHOLERA

Cholera is a severe acute gastrointestinal infection, caused by *Vibrio cholerae*. Its home is in the valleys of the Ganges and other great rivers of the Far East, where high humidity and population density have maintained the disease. In these valleys devastating epidemics have commenced, often following large religious festivals, and pandemics have spread throughout Asia and Europe even to North America. The present, seventh, pandemic began in 1961. Good hygiene has prevented its spread in Europe, but cholera is present in the Near East and Africa, where it has for the first time become endemic. The biotype of *V. cholerae*, El Tor, that is responsible for the pandemic, has replaced the classical vibrio. The organism is passed in stools, or vomit, of patients with cholera and the very much larger number of subclinical cases, who excrete it for a few days. More chronic carriage is rare. The organism survives up to 2 weeks in fresh water and 8 weeks in salt water. Transmission is normally through infected drinking water, though shellfish and contamination of food by flies and hands also occurs.

Pathology. Cholera vibrios multiply in the lumen of the small bowel and are noninvasive. They secrete a powerful exotoxin (enterotoxin) which stimulates the adenyl cyclase-adenosine monophosphate pathway of the mucosa, resulting in an outpouring of normal alkaline, small bowel fluid. Severe dehydration follows rapidly even though absorption of fluid by the bowel is hardly impaired. There may be acidosis and depletion of sodium and potassium with attendant complications, of which renal failure is the most important.

Clinical Features. After an incubation period of a few hours to 5 days severe diarrhoea without pain or colic, followed by vomiting, begins suddenly. Fluid gushes effortlessly from the bowel and stomach. After the faecal contents of the gut have been evacuated the typical 'rice-water' material is passed. This consists of clear fluid with flecks of mucus. In severe cases an enormous quantity of fluid and electrolytes is rapidly lost. This soon leads to intense dehydration with agonising muscular cramps. The skin becomes cold, clammy and wrinkled and the eyes sunken. The blood pressure falls, the pulse becomes imperceptible, and the urine output falls. The patient, however, usually remains mentally clear. Unless fluid and electrolytes are replaced the patient may die from acute circulatory failure within a few hours. With proper treatment, however, improvements is rapid. Rarely anuria persists and may lead to death.

Although this is the classical picture of cholera, the majority of infections cause only a mild illness with slight diarrhoea. Occasionally a very intense illness, 'cholera sicca', occurs in which the patient is overwhelmed by the infection and the rapid loss of fluid into the dilated bowel kills the patient before typical gastrointestinal symptoms appear.

In children under 12 years the mortality rate is higher (15 to 17%) than in adults (4 to 6%). Pulmonary oedema, febrile reactions to therapy, pyrexial convulsions and encephalopathy, tetany, meteorism, hypoglycaemia, hypernatraemia, aci-dosis and water retention and frequently malnutrition are the adverse factors in paediatric practice.

Diagnosis. During a cholera epidemic clinical diagnosis is usually easy. In other situations, it is important to confirm the diagnosis bacteriologically so that an outbreak may be brought rapidly under control. *V. cholerae* has a characteristic movement that can be seen under the microscope. Culture of the stool or a rectal swab is used to isolate and identify the organism. Other diseases such as acute bacillary dysentery, viral enteritis, *P. falciparum* malaria, food poisoning, including *Vibrio parahaemolyticus* infections from eating infected shell fish and certain chemical poisons may produce symptoms like those of cholera. Cholera is notifiable under the International Health Regulations.

Treatment. The chief aim in treatment is to maintain the circulation by replacement of water and electrolytes; the earlier this is started, the better the prognosis. A quick clinical assessment of the state of dehydration is made from the appearance of the patient, the pulse, blood pressure and skin turgor. In severe cases or when there is vomiting, fluids are given intravenously. A large needle is plunged into a large vein (the femoral vein can always be quickly found) and the fluid is run in as fast as possible until pulse and blood pressure return. The rest of the estimated deficit is replaced more slowly. If intravenous fluids or apparatus are unavailable, a nasogastric tube is passed and fluid is poured in remorselessly.

Vomiting usually stops once the patient is rehydrated and fluid should then be given orally every hour. Patients can be made to drink up to 500 ml hourly. The quantity of fluid required is calculated every 8 hours from the output of urine, stool, vomit and estimated insensible loss which may be as much as 5 litres in 24 hours in a hot humid climate. Total fluid requirements can be in excess of 50 litres over a period of 2 to 5 days. Accurate records are essential and are greatly facilitated by the use of a 'cholera cot' which has a reinforced hole under the patient's buttocks beneath which a graded bucket is placed. The ideal solutions are shown in Table 19.2.

Other satisfactory fluids include Ringer lactate

Table 19.2 Ideal solutions for treatment of cholera.

Intravenous			Oral	
	g/l	mmol/l		g/l
Sodium chloride	5	Na 133	Commercial salt	4·2
		Cl 98	(NaCl)	
Potassium chloride	1	K 98	Potassium chloride	1·8
		Cl 98	or citrate	2·7
Sodium bicarbonate	4	HCO₃ 48	Sodium bicarbonate	4
			Glucose	20

(B.P.) or Hartman's solution and Darrow's solution, in which case supplements of potassium are given as 10 mmol/l of intravenous fluid or 2–4 g potassium chloride or citrate three times daily by mouth. Isotonic saline is better than nothing but every 2 litres should be alternated with 1 litre of isotonic sodium lactate (18·7 g/l) or bicarbonate (14 g/l) and added potassium. Acetate is a satisfactory substitute for bicarbonate, and more stable. The presence of glucose in the oral fluid has been shown to promote electrolyte absorption. Chlorpromazine, 50 mg 6 hourly, reduces intestinal secretion and fluid loss.

The use of correct fluids for replacement has done away with the need for estimation of plasma electrolytes or specific gravity. In children, the elderly, the anaemic and those with underlying heart disease overvigorous intravenous rehydration readily causes pulmonary oedema. Children require most careful attention to fluid balance. Ringer lactate is the fluid of choice and it is important that the oral fluids contain glucose. Renal failure is managed in the usual way (p. 401).

Three days' treatment with tetracycline 250 mg 6 hourly or co-trimoxazole one tablet daily reduces the duration of excretion of vibrios and the total volume of fluid needed for replacement.

Prevention and Control. Personal prophylaxis means strict personal hygiene. Water for drinking should come from a clean piped supply or be boiled. Flies must not be allowed access to food. Vaccination with a killed suspension of *V. cholerae*, given in two doses of 0·5 and 1·0 ml 1 to 4 weeks apart may provide some protection (p. 807).

In an epidemic, control of water sources and of population movement and public education are most important. Mass vaccination with a single dose of vaccine and mass treatment with tetracycline are valuable. Disinfection of infective discharges and soiled clothing, the therapeutic use of tetracycline and scrupulous hand washing by medical attendants reduces the danger of spread from treatment centres.

BARTONELLOSIS
(Carrión's Disease, Oroya Fever, Verruga Peruana)

This disease is caused by *Bartonella bacilliformis*, transmitted by sandflies. It is prevalent in narrow hot valleys on the western slopes of the Andes at heights between 2000 and 10 000 ft (600–300 m), in Peru, Ecuador, Bolivia, Colombia and Chile.

Clinical Features. After an incubation period of 14 to 21 days fever and haemolysis develop suddenly, accompanied by pains in muscles and joints, nausea, vomiting and diarrhoea, delirium or coma. The spleen and liver are enlarged and tender. Bartonellae are present in large numbers in the erythrocytes and also in the endothelial cells lining small blood vessels. Untreated the mortality is over 90%. Secondary infection by salmonellae is a frequent cause of death.

The cutaneous form, verruga peruana, usually follows 30 to 40 days later with crops of cherry-red haemangioma-like cutaneous nodules 2 to 10 mm in diameter. They are distributed peripherally on the head and limbs and occasionally on the mucosa of the mouth and pharynx and heal in 2 to 3 months.

The diagnosis is confirmed by the demonstration of bartonellae in the erythrocytes, blood cultures or skin lesions.

Treatment and Prevention. In the early febrile stage penicillin, streptomycin or tetracycline for 5 days give good results. Blood transfusions, fluids and electrolytes may be urgently required. The use of insecticides, insect repellants and sleeping under fine mesh nets are advisable for personal protection.

LEPROSY

Leprosy is the commonest cause of peripheral neuritis in the world. It is a chronic granulomatous disease caused by *Mycobacterium leprae*, an acid-and alcohol-fast bacillus that has a very slow multiplication time of 12–14 days. It is one of the most seriously disabling and economically important diseases of the world and it is estimated that 20 million people are affected. *Myco. leprae* will grow in mice and the armadillo, but not in artificial media. Local multiplication of the organism in the foot-pads of mice is a most useful technique for demonstrating the identity and viability of *Myco. leprae* and the existence of drug-resistant strains, for the screening of drugs and for studying vaccines. The most important mode of spread of *Myco. leprae* is by droplets from the sneezes of lepromatous patients whose nasal mucosa is heavily infected. It is not certain whether the organism enters by inhalation or through the skin. The incubation period is usually between 2 and 5 years.

The disease is common is tropical Asia, the Far East, tropical Africa, Central and South America, and in some Pacific Islands. It is still endemic in southern Europe, North Africa and the Middle East.

Pathology. The organisms show a predilection for peripheral nerves, skin and mucosa of the upper respiratory tract. The response of the host to their presence varies widely. The early infection, usually transient and self-healing, is called '*indeterminate*'. The histological appearances are non-specific. If the infection does not heal it develops into one of the determinate types, whose features reflect the balance between the host cell-mediated immune response and bacillary multiplication.

In *tuberculoid leprosy* there is a marked tuberculoid response, indicative of vigorous cell-mediated immunity, around nerves, sweat glands and hair follicles. Caseation does not occur except occasionally in a nerve. Organisms are scanty, and found mainly in the vicinity of terminal nerve endings in the dermis. They are seen only after prolonged search or by the use of concentration techniques. Tuberculoid leprosy is probably non-infective.

In *lepromatous leprosy*, the infective form of the disease, there is no cell-mediated immune response to *Myco. leprae*. Organisms are present in great abundance in the dermis, eventually replacing the normal architecture. They are mainly grouped in 'globi', which are large macrophages, often showing foamy degeneration, containing 50 or more organisms, and found in nerve tissue, the erectores pilorum muscles and the endothelial cells of blood vessels but rarely in the cells of the epidermis itself. They are carried in the blood stream to the peripheral nerves, eye, and mucosa of the nose and upper respiratory tract, the testes and small muscles and bones of the hands, feet and face, in which they multiply. Nephritis and amyloidosis are common late complications.

Borderline or Dimorphous Leprosy. Between these two 'polar' types of leprosy, there is a spectrum of manifestations grouped under the terms 'borderline' or 'dimorphous'. The host reaction varies from the near-lepromatous to the near-tuberculoid. *Myco. leprae* are demonstrable in varying numbers. In the centre of the spectrum the disease is unstable. Immunity may diminish (downgrading) in untreated patients, especially in pregnancy or other times of stress and the disease becomes more lepromatous. Alternatively immunity may increase (upgrading or reversal), especially in response to successful chemotherapy, and the disease becomes more tuberculoid.

Lepromin Test. Lepromin is a suspension of dead *Myco. leprae*. The lepromin test is performed like the tuberculin test (p. 232), but is read after 4 weeks. The result indicates the degree of cellular hypersensitivity in a patient. Positive reactions are obtained in tuberculoid leprosy, negative responses in lepromatous leprosy and negative or weak positive responses in borderline leprosy. This test is of no value in establishing the diagnosis of leprosy since positive results are also found in many normal people, but it is useful in helping to classify the disease, and so determine treatment and prognosis.

Lepra Reactions. Any determinate form of leprosy may undergo an acute exacerbation or *reaction* which is caused by an episode of acute allergic inflammation. In lepromatous disease the reaction, *lepra reaction type 2*, is due to immune complex mediated vasculitis. In borderline and tuberculoid disease the reaction, *lepra reaction type 1*, is due to a sudden increase in cellular hypersensitivity. Borderline reactions are often associated with upgrading or downgrading.

Leprosy damages the body in three main ways:

1. Peripheral neuritis leads to loss of sensory, motor and autonomic functions. Sensory loss permits trauma from pressure, friction, burns and cuts, the effects of which are intensified if there are abnormal pressures from the contractures following muscular paralysis. Autonomic nerve damage causes dry skin which cracks easily and heals slowly. Secondary bacterial infection in an anaesthetic, unprotected limb leads to cellulitis, osteomyelitis and gross tissue destruction which produces the deformities with which the disease is still, so unnecessarily, associated. Paralyses result in claw hand and dropped foot from damage respectively to the ulnar and peroneal nerves. A combination of fifth and seventh cranial nerve damage exposes an anaesthetic cornea to trauma and sepsis, so the eye is easily blinded.

2. In lepromatous leprosy bacillary growth insidiously damages the infiltrated organs and renders them liable to type 2 lepra reactions. Bones of hands and feet are easily fractured.

3. Acute lepra reactions may destroy nerves overnight, or cause severe eye damage.

Clinical Features. The onset is usually gradual. The most common first symptom is a small but persistent area of impaired sensation or numbness. In other cases the first noticeable feature may be macules, which are usually hypopigmented and erythematous. The disease may also present acutely, in reaction, with neuritis, iritis or erythema nodosum leprosum.

The macule of *indeterminate leprosy* is an inconspicuous lesion 2 to 3 cm in diameter, situated anywhere on the body, exhibiting slight pigmentary and sensory changes. This lesion usually heals spontaneously.

Tuberculoid leprosy is characterised by one or a few solitary lesions in skin and peripheal nerves. Skin lesions are macular or raised as plaques or as rings whose flat centres indicate central healing. The lesion is hypopigmented in dark skins, coppery in pale skins, with a well-defined margin. Its surface is dry, often scaly, and usually anaesthetic unless the lesion is on the face. Lesions are of almost any size and occur anywhere on the body, especially on outer surfaces of arms, legs or buttocks. The nerve twig supplying the skin lesion or a large peripheral nerve at one of the sites of predilection may be enlarged i.e. the ulnar nerve above the elbow, the median above the elbow or at the wrist, radial at the wrist, common peroneal in the popliteal fossa, posterior tibial around the medial malleolus, and great auricular across the sternomastoid muscle.

Tuberculoid leprosy tends spontaneously to heal slowly, often without residual disability. Sometimes its course is punctuated by a reaction and occasionally it downgrades into the borderline part of the spectrum.

Lepromatous lesions of the skin are described as they progress from early to late, as being macular, infiltrative, diffuse or nodular. Lepromatous macules are numerous, hypopigmented and erythematous. They differ from tuberculoid macules in that they are small, widely scattered on the body, usually symmetrically, and with margins that merge imperceptibly with normal skin. Sensation in them is not impaired. They are often inconspicuous except to the trained eye. As the disease advances, the macular lesions become infiltrated and succulent; in advanced lepromatous leprosy nodular lesions appear, especially on the ears and face, and eyebrows are lost. A less common manifestastion of lepromatous leprosy is diffuse symmetrical thickening of the skin, often with thickened lobes of the ear, producing the 'leonine facies'.

Clinical evidence of nerve damage appears relatively late in lepromatous leprosy. Anaesthesia and anhidrosis are first detected in the dorsal aspects of the forearms and lower legs, later in a 'glove and stocking' distribution and eventually over the trunk and face, although the palms, soles, axillae and groins may be spared. Muscular weakness results from bacillary infiltration as well as from nerve damage.

The testes may be destroyed and gynaecomastia ensue. The mucous membranes of the nose, mouth and trachea may ulcerate; necrosis of the cartilage and bones may result in late deformities of the phalanges and of nose and oral cavity and loss of the upper incisor teeth. Adjacent lesions may spread into the eye but, more commonly, this is infected through the blood stream. The most frequent lesions in the eye are miliary lepromata on the iris and superficial punctuate keratitis. Untreated lepromatous leprosy gradually gets worse.

Borderline or dimorphous leprosy may present with lesions intermediate in character between lepromatous and tuberculoid, or as a mixture of them. Skin lesions are often bizarre. The eyes and nose are spared. Nerve lesions are more numerous than in tuberculoid disease. In Asia, the majority of patients have borderline lepromatous leprosy. In Africa the majority have borderline tuberculoid leprosy. If the disease upgrades, nerve damage may increase with severe residual disability. If it downgrades the complications of extensive bacillary multiplication are added to those of widespread nerve damage. In either event the patient is liable to undergo reactions.

LEPRA REACTIONS. These may be defined as episodes of acute inflammation in pre-existing lesions of leprosy. Sometimes a reaction is the first clinical manifestation of the disease. One half of patients with lepromatous leprosy and one quarter with borderline lepromatous disease will be likely to suffer *type 2 lepra reactions* at some time during the course of their disease, most commonly in their second year of treatment. These reactions are characterised by fever and the appearance of crops of painful roseolar papules or nodules, called erythema nodosum leprosum, which may necrose and discharge sterile pus, before subsiding. In addition deeper subcutaneous nodules, iritis, orchitis, lymphadenitis, nerve pain and tenderness, and oedema of hands and feet may develop. Such reactions may threaten eyes and nerves and a succession of them may be extremely debilitating.

Type 1 lepra reactions in borderline disease are especially common in borderland tuberculoid patients. They occur spontaneously or may be precipitated by treatment. Skin and nerve lesions become acutely inflamed, painful and tender. Nerve function is rapidly lost, irretrievably so

unless the reaction is promptly treated. Rarely lesions in the skin ulcerate and nerves caseate.

Diagnosis. Lepromatous and borderline lepromatous disease ('multibacillary leprosy') is diagnosed by demonstration of *Myco. leprae* in material obtained by a skin-slit smear. The skin is pinched between finger and thumb to expel blood, incised with the point of a scalpel and the exposed dermis scraped with the flat of the blade. The tissue juice obtained is smeared on a microscope slide and stained by a modified Ziehl-Neelsen's method. Smears are made from skin lesions, earlobes and dorsum of the ring or middle finger — sites in which bacilli multiply readily and persist. Nasal mucus may also contain the organisms in lepromatous leprosy and this is a good indication of infectivity. *Myco. leprae* are less readily demonstrable in skin smears in borderline tuberculoid disease and are undetectable in tuberculoid disease.

In borderline, and especially tuberculoid disease ('paucibacillary leprosy'), the cardinal signs of leprosy are enlarged nerves and anaesthesia. Nerves are usually enlarged at sites of predilection asymmetrically and irregularly; they may be tender. Loss or diminution of sensation, or misreference (the inability to locate accurately the site stimulated) may be detected in a skin lesion or in the distribution of a large peripheral nerve. Biopsy of skin or nerve is seldom necessary.

There are virtually no other diseases with enlarged peripheral nerves; familial hypertrophic neuritis and primary amyloidosis are rare. A peripheral nerve may become thickened by a neuroma or as the result of trauma. Sometimes leprosy presents as a mono- or polyneuritis without skin lesions.

Treatment of leprosy is long and often complicated. The physician must gain the patient's confidence. The patient must understand the disease and its complications, comply and persevere in the treatment and learn to look after anaesthetic limbs, control fear and cope with any stigma that exists in the community. Admission to hospital for a few days is useful to establish rapport and start education.

SPECIFIC CHEMOTHERAPY. The essential features of the available drugs are given in Table 19.3.

Patients with multi-bacillary disease (leproma-

Table 19.3 Main features of drugs available to treat leprosy.

Drug	Dose (mg)	Peak Serum level × MIC*	Serum level MIC:days	Bactericidal activity
Dapsone	100	100–500	4–12	+
Acedapsone	225	16	200	-
Rifampicin	600	30	1	+ + +
Clofazimine	100	(Stored in R.E. cells, possible depot)		?
Ethionamide	500	60	1	+ +
Thiacetazone	150	8	1	-

*MIC = minimum inhibitory concentration

tous and borderline lepromatous) are preferably isolated until they are rendered non-infectious, which takes only a few days with rifampicin. Ideally treatment should be with three drugs to prevent the emergence of dapsone resistance. Rifampicin, the most expensive but most efficient bactericidal drug need only be given monthly, because of the long generation time of *Myco. leprae*. It is most effective if given for two consecutive days in a daily dose of 600 mg, or 450 mg for patients under 35 kg in weight. Clofazimine is given in a dose of 50 mg daily, or 100 mg three times in the week, (totalling 6 mg/kg/week for children). Dapsone is given in a dose of 2 mg/kg daily, not exceeding 100 mg. For mass treatment campaigns, when compliance is often poor, the World Health Organisation recommends that rifampicin be given in a single supervised monthly dose of 600 mg, and that a supervised monthly dose of clofazimine 300 mg be given in addition to the self administered daily dose of clofazimine and dapsone. Treatment is continued for at least two years, preferably until bacilli can no longer be demonstrated in slit skin smears.

Patients with paucibacillary disease (indeterminate, tuberculoid and borderline tuberculoid) are treated with rifampicin once monthly and dapsone daily for 6 months.

The duration of treatment now recommended with triple therapy is much shorter than with the previous regimes using dapsone alone. Relapse rates are imperfectly known in many parts of the world. Patients should be followed up for 5 years. Side effects of dapsone are rare. They include psychosis, dermatitis and haemolytic anaemia. Should they occur the drug is temporarily withheld, and resumed at half the dose. Thiacetazone is a cheap reserve drug; it is weak, and

cross resistance may develop with the more useful ethionamide. Acedapsone is an injectable repository of dapsone that has sometimes been used in control schemes.

Secondary dapsone resistance occurs in up to 15% of lepromatous patients treated, often intermittently or in low dosage, for 10–20 years with dapsone alone. It presents as the re-emergence of solitary nodules or as a more generalised relapse. In the last 5 years primary dapsone resistance has been emerging as a new and increasing problem in several countries. Resistance is confirmed by mouse footpad inoculation, or by supervised full dose dapsone treatment. It is treated either by clofazimine alone, to which no resistance has yet appeared, or by combined treatment with daily ethionamide and rifampicin given on the first two days of each months. Clofazimine is a red-brown dye that gradually colours the skin and all bodily secretions and is therefore not always acceptable to a pale skinned patient. It does however reduce the incidence of lepra reaction type 2. Doses in excess of those recommended may cause severe abdominal pain.

TREATMENT OF REACTIONS. *Type 1 lepra reactions*, in borderline or tuberculoid disease, causing pain or tenderness in nerves are treated with corticosteroids, such as prednisolone in a dose of 40–80 mg initially, followed by 20 mg daily for a few weeks until the inflammation is settling, then tailing off the drug over several months. Mild reactions, limited to skin lesions, are treated with aspirin 600 mg and chloroquine 150 mg base three times daily or an organic trivalent antimonial, such as stibophen in a dose of 2 ml intramuscularly on alternate days for six doses. Chemotherapy for leprosy is continued.

Type 2 lepra reactions in lepromatous patients

respond rapidly to thalidomide in a dose of 100 mg four times daily. This drug must never be given to premenopausal women because of its disastrous teratogenic effects. If thalidomide is contraindicated or unavailable, the other anti-inflammatory drugs are used; reactions threatening nerve damage or extensive skin ulceration or orchitis require prednisolone in an initial dose of 20–40 mg/day. Increasing the dose of clofazimine to 200 mg or 300 mg daily for a few weeks will help control the reaction and permit prednisolone to be reduced or withdrawn. Iritis is a dangerous complication and can usually be managed by local measures, namely the instillation of 1% hydrocortisone drops or ointment (or the subconjunctival injection of a depot preparation of methyl prednisolone), and the twice daily instillation of 1% atropine drops.

MANAGEMENT OF NERVE DAMAGE. In the event of acute paralysis complicating reactional neuritis, the affected limb is splinted and exercised passively each day until function begins to return when active exercises can be added. A patient with an anaesthetic limb must be taught to accept the limitations it imposes, to adjust life accordingly, to inspect that limb daily for trauma or infection and to learn how not to damage it.

Tarsorrhaphy helps protect an exposed anaesthetic cornea. Secondary sepsis is treated with appropriate antibiotics and osteomyelitis and its sequelae are managed in the most conservative manner possible. Patients with plantar ulcers are confined to bed, or given crutches or a walking plaster until healing is complete. Shoes must fit and protect anaesthetic feet against trauma and must be made specially if there is added deformity.

Prevention and Control. In endemic areas the disease is commonest among intimate contacts of patients, and children and young adults are especially susceptible. *Myco. leprae* is easily spread and two thirds of contacts undergo subclinical immunising infections within 2 years of regular exposure. Of the small proportion of contacts (about 1%) that develop clinical disease only about 2% will be lepromatous. It is at the moment impossible to identify this small group at risk and logical prophylaxis is impossible. No specific vaccine is available. BCG is of some value, especially in Africa, and should be given to all child contacts of lepromatous patients. Dapsone may be given for 2 years to infant contacts of lepromatous patients. Neither measure is a substitute for 6 monthly examination of contacts.

Mass prophylaxis is impossible, but mass treatment and follow-up of all cases identified during a population survey reduces deformity and lowers the incidence of leprosy. With improvement of socioeconomic conditions the disease tends to disappear. The rapid spread of dapsone resistance poses a great problem to existing control schemes.

MYCOBACTERIAL ULCER

This condition, first accurately described in Australia and New Guinea, later named Buruli ulcer from its frequency in the Nile valley of Uganda, is caused by *Mycobacterium ulcerans*. The epidemiology is unknown. It begins as a single small subcutaneous nodule situated commonly on the leg or forearm. The skin over the centre of the nodule ulcerates and, untreated, the ulcer extends to involve a progressively larger area. Histologically there is much necrosis of subcutaneous fat and *Myco. ulcerans* are abundant in the necrotic tissue in the base of the ulcer.

If suspected before ulceration, the nodule should be excised and healing readily follows. Ulcers require to be excised and skin grafted. Antimycobacterial chemotherapy is disappointing.

DISEASES DUE TO SPIROCHAETES

Leptospirosis; Syphilis (p. 409); Yaws; Endemic (non-venereal) syphilis; Pinta; Relapsing fevers; Rat-bite fevers; Tropical ulcer; Cancrum oris; Lyme arthritis (p. 571).

LEPTOSPIROSIS

Although over 100 serotypes of leptospires have been identified only *Leptospira icterohaemorrhagiae* and *L. canicola* have been shown to cause human disease in Britain.

The natural host of *Weil's disease*, caused by *L. icterohaemorrhagiae*, is the rat and other rodents. Infected urine contains spirochaetes which can penetrate the skin or mucosa of man. Abbatoir and farm workers, veterinarians, and vagrants are those most at risk. It has become uncommon in sewer workers, fish cleaners and miners because of better working conditions. Immersion in canals or stagnant water may result in sporadic infection. In patients dying from Weil's disease, there is a combination of hepatic, renal and cardiac failure.

Infection by *L. canicola*, which is contracted from dogs and pigs, usually presents as aseptic meningitis or pyrexia of unknown origin. It is not often associated with jaundice and is less severe than Weil's disease.

Clinical Features. The average incubation period is 10 days, the range being 4 to 21 days. A high proportion of infections are subclinical or cause a mild undiagnosed fever. In the more severe infections the illness begins abruptly with headache, severe myalgia, pyrexia, conjunctival suffusion, anorexia and vomiting. Infrequently, there are rashes or petechiae and enlargement of the liver and spleen.

After about a week leptospiral antibodies appear in the blood. The temperature falls by lysis and is usually normal for 2 or 3 days. In the majority of patients, there is further pyrexia for a few days and transient meningism (p. 637) followed by prompt recovery. In other cases, especially those caused by *L. icterohaemorrhagiae*, during this phase, hepatitis, renal tubular necrosis, myocarditis and meningitis may occur. The condition may progress to acute liver necrosis (p. 349). Renal tubular necrosis may lead to acute renal failure (p. 400). Myocarditis is suggested by tachycardia, fall in blood pressure and cardiac enlargement. The development of profound hypotension, arrhythmias and cardiac failure are ominous signs. Meningitis causes severe headache, neck stiffness and a positive Kernig's sign (p. 638) and is the usual clinical picture in *L. canicola* infections.

By the third and fourth week of the illness, the majority of patients enter the convalescent phase. When there has been serious involvement of the liver, kidneys and heart, mortality in Weil's disease is in the region of 15 to 20%. Those who recover do so completely.

Investigation. Most patients with leptospirosis show a polymorphonuclear leucocytosis. When there is liver involvement, liver function tests indicate a mild hepatocellular jaundice with an intrahepatic obstructive element; bilirubin and urobilinogen are present in the urine. In patients with renal failure the urine contains protein, red blood cells and cellular and granular casts; in severe cases the rise in blood urea is progressive. Meningitis is characterised by an increase of lymphocytes in the cerebrospinal fluid with little or no rise in protein; xanthochromia may be observed in the jaundiced patient.

The diagnosis is made by culturing the organism from the blood in the first week or from the urine in the second and third weeks. Alternatively, blood or urine specimens may be inoculated into a guinea-pig. From the second week onwards, a rising titre of specific leptospiral antibodies is found. The titre may not reach diagnostic levels in those cases treated promptly.

Treatment. Leptospires are sensitive to penicillin *in vitro*. Benzylpenicillin, 600 mg 6 hourly for 7 days is effective provided it is given early enough and in adequate doses; it shortens the average illness and reduces the incidence of complications. Penicillin is of doubtful value if treatment is initiated late in the infection. Appropriate fluid replacement is important during the period of acute illness. In severely affected patients supportive treatment for acute liver necrosis (p. 356), acute renal failure (p. 401), arrhythmias (p. 139) and cardiac failure (p. 154) may be required.

YAWS

Yaws is a granulomatous disease mainly involving the skin and bones and caused by *Treponema pertenue*, morphologically indistinguishable from the causative organisms of syphilis and pinta. The three infections induce similar serological changes and possibly some degree of cross immunity. Organisms are transmitted by bodily contact from a patient with infectious yaws through minor abrasions of the skin of another person, usually a child. Infection is most likely to take place in huts at night when the temperature and humidity are high and families use communal sleeping mats.

Yaws is still to be found among backward indigenous people. Areas of infection exist in Mexico, Panama, the Northern parts of South

America, West Indies, Central, East and West Africa, the Pacific Islands, Malaysia, Burma, Thailand (uncommonly in India and Sri Lanka), and also in Indonesia and the Far East, including China where it extends into temperate zones. The mass campaigns by WHO in 1950–1960 treated over 60 million people and eradicated yaws from many areas.

Pathology. At the site of the inoculation a proliferative granuloma develops containing numerous treponemes. This primary lesion is followed by eruptions, the most characteristic being multiple papillomatous lesions of the skin with a histology similar to the primary lesion. In addition there may be hypertrophic periosteal lesions of many bones with underlying cortical rarefaction. All these lesions of 'early yaws' heal without appreciable scarring or deformity unless there has been secondary infection. After a variable interval 'late yaws' may develop, characterised by destructive lesions which closely resemble the gummas of tertiary syphilis and which heal with much scarring and deformity.

Clinical Features. *Early Yaws.* The incubation period is 3 to 4 weeks. The primary lesion or 'mother yaw' is usually on the leg or buttocks. The secondary eruption usually follows a few weeks or months later, sometimes before the primary lesion has healed. The most typical are the so-called papillomata, often very numerous, consisting of exuberant tissue covered with a whitish-yellow exudate, and more prolific in the moist flexures and around the mouth. There may be successive crops of lesions. The subject, usually a child, may remain active and unconcerned except for the irritation of the sores and from the flies which they attract. These lesions are highly contagious. Sometimes a pathologically similar lesion erupts through the palm or sole, when walking becomes painful, 'wet crab yaws'. The bones of all the fingers distal to the carpus, except the terminal phalanges, particularly in children, may rarify and be surrounded by periosteal deposits. There may be a swelling of a long bone and also of the nasal bones (goundou). The distorted tibia may remain as the 'sabre tibia' but most of the lesions of early yaws will eventually subside, even if untreated.

Latent Yaws. Following the spontaneous resolution of 'early yaws' serological changes may persist, to be followed by further manifestations of 'early yaws', or, after an interval of as much as 5 to 10 years, by the tertiary lesions of 'late yaws'.

Late Yaws. Solitary or multiple nodular lesions develop. They ulcerate and spread superficially and also, in places, penetrate deeply into the underlying tissue. In this way gross disfigurement may be caused with distressing ulceration and deformity. The lesions tend to heal with scarring in one part while the ulcer is extending in another. Osteitis and periostitis present as localised swelling of bones over which tissue may ulcerate giving a picture resembling the gummatous ulceration of tertiary syphilis. Lesions in the hand, skull, nose and palate are common. Gross mutilation making the nose and mouth one open cavity ('gangosa') is one of the most tragic results still compatible with life. Other late lesions include hyperkeratosis with fissuring of the palms and soles 'dry crab yaws', hydrarthrosis, bursitis and juxta-articular nodules consisting of painless, firm, subcutaneous fibrous deposits about the elbows, hips and knees.

Unlike tertiary syphilis, yaws does not affect the internal viscera or the cardiovascular and nervous systems.

Serological tests (VDRL, TPHA and FTA-ABS, p. 410) are positive.

Treatment and Prevention. Lesions of early and late yaws respond rapidly to the intramuscular administration of 750 mg of procaine penicillin on two occasions at an interval of 1 week, or to tetracycline 1 to 2 g daily for 5 days. Early yaws heals completely but late yaws may leave deformity.

With improved housing and increased cleanliness the disease disappears. In few fields of medicine have chemotherapy and improved hygiene achieved such dramatic success as in the control of yaws.

ENDEMIC (NON-VENEREAL) SYPHILIS

In certain tropical countries, where lack of hygiene prevails, this treponematosis occurs as a family disease. The causative organisms are regarded as modified strains of *Treponema pallidum*, with which they are morphologically identical but biologically distinct.

Congenital infections are extremely rare and sexual transmission unusual. The common mode of infection is through an abrasion, the disease being transmitted from one child to another and occasionally from a child to a parent. Sometimes it spreads in a closed community by the use of common drinking vessels and possibly mechanically by flies. The poor social conditions in which the disease prevails are similar to those where yaws is found but the clinical lesions resemble those of juvenile syphilis.

In contrast to venereal syphilis the primary lesion is rarely seen, except when a child has inoculated the nipple of the mother during suckling, in which case the lesion presents as an ulcerative papule without regional adenitis. The secondary and tertiary lesions include all the common types of skin, mucosal and bone manifestations of syphilis but the typical papillomatous lesions of yaws are infrequent. Serological tests cross-react with venereal syphilis and yaws.

The disease responds to treatment by penicillin in the same way as venereal syphilis (p. 411). Prevention depends on the development of improved social and economic conditions and the mass treatment of affected communities with penicillin.

Pinta

Pinta is a clinical and geographic variant of endemic syphilis caused by the related organism *Treponema carateum*. It is endemic in localised areas in Central and South America and in some West Indian and South Pacific Islands.

The incubation period is 14 to 20 days. There is a primary scaly papular lesion on an exposed part, usually the leg. The lesion enlarges slowly, up to 10 cm in diameter and is surrounded by smaller papules. Regional lymph nodes enlarge and like the primary lesion contain treponemes. The second stage is manifest 5 to 12 months later and consists of a generalised eruption of macules and miliary papules, 'pintids', pinkish and slightly scaly. Most of these heal but others coalesce and form hyperpigmented patches, commonly on the face and exposed parts. The secondary lesions may persist for years and may be accompanied by hyperkeratosis of palms and soles. In the tertiary stage the affected patches become atrophic and depigmented. In the second and tertiary stages there are serological changes closely resembling those of syphilis but no effective cross immunity.

Treatment is by a long-acting penicillin (p. 411).

THE RELAPSING FEVERS

The relapsing fevers are a group of diseases due to infections by spirochaetes of the genus *Borrelia* transmitted by body lice or soft (*Argasid*) ticks. The louse-borne *Borrelia recurrentis* infects only man and is not transmitted from a louse to its progeny. This disease appears in epidemics particularly during wars or famine when refugees are crowded together in conditions under which infestation with the human body-louse is frequent and an infected louse is introduced. It may accompany louse-borne typhus. The disease is endemic in Ethiopia from where recently recorded epidemics have probably arisen.

Bor. duttoni, the cause of tick-borne relapsing fever, is transmitted by various species of the genus *Ornithodoros*. Ticks live for years and once infected remain so for life and convey the infection to the offspring. Tick-borne relapsing fever is thus an endemic disease.

Louse-borne Relapsing Fever

Lice cause itching. Borreliae are liberated from the infected louse when it is crushed during scratching which also inoculates the borreliae into the skin.

Pathology. The borreliae multiply in the blood, where they are abundant in the febrile phases, and invade most tissues especially the liver, spleen and meninges. Hepatitis causing jaundice is frequent in severe infections and there may be petechial haemorrhages in the skin, mucous membranes and serous surfaces of internal organs.

Thrombocytopenia is marked. The urine frequently contains protein and sometimes there is frank haematuria.

Clinical Features. After an incubation period varying from 2 to 12 days there is a sudden onset of fever. The temperature rises to 39·5° to 40·5°C and is accompanied by a rapid pulse, headache, generalised aching, injected conjunctivae and frequently a petechial rash, epistaxis and herpes labialis. As the disease progresses, the liver and spleen frequently become tender and palpable and jaundice is common. There may be severe serosal and intestinal haemorrhage. Mental confusion and meningism may occur. The fever ends by crisis between the fourth and tenth day, often associated with profuse sweating, hypotension, circulatory and cardiac failure. There may be no further fever but, in a proportion of cases, after an afebrile period of about 7 days there may be one or more relapses which are usually milder and less prolonged. In the absence of specific treatment the mortality rate may be as high as 40%, especially among the elderly and malnourished.

The organisms are demonstrated in the blood during fever either by dark ground illumination of a wet film or by staining thick and thin films.

Treatment and Prevention. The problems of treatment are to eradicate the infection and to minimise the severe Jarisch-Herxheimer reaction (p. 780) which inevitably follows successful chemotherapy and to prevent relapses. The safest treatment is with procaine penicillin 300 mg intramuscularly followed the next day by 0·5 g tetracycline. Tetracycline alone is effective and prevents relapse, but gives rise to a worse reaction. Doxycycline, 200 mg once by mouth, as an alternative to tetracycline has the advantage of being curative also for typhus, which often accompanies epidemics of relapsing fever.

Treatment is followed within a half to 3 hours by a chill or rigor, a brisk rise of temperature to 40–42°C, tachypnoea, tachycardia and often cough, confusion, distress, delirium and, occasionally, convulsions and coma. This phase is rapidly followed by profound hypotension and vasodilatation which may last from 8–12 hours and may be complicated by cardiac failure. The patient must be confined strictly to bed for 48 hours after treatment, carefully observed and managed as complications demand. Tepid sponging for fever over 41°C, careful attention to hydration, preferably by oral fluids, and prompt treatment of cardiac failure are required.

The patient and the clothing and all contacts must be freed from lice as in epidemic typhus (p. 741).

Tick-borne Relapsing Fever

This disease, due to *Borrelia duttoni*, is conveyed by a variety of soft ticks and its endemicity is governed by the presence of the vector. In the Mediterranean area *Ornithodoros tholozani* is responsible; in the Middle East, Iran, Afghanistan and India and in the New World there are other vectors. These ticks can become infected from rodents or bats as well as by congenital transmission and man is only an incidental host. In Central and East Africa, however, *O. moubata* is the vector and man is probably the only important mammalian host. The disease in these areas is thus confined to old camp sites, old houses and their immediate surroundings, infested with *O. moubata* infected from man or by congenital transmission. *O. moubata* lives in dried mud floors and the cracks of the walls of huts plastered with mud.

The pathological changes resemble those of louse-borne relapsing fever but with late neurological lesions.

Clinical Features. These are similar to those of louse-borne relapsing fever. The febrile bouts, although severe, last usually only for 3 to 5 days, and the apyrexial periods may also be shorter. Relapses are, however, more frequent and may be as numerous as 10. Iritis and neurological complications, including cranial nerve palsies, optic atrophy, localised palsies and spastic paraplegia, may develop during these later relapses.

The methods used in diagnosis are similar to those for louse-borne relapsing fever. *Bor. duttoni* are, however, scantier in the peripheral blood but laboratory animals are readily infected.

Treatment and Prevention. As many strains are resistant to penicillin, tetracycline 1 g daily for 7 days is given and the course repeated after an interval of a week. Except for the Jarisch-Herxheimer reaction, good results follow a single dose of 200 mg doxycycline. Ticks can be killed by lindane (gamma BHC) applied to the inside of the walls, floors and across the entrance to houses.

OTHER SPIROCHAETAL INFECTIONS

Rat-bite Fevers

There are two rat-bite fevers, one caused by *Spirillum minus*, the other by *Streptobacillus moniliformis*. The latter in addition to being transmitted by a rat-bite has also occurred as an epidemic due to infected milk (Haverhill fever) and in other cases also there has been no known contact with rats or mice. Both infections are worldwide in distribution.

Pathological and Clinical Features. The manifestations of both fevers are very similar. In *Sp. minus* infection (Sodoku) the wound usually heals. After 5 to 21 days it suddenly becomes inflamed, indurated, purplish and painful; it may ulcerate and is accompanied by lymphangitis, regional lymphadenitis, leucocytosis, splenomegaly and fever. After a week the local and general reactions subside but recur after a further few days. Periods of fever lasting 24 to 48 hours are followed by a rapid fall of temperature and, without treatment, febrile bouts may continue to recur for weeks and the patient becomes anaemic. A macular or maculopapular dusky red rash, sparse over the trunk and extremities, appears during the febrile phases.

In streptobacillus fever the incubation period is 1 to 5 days. The bite usually heals well but occasionally an abscess forms in the wound. Regional lymphadenopathy is not marked. The general symptoms resemble those of *Sp. minus* infections but there is frequently painful arthritis and it is unusual to have recurrences of fever after the initial bout which only lasts 48 to 72 hours.

Diagnosis and Treatment. *Sp. minus* can be demonstrated in the exudate from the inflamed bite or in fluid aspirated from a lymph node, either by examination under darkground illumination or by inoculation intraperitoneally into an uninfected mouse. Blood inoculated into mice or guinea-pigs will yield *Sp. minus* in the peritoneal fluid 5 to 14 days later. There are serological cross reactions with syphilis. In *Strep. moniliformis* infections specific seroagglutinins are demonstrable after 10 days. A titre of 1 in 80 or a rising titre is considered diagnostic but the serological tests for syphilis are negative. The organism can be re-covered from the blood or, more easily, from an effusion into an inflamed joint. Both infections are readily cured by penicillin, streptomycin or tetracycline.

Tropical Ulcer

Tropical ulcer is a specific infection with *Borrelia vincenti* and an anaerobic bacterium occurring especially in adolescent males. Minor injury in the presence of undernourishment, poor hygiene and debilitating disease are predisposing factors.

Pathological and Clinical Features. The initial lesion of a tropical ulcer is a bleb filled with sanguineous fluid. It may be painful and itchy with some constitutional upset. Soon the bleb ruptures, and a green-grey moist slough is exposed which rapidly spreads in the skin and subcutaneous tissue up to a diameter of 5 cm or more. In a few days these tissues slough and liquefy releasing an offensive discharge. After about a week there is usually no further spread and the necrotic tissue separates, exposing an ulcer. In a chronic ulcer the edges are raised and slope sharply. The damage may be limited to the skin and superficial fascia, but in severe cases deep structures, e.g. tendons, nerves, blood vessels and periosteum, may be invaded. Bone is rarely affected. Tropical ulcers generally affect the parts of the body exposed to trauma, especially the lower third of the leg and the foot. The ulcer is usually solitary.

General constitutional effects of a tropical ulcer are slight, and lymphadenitis is not found except as a result of secondary infection.

The ulcer heals slowly with a tissue-paper-like scar which breaks down easily. Big ulcers lead to scarring and deformity or fail to heal and may develop malignant changes after many years.

Treatment and Prevention. Local treatment consists in thorough cleansing of the ulcer with hypertonic magnesium sulphate. Procaine penicillin 300 mg i.m., metronidazole 400 mg t.i.d., or tetracycline 2 g daily for 7 days gives good results. Chronic ulcers are excised and grafted. Ulcers over 5 cm diameter also need grafting.

Where tropical ulcers are a risk, abrasions should be cleansed and covered. The provision of a good diet, washing facilities and a first-aid service have abolished tropical ulcers from labour forces on well-run estates.

Cancrum Oris

Cancrum oris is now rare except in poorly nourished children in the tropics. It is characteristically preceded by an infective illness, especially measles. The pathology is that of a rapidly developing gangrene, beginning inside the mouth and penetrating through the lips and cheek resulting in severe disfigurement. Untreated it frequently causes death. However, with or without treatment, gangrene becomes demarcated and ulceration follows. *Bor. vincenti* and an anaerobic bacterium are frequently found in the ulcer.

Penicillin or sulphonamides arrest the infection but do not prevent gangrene of already diseased tissue. Coexistent malnutrition, anaemia or dehydration should be corrected. Subsequently skilled plastic surgery may do much to overcome the hideous defects. Prevention depends on improved nutrition and hygiene in the community and on control of acute infectious diseases.

DISEASES DUE TO PROTOZOA

Malaria; Amoebiasis; Giardiasis; Balantidiasis; Leishmaniasis; Trypanosomiasis; Toxoplasmosis

MALARIA

Human malaria results from infection by *Plasmodium falciparum, P. vivax, P. ovale, P. malariae* and rarely other species. The infection may be acquired wherever there are human hosts carrying the parasites and a sufficiency of suitable anopheline mosquitoes, together with conditions of temperature and humidity which favour the development of the parasite in the mosquito. Malaria may also be transmitted by transfusion or inoculation of infected blood, and rarely transplacentally.

Malaria is endemic or sporadic throughout most of the tropics and sub-tropics below an altitude of 1500 m, excluding the Mediterranean littoral, the U.S.A. and Australia. One hundred million people are attacked annually of whom 1% die, mainly children.

As the result of WHO sponsored campaigns of prevention and more effective treatment, the incidence of malaria was greatly reduced in 1950–60 but since 1970 there has been a resurgence. Because of increased travel and neglect of chemoprophylaxis about 2000 cases are imported annually into Britain. Most are due to *P. vivax* from Asia. One in five, usually from Africa, is due to *P. falciparum* and of these 3% die because of late diagnosis. A few people living near airports in Europe have acquired malaria from accidentally imported mosquitoes.

Pathogenesis. The female anopheline mosquito becomes infected when it feeds on human blood containing gametocytes, the sexual forms of the malarial parasite. The further development and multiplication of the parasite is as shown in Figure 19.2.

The development in the mosquito takes from 7–20 days. Sporozoites disappear from human blood within half an hour, but after $5\frac{1}{2}$ days in *P. falciparum* malaria, 8–15 days or occasionally longer for the other species, a greatly increased number of parasites, 'merozoites', leave the liver and invade red cells where further cycles of multiplication of parasites take place producing schizonts. Rupture of the schizont releases more merozoites into the blood and causes fever. Each cycle in the red cells takes 48 hours in the case of *P. vivax* and *P. ovale* and results in a 'tertian' fever, the temperature rising on alternative days; *P. malariae* takes 72 hours resulting in a 'quartan' fever, while the cycle in *P. falciparum* takes rather less than 48 hours, is less well-synchronised and produces a more constant fever.

P. vivax and *P. ovale* may persist in liver cells as dormant forms, hypnozoites, that are capable of developing into merozoites months or years later. Thus the first attack of clinical malaria may occur long after the patient has left the endemic area, and the disease may relapse after treatment with drugs that kill only the erythrocytic stage of the parasite.

P. falciparum and *P. malariae* have no persistent exo-erythrocytic phase but recrudescences of fever may result from multiplication in the red cells of parasites which have not been eliminated by treatment and immune processes.

Malaria is always accompanied by haemolysis

IN MAN

IN ANOPHELINE MOSQUITO

MALE AND FEMALE GAMETOCYTES

SEXUAL CYCLE

BITE

MATURATION OF FEMALE GAMETE

EXFLAGELLATING MALE GAMETOCYTE

FEMALE GAMETE BEING FERTILIZED BY MALE GAMETE

IMMATURE GAMETOCYTES

ZYGOTE

MEROZOITES

STOMACH WALL

SCHIZONT

OÖKINETE

ERYTHROCYTIC (ASEXUAL) CYCLE

YOUNG OÖCYST

SEGMENTING OÖCYST

TROPHOZOITE

RING FORM

MEROZOITES

RUPTURED OÖCYST

SPOROZOITES INVADING SALIVARY GLANDS

PRIMARY EXO-ERYTHROCYTIC

BITE

HYPNOZOOITE

Fig. 19.2 Life cycle of malarial parasites. Adapted from Cruickshank, R., Duguid, J.P., Marmion, B.P. & Swain, R.H.A. (1973) *Medical Microbiology*. Edinburgh: Churchill Livingstone.

and in a severe or prolonged attack anaemia may be profound. Haemolysis is most severe with *P. falciparum* which invades red cells of all ages, but especially young cells, *P. vivax* and *P. ovale* invade reticulocytes, and *P. malariae*, normoblasts, and infections remain lighter. Uninfected red cells are also destroyed by components of complement, activated in the circulation, adhering

to them. Splenomegaly causes red cell sequestration with premature destruction and also haemodilution. Chronic malaria depletes folates stores especially during pregnancy.

In *P. falciparum* malaria, red cells containing schizonts adhere to the lining of capillaries in brain, kidney, liver, lungs and gut. The vessels become congested and the organs, anoxic. Rupture of schizonts liberates toxic and antigenic substances which cause further damage. Thus the main effects of malaria are haemolytic anaemia and, with *P. falciparum*, widespread organ damage.

P. falciparum does not grow well in red cells that contain haemoglobin F, C or especially S. Haemoglobin S heterozygotes (AS) are protected against the lethal complications of malaria. *P. vivax* cannot enter red cells that lack the Duffy blood group. West African negroes and black Americans are protected.

Clinical Features. Malaria is first described as it occurs in the non-immune adult. The interval from the time of biting by the infected mosquito to the onset of detectable fever varies but is often about a week or 10 days for *P. falciparum* infections and somewhat longer for the other species. Occasionally an apparent primary attack of vivax malaria occurs months after the patient has left the tropics, and suppressive drugs may delay the onset for as long as a year after stopping the drug.

P. vivax and P. ovale malaria. In many cases the illness starts with a period of several days of continued fever before the development of classical bouts of fever on alternate days. The malarial paroxysm has three clinical stages: first a cold stage, followed by a hot stage, which ends in a sweating stage. In the cold stage or rigor the patient feels intensely cold and shivers, and frequently the teeth chatter. The temperature is already elevated and rapidly reaches its height, e.g. 40°C. Vomiting is often troublesome and headache severe.

After half an hour or so, the hot stage is reached; the patient feels burning hot and may be delirious. After 1 to 6 hours, profuse perspiration starts, the temperature drops and the patient becomes comfortable, falls asleep and will feel reasonably well on the next day, but fever subsequently recurs on alternate days. Usually the spleen and, especially in children, the liver become palpable and tender, but the absence of detectable splenic enlargement does not exclude malaria. Herpes simplex, usually round the mouth, is a common accompaniment of malaria.

P. malariae infection is usually associated with mild symptoms and bouts of fever every third day. Parasitaemia may persist for many years without producing any symptoms.

P. falciparum infections are more dangerous than other forms of malaria. The onset, especially of primary attacks, is often insidious with malaise, headache and vomiting. Cough and mild diarrhoea are common. The fever has no particular pattern and does not usually rise quite so high as in the other forms. The cold, hot and sweating stages are seldom found. Jaundice is common, due to hepatitis and haemolysis. The liver and spleen enlarge and become tender. Anaemia develops rapidly.

In uncomplicated cases only the ring stage of the parasites and later the gametocytes are found in the peripheral blood, whereas with the other species all stages of the parasites occur in the circulating blood. A patient with falciparum malaria, apparently not seriously ill, may suddenly develop serious complications. Children may die rapidly without any special symptoms other than fever. In pregnancy immunity is impaired, and abortion from parasitisation of the maternal side of the placenta is frequent. Congenital malaria is rare.

Mixed infections with more than one species of malaria parasite may occur.

Relapses are characteristic of vivax, ovale and malariae infections. They seldom occur more than 2 years after the patient has left the malarious area although much longer intervals are recorded with *P. malariae*.

COMPLICATIONS OF FALCIPARUM MALARIA. *Cerebral malaria* is the most urgent complication and is manifested either by the rapid development of coma, usually without localising signs, or by hyperpyrexia or acute mental changes. It is very rare for there to be an increase of cells in the cerebrospinal fluid.

Acute renal failure and less commonly *hepatic failure* may occur, and there may be severe *diarrhoea* and *vomiting*.

Blackwater fever is brought about by a rapid intravascular haemolysis. It is invariably associated with a chronic falciparum malaria, most commonly in those who have taken antimalarial treatment irregularly, or are deficient in glucose-6-phosphate dehydrogenase. The haemolysis may be quite unexpected and very extensive, destroying many uninfected as well as parasitised red cells. The attack may be provoked by administering quinine or by fatigue. The colour of the urine varies from dark red to almost black.

ENDEMIC MALARIA. The manifestations of malaria in unprotected indigenous residents show considerable variation according to the degree of endemicity, and the age of the patient and the development of immunity. In areas of hypoendemicity little immunity is acquired, epidemics of malaria are liable to occur and the disease does not differ materially from that in non-immunes. In mesoendemic areas malaria is frequent but only seasonal. Repeated infections lead to anaemia, considerable enlargement of the spleen with danger of its rupture, and chronic ill-health with bouts of fever. The growth and development of children may be retarded and P. malariae infections may cause immune-complex nephritis and the nephrotic syndrome.

In hyperendemic areas malaria transmission takes place throughout the year, but with seasonal increases, and adults develop considerable immunity. Although they will have palpable spleens and occasional parasitaemia, malaria causes only occasional short bouts of fever. In holoendemic areas malarial transmission is intense throughout the year and adults do not suffer from the infection, although they support a low parasitaemia, and enlargement of the spleen does not usually persist.

In hyperendemic and in holoendemic areas malaria takes a toll of older infants and young children. The regular taking of antimalarial drugs prevents the manifestations of chronic malaria but may impair the development of immunity. People who have been subjected to splenectomy are especially liable to suffer severely from falciparum malaria because of impaired immune responses.

TROPICAL SPLENOMEGALY SYNDROME. In some hyperendemic areas gross splenomegaly is associated with an exaggerated immune response to malaria and is seen, unexpectedly, in adults who have high antibody titres to malaria and low parasitaemias. The condition, which is commoner in females and in certain racial and family groups is characterised by enormous overproduction of IgM, levels reaching 3 to 20 times the local mean value. Much of the IgM is aggregated with other immunoglobulin or complement and precipitates in the cold, in vitro. The IgM aggregates are phagocytosed by reticuloendothelial cells in the spleen and liver, and the demonstration of this by immunofluorescence in a liver biopsy section is diagnostic. Light microscopy of the liver usually shows sinusoidal lymphocytosis. Anaemia and lymphocytosis can be confused with leukaemia. Portal hypertension may develop.

Diagnosis. If a febrile patient is in a malarious locality or has recently left such an area, malaria should be considered. Besides malaria there are many causes for acute febrile splenomegaly in the tropics. Gross enlargement of the spleen may also result from tuberculosis, visceral leishmaniasis, schistosomiasis mansoni and japonicum and chronic brucellosis as well as leukaemia and lymphoma. Well-stained blood films, thick and thin, should be examined and repeated if necessary. P. falciparum parasites may be very scanty, especially in those who have been partially treated. In semi-immunes in endemic areas malaria may co-exist with other diseases and not be the cause of the illness.

Treatment. GENERAL. The acutely ill patient should be put to bed and encouraged to drink fluid freely. Aspirin or paracetamol is useful for the relief of headache. When dehydration is marked and vomiting troublesome, intravenous fluids may be necessary.

SPECIFIC THERAPY OF THE ACUTE ATTACK. The drugs of choice are the 4-aminoquinolines, chloroquine or amodiaquine. The usual course of treatment is 600 g of the effective base (4 tablets) followed by 300 mg base in six hours then 150 mg base twice daily for 3 to 7 more days. The initial dose for children is 5–10 mg/kg. For semi-immunes a single dose is usually adequate. In areas of chloroquine resistance (Table 19.4) P. falciparum may respond poorly and quinine should be used to treat severe infections. Quinine dihydrochloride 650 mg (10 mg/kg) three times daily for 5 days should be given by mouth, followed by a single dose of sulfadoxine 1·5 mg combined with pyrimethamine 75 mg, i.e. 3 tablets of Fansidar.

Treatment of Complicated P. falciparum Malaria. Patients with 'cerebral malaria' or other severe manifestations, or non-immune with more than 1% of red cells infected, are medical emergencies. The immediate administration of chloroquine or quinine is indicated, the drug being given as an intravenous infusion over 2–4 hours to avoid acute circulatory failure or acute encephalopathy. Quinine is indicated if a chloroquine-resistant infection is at all likely. The dose of chloroquine is 5 mg/kg and of quinine 10 mg/kg. The dose should be repeated at intervals of 8 hours until the patient can take drugs orally. The drugs may instead be given intramuscularly but chloroquine may cause convulsions (especially in undernourished children) and quinine may cause necrosis of muscle; the hydrochloride is less irritant than the dihydrochloride. If in the treatment of a comatose patient, return to consciousness is delayed, lumbar puncture is indicated to exclude coexisting bacterial meningitis.

Severe anaemia requires transfusion with packed red cells. In blackwater fever prednisolone (20 mg) may prevent further haemolysis. If oliguria develops, frusemide or an infusion of mannitol may forestall renal failure. Intravenous fluid, if necessary, should be monitored by the central venous pressure, because pulmonary oedema develops easily.

The prognosis is good if correct treatment is given early, but poor if diagnosis is late, parasitaemia is high or organs are failing.

TREATMENT OF TROPICAL SPLENOMEGALY SYNDROME. Splenomegaly and anaemia usually resolve over a period of months of continuous treatment with proguanil 100 mg daily, which should be continued for life to prevent relapse. Complicating folate deficiency is treated with folic acid 5 mg daily.

RADICAL CURE OF MALARIA DUE TO *P. vivax* and *P. ovale*. While relapses can usually be prevented by taking one of the antimalarial drugs in suppressive doses (below), radical cure can be ensured only by a course of one of the 8-aminoquinolines, which destroy the hypnozoite phase in the liver, together with or following a course of chloroquine or amodiaquine. Primaquine given in a dose of 15 mg daily for 14 days produces a high percentage of cures. The patient must be under medical supervision for this period as haemolysis may develop in those who are G6PD deficient. Cyanosis due to the formation of methaemoglobin in the red cells is more common but not dangerous.

Causal Prophylaxis and Suppression. No drug is known which will destroy the sporozoites injected by the mosquito. Clinical attacks of malaria can, however, be prevented by drugs such as proguanil and pyrimethamine which attack the pre-erythrocytic form ('causal prophylaxis'), or by drugs such as chloroquine which act on the parasite after it has entered the erythrocyte ('suppression'). Maloprim (pyrimethamine 12·5 mg and dapsone 100 mg) and Fansidar (pyrimethamine 25 mg and sulfadoxine 500 mg) contain two compounds which block two successive enzymes in the parasite's folate pathway.

Tables 19.4 and 19.5 give the recommended doses for protection of the non-immune. Chemoprophylaxis is begun 1 week before entering the malarious area, and is continued until 4 weeks after leaving it. Resistance to the cheap and well tolerated drugs proguanil and pyrimethamine is increasing and frequently coincides with the much more serious spread of chloroquine resistance. Resistance to Maloprim and Fansidar is also reported. Chloroquine must not be taken continuously as a prophylactic for over 5 years, as it may cause irreversible retinopathy. Infants under 8 weeks of age should not take Maloprim or Fansidar. Pregnant and lactating women may take proguanil or chloroquine safely. Fansidar should be avoided by those sensitive to sulphonamides.

Prevention. Control of anopheline mosquitoes, especially by the spraying of houses with residual insecticides, has greatly reduced or abolished the risk of malaria in many areas. However, unless eradication is complete, all visitors and non-immune residents should take regular prophylactic drugs as detailed above. Chemoprophylaxis alone may not be sufficient to prevent malaria. It is also important to avoid anopheline mosquitoes, which bite at night. Outside the house, long sleeves and trousers should be worn. Repellent creams and sprays can be used. Screened windows and the use of a mosquito net also reduce the risk.

Table 19.4 Chemoprophylaxis of malaria.

Area	Antimalarial tablet	Adult prophylactic dose
Chloroquine resistance present***	Pyrimethamine 12·5 mg plus dapsone 100 mg (Maloprim)*	One tablet weekly
	OR	
	Pyrimethamine 25 mg plus sulphadoxine 500 mg (Fansidar)*	One tablet weekly
Chloroquine resistance absent	Chloroquine 100 mg, 150 mg or 300 mg of base	300 mg weekly
	OR	
	Proguanil 100 mg	100–200 mg daily**

*Chloroquine may be taken in addition where high *P. vivax* transmission is present (East Africa, Brazil, Papua New Guinea, South East Asia, Indian subcontinent).
**200 mg in sub-Saharan Africa.
***South America. South East Asia including Southern China, Indonesia, Malaysia, Phillipines, Papua New Guinea. Bangladesh, N.E. India, Nepal. Kenya, Tanzania, Sudan, Uganda, Zambia, Madagascar.

Table 19.5 Doses of antimalarials for children — weight is preferable to age.

Dose in relation to adult dose	Weight range	Age range
One-quarter	under 5 kg	under 1 year
One-half	5–20 kg	1–5 years
Three-quarters	20–40 kg	6–12 years
Adult dose	over 40 kg	over 12 years

AMOEBIASIS

Amoebiasis is usually caused by *Entamoeba histolytica*, a potentially pathogenic intestinal amoeba that is propagated between humans by its cysts, 10 microns or more in diameter. *Ent. histolytica* must be distinguished from other species which are non-pathogenic, notably *Ent. hartmanii* and *Ent. coli*. In addition two amoebae of genera *Naegleria* and *Acanthamoeba* which inhabit polluted surface water and swimming pools all over the world are causes respectively of fulminating meningitis and granulomatous encephalitis.

Pathogenesis. Cysts of *Ent. histolytica* survive well outside the body and are ingested in water or uncooked food which has been contaminated by human faeces. Lettuce is a common vehicle of infection. The disease is occasionally acquired in Britain.

In the colon the vegetative trophozoite forms emerge from the cysts (Fig. 19.3). While they remain free in the colon the condition is symptomless but under certain circumstances invasion and ulceration of the mucous membrane of the large bowel takes place causing the symptoms of *amoebic dysentery*. The lesions, which are usually maximal in the caecum but may be found as far down as the anal canal, are flask-shaped ulcers varying greatly in size and surrounded by healthy mucosa. A localised granuloma, 'amoeboma', presenting as a palpable mass in the rectum or causing a filling defect in the colon on radiography, is a rare complication. Since it responds well to antiamoebic treatment it is important that it should not be mistaken for a carcinoma. Amoebae may find their way into a vein and be carried to the liver where they multiply rapidly and destroy the parenchyma causing an *amoebic abscess*. The liquid contents at first have a characteristic pinkish colour which later may change to chocolate brown and finally to yellow or green. Amoebic ulcers only rarely penetrate through the muscular coat of the colon. A large vessel may

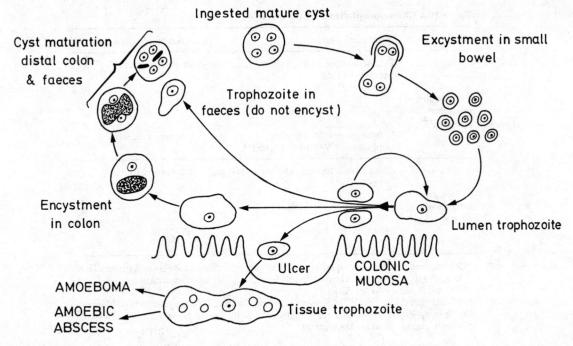

Fig. 19.3 Amoebiasis. Life cycle of *Entamoeba histolytica*. (Adapted from Knight, R., *Parasitic Diseases of Man*).

sometimes be eroded, and severe intestinal hae-morrhage result. Cutaneous amoebiasis presents as progressive genital or perianal ulceration, usu-ally in homosexuals, or around abdominal surgi-cal wounds.

Clinical Features. The incubation period varies from 2 weeks to many years, but is usually several months. *Intestinal amoebiasis*, or *amoebic dysentery* usually runs a chronic course with grumbling pains in the abdomen and two or more rather loose stools a day. Periods of diarrhoea alternating with constipation are a frequent fea-ture. Mucus is usually passed, sometimes with streaks of blood, and the motions often have an offensive odour. On palpation of the abdomen there may be tenderness along the line of the colon, usually more marked over the caecum and pelvic colon. The right iliac pain may simulate acute appendicitis, and if an operation is per-formed the amoebae may cause ulceration of the wound and surrounding tissue. Perforation, when it occurs, is usually in the region of the caecum. Particularly in the aged, in the puerperium and with superadded pyogenic infection of the ulcers there may be more acute bowel symptoms, with very frequent motions and the passage of much blood and mucus, thus simulating bacillary dys-entery or ulcerative colitis.

Hepatic amoebiasis often occurs without a his-tory of recent diarrhoea. It is common in the tropics and an important cause of imported fever in Britain. Early symptoms may be local discom-fort only and malaise; later a swinging tempera-ture, sweating and an enlarged tender liver, cough and pain in the right shoulder are characteristic, but symptoms may remain vague and signs mini-mal. In particular, the less common abscess in the left lobe may not be diagnosed. There is usually a moderate neutrophil leucocytosis and a raised diaphragm with diminished movement on the right side. A large abscess may penetrate the diaphragm and rupture into the lung from where its contents may be coughed up. Rupture into the pleural cavity, the peritoneal cavity or pericardial sac is less common but more serious.

Diagnosis. The signs and symptoms of intesti-nal amoebiasis are often vague. A careful naked-eye inspection of a freshly passed motion should be made. Any exudate is examined at once under the microscope for motile trophozoites which are about 30 microns in diameter, with a clear ecto-plasm and a granular endoplasm, and usually contain red blood cells. Pseudopodia containing clear ectoplasm are protruded and retracted. Movements cease very soon as the preparation cools. Macrophages are sometimes mistaken for amoebae. Sigmoidoscopy may reveal typical ulcers and a scraping should be examined for *Ent. histolytica*. In chronic amoebiasis several stools may need to be examined before cysts are found. The presence of cysts in the faeces does not equate with invasive amoebiasis: in endemic areas one third of the population are symptomless passers of amoebic cysts.

An amoebic abscess of the liver is suspected from the clinical and radiographic appearances and confirmed by radionuclide or ultrasonic scanning. Aspirated pus from an amoebic abcess has a characteristic appearance, as described above, but only rarely contains free amoebae.

Antibodies are detectable by immunofluorescence in over 95% of cases of hepatic amoebiasis and intestinal amoeboma but in only about 60% of dysenteric amoebiasis. Precipitin tests are less sensitive but become negative in a few months after cure.

Treatment and Prevention. Invasive intestinal amoebiasis responds quickly to oral metronidazole, 800 mg three times daily for 5 days, tinidazole in single doses of 2 g orally daily for 3 days, or emetine hydrochloride 60 mg daily, subcutaneously for a few days. Furamide 500 mg should be given orally t.i.d. for 10 days after treatment to eliminate luminal cysts. Stools are reexamined four weeks later.

Early hepatic amoebiasis responds quickly to treatment by metronidazole, tinidazole or emetine as above, or to chloroquine 300 mg base b.d. for 2 days, followed by 150 mg b.d. for 14 days. Emetine should be followed by chloroquine and furamide to eliminate the intestinal infection. If the abscess is large or threatens to burst, or if the response to chemotherapy is not prompt, aspiration is also required and repeated if necessary. If culture of the 'pus' indicates that there is secondary bacterial infection, treatment will be required with an appropriate antibiotic. Rupture of an abscess into the pleural cavity, pericardial sac or peritoneal cavity necessitates immediate aspiration or surgical drainage. Small serous effusions resolve without drainage.

Personal precautions against contracting amoebiasis in the tropics and subtropics consist of not eating fresh uncooked vegetables or drinking unboiled water.

GIARDIASIS

Infection with the flagellate *Giardia intestinalis* (Fig. 19.4), known also as *G. lamblia*, is worldwide but commoner in the tropics. It particularly affects children in endemic areas, tourists and patients in mental hospitals. The flagellates attach to the mucosa of the duodenum and jejunum and cause inflammation and partial villous atrophy. Recurrent attacks of urgent diarrhoea with abdominal discomfort and explosive loose pale stools are characteristic. There may be severe malabsorption. Lethargy, flatulence, abdominal distension, duodenal pain and nausea are frequent. Giardiasis is diagnosed by recognising the cysts in stools or the flagellate form in jejunal juice or mucus.

Fig. 19.4 Giardia intestinalis. Vegetative form ($14 \times 7 \mu$); cystic form ($8 \times 12 \mu$).

Treatment is with a single dose of tinidazole 40 mg/kg in the range 0·5 g to 2 g, repeated after 1 week, or with metronidazole 200–400 mg t.i.d. for 14 days.

BALANTIDIASIS

Balantidium coli is a ciliate that causes dysentery in pigs and occasionally infects man in whom the disease resembles amoebic dysentery.

Treatment is with tetracycline 10 mg/kg four

times daily for 10 days or metronidazole
200–400 mg three times daily according to age for
7 days.

LEISHMANIASIS

This group of diseases is caused by protozoa of
the genus *Leishmania*, conveyed to man by female
phlebotomine sandflies in which the flagellate
(promastigote) forms of leishmania develop. In
man the leishmaniae are found in cells of the
monocyte-macrophage system as oval forms
known as amastigotes or Leishman-Donovan
bodies (Fig. 19.5). Leishmaniasis may take the

form of a generalised visceral infection, kala azar,
or of a purely cutaneous infection, known in the
Old World as oriental sore. In South America
cutaneous leishmaniasis may remain confined to
the skin or metastasise to the nose and mouth.

Visceral Leishmaniasis (Kala Azar)

Kala azar is caused by *Leishmania donovani* and is
prevalent in the Mediterranean and Red Sea
littorals, Sudan, parts of East Africa, Asia Minor,
mountainous regions of Southern Arabia, eastern
parts of India, China and South America. In
India, where the disease is epidemic, man appears

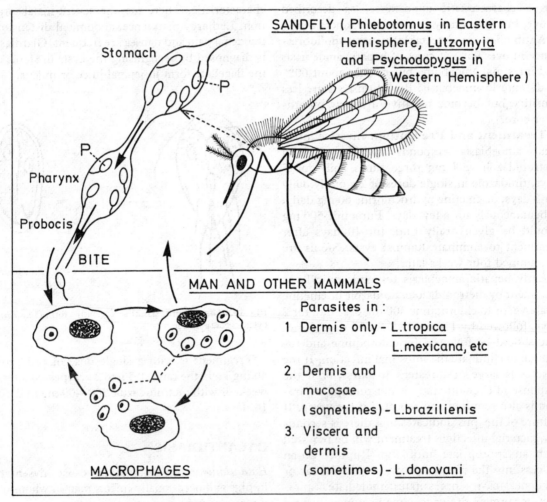

Fig. 19.5 Leishmaniasis. Life cycle of *Leishmania*. A = amastigote (Leishman-Donovan body). P = promastigote.
(Adapted from Knight R., *Parasitic Diseases of Man*).

to be the chief host. In most other areas, including the Mediterranean, dogs and foxes are the main reservoirs of infection. Here the disease is endemic and occurs chiefly in young children or tourists. In Africa various wild rodents provide the reservoir, and the disease is rural occurring in older children and visiting hunters and soldiers. Transmission has also been reported to follow blood transfusion in Northern Europe.

Pathology. Multiplication, by simple fission, of leishmaniae takes place in monocytes and macrophages in various organs, especially the liver and spleen, which becomes greatly enlarged, the bone marrow, lymphoid tissue and the small intestinal submucosa. The disease is accompanied by malnutrition and immunosuppression which is both specific to leishmania and non-specific. Acute intercurrent infection or tuberculosis are common complications. Granulocytopenia and thrombocytopenia occur. Anaemia is due to haemolysis, hypersplenism and marrow depression. Serum albumin is low and globulin, mainly IgG, high, but hepatocellular damage and bleeding are late complications.

Clinical Features. The incubation period is usually about 1 or 2 months but up to 10 years has been recorded. The onset is usually insidious with a low grade fever, the patient remaining ambulant, or it may be abrupt with sweating and high intermittent fever, sometimes showing a double rise of temperature in the 24 hours. The spleen soon becomes enlarged, often massively. Hepatomegaly is less marked. If not treated, the patient will become anaemic and wasted, frequently with increased pigmentation especially on the face. Lymphadenopathy is common and rarely is the only clinical finding.

After recovery dermal leishmaniasis sometimes develops. It may present first as hypopigmented or erythematous macules on any part of the body and later a nodular eruption may appear, especially on the face. In macular lesions intracellular amastigotes are scanty; in nodules they are more abundant.

Diagnosis is established by demonstrating the parasite in stained smears of aspirates of bone marrow, lymph node, spleen or liver, or by culture of these aspirates. Antibody is detected by immunofluorescence or complement-fixation early in the disease. The leishmanin skin test is negative. The test is performed and read in the same way as the tuberculin test, using a suspension of killed promastigotes as antigen.

Treatment and Prevention. The response to treatment varies with the geographical area in which the disease has been acquired. In Europe and Asia the disease is readily cured, but in the Sudan and East Africa it is more resistant. Pentavalent antimonials are the drugs of choice. Sodium stibogluconate contains 100 mg Sb/ml, meglumine antimoniate contains 85 mg Sb/ml. Children are given 20 mg Sb/kg i.v. or i.m. daily for 20 to 30 days. The adult dose is 10–20 mg Sb/kg to a maximum of 850 mg.

Intercurrent infection is sought and treated. Rarely blood transfusion is needed for anaemia or bleeding. Measurement of spleen size, haemoglobin and serum albumin are useful in assessing progress. A small proportion of patients relapse, and should be re-treated for two months. Second line drugs for patients who fail to respond to antimonials include pentamidine (p. 780) and amphotericin (p. 804).

In an endemic area where they are the reservoir, infected or stray dogs should be destroyed. Sandflies should be combated. They are extremely sensitive to insecticides and combined with repellants useful protection is obtained. The ordinary mosquito net sprayed with an insecticide will keep out the tiny sandfly.

Early diagnosis and treatment of human infections reduces the reservoir and controls epidemic kala azar in India. Serology is useful for case detection in the field. There is no vaccine.

Cutaneous Leishmaniasis of the Old World (Oriental Sore)

In the Old World, cutaneous leishmaniasis is found around the Mediterranean littoral, throughout the Middle East and Central Asia, as far as Pakistan, and in Subsaharan West Africa and Sudan. It is caused either by zoonotic *L. major*, a parasite of gerbils and other desert rodents, or by the arthroponotic *L. tropica*, in towns. In the highlands of Ethiopia and Kenya a third parasite, of hyraxes, *L. aethiopica* is the cause. The disease is commonly imported into

Britain. On inoculation the parasites are taken up by dermal histiocytes in which they multiply and around which lymphocytes and plasma cells accumulate. With time, the histology becomes more tuberculoid and the overlying epidermis crusts and may ulcerate centrally. Healing is accompanied by subepidermal fibrosis.

Clinical Features. The incubation period is from 2 weeks to 5 or more years but usually is from 2 to 3 months. Lesions, single or multiple on exposed parts of the body, start as small red papules which increase gradually in size, reaching 2–10 cm in diameter. A crust forms, overlying an ulcer with a granular base. Tiny satellite papules are characteristic. Untreated, the lesion heals in 3 months to 3 years, or longer. Healing produces a depressed mottled scar which may be disfiguring or disabling.

Forms of cutaneous leishmaniasis occur that do not heal spontaneously. In diffuse cutaneous leishmaniasis (*L. aethiopica*) an immune defect permits the disease to spread all over the skin, and in recidivans (lupoid) leishmaniasis (*L. tropica*) apparently healed sores relapse persistently.

The appearance of a typical lesion in a patient from an endemic area suggests the diagnosis. Leishman-Donovan bodies can be demonstrated by inserting a dry needle into the margin of the ulcer, or making a skin slit smear (p. 758) and staining the material obtained with Giemsa's stain or culturing it. The leishmanin skin test is positive except in diffuse cutaneous leishmaniasis. Serology is unhelpful.

Treatment and Prevention. The local application of heat by infra-red, hot water or a thermostatically controlled pad at 40°C may accelerate healing. Cryotherapy is said to be effective.

When the lesions are multiple or in a disfiguring site it is better to treat the patient by parenteral injections of pentavalent antimonials (p. 777), but *L. aethiopica* is not sensitive to antimonials. Diffuse cutaneous leishmaniasis is treated with pentamidine (p. 780).

In addition to those prophylactic measures described under visceral leishmaniasis against animals and sandflies, a lasting immunity can be achieved by deliberate inoculation of a living culture of *L. major* on the upper arm, which produces a typical sore but protects against a subsequent, possibly disfiguring, lesion.

Cutaneous and Mucocutaneous Leishmaniasis of the New World

In South and Central America, cutaneous leishmaniasis is endemic and mostly caused by parasites of the *L. mexicana* and *L. brasiliensis* groups, which occur in hot, moist, forest regions and are conveyed to man from a variety of rodents by several species of sandflies (Fig. 19.5). *L. mexicana* is responsible for chicleros ulcer, the self-healing sores of Mexico, Guatemala and Honduras, and for some of the sores in the north of South America, including diffuse cutaneous leishmaniasis. *L. braziliensis* extends widely from the Amazon basin as far as Paraguay and Costa Rica and is responsible for self-healing sores and for muco-cutaneous leishmaniasis. A third variety of the disease occurring in the Peruvian Andes is known as 'uta' and is caused by *L. peruviana*, dogs providing the reservoir.

Pathological and Clinical Features. The microscopic appearances of the skin lesions may be similar to oriental sore but are not always characteristic. The mucocutaneous lesions begin as a perivascular infiltration; later endarteritis may lead to destruction of the surrounding tissues (see below). Clinically, lesions of *L. mexicana* and *L. peruviana* closely resemble those seen in the Old World, but lesions on the pinna of the ear are common and are chronic and destructive.

The primary lesions of *L. braziliensis* are similar but in some areas up to 80% develop 'espundia' i.e. metastatic lesions in the mucosa of the nose or mouth. Mucosal lesions either accompany the skin lesions or appear some years later. The nasal mucosa becomes congested and later all tissues of the nose ulcerate except for the bone. The lips, soft palate and fauces may be invaded and destroyed leading to terrible suffering and deformity. Secondary bacterial infection is common.

Diagnosis depends on the history and clinical appearance, confirmed by demonstration of the parasites in smears, culture or histological section. As parasites are not easily found the Leishmanin test is of value.

Treatment. Purely cutaneous disease may be

successfully treated by sodium stibogluconate given as recommended for visceral leishmaniasis (p. 777) but in established espundia amphotericin (p. 804) may be necessary.

AFRICAN TRYPANOSOMIASIS (SLEEPING SICKNESS)

African sleeping sickness is caused by trypanosomes conveyed to man by the bites of infected tsetse flies of either sex. The disease is naturally acquired only in Africa between 12°N and 25°S. Two trypanosomes affect man, *Trypanosoma brucei gambiense* conveyed by *Glossina palpalis* and *G. tachinoides* and *T. b. rhodesiense* transmitted by *G. morsitans*, *G. pallidipes*, *G. swynnertoni* and *G. palpalis*.

Gambiense trypanosomiasis has a wide distribution in West and Central Africa reaching to Uganda and Kenya; rhodesiense trypanosomiasis is found in parts of East and Central Africa where it is currently on the increase. In West Africa trypanosomiasis transmission is mainly at the riverside, where the fly rests in the shade of trees. Animal reservoirs of *T. b. gambiense* have not been identified although pigs may harbour it. *T. b. rhodesiense* has a large reservoir in numerous wild animals and transmission takes place in the shade of woods bordering grasslands. Devastating epidemics of both types have occurred. Trypanosomiasis of cattle, caused mainly by *T. b. brucei*, is also widespread and seriously reduces grazing land and the production of meat and milk.

Pathological and Clinical Features. Only a low percentage of tsetse flies are infected. A bite by a tsetse fly is painful and commonly becomes inflamed but, if trypanosomes are introduced, the site of the bite may again become painful and swollen about 10 days later, ('trypanosomal chancre') and the regional lymph nodes enlarge. Within 2 to 3 weeks of infection the trypanosomes invade the blood stream.

In *gambiense infections* the disease usually runs a slow course over months or years with irregular bouts of fever and enlargement of lymph nodes. These are characteristically firm, discrete, rubbery and painless and are particularly prominent in the posterior triangle of the neck. Sometimes during these early weeks transient circinate erythematous eruptions can be seen and there is tachycardia. The spleen and liver may become palpable. After some months, in the absence of treatment, the central nervous system is invaded. This is shown clinically by headaches and changed behaviour, insomnia by night and sleepiness by day, mental confusion and eventually tremors, pareses, wasting, coma and death. The histological changes in the brain are similar to those found in viral encephalitis but trypanosomes are scattered in the substance of the brain and large mononuclear (morula) cells are found whose cytoplasm is eosinophilic and contains globules of IgM.

In *rhodesiense infections* fever is higher and more constant than in gambiense infections, so that within days or a few weeks the patient is usually severely ill and may have developed pleural effusions and signs of myocarditis or hepatitis. There may be a petechial rash. Enlargement of lymph nodes is usually less than in gambiense infections. The clinical manifestations of involvement of the nervous system may not be obvious but within a few weeks of infection the cerebrospinal fluid will be abnormal and in the untreated case death ensues from toxaemia or heart failure. If the illness is less acute, drowsiness, tremors, and coma may be prominent.

Diagnosis. In any febrile patient from an endemic area trypanosomiasis should be considered. In rhodesiense infections the trypanosomes can often be detected by microscopic examination of a wet blood film in which agitation of red cells by the trypanosomes is seen. Thick and thin blood films stained as for the detection of malaria, will reveal trypanosomes (Fig. 19.6).

In the earliest stages of gambiense infections

Fig. 19.6 Trypanosome in blood film.

the trypanosomes may be seen in the blood or from puncture of the primary lesion but it is usually easier to demonstrate them by puncture of a lymph node. Using a medium sized dry needle, the node, held between finger and thumb, is punctured and the node moved on the needle and the material aspirated and examined in a similar way to the blood.

Concentration methods include microhaematocrit, buffy coat microscopy and miniature anion exchange chromotography. Animal inoculation is sometimes used for the detection of rhodesiense infections. Serological tests are also employed especially in field work. If the central nervous system is affected the cell count and protein content of the cerebrospinal fluid are increased and the glucose diminished and sometimes trypanosomes may be found by centrifugation. Very high levels of serum IgM or the presence of IgM in the cerebrospinal fluid are suggestive of trypanosomiasis.

Treatment. If treatment is begun early, before the brain has been invaded, the prognosis is good. For this purpose either suramin or pentamidine isethionate may be used, the latter being employed only for gambiense infections. After the nervous system is affected an arsenical will be required to penetrate into the brain.

Suramin is usually given intravenously. An initial trial dose of 200 mg is given to test for sensitivity. This is followed on the next day by 1 g dissolved in 10 ml of distilled water repeated at intervals of 3 to 5 days to a total dosage of 5 to 10 g. Children are given doses according to weight. Toxic effects include dermatitis, nausea, vomiting, diarrhoea, peripheral neuritis and nephritis. The urine should be examined before each injection and the drug temporarily discontinued if red cells and casts appear.

Pentamidine isethionate is less toxic than suramin, but may cause diabetes. It is painful when administered intramuscularly but intravenous administration causes profound hypotension. The intramuscular dose is 3 to 5 mg/kg to a maximum of 250 mg dissolved in 5 ml distilled water, on alternate days for 10 injections. When used to treat leishmaniasis (p. 777), less frequent injections for a longer period are preferred.

Melarsoprol is a chemical combination of the trivalent melarsan oxide and dimercaprol. It is presented as 3·6% w/v solution in glycolpropylene and is administered intravenously. It has proved highly efficacious in advanced rhodesiense infections, which were formerly fatal, and for other resistant and relapsing cases. The main danger is encephalopathy due to a Jarisch-Herxheimer reaction following the death of many trypanosomes and encephalopathy due to arsenic which kills 10% of cases.

Before commencing treatment with melarsoprol the patient's general condition may be improved by a few preliminary injections of suramin. The initial dose of melarsoprol is assessed on the patient's general condition rather than on the weight. Patients who are severely ill may only tolerate 0·5 ml and the initial dose must never exceed 2 ml. Further injections are given on the second and third days. The maximum dose is 3·6 mg/kg, i.e. 5 ml for a man of 50 kg. There then follows a rest period of 1 to 2 weeks followed by a second series of three injections. If the initial dose was very small, additional courses may be required during the next 4 or 5 weeks. The total dosage aimed at is 30 ml.

Nitrofurazone is liable to produce haemolytic anaemia in those whose red cells are deficient in G6PD and peripheral neuritis, but it has been used successfully in cerebral trypanosomiasis in a dose of 10 mg/kg t.i.d. for 10 days.

Prevention. Against *T. b. gambiense* a single intramuscular injection of 250 mg pentamidine gives protection for six months because of the slow excretion of the drug. As the protection against *T. b. rhodesiense* is less sure and shorter in duration, chemoprophylaxis is not advised in rhodesiense areas. In such areas it is safer to have no protection but to ensure early recognition of the 'trypanosomal chancre' and to have the blood examined whenever there is any fever. In endemic gambiense areas various measures may be taken against tsetse flies and field teams detect and treat early human infection. In rhodesiense areas control is more difficult.

AMERICAN TRYPANOSOMIASIS (CHAGAS' DISEASE)

The cause of Chagas' disease is *Trypanosoma cruzi* transmitted to man from the faeces of a reduviid bug in which the trypanosomes have a cycle of development before becoming infective to man. The bugs are liable to fly down from the ceilings of primitive houses on to the faces of those sleeping below. Infected faeces from the bug are rubbed in through the conjunctiva, mucosa of mouth or nose or through an abrasion of the skin. Dogs and cats are the sources of infection for bugs in houses although in nature opposums and armadillos and other animals are commonly infected. Acute illness has also followed blood transfusion.

The trypanosomes travel by the blood stream and develop into amastigote forms in the tissues. These multiply in many sites, especially in the myocardium causing pseudocysts, in muscle fibres, and also in the ganglion cells of the autonomic nervous system, giving rise to the changes described below. Chagas' disease occurs widely in South and Central America.

Clinical Features. The entrance of *T. cruzi* through an abrasion produces a dusky-red firm swelling with enlargement of regional lymph nodes. A conjunctival lesion, though less common, is more characteristic; the unilateral firm reddish swelling of the lids may close the eye and constitutes 'Romana's sign'. Young children are most commonly affected. Evidence of a generalised infection soon appears, with fever, generalised lymphadenopathy and enlargement of the spleen and liver. Neurological features include insomnia, personality changes and signs of meningo-encephalitis.

Most survive but may later develop features of the chronic infection. Indeed in most cases the early infection is silent. Only infants die readily from the acute infection, death being caused in the first few days of the illness by encephalitis or a few weeks later by myocarditis or overwhelming infection. Chronic infections frequently damage Auerbach's plexus with resulting dilatation of various parts of the alimentary canal, especially the colon and oesophagus. Dilatation of the bile ducts and bronchi are also recognised sequelae. Invasion of the myocardium causes a cardiomyopathy characterised by cardiac dilatation, arrhythmias, partial or complete heart block and sudden death. Autoimmune processes are responsible for much of the damage.

Diagnosis. In the acute illness *T. cruzi* may be seen in a blood film; in chronic disease it may be recovered by xenodiagnosis. In the latter method infection-free, laboratory-bred, reduviid bugs are fed on the patient and subsequently the hind gut or faeces of the bug are examined for parasites. Complement-fixation, direct agglutination and fluorescent antibody tests are positive in 95% of cases.

Treatment and Prevention. Nifurtimox is given orally. The dosage, which has to be carefully supervised to minimise toxicity while preserving parasiticidal activity, is: under 10 years, 15–20 mg/kg and 10–17 years, 12·5–15 mg/kg for 90 days; over 17 years, 8–10 mg/kg for 120 days. Cure rates of 80% in acute disease and 90% in chronic disease are obtained. Temporary side-effects include anorexia, nausea, vomiting and epigastric pain; insomnia, headache, vertigo and excitability; myalgia and arthralgia.

Preventive measures include improved housing and destruction of reduviid bugs by spraying of houses with lindane (gamma benzylhexachloride), or other suitable insecticides. Blood taken for transfusion in endemic areas is treated with gentian violet.

TOXOPLASMOSIS

Toxoplasmosis is caused by *Toxoplasma gondii*. It is probable that human infection after birth results from the ingestion of cysts excreted in the faeces of infected cats or from eating undercooked beef or lamb. Transmission from a mother infected during pregnancy to the fetus causes congenital toxoplasmosis. Human toxoplasmosis is worldwide. Immunocompromised patients are particularly at risk.

Pathology. In the congenital form the organism is widespread in the central nervous system, eyes, heart, lungs and adrenals. If the infant survives, the parasite soon disappears from most organs except the central nervous system and retina. The brain shows large areas of necrosis with cyst formation and patchy calcification; the spinal cord may be similarly affected. In the acquired disease the organism commonly invades lymph nodes and spleen and less commonly liver and myocardium.

Clinical Features. The manifestations in congenital infections are mainly cerebral. There may be hydrocephalus or microcephaly associated with convulsions, tremors or paralysis. Radiological examination may show patches of calcification in the brain. Microphthalmos, nystagmus and chorioretinitis are common. The cerebrospinal fluid is often xanthochromic with increased protein and mononuclear cells. An enlarged liver, jaundice, diminished thrombocytes and purpura may also be found. Congenital infections are usually fatal, and if the child survives it is usually gravely incapacitated.

Many acquired infections are symptomless. In the acute form there may be pneumonia with fever, cough, generalised aches and pains, profound malaise, a maculopapular rash and rarely jaundice and myocarditis. In the more chronic infections, often afebrile, there may be only enlargement of the lymph nodes with a lymphocytosis showing atypical mononuclear cells similar to those present in infectious mononucleosis. Toxoplasmosis is recognised as a cause of chorioretinitis and uveitis in adults.

Diagnosis. Serological tests are of value. Antibodies detectable by fluorescence or the dye test appear early in the disease and persist for years. Complement fixing antibodies are late to appear and decline more quickly. A rise in titre indicates acute infection. Antibodies may not be detectable in adult ocular toxoplasmosis. Biopsy material from a lymph node may be inoculated into a laboratory animal, or show characteristic histological changes.

Treatment. Most patients with toxoplasmosis do not require specific therapy as the infection usually resolves spontaneously. Patients for whom treatment is essential include the immunosuppressed and those with eye involvement. A combination of a sulphonamide 1 g 6-hourly and pyrimethamine 25 mg daily for 2–6 weeks should be administered. If this fails or causes adverse effects such as a rash, an alternative treatment is tetracycline (250 mg 6 hourly) is given for 4 weeks. For uveitis and choroidoretinitis corticosteroids are given in addition.

DISEASES DUE TO HELMINTHS

Infections caused by the commoner helminths, or worms, are described in this section, grouped according to the three zoological classes which parasitise man: (1) trematodes or flukes, (2) cestodes or tapeworms and (3) nematodes or roundworms. Much morbidity is caused in the tropics by helminths, and they are an important cause of imported disease in temperate countries.

The only prevalent parasitic helminth of humans in Britain is the nematode *Enterobius (Oxyuris) vermicularis* or threadworm. Other worms which may be acquired in Britain include the roundworms, *Ascaris lumbricoides*, *Toxocara canis*, *Trichuris trichiura* (whipworm) and *Trichinella spiralis*. *Taenia saginata* (beef tapeworm), *Echinococcus granulosus* causing hydatid disease and *Fasciola hepatica*, an endemic fluke infecting sheep, are occasionally acquired in Britain.

Many helminths have a complicated life cycle, often involving one or more intermediate host. Only *Strongyloides stercoralis* can complete its life cycle within man. Disease may be caused by invasive larval stages (e.g. Löeffler's syndrome), adult worms (e.g. hookworms) or their progeny, either eggs (e.g. schistosomiasis) or microfilariae (e.g. onchocerciasis). Adult worms may be present in the body before, or without, producing disease. Sometimes larval stages that normally develop in intermediate hosts cause disease in man (e.g. cysticercosis). Man may also suffer from invasion by larval stages of worms that normally only infect other animals (e.g. hydatid disease).

1. DISEASES DUE TO TREMATODES (FLUKES)

Schistosomiasis; Paragonimiasis; Liver Flukes; Fasciolopsiasis

Schistosomiasis (Bilharziasis)

Schistosomiasis is one of the most important causes of morbidity in the tropics and is being spread by irrigation schemes. Schistosome eggs have been found in Egyptian mummies dated 1250 B.C.

There are three species of the genus *Schistosoma* which commonly cause disease in man, *S.*

haematobium, *S. mansoni* and *S. japonicum*. *S. haematobium* was discovered by Theodor Bilharz in Cairo in 1861 and the genus is sometimes called *Bilharzia* and the disease bilharziasis. The ovum is passed in the urine or faeces and gains access to fresh water where the ciliated miracidium inside it is liberated and enters its intermediate host, a certain species of fresh water snail, in which it multiplies. Large numbers of fork-tailed cercariae are then liberated into the water where they may survive for 2 to 3 days. Cercariae can penetrate the skin if there is only a thin film of water next to it, or the mucous membrane of the mouth of their definitive host, man. They transform into schistosomulae and moult as they pass through the lungs and are carried by the blood stream to the liver and so to the portal vein where they mature. The male worm is up to 20 mm in length and the more slender cylindrical female, usually enfolded longitudinally by the male, is rather longer (Fig. 19.7). Within 4 to 6 weeks of infection they migrate to the venules draining the pelvic viscera where the females deposit their ova. The eggs of *S. haematobium* pass mainly through the walls of the bladder and rectum. The eggs of *S. mansoni* and *S. japonicum* pass mainly through the lower bowel wall.

Fig. 19.7 Schistosoma. i. *S. haematobium*, ii. *S. mansoni*, iii. *S. japonicum* (80–160 × 50–70 μ).

Pathology. Penetration of the skin by the cercariae may produce a papular eruption which may later become vesicular. A similar cutaneous eruption may follow invasion of the skin by cercariae of non-human schistosomes. During the migration of the immature schistosomes, transitory lesions may be produced, including areas of pneumonia. At this stage there is usually an eosinophilia but the count falls progressively after the disease is established. Adult worms do not normally cause disease, unless they lodge in unusual sites. Schistosome eggs are responsible for most of the lesions. In a heavy infection ova may be found widely distributed in many tissues, but each species has a special territory for maximum egg deposition (see below). After the egg has escaped from the vein, a granuloma forms around it consisting of epithelioid cells, fibroblasts and giant cells surrounded by a zone of plasma cells and eosinophils. When the egg is near a mucosal surface, aided by the cytolytic enzyme excreted by the miracidium, it may be discharged into the bowel or bladder. If, however, the ovum is retained in the tissues the miracidium soon dies and the egg then either disintegrates or becomes calcified, and fibrous tissue forms at the site. The degree of fibrosis depends on the intensity of the infection and the frequency of re-infection. In endemic areas the immune response to an established infection may limit re-infections.

Clinical Features of the Early Infection. Occasionally there may be itching at the site of cercarial penetration, lasting 1–2 days. After a symptom-free period of 3 to 5 weeks allergic manifestations may develop such as urticaria, eosinophilia, fever, aches in the muscles, abdominal pain, splenomegaly, headaches, cough and sweating. Patches of pneumonia may be present. These allergic phenomena (*Katayama syndrome*) may be severe in infections with *S. mansoni* and *S. japonicum* but are rare with *S. haematobium*. After 1 to 2 weeks these features subside and for 2 or 3 months there may be no further symptoms until the deposition of eggs causes fresh ones to develop. The symptoms then depend on the intensity of the infection and the species of the infecting schistosome. In addition, schistosomiasis may cause glomerulonephritis, through the deposition of immune complexes.

Diagnosis and treatment are discussed on page 785.

Schistosoma haematobium

This species of schistosome affects mainly the urinary bladder, ureters and genitalia. Man is the only natural host. *S. haematobium* is highly endemic in Egypt, the east coast of Africa and the adjacent islands and occurs throughout most of

Africa, in Iran, Iraq, Syria, Yemen, South Arabia, Lebanon and Israel. It also occurs in Turkey, Cyprus and in solitary foci in Portugal and the Maharashtra State of India.

Pathology. The early changes are hyperaemia and petechiae of the bladder mucosa, followed by papilloma formation, ulceration and fibrosis. Calcification of ova produces, in intense infections, sandy patches at the base of the bladder. The lower third of the ureter is liable to fibrosis, calcification, dilatation with reflux, or stenosis. The capacity of the bladder decreases. Hydronephrosis and renal failure follow, often complicated by secondary bacterial infection of the urinary tract and the formation of calculi and sometimes amyloid disease. Squamous cell carcinoma of the bladder in relatively young males is of common occurrence in some areas of high endemicity of S. haematobium.

Egg deposition may damage the urethra, with sinus formation, the seminal vesicles, vagina, cervix, Fallopian tubes and rectum. Deposition of ova in the pulmonary arterioles may lead to pulmonary hypertension and cor pulmonale. These lung changes are especially frequent in combined infections with S. haematobium and S. mansoni. Discrete granulomas in the lung may be large enough to be visible radiologically. Ova may also be carried to the central nervous system, skin and elsewhere.

Clinical Features. Painless terminal haematuria is usually the first symptom. Frequency of micturition follows when the disease is long established, due largely to the contracted fibrosed or calcified bladder. Pain is often felt in the iliac fossa or in the loin, passing down to the groin. In advanced cases pyelonephritis, hydronephrosis or pyonephrosis may be accompanied by hypertension or uraemia. Disease of the seminal vesicles may lead to haemospermia. Females may be sterile and schistosomal lesions of the cervix may be mistaken for carcinoma. Intestinal symptoms may result from lesions in the bowel wall.

The severity of S. haematobium infection varies greatly, and many with light infections suffer a minimum of discomfort. However, as the adult worms can live for 20 years or more and progressive lesions may develop, treatment should always be given (p. 785).

Schistosoma mansoni

This species of schistosome affects particularly the large bowel. Man is the only natural host of importance although the infection is also found in baboons. S. mansoni is endemic in the Nile Delta and Libya, Southern Sudan, East Africa continuing as far south as the Transvaal and in West Africa from Sénégal and Gambia to Cameroun, throughout Zaïre and also Arabia. It is also found in South America in Venezuela, Brazil and in the West Indian Islands of the lesser Antilles, Puerto Rico and Dominica.

Pathology. The early lesions are congestion and petechiae of the large bowel mucosa, followed by papillomas, which become pedunculated, and fibrosis. The rectum is first and most affected but later the whole colon may be involved. Occasionally a segment of bowel becomes thickened and stenosed but malignant change is not a feature.

Granulomatous hepatitis, in response to eggs deposited in the liver, causes hepatomegaly and mild splenomegaly. In heavy infections, periportal fibrosis (pipe stem cirrhosis) is followed by portal hypertension and massive splenomegaly, oesophageal varices and ascites. The portal shunt provided by these varices enables ova to reach the lungs and cause disease. Ectopic deposition of ova into the central nervous system is commoner than with S. haematobium.

Clinical Features. The early manifestations are described on page 783. The characteristic symptoms of local disease begin 2 months or longer after infection. They may be slight or consist of abdominal pain and frequent stools which contain blood stained mucus. With severe advanced disease increased discomfort from rectal polypi may be experienced. The early hepatomegaly is reversible but portal hypertension may cause fatal haematemesis or progressive ascites. Jaundice and hepatic failure is uncommon. Paraplegia rarely occurs from migrating worms, being more commonly due to a granuloma compressing the cord. S. mansoni infections predispose to the carrier state of Salm. typhi.

Diagnosis and treatment are described on page 785.

Schistosoma japonicum

S. japonicum infects particularly the portal drainage of the small intestine and upper part of the large bowel. The adult worm parasitises, in addition to man, the dog, rat, field mouse, water buffalo, ox, cat, pig, horse and sheep. *S. japonicum* is prevalent in the Yellow River and Yangste-Kiang basins in China where the infection is a major public health problem. It also has a focal distribution in Japan, the Philippines, Celebes, Laos, Thailand, Vietnam and the Shan States of Burma.

Pathology and Clinical Features. The histopathology of *S. japonicum* is similar to that of *S. mansoni* but as this worm produces more eggs the lesions tend to be more extensive and widespread. The small bowel as well as the large may be affected, and hepatic fibrosis with splenic enlargement is usual. Deposition of eggs or worms in the central nervous system, especially in the brain, causes symptoms of cerebral irritation or compression in about 5% of infections.

The clinical features of schistosomiasis due to *S. japonicum* resemble those of very severe infection with *S. mansoni*. Evidence of cerebral involvement includes Jacksonian epilepsy, hemiplegia, blindness and terminal coma. Paraplegia from compression of the cord may also occur. The morbidity and mortality rate in *S. japonicum* infections is greater than from either of the other species.

Diagnosis of Schistosomiasis

A history of residence in an endemic area with symptoms as described will indicate the need for investigation. In *S. haematobium* infection the terminal spined egg can usually be found by microscopical examination of the centrifuged deposit of terminal stream urine, especially late in the morning or after exercise. The eggs may also be found by microscopic examination of the stools or of a rectal snip: a fragment of unstained rectal mucosa removed through a proctoscope. In a case of some duration a radiograph may show calcification in the wall of the bladder while intravenous urography may show stenosis or dilatation of the ureters, reduction in capacity of the bladder, or hydronephrosis. Such changes are found in endemic areas even in children, in whom large intravesical granulomas are common. In a heavy infection with *S. mansoni* or *S. japonicum* the characteristic egg with its lateral spine can usually be found in the stool. When, however, the infection is light it may be necessary to repeat the examinations over a number of days or to perform a rectal snip. Cystoscopy or sigmoidoscopy may show characteristic changes. Biopsies should be examined for ova. Serological tests (enzyme-linked immunosorbent assay or immunofluorescence) are useful as screening tests, but diagnosis rests on demonstration of ova.

The bowel symptoms and barium enema appearances of *S. mansoni* and *S. japonicum* infection may be very like those associated with intestinal amoebiasis or with a neoplasm of the large bowel, so steps should be taken to exclude these.

Treatment of Schistosomiasis

The object of specific treatment is to kill the adult schisotosomes and stop egg laying. In mass treatment campaigns in communities where reinfection is likely, it may not be possible or desirable to kill all adult worms, but a reduction in egg output of around 90% is often achieved and this significantly reduces morbidity, and possibly transmission, without impairing what little acquired immunity there may be.

Niridazole, 25 mg/kg daily, orally in 3 divided doses, for 7 days is highly effective in haematobium schistosomiasis but rather less so in mansoni schistosomiasis. The drug colours the urine brown and may cause anorexia, vomiting, headache and psychosis, especially in the presence of portal hypertension. It has largely been replaced by the following three newer but more expensive drugs.

Praziquantel is normally the drug of choice for all forms of schistosomiasis. For *S. haematobium* and *S. mansoni* a single dose (40 mg/kg) is given by mouth. Cure rates are of the order 90–100% in the former and 60–90% in the latter, depending to some extent on the intensity of infection. Egg production is reduced by over 99%. For *S japonicum* infections 2 doses each of 30 mg/kg are given in one day, or better 10 mg/kg thrice daily for two days. Side effects are uncommon and mild, and include nausea, headache, giddiness and drowsiness.

Oxamniquine orally in a dose of 15 mg/kg twice daily for 2 days cures over 95% of cases of *S. mansoni*. It is safe in the chronic hepatic forms of the disease, though it may cause fever for a few days. In uncomplicated patients only mild dizziness has been noted.

Metrifonate is an organophosphorus inhibitor of cholinesterase, and paralyses the worm. It is effective against *S. haematobium* only, and is given in a dose of 7·5 mg/kg once every 2 weeks for three doses. Higher or more frequent doses cause abdominal pain, nausea or vomiting. A simple, cheap and efficient treatment for *S. haematobium* is a single dose of metrifonate 10 mg/kg, combined with a single dose of niridazole 25 mg/kg; this reduces the egg output of *S. haematobium* by over 90%.

Surgery may be required to deal with residual lesions but large vesical granulomas usually respond well to chemotherapy. In cases of chronic *S. haematobium* infection, ureteric stricture and the small fibrotic urinary bladder may require plastic procedures. For rectal papillomas removal by diathermy or by other means may give the patient relief. Granulomatous masses in the brain or spinal cord may call for neurosurgery if the manifestations do not yield to chemotherapy.

Prevention. This presents great difficulties, and so far no really satisfactory means of controlling schistosomiasis has been established. If the ova of the schistosome in the urine or faeces are not allowed to contaminate fresh water containing the required snail host, then the life cycle is terminated.

The provision of latrines and of a safe water supply remains a major problem in rural areas throughout the tropics. In the case of *S. japonicum*, moreover, there are so many hosts besides man that the proper use of latrines would be of little avail. Mass treatment of the population helps against *S. haematobium* and *S. mansoni* but this method has so far had little success against *S japonicum*.

Attack on the intermediate host, the snail, presents many difficulties and has not on its own proved successful on any scale.

Personal Protection. Contact with infected water must be avoided. Accidental immersion or contact should be followed by a shower and vigorous towelling. Storage of water, free of snails, for three days will usually kill cercariae.

Paragonimiasis (Endemic Haemoptysis)

There are several species of the flukes of the genus *Paragonimus* which may affect man, the commonest being *P. westermani*. The adult worms measuring 10 × 6 mm live in small cysts in the lung and elsewhere. If a pulmonary cyst ruptures, the sputum of the patient contains ova, some of which may be expectorated and the others swallowed and passed in the faeces. From these eggs the larval worms emerge in water and seek the first intermediate host, a freshwater snail. Larvae emerging from the snail enter freshwater crabs or crayfish. If man or certain other mammals eat these crustacea raw or inadequately cooked, infection takes place. Human infections are most frequent in the Far East but there are also endemic foci in South America, West Africa, Somalia and India.

Pathological and Clinical Features. The adults lie in cysts up to 1 cm in diameter, containing reddish brown fluid, situated chiefly in the lung. There are seldom more than 20 such cysts present. In heavy infections, cysts may also be present in the pleural or peritoneal cavities, in the brain, muscles, skin or elsewhere.

The first symptoms are slight fever, cough and the expectoration of brown sputum. Occasionally there are bouts of frank haemoptysis with severe pain in the chest. Increasing signs in the chest may simulate pneumonia or pulmonary tuberculosis which frequently co-exists. When the parasites lodge in the abdomen there may be symptoms of enteritis or hepatitis. If they settle in the abdominal wall they may produce sinuses with a discharge through the skin. Development in the central nervous system may cause signs of cerebral irritation, encephalitis or myelitis. The disease may be very chronic and the adult worms may survive for 20 years.

Ova may be found on microscopic examination of the faeces, sputum, or a discharge. The radiological appearances of affected lungs are variable but the lesions are usually situated close to the pleural surfaces. Extrapulmonary lesions are diagnosed in life by biopsy.

Treatment and Prevention. Praziquantel is given in a dose of 25 mg/kg twice daily for 2 days. Less effective is bithionol given in a dose of 50 mg/kg daily in three divided doses on alternate days for 15 days. Lesions localised to or maximal in one lobe of a lung may be treated surgically.

In an endemic area crab or crayfish should not be eaten unless adequately cooked. Immersion of crustaceans in wine, vinegar or brine does not kill the parasites.

Liver Flukes

Table 19.6 sets out the main features of the diseases caused by flukes which infect the bile ducts of man. In the Far East and South East Asia, liver flukes are an important cause of ill health. Severe acute infections cause anorexia, abdominal pain, diarrhoea, eosinophila and increased serum levels of liver enzymes. Chronic infections cause recurrent febrile jaundice from cholangitis, and rarely cirrhosis and biliary carcinoma. Many people with light infections remain symptom free.

Fasciolopsiasis

Fasciolopsis buski is the largest fluke to infect man. The adults, 2–7.5 cm long, inhabit the small intestine of man, pigs and dogs. It is common in Central and S. China and among Chinese in S.E. Asia. The infection is spread from ova passed in the faeces into water. The intermediate hosts are snails. Man becomes infected by ingesting metacercariae encysted on water plants, particularly when he uses his teeth to peel them.

Light infections are symptomless. Heavy infections give rise to epigastric pain and loose motions. Very heavy infections may be fatal. The diagnosis is made by detecting ova or adult worms in the faeces.

Tetrachloroethylene (0.1 ml/kg with a maximum of 4 ml) is given orally on 2 or more occasions not more frequently than on alternate days. This drug rapidly deteriorates in warm climates and so must be stored in a cool dark place. Alternative treatment is with dichlorophen 100 mg/kg, repeated after one week.

Prevention is by the proper disposal of faeces. Edible water plants can be made safe by immersing them in boiling water.

Table 19.6 Diseases caused by flukes in the bile ducts.

Disease	Clonorchiasis	Opisthorciasis	Fascioliasis
Parasite	*Clonorchis sinensis*	*Opisthorcis felineus*	*Fasciola hepatica*
Other mammalian hosts	Dogs, cats, pigs	Dogs, cats, foxes, pigs	Sheep, cattle
Mode of spread	Ova in faeces into water	As for *C. sinensis*	Ova in faeces on to wet pasture
1st intermediate host	Snails	Snails	Snails
2nd intermediate host	Freshwater fish	Freshwater fish	Nil (encysts on vegetation)
Geographical distribution	Far East, esp. S. China	Far East, esp. N.E. Thailand	Cosmopolitan incl. Britain
Pathology	*Esch. coli* cholangitis, liver abscesses, biliary carcinoma	As for *C. sinensis*	Toxaemia, cholangitis, eosinophilia
Symptoms	Often symptom-free, recurrent jaundice	As for *C. sinensis*	Obscure fever, tender liver, may be ectopic subcut. fluke
Diagnosis	Ova in stool or duodenal aspirate	As for *C. sinensis*	As for *C. sinensis* also immunofluorescence
Prevention	Cook fish	Cook fish	Avoid contaminated watercress
Treatment	Praziquantel 25 mg/kg in one day		Bithionol 30 mg/kg daily for 10–15 days

2. DISEASES DUE TO CESTODES (TAPEWORMS)

Taenia saginata; Taenia solium and Cysticercosis; Echinococcus granulosus and hydatid disease; Multiceps multiceps; Diphyllobothrium latum; Diphyllobothrium mansoni; Dipylidium caninum; Hymenolepis nana.

Cestodes are ribbon-shaped worms which inhabit the human intestinal tract. They have no alimentary system and absorb nutrients through the surface. The anterior end, or scolex, is provided with suckers for attachment to the host. From the scolex arises a series of progressively developing segments, the proglottides, which when shed may continue to show active movements for some time. Cross-fertilisation takes place between segments. Ova, present in large numbers in mature proglottides, remain viable for weeks and during this period they may be consumed by the intermediate host. The larvae liberated from the ova pass into the tissues of the intermediate host, and the human disease is acquired by eating undercooked beef infected with *Cysticercus bovis*, the larval stage of *Taenia saginata* (beef tapeworm), undercooked pork containing *Cysticercus cellulosae*, the larval stage of *T. solium* (pork tapeworm), or undercooked freshwater fish containing larvae of *Diphyllobothrium latum* (fish tapeworm). Usually only one adult tapeworm is present but up to 10 have been reported.

The adult worm produces little or no intestinal upset in human beings, but knowledge of its presence, by noting segments from it in the faeces or on underclothing, may distress the patient. The life-cyles of *Diphyllobothrium mansoni, Dipylidium caninum* and *Hymenolepsis nana* are different (p. 790).

Taenia saginata

This worm may be several metres long. The scolex, the size of a pin head, has four suckers; mature segments 1·3 cm × 1 cm, contain a central-stemmed uterus with 15 to 20 lateral branches which are easily seen if the segments are left in water for 24 hours (Fig. 19.8). The ova of both *T. saginata* and *T. solium* are spherical and indistinguishable microscopically. The thick outer

Fig. 19.8 Taenia saginata (Ova 30–40 μ).

shell has radial striations and the ovum contains six hooklets.

Infection with *T. saginata* occurs in all parts of the world, including Britain. The patient usually notices segments on underclothing or in stools. The segments should be identified. Ova may also be found in the stool.

Treatment and Prevention. Praziquantel is the drug of choice, in a single dose of 10 mg/kg. Less effective is niclosamide; 2 tablets of the drug, each containing 0·5 g, are chewed and swallowed with a little water. One hour later a further 2 tablets are similarly taken. There are no side-effects. Prevention depends on efficient meat inspection or the thorough cooking of beef.

Taenia solium and Cysticercosis

T. solium, the pork tapeworm, was formerly cosmopolitan in distribution but is now rare except in Central Europe, Ethiopia, South Africa, the Andes and in parts of Asia. It is not so large as *T. saginata*, and the uterus usually has less than 14 lateral branches. The scolex has, in addition to suckers, two circular rows of hooklets anterior to the suckers. The adult worm is found only in man following the eating of undercooked pork containing cysticerci.

Human cysticercosis results from ova being swallowed or gaining access to the human stomach by regurgitation from the intestine harbouring an adult worm (Fig. 19.9). In the stomach the larvae are liberated from the eggs, penetrate the intestinal mucosa and are carried to many parts of the body where they develop and form cysticerci. The most common locations are the subcutaneous tissue and skeletal muscles; when superficially placed they can be palpated under the skin or mucosa as pea-like ovoid bodies. Here they cause few or no symptoms; however cysts may also develop in the brain.

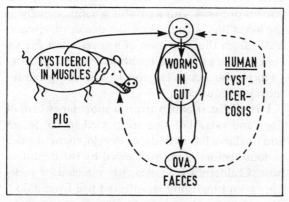

Fig. 19.9 Cysticercosis. Life cycle of *Taenia solium.*

About 5 to 20 years later the larvae die; in the brain the tissue reaction may cause epileptic fits, obscure neurological disorders, personality changes and occasionally internal hydrocephalus. After death of the larvae in muscles the cysts calcify and this enables them to be recognised radiologically. In the brain, however, much less calcification takes place and larvae are only occasionally demonstrated radiologically. Epileptic fits starting in adult life should suggest the possibility of cysticercosis if the patient has lived in an endemic area. The subcutaneous tissue should be palpated and any nodule excised for histology. Radiological examination of the skeletal muscles for calcified cysts must be made and repeated after intervals of 6 months if at first negative.

Treatment and Prevention. *T. solium* can be destroyed by praziquantel or niclosamide (p. 788).

Praziquantel improves the prognosis of cerebral cysticercosis — 50 mg/kg in 3 divided doses daily for 10 days. Prednisone, 10 mg every 8 hours is also given for 14 days, starting one day before the praziquantel. In addition antiepileptic drugs should be given to tide the patient over the period until the reaction in the brain has subsided. Operative intervention is indicated if hydrocephalus develops.

Prevention of *T. solium* infection consists in cooking pork well before eating it. Cysticercosis is avoided if food is not contaminated by ova or segments. Patients with pork tapeworm probably get cysticercosis from ingesting ova from contaminated fingers, rather than from regurgitation of segments. Great care must be taken by nurses and others while attending to a patient harbouring an adult worm.

Echinococcus granulosus (Taenia echinococcus) and Hydatid Disease

The dog, and certain wild canines, are the definitive host of the tiny tapeworm *E. granulosus*. The larval stage, a hydatid cyst, normally occurs in sheep, cattle and other animals, including camels, that are infected from contaminated pastures or water. Man, by handling a dog or drinking contaminated water may ingest eggs (Fig. 19.10). The embryo is liberated from the ovum in the small intestine and gains access to the blood stream and thus to the liver. The resultant cyst grows very slowly. It may calcify or may rupture giving rise to multiple cysts. A variant, *E. multilocularis* which has a cycle between foxes and

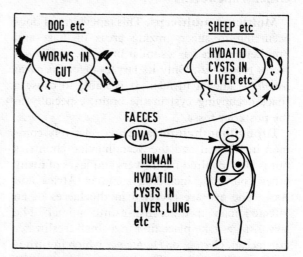

Fig. 19.10 Hydatid disease. Life cycle of *Echinococcus granulosus.*

voles, causes a similar but more severe infection, 'alveococcosis' which invades the liver like cancer.

In man a hydatid cyst is typically acquired in childhood and it may, after growing for some years, cause pressure symptons. These will vary, depending on the organ or tissue involved. In nearly 75% of patients with hydatid disease the right lobe of the liver is invaded and contains a single cyst. In others a cyst may be found in lung, brain, or elsewhere. The diagnosis depends on the clinical, radiological, and ultrasound findings in a patient who has lived in close contact with dogs. Intradermal (Casoni), complement-fixation, and immunofluorescent tests usually give support to the diagnosis.

Treatment and Prevention of hydatid disease is surgical. Great care is taken to avoid spillage and cavities are sterilised with 2% formalin, 0·5% silver nitrate or 30% sodium chloride. Mebendazole in a dose of 40–200 mg/kg/d has been used for inoperable disease. The drug is extremely expensive and the results generally discouraging. It may have a role, however, in alveolar hydatid disease.

Prevention is difficult when man lives in close association with dogs and sheep. Better personal hygiene, meat inspection and deworming of dogs can greatly reduce the prevalence of disease.

Other Tapeworms

Multiceps multiceps. This tapeworm of dogs occurring in sheep-grazing areas of East and Southern Africa has a similar life cycle to *Echinococcus granulosus*. Only its larval stage, *Coenurus serialis* is known in man. It is liable to cause a space occupying cyst in the brain, especially in the posterior fossa.

Diphyllobothrium latum is relatively common in Finland and the Scandinavian countries but is also acquired from rivers and lakes of many other countries, including some in Africa and Asia. The ova are excreted in the faeces of an infected man or other fish-eating animal. The larval stages take place first in a small freshwater crustacean, *Cyclops* or *Diaptomus* which in turn is swallowed by a fish. The infections are usually symptomless. Occasionally there are signs of allergy and in a small percentage of cases a megaloblastic anaemia develops, the worm competing with the host for vitamin B_{12}. The diagnosis is made by finding ova in the stool and treatment is by praziquantel or niclosamide (p. 788).

Diphyllobothrium mansoni (Spirometra erinacei). The adult worms are harboured by cats and dogs. The second larval stage, a sparganum, is occasionally found in the subcutaneous tissues of man. The Masai in East Africa probably become infected by ingestion of the first intermediate host, a *Cyclops*, from well water and the patient presents with a painful swelling usually in the lower limbs. In the Far East ocular *sparganosis* arises from the migration of a sparganum from a split frog applied as a traditional poultice. Sparganosis also occurs in the U.S.A. Surgical removal is required.

Dipylidium caninum is a short tapeworm of dogs and cats. The ova are passed in the faeces and the larva has to undergo development in a flea or louse before being swallowed by the definitive host. Children are occasionally infected by picking up and ingesting an infected flea from a dog. The diagnosis is made by finding segments or ova in the stools. Treatment, in appropriate doses for a child, is by niclosamide in a single dose of 1–2 g depending on age.

Hymenolepis nana. This dwarf tapeworm is unusual in not requiring an intermediate host. It is a common infection in children living in insanitary conditions in the tropics and subtropics. Apart from an eosinophilia, no signs or symptoms are present except in the presence of numerous worms, when enteritis and allergic phenomena may be encountered. The diagnosis is made by recognising the ova in the faeces. Treatment is with praziquantel in a dose of 20 mg/kg once or niclosamide 0·5–2 g, depending on age, daily for a week.

3. DISEASES DUE TO NEMATODES (ROUNDWORMS)

Nematode infections of man may be divided into three groups:

1. INTESTINAL NEMATODES. The commonest that cause disease are *Enterobius vermicularis, Ascaris lumbricoides, Trichuris trichiura, Necator*

americanus and *Ancylostoma duodenale, Strongyloides stercloralis, Capillaria phillippinensis.* Others, notably *Trichostrongylus*, are not pathogenic.

Adult male and female worms live in the lumen of the gut and do not normally invade tissues. They often have complex life cycles and may cause a syndrome of fever, cough and eosinophilia during the stage of larval invasion. Eggs or larvae are passed in the faeces and the worm does not normally complete its life cycle in man. *Strongyloides*, however, breaks both these rules and is potentially the most dangerous.

2. TISSUE-DWELLING HUMAN NEMATODES. These are the filarial worms (*Wuchereria bancrofti, Brugia malayi, Loa loa, Onchocerca volvulus*, and some others with a more restricted distribution), and the guinea worm *Drancunculus medinensis.*

These worms have complex life cycles, with an intermediate host that is also a vector. Disease may be due to the presence of the adult viviparous worms or to their progeny, the microfilariae, which migrate in the blood or tissues, provoking a massive eosinophilia; but often the infection is long lived and well tolerated.

3. NEMATODES OF OTHER ANIMALS that cause ectopic infections in man. The most important are *Toxocara canis, Ancylostoma brasiliensis, Oesophagostomum* species, *Angiostrongylus cantonensis, Trichinella spiralis, Gnasthostoma spinigerum* and *Anisakis marina.*

The infective larvae of these worms are unable to 'home' to their normal site for development into adults, in their abnormal host. They may wander or may become trapped in a particular organ. They tend to provoke severe inflammatory reactions characterised by eosinophilic granulomas.

1. DISEASES DUE TO INTESTINAL NEMATODES

Enterobius vermicularis (Threadworm)

This helminth is common throughout the world, including Britain. It affects children especially. The male worm is 2–5 mm long and the female 8–13 mm (Fig. 19.11). After the ova are swallowed, development takes place in the small intestine, but the adult worms are found chiefly in the colon. The gravid female worm lays ova

around the anal orifice, and causes intense itching, especially at night. The ova are often carried to the mouth on the fingers and so reinfection takes place. In female patients the genitalia may be invaded. The adult worms may be seen moving on the buttocks or in the stool. Ova are detected by applying the adhesive surface of cellophane tape to the perianal skin in the morning. This is then examined on a glass slide under the microscope.

Fig. 19.11 Threadworm. *Enterobius vermicularis* (Ova 55 × 25 μ).

Treatment. A single dose of one of the drugs in Table 19.7 is given and repeated after 2 weeks to control auto-reinfection. Where infection constantly recurs in a family, all members should be treated with mebendazole 100 mg twice daily for 3 days repeated after 10 days. During this period all night clothes and bed linen are laundered and finger nails are scrubbed before meals.

Ascaris lumbricoides ('Roundworm')

This is a large, pale yellow roundworm 20–35 cm long, something like an earthworm, but not segmented.

Man is infected by ingesting food contaminated with mature ova. The larvae escape from the ova in the duodenum and find their way to the lungs where they develop further. After invading the alveoli they then ascend the bronchi and trachea and are swallowed, thus entering the small intestine where they reach maturity. In heavy infections, migration of larvae through the lung may cause pulmonary eosinophilia (p. 247).

Symptoms due to adult worms may be absent or consist of nausea, colicky abdominal pain and irregular motions. Sometimes a worm is vomited or passed *per rectum*. In children with severe infections a tangled mass of worms may cause intestinal obstruction. Many worms competing with the host for nourishment may contribute to malnutrition. Other complications include block-

Table 19.7 Relative activity of drugs used for the common gut nematodes.

	Ascaris	Hookworm	Enterobius	Trichuris	Strongyloides
Piperazine salts 100 mg/kg	+ + +	+	+ + +	--	--
Pyrantel pamoate 10 mg/kg	+ + +	+ +	+ + +	--	--
Oxantel pamoate 10 mg/kg	--	--	--	+ + +	--
Mebendazole 100 mg (any age)	+ +	+ +	+ + +	+ +	+
Thiabendazole 25 mg/kg	(+ +)	(+ +)	(+ +)	(+)	+ + +
Levamisole 5 mg/kg	+ + +	+	+	--	--
Pyrvinium 5 mg/kg	+	--	+ + +	--	--

Size of single dose is given. Activities given in parenthesis indicate that the drug is not used for that species. Piperazine is cheap and safe, but with a limited range. Mebendazole given twice daily for 3 days is completely safe and eradicates most infections. Thiabendazole has a wide spectrum; it is absorbed and effective against many tissue dwelling nematodes, but toxic, causing dizziness, headache, anorexia, vomiting and drowsiness. A single dose antihelminthic is ideal for mass treatment and control schemes. Levamisole is the first choice for roundworms, and has a useful action against hookworms. A single dose of pyrantel pamoate and oxantel pamoate is used for multiple infections.

(Adapted from Knight, R. p. 807)

age of the bile or pancreatic duct and obstruction of the appendix by adult worms.

The diagnosis is made by finding ova in the faeces or by observing an adult worm (Fig. 19.12). A solely male infection is usually revealed only after the giving of an anthelmintic to a patient with an unexplained eosinophilia. Occasionally the worms are demonstrated radiographically by barium.

FERTILIZED UNFERTILIZED
OVA

Fig. 19.12 Roundworm. *Ascaris lumbricoides* (Ova 16 × 45 μ fertilised; 90 × 40 μ unfertilised)

Treatment. See Table 19.7. Single doses of piperazine, levamisole or pyrantel are effective, but mebendazole should be given twice daily for 3 days. If obstruction occurs and fails to respond to nasogastric suction and sedation, surgery is required, when the worms are 'milked' past the obstruction, or removed by enterostomy.

Trichuris trichiura (Whipworm).

Under unhygienic conditions, infections with whipworm are common all over the world. Man is the only host. Infection takes place by the ingestion of earth or food contaminated with ova which have become infective after lying for 3 weeks or more in moist soil. The adult worm is 3–5 cm long and has a coiled anterior end resembling a whip (Fig. 19.13).

OVUM

Fig. 19.13 Whipworm. *Trichuris trichiura* (Ova 50 × 22 μ).

Whipworms inhabit chiefly the caecum but occasionally also the lower ileum, appendix, colon and anal canal. There are usually no symptoms, but intense infections in children may cause persistent diarrhoea or rectal prolapse. The diagnosis is readily made by identifying ova in faeces. In heavy infections adult whipworms are found in the anal canal. Treatment is with mebendazole in doses of 100 mg twice daily for 3–5 days or a single dose of oxantel (Table 19.7).

Ancylostomiasis (Hookworm Infection)

Ancylostomiasis is caused by parasitisation of the small intestine with *Ancylostoma duodenale* or *Necator americanus*. The adult hookworm is a greyish-white nematode about 1 cm long (Fig. 19.14) which lives, often in large numbers, in the duodenum and upper jejunum. Eggs are passed in the faeces. In warm, moist, shady soil the larvae develop and reach the filariform infective stage. On coming in contact with human skin they penetrate it and are carried to the lungs. After entering the alveoli they ascend the bronchi, are swallowed and develop in the small intestine, reaching maturity in 4 to 7 weeks after infection. The larvae may also enter through the mucous membrane of the mouth. Man is the only host.

Hookworm infection is widespread under insanitary conditions in the tropics and subtropics and occurs in certain mines in Europe. *A. duodenale* is endemic in the Far East and Mediterranean coastal regions and is also present in Africa. *N. americanus* is endemic in West, East and Central Africa and Central and South America as well as in the Far East.

Pathology. At the site of entry the larvae may cause allergic inflammation. When infection is heavy, the passage through the lungs may cause pulmonary eosinophilia (p. 247). In the small intestine the worms attach themselves to the mucosa by their buccal capsule and withdraw blood. The mean daily loss of blood from one *A. duodenale* is 0·15 ml and for *N. americanus* 0·03 ml. The degree of iron and protein deficiency which develops depends not only on the load of worms but also on the nutrition of the patient and especially on the stores of iron, so that in a light infection there may be no anaemia. In the early stage of infection eosinophilia is common.

Clinical Features. In a well nourished person with a light established infection there may be no symptoms. At the time of infection hookworm dermatitis (ground itch) may be experienced, usually on the feet. An itchy erythema appears first and soon develops through papules and vesicles to the pustular stage. In a heavy infection the passage of the larvae through the lungs causes a paroxysmal cough with blood-stained sputum, associated with patchy pulmonary consolidation. When the worms have reached the small intestine, vomiting and epigastric pain, like that of a duodenal ulcer, may ensue. Sometimes frequent loose stools are passed, the condition then resembling early sprue (p. 719) or giardiasis (p. 775). In the undernourished, anaemia and hypoproteinaemia may develop with a puffy face, peripheral oedema or ascites, tachycardia, breathlessness and signs of cardiac failure. In children mental and physical development may be retarded.

Diagnosis. The characteristic egg can be recognised in the stool (Fig. 19.14). The oedema with anaemia has to be differentiated from that due to kwashiorkor, heart failure or nephritis. If hookworms are present in numbers sufficient to cause anaemia, tests of the stool for occult blood will be positive and ova will be present in large numbers.

ADULTS   OVUM

Fig. 19.14 Hookworm. Ancylostoma duodenale (Ova 60 × 40 μ).

Treatment. See Table 19.7. Mebendazole twice daily for 3 days is preferred, but for single dose treatment pyrantel is more effective.

Anaemia associated with hookworm infection responds well to oral iron. When it is severe enough to cause heart failure blood should be transfused slowly, with frusemide 20 mg in each unit.

Stronglyoidiasis

Strongyloides stercoralis is a very small nematode (2 mm × 0·4 mm) which parasitises the mucosa of the upper part of the small intestine in large numbers. The eggs hatch in the bowel and only larvae are passed in the faeces. In moist soil they moult and become the infective filariform larvae. These, on penetrating the tissues of man, undergo a development cycle similar to that of hookworms but the female worms burrow into the mucosa and submucosa. In the intestine some larvae may develop into filariform larvae which may then penetrate the mucosa or the perianal skin and lead to auto-infection and a very persistent infection, still seen in some ex-prisoners of the Second World War. Man is the natural host, but dogs may also be infected.

Stronglyoidiasis is worldwide in the tropics and subtropics and is especially prevalent in the Far East.

Pathology. There may be a dermatitis at the time of entry of the larval worms. In the intestine the female worm burrows into the mucosa and sets up an inflammatory reaction; with very heavy infections the mucosa may be severely damaged leading to malabsorption. Granulomatous changes, necrosis, and even perforation and peritonitis may also occur. Eosinophilia commonly persists. Actively motile larvae are passed in the faeces. Immunosuppression due to disease or drugs such as corticosteroids, may lead to fatal systemic strongyloidiasis.

Clinical Features. An itch may be produced during invasion of the skin. With slight infections there will be no intestinal symptoms, but in more severe cases abdominal pain and diarrhoea may be produced, which is on occasion severe. Urticaria, arthralgia, wheeze, anaemia, weakness and emaciation may also be present as well as signs of malabsorption, ileus or volvulus. Penetration of the skin about the anus or the intestinal wall by filariform larvae may lead to extremely itchy, linear, urticarial weals. These usually subside in a few hours but tend to keep on recurring. The eruptions may extend 3 or 4 cm in an hour.

This rapid progress has led to the term 'larva currens' being used rather than 'larve migrans' or creeping eruption. In addition there are frequently urticarial weals or less well defined areas of erythema. These skin lesions may persist for years without there being any intestinal symptoms.

Systemic strongyloidiasis causes diarrhoea and pneumonia and is rapidly fatal unless diagnosed and promptly treated.

Diagnosis and Treatment. Motile rod-shaped larvae can be seen on microscopic examination of the faeces and occasionally in the sputum, urine or bile. Excretion of them is intermittent so repeated examinations may be necessary. In ancylostomiasis, ova, not larvae, are found in a fresh stool. Filarial serology is positive in 15% of patients.

Thiabendazole is given orally in a dose of 25 mg/kg body weight twice daily for 2 to 4 days, according to tolerance. A second similar course may be required.

Capillariasis

Infection with *C. phillippinensis* suddenly appeared as an epidemic in the Philippines in the 1960s and in Thailand. Adult worms 2–4 mm long invade the jejunal mucosa, causing abdominal pain with severe diarrhoea and malabsorption. Eggs resembling those of *Trichuris* are passed in the faeces. Migrating fish are intermediate hosts. Untreated, mortality is high, but thiabendazole 25 mg b.d. for 3 weeks or mebendazole 200 mg b.d. for 2 weeks, is effective.

Control of Intestinal Nematode Infections

Most of these worms are transmitted through contaminated soil or unwashed hands. Safe disposal of faeces, the provision of clean drinking water and strict personal hygiene form the basis of control. Mass treatment at yearly intervals is also useful (Table 19.7). Capillariasis is controlled by cooking fish.

2. DISEASES DUE TO TISSUE-DWELLING HUMAN NEMATODES

Filariases

A number of different nematodes of the family *Filariidae* affect man. The adults are thin worms varying from 2 to 50 cm in length and the larvae, or microfilariae, are easily visible under the low power of the microscope. The mature females are viviparous. The adults of the species *Wuchereria bancrofti* and *Brugia malayi* inhabit and tend to block lymphatic vessels. Adult filariae of the species *Loa loa* wander in the subcutaneous tissue and cause 'Calabar' swellings. The adults of *Onchocerca volvulus* may be surrounded by fibrous tissue in subcutaneous nodules but it is their larvae which cause a dermatosis and eye lesions. The larvae of *Dipetalonema streptocerca* may produce a similar but milder dermatosis but *Dipetalonema perstans* and *Mansonella ozzardi*, the larvae of which circulate in the blood, are non-pathogenic. The microflariae have distinguishing morphological appearances (Fig. 19.15). Filarial infections are commonly associated with a marked eosinophilia.

Bancroftian Filariasis

Wuchereria bancrofti is conveyed to man by the bites of infected mosquitoes of a number of

W. bancrofti   B. malayi   Loa loa

O. volvulus   D. streptocerca   M. ozzardi   D. perstans

Fig. 19.15 Microfilariae (170–320 × 3–10 μ) Second and fourth rows show tails (greatly enlarged).

different species, the most common being *Culex fatigans*. The adult worms, 4 to 10 cm in length, live in the lymphatics of man, and the females produce microfilariae which at night circulate in large numbers in the peripheral blood. In the mosquito the microfilaria develop and enlarge and the surviving few are able to infect man when the mosquito again bites. As *Culex fatigans* bites at night the nocturnal periodicity of the microfilariae facilitates the spread of the infection. In some of the Pacific islands there is a non-periodic strain of *W. bancrofti* maintained by mosquitoes which bite in the day-time. When not circulating in the peripheral blood, the microfilariae are chiefly in the capillaries in the lungs. The infection is widespread in tropical Africa, the North African coast, coastal areas of Asia, Indonesia and Northern Australia, South Pacific Islands, West Indies and also in North and South America.

Pathology. The microfilariae do not harm the human host. Light infections may remain symptomless but are likely to be associated with an eosinophilia. In more intense and repeated infections the presence of mature worms in the lymphatic vessels and nodes leads to allergic inflammation around the lymphatics and to temporary lymphatic obstruction. Eventually, after repeated attacks, in some of which secondary bacterial infections may play a part, permanent obstruction of a main lymphatic trunk may be produced. Lymphatics rupture and lymph spills into tissues. Progressive enlargement of the limb or region below the obstruction then follows with thickening and fibrosis of the tissues.

Clinical Features. After an incubation period of not less than 3 months there are bouts of fever accompanied by pain, tenderness and erythema along the course of inflamed lymphatic vessels. In addition there may be urticaria. Inflammation of the spermatic cord, epididymitis and orchitis are common. After a few days the fever abates and the symptoms and signs subside.

Further attacks are likely to follow and temporary oedema from obstructed lymphatics tends to become more persistent, and some enlargement of regional lymph nodes may remain. The lymphatics draining the lower limbs, the scrotum and the upper limbs are those most frequently affected, mainly or only on one side, and often accompanied by the formation of superficial lymph varices and the production of hydroceles. Progressive enlargement, coarsening, corrugation and fissuring of the skin and subcutaneous tissue, with warty superficial excrescences, develops gradually until a leg resembles that of an elephant. The name 'elephantiasis' is thus applied to this condition which may also occur in an upper limb, the scrotum, vulva or breast. The scrotum may reach an enormous size. Obstruction of the abdominal or thoracic lymphatics may lead to chyluria, chylous ascites or a chylous pleural effusion (p. 271).

The interval between infection and the onset of elephantiasis is usually not less than 10 years, after which the condition tends to be slowly but remorselessly progressive. Gross elephantiasis develops only in association with repeated infections in highly endemic areas.

Diagnosis. In the earliest stages of lymphangitis the diagnosis is made on clinical grounds, supported usually by an eosinophilia and sometimes by a positive complement-fixation or intradermal test. After about a year from the time of infection microfilariae appear in the blood at night and can be seen moving in a wet blood film or a sample of lysed blood passed through a microfilter and identified after staining. They are usually present in hydrocele fluid which may on occasion yield an adult filaria. With the establishment of permanent elephantiasis it becomes unusual for microfilariae to reach the blood stream and eventually the adult worms may die but the lymphatics remain obstructed. Shadows of calcified filariae may sometimes be demonstrable by radiography. An initial exaggeration of symptoms following the administration of diethylcarbamazine is indicative of a filarial infection.

Immunodiagnosis. Indirect fluorescence detects antibody in over 95% of active cases and 70% of established elephantiasis. Cross reactions occur in 15% of cases of strongyloidiasis and 5% of other intestinal nematodes. The test becomes negative 1–2 years after cure. Complement fixation is rather less specific and sensitive. Intradermal tests of immediate hypersensitivity are positive and persist for life. None of these tests distinguishes between the different filarial infections.

Non-filarial elephantiasis, usually affecting only one lower limb, occurs in certain geographical areas which are free from filariasis. It is attributable to damage to lymphatics by silicates absorbed from soil derived from volcanic rocks.

Treatment. Diethylcarbamazine, given orally, has a rapid destructive effect on microfilariae and a slower action against adult filariae. The dosage is 9 to 12 mg/kg daily in three divided doses for 21 days. The full dosage should, however, only be reached slowly, starting with 50 mg (one tablet) and doubling daily if no untoward allergic responses ensue. This course may be repeated twice at intervals of 4 to 6 weeks. To control allergic phenomena antihistamines or corticosteroids may be required. In established elephantiasis plastic surgery, perferably after preliminary radiological investigation of the lymphatics, is indicated. Great relief may be obtained by removal of excess tissue but recurrences are probable unless new lymphatic drainage is established. Tight bandaging, or bed rest with suspension or raising of the affected part or the nightly use of pneumatic stockings, may control the swelling to some extent.

Prevention. In endemic areas treatment of the whole population with diethylcarbamazine, 100 mg for adults (50 mg for children) three times daily for 7 days, has reduced but not eliminated the infection. Children are given such a course on starting and just before leaving school. This mass treatment should be combined with control of the vector by insecticides. Personal protection is obtained by the wearing of protective clothing and the use of insect repellants. Where the vector is a night-biting mosquito wire-screening of the house or the use of mosquito nets prevent infection. Early chemotherapy prevents later elephantiasis.

Brugia Filariasis

Brugia malayi resembles *W. bancrofti* closely (Fig. 19.15). The microfilariae usually exhibit nocturnal periodicity but a semiperiodic form, which may affect man, commonly infects animals. A similar filaria, *Brugia pahangi,* is found chiefly in animals but has been transmitted to man. It, or a similar filaria, may be responsible for some cases of tropical pulmonary eosinophilia (p. 799). The vectors of *B. malayi* are mosquitoes mostly belonging to the genus *Mansonioides*. *B. malayi* is found in Indonesia, Borneo, Malaysia, Vietnam, South China, South India and Sri Lanka. A distinct, closely related, species, *B. timori* occurs in Timor.

The pathology, clinical manifestations, treatment and personal prophylaxis are the same as those recorded for *W. bancrofti* except that elephantiasis is usually limited to the legs. A selective ´weed-killer, phenoxylene, has been used with success to rid ponds of the water hyacinth upon which the larvae of *Mansonioides* are dependent.

Loiasis

Loiasis is caused by infection with the filaria *Loa loa* (Fig. 19.15). The adults, 3 to 7 cm × 0·4 mm, parasitise chiefly the subcutaneous tissue of man. The larval microfilariae circulate harmlessly in the peripheral blood in the day-time. The vector is *Chrysops*, a day biting, forest dwelling, fly.

Pathology. The adult worms move about in the subcutaneous tissues and other interstitial planes. Usually there is little evidence, apart from an eosinophilia, of a reaction of the host's tissues but from time to time a short-lived, inflammatory, oedematous swelling (a 'Calabar' swelling) is produced, presumably around an adult worm. Heavy infections may rarely cause encephalitis, especially when treated.

Clinical Features. The incubation period is commonly over a year but is often as short as 3 months. The infection is often symptomless. The first sign is usually a Calabar swelling. This is an irritating tense localised swelling which is painful if it is near a joint. The swelling is generally on a limb; it measures a few centimetres in diameter but sometimes is more diffuse and extensive. It usually disappears after a few days but may persist for 2 or 3 weeks. A succession of such swellings may appear at irregular intervals, often in near-by sites. Sometimes there is some urticaria and pruritus elsewhere. Occasionally a worm may be distinctly seen wriggling under the skin, especially of an eyelid and may cross the eye under the conjunctiva, taking many minutes to do so. When an adult worm is moving in retro-orbital tissues, severe unilateral headache resembling migraine is experienced.

A worm crossing the eye or penetrating the skin enables a clinical diagnosis to be made. Also characteristic are Calabar swellings in one who has resided in an endemic area. Usually microfilariae of *Loa loa* can be demonstrated in the blood. The filarial indirect fluorescent antibody test is positive in 95% of cases, complement fixation in 80%, the intradermal test is usually positive and there is an eosinophilia. Occasionally a calcified dead worm may be seen on a radiograph.

Treatment and Prevention. Diethylcarbamazine (p. 796) is curative, given orally, gradually increased to a dose of 9 to 12 mg/kg body weight daily and continued at that dosage for 21 days. Treatment may precipitate a severe reaction characterised by fever, malaise, joint and muscle pain and rarely encephalitis.

Protection is afforded by siting houses away from trees and by having dwellings wire-screened against the fly. Protective clothing and repellents are also useful. Mud flats where *Chrysops* is breeding should be treated with Dieldrin or other chemicals to destroy the larvae and pupae. Treatment of the population with diethylcarbamazine will diminish the infective rate of the potential vector.

Onchocerciasis (River Blindness)

Onchocerciasis is the result of infection by the filaria *Onchocerca volvulus* (Fig. 19.15). Although only about 0·3 mm in diameter, the adult female may be as long as 50 cm, the male being much shorter. The infection is conveyed by flies of the genus *Simulium* which inflict a painful bite. In West Africa the vector is *S. damnosum*, in northern Nigeria also *S. bovis* and in East Africa and Zaïre *S. neavei*. The flies breed in rapidly flowing well aerated water, the larvae being attached to submerged vegetation and rocks. The larvae of *S. neavei* may be attached to crabs and mayfly nymphs. Adult flies bite during the day-time both inside and outside houses. Man is the only known definitive host.

Onchocerciasis is endemic in well defined areas throughout tropical Africa, in Southern Arabia and also in South Mexico, Guatemala, Colombia, Venezuela and Brazil. It is estimated that over 20 million people are infected. In parts of West and Central Africa it affects the whole adult population and blindness rates of 10% are common, reaching 35% in some parts of Ghana. Because of onchocerciasis huge tracts of fertile land lie virtually untilled.

Pathology. Infective larvae of *O. volvulus* are introduced into the skin by the bite of an infected *Simulium*. The worms mature in 2 to 4 months and live for up to 17 years in small colonies in subcutaneous and connective tissue. At sites of trauma, over bony prominences and around joints, fibrosis may form nodules around adult worms which otherwise cause no direct damage. In these nodules, in the adjacent tissues and widely distributed in the skin, innumerable microfilariae, discharged by the female *O. volvulus*, move actively and may invade the eye.

Live microfilariae elicit little tissue reaction, but dead microfilariae may cause severe allergic inflammation leading to hyaline necrosis and loss of collagen and elastin. In the eye, death of microfilariae causes conjunctivitis, sclerosing keratitis with pannus formation, iritis which may lead to glaucoma and cataract and, less commonly, choroidoretinitis and optic neuritis.

Clinical Features. The infection may remain symptomless for months or years. The first symptom is usually itching at first localised to one quadrant of the body and later becoming generalised and involving the eyes. In Europeans evanescent oedema of part or all of a limb is an early sign, followed by papular urticaria spreading gradually from the site of infection. This is difficult to see on dark skins in which the commonest signs are papules excoriated by scratching, spotty hyperpigmentation from resolving inflammation and more chronic changes of a rough, thickened skin or inelastic wrinkled skin. Superficial lymph nodes enlarge and may hang down in folds of loose skin at the groins. Hydrocele, femoral hernias and scrotal elephantiasis occur. In chronic infections, firm subcutaneous nodules (onchocercomas) are palpable, one or more cm in diameter.

Eye disease is commonest in some highly endemic areas and is associated with chronic heavy infections and nodules on the head. Early manifestations include itching, lachrymation, conjunctival injection and evidence of the features listed under pathology. Classically, 'snow flake' deposits are seen in the edges of the cornea.

Diagnosis. The finding of nodules or characteristic lesions of the skin or eyes, in a patient from an endemic area, associated with eosinophilia is suggestive. Aggravation of the dermatosis after a test dose of 50 mg of diethylcarbamazine supports the diagnosis. A skin snip or shaving, repeated if necessary from calf, buttock and shoulder is placed in saline under a cover slip on a microscope slide and examined after one hour. In all but the lightest infections microfilariae are seen wriggling free. Microfilariae can also sometimes be seen moving in the anterior chamber of the eye examined with a slit-lamp or identified in a conjunctival snip. A nodule may be removed and incised, showing the coiled threadlike adult worm. Filarial antibodies may be detected by immunofluorescence in 95% of cases and by complement fixation in 50%. The intradermal test is usually positive.

Treatment and Prevention. Any nodules detected should be removed.

Diethylcarbamazine (p. 796) rapidly kills the microfilariae and this causes an allergic reaction for the first few days of treatment. The itch increases, eye lesions are aggravated and there may be accompanying fever with pain in the joints. Other reactions include hypotension and respiratory distress. Only a small dose should be given initially, 25 mg on the first day, this being gradually increased as the drug is tolerated until, if possible, a dose of 12 mg/kg is reached. This dose should be continued for 21 days. An antihistamine, such as chlorpheniramine maleate, may alleviate mild reactions but corticosteroids, locally as drops to the eyes and systemically, are needed to control severe reactions. Ideally the patient should be in bed for the first 24 hours of treatment.

Adult worms are killed by suramin (p. 780), the intervals between intravenous injections of 1 g should be 5 to 7 days and the maximum total dose 6 g. In endemic areas where reinfection is inevitable, and in patients with little or no eye involvement, repeated courses of diethylcarbamazine or long-term suppression with 50 mg daily may be preferred to the potential toxicity of suramin.

Mass treatment is impossible at present. The *Simulium* can be destroyed in its larval stage by the application of insecticide to streams or the adult flies can be attacked by spraying vegetation near streams. Dimethylphthalate applied to skin or clothing will repel the fly for several hours. Long trousers or skirts and sleeves discourage the fly from biting.

Other Filariases

Dipetalonema streptocerca. Microfilariae and adult worms of this parasite have been identified in the skin of man and chimpanzees in Ghana, Cameroun and Zaïre. The intermediate host and vector is the midge *Culicoides grahami*. The microfilariae may produce a mild dermatosis of the trunk, usually less irritating than the dermatosis of onchocerciasis. This filariasis also responds to a course of diethylcarbamazine.

Dipetalonema perstans is a filarial parasite of man which is usually non-pathogenic. In endemic areas microfilariae of *D. perstans* are commonly found in the peripheral blood in which they circulate both by day and night. The adults inhabit chiefly the retroperitoneal and perirenal tissues and have been found in the pericardial sac. The intermediate hosts and vectors are the midges *Culicoides austeni* and *C. grahami*. This filaria is found throughout equatorial Africa as far south as Zambia, and also in Trinidad and parts of northern and eastern South America.

D. perstans has never been shown to cause disease but it may be responsible for a persistent eosinophilia and occasional allergic manifestations. *D. perstans* is resistant to diethylcarbamazine and the infection may persist for many years.

Mansonella ozzardi. This filaria of man is non-pathogenic and is found in the West Indies and central and northern parts of South America. The adults inhabit the mesentery and subperitoneal tissues. The microfilariae circulate in the blood. The intermediate hosts are species of *Culicoides*. Diethylcarbamazine is ineffective.

Tropical pulmonary eosinophilia is attributable to an infection with a filarial worm such as *Dirofilaria* or *Brugia pahangi*, which is unable to mature in man. Alternatively it may be an unusual host reaction to the microfilariae of *Wuchereria bancrofti* or *Brugia malayi*. The disease is found in many tropical regions including India, Sri Lanka, Malaysia, China, Philippines, Australia, South America and uncommonly in Africa. Clinical features are discussed on page 247. It is successfully treated by diethylcarbamazine 12 mg/kg daily for 10 days.

Dracontiasis (Guinea Worm Infection)

The female *Dracunculus medinensis*, which measures over a metre in length, 0·9 to 1·7 mm in diameter, lives in the interstitial and subcutaneous tissues of man. The male worm, which is rarely seen, is only 2·5 cm long and dies earlier. Man is infected by ingesting a small crustacean, *Cyclops*, which inhabits the bottom of wells and ponds and which contains the infective larval stage of the worm.

When the cyclops is ingested by man the mature larvae penetrate the intestinal wall and migrate through the connective tissue of the host. After 9 to 18 months the fully mature female seeks the surface of the skin where a vesicle is raised, soon ruptures and exposes the anterior end of the worm. The distended uterus then ruptures and discharges its larvae externally. The worm is attracted to the surface by cooling, hence the larvae are likely to be expelled into water and complete the life cycle. Man is the most important host but *D. medinensis* has been found in dogs and cats.

The disease can be extremely disabling and is especially liable to affect farmers at the beginning of the rains and thus seriously interfere with planting. It is found in West, Central and East Africa, the Sudan, Arabia, Iran, Turkey, Pakistan, Central India, Burma, the Caribbean Islands and the northern parts of South America.

Clinical Features. When mature the adult may sometimes be felt beneath the skin. Some hours before the head of the worm emerges from the skin there is usually some local redness and tenderness. There may also be general allergic symptoms, erythema, giant urticaria, nausea, vomiting and diarrhoea. These symptoms usually subside as soon as the vesicle has ruptured and the larvae begin to be discharged. This is usually complete in 3 to 4 weeks, after which the worm is often spontaneously extruded and healing takes place.

The vesicle commonly appears in the lower part of the leg or in any area which has been kept moist and relatively cool. If the worm dies or is broken during extraction there will be a marked allergic inflammation. The patient is immobilised by pain and swelling. Secondary infection is common and causes severe cellulitis, septicaemia, aseptic or pyogenic arthritis. Tetanus is a well recognised complication. Multiple infections may occur and reactions around aberrant worms may cause serious lesions, exceptionally spinal cord compression.

Diagnosis is usually easy from the appearance of a vesicle, the protrusion of a worm and the recognition of the discharged larvae. A radiograph occasionally shows calcified worms.

Treatment and Prevention. Traditionally the protruding worm has been extracted by winding it out gently over several days on a sterile match stick. Niridazole in doses of 25 mg/kg daily in 2 divided doses for 10 days, or mebendazole 100 mg b.d. for 7 days, may reduce inflammation and aid the extraction of the worm. Antibiotics and prophylaxis of tetanus are required for secondary infection.

The provision of a satisfactory water supply would eradicate the infection. Where this is impracticable, wells and ponds may be protected or treated chemically.

3. DISEASES DUE TO ANIMAL NEMATODES

Toxocara canis. This is a common intestinal ascarid of dogs. The eggs are passed in the animal's faeces. Children who are in close contact with infected puppies are particularly liable to ingest ova of *Toxocara canis*. Larvae, liberated in the stomach, then migrate through the body and may cause allergic phenomena such as asthma, eosinophilia and also splenomegaly ('visceral larva migrans'). The worms do not usually mature in the human host. Occasionally a granuloma develops around a dead larva in the eye, resembling a neoplasm and causes blindness. Serology may aid diagnosis.

Larval worms can be killed by diethylcarbamazine (9–12 mg/kg daily for 3 weeks). Granulomas may require surgical treatment.

Hookworms causing Larva Migrans. *Ancylostoma braziliense and A. caninum* are intestinal parasites of dogs with a similar life cycle to *A. duodenale*, but in man they cause a creeping eruption or cutaneous larva migrans. The larva burrows between the corium and stratum granulosum and progresses irregularly at about 1 cm in 24 hours. The skin at the advancing end is erythematous and the older part of the burrow discoloured and scaly. Itching may be intense. The larva may remain active for some weeks or months. Treatment is topical. One 0·5 g tablet of thiabendazole is ground into 5 g petroleum jelly and rubbed in twice daily. Symptoms are relieved and the larva dies in a day or two.

Oesophagostomiasis. Species of the genus *Oesophagostomum*, a nematode related to hookworms, may cause a granuloma of the wall of the small intestine resembling a neoplasm. It has been reported chiefly from Uganda and is diagnosed at laparotomy.

Angiostrongylus. *A. cantonensis*, a nematode affecting the lungs of rodents, has a larval stage in molluscs and freshwater shrimps. In the Far East and the Pacific, where infected crustacea are eaten or infected slugs on vegetables are inadvertently swallowed, the larvae may cause a serious eosinophilic meningitis and immature worms may be found in the cerebrospinal fluid. Thiabendazole is effective but patients often recover spontaneously.

Trichinella spiralis. This parasite of rats and pigs is transmitted to man by eating partially cooked infected pork, usually as sausage or ham. Symptoms result from invasion of the body by larvae produced by the adult female worm in the small intestine and from their encystment in striated muscles. Outbreaks have occurred in Britain as well as in other countries where pork is eaten. Polar bear meat is another source.

The clinical course of trichinosis depends largely on the number of larvae. If there are only a few worms present there may be no symptoms but many worms may cause nausea and diarrhoea 24 to 48 hours after the infected meal. Soon, however, these symptoms are overshadowed by those associated with larval invasion, namely fever and oedema of the face, eyelids and conjunctivae. Invasion of the diaphragm may lead to pain, cough and dyspnoea; involvement of the muscles of the limbs, chest and mouth causes stiffness, pain and tenderness in the affected muscle groups. Pyrexia may reach 40°C with daily remissions. Larval migration may cause acute myocarditis and encephalitis. An eosinophilia is usually found after the second week. An intense infection may prove fatal, but those who survive recover completely.

It is not uncommon for a group of persons who have eaten infected pork from a common source to develop symptoms about the same time. When suspected, biopsy from the deltoid or gastrocnemius after the third week of symptoms may reveal encysted larvae. Precipitin and intradermal tests are also helpful.

Thiabendazole, 25 mg/kg b.d. for 2 days, may relieve muscle pain. Given early in the infection it may kill adult worms in the gut. Corticosteroids are given to control the serious effects of acute inflammation.

Gnathostomiasis. *G. spinigerum* is a nematode of dogs and cats. In the Far East the third stage larva is acquired by man eating inadequately cooked infected fish or by swallowing water containing infected *Cyclops*. The immature worm usually migrates to the subcutaneous tissue where it causes recurrent swellings. The full grown adult worm, which may be as long as 3 cm, may be visible through the skin when it can be removed surgically. In deeper tissues the worm may cause injury to the brain, kidney, lung, eye or other organs. Eosinophilia is usually pronounced. Diagnosis is easy when the adult worm is visible. Otherwise serological tests are performed. Treatment is not satisfactory but some success has been obtained with bithionol used as for paragonimiasis (p. 787).

Anisakiasis (Herring Worm Disease). *A. marina* is an ascarid which parasitises herrings and other marine animals. Human infections occur in Holland and Japan from the consumption of raw herrings. An eosinophilic granuloma forms in the intestine and may give rise to colic, fever and intestinal obstruction. An indirect haemagglutination test has been used for diagnosis. Surgery may be required.

DISEASES DUE TO FUNGI (MYCOSES)

Dermatophytes; Pityriasis versicolor; Candidiasis; Mycetoma; Zygomycosis; Chromomycosis; Rhinosporidiosis; Sporotrichosis; Histoplasmosis; Coccidioidomycosis; Paracoccidioidomycosis; Blastomycosis; Cryptococcosis.

Pathogenic fungi are ubiquitous; their importance varies between different parts of the world. Some fungi are opportunistic and will not normally invade unless the defence mechanisms are impaired, as in the immunocompromised host (p. 38). Fungal infections are transmitted by spores or hyphae, and normally enter the body through the lungs or skin, where they may cause disease, or from where they may disseminate to other parts of the body. Fungal infections tend to be chronic, and often require prolonged chemotherapy. For some infections there is still no effective treatment. Fungi also cause disease through allergy (p. 240) and toxins such as ergot, muscarine and aflatoxin (p. 720).

Fungal infections commonly present as skin disease, as subcutaneous swellings or as systemic infections.

CUTANEOUS FUNGAL INFECTIONS

An intact healthy skin is especially important in the tropics, where fungal infections are common. Extensive infections may impair sweating and heat loss, and cause great misery through irritation. Scratching leads to secondary pyogenic infection.

Dermatophytes. This large group of fungi infect keratinised tissues and are responsible for ringworm of the body and scalp, 'dhobi's itch' in the inguinal folds, and infection of the hair and nails. *Trichophyton rubrum* is the commonest cause and most difficult to treat. Tinea imbricata (*T. concentricum*), characterised by multiple concentric rings, causes widespread disabling infections in some Pacific Islands and in South East Asia. *Trichphyton schoenleinii* produces a mass of creamy white material, with an offensive odour, on the scalp, known as favus. Many dermatophytes are primarily parasites of domestic and farm animals. Dermatophytes are treated with topical antifungal ointments if mild, or if severe with griseofulvin 500 mg twice daily or ketoconazole 200–400 mg daily, by mouth.

Pityriasis versicolor is due to a yeast that causes a widespread very superficial infection, especially of the chest, back and upper arms.

Candidiasis (Moniliasis). A yeast, *Candida albicans* is the commonest fungus of medical importance. Infections of skin or nails may resemble those caused by dermatophytes. Infections of skin folds and on the buttocks of babies are common. Mucosal infection (thrush) is also frequent, especially in the mouth (p. 286) and, in diabetic women, on the vulvae (p. 480). Chronic mucocutaneous or disseminated candidiasis occurs in immunocompromised individuals. Superficial infections may respond to topical treatment with gentian violet or nystatin, but otherwise ketoconazole (p. 48) is given orally in a dose of 200–600 mg daily according to severity. Amphotericin (p. 804) is required for systemic infections.

SUBCUTANEOUS FUNGAL INFECTIONS

Mycetoma (Madura Foot)

Mycetoma, in this restricted sense, is a chronic fungal infection of the deep soft tissues and bones, most commonly of the limbs, but also of the abdominal or chest wall or head. It is produced by members of two groups of organisms classified as *Eumycetes* and aerobic *Actinomycetes*. A feature common to both groups is the formation by the fungus of grains, with characteristic colours, ranging from 60 microns to 3 mm in diameter. The incidence appears to be related to climate, being especially high when an arid hot season ends in rains. The more common species of fungi causing mycetoma, as defined above, are shown in Table 19.8. The fungus can be identified by the microscopic appearances of the tissue and grains and confirmed by culture. Antibodies can usually be demonstrated by precipitation.

Pathological and Clinical Features. The lesions may occur in any part of the body but as the fungus is usually introduced by a thorn they are more common in the foot and leg in those who walk bare-footed. At the site of implantation the mycetoma begins as a painless swelling which grows and spreads inexorably within the soft

Table 19.8 Fungi causing mycetoma

Species	Type of Grains
Eumycetoma	
Madurella mycetomatis	brown or black (big)
Madurella grisea	black or brown (big)
Exophiala jeanselmei	black
Pseudoallescheria boydii	white or yellow (big)
Acremonium spp.	white or yellow
Actinomycetoma	
Actinomadura madurae	white, yellow, red (big)
Actinomadura pelletieri	red (small)
Streptomyces somaliensis	white or yellow (big)
Nocardia brasiliensis	white, yellow (microscopic)

tissues causing swelling and eventually penetrates bones.

The histology is that of a chronic granuloma with a fibrous stroma and cyst-like spaces in which lie the characteristic grains. Nodules develop under the epidermis and these rupture revealing sinuses through which mucopus containing the coloured grains is discharged. Some sinuses may heal with scarring while fresh sinuses appear elsewhere.

There is little pain and usually no fever, but progressive disability. Secondary pyogenic infection does not usually penetrate far down the sinuses, possibly because of antibiotic activity of the fungi. It is unusual for the fungus to reach the lymph nodes unless there has been surgical interference. When the lesion is in the scalp, the skull may be affected but the dura mater appears to be an effective barrier. Apart from involvement of bones by a spreading mycetoma, intraosseous lesions may be found in the metaphysis of a long bone, especially at the upper end of the tibia and sometimes there may be an encapsulated periosteal mass. *Nocardia brasiliensis* often affects the skin of the back. It is seldom localised and may spread widely.

Diagnosis is confirmed by demonstration of fungal grains in pus or tissue biopsy. Culture is usually necessary for species identification, although serology may be helpful.

Treatment. The difference between *Eumycetes* and *Actinomycetes* is crucial in that there is no drug of proven efficacy for the former. Sporadic successes with griseofulvin against *Eumycetes* have been reported, but the results have been mostly disappointing and up to the present eumycetoma requires to be surgically removed. It has a strong tendency to recur locally unless the excision has been adequate or the amputation high enough.

The treatment of actinomycetoma is more hopeful. It consists of rifampicin (4 mg/kg daily by mouth) or streptomycin (14 mg/kg daily i.m.) for 3 months plus oral dapsone (1·5 mg/kg b.d.) or oral co-trimoxazole for 4–24 months. *Nocardia* infection may respond to dapsone alone. Precipitating antibodies disappear if treatment is successful.

Other Subcutaneous Mycoses

Zygomycosis (phycomycosis) is caused by one of several species of fungi. Subcutaneous swellings of the face or proximal limbs are the commonest presentations. Systemic infections are occasionally seen in immunocompromised or diabetic patients. According to the species of fungus isolated, treatment is with potassium iodide 1·5–3·5 g daily.

Chromoblastomycosis is one of the causes of mossy foot and is to be distinguished from the warty excrescences which accompany the chronic lymphatic obstruction of elephantiasis, and also from mycetoma.

These pigmented fungi are acquired on splinters from decaying timber and give rise to a warty condition of the foot and also rarely affect the face, and upper limbs. The diagnosis is confirmed by the recognition of dark brown spheroid bodies 4 to 8 microns in diameter in biopsy specimens or by culture.

Treatment is oral flucytosine 30–50 mg/kg body weight 6 hourly for several months. Blood levels are monitored, especially when renal function is poor. In stubborn cases amphotericin is added.

Rhinosporidiosis is caused by *Rhinosporidium seeberi* and occurs in South America, India, Sri Lanka, and East Africa. This organism forms a cyst which on rupture discharges spores which spread by lymphatics to connective tissue. It produces polypi in the nose and localised swellings on the cheek and elsewhere. The characteristic sporangia and spores are recognised

histologically. The organism has not yet been cultured. Treatment is surgical.

Sporotrichosis is caused by *Sporothrix schenckii*. The infection occurs throughout the world and is prevalent in Central and Southern Africa. It causes swellings resembling a gumma or a chancroid type of ulcer. Affected lymphatic vessels may be thickened and palpable as a chain of nodules. Uncommonly dissemination takes place into lungs, bones, the central nervous system and elsewhere. The fungus can be cultured from discharges or biopsy material.

Potassium iodide up to 10 g daily should be given orally until some time after apparent clinical cure. Widely disseminated infections respond to amphotericin.

SYSTEMIC FUNGAL INFECTIONS

Histoplasmosis

Histoplasmosis is caused by *Histoplasma capsulatum (Darling)* which is a yeast in its parasitic phase but is a filamentous fungus of soil at other times. A variant, *Histoplasma duboisii*, is found in parts of tropical Africa. The spores of *Histoplasma* remain viable for years in the soil and infection is by inhalation of infected dust. Occasionally infection passes through the buccal or intestinal mucosa or through the skin. The disease attacks dogs, rats and mice, and the fungus multiplies in soil enriched by the droppings of chickens, pigeons and bats. The infection is thus a hazard for explorers of caves.

Histoplasma capsulatum

This is found in all parts of the United States of America, especially in the East Central States, and less commonly in Latin America from Mexico to Argentina, in Europe, North, South and East Africa, Nigeria, Malaysia, Indonesia and Australia.

Pathological and Clinical Features. The parasite in its yeast phase multiplies mainly in monocytes and macrophages and produces areas of necrosis in which the parasites may abound. From these foci the blood stream may be invaded leading to metastatic lesions in the liver, spleen and lymph nodes. Pulmonary histoplasmosis may produce pathological changes similar to those of tuberculosis.

Probably 90% of pulmonary infections are benign producing no symptoms, but more severe infections may closely simulate pulmonary tuberculosis, including the production of a primary complex with enlarged satellite lymph nodes, multiple small discrete lesions and occasionally cavitation. Healed lesions may calcify. Lesions of the skin or mucosa may be found on the rare occasions when infection has entered that way. They are common in disseminated histoplasmosis which is characterised by enlargement of the liver, spleen and lymph nodes, irregular pyrexia, anaemia and leucopenia. Addison's disease may be produced by caseation in the adrenals. Endocarditis is rare. When the mucosa of the mouth and gastrointestinal tract become infected, the predominant symptoms may be vomiting and diarrhoea. Occasionally the central nervous system is invaded. The severity of the symptoms of histoplasmosis varies from, in the majority of cases, a slight fever of short duration, like influenza, to a severe and prolonged pyrexial illness which ultimately proves fatal.

Diagnosis. In an area where the disease occurs, histoplasmosis should be suspected in every obscure infection in which there are pulmonary signs or where there are enlarged lymph nodes with or without hepatosplenomegaly. Tissue is obtained by biopsy for impression smear, histology, culture and animal inoculation. Radiological examination in long standing cases may show calcified lesions in the lungs, spleen or other organs. In the more acute phases of the disease single or multiple soft pulmonary shadows with enlarged tracheo-bronchial nodes may be seen.

Delayed hypersensitivity to the intradermal injection of histoplasmin develops in patients with either active or healed infections but is usually negative in the rapidly progressive form of the disease. Complement fixing antibodies are detected within 3 weeks of the onset of an acute primary infection and increase in titre as the disease progresses. Precipitating antibodies may also be detected.

Treatment. Specific treatment with amphotericin is indicated only in severe infections. The dosage is 0·5 mg/kg, in 500 ml of 5% glucose given intraveneously over a 6-hour period, gradually increasing to a maximum of 1·0 mg/kg. Treatment is given on alternate days. If badly tolerated, the dosage may have to be reduced. Side-effects are malaise, anorexia, nausea, fever, headache and venous thrombosis. These may be controlled to a considerable extent by the addition of 10 mg prednisolone to the intravenous solution. Plasma urea rises and haemoglobin falls during treatment, but later return to normal. Amphotericin may have to be continued for up to a month or longer, depending on the clinical response. Recovery from generalised histoplasmosis is rare.

Histoplasma duboisii

Histoplasma duboisii, the fungus of African histoplasmosis, is considerably larger than the classical *H. capsulatum*. It is found in Ghana, Uganda, Nigeria, Sénégal, Sudan and Zaïre.

This disease differs in several ways from *H. capsulatum* infection. The bones, skin, lymph nodes and liver develop granulomatous lesions or cold abscesses resembling tuberculosis, but the lungs are seldom involved. The visceral form with liver and splenic invasion is often fatal, while ulcerative skin lesions and bone abscesses follow a more benign course.

Radiological examination may show rounded foci of bone destruction sometimes associated with abscess formation. Multiple lesions of the ribs are common and the bones of the limbs may also be involved. Diagnosis is by isolation of the fungus. Immunodiagnostic tests are helpful.

The disease is treated in the same way as *H. capsulatum* infections. A solitary lesion in bone may require only local surgical treatment.

Other Systemic Mycoses

Aspergillosis is the most common respiratory mycosis in Britain and is discussed on page 240.

Coccidioidomycosis is caused by *Coccidioides immitis*. This infection is found in Southern United States, and in Central and South America. The disease is acquired by inhalation. In 40% of cases if affects the lungs, lymph nodes and skin. Rarely it may be carried by the blood stream to the bones, adrenals, meninges and other organs. In 60% of cases the infection is asymptomatic. Infections, including subclinical attacks, are followed by immunity.

The fungi grow readily on culture media but as they are highly infective, diagnostic investigations are usually limited to intradermal, complement-fixation and precipitin tests.

Some localised pulmonary lesions can be successfully treated by surgery. Amphotericin or ketoconazole may be used.

Paracoccidiodomycosis is caused by *Paracoccicidiodes brasiliensis* and occurs in South America. Mucocutaneous lesions occur early. Involvement of lymphatic nodes and the lungs is prominent and the gastrointestinal tract may also be attacked. Most cases respond to ketoconazole 600 mg/day. Otherwise sulphonamides or amphotericin may be used.

Blastomycosis. *North American blastomycosis* is caused by *Blastomyces dermatitidis*. It also occurs in Africa. Systemic infection begins in the lungs and mediastinal lymph nodes and resembles pulmonary tuberculosis. Bones, skin and the genito-urinary tract may also be affected. Treatment is with amphotericin (p. 804).

Cryptococcosis is caused by *Cryptococcus neoformans*. Its distribution is worldwide. It causes local gummatous-like tumours and granulomatous lesions of the lung, bones, brain and

meninges. The cerebrospinal fluid often contains the fungus when the nervous system is affected. The diagnosis is made by culture or recognition of spores in the cerebrospinal fluid, biopsy and serological detection of antigen.

Amphotericin should be given intravenously or flucytosine orally (p. 48). Surgical removal of local pulmonary lesions may be necessary. Recovery may be monitored by fall in antigen titre.

DISEASES DUE TO ARTHROPODS

Infections Conveyed by Arthropods; Lice Infestation; Scabies; Tungiasis; Myiasis; Porocephalosis.

Arthropods may be responsible for disease in three ways. They may act as vectors of infectious agents (Table 19.9). They may envenomate through stings or bites (p. 706), or they may infest or even infect the human body directly.

Lice. As well as transmitting serious diseases, the body louse *Pediculus humanus corporis* causes dermatitis and sleeplessness through itching, especially in poor crowded communities in cold countries (for control see p. 741). The head louse, *Pediculus humanus capitis*, is cosmopolitan and increasing in prevalence in British schools. It makes the child itch and alarms parents and teachers. Tiny white oval eggs, 'nits', are seen attached to the base of hairs on the scalp. The

Table 19.9 Infections conveyed by arthropods

Name	Genus	Disease
House fly	*Musca*	Dysenteries, enteric fevers, salmonelloses, ?cholera, ?trachoma, ?tropical ulcer.
Horse fly	*Tabanidae*	?anthrax, tularaemia
Oscinid fly	*Hippelates*	?yaws, streptococcal dermatitis and nephritis
Tsetse fly	*Glossina*	African trypanosomiasis
Mosquito	*Anopheles*	Malaria, some arboviruses, Bancroftian and Brugia filariasis in some areas.
	Aedes	Yellow fever, dengue, and other arboviruses.
	Culex	Bancroftian and Brugia filariasis, Japanese B encephalitis and other arboviruses
Black fly	*Simulium*	Onchocerciasis.
Midges	*Culicoides*	*Dipetolema perstans, D. streptocerca, Mansonella ozzardi.*
Soft ticks	*Ornithodoros*	Tick-borne relapsing fever
Hard ticks	*(Ixodidae)*, *Rhipicephalus* etc.	Some typhus fevers, ?Q fever, Kyasanur Forest disease, tularaemia.
Sandflies	*Phebotomus*	Leishmaniases, sandfly fever, bartonellosis.
Lice	*Pediculus*	Epidemic typhus fever, louse-borne relapsing fever, trench fever, *Dipylidium caninum.*
Mites	*Leptotrombidium*	Scrub typhus fever
	Allodermanyssus	Rickettsialpox
Winged Bug	*Triatoma*	Chagas' disease.
Fleas	*Xenopsylla*	Plague, endemic typhus fever.
	Ctenocephalides	*Dipylidium caninum.*

crab louse (p. 415) is transmitted while sharing beds. A single treatment with gammabenzene hexachloride (BHC) shampoo or lotion is usually curative. In countries, such as Britain, where resistance is developing to BHC, malathion or carbaryl is preferred.

Scabies is due to the mite *Sarcoptes scabei*; it is common all over the world. It causes itching, initially between the fingers or on the buttocks or genitals where the mite burrows, and later all over the body. In the tropics secondary streptococcal infection is an important cause of rheumatic fever and glomerulonephritis. The diagnosis of scabies is confirmed by finding the causative mite in a burrow. Scabies is treated by a single application of gammabenzene hexachloride 1% to the whole body below the neck or by three daily applications of benzyl benzoate 15%.

Tungiasis (Jiggers) is due to infestation with *Tunga penetrans* (the chigoe or jigger flea). It is widespread in tropical America and Africa. Man and pigs are important hosts. The pregnant female flea burrows into the skin about the toes and soles and grows as large as a pea, packed with eggs which are subsequently discharged on to the surface. The burrows irritate and become inflamed but the chief danger is from secondary pyogenic infection or tetanus. The chigoe and egg sac should be removed with a sterile needle and a mild antiseptic ointment applied. Massive infestations, such as may be seen in neglected children and in senile persons, may be treated by immersing the feet in an aqueous solution containing benzene hexachloride 5% and cetrimide 0·8%.

Myiasis is an infestation of various tissues of man by the larvae of flies.

CUTANEOUS MYIASIS. A common cause of cutaneous myiasis is *Cordylobia anthropophaga* (Tumbu fly) which lays its eggs on laundry spread on grass. The larvae penetrate the skin and produce lesions like boils with central orifices through which they breathe. On reaching maturity they emerge. A drop of thick oil or petroleum jelly usually brings a larva out in search of air and facilitates its removal. Occasionally the common warble fly (*Hypoderma bovis*) may infest man.

MYIASIS OF WOUNDS, SORES AND CAVITIES. The larvae of many flies may infest necrotic tissue in open wounds or ulcers and occasionally invade living tissue. *Chrysomya bezziana* is found in Africa, India and South Vietnam. It may penetrate the nasal sinuses and cause great destruction. The application of 10% chloroform in a light vegetable oil is the treatment of choice for infested wounds.

INTESTINAL MYIASIS. In the tropics especially, vague digestive disturbances or abdominal cramps with diarrhoea and vomiting may be caused by fly larvae in the intestinal canal, the eggs having been ingested with food.

Porocephalosis is invasion of the body by 'tongue worms', degenerate arthropods of which *Armillifer armillatus*, *A. moniliformis* and *Linguatula serrata* occur in man. Adult *Armillifer* parasitise the trachea and bronchi of snakes. Man is infected by ingesting ova on uncooked vegetables or by eating undercooked snakes. The condition is usually symptomless in man but calcified nymphs may be seen in the radiographs of the chest and abdomen.

Halzoun is the name given in the Middle East to a form of acute dysphagia and laryngeal obstruction from pharyngitis and oedema of the larynx. It is due to the ingestion of nymphs of *Linguatula serrata* in undercooked liver and lymph nodes of sheep and goats. Foxes and dogs are the definitive hosts. Antihistamines and a local anaesthetic spray are suggested for treatment.

ADVICE TO TRAVELLERS

Yellow fever is the only infection for which immunisation is currently required by International Health Regulations. Information about this and about other medically recommended immunisations is given in Table 19.10.

In addition, it is very important that all visitors to the tropics and subtropics should take all appropriate measures to avoid malaria and also take prophylactic antimalarial drugs regularly from the week before travel and continue until 4 weeks after returning to a non-malarious area. Details are given on page 772. Neglect of this advice has been responsible for fatalities. Other common problems that the traveller should take steps to avoid include diarrhoea, hepatitis, insect bites, venereal disease, disorders due to climate and jet lag.

Table 19.10 Medically recommended immunisations for travellers

Inoculation	Where advised	Course Programme	Validity	Minimum age advised	Other comments
Yellow fever	Central Africa 15°N to 10°S Panama State to 15°S	1 subcutaneous injection	After 10 days for 10 years	1 year	The only immunisation currently *required* by International Health Regulations
Cholera	Entering or transiting a cholera zone	2 subcutaneous injections, 4–6 weeks apart	After 6 days for 6 months	1 year	Poor protection. Very few countries *require* it
Typhoid	Everywhere	2 subcutaneous injections, 4–6 weeks apart	Booster injection every 3 years	2 years	0.1 ml intradermal adequate for booster, less toxic
Tetanus	Everywhere	3 subcutaneous injections, 4–6 weeks and 6 months apart	Booster injection every 5 years	None	See also page 41
Poliomyelitis	Everywhere	3 oral doses of attenuated virus at monthly intervals	Booster every 5 years, 3 doses better than 1	None	See also page 41
Rabies	Endemic countries	3 subcutaneous or intradermal injections 4 weeks and 4–6 months apart	Over 5 years	1 year	Groups at risk, using human diploid cell vaccine
Plague	Parts of S.E Asia, E. Africa, U.S.A.	2 injections at 10–20 day intervals, 3rd 6 months later	6 months	1 year	Only special groups at risk.
Typhus	Parts of S.E Asia, Ethiopia, etc	2 injections at 7–10 day intervals 3rd 6 months later	1 year		Only special groups at risk.
Gamma Globulin for type A hepatitis	Countries where sanitation is poor	Intramuscular injection 250 mg or 500 mg. Age under 10 years, halfdose	4–6 months	10 years	Also protects against measles, rubella

Malaria prophylaxis, see page 772.
Diphtheria and pertussis, see page 41.

A map illustrating the distribution of the most serious tropical diseases is shown in Figure 18.1. Much useful advice may be found in *Preservation of Health in Warm Climates*, The Ross Institute, London and in *Travel Medicine* by Turner, A.C. Edinburgh: Churchill Livingstone.

Global aspects of the prevention of disease and the promotion of health are discussed in the next chapter.

A.D.M. BRYCESON
A.M. GEDDES

FURTHER READING:

Infectious and parasitic diseases:
Christie, A.B. (1980) *Infectious Diseases: Epidemiology and Clinical Practice*, 3rd edn. Edinburgh: Churchill Livingstone.
Knight, R. (1982) *Parasitic Disease in Man*. Edinburgh: Churchill Livingstone.
Manson-Bahr, P.E.C., Apted, F.I.C. (1982) *Manson's Tropical Diseases*, 18th edn. London: Biallière Tindall.

Muller, R. (1975) *Worms and Disease*. London: William Heinemann.

Rabies:
Symposium on Rabies (1976) *Transactions of the Royal Society of Tropical Medicine and Hygiene*, 70, 175–205.

Plague:
Ziegler, P. (1969) *The Black Death*. London: Collins.

Leprosy:
Bryceson, A.D.M. & Pfaltzgraff, R.E. (1979) *Leprosy*, 2nd edn. Edinburgh: Churchill Livingstone.

Malaria:
Cohen S. (Ed.) (1982) Malaria. *British Medical Bulletin*, 38, 115–218.
Hall, A.P. (1977) The treatment of severe falciparum malaria. *Transactions of the Royal Society of Tropical Medicine and Hygiene*, 71, 80.

Amoebiasis:
Stamm, W.P. (1976) Amoebiasis: a neglected diagnosis. *Journal of the Royal College of Physicians of London*, 10, 294–298.

20. The Promotion of Health and Prevention of Disease

Physicians of the utmost fame,
Were called at once; but when they came,
They answered as they took their fees,
'There is no cure for this disease.'

Hilaire Belloc

Unfortunately most doctors see their role as curing rather than preventing disease. However, despite the major advances that have occurred in medicine, there are still many diseases for which there is no cure and where immediate hope for the future lies in prevention. An example of this is the antenatal diagnosis of diseases such as Down's syndrome or neural tube defects. It is likely that major advances in the field of prevention will markedly affect the pattern of diseases that doctors will face in the next decade. Throughout this book special attention has been paid to prevention when individual diseases have been discussed. However, the importance of the topic is such that it is appropriate to conclude by giving a broader consideration to the allied questions of the promotion of health and prevention of disease. In this context we must obviously consider not just the problems of an affluent society but also put diseases into a global perspective. Physicians would do well to remember Sir Thomas Browne's full quotation:
'Charity begins at home, is the voice of the world'.

Needs of Tropical and Developing Countries

A survey of patterns of disease in the tropics and developing countries has been made in Chapter 18 and methods of prevention of individual diseases have been discussed. The promotion of health and the prevention of disease are, however, related to fundamental principles sometimes far removed from medical therapeutics and prophylaxis.

Whereas obesity is a major problem in affluent communities, undernutrition and malnutrition are dominant in underdeveloped countries. Adequate nutrition depends primarily on preserving the fertility of the soil and making good use of its vegetable products and, if customs permit, of the animals which are themselves dependent on the vegetation. Preservation or construction of water supplies is also a fundamental need and afforestation and contour terracing may help to prevent the land becoming denuded by floods. Only if a poor country can become richer, can sustained improvement in health be expected. More efficient agriculture and animal husbandry will tend to lead to improved health and economy; further progress may follow the utilisation of mineral resources and the development of productive industries and tourism.

Much help has been given in starting these processes by outside agencies but in order that lasting benefit should accrue it must be accompanied by better education. It is of paramount importance that the people concerned must themselves be fully convinced of the value and practicability of the projects and desire their benefits. Progress may be slow when improvements in health necessitate changes in food habits and other traditional practices, and will be maintained only when projects become an integral part of the development programme of the country and are operated largely by local personnel. Training of local nationals is, therefore, essential.

Increases in food supplies may be outstripped by increases in population. Family planning is, thus, a priority in many developing countries and emphasis should be laid both on the successful rearing of healthy children and on the reduction of the population growth. Any progress can be vitiated by war or other political disturbance, hence the preservation of peace and law and order are crucial.

It will be clear that the medical practitioner's role in these measures will be chiefly that of an informed adviser. The relative values to community health of money spent, for example, on improved schooling as compared with eradication of malaria may be very difficult to assess, yet governments with limited resources have frequently to decide between such priorities. It has been shown in some areas that the provision of a protected water supply is the most economical way of improving health. Irrigation schemes may be essential to increase the areas of fertile land but expert advice may be required to prevent the spread thereby of malaria, schistosomiasis and onchocerciasis. The eradication of onchocerciasis and animal trypanosomiasis would lead, but at great expense, to the conversion of vast tracts of unused fertile land to pastoral and agricultural use.

In developing countries the provision of curative measures, which may also be important factors in prevention, involves the same principles as in affluent societies but their application is modified by the limitations of available finance and personnel. Priority should be given to measures which will improve the health and prospects of children and wage earners.

In order to reach the scattered rural population a chain of health centres, under-5-year-old clinics and peripheral aid posts have proved of great value. At the health centres, maternity and child welfare have priority and at all levels health education is actively pursued. Breast feeding of all children for at least the first 6 months should be the rule and importation of expensive foreign baby foods should be kept to a minimum. Breast feeding is probably the most important contraceptive in the world. Frequent suckling maintains high levels of prolactin and hence continuing secondary amenorrhoea and infertility. Thus the introduction of free milk powder with cessation of breast feeding has produced a population explosion in some countries.

Immunisation of children and, in the case of tetanus, of expectant mothers also, may do much to reduce mortality rates. Domiciliary visits from the centres increase the contact with outlying homesteads. The vulnerability of small children to gastroenteritis underlines the importance of education in cleanliness and the provision of pure water supplies, but may also necessitate the organisation of local facilities for rapid rehydration.

Making the best use of medical auxiliaries is essential if the health services are to become widely available. Peripheral clinics have to be related to district and central hospitals from which some degree of supervision can be exercised and to which patients can be referred if transport is available. Only minimal curative medicine is carried out at the peripheral clinics, but preventive measures must be seen to be related to curative medicine, otherwise little support for them will be forthcoming. The provision of specialised care, even in the central hospitals, should not be out of proportion to the general standard of medical care and medical education should include experience in both categories. Political pressure to divert effort and money into prestige units should be resisted.

The misuse of drugs in the developed countries is more than matched by that in the developing world. Thus scarce resources are often wasted because people are prescribed drugs which are not required and many expensive combinations are used. Because of this antibiotic resistance is common and drug side effects present a major problem. What is tragic is that this abuse of drugs by one section of the population is associated with the lack of essential drugs for the majority. These problems can be solved only by educating doctors so that prescribing is improved, and by informing patients so that their demands for polypharmacy are reduced. Only then will all pharmaceutical companies realise that the Third World can no longer be used as a dumping ground for drugs with toxicity that has severely limited their use in more developed countries, or as an area to be exploited to maintain profit margins.

Organisation in Disaster Situations

If earthquakes, floods, drought or other disasters strike an area, help from outside is urgently needed to maintain food supplies and to prevent the spread of disease from sudden impairment of hygiene. When the disaster is war, a nuclear accident (p. 528), earthquakes or volcanic eruptions it may be difficult and dangerous to get supplies to the stricken areas. Failure of food and medicines to reach the people is often more the result of disorganisation than unavailability of supplies that can be flown in from international donors. Relief agencies from different countries often try to operate without adequate communication with local community leaders or with one another. Governments in countries where famine is recurrent should have civil servants permanently employed in keeping plans for famine relief up to date.

Needs of Developed Countries

The term 'developed' is used to denote wealthy communities, mainly industrial. It is not intended to imply that the acquisition of more material possessions is necessarily a desirable goal or that the way of life in developed societies does not contain defects, some of which are deleterious to health.

The Role of the Family Doctor. National and local government bodies assume the responsibility for ensuring the availability of adequate food supplies, education, housing, health services and the prevention of environmental pollution but the family doctor plays an important role in encouraging people to make full use of preventive services and in advising them about healthy living. All doctors must give much thought to finding means of enhancing the acceptance of health advice by individual patients.

Genetic counselling (p. 17), immunisation programmes and the early recognition and treatment of disease, the provision of iron and folic acid for expectant mothers and vitamins C and D for young children do much to ensure a good beginning in the building of a healthy nation. Where local mineral deficiencies exist, fluoridation of water to prevent dental caries and iodised salt to prevent goitre have proved their value.

The medical profession must continue to seek improvement in the working conditions in mines and factories and to draw attention to the special needs of persons in stressful occupations or doing repetitive work on mass production assembly lines. Industrial hazards and environmental risk factors such as lead must be identified and eliminated.

Screening for disease, such as tuberculosis, hypertension and diabetes mellitus, can be carried out readily by the family doctor and can be supplemented by the use of mass miniature chest radiography. Malignant disease of the breast and cervix can be detected at a very early stage, if apparently healthy young women are examined regularly. Self-examination of the breasts can be taught. For those in the middle years of life, medical reviews, at intervals of no longer than 2 years, facilitate the early recognition of disease such as hypertension, diabetes and malignancy.

The needs of the elderly may include prophylactic measures such as the use of vitamins C and D. There is also a requirement to assess and treat the multiple disabilities frequently overlooked in this age group, to provide social support and community services for the isolated and to find suitable accommodation for those whose need is for continuing care.

For patients of all ages it is the doctor's duty to encourage healthy living habits in matters such as exercise and diet with emphasis on an energy value appropriate to the needs of the individual, an ample content of dietary fibre, and, more contentiously, moderation in the intake of saturated fat.

The dietary guidelines in Scandinavia for the general public were introduced in 1968 and have since been followed, with local modifications, in several major industrial countries: 'The supply of calories (energy) in the diet should in many cases be reduced to prevent overweight. The total consumption of fat should be reduced from 40% (the present figure) to between 25 and 35% of energy. The use of saturated fat should be reduced and consumption of polyunsaturated fats increased (p. 814). Consumption of sugar and sugar-rich products should be reduced. The consumption of vegetables, fruit, potatoes, skimmed milk, fish, lean meat and cereal products should be increased'. Food additives are rightly kept under regular and careful review by responsible governments.

From the medical and nutritional standpoint the importance of taking regular exercise from an early age, particularly for those who have mainly sedentary occupations, should also be emphasised. What has been lightheartedly called the runner's 'high' or the daily exercise 'fix' may well be due to a surge of opioid peptides. Regular exercise is also beneficial for the elderly.

There must be a constant awareness of the dangers of tobacco smoking and of excessive consumption of alcohol or other addictive drugs.

Much can be done to promote mental health by doctors listening attentively to patients and thus helping individuals to contend with their psychological problems while also detecting those with psychiatric disturbances. In this area the prevention of intentional self-poisoning in modern society presents a major challenge (p. 711). There is increasing evidence that good mental health retards physical deterioration in mid-life. Many people think that for full health some form of 'belief' may be necessary to satisfy man's need to feel he belongs to the cosmos and is part of something outside himself. In the words of John Donne, 'No man is an island, entire of itself'.

Conclusion

In all communities, there should be continuing demands for improvement in housing standards and in food hygiene particularly for those in the lower socio-economic group whose vulnerability is often increased by unemployment and by inadequate access to health resources. In many societies the morbidity and mortality from road traffic accidents is rapidly increasing and is related to the abuse of alcohol and drugs. In urban areas there are growing problems in regard to corruption, crime, violence, baby and wife battering, rape, sexual promiscuity and heroin addiction. But there are even greater potential hazards. Man has now the capacity to destroy himself not only with nuclear weapons but by using up the natural resources of the planet so fast and by polluting the environment so thoroughly that he is in danger of precipitating his own doom. Everyone, especially doctors, economists, agriculturists and statesmen, is involved in this challenge and the response to it is vital.

C. R. W. EDWARDS

FURTHER READING:

Black, D., Morris, J. N., Smith, C. & Townsend, P. (1982) In: Townsend, P., Davidson, N., (Eds.) *Inequalities in Health: the Black Report*. Harmondsworth: Penguin Books. A critical analysis of health in Britain in comparison with other industrialised countries, containing many recommendations for improvement.

Howe, G. M. & Lorraine, J. A. (Eds.) (1980) *Environmental Medicine*, 2nd edn. London: William Heinemann. Wide-ranging reviews by experts on environmental and social threats to health.

Morley, D. (1973) *Paediatric Priorities in the Developing World*. Obtainable at low cost from Institute of Child Health, 30 Guildford Street, London WC1.

Robinson, D. A. (Ed.) (1984) *Epidemiology and Community Control of Disease in Warm Climate Countries*, 2nd edn. Edinburgh: Churchill Livingstone.

21. Appendices

CONTENTS

Diets

1. Low Energy Diet
2. Measured Diabetic Diet
3. Unmeasured Diabetic Diet
4. Fat-Modified Diet

Desirable Weights

Notes on SI Units

Biochemical Values

Venous Blood
Arterial Blood
Miscellaneous Values
  CSF
  Gastrointestinal, Pancreas & Liver
  Sweat
  Urine
Hormone Concentrations in Plasma
Therapeutic Blood Concentration of Drugs

Haematological Values

Drug Nomenclature and Prescription

DIETS

The diet sheets that follow have been constructed to illustrate the quantitative and qualitative aspects of diets required for the treatment of obesity and diabetes mellitus. The quantities given in a standard diet sheet will obviously require some modification in relation to the size, age, sex, and occupation of the patient. In the dietetic treatment of most diseases it is unnecessary to weigh accurately the amounts of the different foods eaten. Under these circumstances sufficient accuracy will be secured by the use of household measures as illustrated in Diet 1 and by the terms 'small', 'medium' or 'large' helping for meat, fish or chicken. A small helping weighs approximately 30–60 g (1 to 2 oz), a medium helping 60–90 g (2 to 3 oz) and a large helping 120 g (4 oz) or more.

The qualitative content of the diet, i.e. the actual food consumed, will vary widely. The examples detailed here are suitable for persons whose food habits are those of the Western world. If they are to be effective therapeutically, diet prescriptions must be carefully adapted to take account of national, cultural and local eating habits.

The subcommittee on Metrication of the British National Committee for Nutritional Sciences of the Royal Society recommended in 1972 that kilojoules should be used in place of the kilocalories. 1 kcal = 4·184 kJ, so that the calorie conversion factors (heat of combustion; available energy) for carbohydrate, fat, protein and alcohol are 16, 37, 17 and 29 kJ/g. Useful practical approximations are: 950 kcal = 4000 kJ; 1450 kcal = 6000 kJ; 2850 kcal = 12 000 kJ

1. LOW ENERGY (CALORIE) DIET
suitable for adults with obesity with or without diabetes

Approximately: Protein 60 g. Carbohydrate 100 g. Fat 40 g. Energy 1000 kcal (4184 kJ)

Early morning	Cup of tea, milk from allowance, if desired.
Breakfast	1 egg or 30 g (1 oz) grilled lean bacon (2 rashers) *or* cold ham *or* breakfast fish. 20 g (⅔ oz) white or brown bread, *or* exchange, with butter from allowance. Tea or coffee, with milk from allowance.
Mid-morning	Tea or coffee, with milk from allowance, or 'free' drink from Group A3. 1 cream cracker or water biscuit
Mid-day meal	Clear soup, tomato juice or grapefruit, if desired. Small helping, 60 g (2 oz) lean meat, ham, poultry, game or offal *or* 90 g (3 oz) white fish (steamed, baked or grilled) *or* 2 eggs *or* 45 g (1½ oz) cheese. Salad or vegetables from Group A1 as desired. 40 g (1⅓ oz) bread (white or brown) *or* exchange, with butter from allowance if desired. 1 portion of fruit from bread exchange list below. Tea or coffee with milk from allowance.
Mid-afternoon	20 g (⅔ oz) white or brown bread, *or* exchange, with butter from allowance.

Evening Meal   Clear soup, meat or yeast extracts, tomato juice or grapefruit, if desired.

Small helping, 60 g (2 oz) lean meat, ham, poultry, game or offal *or* 90 g (3 oz) white fish (steamed, baked or grilled) *or* 1 egg *or* 45 g (1½ oz) cheese.

Salad or vegetables from Group A1 as desired.

40 g (1½ oz) bread (white or brown) *or* exchange, with butter from allowance if desired.

1 portion of fruit from list below.

Tea or coffee with milk from allowance.

Before bed   Tea or coffee with milk from allowance.
1 cream cracker or water biscuit.

Allowance for day: 200 ml (⅓ pint) milk with the cream poured off the top.
15 g (½ oz) butter or margarine.

Exchanges for 20 g (⅔ oz) bread (½ slice from a large cut loaf):
2 cream crackers   1 potato (the size of a hen's egg)
1½ of any crispbread   1 portion of fruit (from list below)
2 water biscuits
1 oatcake

Exchanges for 40 g (1⅓ oz) bread (1 slice from a large cut loaf):
4 cream crackers   2 potatoes
3 Ryvita   4 water biscuits
2 oatcakes

Fruit list: 1 medium apple, 1 orange, 1 pear, 1 small banana, 10 grapes.

Group A: Foods Which May be Taken as Desired
1. *Vegetables*
Artichoke, asparagus, aubergine, French beans, runner beans, broccoli, Brussels sprouts, cabbage, carrots, cauliflower, celeriac, celery, chicory, courgette, cucumber, endive, leeks, lettuce, mushrooms, mustard and cress, onions, parsley, pumpkin, radishes, salsify, seakale, spinach, swede, tomatoes, turnip tops, vegetable marrow, watercress.

2. *Fruits* (stewed without sugar, or raw)
Gooseberries, grapefruit, lemon, melons (cantaloupe, water or honeydew), rhubarb, blackcurrants, red currants, blackberries, strawberries and raspberries.

3. *Drinks*
Water, soda water, tea or coffee (without milk or sugar) lemon juice, tomato juice, diabetic fruit squash, Marmite, Bovril, Oxo, clear soup (chicken or beef cubes may be used).

4. *Miscellaneous*
Saxine, saccharine or any proprietary sweetening agents (except Sucron and sorbitol) salt, pepper, mustard, vinegar, herbs, spices, gelatine. Worcester Sauce, flavourings and colourings may be used.

Group B: Foods to be Avoided
All fried foods.
Sugar (brown or white), glucose, sorbitol.
Sweets, toffees, chocolates, cornflour, custard powder.
Jam, marmalade, lemon curd, syrup, honey, treacle.
Tinned, frozen or bottled fruits.
Dried fruits, e.g. dates, figs, prunes, apricots, sultanas, currants, raisins, bananas, grapes.
Cakes, buns, pastries, pies, steamed or milk puddings.
Sweet or chocolate biscuits, scones.
Cereals, e.g. rice, sago, macaroni, barley, spaghetti.
Breakfast cereal, porridge.
Cocoa, Ovaltine, Horlicks.
Ice cream, fresh or synthetic cream. Table jelly.
Evaporated or condensed milk.
Peas, parsnips, beetroot, sweetcorn, haricot beans, butter beans, broad beans, lentils.
Nuts.
Salad cream, salad dressing, mayonnaise.
Tomato and brown sauce or any thickened sauce.
Sweet pickles and chutney.
Thickened soups, gravies, Bisto.
Alcoholic drinks, e.g. beer, wine, sherry, spirits.
Sweetened fruit juices, fruit squash, Coca Cola and other sweet, fizzy, 'soft drinks'.
Lemonades, Lucozade, Ribena.
Starch-reduced products, 'diabetic' foodstuffs.
Sausages.

All foods must be served without thickened gravies and sauces. All foods may be baked, grilled, boiled or steamed — *but not fried.*

2. MEASURED DIABETIC DIET
Method of constructing a diet restricted in carbohydrate containing approximately 1800 kcal (7560 kJ) with 210 g carbohydrate 80 g protein and 70 g fat suitable for adults with diabetes mellitus

Use is made of the Atwater calorie conversion factors of 4, 4 and 9 kcal/g for carbohydrate, protein and fat respectively. Each *carbohydrate exchange* contains approximately 10 g carbohydrate, 1·5 g protein and 0·3 fat. Calorie value is about 50 (equivalent to 20 g bread).

Each *protein exchange* contains approximately 7 g protein and 5 g fat. Calorie value is about 70 (equivalent to 30 g meat).

Each *fat exchange* contains approximately 12 g fat and almost no carbohydratge or protein. Calorie value is about 110 (equivalent to ½ oz butter). One pint of milk contains approximately 30 g carbohydrate, 18 g protein and 24 g fat. Calorie value is about 410.

In practice, for quick construction of a diabetic diet it is usually only necessary to work in terms of grams of carbohydrate and total calories. Thus, a diet prescription for 210 g carbohydrate, 1800 kcal would be calculated as follows:

1. The daily intake of carbohydrate (210 g) represents 21 carbohydrate exchanges.

2. The daily allowance of milk is decided, either on the basis of the patient's food habits or special requirements. In this example it is 400 ml (⅔ pint), which contains 2 carbohydrate exchanges, leaving 19 for distribution throughout the day.

3. The daily allowance of protein is then decided. Five protein exchanges will provide 350 kcal.

4. The calories allocated so far amount to 1580; a further 220 kcal are needed to bring the total up to 1800 kcal. This must be provided by fat. As one fat exchange provides 110 kcal, two are needed.

Exchanges	Grams of carbohydrate	kcal
400 ml (⅔ pint) milk = 2 carbo-hydrate exchange	20	280
19 carbohydrate exchanges	190	950
5 protein exchanges	—	350
Total	210	1580
2 fat exchanges	—	220
GRAND TOTAL	210	1800

5. Finally, the exchanges (21 carbohydrate, 5 protein and 2 fat) are distributed throughout the day according to the eating habits and daily routine of the patient.

Useful CHO exchanges

Each item on this list = 1 CHO exchange (10 g CHO): ½ slice bread from a large loaf, 1 large digestive biscuit, 2 Rich Tea biscuits, 2 cream crackers, 2 heaped teaspoons Ovaltine or Horlicks, 8 tablespoons natural unsweetened orange juice or grapefruit juice, 1 medium sized eating apple or orange, 10 grapes, 1 small banana, ⅓ pint milk, 1 teacup cooked porridge, 1 teacup of cream or tinned soup, ⅔ teacup cornflakes, 1 small packet of crisps, one small potato.

3. UNMEASURED DIABETIC DIET

Patients who are unable to measure their diet or for whom this is unnecessary, are given a list of foods which are grouped into three categories.

I. *Foods to be avoided altogether:*

1. Suger, glucose, jam, marmalade, honey, syrup, treacle, tinned fruits, sweets, chocolate, lemonade, glucose drinks, proprietary milk preparations and similar foods which are sweetened with sugar.

2. Cakes, sweet biscuits, chocolate biscuits, pies, puddings, thick sauces.

3. Alcoholic drinks unless permission has been given by the doctor.

II. *Foods to be eaten in moderation only:*

1. Breads of all kinds (including so-called 'slimming' and 'starch-reduced' breads, brown or white, plain or toasted).

2. Rolls, scones, biscuits and crispbreads.

3. Potatoes, peas and baked beans.

4. Breakfast cereals and porridge.

5. All fresh or dried fruit.

6. Macaroni, spaghetti, custard and foods with much flour.

7. Thick soups.

8. Diabetic foods.

9. Milk.

III *Foods to be eaten as desired:*

1. All meats, fish, eggs.

2. Cheese.

3. Clear soups or meat extracts, tomato or lemon juice.

4. Tea or coffee.

5. Cabbage, Brussels sprouts, broccoli, cauliflower, spinach, turnip, runner or French beans, onions, leeks or mushrooms, lettuce, cucumber, tomatoes, spring onions, radishes, mustard and cress, asparagus, parsley, rhubarb.

6. Herbs, spices, salt, pepper and mustard.

7. Saccharine preparations for sweetening.

For overweight diabetics butter, margarine, fatty and dried foods must be restricted.

4. FAT-MODIFIED DIET

Low in saturated fats and cholesterol with increased amounts of polyunsaturated fat.

Foods to be avoided:

Butter and hydrogenated margarines. Use polyunsaturated margarine, e.g. 'Flora'.

Lard, suet, shortenings and cakes, biscuits and pastries made with these.

Fatty meat and visible fat on meat. Meat pieces, sausages and luncheon meats.

Whole milk and cream.

Chocolate, ice cream (except water ices). Cheese, except low fat cottage cheese.

Coconut, coconut oil and 'Coffee mate'.

Eggs — no more than 1 to 2 eggs yolks per week, including that used in cooking.

Organ meats — liver, kidneys and brain.

Shellfish and fish roes.

Fried foods unless fried in polyunsaturated oil (like sunflower or corn oil).

Potato crisps and most nuts.

Gravy unless made with polyunsaturated oil, and tinned soups.

Salad dressing unless made with polyunsaturated oil.

Use:

Polyunsaturated margarine, e.g. Flora instead of butter.
Polyunsaturated oil, e.g. Sunflower or corn oil in place of lard.

Further reading about dietetics and additional diets:

Davidson, Sir Stanley, Passmore, R., Brock, J.F. & Truswell, A.S. (1979) *Human Nutrition and Dietetics*, 7th edn. Edinburgh: Churchill Livingstone.

DESIRABLE WEIGHTS

Table 21.1 Weight for Age: Birth to 5 Years[1]. Sexes combined[2]

Age (months)	Weight (kg) Standard	80% Std	60% Std	Age (months)	Weight (kg) Standard	80% Std	60% Std
0	3·25	2·6	1·95	31	13·45	10·8	8·1
1	4·15	3·3	2·5	32	13·65	10·9	8·2
2	4·95	4·0	3·0	33	13·85	11·1	8·3
3	5·7	4·6	3·4	34	14·05	11·2	8·4
4	6·35	5·1	3·8	35	14·15	11·3	8·5
5	7·0	5·6	4·2	36	14·35	11·5	8·6
6	7·5	6·0	4·5	37	14·55	11·6	8·7
7	8·0	6·4	4·8	38	14·7	11·8	8·8
8	8·5	6·8	5·1	39	14·9	11·9	8·9
9	8·9	7·1	5·3	40	15·05	12·0	9·0
10	9·2	7·4	5·5	41	15·2	12·2	9·1
11	9·55	7·6	5·7	42	15·4	12·3	9·2
12	9·85	7·9	5·9	43	15·5	12·4	9·3
13	10·1	8·1	6·1	44	15·7	12·6	9·4
14	10·35	8·3	6·2	45	15·85	12·7	9·5
15	10·55	8·4	6·3	46	16·05	12·8	9.6
16	10·75	8·6	6·45	47	16·15	12·9	9·7
17	10·95	8·8	6·6	48	16·35	13·1	9·8
18	11·15	8·9	6·7	49	16·5	13·2	9·9
19	11·35	9·1	6·8	50	16·6	13·3	10·0
20	11·5	9·2	6·9	51	16·8	13·4	10·1
21	11·7	9·4	7·0	52	16·95	13·6	10·2
22	11·85	9·5	7·1	53	17·1	13·7	10·3
23	12·05	9·6	7·2	54	17·25	13·8	10·4
24	12·25	9·8	7·35	55	17·45	14·0	10·5
25	12·25	9·8	7·35	56	17·55	14·1	10·5
26	12·45	10·0	7·47	57	17·7	14·2	10·6
27	12·65	10·1	7·6	58	17·85	14·3	10·7
28	12·85	10·3	7·7	59	18·0	14·4	10·8
29	13·05	10·4	7·8	60	18·2	14·6	10·9
30	13·25	10·6	7·95				

[1] Based on *A growth chart for international use in maternal and child health care*. WHO, Geneva (1978).

[2] On average boys are 0·3 kg heavier and girls 0·3 kg lighter than the mean standard but the differences are smaller than this in the first 2 months and from 50–60 months.

Table 21.2 Desirable Weights of Adults. According to height and frame

Height without shoes (approximate equivalents)			Desirable weight in kilograms and pounds in indoor clothing, ages 25 and over					
metres	Ft	in	Small frame kg	lb	Medium frame kg	lb	Large frame kg	lb
			MEN					
1·550	5	1	58·2–60·9	128–134	59·5–64·1	131–141	62·7–68·2	138–150
1·575	5	2	59·1–61·8	130–136	60·4–65·0	133–143	63·6–60·5	140–153
1·600	5	3	60·0–62·7	132–138	6·14–65·9	135–145	64·5–70·9	142–156
1·625	5	4	60·9–63·6	134–140	62·2–67·3	137–148	65·4–72·7	144–160
1·650	5	5	61·8–64·5	136–142	63·2–68·6	139–151	66·4–74·5	146–164
1·675	5	6	62·7–65·9	138–145	64·5–70·0	142–154	67·6–76·4	149–168
1·700	5	7	63·6–67·3	140–148	65·9–71·4	145–157	69·0–78·2	152–172
1·725	5	8	64·5–68·6	142–151	67·3–72·7	148–160	70·5–80·0	155–176
1·750	5	9	65·4–70·0	144–154	68·6–74·1	151–163	71·8–81·8	158–180
1·775	5	10	64·4–71·4	146–157	70·0–75·4	154–166	73·2–83·6	161–184
1·800	5	11	67·7–72·7	149–160	71·4–77·3	157–170	74·5–85·4	164–188
1·825	6	0	69·1–74·5	152–164	72·7–79·1	160–174	76·4–87·3	168–192
1·850	6	1	70·5–76·4	155–168	74·5–80·9	164–178	78·2–89·5	172–197
1·875	6	2	71·8–78·2	158–172	75·9–82·7	167–182	80·0–91·8	176–202
1·900	6	3	73·6–80·0	162–176	77·7–85·0	171–187	82·5–94·1	181–207
			WOMEN					
1·450	4	9	46·4–50·4	102–111	49·5–55·0	109–121	53·6–59·5	118–131
1·475	4	10	46·8–51·4	103–113	50·4–55·9	111–123	54·5–60·9	120–134
1·500	4	11	47·3–52·3	104–115	51·4–57·3	113–126	55·4–62·3	133–137
1·525	5	0	48·2–53·6	106–118	52·3–58·6	115–129	56·8–63·6	125–140
1·550	5	1	49·1–55·0	108–121	53·6–60·0	118–132	58·2–65·0	128–143
1·575	5	2	50·4–56·4	111–124	55·0–61·4	121–135	59·5–66·8	131–147
1·600	5	3	51·8–57·5	114–127	56·4–62·7	124–138	60·9–68·6	134–151
1·625	5	4	53·2–59·0	117–130	57·5–64·1	127–141	62·3–70·4	137–155
1·650	5	5	54·5–60·4	120–133	59·1–65·4	130–144	63·6–72·8	140–159
1·675	5	6	55·9–61·8	123–136	60·4–66·8	133–147	65·0–74·1	143–163
1·700	5	7	57·3–63·2	126–139	61·8–68·2	136–150	66·4–75·9	146–167
1·725	5	8	58·6–64·5	129–142	63·2–69·5	139–153	67·7–77·3	149–170
1·750	5	9	60·0–65·9	132–145	64·5–70·9	142–156	69·1–78·4	152–173
1·775	5	10	61·4–67·3	135–148	65·9–72·3	145–159	70·4–80·0	155–176
1·800	5	11	62·7–68·6	138–151	67·3–73·6	148–162	71·8–81·4	158–179

Based on weights of insured persons in the United States associated with lowest mortality (1983 Metropolitan Height and Weight Tables. Source of basic data 1979 Build Study Society of Actuaries and Association of Life Insurance Medical Directors of America 1980).

Table 21.3 BIOCHEMICAL VALUES

Venous Blood: Approximate Adult Reference Values

Analysis	Reference Values	
	S.I. Units	Other Units
Acid phosphatase (unstable enzyme)		0·1–0·4 u/l
Alanine aminotransferase (ALT) (glutamic-pyruvic transaminase (GPT)		10–40 u/l
Alkaline phosphatase		40–100 u/l
Amylase		50–300 u/l
α_1-antitrypsin	2–4 g/l	
Ascorbic acid — serum	23–57 μmol/l	0·4–1·0 mg/dl
— leukocytes	1420–2270 μmol/l	25–40 mg/dl
Aspartate aminotransferase (AST) (glutamic-oxaloacetic transaminase (GOT)		10–35 u/l
Bile acids		
Cholate — fasting	<3 μmol/l	
— 2 h post prandial	<9 μmol/l	
Chenodeoxycholate — fasting	<3 μmol/l	
— 2 h post prandial	<13 μmol/l	
Bilirubin (total)	2–17 μmol/l	0·3–1·0 mg/dl
Caeruloplasmin	150–400 mg/l	15–40 mg/dl
Calcium (total)	2·12–2·62 mmol/l	8·5–10·5 mg/dl
Carbon dioxide (total)	24–30 mmol/l	
β-Carotene	0·9–5·6 μmol/l	50–300 μg/dl
Chloride	95–105 mmol/l	
Cholesterol (fasting)	3·6–6·7 mmol/l	145–270 mg/dl
Copper	11–24 μmol/l	100–128 μg/dl
Creatinine	55–150 μmol/l	0·6–1·7 mg/dl
Creatinine clearance		90–130 ml/min
Creatine kinase (CK) — males		30–200 u/l
— females		30–150 u/l
Ethanol — marked intoxication	65–87 mmol/l	0·3–0·4 g/dl
— stupor	87–109 mmol/l	0·4–0·5 g/dl
— coma	>109 mmol/l	>0·5 g/dl
Ferritin — males		6–186 μg/ml
— females	*	3–162 μg/ml
α-Fetoprotein	2–6 units/ml	<30 ng/ml
γ-Glutamyl transferase (γ-GT) — males		10–55 u/l
— females		5–35 u/l
Glucose (fasting)	<5·5 mmol/l	<100 mg/dl
Immunoglobulins (Ig): IgA	0·5–4·0 g/l (40–300 i.u./l)	
IgG	5·0–13·0 g/l (60–160 i.u./l)	
IgM — males	0·3–2·2 g/l (40–270 i.u./l)	
— females	0·4–2·5 g/l (50–300 i.u./l)	
Iron — males	14–32 μmol/l	77–178 μg/dl
— females	10–28 μmol/l	56–156 μg/dl
Iron binding capacity (total)	45–72 μmol/l	250–400 μg/dl
Iron binding capacity (saturation)		14–47%
Lactate	0·4–1·4 mmol/l	3·6–13·0 mg/dl
Lactate dehydrogenase (LD)		100–300 u/l
Lead	0·5–1·9 μmol./l	10–40 μg/dl
Magnesium	0·75–1·0 mmol/l	1·8–2·4 mg/dl
Osmolality	285–295 mosm/kg	

*Measured against a British standard preparation

BIOCHEMICAL VALUES (*continued*)

Analysis	Reference Values	
	S.I. Units	Other Units
Phosphatase *see* acid and alkaline		
Phosphate	0·8–1·4 mmol/l	2·5–4·5 mg/dl
Potassium	3·3–4·7 mmol/l	
Proteins — total	62–82 g/l	6·2–8·2 g/dl
— albumin	36–52 g/l	3·6–5·2 g/dl
— globulins	24–37 g/l	2·4–3·7 g/dl
Pyruvate — fasting	35–80 μmol/l	
— after 50g glucose — 60m	<110 μmol/l	
— 90m	<120 μmol/l	
Sodium	132–144 mmol/l	
Triglyceride (fasting)	0·6–1·7 mmol/l	40–145 mg/dl
Urate — males	0·12–0·42 mmol/l	2–7 mg/dl
— females	0·12–0·36 mmol/l	2–6 mg/dl
Urea**	2·5–6·6 mmol/l	15–40 mg/dl
Vitamin A	0·7–1·7 μmol/l	20–50 μg/dl

**Urea × 0·4665 = Urea Nitrogen   Urea Nitrogen × 2·14 = Urea

Note. The normal adult reference values given above are largely those of the Department of Clinical Chemistry, Royal Infirmary, Edinburgh. Methodology varies between laboratories, and clinicians should be guided by the normal reference ranges for the laboratories they use; this applies especially to the results of enzyme assays. The above estimations can be made in plasma or serum; serum is required for plasma protein electrophoresis and is preferable for radioimmunoassays.

NOTES ON INTERNATIONAL SYSTEM OF UNITS (SI UNITS)

Examples of Basic SI Units

Length	metre (m)
Mass	kilogram (kg)
Amount of substance	mole (mol)
Energy	joule (J)
Pressure	pascal (pa)

Examples of Decimal Multiples and Submultiples of SI Units

Factor	Name	Symbol
10^6	mega-	M
10^3	kilo-	k
10^{-1}	deci-	d
10^{-2}	centi-	c
10^{-3}	milli-	m
10^{-6}	micro-	μ
10^{-9}	nano-	n
10^{-12}	pico-	p
10^{-15}	femto-	f

Volume. The basic SI unit of volume is the cubic metre (1000 litre). Because of its convenience the litre is used as the unit of volume in laboratory work.

Amount of Substance ('Molar') Concentration (e.g., mol/*l*, μmol/*l*) is used for substances of defined chemical composition. It replaces equivalent concentration (mEq/*l*), which is not part of the SI system. For univalent ions such as sodium, potassium, chloride and bicarbonate the numerical value is unchanged. For divalent ions such as calcium and magnesium the numerical value is halved.

Mass Concentration (e.g. g/*l*, μg/*l*) is used for all protein measurements, for substances which do not have a sufficiently well defined composition and for serum vitamin B_{12} and folate measurements. The numerical value in SI units will change by a factor of 10 in those instances previously expressed in terms of 100 ml.

Haemoglobin is an exception. It is generally expressed in terms of g/dl although the International Committee for standardisation in Haematology recommended in 1982 that the unit for haemoglobin should be g/*l*.

SI units are not employed for enzymes nor usually for immunoglobulins.

Table 21.4 MISCELLANEOUS APPROXIMATE ADULT REFERENCE VALUES

Arterial Blood Analyses

Analysis	Reference Values	
	S.I. Units	Other Units
Ammonia	11–35 μmol/l	20–63 μg/dl
Hydrogen ion	36–44 nmol/l	pH 7·37–7·45
Carbon dioxide (P_aCO_2)	4·8–6·0 kPa	36–45 mmHg
Plasma bicarbonate	21–27·5 mmol/l	21–27·5 mEq/L
Oxygen (P_aO_2)	11–13 kPa	83–98 mmHg

Cerebrospinal Fluid (Lumbar puncture)
Cells: 5/mm³ (all lymphocytes)
Glucose: 2·5–4·0 mmol/l (45–72 mg/dl) — 50 to 70% of plasma concentration
Immunoglobulin G: 20–50 mg/l
Protein (total): 100–400 mg/l
Pressure: 5–15 cmCSF

Gastrointestinal, Pancreas and Liver
Faecal Fat: <18 mmol/24 h (<5 g/24 h)
Stool Weight (Wet): <200 g/24 h
D-Xylose excretion (25g dose): 33–53 mmol/5 h (5–8 g/5 h)
    Serum Xylose: 1·7–2·7 mmol/l at 1 h (25–40 mg/dl)
Pancreatic Exocrine Function (secretion stimulation 1 u/kg i.v.)
  Juice volume: >2 mg/kg/h
  Bicarbonate — output: >10 mmol/h
          — concentration: >80 mmol/l
Liver: Copper <50 μg/g dry weight
(Wilson's disease >250 μg/g dry weight)

Sweat (pilocarpine iontophoresis)
Sodium <85 mmol/l
Potassium <25 mmol/l
NB Minimum sweat sample 50 mg

Table 21.5 Hormone Concentrations in Plasma; Approximate Adult Reference Values

Analysis	Conditions	Reference Values	
		S.I. Units	Other Units
Adrenocorticotrophin (ACTH) 0900 h	Avoid stressful venepuncture	10–80 ng/l	
2200 h	Separate and store at −20°C immediately	<10	
Cortisol			
(fluorimetry) 0900 h	Avoid stressful venepuncture	220–720 nmol/l	8·0–26 μg/100 ml
2200 h		<275	<10
(RIA) 0900 h		190–550	7·0–20
2200 h		<190	<190
Follicle-stimulating hormone (FSH)			
Male			1·5–9·0 U/l
Female, early follicular			3·0–15·0 U/l
Female, post-menopausal			30–115 U/l
Gastrin	Collect after overnight fast. Separate and store immediately at −20°C	60–200 pg/ml	
Growth hormone (GH)	Avoid stressful venepuncture		often <1·0 mU/l but variable
Insulin	Collect after overnight fast Separate and store immediately at −20°C		5–25 mU/l, but variable
Luteinising hormone (LH)			
Male			1·5–9·0 U/l
Female, early follicular			2·5–9·0 U/l
Female, post menopausal			30–115 U/l
Parathryoid hormone (PTH)	Separate and store at −20°C immediately	Values depend upon antiserum specificity	
Prolactin (PRL)	Avoid stressful venepuncture		60–390 mU/l
Testosterone			
Male		10–30 nmol/l	290–860 ng/100 ml
Female		0·8–2·8 nmol/l	23–81 ng/100 ml
Thyroid-stimulating hormone (TSH)			<5·7 mU/l
Thyroxine		70–150 nmol/l	5·5–12 μg 100 ml variable
Triiodothyrone		1·1–2·8 nmol/l	70–180 ng 100 ml

Table 21.6 Urine: Approximate Adult Reference Values

Analysis	Reference Values	
	S.I. Units	Other Units
Amylase		35–260 Somogyi units/h
Calcium (low calcium diet)	1·2–3·7 mmol/24 h	50–150 mg/24 h
Copper	<1 μmol/24 h	<100 μg/24 h
5-Hydroxyindole-3-acetic acid	10–45 μmol/24 h	2–9 mg/24 h
4-Hydroxy, 3-methoxy mandelic acid	<30 μmol/24 h	8 mg/24 h
Metadrenalines	<7 μmol/24 h	
Osmolality	70–1200 mosm/kg	
Phosphate (normal diet)	15–50 mmol/24 h	
Porphyrins — coproporphyrins	150–230 nmol/24 h	
— uroporphyrins	<40 nmol/24 h	
Potassium	25–100 mmol/24 h	
Protein	<100 mg/24 h	
Sodium	100–200 mmol/24 h	

Table 21.7 Therapeutic Blood Concentration of Drugs

Drug	Blood Concentration		Conditions
	S.I. Units	Other Units	
Antiepileptic drugs			
Carbamazepine	34–51 μmol/l	4–10 μg/ml	4–6 h after last dose
Ethosuximide		50–85 μg/ml	
Phenobarbitone	65–170 μmol/l	15–40 μg/ml	
Phenytoin	40–80 μmol/l	10–20 μg/ml	>10 d after start of therapy
Digoxin		1–2·6 ng/ml	>8 h after last dose
Gentamicin		Peak: >5 μg/ml	Immediately after intravenous injection
		Trough: 4 μg/ml	6–8 h after last dose
Lithium	0·8–1·2 mmol/l		10–12 h after last dose

Note: Monitoring the concentration of a drug in the blood is not a substitute for a careful clinical assessment but is helpful (1) if toxic effects occur when dosage is only slightly greater than that required for a therapeutic effect as in the case of phenytoin or digoxin, (2) when renal function is impaired, and (3) if there is uncertainty about the patient taking the drug. Peak and trough measurements are helpful if there is a risk of accumulation of a drug as in the case of gentamicin. Lithium can be measured as easily as other electrolytes and its level should be monitored regularly when it is used in the treatment of manic-depressive states.

Table 21.8 Haematological Values

	S.I. Units	Other Units
Bleeding time (Ivy)	Up to 11 min	
Body fluid (total)		50% (obese)–70% (lean) of body weight
Intracellular		30–40% of body weight
Extracellular		20–30% of body weight
Blood volume		
Red cell mass, men	30 ± 5 ml/kg	
women	25 ± 5 ml/kg	
Plasma volume (both sexes)	45 ± 5 ml/kg	
Total blood volume, men	75 ± 10 ml/kg	
women	70 ± 10 ml/kg	
Erythrocyte Sedimentation Rate (Westergren) (Figures given are for patients under 60 years of age. Higher values in older persons are not necessarily abnormal).		0–6 mm in 1 h normal 7–20 mm in 1 h doubtful >20 mm in 1 h abnormal
Fibrinogen	1·5–4·0 g/l	150–400 mg/dl
*Folate — serum	2–20 μg/l	2–20 ng/ml
— red cell	>100 μg/l	>100 ng/ml
Haemoglobin — men	13–18 g/dl	13–18 g/100 ml
— women	11·5–16·5 g/dl	11·5–16·5 g/100 ml
Haptoglobin	0·3–2·0 g/l	30–200 mg/dl
Leucocytes — adults	$4·0–11·0 \times 10^9$/l	4000–11000/μl $4·0–11·0 \times 10^3$/mm^3
Differential white cell count		
Neutrophil granulocytes	$2·5–7·5 \times 10^9$/l	40–75%
Lymphocytes	$1·0–3·5 \times 10^9$/l	20–45%
Monocytes	$0·2–0·8 \times 10^9$/l	2–10%
Eosinophil granulocytes	$0·04–0·4 \times 10^9$/l	1–6%
Basophil granulocytes	$0·01–0·1 \times 10^9$/l	0–1%
Mean corpuscular haemoglobin (MCH)	27–32 pg	27–32 $\mu\mu$g
Mean corpuscular haemoglobin concentration (MCHC)	30–35 g/dl	30–35%
Mean corpuscular volume (MCV)	78–98 fl	78–98 μ^3 or μm^3
Packed cell volume (PCV) or haematocrit — men	0·40–0·54	40–54%
— women	0·35–0·47	35–47%
Platelets	$150–400 \times 10^9$/l	150 000–400 000/μl or/mm^3
Prothrombin Time	11–15 s	
Red cell count — men	$4·5–6·5 \times 10^{12}$/l	$4·5–6·5 \times 10^6$/μl or mm
— women	$3·8–5·8 \times 10^{12}$/l	$3·8–5·8 \times 10^6$/μl or mm
Red cell life span (mean)	120 d	
Red cell life span $T_{\frac{1}{2}}$ (^{51}Cr)	25–35 days	
Reticulocytes (adults)	$10–100 \times 10^9$/l	0·2–2%
*Vitamin B_{12} (in serum as cyanocobalamin)	160–925 ng/l	160–925 pg/ml or $\mu\mu$g/ml

*also measured by radioassay; normal range of reference values should be obtained from the laboratory carrying out the estimation.

DRUG NOMENCLATURE AND PRESCRIPTION

In this book the names that have been given for drugs have almost invariably been those approved for use in Britain. These are devised or selected by the British Pharmacopoeia Commission and published by the Health Ministers at regular intervals. It must be realised, however, that many countries have their national non-proprietary names, and that the World Health Organisation also has its own list. Usually these various names are similar, but there are significant differences; for example, paracetamol (B.P.) is listed as acetaminophen in the United States Pharmacopeia. Proprietary names are given in this book only in exceptional circumstances, but can usually be found in the British National Formulary, the Data Sheet Compendium and as an addendum to some text books. There may be many totally different names for the same substance and this can cause confusion.

Abbreviations used in relationship to the administration of drugs are i.m. (intramuscular injection), i.v. (intravenous injection), s.c. (subcutaneous injection), b.d. (twice daily) and t.i.d. (thrice daily). The dosage given is a guide for use in adults of average build and should be checked against that in a national formulary or in the manufacturer's instructions. It is particularly important to confirm that a dosage given in mg/kg body weight is, indeed, correct, and great care must be taken to ensure that no error occurs in the quantity of a drug prescribed for an infant or child.

Some drugs, e.g. in the chemotherapy of malignant disease, are prescribed in weight of drug per square metre of body surface. With the use of a nomogram, the body surface area can be calculated from the height in centimetres and the weight in kilograms.

Patient compliance (i.e. the taking of medicines as prescribed) is improved if instructions are simple and specific, especially for the elderly. Polypharmacy should be avoided if possible, one reason being the danger of interaction between drugs. Some (e.g. rifampicin) induce liver enzymes (p. 000) which may increase the metabolism of concurrently administered preparations (e.g. corticosteroids, oral contraceptives, oral anticoagulants, oral hypoglycaemic drugs, dapsone and phenytoin). Conversely elimination of compounds metabolised in the liver by oxidation (e.g. oral anticoagulants, phenytoin and diazepam) can be prolonged by the action of other drugs (e.g. cimetidine). All drugs, whenever possible, should be avoided during the early months of pregnancy.

STANDARD REFERENCE BOOKS:

British National Formulary (1984) London: The British Medical Association and The Pharmaceutical Society of Great Britain.
Martindale — The Extra Pharmacopoeia (1983), 28th edn. London: The Pharmaceutical Press.

FURTHER READING ABOUT DRUGS:

Avery, G.S. (Ed.) (1980) *Drug Treatment*, 2nd edn. Edinburgh: Churchill Livingstone.
Girdwood, R.H. (Ed.) (1984) *Clinical Pharmacology*, 25th edn. London: Baillière Tindall.

Index

Abdomen, examination of, 281
  ultrasonography, 282
Abducent nerve, 609
Abortion, genetic factors in, 7
  selective, 17
Abortus fever, 748
Abram's pleural biopsy, 213
Abscess, amoebic, 773
  Brodie's 587
  cerebral, 636
  cold, 231
  ischiorectal, 236
  liver, 368
  pelvic, 320
  perinephric, 396
  pulmonary, 226
  spinal epidural, 637
  subphrenic, 320
'Absences', 617
Acanthosis nigricans, 109
Acclimatisation, to altitude, 725
  to heat, 722
Acedapsone, 761
Acetaminophen, poisoning, 709
Acetic acids, 559
Acetohexamide, 468
Acetone, in urine, 461, 463
Acetylcysteine, 709
Achalasia of the cardia, 290
Achlorhydria, 284
Achondroplasia, 10, 424
Acid-base equilibrium, 98, 378
Acid excretion, by kidney, 381
Acidosis, in shock, 100
  lactic, 100, 469, 477
  metabolic, 100
  renal tubular, 379
  respiratory, 102
Ackee poisoning, 711
Aclasis, diaphyseal, 588
Acne vulgaris, tetracyclines in, 45
Acromegaly, 423
ACTH, 419, 443
  test, 450
Actinomycetoma, 802
Actinomycin, 113
Actinomycosis, 224
Acyclovir, 48
Acylureidopenicillins, 44

Adams-Stokes attacks, 144
ADCC, 28
Adder bite, 710
Addiction to drugs, 694
Addisonian pernicious anaemia, 501
Addison's disease, 447
Adenoma, bronchial, 262
  pituitary, 421
  sebaceum, 11
Adenomatosis, multiple endocrine, 440
Adenomyomatosis of gall bladder, 373
Adenoviruses, 726
ADH, 420
Adolescence, psychiatric illness in, 698
Adrenal gland, anatomy and
    physiology, 443
  hyperfunction of, 444
Adrenal hyperplasia, congenital, 449
Adrenaline, 32
Adrenoceptor agonists and
    antagonists, see Beta-
    adrenoceptor
Adrenocorticotrophic hormone, 419,
    443
  ectopic, 444
Adrianmycin, 113, 118
Adult respiratory distress syndrome,
  210
Adulthood, psychiatric illness in, 699
Aerophagy, 281
Aflatoxin, 720
Afterload, cardiac, 152
Agammaglobulinaemia, 34
Agglutination tests, 26
Agglutinin, cold and warm, 512
Agnosia, 604
Agoraphobia, 691
Agranulocytosis, 519
AIDS, 35
Albinism, 14
Albumin, plasma, 341
Alcohol and, anaemia, 503
  blood levels of, 817
  cardiomyopathy, 186
  chlorpropamide, 468
  fetal syndrome, 695
  gastritis, 302
  Hodgkin's lymphoma, 530
  hypertension, 181

Alcohol (contd)
  liver disease, 356
  metabolism of, 338
  myelopathy, 656
  myocardium, 186
  neuropathy, 661
  pancreatitis, 306
  pregnancy, 695
  psychosis, 75
Alcoholism, 694
  self poisoning and, 702
Aldosterone, 443
Alfacalcidol, 67
Alimentary disease, in the tropics, 718
  tract, 278
    absorptive system, 280
    defence mechanisms, 280
    endoscopy, 282
    infections, 330
    investigation, 281
    ischaemia, 330
    motility, 279
    psychogenic disorders, 331
    radionuclide scan, 282
    secretion, 280
Alkaloids, plant, 113
Alkalosis, hypokalaemic, 92
  metabolic, 101
  respiratory, 103
Alkaptonuria, 582
Alkylating agents, 113
Allergy, 19
  of respiratory tract, 241
  to food, 25
Allele, 10
Alleleic association, 31
Allopurinol, 525, 581
Alopecia, 117
Aloxiprin, 559
Alpha$_1$-antitrypsin deficiency, 344
Alpha-fetoprotein, 344
  in anencephaly and spina bifida, 17
  in hepatoma, 368
  in testicular teratoma, 107
Alpha-tocopherol, 71
Altitude, acclimatisation to, 725
Alveococcosis, 790
Alveolitis, extrinsic allergic, 249
  fibrosing, 265

Alzheimer's disease, 680
Amantadine, 650
Amastigote, 776
Amaurosis fugax, 629
Amblyopia, 609
Amikacin, 47
Amiloride, 97
Amino acids, essential, 53
Aminocaproic acid, 545
Aminoglutethamide, 118
Aminoglycosides, 46
Aminophylline, 246
Aminoquinolines, 771
Aminotransferase, 340
  in myocardial infarction, 175
Amiodarone, 141
Amitriptyline, 682
Amnesia, 680
Amniocentesis, 17
Amodiaquine, 772
Amoebiasis, 773
Amoeboma, 773
Amoxycillin, 44
Amphetamine, addiction, 696
  poisoning, 706
Amphotericin, 48, 804
Ampicillin, 44
Amylase, serum, 306
Amyloidosis, 390
  of heart, 186
  of joints, 572
Amyotrophic lateral sclerosis, 652
Amyotrophy, diabetic, 663
  neuralgic, 662
Anaemia, after gastric operation, 301
  aplastic, 504
  classification of, 494
  clinical features of, 494
  dimorphic, 502
  haemolytic, 505
    and methyldopa, 29
    autoimmune, 512
    of newborn, 513
  hypochromic, 497
  in blood loss, 495
  in chronic disease, 499
  in iron deficiency, 495
  in the tropics, 720
  megaloblastic, 500
    in haemolytic anaemia, 503
    in leukaemia, 503
    in pregnancy, 503
    nutritional, 503
  pernicious, 501
  sideroblastic, 499
Analeptic therapy, 217
Analgesics, 219, 558
  and nephropathy, 406
Anaphase, 4
Anaphylaxis, 24
Ancylostomiasis, 793
Anencephaly, 16
Aneuploidy, 7
Aneurysm, aortic,197
  cerebral, 632
  dissecting, 197

Aneurysm (contd)
  mycotic, 165
  saccular, 632
  syphilitic, 198
  ventricular, 172
Angina, abdominal, 331
  decubitus, 167
  pectoris, 167
  Prinzmetal's, 167
  unstable, 117
  variant, 167
Angiodysplasia, 327
Angiography, cardiac, 132
  cerebral, 607
  mesenteric, 327
  pulmonary, 185
Angio-oedema, 388
Angioplasty, coronary, 170
Angiostrongylus cantonensis, 800
Angiotensin, 379
  and hypertension, 179
Anisakiasis, 801
Anisocytosis, 493
Ankylosing spondylitis, 564
Ann Arbor classification, 531
Anogenital herpes infection, 414
Anorectic drugs, 86
Anorexia, 281
  nervosa, 425, 688
Anosmia, 608
Antacids, 295
Antenatal diagnosis, 17
Anthranilic acids, 559
Anthrax, 746
Anti-arrhythmic drugs, 139
Antibiotics, 42
  combinations of, 49
  in oncology, 113
  prophylactic use of, 50
Antibody(ies), 19
  antimicrosomal, 343
  antimitochondrial, 343
  antinuclear, 343, 572
  blocking, 28
  erythrocyte, 25
  gastric, 25
  glomerular basement membrane, 25
  intrinsic factor, 25
  mediated cytotoxic reactions, 25
  monoclonal, 550
  tests for, 26
  thyroid, 26
Anticancer drugs, 113
Anticholinergic drugs, 650
Anticholinesterase drugs, 665
Anticoagulants, 547
  bleeding from 548
  in cerebral arterial disease, 635
  in myocardial infarction, 176
  in pulmonary embolism, 185
  in venous thrombosis, 200
Antidepressants, 681
Antidiuretic hormone (ADH), 420
  drugs and, 95
  inappropriate secretion of, 261, 427
Antidotes, in poisoning, 706

Antiemetics, 532
Antiepileptic drugs, 618
  megaloblastic anaemia due to, 503
  osteomalacia due to, 67
Antifungal agents, 48
Antigen, 19
  hepatitis associated, 342
Antihaemophilic globulin, 540, 544
Antihistamines, 32, 241
Antihypertensive drugs, 181
Anti-inflammatory drugs, 33, 558
Antimetabolites, 113
Antimicrobial agents, 41
  adverse effects, 49
Antimongolism, 9
Antimonials, pentavalent, 777
Antineoplastic drugs, 113
Antinuclear factor, 574
Antiplatelet drugs, 176
Antiserum, precautions in use, 744
Antisocial disorder, 693
Antistreptolysin titre, 157, 388
Antitetanus serum, 745
Antithrombin, 541
Antithyroid drugs, 431
Antitrypsin (α_1), 344
Antivenom, 710
Antiviral agents, 48
Antivitamins, 64
Anuria, 380
Anxiety neurosis, 685
Aorta, coarctation of, 190
  cystic medial necrosis of, 163
  dissection of, 197
Aortic arch syndrome, 199
Aortic valve, bicuspid, 161
  see also Stenosis and Regurgitation,
Aortitis, syphilitic, 198
Apex beat, 126
Apheresis, 33
Aplasia, of marrow, 504
Apoferritin, 496
Appendicitis, 320
Apraxia, 604
Arbovirus, 733
Arenavirus, 726
Argemone poisoning, 711
Arginine vasopressin, 420
Argyll Robertson pupil, 639
Arnold-Chiari syndrome, 654
Arrest, cardiac, 138
Arrhythmia, sinus, 133, 139
  in myocardial infarction, 172, 175
Arteriography, cerebral, 634
  coronary, 168
  renal, 383
Arteriosclerosis, 196
Arteriovenous malformation, 632
Arteritis, 577
  cerebral, 630
  cranial (giant cell; temporal), 199
Artery(ies), diseases of, 196
  occlusion of, 197
  ultrasonography of, 197
Arthritis, enteropathic, 567
  gonococcal, 570

Arthritis (*contd*)
  in acromegaly, 571
  in amyloidosis, 572
  in brucellosis, 571
  in hyperlipidaemia, 572
  in sarcoidosis, 572
  in viral infection, 571
  infective, 570
  juvenile, 568
  meningococcal, 570
  mutilans, 556
  psoriatic, 567
  reactive, 565
  rheumatoid, 551
  septic, 556, 570
  syphilitic, 571
  seronegative, 563
  tropical, acute, 721
  tuberculous, 571
  Yersinia, 563
Arthroscopy, 557
Arthropods, diseases due to, 805
Arthrosis, 582
Arthus reaction, 26
Asbestosis, 267
Ascariasis, 791
Aschoff nodule, 156
Ascites, 360
  chylous, 796
  in constrictive pericarditis, 189
  malignant, 304
  treatment of, 363
Ascorbic acid, 72
Aspartate aminotransferase, 175
Aspergillosis, 240
Aspirin, and haematemesis, 297
  and thrombosis, 547
  in rheumatoid arthritis, 558
Astereognosis, 598
Asthenia, tropical, anhidrotic, 723
Asthma, bronchial, 241
  cardiac, 122
  exercise induced, 243
Astrocytoma, 620, 623
Asystole, ventricular, 138
Ataxia, cerebellar, 595
  hereditary, 654
  sensory, 597
  tropical spinal, 656
Atenolol, 141
  in hypertension, 182
Atheroma, 196
Atherosclerosis, 196
  cerebral, 628
  in diabetes, 477
  obliterans, 196
Athetosis, 651
Atlanto-axial subluxation, 555
Atomic explosion, 528
Atopy, 242
Atrial septal defect, 191
Atrophy, cerebral, 680
  optic, 609
  progressive muscular, 652
  spinal muscular, 653

Atropine, 176
Auditory nerve, 614
Autoimmunity, 28
  and adrenal failure, 447
  and diabetes mellitus, 458
  and haemolytic anaemia, 512
  and liver disease, 343
  and myasthenia, 665
  and rheumatoid arthritis, 552
  and thyroid disease, 430
  genetic factors, 29
Automatism, 617
Autosome, abnormalities of, 7
AVP, 420
Azapropazone, 559
Azathioprine, 32
  in rheumatoid arthritis, 561
  in ulcerative colitis, 325
Azlocillin, 44
Azoospermia, 456

B lymphocytes, 20
Babinski reflex, 599
Bacampicillin, 44
Bacillus cereus food poisoning, 753
Bacteraemia, 50
Bacteria, diseases due to, 742
Bacteriuria, 382
Bacteroides fragilis infections, 330
Baculovirus, 726
Bagassosis, 249, 266
Baker's cyst, 554
Balanitis, 415
Balantidiasis, 775
Ballism, 651
Barbiturate addiction, 696
  and enzyme induction, 339
  poisoning, 706
Barium enema, and meal, 282
Barr-body, 6
Bartonellosis, 757
Basophil granulocyte, 492
Basophilia, punctate, 493
BCG vaccination, 239
  in leprosy, 762
Beclomethasone, 246
Bee stings, 707
Behaviour therapy, 691
Behçet's disease, 568
Bell's palsy, 613
Bence-Jones protein, 536
Benorylate, 559
Benserazide, 650
Benzathine penicillin, 43
Benzodiazepine poisoning, 706
Benzylpenicillin, 43
Beriberi, 74
  infantile, 75
Berylliosis, 266
Beta-adrenoceptor (adrenergic)
    agonists, 246
  antagonists, (beta-blockers)
    adverse effects, 181
    cardioselective, 182
    in angina pectoris, 170

Beta-adrenoceptor antagonists (*contd*)
    in arrhythmias, 141
    in hypertension, 182
    in hyperthyroidism, 432
    in myocardial infarction, 176
    in psychoneurosis, 687
    poisoning from, 706
Beta-endorphin, 420
Betahistine, 615
Beta-lactam antibiotics, 42
Beta-lipotrophin, 419
Betamethasone, 451
Bicarbonate, buffer system, 99
Biguanides, 469
Bile acids, metabolism of, 338
Bile ducts, anatomy of, 369
Bilharziasis, 782
Biliary cirrhosis, 362
Biligraphin, 370
Bilirubin, and liver function, 339
  metabolism of, 336
Biochemical values, 817
Biopsy, alimentary tract, 284
  jejunal, 284
  liver, 344
  lung, 213
  lymph node, 213
  needle, 106
  pleural, 213
  rectal, 316, 323
  renal, 384
  synovial, 557
Biotin, 79
Bird fancier's lung, 249
Bismuth, colloidal, 296
Bithionol, 787
Bitôt's spots, 65
Black death, 749
Blackwater fever, 770
Bladder, urinary, control of, 600
  paralysis of, 659
  tumours of, 407
Blalock-Taussig operation, 194
Blastomycoses, 805
Bleach poisoning, 707
Bleeding, arrest of, in haemophilia, 545
  oesophagogastric, treatment of, 364
  time, 541
Bleomycin, 118
Blind loop syndrome, 314
Blindness, causes of, 64
  in diabetes mellitus, 479
  in onchocerciasis, 797
  in trachoma, 737
  river, 797
Block, atrioventricular, 143
  bundle branch, 144
  sino-atrial, 142
Blood, destruction, 492
  diseases, in tropics, 720
  formation, 488
  in urine, 381
  pressure, 128
  transfusion of, incompatible, 515
Blood-gas analysis, 213

Blood pool scanning, 132
Bone, diseases of, 586
  metastases, 587
  physiology of, 585
  radionuclide scan, 565
Bornholm disease, 270
Botulism, 754
Bowel, inflammatory disease of, 314
  irritable, 332
Brachytherapy, 112
Bradycardia, in myocardial infarction, 176
  sinus, 133
Brain, computed tomography, 606
  infections of, 636
  localising signs of disease, 603
  nuclear magnetic resonance, 607
  radiological examination, 604
  radionuclide scan, 606
  stem, signs, 593, 598, 629
  tumours of, 619
  ultrasonography, 607
Breast, carcinoma of, 105, 118
Breath sounds, 211
  test, glychocolic, 314
    hydrogen, 311
Breathing, control of, 205
  periodic, 122
Bromocriptine, 423, 650
Bromsulphthalein excretion, 342
Bronchi, 202
Bronchiectasis, 256
Bronchitis, acute, 222
  chronic, 252
Bronchodilator drugs, 245
Bronchography, 211
Bronchopneumonia, 225
Bronchoscopy, 212
Bronchus, obstruction of, 257
  tumours of, 260
Bronzed diabetes, 366
Brown-Séquard syndrome, 657
Brucellosis, 748
Brugia filariasis, 796
Bruits, arterial, 125
Buccal smear, 6
Budd-Chiari syndrome, 367
Buerger's disease, 198
Buffer system of blood, 99
Bulbar palsy, progressive, 652
Bulima, 688
Bullae, pulmonary, 255
Bumetanide, 96
Bundle branch block, 144
Bunyavirus, 726
Burkitt's lymphoma, 535
Burning feet syndrome, 657
Bursa of Fabricius, 20
Busitis, 554
  subacromial, 585
Buruli ulcer, 762
Bush tea and liver disease, 367
Busulphan, 517, 525
  lung, 525
Butyrophenones, 683

Bypass, cardiopulmonary, 194
Byssinosis, 268

Cachexia in malignant disease, 108
Caeruloplasmin, 344
Calabar swelling, 795
Calciferol, 66
  in tetany, 443
Calcitonin, 439
Calcium, channel blockers, 170,
    in hypertension, 182
  dietary sources of, 61
Calculi, biliary, 370
  renal, 403
  salivary, 287
  vesical, 403
Calorie, 54
Campylobacter enteritis, 753
Cancer, aetiology and epidemiology, 104
  embryonic antigen (CEA), 107
  immunology, 33
  performance status in, 110
  staging of, 110
  see also carcinoma and tumours
Cancerophobia, 685
Cancrum oris, 768
Candidiasis, 286, 802
Canicola infection, 763
Cannabis addiction, 696
Cannon waves, 125
Capillariasis, 794
Caplan's syndrome, 267
Capreomycin, 238
Captopril, 155, 183
Caput medusae, 360
Carbamazepine, 612, 618
Carbenicillin, 44
Carbenoxolone, 296
Carbidopa, 650
Carbimazole, 432
Carbimide, calcium, 695
Carbohydrate, 53
  absorption, 310
  metabolism, in diabetes mellitus, 460
  in liver, 336
Carbon dioxide, 98, 204
Carbon monoxide poisoning, 701
Carbonic acid, buffer system, 99
Carboxylic acids, 559
Carbuncle, 480
Carcinoid tumour, 321
Carcinoma, 106
  in tropics, 722
  neurological complications of, 668
  see also individual organs
Cardiac, arrest, 138
  catheterisation, 132
  failure, 151
  output, 132
  rhythm, 133
  see also Heart
Cardiomyopathy, 186
Cardiospasm, 290

Cardiovascular disease in the tropics, 716
Cardioversion, 145
Carditis, in rheumatic fever, 157
Carey-Coombs murmur, 157
Caries, dental, 63
Carotene, 65
Carotid, artery stenosis, 630
  kinked, 125
Carpal tunnel syndrome, 661
Carrión's disease, 757
Casoni test, 790
Cassava, toxic effects of, 656
Casts, in urine, 382
Cataplexy, 619
Cataract, 480
Cavernous sinus thrombosis, 636
Cefaclor, 45
Cefotaxime, 45
Cefoxitin, 45
Cefsulodin, 45
Ceftazidime, 45
Ceftizoxime, 45
Cefuroxime, 45
Centigray, 112
Centromere, of chromosome, 3
Cephalexin, 45
Cephalosporins, 45
Cephamandole, 45
Cephamycin antibiotic, 45
Cephazolin, 45
Cephradine, 45
Cerebellum, signs, 594
Cerebrospinal fluid, 605
  reference values, 819
Cerebrovascular disease, causes, 627
  diagnosis, 632
  investigation, 633
  treatment, 634
Cerebrum, signs, 603
Cestodes, 788
Chagas' disease, 780
  and megacolon, 329
  of oesophagus, 290
Chancre, 409
  trypanosomal, 779
Chancroid, 413
Charcot-Marie-Tooth syndrome, 653
Charcot's joints, 640, 663
Cheilosis, 79
Chemoreceptors, respiratory, 206
Chemotherapy, of infections, 41
  of tumours, 113, 116
Chenodeoxycholic (chenic) acid, 371
Chest, examination of, 210
  physical signs in, 211
  radiological examination of, 211
  wall, deformitis of, 276
Cheyne-Stokes respiration, 122
Chickenpox, 730
Chicleros ulcer, 778
Chikungunya fever, 733
Childhood, diabetes in, 481
  psychiatric illness in, 698

Chlamydia infection, 737
  genital, 412
  of lung, 225
Chlorambucil, 528, 532, 534
Chloramphenicol, 46
Chlordiazepoxide, 687
Chlormethiazole, 695
Chloroquine, 771
  in rheumatoid arthritis, 559
Chlorpromazine, 679, 683
Chlorpropamide, 468
Chlortetracycline, 45
Chlorthalidone, 96
Cholangiocarcinoma, 374
Cholangiography, 370
Cholangitis, ascending, 363
  sclerosing, 373
Cholecalciferol, 66
Cholecystitis, acute, 372
  non-calculus, 373
Cholecystography, 369
Cholecystokinin, 280
Cholelithiasis, 370
Cholera, 755
Cholescintigraphy, 370
Cholestasis, 346
  and viral hepatitis, 350
Cholesterol, 485
  and atherosclerosis, 178
Cholesterosis of gall bladder, 373
Cholestyramine, 486
  for pruritus, 365
Cholinergic crisis, 666
Chondrocalcinosis, 581
Chondroma, 588
Chorea, 651
  and rheumatic fever, 157
Choriomeningitis, acute lymphocytic, 641
Christmas disease, 545
Chromium, deficiency of, 64
Chromoblastomycosis, 803
Chromosome(s), 2
  deletions, 8
  disorders, 6
  nomenclature, 6
  Philadelphia, 8
  ring, 8
Chrysotherapy, 560
Chvostek's sign, 442
Chyluria, 796
Cigarette smoking, and bronchial
    carcinoma, 260
  and chronic bronchitis, 252
  and ischaemic heart disease, 178
  and optic neuritis, 609
  and peptic ulceration, 292
  and thrombo-angiitis obliterans, 198
Ciguatera poisoning, 707
Cimetidine, 296
Cinnarizine, 614
Circulation, failure of, 147
Cirrhosis, biliary, 362
  Laënnec's, 358
  macronodular, 358
  micronodular, 358

Cirrhosis (contd)
  of liver, 360
Cis-diammine-dichloroplatinum,
    (cisplastin), 118
Claudication, intermittent, 196
Claustrophobia, 691
Clavulanic acid, 44
Clearance, renal, 382
Cleft lip and palate, heritability, 14
Click, systolic, 127
Climate, disorders due to, 722
Clindamycin, 46
Clinistix and Clinitest, 463
Clofazimine, 761
Clofibrate, 486
Clomiphene, 421
Clonazepam, 612
Clonorchiasis, 787
Clonus, 593
Clostridium difficile infection, 46
  welchii food poisoning, 753
Clotrimazole, 48
Cloxacillin, 44
Club foot heritability, 15
Clubbing of the fingers, 210
Cluster headache, 625
Clutton's joints, 571
Coagulation, disseminated
    intravascular, 548
  factors, and liver, 342
  inhibitors, 541
  of blood, 539
Coal-workers' pneumoconiosis, 267
Coarctation of aorta, 190
Cobalamin, 500
Cobalt in radiotherapy, 112
Cocaine addiction, 696
Coccidioidomycosis, 804
Codeine phosphate, 219
Coelenterata, venomous, 708
Coeliac disease, 313
Colchicine, 580
Cold injury, 724
Colectomy, 325, 329
Colic, biliary, 372
  renal, 404
Colitis, antibiotic associated, 46
  ischaemic, 331
  pseudomembranous, 46
  ulcerative, 321
Collapse of lung, 257
Colon, carcinoma of, 327
  polyposis of, 329
  toxic dilitation of, 322
Colonoscopy, 284
Colostomy, 329
Coma, diabetic, 475
  hepatic, 353, 361
  hyperosmolar diabetic, 475
  hypoglycaemic, 478
  in hypercapnoea, 209
  in hypopituitarism, 425
  in lactic acidosis, 477
  in malaria, 770
  in myxoedema, 436

Complement, 23
  deficiency, 35
  fixation tests, 26
  in glomerulonephritis, 386
Compliance, of lung, 205
  of patient, 822
Compromised host, 37
Compulsion, 689
Computed tomography, see individual
    organs
Condylomata, 410
Cone shell, stings, 708
Confabulation, 679
Connective tissue diseases, 551
  in the tropics, 721
Conn's syndrome, 446
Consciousness, grading of, 704
Constipation, 281
Contraception, oral, and hypertension,
    179
  and jaundice, 348
  and pyridoxine, 79
  and venous thrombosis, 200
  risks of, 456
Conversion neurosis, 687
Coombs' test, 25
Copper, deficiency of, 63
  metabolism, 366
Cord, spinal, compression of, 657
  infections of, 637
  transverse section of, 598
  tumour of, 657
Coronavirus, 726
Coronary heart disease, 166
Cor pulmonale, 184
Corrosive poisoning, 707
Cortex, cerebral, signs, 593, 598
Corticospinal tract, 592
Corticosteroids, in bronchial asthma,
    245
  in Crohn's disease, 316
  in glomerulonephritis, 391
  in rheumatoid arthritis, 561
  in tuberculosis, 238
  in ulcerative colitis, 324
  uses and dangers of, 452
Corticotrophin, 419, 443
  in rheumatoid arthritis, 561
  releasing factor, 419
Cortisol, 450, 451
Cortisone, 451
Coryza, 219
  and ascorbic acid, 73
Cosmos, man and the, 811
Co-trifamole, 42
Co-trimoxazole, 42
Cough, 207
  bovine, 250
  syncope, 123
  treatment of, 219
Coughing, postural, 219
Coultercounter, 497
Councilman bodies, 349
Counter current
    immunoelectrophoresis, 638

Coxsackie infection, 726
of heart, 186, 187
of meninges, 641
of muscles, 584
respiratory, 220, 270
CPPD, 581
Crab louse, 415
Craniopharyngioma, 421
C-reactive protein, 556
Creatine kinase, 175
Creatinine clearance, 383
Crepitations, 211
CR(E) ST syndrome, 576
Cretinism, 436
Creutzfeldt-Jakob disease, 641
Cri du chat syndrome, 9
Crigler-Najjar syndrome, 347
Crisis, adrenal, 448
aplastic, 506
cholinergic, 666
oculogyric, 649
thyrotoxic, 431
Crohn's disease, 314
Cromoglycate, 245
in ulcerative colitis, 325
Croup, 220
Cryoprecipitate, 544
Cryptococcosis, 805
Cryptorchidism, 455
Crystal deposition disease, 578
Cushing's disease and syndrome, 444
Cyanide poisoning, 707
Cyanosis, central and peripheral, 124
Cyclophosphamide, 532, 561
Cycloserine, 238
Cyclosporin, 33
Cyst, choledochal, 373
popliteal, 554
see also individual organs
Cysternography, 422
Cystic fibrosis, 308
Cysticercosis, 788
Cystinuria, 379
Cystitis, 398
Cystogram, micturating, 383
Cytarabine, 522
Cytomegalovirus, 729
Cytotoxic drugs, 113

D antigen, 514
Dactylitis, in sickle-cell anaemia, 509
Dapsone, 761
Dark adaptation, 65
Daunorubicin, 522
DDAVP, 427
Death, cap poisoning, 709
sudden, 177
Defence, mental mechanisms of, 672
Defibrillation, 145
De Grouchy's syndrome, 9
Dehydration, 91
Déjà vu, 617
Delirium, 679
tremens, 695
Delusion, 676

Dementia, 680
multi-infarct, 630
Demyelinating disease, 644
Dengue, 736
Dependency, drug, 694
Depression, agitated, 699
major illness, 681
psychoneurotic (reactive), 690
psychotic (endogenous), 681
de Quervain's thyroiditis, 438
Dermatitis, contact, 28
herpetiformis, 313
Dermatomyositis, 576
Dermatophytosis, 801
Desmopressin, 427
in haemophilia, 545
Developing countries, pattern of
disease in, 714
Deviation, sexual, 697
Dexamethasone, in raised intracranial
pressure, 622
Dextropropoxyphene poisoning, 707
Dextrostix, 472
Dhobi's itch, 801
Diflunisal, 559
Di George syndrome, 34
Diabetes insipidus, 426
nephrogenic, 426
Diabetes mellitus, 457
aetiology, 457
cataract in, 480
chemical pathology, 460
clinical features, 461
coma, 478
complications, 474
corticosteroids and, 458
diet in, 465, 813
genetic counselling, 484
gestational, 458
in children, 481
in pregnancy, 481
infections in, 480
insulin dependent, 458
latent, 462
nephropathy, 478
neuropathy in, 480
non-insulin dependent, 458
pathology, 461
potential, 461
prevention, 483
retinopathy, 478
screening, 484
secondary, 458
surgery in, 482
treatment, 465
urine testing, 463, 472
vascular disorders in 477
Dialysis, haemo- and peritoneal, 394
in poisoning, 706
Diamorphine in myocardial infarction,
175
Diaphragm, hernia of, 288
paralysis of, 262
Diarrhoea, 281
idiopathic, 332

Diarrhoea (contd)
postoperative, 301
travellers', 330
Diazepam, 687
in status epilepticus, 619
Dibromomanitol, 525
Dichloralphenazone, 680
Diclofenac, 559
Diet, elemental, 316
guidelines, 810
Diet, in, coronary disease, 178
diabetes mellitus, 465, 813
diverticular disease, 327
glomerulonephritis, 388
gluten enteropathy, 313
gout, 581
hepatic encephalopathy, 364
hepatitis, 355
hypercholesterolaemia, 485
hyperlipoproteinaemia, 485
hypertension, 181
ischaemic heart disease, 178
nephrotic syndrome, 391
obesity, 85, 812
pancreatitis, chronic, 308
peptic ulcer, 295
renal calculi, 405
renal failure, 401
tropical sprue, 720
Diethylcarbamazine, 796
Diethylpropion, 86
Diffusion of gases in lungs, 206
Diflunisal, 559
Digitalis, 142, 154
Digoxin, 141, 154
Dimercaprol, 560
Dinitro-ortho-cresyl poisoning, 707
Dipetalonema perstans, and
streptocerca, 799
Diphenoxylate, 330
Diphtheria, 743
Diphyllobothrium latum and mansoni,
790
Diploid, 3
Diplopia, 609
Dipstix, 381
Dipylidium caninum, 790
Dipyridamole, 176, 635
Disaster situations, 810
Disc, intervertebral, lesions of,
659
Discrimination, sensory, 598
Disease, prevention of, 808
Disopyramide, 140
Dissection of aorta, 197
Disseminated intravascular
coagulation, 548
Disseminated sclerosis, 645
Dissociative disorder, 688
Distribution, of gas in lungs, 206
Disulfiram, 695
Diuretics, 96
in cardiac failure, 154
in hypertension, 181
Diverticular disease, 326

DNA, 1
  antibodies, 572
  recombinant, 18
Dolbutamide, 150
Dominant inheritance, 10, 12
Donovan bodies, 413
Dopamine, 150
  agonists, 423, 650
Doppler ultrasound, 197
Down's syndrome, 7
Doxapram, 217
Doxorubicin, 528, 535, 538
Doxycycline, 45
Dracontiasis, 799
Dressler's syndrome, 172
Dropsy, epidemic 711
Drugs, and agranulocytosis, 519
  and autoimmunity, 29
  and bilirubin metabolism, 348
  and G6PD, 507
  and haemolysis, 515
  and hepatitis, 355
  and megaloblastic anaemia, 503
  and pancytopenia, 505
  and parkinsonism, 648
  and purpura, 542
  and renal disease, 406
  and thrombocytopenia, 543
  and tics, 652
  clinical trials of, 116
  dependence on, 675, 694
  idiosyncracy to, 349
  metabolism in liver, 338
  nomenclature of, 822
  prescription of, 822
  therapeutic blood concentrations, 820
DSM III, 679
Dubin-Johnson syndrome, 347
Duchenne muscular dystrophy, 666
Duckett Jones criteria, 157
Ductus arteriosus, persistent, 189
Dumping syndrome, 301
Duodenocopy, 283
Duodenum, diseases of, 292
Dupuytren's contracture, 361
Dusts, causing lung disease, 266
Dwarfism, differential diagnosis, 424
  nutritional, 60
Dyes, in urine, 382
Dysarthria, 601
Dysdiadochokinesis, 595
Dysentery, amoebic, 773
  bacillary, 755
Dyshormonogenesis, 438
Dyskinesia, biliary, 373
  tardive, 684
Dysmetria, 595
Dyspepsia, psychogenic, 331
Dysphagia, 287
  sideropenic, 288
Dysphasia, 601
Dysphonia, 601
Dysplasia, skeletal, 589

Dyspnoea, 208
  in heart failure, 122
  paroxysmal nocturnal, 122
Dyssebacea, 79
Dyssynergia, 595
Dystrophy, myotonic, 667
  progressive muscular, 666

Ebola virus disease, 782
Echinococcal disease, 789
Echocardiography, 131
Echoencephalography, 607
Echovirus, 726
Econazole, 48
Ectopic beats, atrial, 134
  ventricular, 136
Edrophonium, 665
Edwards' syndrome, 8
Effusion, pericardial, 187
  pleural, 270
    malignant, 271
    postpneumonic, 272
    tuberculous, 271
Eisenmenger's syndrome, 193
Ejaculation premature, 697
Ejection, fraction, 152
  sound, 127
Electrocardiography, 128
  ambulatory, 129
  see also individual diseases
Electroconvulsive therapy, 682
Electroencephalography, 606, 617
Electrolyte balance, 88
Electrolytes, in urine, 98
  regulation of, 376
Electromyography, 607
Electrophoresis of plasma proteins, 342
Elements, in nutrition, 61
Elephantiasis, 796
Elliptocytosis, 493
Embolectomy, pulmonary, 185
Embolism, arterial, 197
  cerebral, 630
  in infective endocarditis, 165
  peripheral, 197
  pulmonary, 184
  therapeutic, 327
Emetine, 775
Emotion and disease, 698
Emphysema, mediastinal, 254
  obstructive, 258
  pulmonary, 254
  subcutaneous, 254
Empiric risk, 16
Empyema, of gall bladder, 372
  thoracis, 272
Encephalitis, arboviral, 733
  Californian, 734
  Japanese B, 737
  lethargica, 642
  Russian and European, 733
  sclerosing, 643
  suppurative, 636
  viral, 642

Encephalomyelitis, acute
    demyelinating, 647
  epidemic myalgic, 642
  post-vaccinial, 647
Encephalopathy, hepatic, 353, 361, 364
  hypertensive, 179
  in acute nephritis, 386
  Wernicke's, 75
Endemic typhus fever, 739
Endocarditis, infective, 165
Endocrine, adenomatosis, 440
  disease in the tropics, 720
  therapy in cancer, 118
Endomyocardial fibrosis, 716
Endorphin, 420
Endoscopic cholangiopancreatography (ERCP), 283
Endoscopy, of alimentary tract, 282
Energy, requirements, 53
  yielding nutrients, 53
Engineering, genetic, 18
Enolic acids, 559
Enteric fever, 751
Enteritis, infective, 330
  regional, 314
  tuberculous, 236
Enterobiasis, 791
Enterocolitis, 330
Enterohepatic circulation of bile salts, 338
Enteropathy, tropical, 719
Enterovirus, 726
Enthesopathy, 564
Entrapment neuropathy, 661
Environment, perception of, 676
Enzyme(s), and liver function, 340
  induction, 339
  plasma in myocardial infarction, 173
Eosinophil, granulocyte, 492, 494
  leukaemia, 527
Eosinophilia, bronchopulmonary, 247
  endocardial, 187
  tropical pulmonary, 249, 799
Ependymoma, 620
Epidemic typhus fever, 738
Epidemiology, and tropical disease, 715
  of cancer, 104
  of infection, 37
Epididymitis, 232, 411
Epiglottitis, 220
Epilepsy, 615
  focal, 617
  Jacksonian, 617
  temporal lobe, 617
Epiloia, 11
Episcleritis, 554
Epoprostenol, 547
Epstein Barr virus, 519, 535
Erb's muscular dystrophy, 667
Ergocalciferol, 66
Ergotamine, 626
Erysipelas, 743

Erythema, chronicum migrans, 571
  marginatum, (annulare), 157
Erythema nodosum, in sarcoidosis, 269
  in tuberculosis, 232
  in ulcerative colitis, 324
  leprosum, 759
Erythroblastosis fetalis, 513
Erythrocyte, 488
  sedimentation rate, 821
Erythrocytosis, 516
Erythromycin, 45
Erythropoietin, 490
Ethambutol, 237
Ethanol, 339
  in venous blood, 817
  see also Alcohol
Ethionamide, 238
Ethosuximide, 619
Eumycetoma, 802
Eunuch, 455
Evoked potentials, 606
Ewing's tumour, 588
Exchange transfusion, 514
Exercise, and coronary disease, 178
  and obesity, 83
  syncope, 123
Exhibitionism, 697
Exophthalmos, 435
Exostosis, 588
Expressivity (genetic), 11
Extrapyramidal system, diseases of, 648
  signs, 594
Extrasystoles, atrial, 134
  ventricular, 136

F body, 6
Facial nerve, 612
Facio-scapulo-humeral dystrophy, 667
Factors, coagulation, 539
Factor VIII, 540, 544
Factor IX, 545
Failure, acute intestinal, 331
  adrenal, 448
  cardiac, 151
  circulatory, 147
  hepatic, 353
  renal, 399
  respiratory, 210
  ventilatory, 210
Fainting, 123
Fallot's tetralogy, 193
Familial periodic paralysis, 667
Family doctor, role of, 810
Famine oedema, 54
Fanconi syndrome, 379
Fansidar, 771
Farmer's lung, 249, 266
Fasciculation, 593
Fasciitis, eosinophilic, 576
Fascioliasis, 787
Fasciolopsiasis, 787
Fat(s), 53
  absorption, 310

Fat(s) (contd)
  brown, 83
  metabolism, in diabetes mellitus, 460
  satuated and polyunsaturated, 814
Favism, 507
Favus, 801
Felty's syndrome, 556
Feminisation 445
Fenbufen, 559
Fenclofenac, 559
Fenfluramine, 86
Fenoprofen, 559
Fenoterol, 246
Ferritin, 344, 498
Fertility, and antineoplastic drugs, 117
Fetishism, 697
Fetor hepaticus, 354
Fever, abortus, 748
  blackwater, 770
  cerebrospinal, 637
  enteric, 751
  factitious, 39
  haemorrhagic, 733
  Lassa, 732
  nursing (in Typhus), 740
  of unknown origin, 39
  Oroya, 757
  Q, 741
  rat-bite, 767
  relapsing, 765
  rheumatic, 156
  Rocky Mountain spotted, 739
  sandfly, 734
  scarlet, 742
  trench, 740
  typhoid, 751
  typhus, 738
  yellow, 734
FEV/FVC%, 213
Fibre, in diet, 80, 327
Fibrillation, atrial, 135
  ventricular, 137
  and diabetes, 469
Fibrin, 540
  degradation products, 385
Fibrinogen, 540
  ^{125}I, in venous thrombosis, 200
Fibrinolysis, 541
Fibrosarcoma, 588
Fibrosis, hepatic, congenital, 367
  pulmonary, 264
Filariasis, 794
Fish, poisonous and venomous, 707
Fistula, biliary, 371
  bronchopleural, 274
  gastro-jejuno-colic, 301
  tracheo-oesophageal, 252
Fit, epileptic, 616
  hysterical, 688
Flatulence, 281
Flea, disease conveyed by, 805
Flucloxacillin, 44
Flucytosine, 48
Fludrocortisone, 451

Flufenamic acid, 559
Flukes, 787
Fluoride, 63
Fluorocytosine, 803
Fluphenazine decanoate, 684
Flurbiprofen, 559
Flutter, atrial, 135
Fly, disease conveyed by, 805
Fogarty catheter, 197
Folate(s), 500
  absorption of, 500
  deficiency of, 503
Folic acid, 504
Follicle stimulating hormone, 419
Food allergy, 25
  poisoning, 753
Forced expiratory time, 213
Forced expiratory volume, 213
Forced vital capacity, 213
Foreign body, in bronchus, 260
  in larynx, 251
Formication, 696
Foster Kennedy syndrome, 622
Friction, pericardial, 187
  pleural, 211
Friedreich's ataxia, 654
Froin's syndrome, 658
Frostbite, 725
Fructosuria, 485
Frusemide, 96
FTA-ABS test, 410
Fugues, hysterical, 688
Fundus, ocular, 608
Fungi, diseases due to, 240, 801
Funnel chest, 276
Furamide, 775
Fusidic acid, 46

GABA, 619
Galactosaemia, 485
Gall bladder, anatomy and physiology, 369
  carcinoma, 374
  tumours of, 374
Gallstone, 370
Gammaglobulin, in hepatitis, 351, 353
Gamma-glutamyl transferase, 341
Gangosa, 764
Gangrene, in atherosclerosis, 196
  in diabetes mellitus, 478
Gargoylism, 17
Gas, exchange in lungs, 206
  gangrene, penicillin in, 43
  in blood, 205
  transfer factor, 207
Gastrectomy, 296
  and anaemia, 503
Gastric outlet obstruction, 299
Gastrin, 280
Gastritis, 302
  biliary, 301
  acute haemorrhagic, 297
Gastroenteritis acute, 330, 718
Gastroenterostomy, 297

Gastrointestinal tract, *see* alimentary tract
Gastroscopy, 283
General paralysis of the insane, 639
Genes, structural and control, 2
Genetic advice, 17
  engineering, 18
  in diabetes mellitus, 484
Genitalia, miscellaneous lesions of, 415
Gentamicin, 47
Geography of disease, 717
Geriatric patients, digoxin in, 142
  heart block in, 143
  hyperparathyroidism in, 441
  hypertension in, 181
  hypothermia in 805
  infective endocarditis in, 165
  intestinal obstruction in, 317
  medial sclerosis in, 196
  osteomalacia in, 69
  osteoporosis in, 70
  psychiatric disorders in, 699
  scurvy in, 73
German measles, 728
GH, 419
GHRF, 419
GHRIH, 419
Giant cell tumour of bone, 588
Gigantism, 423
Giardiasis, 775
Gilbert's syndrome, 347
Gingivitis, 286
Glanders, 750
Glandular fever, 519
Glibenclamide, 468
Glioma, 620, 623
Glipizide, 468
Globulin, antihaemophilic, 540, 544
  immune serum, in hepatitis, 351, 353
  plasma, 341
Globus hystericus, 331
Glomerulonephritis, 384
  chronic, 391
  crescentic, 385
  focal (segmental), 384
  immune complexes and, 26
  membranous, 389
  mesangiocapillary, 386
  minimal lesion, 389
  proliferative, 384
Glomerulosclerosis, diabetic, 478
Glossitis, 287
Glossopharyngeal nerve, 615
Glottis, oedema of, 251
Glucagon, 304, 473
Glucocorticoids, 443
Gluconeogenesis, 460
Glucose 6PD deficiency, 507
Glucose tolerance test, 463
Glue sniffing, 696
Gluten-free diet, 313
Gluten-induced enteropathy, 313
Glyceryl trinitrate, 169
Glycogenolysis, 460

Glycogen storage disease, 485
Glycosuria, alimentary, 464
  in diabetes mellitus, 463
  'lag-storage', 464
  renal, 463
Glycosylated haemoglobin, 473
Glymidine, 468
Glypressin, 364
Gnathostomiasis, 801
Goitre, 437
  endemic, 62
  investigation of, 429
  simple, 439
Gold therapy, 560
Golfer's elbow, 585
Gonadotrophin, chorionic, 419
  in testicular tumours, 107
Gonorrhoea, 411
Goodpasture's syndrome, 385
Gout, 578
Graft rejection, 28
  versus-host (GVH) disease, 526
Graham Steel murmur, 165
Grand mal, 616
Granulocytes, 491
Granuloma inguinale, 413
Graves' disease, 430
Gray unit, 111
Grey baby syndrome, 46
Griseofulvin, 48
Growth hormone, 419
  and diabetes, 458
Guillain-Barré syndrome, 663
Guinea worm, 799
Gumma, 410
Gums, scurvy in, 72
Gynaecomastia, in liver disease 361

Haemarthrosis, in haemophilia, 545
Haematemesis, 297
  in portal hypertension, 360
Haematological values, 821
Haematoma, extradural and subdural, 632
Haematopoiesis, extramedullary, 494
Haematuria, 381
Haemochromatosis, 365
Haemodialysis, 394
  in acute tubular necrosis, 401
Haemoglobin, 490
  C disease, 511
  glycosylated, 473
  SC disease, 511
Haemoglobinopathy, 508
Haemoglobinuria, 382
  paroxysmal nocturnal, 515
Haemolysis, causes of, 514
Haemolytic anaemia, 505
  autoimmune, 512
  isoimmune, 513
Haemolytic uraemic syndrome, 399
Haemoperfusion, 706
Haemophilia, 543
Haemophilus influenzae, 219, 637
Haemopneumothorax, 204

Haemoptysis, 208
  endemic, 786
  treatment of, 219
Haemorrhage, from lower bowel, 327
  gastroduodenal, 297
  in liver disease, 361
Haemorrhage,
  intracerebral, 631
  subarachnoid, 631
Haemorrhagic disease, 539
  classification, 541
  investigation, 541
  of newborn, 546
Haemorrhagic fever, Argentine, 733
  Bolivian, 733
  with renal syndrome, 733
Haemosiderin, 496
Haemosiderinuria, 506
Haemosiderosis, pulmonary, 265
  secondary, 366
Haemothorax, 204
Hair, in malnutrition, 56
Halitosis, 287
Hallucinations, 604, 619, 676, 679
Haloperidal, 695
Halzoun, 806
Haploid, 3
Haplotype, 31
Haptoglobin, 506
Hartnup disease, 77
Hashimoto's thyroiditis, 437
Hashish addiction, 696
Haverhill fever, 767
Hay fever, 241
Headache, causes of, 624
Heaf test, 233
Health, promotion of, 808
  regulations, 806
Heart, auscultation of, 126
  block, 142
  disease, congenital, 189
    in pregnancy, 195
    in tropics, 716
    ischaemic, 166
    rheumatic, 156
    valvular, 158
  examination of, 126
  failure, 151
    high output, 153
    in beriberi, 75
  murmurs, 127
  palpation of, 126
  percussion of, 126
  radiological examination of, 130
  radionuclide scan, 132
  rhythm, 133
  sounds, 126
  thrills, 126
Heartburn, 281
Heat, acclimatisation to, 722
  exhaustion, 723
  hyperpyrexia, 724
  prickly, 723
  stroke, 723
  syncope, 722

Heberden's nodes, 583
Heimlich, manoeuvre, 251
  valve, 275
Helminths, diseases due to, 782
  liver diseases due to, 367
Hemianopia, 603
Hemiblock, 144
Hemiplegia, 629
  due to migraine, 626
Hemisphere, dominant, 598
Henoch-Schönlein purpura, 569
Heparin, 547
Hepatitis, aggressive, 358
  carriers, 352
  causes of, 348
  chronic, 358
  chronic active, 358
  chronic persistent, 358
  due to infections, 349
  non A, non B, 353
  persistent, 357
  toxic, 349
  treatment of, 355
  type A, 349
  type B, 351
  vaccination, 353
Hepatocyte, 334
Hepato-jugular reflux, 125
Hepato-lenticular degeneration, 366
Hepatoma, 368
Hepatomegaly, causes of, 362
Hepatorenal syndrome, 361
Hering-Breuer reflexes, 206
Heritability, 15
Hermaphroditism, 454
Hernia, oesophageal, 288
Heroin dependence, 696
Herpangina, 220
Herpes, labialis, 729
  simplex, 729
    anogenital, 414
    encephalitis, 642
  zoster, 644
Herpesvirus, 726
Herring worm disease, 801
Herxheimer reaction, 780
Heterocyclic acetic acids, 559
Heterozygote, 10
HGPRT deficiency, 579
Hiatus hernia, 288
Hip, congenital dislocation,
    heritability, 15
Hirschprung's disease, 329
Hirsutism, 444
Histamine, 24
  H_2 receptor antagonist drugs, 295
Histiocytosis X, 265
Histoplasmosis, 803
Histrionic pesonality disorder, 693
HLA, 30
  restriction, 31
Hodgkin's lymphoma, 530
Holter monitoring, 130
Homosexuality, 697
  and liver disease, 351
  infection in, 415

Homozygote, 10
Honeycomb lung, 265
Hookworm infection, 793
Hormone(s), concentrations in plasma,
    819
  ectopic, as tumour markers, 107
  gastrointestinal, 279
  metabolism in liver, 338
Horner's syndrome, 615
Humidifier (oxygen), 216
'Hungry bones' syndrome, 441
Hunter's syndrome, 17
Huntington's chorea, 651
Hurler's syndrome, 17
Hyaluronidase, in myocardial
    infarction, 176
Hydatid disease, 789
Hydralazine, 183
Hydrocephalus, 623
Hydrochloric acid, gastric, 293
Hydrocortisone, 451
Hydrogen ion concentration, 98
  disturbances in, 100
Hydroid stings, 708
Hydronephrosis, 403
Hydrophobia, 731
Hydropneumothorax, 204
Hydrops fetalis, 513
Hydroxocobalamin, 502
Hydroxycholecalciferol, 66
5-Hydroxytryptamine, 321
Hydroxyurea, 525
Hymenolepis nana, 790
Hyperacusis, 613
Hyperaldosteronism, 446
Hyperbilirubinaemia, 339
  congenital non-haemolytic, 347
Hypercalcaemia, 441
  due to vitamin D, 69
Hypercalciuria, causes, 404
Hypercapnia, 209
Hypercholesterolaemia, 485
Hypergammaglobulinaemia, 341
  benign monoclonal, 537
Hyperglycaemia, 460
Hyperkalaemia, 94
Hyperlipidaemia, 485
Hyperlipoproteinaemia, 485
Hypermobility syndrome, 584
Hypernephroma, 407
Hyperosmolar diabetic coma, 475
Hyperostosis, 565
Hyperparathyroidism, 440
Hyperprolactinaemia, 423
Hyperpyrexia, 724
Hypersensitivity, 19
  delayed, 28
  immediate, 24
Hypersplenism, 538
Hypertension, accelerated, 180
  benign intracranial, 625
  emergency treatment, 183
  essential, 179
  malignant, 180
  portal, 360

Hypertension (contd)
  non-cirrhotic, 367
  pulmonary, 183
  refractory, 183
  secondary, 178
  systemic, 178
Hyperthyroidism, 430
  in children, 434
  in pregnancy, 434
  neonatal, 28
Hyperuricaemia, 578
Hyperventilation and tetany, 442
Hypervitaminosis D, 69
Hypnotics, 680
Hypocalcaemia, causes of, 442
Hypochondriasis, 685
Hypochromia, 493
Hypogammaglobulinaemia, 34
Hypoglossal nerve, 615
Hypoglycaemia, 473
  following gastrectomy, 301
Hypoglycaemic drugs, 468
  and coronary disease, 469
Hypogonadism, male, 454
Hypokalaemia, 92
  in cardiac failure, 156
Hyponatraemia, 89, 97
  in cardiac failure, 156
Hypoparathyroidism, 441
Hypophosphataemia, familial, 379
Hypopituitarism, 424
Hypoprothrombinaemia, 546
Hyposensitisation, 32, 245
Hypotension, postural, 123
Hypothalamic-pituitary-adrenal
    function, tests of, 449
Hypothalamus, physiology of, 418
  tumour of, 422
Hypothermia, accidental, 725
  in hypopituitarism, 425
  in hypothyroidism, 436
  in poisoning, 706
Hypothyroidism, 435
Hypotonia, 595
Hypoxaemia, 209
Hysteria, 687

Ibuprofen, 559
Icterus gravis neonatorum, 513
Idiotype, 22
Idoxuridine, 48
Ig A nephropathy, 384
Ileitis, regional, 314
Ileostomy, 325
Ileus, 317
Illusion, 676
Imaging, diagnostic, see,
    nuclear magnetic resonance,
    radiological examination,
    radionuclide scan,
    tomography, computed,
      emission computed,
    ultrasonography.
    under individual organs
Imidazole, 48
Imipramine, 682

Immune complex, 26
  reactions, 24
  response, 19
Immunisation, 40, 807
  see also individual diseases
Immunity, and tropical disease, 716
  and tuberculosis, 230
  cellular, 19
  humoral, 19
Immunocompromised host, 38
Immunodeficiency disorders, 33
  acquired (AIDS), 35
  common, unclassifiable, 34
Immunoelectrophoresis, counter
    current, 638
Immunofluorescence, for antibody
    detection, 26
Immunoglobulin, 21
  thyroid stimulating, 28
Immunological memory, 21
Immunology, and liver disease, 357
Immunomodulation, in rheumatoid
    arthritis, 561
Immunosuppression, 32
  in glomerulonephritis, 391
Immunotherapy, in cancer, 120
Impotence, 455
Inattention, sensory, 604
Incompetence, valvular, *see*
    Regurgitation
Incontinence of faeces, 330
  of urine, 600
Incubation period, 39
Indole acetic acids, 559
Indomethacin, 559
Infantilism, pituitary, 423
Infants, beriberi in, 75
  scurvy in, 73
Infarction, cerebral, 627
  crisis, 509
  myocardial, 171
  pulmonary, 184
Infection, communicable (contagious),
    37
  diagnosis, 39
  diseases due to, 40
  in compromised host, 37
  in the tropics, 715
  nosocomial, 37
  opportunist, 38
    of lung, 225
  prevention, 40
  respiratory, treatment of, 214
  sources and spread of, 38
Infectious mononucleosis, 519
Infertility, male, 456
Infestation, genital, 415
Inflammatory bowel disease, 314
Influenza, 221
Inhalers, in asthma, 245
Inheritance, multifactorial, 13
  unifactorial, 9
Inotropic agents, 150
Insect repellant, 741
  stings, 707

Insulin, antagonists, 458
  binding antibodies, 469
  depot, 470
  induced hypoglycaemia, 450
  isophane, 470
  lente and ultralente, 470
  preparations of, 469
  protamine zinc, 470
  reactions to, 473
  semilente, 470
  soluble, 470
  synthesis of, 18
  test, of gastric secretion, 284
  types of, 469
  zinc suspensions, 470
Intelligence, assessment, 676
Interferon, 48
International System of Units, 818
International Health Regulations, 806
Interphase, 3
Intersex, 454
Interview, psychiatric, 677
Intestine, large, diseases of, 321
    tumours of, 327, 329
  small, diseases of, 310
    tumours of, 321
Introversion, 692
Intussusception, 317
Iodine, 62
  deficient intake, 439
  dietary sources, 62
  radioactive, 433
  uptake, 429
I.Q., 675
Iridovirus, 726
Iritis, in Reiter's disease, 566
  in sarcoidosis, 269
  in tuberculosis, 232
Iron, binding capacity, 344, 498
  deficiency, 495
  dietary sources of, 62
  metabolism of, 495
  poisoning, 707
  serum, 344
  therapy, 498
Iron-dextran, 499
Iron-sorbitol, 498
Irritable bowel syndrome, 332
Ischaemia of, bowel 330
  brain, 627
  kidneys, 379
  legs, 196
  myocardium, 166
Islet-cell tumours of pancreas, 310
Isochromosome, 8
Isoimmune haemolytic disease, 513
Isoniazid, 237
Isophane insulin, 470
Isoprenaline, 32, 144
Isosorbide dinitrate, 150, 170, 172, 185
Ito cell, 334

Jacksonian epilepsy, 617
Jacob and Jandl test, 508
Jamaica, vomiting sickness of, 711

Japanese B encephalitis, 737
Jarisch-Herxheimer reaction, 780
Jaundice, 345
  cholestatic, 346
  differential diagnosis, 354
  haemolytic, 345
  hepatocellular, 346
  obstructive, 346
  ultrasonography in, 370
Jaws, wiring of, 86
Jejunum, biopsy of, 284
  ulcer of, 301
Jellyfish stings, 708
Jigger flea, 806
Joints, diseases of, 551
  intra-articular corticosteroids, 558
Joule, 54
Jugular venous pulse, 125
Juvenile chronic arthritis, 568
Juxtaglomerular apparatus, 376

Kala azar, 776
Kanamycin, 47
Kaposi's sarcoma, 722
Kartagener's syndrome, 256
Karyotype, 5
Katayama syndrome, 783
Kayser-Fleischer ring, 366
Keratoconjunctivitis, 554
Keratoderma blennorrhagica, 566
Keratomalacia, 66
Keratosis, follicular, 66
  solar, 723
Kernicterus, 651
Kernig's sign, 638
Ketoacidosis, 474
Ketoconazole, 48
Ketone bodies, detection in urine, 463
Ketoprofen, 559
Ketosis, 102
Ketostix, 463
Ketotifen, 245
Kidney(s), anatomy and physiology,
    376
  arteriography, 383
  biopsy, 384
  computed tomography, 384
  congenital abnormalities, 405
  disease in tropics, 720
  drug induced disease, 406
  enlargement, 406
  failure, 399
  infection, 395
  medullary sponge, 406
  polycystic, 405
  radiological examination, 383
  radionuclide scan, 384
  transplantation, 394
  tumours, 407
  ultrasonography, 383
K (killer) cells, 21
Kilocalorie (kcal), 812
Kilojoule (kJ), 812
Kimmelstiel-Wilson bodies, 478
Kinins, plasma, 24

Klebsiella pneumonia, 224
Klinefelter's syndrome, 9
Koilonychia, 497
Koplik's spots, 727
Korotkov sounds, 128
Korsakoff's psychosis, 75
Kupffer cell, 334
Kuru, 641
Kussmaul's respiration, 392
Kveim test, 269
Kwashiorkor, 56
Kyasanur Forest disease, 733
Kyphoscoliosis, 276

Labetalol, 182
Labyrinthitis, 614
Lactate dehydrogenase, 175
Lactic acidosis, 100
  in diabetes, 469, 477
Lactose intolerance, 314
  tolerance test, 311
Lactulose, 364
Laënnec's cirrhosis, 358
Landouzy-Déjerine dystrophy, 667
Laparoscopy, 345
Laplace's law, 152
Larva migrans, 800
Laryngitis, acute, 220
  chronic, 250
Laryngoscopy, 212
Laryngotracheobronchitis, 220
Larynx, obstruction of, 251
  paralysis of, 250
Lasègue's sign, 661
Lassa fever, 732
Latamoxef, 45
Latex test, 556
Lathyrism, 656
Laxatives, and potassium depletion,
  92
LE cells, 574
Lead poisoning, 493
  gums in, 286
Legionnaires' disease, 224
Leishmaniasis, 776
  cutaneous, 777
  visceral, 815
Leishman-Donovan bodies, 776
Lepromin test, 758
Leprosy, 758
  reactions in, 758
Leptospirosis, 762
Lesch-Nyhan syndrome, 579
Leucapheresis, 523
Leucocytes, 491
Leucocytosis, 493
Leucoencephalopathy, progressive,
  643
Leucoerythroblastosis, 494
Leucopenia, 493
Leukaemia, 520
  acute, 521
  aleukaemic, 521
  chronic lymphatic, 527
  chronic monocytic, 527

Leukaemia (contd)
  chronic myeloid, 524
  hairy cell, 528
  plasma cell, 537
  prolymphocytic, 528
  subleukaemic, 520
Leukoplakia, of the tongue, 287
  vulvae, 457
Leukotrienes, 24
Levamisole, 562, 792
LeVeen shunt, 363
Levodopa, 650
LH, 419
LHRH, 419
Liability (genetic), 13
Libido, and oral contraception, 456
Libman-Sach's endocarditis, 573
Lice, diseases due to, 805
Lightning pains, 640
Lignocaine, 140
Linear accelator, 112
Linkage disequilibrium, 31
Lipid metabolism, in liver, 336
Lipolysis, 460
Lipoprotein, 336, 485
  in ischaemic heart disease, 178
Lipotrophin, 419
Lithium carbonate, 682
Liver, adenoma 369
  aetiology of chronic disease, 357
  anatomy, 334
  biopsy, 345
  carcinoma, 368
  cirrhosis, 360
  congestion and cirrhosis, 357
  cysts, 368
  diseases due to flukes, 787
  disease, in tropics, 720
  failure, treatment, 356
  function tests, 339
  imaging, 345
  infections, 349
  massive necrosis, 349
  metastatic carcinoma of, 368
  parenchymal disease, 348
  physiology, 335
  radiological examination, 345
  transplantation, 375
  ultrasonography, 345
  venography, 345
  viral disease 349
Lockjaw, 745
Loiasis, 797
Loop diuretic, 96
Looser's zones, 70
Loperamide, 330
Louping ill, 733
Louse-borne relapsing fever, 765
  typhus fever, 738
LPH, 419
Lumbago-sciatica syndrome, 660
Lundh test, 305
Lung, abscess, 226
  anatomy, 202
  collapse, 257

Lung (contd)
  diffusing capacity, 207
  disease in tropics, 718
  fibrosis, 264
  interstitial disease, 264
  lymphatic carcinomatosis, 263
  occupational diseases, 265
  radionuclide scan, 132
  tests of function, 213
  tuberculosis, 230
  tumours, 260
Lupus erythematosus, systemic, 572
  pernio, 269
Luteinising hormone, 419
Lyme arthritis, 571
Lymphadenopathy, causes of, 531
  in rheumatoid arthritis, 553
Lymphangiectasia, primary, 312
Lymphoblasts, 20, 521
Lymphocyte, 492
  and immune response, 20
  B and T cells, 20
Lymphocytapheresis, in rheumatoid
  arthritis, 562
Lymphogranuloma venereum, 413
Lymphokines, 20
Lymphoma, Burkitt's, 535
  Hodgkins, 530
  non-Hodgkin, 533
Lysergic acid, addiction, 696
Lysine vasopressin, 364

Macrocytosis, 493
Macroglobulinaemia, Waldenström's,
  538
Macrophage, and immunity, 20
Madura foot, 802
Magnesium deficiency, 94
  excess, 95
Malabsorption syndrome, causes of,
  311
  tests for, 310
Malaria, 768
  and haemolysis, 515
  cerebral, 770
  protection against, 772
  treatment, 771
Malignant disease, in tropics, 722
Mallory-Weiss syndrome, 297
Malnutrition, 52
  and cirrhosis of liver, 357
Maloprim, 772
Malta fever, 748
Maltworker's lung, 249, 266
Manic-depressive psychosis, 681
Mansonella ozzardi, 799
Mantoux test, 232
Maple bark disease, 249
Marasmus, nutritional, 59
Marburg disease, 732
Marfan's syndrome, 198
Margarine, and vitamin D, 67
Marihuana addiction, 696
Marine animals, poisoning due to, 707
Massage, cardiac, 138

Mast cells, and IgE, 24
M.C. mask, 216
Measles, 727
Mebanazine, 681
Mebendazole, 792
Median nerve paralysis, 661
Mediastinoscopy, 213
Mediastinum, tumours of, 263
Meditation, in hypertension, 181
Medullary cystic disease, 406
  sponge kidney, 406
Medulloblastoma, 620
Mefenamic acid, 559
Meiosis, 5
Megacolon, 329
Megakaryocyte, 492
Melaena, 297
Melanocyte stimulating hormones, 419
Melanoma, malignant, 105
Melarsoprol, 780
Melioidosis, 750
Melphalan, 517, 525, 537
Ménière's syndrome, 614
Meninges, carcinoma of, 637
  infections of, 637
  irritation of, 624, 637
Meningioma, 620, 623
Meningism, 637
Meningitis, 637
  amoebic, 773
  bacterial, 637
  lymphocytic, 641
  meningococcal, 637
  syphilitic, 639
  tuberculous, 638
  viral, 641
Meningococcal infections, 747
Menopause, disorders of, 457
Mental handicap, 675
  health, 670
  state, examination of, 676
Meralgia paraesthetica, 662
Mercaptopurine, 522, 525
Mesenteric lymphadenitis, 321
Mesothelioma, pleural, 268
Metabolism, disorders of, 484
Metaphase, 4
Metaplasia, myeloid, 517
Metenkephalin, 420
Metformin, 469
Methadone, 219, 696
Methaemoglobinaemia, 772
Methimazole, 432
Methotrexate, 113, 522
Methyl cellulose, 86
Methyldopa, 182
Methyltestosterone, 348
  for pruritus, 365
Methylxanthine, 246
Methysergide, 626
Metoclopramide, 289
Metoprolol, 141, 182
Metrifonate, 786
Metronidazole, 47
Mexiletine, 140

Mezlocillin, 44
Micelle, 310
Miconazole, 48
Microangiopathy, diabetic, 479
Microcytosis, 493
Micturition, control of, 600
  syncope, 123
Migraine, 625
Miliary tuberculosis, 233
Mineralocorticoids, 443
Minerals, 61
Minnesota tube, 364
Minocycline, 747
Minoxidil, 183
Mitosis, 3
Mitral valve disease, 158
  see also Stenosis and Regurgitation
Mixed connective tissue disease, 575
Molluscum contagiosum, 414
Mollux, venomous, 708
Mönckeberg's sclerosis, 196
Mongolism, 7
Moniliasis, 802
Monkeypox, 731
Monoamine oxidase inhibitors, 681, 682
Monocyte, 492
  leukaemia, 527
Monocyte-macrophage system, 339, 492
Monocytosis, 494
Mononeuritis multiplex, 662
Mononeuropathy, 661
Mononucleosis, infectious, 519
Monosomy, 7
Monospot test, 520
Mood, assessment of 676
Moon-face, 444
Morphine, dependence, 695
  in myocardial infarction, 175
  in pulmonary oedema, 150
Morphoea, 576
Mosaic, 7
Mossy foot, 803
Motility, of alimentary tract, 279, 284
Motor neurone disease, 652
Motor system, 591
Mountain sickness, 725
Mouth, diseases of, 285
  nutritional disorders of, 79
Movement, involuntary, 594
Mucocele, of gall bladder, 372
Mucous patches, 410
Multiceps multiceps, 790
Multiple myeloma, 536
Multiple sclerosis, 645
Mumps, 729
Murphy's sign, 372
Murray Valley fever, 733
Muscle, diseases of, 665
Mushroom poisoning, 708
  worker's lung, 249, 266
Myalgia, epidemic, 584
  and encephalitis, 642

Myasthenia, carcinomatous, 668
  gravis, 665
Mycetoma, 240, 802
Mycobacteria, 230
Mycobacterial ulcer, 762
Mycoplasma infections, respiratory, 225
Mycoses, 801
  pulmonary, 240
  treatment of 48
Mycosis fungoides, 533
Myelinolysis, pontine, 656
Myelodysplastic syndrome, 518
Myelofibrosis, 517
Myelography, 607
Myelomatosis, 536
Myeloproliferative disorders, 517
Myiasis, 806
Myocarditis, 186
Myocardium, diseases of, 185
  infarction of, 171
    and diabetes, 469
  rupture of, 172
  scanning of, 132
Myopathy, 666
Myositis, carcinomatous, 668
  tropical, 721
Myotonia, atrophica, 667
  congenita, 667
Mythramycin, 538
Myxoedema, 435
  coma, 436
  madness, 436
  pretibial, 431

Nalidixic acid, 397
Naloxone, 709
Nandrolone deconate, 504
Naproxen, 559
Narcolepsy, 619
Nasal cannulae, for oxygen, 216
Nebuliser, in asthma, 247
Neck rigidity, 638
Necrosis, acute tubular, 400
  hepatic, massive, 349
  of renal cortex, 400
  of papillae, 396, 407
Nelson's syndrome, 423, 445
Nematodes, 790
Neomycin, 47
Neoplasia, 104
Neostigmine, 666
Nephritis, acute, 385
  chronic, 391
  focal, 388
  interstitial, 397
  pathology, 387
  salt-losing, 89
Nephroblastoma, 407
Nephrocalcinosis, 403
Nephropathy, analgesic, 406
  and antibiotics, 406
  diabetic, 478
Nephrotic syndrome, 390

Nerve, cranial, first, 608
  second, 608
  third, 609
  fourth, 609
  fifth, 611
  sixth, 609
  seventh, 612
  eighth, 614
  ninth to twelfth, 615
  peripheral, signs, 597
Netilmicin, 47
Neuralgia, brachial, 662
  cranial, 624
glossopharangeal, 624
  post-herpetic, 644
  temporomandibular, 624
  trigeminal, 612
Neuritis, optic, 609
  retrobulbar, 609, 645
Neurofibromatosis, 655
Neurology, in tropics, 721
Neuroma, acoustic, 614
Neuromyelitis optica, 648
Neurone, lower motor, 593
  upper motor, 592
Neuropathy, autonomic, 123, 663
  carcinomatous, 668
  diabetic, 663
  entrapment, 661
  in leprosy, 759
  nutritional, 655
  peripheral, 661
  vitamin B_{12}, 656
Neurophysiology, clinical, 607
Neurosis, see Psychoneurosis
Neurosyphilis, 639
Neutropenia, 519
  cyclic, 519
Neutrophil granulocyte, 491
Niacin, 76
Niclosamide, 788
Nicotinamide, 76
Nicotinic acid, 76
  in hyperlipidaemia, 486
Nifedipine, 170, 199
Nifurtimox, 781
Night blindness, 65
Nikethamide, 217
Niridazole, 785
Nitrazepam, 680
Nitrofurazone, 780
Nitrogen mustard, 113, 532
Niroprusside, sodium, 183
Nitrosoureas, 113
Nocardiosis, 802
Nocturia, in cardiac failure, 124
Nodules, in rheumatic fever, 157
  in rheumatoid arthritis, 553, 554
Non-gonococcal infection, 412
Noradrenaline, 454
Norethandrolone, for pruritus, 365
Normality, psychological, 673
Novobiocin, 348
NSAID, 558
Nuclear magnetic resonance, 607

Nutrients, classification of, 52
Nutrition, and disorders of hair, 56
  and disorders of mouth, 79
  and disorders of skin, 57
  and neurological disorders, 655
  deficiencies, 52
    aetiology, 52
    biochemical diagnosis, 80
    classification, 52
    prevention, 80
  enteral, 285
  in the tropics, 715
  parenteral, 285
Nystagmus, 610
Nystatin, 48

Obesity, 82
Obsession, 676
Obstruction, intestinal, 317
  of hepatic venous outflow, 367
  urinary, 402
Obstructive airways disease, 252
Occupation and lung disease, 265
Ochronosis, 582
Octopus poisoning, 708
Oculogyric crisis, 649
Oculomotor nerve, 609
Oedema, causes of, 95
  cerebral, 622
  famine, 54
  pitting, 123
  pulmonary, 122
    treatment of, 150
  treatment of, 96
Oesophagitis, reflux, 288
Oesophagoscopy, 283
Oesophagostomiasis, 800
Oesophagus, carcinoma of, 291
  'corkscrew', 291
  diverticulum of, 289
  motility of, 284
  spasm of, 291
  varices of, 360
Oestrogen, in menopause, 457
  in cancer, 119
Okuda needle, 370
Olfactory nerve, 608
Oligodendroglioma, 620, 623
Oligospermia, 456
Oliguria, 380
Omsk haemorrhagic fever, 733
Onchocerciasis, 797
Oncogene, 106
Oncology, 104
  prospects in, 120
Onyalai, 543
O'nyong-nyong fever, 733
Ophthalmia neonatorum, 712
Ophthalmic disease, in the tropics, 721
Ophthalmoplegia, 435
Opisthorciasis, 787
Opium, poisoning with, 709
Optic nerve, 608
Optic tract, 603
Orbivirus, 726

Orchitis, in mumps, 729
Organophosphorus poisoning, 709
Oriental sore, 777
Ornithosis, 225
Oroya fever, 757
Orthomyxovirus, 726
Orthopnoea, 122
Osler's nodes, 165
Osmolality of plasma, 426
Osteitis deformans, 587
  fibrosa, 440
Osteoarthritis, 582
Osteoarthrosis, 582
Osteodystrophy, renal, 392
Osteogenesis impefecta, 11
Osteolyses, hereditary, 589
Osteoma, 588
Osteomalacia, 69
Osteomyelitis, 586
Osteopetrosis, 589
Osteoporosis, 70
  idiopathic juvenile, 589
  postmenopausal and senile, 70
Osteosarcoma, 588
Otitis media, and cerebral abscess, 636
Ovalocytosis, 493
Oxamniquine, 786
Oxantel, 792
Oxicams, 559
Oxygen therapy, 214
Oxymetholone, 504, 534
Oxyphenbutazone, 505
Oxytetracycline, 45
Oxytocin, 420

Pacemaker, artificial, 146
Pachymeningitis, hypertrophic, 639
Paedophilia, 697
Paget's disease, 587
Pain, abdominal, 280
  cardiac, 123
  facial, 624
  in malignant disease, 108
  pleural, 208
Palpitation, 123
Pancreas, anatomy and physiology, 304
  'artificial', 487
  carcinoma, 309
  cystic fibrosis, 308
  cysts, 308
  disease, in tropics, 718
  investigation, 305
  pseudocyst, 308
  radiological examination, 305
  scanning, 305
  transplantation, 487
  tumours, 309
Pancreatitis, acute, 305
  chronic, 307
Pancreozymin, 278
Pancytopenia, 505
Panencephalitis, subacute sclerosing, 643
Panic disorder, 685
Pantothenic acid, 64

Papillary muscle, infarction of, 172
Papillitis, 608
  acute necrotising, 396
Papilloedema, 608
Papilloma of bladder, 408
Papovavirus, 726
Para-aminosalicylic acid, 238
Paracentesis abdominis, 345
Paracetamol, 558
  poisoning, 709
Paracoccidioidomycosis, 805
Paracrine substances, 278
Paraffin poisoning, 709
Paragonimiasis, 786
Paraldehyde, 619
Paralysis agitans, 648
  bulbar, 652
  facial, 613
  laryngeal, 250
Paramyxovirus, 792
Paraneoplastic syndromes, 108
Paranoia, 682
Paraphilia, 697
Paraplegia, 658
Paraprotein, 536
Parasuicide, 702
Parathyroid glands, anatomy and
        physiology, 439
  adenoma of, 440
Paratyphoid fever, 752
Parkinsonism, 648
Parotitis, 287
Parvovirus, 726
Past-pointing, 595
Pateau's syndrome, 8
Patient, communication of diagnosis
        and prognosis to, 119
Paul-Bunnell test, 520
PCo₂, 204
Peak expiratory flow, 213
Pectus carinatum, 276
  excavatum, 276
Pediculus humanus infections, 805
Pel-Ebstein fever, 530
Pellagra, 77
Pendred's syndrome, 438
Penetrance (genetic), 11
Penicillamine, 367, 560
Penicillin, 43
Pentagastrin test, 284
Pentamidine isethionate, 780
Peptic ulcer, 292
Peptides, gastrointestinal, 278
Perforation of ulcer, 298, 752
Perfusion of lungs, 206
Pergolide, 423
Pericarditis, acute, 187
  constrictive, 188
Perihepatitis, gonococcal, 411
Peritonitis, 319
  tuberculous, 320
Pernicious anaemia, 501
Peroneal muscular atrophy, 653
  peripheral type, 662
  spinal type, 653

Personality, development, 670
  disorders, 674, 691
    hysterical, 693
    obsessional, 692
    schizoid, 692
    sociopathy, 693
Pertussis, 748
Petit mal, 617
Petroleum poisoning, 709
pH, see Hydrogen ion concentration,
        98
Phaeochromocytoma, 454
Pharyngoconjunctival fever, 220
Pharynx, pouch of, 290
Phenacetin nephropathy, 406
Phenelzine, 681
Phenformin, 469
Phenindione, 548
Phenocopy, 17
Phenolphthalein, in urine, 382
Phenoxybenzamine, 454
Phenoxymethylpenicillin, 43
Phentermine, 86
Phentolamine, 454
Phenylbutazone, 559
Phenylketonuria, 14, 485
Phenytoin, 140, 618
Philadelphia chromosome, 8
Phlebitis, tropical, 718
Phlebography, 200
Phlebothrombosis, 199
Phobia, 685, 690
Pholcodine, 219
Phonocardiography, 132
Phosphatase, acid, 408
  alkaline, and liver, 341
    in neutrophils, 525
    in rickets, 68
    placental, 107
Phosphorus, 62
  radioactive, 517
Phrenic nerve, paralysis of, 262
Physical signs, in chest, 211
Physiotherapy, after stroke, 635
  in emphysema, 255
  in rheumatoid arthritis, 557
Phytic acid, in flour, 62
Phytomenadione, 72
Pica, 497
Picornavirus, 726
Pigeon chest, 276
Pigmentation, in Addison's disease,
        448
  in liver disease, 361
Pinta, 765
Piperacillin, 44
Piperazine, 792
Piroxicam, 559
Pituitary gland, anatomy and
        physiology, 418
  hormones, 418
  tumours, 421
Pityriasis versicolor, 802
Pivampicillin, 44
Pizotifen, 626

Plague, 749
Plasma cell, 19, 536
  leukaemia, 537
  exchange, 33, 666
Plasmapheresis, 33
Plasmid, and betalactams, 43
  in genetic engineering, 18
Platelets, 492
  in blood coagulation, 539, 542
  inhibitors, 548, 635
Pleura, tumours of, 271
Pleurisy, diaphragmatic, 208
  fibrinous, 269
  with effusion, 270
Pleurodesis, 275
Plummer-Vinson syndrome, 288
Pneumoconiosis, 267
Pneumoencephalography, 607
Pneumonia, aspiration, 226
  broncho-, 225
  coxiella, 225
  due to small bacteria, 224
  hypostatic, 225
  klebsiella, 224
  legionella, 224
  lobar, 223
  mycoplasma, 225
  plague and, 749
  pneumococcal, 223
  Pneumocystis carinii, 225
  post-operative, 225
  primary, 223
  secondary, 225
  staphylococcal, 223
  suppurative, 226
  treatment of, 228
  tuberculous, 234
  viral, 224
Pneumothorax, spontaneous, 273
  tension, 274
Po₂, 204
Poikilocytosis, 493
Poisoning, acute, 701
  agricultural, 711
  classification and causes, 702
  food, 753
  identification of, 704
  industrial, 711
  Information Service, 703
  prevention of, 711
  therapeutic measures, 704
  see also individual drugs
Poisons, affecting liver, 349
Poliomyelitis, 643
Polyarteritis nodosa, 198
  and kidney, 388
Polychromasia, 493
Polycystic disease of kidneys, 405
Polycythaemia, stress or spurious, 516
  vera, 516
Polydipsia, psychogenic, 426
Polymyalgia rheumatica, 578
Polymyositis, 576
Polyneuropathy, acute post-infection,
        663

Polyneuropathy (contd)
  causes of, 662
  diabetic, 663
  diagnosis and treatment, 664
  nutritional, 657
Polypharmacy, 822
Polyploidy, 7
Polyposis, multiple, of colon, 329
Polyuria, 380
Population explosion, 51
Porocephalosis, 806
Porphobilinogen, 382
Porphyria, acute intermittent, 382,
    664
Porphyrin, 490
Post-cholecystectomy syndrome, 373
Post-cibal syndrome, 301
Post-hepatitis syndrome, 351
Post-myocardial infarction syndrome,
    172
Potassium depletion, 91
  excess, 94
  iodide, 433
  perchlorate, 432
Poxvirus, 726
Praziquantel, 785, 787
Prazosin, 155, 182
Precipitation test, for antibodies, 26
Precocity, sexual, 449
Prednisolone, in bronchial asthma,
    246
  in haemolytic anaemia, 513
  in leukaemia, 522, 528
  in Hodgkin's lymphoma, 532
  in multiple myeloma, 538
  in rheumatic fever, 157
  in rheumatoid arthritis, 561
  in ulcerative colitis, 324
  uses and side-effects of, 452
Pregnancy, and rubella, 728
  and sickle-cell disease, 510
  diabetes in, 481
  heart disease in, 195
  hyperthyroidism in, 435
  immunology in relation to, 20
  megaloblastic anaemia in, 503
Preload, cardiac, 152
Pressure, arterial, 128
  central venous, 150
  jugular venous, 125
Prevention of, disease, 808
  diabetes mellitus, 483
  genetic disease, 15
  infectious disease, 40
  ischaemic heart disease, 176, 177
  nutritional disorders, 80
  tuberculosis, 239
  see also individual diseases
Prickly heat, 723
Primaquine, 772
Primidone, 618
Prinzmetal's angina, 167
PRL, 419
Probenecid, 43, 581
Procainamide, 140

Procaine penicillin, 43
Procarbazine, 532
Prochlorperazine, 614
Proctitis, 322
Proctoscopy, 283
Professional attitudes, 678
Progestogens in cancer, 119
Proguanil, 772
Prolactin, 419
Prolapse of mitral valve, 160
Prophase, 4
Propionic acid drugs, 559
Propranolol, 141, 182
  in hyperthyroidism, 433
Prospects in, alimentary disease,
    333
  cardiology, 201
  diabetes mellitus, 486
  genetics, 18
  haematology, 549
  immunology, 36
  liver disease, 374
  nephrology, 415
  neurology, 669
  respiratory medicine, 276
  rheumatology, 589
Prostacyclin, 547
Prostaglandin, and anti-inflammatory
    drugs, 558
  and kidney, 379
Prostate gland, benign enlargement,
    408
  carcinoma, 408
Prostatitis, 398
Protamine zinc insulin, 470
Protein, absorption of, 311
  losing enteropathy, 311
  metabolism, in liver, 336
Protein energy (calorie) malnutrition,
    55
  classification, 55
  in adults, 61
  mild to moderate, 60
Proteins, plasma, 341
Proteinuria, 381
  postural (orthostatic), 381
Prothrombin, 546
  time, 548
    and liver function, 342
Protozoa, diseases due to, 768
  infection of liver, 367
Proviamins, 64
PRPP overactivity, 579
Pruritus, in cholestasis, 365
  vulvae, 457, 462
Pseudobulbar palsy, 630
Pseudodementia, 688
Pseudo-gout, 581
Pseudohypertrophic muscular
    dystrophy, 666
Pseudohypoparathyroidism, 442
Pseudomonas infections, 44
Pseudoscleroderma, 576
Psittacosis, 225
Psoriasis and arthritis, 567

Psychiatric assessment, in poisoning,
    706
  disorders, classification, 678
  examination, 675
Psychiatry, diagnosis in, 673
  in tropics, 721
Psychogenic disorders, of alimentary
    tract, 331
Psychoneurosis, 674, 684
  anxiety, 685
  cardiac, 685
  depressive, 690
  hysterical, 687
  obsessive, 689
  phobic, 690
Psychoses, 674
  functional, 674, 681
  organic, 674, 679
Psychosexual disorders, 675, 697
Psychosomatic disorders, 698
Psychotherapy, 686
Ptosis, 609
Puffer fish poisoning, 708
Pulmonary, see Lung
  valve disease, 164
Pulse, arterial, 124
  collapsing, 124
  jugular venous, 125
  pressure, 128
Pulseless disease, 199
Pulsus alternans, 124
  bisferiens, 124
  paradoxus, 124
Pump, ionic, 89
Pupils, abnormalities of, 609
Purpura, 541
  anaphylactoid, 542
  Henoch Schönlein, 569
  idiopathic thrombocytopenic, 542
  simplex, 542
Pyelography, 383
Pyelonephritis, acute, 395
  chronic, 396
Pyloric stenosis, 299
Pyloroplasty, 297
Pyoderma gangrenosum, 324
Pyomyositis, 721
Pyonephrosis, 397
Pyopneumothorax, 272
Pyramidal tract, signs, 593
Pyrantel, 792
Pyrazinamide, 237
Pyrazolones, 559
Pyrexia, of unknown origin, 39
Pyridostigmine, 666
Pyridoxine, 79
Pyrimethamine, 772
Pyrophosphate arthropathy, 581
Pyruvic acid, in beriberi, 76
Pyrvinium, 792
Pyuria, 382

Q fever, 741
Quinidine, 140
Quinine, 771

Rabies, 731
Radial neve paralysis, 661
Radiation, ionising, 528
Radiculopathy, 662
Radiocolloids, in arthritis, 562
Radioimmunoassay, in adrenal disease, 445
Radiological examination, *see individual organs*
Radionuclide (radioisotope) scan, *see individual organs*
Radioscopy, of heart, 131
Radiotherapy, 111
    in ankylosing spondylitis, 565
    in bronchial carcinoma, 262
    in leukaemia, 528
    in lymphoma, 531, 534
    lymphoid irradiation, 562
Ranitidine, 296
Rappaport classification, 533
Rat-bite fevers, 767
Raynaud's disease and phenomenon, 199
Reagin, 242
Rebound phenomenon, 595
Recessive inheritance, autosomal, 11
    X-linked, 12
Recombinant DNA technology, 18
Rectum, carcinoma of, 327
    nervous control of, 600
Red blood cell, 488
    diseases of, 494
    nucleated, 493
Reed Sternberg cell, 530
Re-entry circuit, 133
Reflex, abdominal, 600
    corneal, 600
    plantar, 599
    superficial, 599
    tendon, 599
Regurgitation, aortic, 163
    mitral, 160
    oesophageal, 281
    pulmonary, 165
    tricuspid, 164
Rehabilitation, after myocardial infarction, 176
    after paraplegia, 659
    after stroke, 635
    centre, nutritional, 58
    in depression, 682
    of arthritis, 562
Rehydration, in cholera, 756
Reiter's disease, 565
Relapsing fevers, 765
Renin, 379
    and hypertension, 179
    -angiotensin system, 379
Reovirus, 726
Resonance, vocal, 211
Respiratory, disease, investigation of, 210
        treatment of, 214
    distress syndrome, 210
    failure, 210, 217

Respiratory (*contd*)
    system, anatomy, 202
        physiology, 204
Resuscitation, cardiopulmonary, 138
Reticulocyte, 489
Reticulo-endothelial system, 492
Retinitis proliferans, 479
Retinol, 64
Retinopathy, diabetic, 478
    hypertensive, 180
Retrovirus, 726
Reverse T3, 428
Reye's syndrome, 349
Rhabdomyolysis, 400
Rhabdovirus, 726
Rhesus factor, 514
Rheumatic disease, 551
    fever, 156
Rheumatism, non-articular, 584
Rheumatoid arthritis, 551
    factor, 556
Rhinitis, allergic, 241
Rhinosporidiosis, 803
Rhinovirus, 726
Rhodiascit machine, 364
Rhonchi, 211
Rib, cervical, 662
Riboflavin, 78
Rickets, 67
    renal, 69
    vitamin D resistant, 69
Rickettsiae, diseases due to, 737
Rickettsialpox, 740
Rifampicin, 237
    in leprosy, 761
Rift Valley fever, 736
Rigidity, clasp-knife, 593
    cog-wheel, 594
    lead-pipe, 594
Ringworm, 801
    griseofulvin, in 48
Risus sardonicus, 745
Rivalry, perceptual, 604
River blindness, 797
RNA, 2
Rocky Mountain spotted fever, 739
Romana's sign, 781
Romberg's test, 597
Rosacea, tetracyclines in, 45
Rose-Waaler test, 556
Ross River fever, 733
Rotator cuff syndrome, 584
Rotavirus, 726
Rotor syndrome, 347
Roundworms, 791
Rubella, 728
Rumination, 690

Saccharin, 468
Sacroiliitis, 568
Sadism, 697
Saint Vitus dance, 651
Salbutamol, 246
Salicylate in rheumatic fever, 157
    poisoning, 709

Salivary glands, diseases of, 287
Salmonella infections, 751
Salpingitis, gonococcal, 411
    tuberculous, 232
Salsalate, 559
Salt, depletion, 89
    in hypertension, 181
    -losing nephritis, 89
    reduction in diet, 363
Sandflies, 757, 776
Sarcoidosis, 268
Sarcoma, 106
Scabies, 806
Scan, *see* radionuclide, tomography, ultrasonography
Scarlet fever, 742
Schilling test, 502
Schirmer test, 554
Schistosomiasis, 782
Schizophrenia, 682
Schum's test, 505
Sciatica, 660
Scleritis, 554
Scleroderma, 576
Scleromalacia, 554
Sclerosis, amyotrophic lateral, 652
    multiple (disseminated), 645
    systemic, 575
Sclerosteosis, 589
Scorpion stings, 709
Scotoma, 603
Scromboid fish poisoning, 708
Scrub typhus fever, 740
Scurvy, 72
Sea anemone stings, 708
    wasp stings, 708
Seborrhoea, nasolabial, 79
Self-poisoning, 702
Semiliki forest fever, 733
Seminoma, 408
Sengstaken tube, 364
Sensory system, 595
Septicaemia, 50
Septum, interventricular, defect of, 192
    rupture of, 172
Serotonin, 24, 321, 626
Serum sickness, 27
Sex, chromosome, abnormalities of, 8
    disorders of, in male, 454
        in female, 456
    -linked inheritance, 12
Sexual deviation, 697
    intercourse, and urinary infection, 398
    orientation disturbances, 697
    precocity, 449
Sexually transmitted disease, 408
Sheehan's syndrome, 424
Shellfish poisoning, 708
Shingles, 644
Shock, anaphylactic, 24
    bacteraemic, 50
    cardiogenic, 147
    hypovolaemic, 148
    septic, 50

Shoulder, frozen, 585
  hand syndrome, 585
Shunt, cardiac, 189
  porto-systemic, 365
SI units, 818
Sicca syndrome, 554
Sick sinus syndrome, 133
Sickle-cell anaemia, 508
  trait, 511
Sickling test, 510
Sideroblast, 499
Siderosis, 62
Sigmoidoscopy, 283
Silicosis, 267
Simulator, in radiotherapy, 112
Sindbis fever, 733
Sinoatrial disease, 133
Sinus rhythms, 133
Sinuses, nasal, 202
  venous, thrombosis, 636
Sinusitis, 220
Sjögren's syndrome, 554
Skin, diseases affecting genitalia,
      415
    involving mouth, 286
    nutritional disorders, 57
    sensitivity tests, 244
Skull, radiograph of, 604
Sleep, apnoea, 253
  paralysis, 619
Sleeping sickness, 779
Slow viral infection, 641
Smallpox, 730
Smoking, see Cigarette smoking
Snake bite, 710
Snap, opening, 127
Sociopathy, 693
Sodium and water excess, 95
  depletion, 89
  fusidate, 46
Sodoku, 767
Solvent abuse, 697
Somatiform disorder, 688
Somatostatin, 419
Sorbitol, 468
Sotalol, 141
Southern blot, 18
Sparganosis, 790
Spasm, cerebrovascular, 628
  coronary, 167, 171
Spastic colon, 332
Spasticity, 593
Spectinomycin, 47
Speech, 600
Sperm, antibodies to, 29
  storage of, 532
Spherocytosis, hereditary, 506
Spider bite, 710
Spina bifida, 17
Spinal accessory nerve, 615
  muscular atrophy, 653
Spinothalamic tract, signs, 597
Spirochaetes, diseases due to, 762
Spirometra erinacei, 790
Spironolactone, 97

Splenectomy in, autoimmune
      haemolytic anaemia, 513
  hereditary spherocytosis, 507
  Hodgkin's disease, 532
  thrombocytopenic purpura, 543
Splenomegaly in, cirrhosis of liver, 360
  infective endocarditis, 165
  kala azar, 777
  leukaemia, 525
  malaria, 771
Splinter haemorrhages, 124
Spondarthritis, 563
Spondylitis, ankylosing, 564
Spondylosis, cervical, 659
Sporotrichosis, 803
Sprue, tropical, 719
Sputum, 208
  examination of, 212
Squint, concomitant and paralytic, 610
St Louis fever, 733
Stannosis, 266
Staphylococcal infection, 743
Starvation, 54
  therapeutic, 85
Stature, 423
Status asthmaticus, 243
  epilepticus, 619
Steatorrhoea, 312
  in cholestasis, 365
Stenosis, aortic, 161
  mitral, 158
  pulmonary, 164
    congenital, 193
  tricuspid, 164
Stereotactic thalamotomy, 650
Steroids, anabolic, 348
  androgenic, 504
Stethoscope, 126
Stevens-Johnson syndrome, 42
Still's disease, 568
Stomach, aspiration of, 300
  carcinoma of, 302
  investigation of, 282
  lavage of, 705
  peptic ulcer of, 292
Stomatitis, angular, 79
  aphthous, 286
  ulcerative, 286
Stones, see calculi
Stool, examination of, 284
Strabismus, 610
Streptococcal infection, 742
Streptokinase, 201, 548
Streptomycin, 46, 237
Stress disorders, 698
Stridor, 209
Stroke, 628
  diagnosis of, 632
  treatment of, 634
Strongyloidiasis, 793
Stupor, hysterical, 688
Subacute combined degeneration of
      the cord, 656
Subclavian steal syndrome, 629
Subarachnoid haemorrhage, 631

Substance use disorder, 694
Suicide, 681, 702
Sulfadoxine, 772
Sulindac, 559
Sulphadimidine, 42
Sulphasalazine, 325
Sulphinpyrazone, 176, 581
Sulphonamides, 42
Sulphonylurea, 468
Sulphur, dietary sources of, 63
Sunburn, 722
Sunlight, exposure to, 722
Suramin, 780
Surfactant, 203
Surgery in, angina pectoris, 170
  arthritis, 562
  cerebral tumours, 622
  diabetes, 482
  heart disease, 194
  obesity, 86
  peptic ulcer, 296
  thyrotoxicosis, 432
  ulcerative colitis, 325
  see also individual diseases
Surveillance, immunological, 33
Swan-Ganz catheter, 150
Sweat, reference values, 819
Sydenham's chorea, 651
Sympathetic nerves, cervical, 615
Syncope, 123
  due to heat, 722
Synovectomy, 562
Synovial fluid, examination of, 557
Syphilis, 409
  endemic (non-venereal), 764
  of aorta, 198
  of nervous system, 639
Syringobulbia, 655
Syringomyelia, 654
Systemic lupus erythematosus, 572
Systemic sclerosis, 575

T_3, 428
T_3, resin uptake, 429
  thyrotoxicosis, 429
T_4, 428
TAB vaccine, 807
Tabes dorsalis, 640
Tachyarrhythmia, paroxysmal, 133
Tachycardia, atrial, 134
  sinus, 133
  supraventricular, 134
  ventricular, 137
Taeniasis, 788
Takayasu's syndrome, 199
Talampicillin, 44
Tamoxifen, 119
Tamponade, cardiac, 187
Tapeworms, 788
Tarsal tunnel syndrome, 555
Taste, 613, 615
Tay-Sachs disease, 14
Teeth, disorders of, 285
  extraction of, in haemophilia, 545
  fluoride and caries, 63

Telangiectasia, hereditary haemorrhagic, 542
Teletherapy, 112
Television, and epilepsy, 616
Telophase, 4
Ten day rule, 282
Tendinitis, bicipital, 585
   supraspinatus, 584
Tennis elbow, 585
Tenosynovitis, 554
Teratoma of testis, 408
Terbutaline, 246
Terfenadine, 241
Terminal care, 119
Testis, tumours of, 408
Testosterone, 426, 455
Tests of function, see individual organs
Tetanus, 745
Tetany, 442
   in rickets, 68
Tetrachloroethylene, 787
Tetracosactrin, 450
Tetracyclines, 45
Tetrodotoxic poisoning, 708
Thalamus, signs, 598
Thalassaemia, 511
Thalidomide, 762
Theophylline, 246
Thiabendazole, 792
Thiacetazone, 238
Thiazide diuretics, 96
   in hypertension, 181
Thiamin, 73
Thioguanine, 522, 525
Thiopentone, 619
Thioridazine, 679
Thiouracil, 432
Thomsen's disease, 667
Threadworm, 791
Threshold (genetic), 14
Thrombasthenia, 543
Thromboangiitis obliterans, 198
Thrombocyte, 492
Thrombocythaemia, 543
   essential, 518
Thrombocytopenia, 494
Thrombolysis, 200
Thrombophlebitis, 199
Thromboplastin, 539
   time, 541
Thrombosis, 546
   cerebral, arterial, 628
      venous, 636
   mesenteric, 331
   of axillary vein, 200
   of peripheral arteries, 196
   of renal vein, 390
   of veins of legs, 199
   ventricular, 172
Thrombotest, 548
Thromboxane, 547
Thrush, 286
Thymectomy, 33, 666
Thymic hypoplasia, 34
Thymus gland, 20

Thyroid gland, anatomy and physiology, 427
   biopsy, 430
   function tests, 428
   radiological examination, 429
   radionuclide uptake and scan, 429
   tumours, 438
   ultrasonography, 430
Thyroid stimulating hormone, 419, 429, 437
Thyroidectomy, 432
Thyroiditis, de Quervain's, 438
   Hashimoto's, 437
   subacute, 438
Thyrotoxic crisis, 431, 434
Thyrotoxicosis, 430
Thyrotrophin, 419
Thyroxine (T4), 428, 437
   index and ratio, 429
   total plasma, 428
Tiaprofenic acid, 559
Tic, 652
Ticarcillin, 44
Tick-borne relapsing fever, 766
   typhus fever, 739
Tine test, 233
Tinidazole, 48
Tissue typing, 30
T lymphocytre, 20
   subsets, 21
TNM classification, 110
Tobacco, see Cigarette smoking
   amblyopia, 609
Tobramycin, 47
Todd's paralysis, 617
Togavirus, 726
Tolazamide, 468
Tolbutamide, 468
Tolerance, immune, 23
   defect in, 29
Tolmetin, 559
Tomography, computed, see individual organs
   emission computed, 607
Tone, disturbance of, 593, 594
Tongue, carcinoma of, 287
   diseases of, 287
   geographical, 287
Tonsillitis, streptococcal, 742
Tophus, 580
Torticollis, 652
Toxic shock syndrome, 743
Toxocara canis, 800
Toxoplasmosis, 781
TPHA test for syphilis, 410
Trachea, obstruction of, 251
Tracheitis, acute, 251
Tracheo-oesophageal fistula, 252
Tracheostomy, 218
Trachoma, 737
Tranexamic acid, 545
Transaminase and myocardial infarction, 175
   and liver, 340
Transfer factor, 20

Transferrin, 496
Transient ischaemic attack, 629
Transketolase, in beriberi, 76
Translocation, 7
Transplantation, of bone marrow, 525
   of heart, 194
   of kidney, 394
   of liver, 375
   of pancreas, 487
Transvestism, 697
Tranylcypromine, 681
Travellers, advice to, 806
   diarrhoea, 330
Trematodes, 782
Tremor, causes of, 649
   intention, 595
Trench fever, 740
TRH, 419, 437
   test, 429
Triamterene, 97
Trichinella spiralis, 800
Trichomoniasis, 415
Trichuris trichiura, 792
Tricustid valve disease, 164
Tricyclic drugs, 681
   poisoning by, 711
Trigeminal nerve, 611
Triglyceride, 485
Triiodothyronine, 428
Trilisate, 559
Trilostane, 446
Trimethoprim, 42
Trimipramine, 682
Trisomy, 7
Trochlear nerve, 609
Tropical, anhidrotic asthenia, 723
   countries, pattern of disease, 714
   diseases, 714
   spinal ataxia, 656
   splenomegaly syndrome, 771
   sprue, 719
   ulcer, 767
Trousseau's sign, 442
Trypanosomiasis, African, 779
   American, 780
Tsetse flies, 779
TSH, 419
Tuberculin test, 232
Tuberculosis, 230
   chemoprophylaxis, 239
   clinical features, 231
   cryptic, 234
   diagnosis of, 235
   drug-resistant, 238
   in diabetes, 480
   miliary, 233
   of bone, 587
   of intestine, 236
   of joints, 571
   of kidney, 399
   of lymph nodes, 232
   of meninges, 638
   of pericardium, 188
   of peritoneum, 320
   of pleura, 271

Tuberculosis (contd)
  pathology, 230
  prevention, 239
  primary pulmonary, 232
  pulmonary, 230
    post-primary, 234
  P.U.O. due to, 39, 234
  therapeutic regimens, 237
  treatment, 236
Tuberous sclerosis, 11, 265
Tularaemia, 750
Tumour(s),
  clinical features, 107
  markers, 106
  pathology, 106
  treatment, 109
  see also individual organs
Tungiasis, 806
Turner's syndrome, 9
Typhoid fever, 751
Typhus fever, 738

Ulcer, genital, 415
  jejunal, 301
  mycobacterial, 762
  peptic, aetiology, 292
    complications of, 297
    perforation of, 298
    recurrent, 301
    surgery in, 296
    tropical, 767
Ulcerative colitis, 321
Ultrasonography, see individual organs
Undernutrition, 54
Undulant fever, 748
Uraemia, 399
  in cardiac failure, 156
  postrenal, 402
  prerenal, 399
  renal, 399
Urethral syndrome, 398
Urethritis, 398
  non-gonococcal, 412
Uricosuric agents, 581
Urinary tract, infection, 395
  obstruction, 402
  tumours, 407
Urine, abnormal constituents, 381
  formation of, 377
  reaction of, 381
  reference values, 820
  specific gravity of, 380
  testing, in diabetes mellitus, 463
  volume of, 380
Urobilinogen, 340
  in haemolytic anaemia, 505
Urography, 583
  in hypertension, 180
Urokinase, 548
Ursodeoxycholic acid, 371
Urticaria, 25
Uta, 778
Uterus, cancer of, 105
Uveitis, 564

V̇A/Q̇, 206
Vaccination, 40, 807
  BCG, 239
  hepatitis B, 353
  see also individual diseases
Vagina, discharge from, 415
Vaginismus, 697
Vaginitis, senile, 457
Vagotomy, 296
Vagus nerve, 615
Valproate, sodium, 619
Valsalva manoeuvre, and syncope, 123
Valvotomy mitral, 194
Valvular heart disease, 158
  see also Stenosis and Regurgitation
Vancomycin, 46
Varicella, 730
Varices, oesophageal, 360
Vasculitis, in rheumatoid arthritis, 555
Vasodilators, in cardiac failure, 155
  in circulatory failure, 150
  in hypertension, 182
Vasopressin, 420
  in diabetes insipidus, 427
  in portal hypertension, 364
Vasovagal syncope, 123
VDRL, 410
Vegetable toxins, 711
Veins, diseases of, 199
  radionuclide and ultrasound
    scanning, 200
  venography, 200
Vena cava, obstruction of, 264
Venereal disease, 408
Venesection in haemochromatosis, 366
  in polycythaemia, 517
Veno-occlusive disease, 367
Ventilation, 204
  mechanical, 217
  perfusion ratio, 206
Ventilatory capacity, estimation of, 213
  failure, 210
Ventimask, 216
Ventricular septal defect, 192
Verapamil, 141, 170
Verruga peruana, 757
Vertebro-basilar ischaemia, 629
Vertigo, 614
Vesico-ureteric reflux, 395
Vestibular nerve, 614
Vidarabine, 48
Vinblastine, 532
Vinca alkaloid, 532
Vincent's infection, 286
Vincristine, 532
Vindesine, 532
Viper bite, 710
Virilisation, 445
Virus(es) and cancer, 105
  classification, 726
  infection, of alimentary tract, 330
    of nervous system, 641
    of respiratory system, 220, 224
  oncogenic, 33
  therapy, 48

Viscosity of blood, and thrombosis,
    547
  in multiple myeloma, 537
  in polycythaemia, 517
Vision, impairment of, 601
Visual evoked response, 609
Visual pathway, 601
Vitamin A, 64
  B complex, 64
  B₁, 73
  B₆, 79
  B₁₂, 500
    neuropathy, 656
  C, 72
  D, 66
    dangers of excessive intake of, 69
  E, 71
  K, 71
    in hypoprothrombinaemia, 546
Vitamins, biosynthesis in the gut, 64
  deficiency, biochemical diagnosis,
    80
  metabolism, in liver, 338
Vitiligo, 448
Volvulus of intestine, 317
Vomiting, 281
  psychogenic, 331
  sickness of Jamaica, 711
von Gierke's disease, 579
von Recklinghausen's disease,
    (neurofibromatosis), 655
von Recklinghausen's disease of bone,
    440
von Willebrand's disease, 545

Waldenström's macroglobulinaemia,
    538
Warfarin, 548
Warts, genital, 414
Wasp sting, 707
Wassermann reaction, 410
Water, balance, 88
  depletion, 90
  excess, 95
  regulation of, 376
Waterbrash, 281
Weedkiller poisoning, 707
Weight(s), desirable for adults, 816
  for age, birth to 5 years, 815
  reduction of, 84
Weil's disease, 762
Weil-Felix reaction, 738
Wenckebach phenomenon, 143
Werdnig-Hoffman disease, 654
Wernicke's encephalopathy, 75
West Nile fever, 733
Wheeze, 209
Whipple's disease, 568
Whipworm, 792
White blood cell, 491
Whooping cough, 748
Widal reaction, 752
Wilms' tumour, 407
Wilson's disease, 366
Wiskott-Aldrich syndrome, 35

Wolff-Parkinson-White syndrome, 134
'Woody leg' in scurvy, 73
Wool-sorter's disease, 746
World, distribution of disease in, 717
Worms, diseases due to, 782

Xenodiagnosis, 781
Xerophthalmia, 65
Xerosis conjuctivae, 65

Xerostomia, 287
Xylose absorption, 310
XXX constitution, 9
XYY constitution, 9

Yaws, 763
Yellow fever, 734
Yersiniosis, 330, 563, 749
Yttrium, 422, 562

Zinc deficiency, 63
Zollinger-Ellison syndrome, 300
Zona fascilulata/reticularis,
    overactivity, 445
Zona glomerulosa, overactivity, 446
Zoster, 644
Zygomycosis, 803

NOTES